Standards of Psychiatric and Mental Health Nursing Practice

STANDARD I. ASSESSMENT

The Psychiatric–Mental Health Nurse Collects Client Health Data.

Rationale: The assessment interview—which requires linguistically and culturally effective communication skills, interviewing, behavioral observation, database record review, and comprehensive assessment of the client and relevant systems—enables the psychiatric–mental health nurse to make sound clinical judgments and plan appropriate interventions with the client.

STANDARD II. DIAGNOSIS

The Psychiatric–Mental Health Nurse Analyzes the Assessment Data in Determining Diagnoses.

Rationale: The basis for providing psychiatric–mental health nursing care is the recognition and identification of patterns of response to actual or potential psychiatric illnesses and mental health problems.

STANDARD III. OUTCOME IDENTIFICATION

The Psychiatric–Mental Health Nurse Identifies Expected Outcomes Individualized to the Client.

Rationale: Within the context of providing nursing care, the ultimate goal is to influence health outcomes and improve the client's health status.

STANDARD IV. PLANNING

The Psychiatric–Mental Health Nurse Develops a Plan of Care that Prescribes Interventions to Attain Expected Outcomes.

Rationale: A plan of care is used to guide therapeutic intervention systematically and achieve the expected client outcomes.

STANDARD V. IMPLEMENTATION

The Psychiatric–Mental Health Nurse Implements the Interventions Identified in the Plan of Care.

Rationale: **At the basic level,** the nurse may select counseling, milieu therapy, self-care activities, psychobiological interventions, health teaching, case management, health promotion and health maintenance, and a variety of other approaches to meet the mental health needs of clients. In addition to the intervention options available to the basic-level psychiatric–mental health nurse, **at the advanced level,** the certified specialist may provide consultation, engage in psychotherapy, and prescribe pharmacological agents where permitted by state statutes or regulations.

STANDARD Va. COUNSELING
STANDARD Vb. MILIEU THERAPY
STANDARD Vc. SELF-CARE ACTIVITIES
STANDARD Vd. PSYCHOBIOLOGICAL INTERVENTIONS
STANDARD Ve. HEALTH TEACHING
STANDARD Vf. CASE MANAGEMENT
STANDARD Vg. HEALTH PROMOTION AND HEALTH MAINTENANCE

Advanced Practice Interventions Vh–Vj

The following interventions (Vh–Vj) may be performed only by the certified specialist in psychiatric–mental health nursing.

STANDARD Vh. PSYCHOTHERAPY
STANDARD Vi. PRESCRIPTION OF PHARMACOLOGICAL AGENTS
STANDARD Vj. CONSULTATION

STANDARD VI. EVALUATION

The Psychiatric–Mental Health Nurse Evaluates the Client's Progress in Attaining Expected Outcomes.

Rationale: Nursing care is a dynamic process involving change in the client's health status over time, giving rise to the need for new data, different diagnoses, and modifications in the plan of care. Therefore, evaluation is a continuous process of appraising the effect of nursing interventions and the treatment regimen on the client's health status and expected health outcomes.

Foundations of Psychiatric Mental Health Nursing

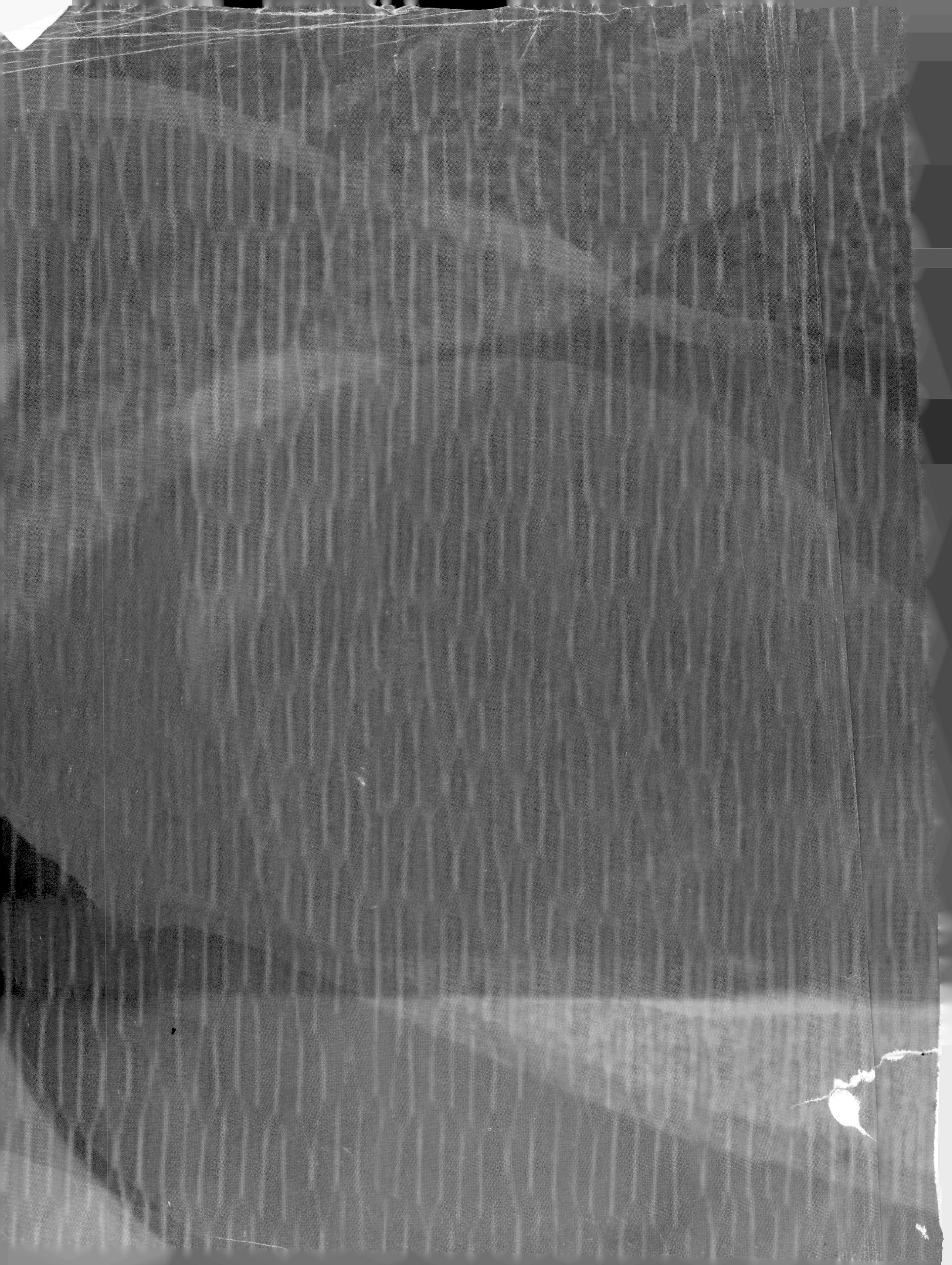

Foundations of Psychiatric Mental Health Nursing

Third Edition

Elizabeth M. Varcarolis, R.N., M.A.

Professor Emeritus
Formerly Deputy Chairperson, Department of Nursing
Borough of Manhattan Community College
New York, New York

Associate Fellow
Albert Ellis Institute for Rational
Emotive Behavioral Therapy (REBT)
New York, New York

W.B. Saunders Company
A Division of Harcourt Brace & Company

Philadelphia London Toronto Montreal Sydney Tokyo

W.B. SAUNDERS COMPANY
A Division of Harcourt Brace & Company

The Curtis Center
Independence Square West
Philadelphia, Pennsylvania 19106

Library of Congress Cataloging-in-Publication Data

Varcarolis, Elizabeth M.
Foundations of psychiatric mental health nursing / Elizabeth M. Varcarolis.—3rd ed.

p. cm.

Includes bibliographical references and index.

ISBN 0–7216–8643–5

1. Psychiatric nursing. I. Title.
[DNLM: 1. Mental Disorders—nursing. 2. Psychiatric Nursing. WY 160 V278f 1998]

RC440.F58 1998 610.73′68
—dc21
DNLM/DLC 97-7150

FOUNDATIONS OF PSYCHIATRIC MENTAL HEALTH NURSING ISBN 0–7216–8643–5

Printed in the United States of America.

Last digit is the print number: 9 8 7 6 5 4 3 2 1

NOTICE

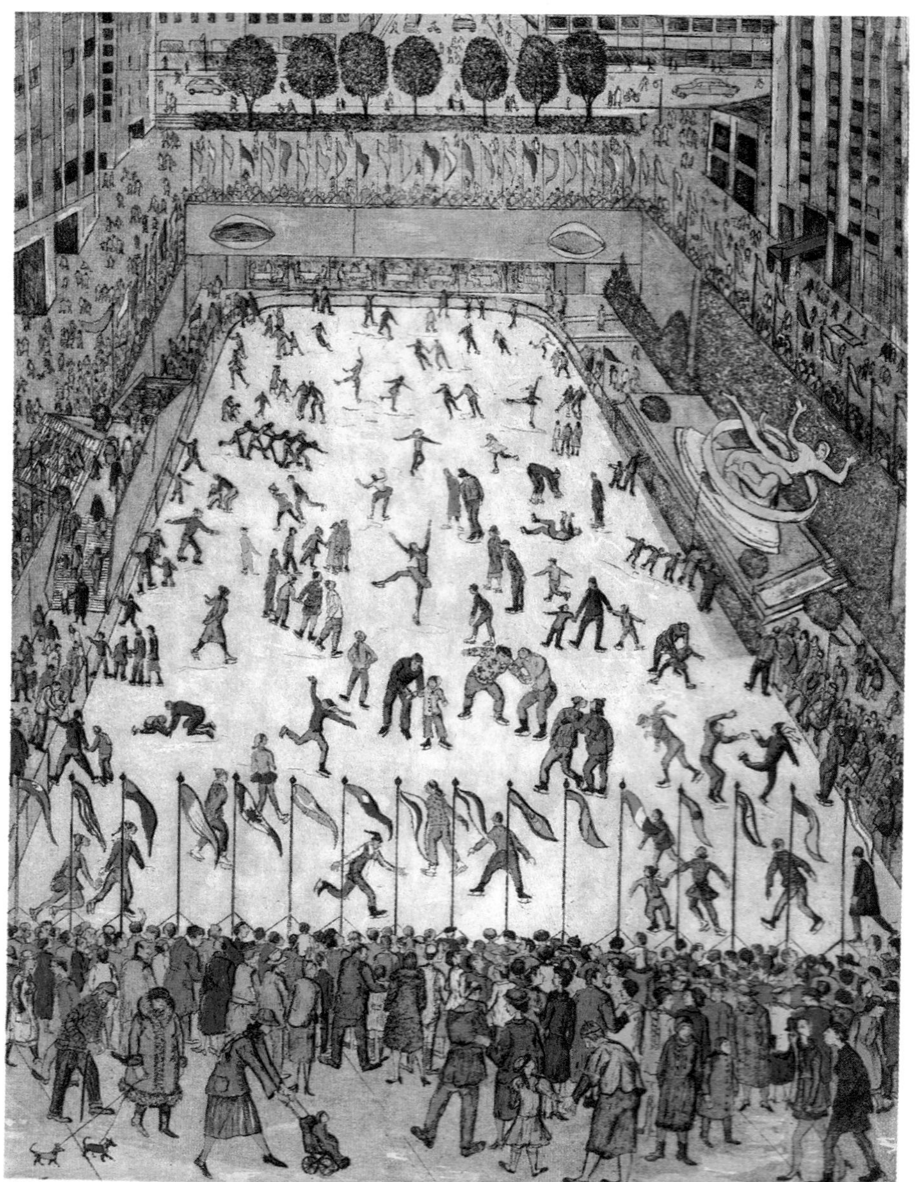

Scating Rink

for Betsy and Paul

Lida Whedon

To the memory of

Josiah and Ruth Merrill,

who I owe so much and think of every day.

Always to my husband

Paul,

whose pride and pleasure, interest and enthusiasm,
help and encouragement, love and companionship mean everything to me.

To

Ilze Rader,

my editor for three editions,
thank you for your creative energy,
imaginative contributions, and restorative humor.

The etching on the left was done by Aida Whedon, who was part of my extended family growing up. Aida, a renowned artist, was a loving and gracious woman. She encouraged creativity in hundreds of young people of all ages, myself included. The others in my extended family included Aida's husband Dan, Jane and George Nogle, Patty and Allen Wile, Helen and Bill Hickey, and Lila and George Wiley. I am blest for their being an important part of my life.

CONTRIBUTORS

Carrol Alvarez, BS, MS, CS
Clinical Faculty, University of Washington; Clinical Nurse Specialist, Psychiatry, Harborview Medical Center, Seattle, Washington
Communication with Angry and Aggressive Clients

Jeannemarie G. Baker, MSN, APRN, CS
Adjunct Professor, Family Theory and Therapy, Columbia University School of Nursing, New York, New York
Communication Within Families

Penny S. Brooke, RN, MS, JD
Associate Professor and Assistant Dean, University of Utah College of Nursing, Salt Lake City, Utah
Legal and Ethical Aspects of Mental Health Care

Jane Bruker, MSN, RNCS
Health Careers, Department Chair, University of New Mexico–Gallup, Gallup, New Mexico
A Nurse Speaks, Unit IV

Susan Caverly, ARNP, MA, CS
Clinical Instructor/Researcher, Department of Psychosocial and Community Health, School of Nursing, University of Washington; Psychiatric Nurse Practitioner, Seattle Counseling Services for Sexual Minorities and Therapeutic Health Services, Seattle, Washington
Psychiatric Mental Health Nursing in Community Settings

Helene S. (Kay) Charron, MS, RN
Professor Emeritus, Monroe Community College, Rochester, New York
Anxiety Disorders; Somatoform and Dissociative Disorders

Cherrill W. Colson, BSN, MA, EdD
Assistant Professor, Department of Nursing, Lehman College, City University of New York, Bronx, New York
Children and Adolescents

Michelle Conant Dan-El, RN, MSN, CS
Former Adjunct Professor, Nursing Faculty Department of Nursing, Borough of Manhattan Community College, New York, New York; Lehman College, New York, New York; Fairleigh Dickinson University, Madison, New Jersey; Private Practice, Livingston, New Jersey and New York, New York
Psychosocial Issues of People with Physical Illness

Anne Cowley Herzog, RN, MSN
Assistant Professor, RN Program, Cypress College at Cypress; Instructor, Nursing Program, California State University, Fullerton at Fullerton; Clinical Nurse Educator, University of California Medical Center at Orange, California
The Severely and Persistently Mentally Ill

Sally K. Holzapfel, RN, MSN, CS, CETN, CGNP
Nurse Practitioner, Geriatric and Enterostomal Therapy, Department of Veterans Affairs, New Jersey Health Care System, Lyons; Clinical Assistant Professor, University of Medicine and Dentistry of New Jersey, Newark, New Jersey
The Elderly

Kathleen Ibrahim, MA, RN, CS
Assistant to Director of Nursing for Staff Development, New York State Psychiatric Institute, New York, New York
People with Eating Disorders

Catherine M. Lala, MSN, CS
Adjunctive Clinical Professor, Russell Sage College, Troy, and Dominican College, Orangeburg; Adult Psychiatric Mental Health Clinical Nurse Specialist, Albany Medical Center, Albany, New York
Communication Within Groups

Kem B. Louie, PhD, RN, CS, FAAN
Professor and Chairperson, Graduate Nursing Program, College of Mount Saint Vincent, Riverdale; Visiting Assistant Professor, Department of Psychiatry, Einstein Medical School, Bronx, New York
A Nurse Speaks, Unit VIII

Maureen H. McCracken, RN, CS, CHTI
Certified Healing Touch Instructor, Colorado Center for Healing Touch; McCracken and Associates, P.C., Healing Touch of North Virginia; Allied Staff, Columbia Dominion Hospital, Falls Church, Virginia
A Nurse Speaks, Unit III

Susan Mejo, ARNP, CS, PsyD
Private Practice
Longview, Washington
Psychiatric Mental Health Nursing in Community Settings

Peggy H. Miller, RN, MSN
Associate Professor, Health Science Division, Cypress College, Cypress; Clinical Instructor, Woodruff Hospital, Long Beach, and University of California at Irvine Medical Center, Irvine, California
The Severely and Persistently Mentally Ill

Mary D. Moller, MSN, ARNP, CS
Adjunct Faculty, Washington State University and Gonzaga University; Administrator, The Suncrest Wellness Center, Spokane, Washington
A Nurse Speaks, Unit V

John A. Payne, RN, BS, MA
Formerly Assistant Professor of Psychiatric Nursing, Borough of Manhattan Community College, New York; Retired NYC Department of Hospitals, Senior Management Consult, Director of Nursing for Long Term Care and Psychiatry, New York; Formerly Director of Nursing Services, Harlem Hospital, New York
A Nurse Speaks, Unit I

Francesca Profiri, ARNP, MEd
Private Practice, Seattle, Washington
Personality Disorders

Carla E. Randall, RN, MSN
Doctoral Student, University of British Columbia, Vancouver, British Columbia, Canada
Adult Relationships and Sexuality

John Raynor, PhD
Professor, Department of Science, Borough of Manhattan Community College, City University of New York, New York, New York
Psychobiology of Mental Disorders

Denise Saint Arnault, MS, RN
Assistant Professor of Nursing, Madonna University, Livonia, Michigan
Framework for Culturally Relevant Psychiatric Nursing

Sharon Shisler, RN, MA, CS
Adjunct Professor, Herbert Lehman College; Psychiatric Liaison Coordinator, Greenwich Hospital; Group Facilitator for AIDS Alliance of Greenwich, Greenwich, Connecticut
A Nurse Speaks, Unit VI

Kathleen Smith-DiJulio, BSN, MA
Clinical Assistant Professor, University of Washington; Director, Ambulatory Practice Improvement and Service Quality, Group Health Cooperative, Seattle, Washington
Families in Crisis: Family Violence; Rape; People Who Depend Upon Substances of Abuse

Margaret Swisher, MSN, RN
Nursing Instructor, Mental Health, Montgomery County Community College, Blue Bell, Pennsylvania
Psychiatric Nursing in the Acute Psychiatric Hospital Setting

Constance Kolva Taylor, MSN, RN
President, Kolva Consulting, Harrisburg, Pennsylvania
A Nurse Speaks, Unit II

Rosie Gooden Taylor, MS, RN, CNS
Lecturer, Clinical Faculty, Baylor University School of Nursing, Dallas, Texas
A Nurse Speaks, Unit VII

Julius Trubowitz, EdD
Assistant Professor, Queens College, Flushing, Private Practice, New York, New York
Mental Health: Theories and Therapies

Elizabeth M. Varcarolis, RN, MA
Professor Emeritus, Formerly Deputy Chairperson, Department of Nursing, Borough of Manhattan Community College; Associate Fellow, Albert Ellis Institute for Rational Emotive Behavioral Therapy (REBT), New York, New York
Psychiatric Nursing: Past, Present, Future; The Nurse-Client Relationship and the Nursing Process; Communication and the Clinical Interview; Reducing Stress and Anxiety; Crisis and Crisis Intervention; Alterations in Mood: Grief and Depression; Alterations in Mood: Elation in Bipolar Disorders; Schizophrenic Disorders; Cognitive Disorders; People Who Contemplate Suicide

Thomas Wenzka, MSN
Assistant Professor, Nursing Department, Coastal Georgia Community College, Brunswick, Georgia
Psychiatric Nursing in the Acute Psychiatric Hospital Setting

PREFACE

Nursing steps into the twenty-first century amidst continued changes in the health care system and ever-emerging managed care environment, and faces complex challenges. Because of these changes, nursing roles have the opportunity for expansion while at the same time many nursing tasks are being taken over by other health care workers. Clear delineation of nursing levels and functions is vital if we are to survive and thrive in this new century. The *Standards of Psychiatric–Mental Health Clinical Nursing Practice* and *Statement on Psychiatric–Mental Health Clinical Nursing Practice* (ANA, APNA, ACAPN, SERPN 1994) have clearly addressed the trends and developments and responsibilities of nurses in the practice of mental health care. The *Standards* delineate the roles, functions, and scope of psychiatric mental health clinical nursing for both the basic and advanced practice level.

Nursing's clinical arena is becoming predominantly community settings while the acute phase of illness is addressed in short-stay hospital settings. Our population is becoming more diverse: therefore, becoming aware of alternative ways of viewing illness and alternative ways to intervene is more important than at any other time in our history, if we are to be competent healers who help ameliorate the emotional turmoil of others. To be effective practitioners, we are best served if we become sensitive to the differences in our colleagues as well as in our clients. To be proficient practitioners, it is best if we increase our critical thinking skills and learn to apply our knowledge in diverse settings among various cultural groups.

Many of the issues we grapple with as nurses accompany us into the new millennium: AIDS, Alzheimer's disease, addictions, domestic violence, homelessness, impaired colleagues, and uninsured children, adults, and elderly. Along with those challenges, however, come new biological and neurobiological findings, exciting breakthroughs in psychopharmacology, and expanded roles for nurses in clinical settings to address these and many other issues and conditions.

Therefore, this third edition incorporates these issues throughout all of the clinical chapters:

*The diversity in the settings in which nursing in general, and psychiatric mental health nursing in particular, is practiced.

*The levels of clinical practice (basic and advanced practice) and the interventions each is prepared for—for example, case finding, counseling (basic level), and prescriptive authority and psychotherapy (advanced practice level).

*Awareness of cultural differences in thinking and approaches to illness.

*The newest psychopharmacological aids and neurobiological findings.

*Critical thinking questions and exercises at the end of each chapter.

*The latest in psychobiological research and pharmacology.

FAMILIAR FEATURES RETAINED AND UPDATED

The third edition retains the basic nursing process format and uses the Mental Health Continuum in place of the anxiety continuum as the organizing framework. Clinical treatments, clinical settings, psychopharmacology, and changes in social issues have been profoundly updated.

The clinical chapters (14 to 27) continue to use the following format: Theory, Nursing Process, Case Study, Nursing Care Plan, and Self-Study Questions, now including Critical Thinking exercises.

*The *Assessment* section now includes a variety of standard assessment tools.

**Planning* includes Identifying Outcome Criteria as well as Nurse's Self-Assessment of personal thoughts and feelings.

Intervention* includes Counseling, Milieu Therapy, Self-Care Activities, Psychobiological Interventions, Health Teaching, Case Management, and Health Promotion and Health Maintenance for the **basic level, and Psychotherapy, Prescription of Pharmacological Agents, and Consultation for the **advanced practice level.**

**Intervention* also includes in selected chapters examples of clinical/critical pathways that are being incorporated in both inpatient and outpatient clinical settings increasingly across the United States.

*Case Studies and Nursing Care Plans help students to translate theoretical material into clinical practice.

*A Glossary and relevant Appendices include pertinent health care resources and nursing web sites.

NEW TO THIRD EDITION

A dynamic new chapter on Psychobiology and Psychopharmacology with PET scans is included in this edition. In clear and straightforward language, this chapter helps the reader understand how specific changes in the neurophysiology of the brain contribute to the symptoms of various mental disorders and how medications work to ameliorate these symptoms.

An emerging model in mental health care suggests that certain psychiatric illnesses (schizophrenia, bipolar disorder, and obsessive-compulsive disorder) may be viewed as brain diseases along a neurological continuum that includes other neurological diseases such as Parkinson's disease and multiple sclerosis (refer to chapter 9).

Integration of the newest medications, protocols, and medication teaching tools are found in each of the appropriate clinical chapters.

Other chapters new to this edition include

- Psychiatric Nursing: Past, Present, Future
- Psychiatric Nursing in Acute Psychiatric Hospital Setting
- Psychiatric Nursing in Community Settings
- Communication Within Families

All chapters have been thoroughly updated and have undergone significant revisions to reflect today's health care system, the times we live in, and the tools and knowledge at our disposal.

Readers are encouraged to take advantage of the tremendous resources on the Internet both for increasing their own knowledge and for obtaining health teaching aids for their clients. Selected web sites have been included to help students get involved with nursing groups and student groups, and find useful self-help groups for their clients.

AIDS TO LEARNING

The **Instructor's Manual** has been updated to include chapter outlines and critical thinking questions while learning exercises and games remain. This should prove to be an invaluable tool for all instructors.

A **Clinical Companion** booklet has been devised for students' use in the clinical area with assessment guides, identification of nursing problems, helpful interventions, and medication information in a clear, coherent format that will be clinically useful and relevant. The medication cards originally in the back of the first and second editions are found in the back of the **Companion,** although not to be torn out, but rather as part of the whole booklet, which fits nicely into the student's pocket for easy reference in the clinical area.

A set of 30 **Transparencies** are included to facilitate student learning and clarify important information.

Multiple choice and critical thinking questions have been updated and are included in the **NCLEX test bank.**

I remain grateful for all the positive feedback and the invaluable suggestions and comments by faculty and students from all parts of the country. You will find that the additions and changes reflect your suggestions and ideas. I continue to welcome your comments and ideas and am warmed by the support of those of you who have adopted this text. Thank you.

ELIZABETH M. VARCAROLIS

ACKNOWLEDGMENTS

First, I wish to thank the authors who helped to take this edition into the twenty-first century. They brought with them their clinical expertise, knowledge, and clarity of thought that for many included gracious rewrites and bold last-minute updates.

My thanks to previous authors of the second edition, who helped shape and expand this text: Margie Lovett-Scott and Marcia A. Ullman, Hildegard E. Peplau, Suzanne Lego, Kem B. Louie, Brenda Lewis Cleary, Barbara B. Bauer, Signe S. Hill, Mary McAndrew, Jane Bryant Neese, Beth Bonham, Mary Jane Herron, and William G. Herron.

I bow to the contributors of *A Nurse Speaks*, who keep me mindful of the purpose of such a text with their warm and wonderful stories. This remains one of my favorite parts of the text.

My special thanks again to Kay Charron for her creative work for the *Instructor's Manual* with the addition of chapter outlines and critical thinking exercises. I thank Kay also for the excellent comprehensive test bank. Special thanks as well go to my nephew, James Varcarolis, who took the right pictures for the Unit openings, except for the one for Unit II, by Ed Leopold.

Never would this book have taken shape without some pretty remarkable people. First, to Ilze Rader, my editor, who has seen this text through three editions, and whose mark is on every one. Her creative energy, constant vigilance, and timely suggestions have guaranteed the success of *Foundations*. I will miss you, Ilze. Thanks to Marie Thomas, Editorial Assistant, who remains cheerful, gracious, always helpful, and efficient in the midst of chaos. My gratitude for your prompt response to my myriad requests.

To Judy Johnstone, my developmental editor. Thanks for the sharing, caring, humor, and oh yes—the brilliant smoothing out, pulling together, and keeping organized and coherent the many inevitable loose ends, and problem-solving the many inevitable manuscript dilemmas. To Patty Romo, literally my right hand, who types, retypes, and then revamps and updates the same manuscript over and over and manages to do it just how I wish it to be done. And finally, to David Harvey, a truly incredible copy editor whose eyes miss not a thing. If there is a mistake in this text, it is not a mistake, it is supposed to be there.

Again—I have to give so much credit and so much appreciation to the educators who have reviewed these chapters, so many of which are new or completely revised. They offered valuable suggestions and ideas, shared their experiences and opinions, and have broadened and strengthened this edition to a remarkable level. I thank you all.

Wilda K. Arnold, RN, BSN, MSN, EdD
Texas Women's University
School of Nursing
Dallas, Texas

Karen S. Bloomfield, RN, MS, CS
Piedmont Virginia Community College
School of Nursing
Charlottesville, Virginia

Linda L. Reeder Breidigam, RN, MSN, CCE
Alvernia College
School of Nursing
Reading, Pennsylvania

Vicki L. Britt, RN, MSN, CS
Coordinator, Psychiatric Nursing
Community Nursing Service at Lee Hospital
Johnstown, Pennsylvania
Adjunct Clinical Instructor
Mt. Aloysius College
Cresson, Pennsylvania

Jane Bruker, MSN, RNCS
Department Chair, Health Careers
University of New Mexico
Gallup, New Mexico

Carolyn R. Pierce Buckelew, BSN, MA, NCC, CS
Charles E. Gregory School of Nursing
Raritan Bay Medical Center
Perth Amboy, New Jersey

Kathy Lynn Burlingame, MS, BSN, CCRN
Northland Community and Technical College
School of Nursing
Thief River Falls, Minnesota

Corinne L. Conlon, MSN, RN, CS
Associate Professor of Nursing
Piedmont Virginia Community College
Charlottesville, Virginia

Sandra R. DeLuca, MSN, RN
The Western Pennsylvania Hospital
School of Nursing
Pittsburgh, Pennsylvania

Judith M. Dempsey, RN, EdD
The Dorothea Hopfer School of Nursing
Mt. Vernon Hospital
Mt. Vernon, New York

Rebecca Crews Gruener, RN, MSN
Associate Professor, Division of Nursing
Louisiana State University
Alexandria, Louisiana

Mary E. Halupa, RN, MSN
Pottsville Hospital
School of Nursing
Pottsville, Pennsylvania

Dorothy J. Irvin, DNS, RN, CS
St. John's College
Department of Nursing
Springfield, Illinois

Bonita Jackson, MSN, RN
Indiana University
School of Nursing
Kokomo, Indiana

Phyllis M. Jacobs, RN, MSN
Wichita State University
School of Nursing
Wichita, Kansas

Alica B. Jehle, RN, MS, FNP
Professor of Nursing
Berkshire Community College
Pittsfield, Massachusetts

Alice R. Kempe, PhD, RN, CS
Associate Professor, School of Nursing
Ursuline College
Pepper Pike, Ohio

Barbara B. Marckx, MS, RN
Broome Community College
School of Nursing
Binghamton, New York

Elizabeth A. Peterson, RN, MA, MS
Associate Professor of Nursing
Bethel College
St. Paul, Minnesota

Sandra J. Peterson, PhD, RN
Associate Professor of Nursing
Bethel College
St. Paul, Minnesota

Yvette M. Pryse, RN, MSN
IVY Technical State College
School of Nursing
Madison, Indiana

Patricia A. Rahe, MS, BSN, RN, CNA
Chair, School of Nursing
IVY Technical State College
Lawrenceburg, Indiana

Carla E. Randall, RN, MSN
Doctoral Student
University of British Columbia
Vancouver, British Columbia
Canada

Mary Ann Bulwicz Ruiz, RNCS, BS, MA
Charles E. Gregory School of Nursing
Raritan Bay Medical Center
Perth Amboy, New Jersey

Elizabeth Savaria-Porter, MS, RN
St. Joseph Hospital
School of Nursing
North Providence, Rhode Island

Cynthia Ann Schaeffer, MSN, RN
Pottsville Hospital
School of Nursing
Pottsville, Pennsylvania

Dawn Margaret Scheick, MS, RN, CS
Associate Professor of Nursing
Alderson-Broaddus College
Philippi, West Virginia
Consultant/Educator
William R. Shapre, Jr. State Psychiatric Hospital
Philippi, West Virginia

Linda S. Smith, MSN, RN
Assistant Professor, School of Nursing
State University of West Georgia
Carrollton, Georgia

Jeanne Venhaus Stein, RN, MSN
St. Louis Community College at Meramec
School of Nursing
Kirkwood, Missouri

Susan Stocker, RN, MSN
Kent State University
School of Nursing
Ashtabula, Ohio

Margaret R. Swisher, MSN, RN
Montgomery County Community College
School of Nursing
Blue Bell, Pennsylvania

B. Gayle Twiname, PhD, RN, CS, CGP
Lamar University
School of Nursing
Beaumont, Texas

Karen S. Ward, PhD, RN
Middle Tennessee State University
School of Nursing
Murfreesboro, Tennessee

Wanda May Webb, MSN, RN, CS
Brandywine School of Nursing
Coatesville, Pennsylvania

Dixie R. Whong, RN, MSN
Alvernia College
School of Nursing
Reading, Pennsylvania

CONTENTS

KEY TO SPECIAL FEATURES

DIAGNOSTIC CRITERIA

DRUG INFORMATION

MENTAL HEALTH CONTINUUM

NURSING ASSESSMENT

NURSING INTERVENTIONS AND RATIONALES

Foundations of Psychiatric Mental Health Nursing

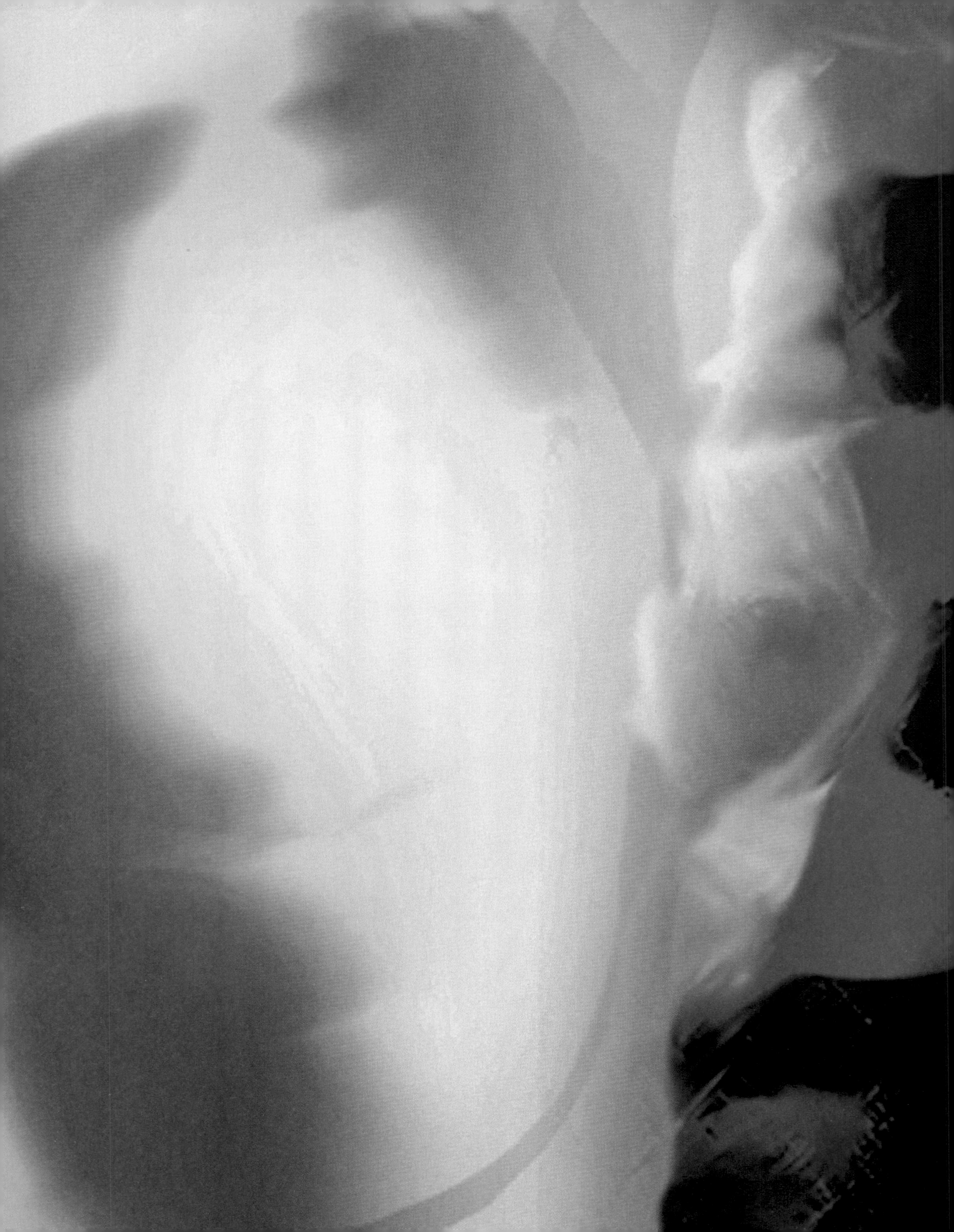

PART I

FOUNDATIONS IN THEORY

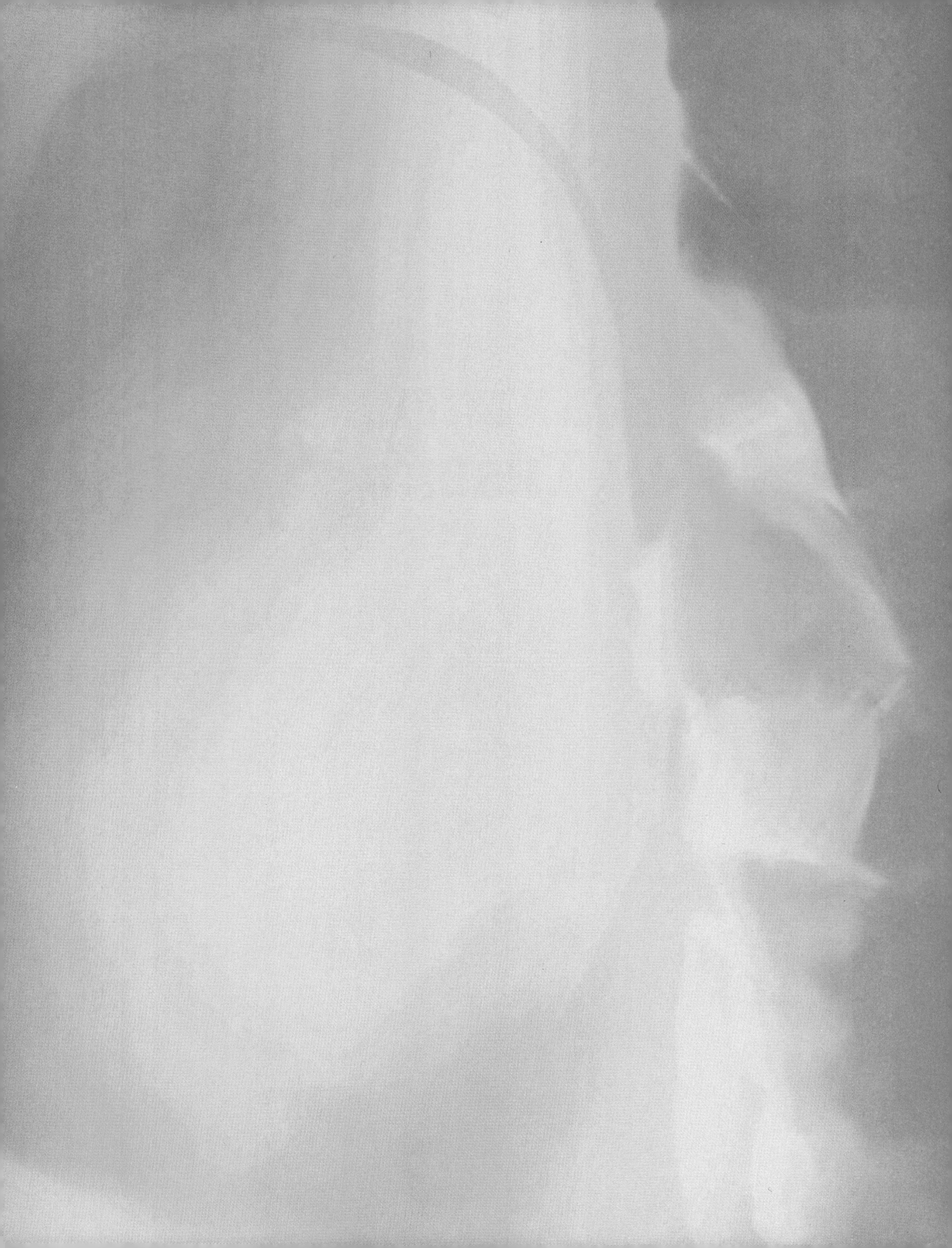

UNIT ONE

Frameworks for the Practice of Psychosocial Nursing

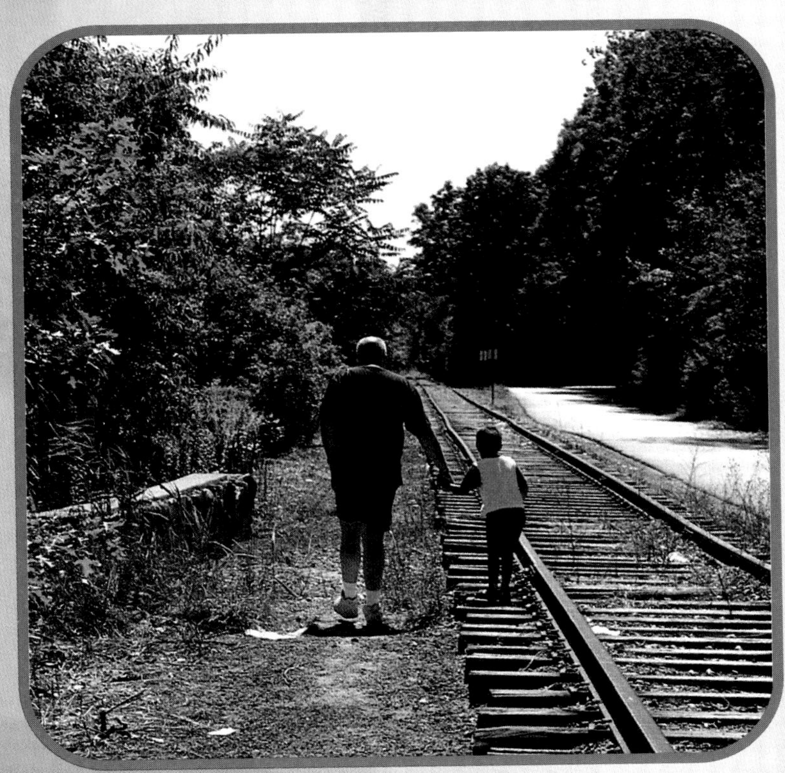

If a child is to keep alive his inborn sense of wonder, he needs the companionship of at least one adult who can share it, rediscovering with him the joy, excitement and mystery of the world we live in.

RACHEL CARSON,
THE SENSE OF WONDER, 1965

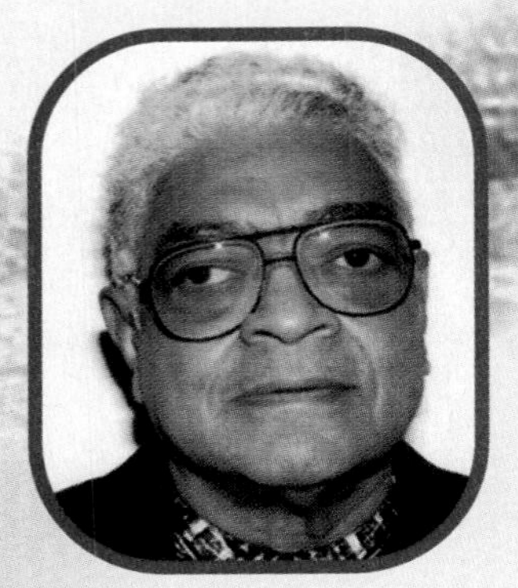

A Nurse Speaks

John A. Payne

Fifty years ago psychiatry was practiced in an environment vastly different from the one in which it is practiced today. Most clients were treated in large state hospitals, which were like small towns with their own store, restaurant, churches, farms, power plants, carpentry shop, and buildings housing thousands of clients and staff. There were buildings for admission and for treatment, infirmaries, chronic quiet units, and chronic disturbed units.

As nursing students, we were taught to care for clients who were receiving sedation, insulin shock, electric shock, malaria therapy, continuous hydrotherapy, wet packs, supraorbital lobotomies, physical restraints, and seclusion. All of these treatments were designed to make the clients more amenable to psychotherapy, to calm them, or for the safety of themselves or others. The disturbed wards were usually noisy and very active places in which clients acted out their psychoses both physically and vocally. Care for these clients was mostly custodial and involved keeping them clean, fed, safe, and calm.

I distinctly remember one client who was almost continuously kept in seclusion because of bizarre and aggressive behavior. He would not keep his clothes on, could not safely use eating utensils, and roared like a lion. Because of his behavior, he was frequently referred to as the Lion Man.

Keeping him clean and fed was a major project for the staff and always required several people. It was a frustrating experience because we all wanted to help him and see him behave in a more acceptable manner.

During the Korean War, I was away in the Air Force for four years. For three years I was a part of a system that treated young men for psychiatric problems by using many of the same modalities that were used in the state hopitals. The treatment there was somewhat more successful than that provided in the state hospitals because most of the men's visible signs of psychoses were of recent origin, having been caused by the stress of basic training or the stress of being in battle.

During my fourth year in the Air Force, psychotropic drugs were introduced. We began to use them very cautiously on our clients, with very limited success. As the doctors became more familiar with the drugs and increased the dosages, the results showed much improved behavior with most clients. Gradually no clients were being put into packs, and the hydrotherapy room was seldom used.

After being discharged from the Air Force, I returned to the hospital in which I had trained. As I went to the different buildings, I was surprised to see that here too there had been a decrease in the use of the old treatment modalities. Clients for the most part appeared much calmer; no clients were in seclusion all of the time, not even the Lion Man.

One day, while I was walking on the grounds with one of the charge attendants, he asked me if I knew who a client sitting on a bench talking with another client was. I said, "No. Who is he?" "That is the guy we used to call the Lion Man." What a change! The attendant told me that they had given him Thorazine and that within one week he was out of seclusion and keeping his clothes on. Gradually he began to socialize with staff and other clients. Within 1 month he was playing checkers, and within one year he was granted ground privileges. Truly, the psychotropic drugs revolutionized the treatment of psychiatric clients.

Some psychotherapeutic modalities that had been used in smaller settings began to be used in the state hospitals. Group therapy, milieu therapy, and remotivation therapy became the vogue, and with this the role of nursing became a more therapeutic one.

During President Kennedy's tenure in office, the Community Mental Health Bill was passed. This provided funds for moving the treatment of clients from the large state hospitals to the local hospital. Two things were significant about this legislation. First, all levels and modalities of treatment had to be provided to all residents within a specific "catchment area." Second, all disciplines (including nursing) had to be represented on the treatment team.

States passed clients' bills of rights that released into the community thousands of clients who had spent many years in state hospitals. A part of the movement that was never adequate was the provision of group homes and follow-up supervision. This has led to our present situation of many actively psychotic ex-clients wandering our streets as homeless citizens. A change is going to come, and nursing is going to be an important part of that change. For now we have nurses in ever-increasing numbers who are becoming psychotherapists and psychiatric nurse practioners. They will be leaders in providing care themselves and through mental health or psychiatric technicians—for nursing is still the only discipline that is proficient in providing 24-hour care to people in need.

1

Psychiatric Nursing: PAST, PRESENT, FUTURE

ELIZABETH M. VARCAROLIS

OUTLINE

KEY TERMS AND CONCEPTS

The key terms and concepts listed here also appear in bold where they are defined or discussed in this chapter.

basic level, psychiatric mental health registered nurse (RN, C)

advanced level, psychiatric mental health advanced practice registered nurse (RN, CS)

critical (or clinical) pathways

case management

nursing informatics

computer-based client records (CPRs)

advocacy role in nursing

community nursing centers (CNCs)

OBJECTIVES

After studying this chapter, the reader will be able to:

1. Identify at least five arenas in which psychiatric mental health nurses work.
2. Compare and contrast the preparation and requirements for a psychiatric mental health nurse at the basic level with one prepared at the advanced practice level.
3. Describe at least five interventions that the basic level psychiatric mental health nurse is prepared to perform, and the additional three interventions that the advanced practice level psychiatric mental health nurse is prepared to perform.
4. Identify at least eight painful, frightening, or dysfunctional phenomena that psychiatric mental health nurses target and ameliorate.
5. Discuss two political and social trends that led to the growing role of the psychiatric mental health nurse, and state how they continue to do so.
6. Explain what clinical/critical pathways are and how they can be effective for client care.
7. Describe the role(s) of a case manager.
8. Analyze the pros and cons of using computer-based records (CPRs) for the hospital and community and computer-assisted instruction (CAI) for student and client learning.
9. Assess some of the ways that continuing ethnic and cultural changes can affect the delivery of health care in the United States.
10. Identify and discuss three trends in psychiatric mental health nursing.
11. Apply information from this text to access a nursing network on the Internet.

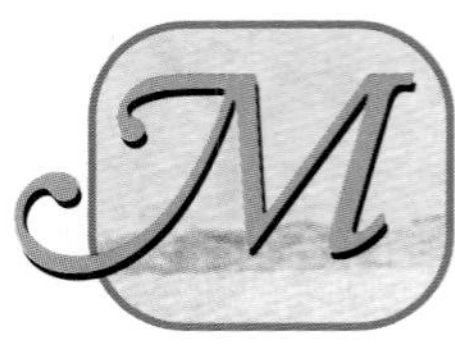

Most of you will probably never work on a psychiatric unit or in a mental health community center. However, all of you will be working with people who are going through crises, suffering periods of intense anxiety and fear, experiencing loss, or facing a life-altering event. Most of you will encounter clients who are experiencing feelings of hopelessness, helplessness, anxiety, anger, low self-esteem, or confusion. No matter what work setting you choose as a registered nurse, you will encounter people who are withdrawn, suspicious, elated, depressed, hostile, manipulative, suicidal, intoxicated, or withdrawing from a substance. Many of you have already come across people who are going through difficult times in their lives. At times you may have handled these situations skillfully, and at other times you may have wished you had additional skills and knowledge.

Basic concepts of psychosocial nursing will become central to your practice of nursing and increase your competency as a practitioner in all clinical settings. Your experience in the psychiatric nursing rotation can help you gain insight into yourself and greatly increase your insight into the experiences of others. This part of your nursing education can also give you guidelines and the opportunity to learn new skills for dealing with a variety of challenging behaviors. Therefore, psychosocial skills are relevant to anything you choose to do both inside and outside your nursing profession. I hope this is an enjoyable, exciting, and gratifying experience for you. I hope some of you may even choose to become psychiatric nurses.

This chapter presents a brief overview of what professional psychatric nurses do. It will acquaint you with some of the history of psychatric nursing and, within the social climate of the times, some of the issues dominating our current health care practices. Finally, it looks at the direction that nursing is taking into the future.

WHAT IS A PSYCHIATRIC MENTAL HEALTH NURSE?

About 28% of Americans over 18 years of age suffer from a mental or addictive disorder in any 1-year period. A partial classification is as follows (Goldberg 1995):

- Addictive disorders, 9.5%
- Anxiety disorders, 12.6%
- Schizophrenia, 1.1%
- Affective disorders, 9.5%
- Antisocial personality disorders, 1.5%
- Cognitive disorders, 2.7%

Psychiatric mental health nurses work with children, adults, and the elderly who have acute or long-term mental health problems. Their clients may include people with dual diagnoses (a mental disorder and a coexisting substance disorder), homeless persons and families, people in jail (forensic nursing), people who have survived abusive situations, people with acquired immunodeficiency syndrome (AIDS), and people in crisis. Psychiatric nurses work with individuals, families, and groups. They work with clients in hospitals, in their homes, in halfway houses, in shelters, in clinics, in storefronts, on the street—virtually wherever there are people.

The *Statement on psychiatric–mental health clinical nursing practice* (ANA et al. 1994a) defines the psychiatric mental health nurse as one who "diagnoses and treats human responses to actual or potential mental health problems." Psychiatric mental health nursing is a specialized area of nursing practice that draws on accepted theories for its base of care. The theories are derived from nursing, as well as from the "biological, cultural, environmental, psychological, and sociological sciences," and "these theories provide a basis for psychiatric mental health nursing" (ANA et al. 1994a, pp. 7, 9). Psychiatric mental health nurses, like all nurses, use both primary sources (client interview and client observation) and secondary sources (chart, family/friends/others, staff) to make their assessment and formulate their nursing diagnoses. Psychiatric mental health nurses also make use of the standard classifications of mental disorders such as the *Diagnostic and statistical manual of mental disorders* of the American Psychiatric Association (DSM-IV 1994). In Chapter 2 you will find an overview of DSM-IV. In the clinical chapters of this text we present the criteria for discrete diagnostic DSM-IV categories (e.g., schizophrenia, depression, anxiety disorders). Many psychiatric mental health nurses also use the *International Classification of Disease* (ICD 10) developed by the World Health Organization, the latest update of which was in 1993.

LEVELS OF CLINICAL PRACTICE

Many nurses who work on psychiatric units are not certified as psychiatric nurses. They may be staff nurses who have chosen, or been asked to work on, a psychiatric unit and perform the necessary nursing duties to help the unit function smoothly. Some staff nurses may have excellent communication skills; others may not. Some may have a sound understanding of how to approach clients with specific behaviors (clients who are hallucinating, paranoid, delusional, withdrawn, suicidal, depressed, manic), while others may not. Some may have an affinity for relieving emotional pain; others may not. The *Statement on psychiatric–mental health clinical nursing practice* (ANA et al. 1994a) identifies the criteria and definition specific for the title of professional psychiatric mental health nurse.

There are two levels of psychiatric mental health nurses: basic and advanced. The two levels are clearly delineated by educational preparation, professional experience, type of practice, and certification. The above-mentioned statement (ANA et al. 1994a, pp. 10–11) formally distinguishes between the two.

Basic Level, Psychiatric Mental Health Registered Nurse

Currently, there are many associate-degree nurses (ADNs) with certification at this basic level who are working as psychiatric mental health registered nurses. However, beginning in 1998, a minimum of a bachelor of science (BS) degree in nursing will be a prerequisite for initial certification as a generalist in this field.

The basic level as of 1998 will have two requirements: (1) a baccalaureate degree in nursing and demonstration of clinical skills within the specialty, exceeding those of a beginning RN or novice; (2) certification that attests to having met the profession's standards of knowledge and experience. Certification is a formal process that validates the nurse's competence at this level of psychiatric nursing. To show certification as a psychiatric mental health registered nurse, a nurse would place a "C" after the RN (e.g., Tom Smith, RN, C).

Advanced Level, Psychiatric Mental Health Advanced Practice Registered Nurse

The psychiatric mental health advanced practice registered nurse (APRN) is prepared, at a minimum, with a master's degree. Certification is national and requires a "depth of knowledge of theory and practice, supervised clinical practice, and competence in advanced clinical nursing skills" (ANA et al. 1994a, p. 11). The nurse who meets the above criteria and passes the national certifying examination is awarded certification for 5 years as a specialist in either adult or child and adolescent psychiatric nursing (CS). At the end of the 5-year period, the nurse must complete the certification renewal process. The nurse who is a certified specialist in psychiatric and mental health nursing is identified with a CS following the RN (e.g., Nancy Rivera, RN, CS).

The rapid changes in the health care system are reflected in the expanding scope of nursing practice. "Many state legislators and Congress have acknowledged the unique role of advanced practice psychiatric nursing in the delivery of mental health services by passing legislation which makes them eligible for prescriptive authority (ordering medications), hospital admissions privileges, and third-party reimbursement" (ANA et al. 1994a, p. 11). Not every state has passed legislation covering all of these privileges at this time.

At this writing there are about 40,000 clinical nurse specialists in the United States, and nearly 700 of them are credentialed at the national level by the American Nurses Credentialing Center (ANCC) as certified specialists (RN, CS) (APNA 1995).

WHAT DO PSYCHIATRIC NURSES DO?

The main focus of the psychiatric mental health nurse is to promote and maintain optimal mental functioning, to prevent mental illness (or prevent further dysfunction), and to help clients regain or improve their coping abilities. These goals are realized through a variety of nursing activities in all sorts of hospital and community settings.

Standards of psychiatric–mental health clinical nursing practice (ANA et al. 1994a) clearly defines nursing actions for the professional nurse, distinguishing those nursing activities appropriate for the basic level psychiatric nurse (RN, C) and those for the advanced practice clinical nurse specialist (RN, CS). These guidelines are used by the nurse throughout the nursing process, which "is the foundation of decision making and encompasses all significant action taken by nurses in providing psychiatric–mental health nursing care" (ANA et al. 1994a, p. 25). *Standards of psychiatric–mental health clinical nursing practice* will be utilized throughout the clinical chapters (Chapters 11 to 27) when presenting the appropriate interventions for each specific diagnostic category.

Essentially, the interventions of the **basic level, psychiatric mental health registered nurse (RN, C)** focus on

- Counseling, including crisis intervention
- Management of the therapeutic environment (milieu management)
- Assisting clients with self-care activities
- Administrating and monitoring psychobiological treatments
- Health teaching, including psychoeducation
- Providing culturally relevant health promotion and disease prevention strategies
- Case management

The specialist at the **advanced level, psychiatric mental health advanced practice registered nurse (RN, CS),** in addition to the above nursing activities, is qualified to provide

- Psychotherapy (individual, group, family, and other therapeutic treatments)
- Prescription of pharmacological agents (in accordance with the State Nursing Practice Act)
- Consultation (to health care providers and others)

The standards of care are outlined on the inside front cover of *Standards of psychiatric–mental health clinical nursing practice* (ANA et al. 1994a). Refer to Table 1–1 for a more comprehensive understanding of the nursing activities provided by psychiatric mental health nurses as outlined in the *Standards*.

IN WHAT PHENOMENA DO PSYCHIATRIC MENTAL HEALTH NURSES INTERVENE?

Psychiatric mental health nurses plan intervention strategies through the nursing process. "Diagnosis of human responses to actual or potential mental health problems involves the application of theory to human phenomena, through the process of assessment, diagnosis, planning, intervention or treatment, and evaluation" (ANA et al. 1994a, p. 9). Psychiatric mental health nurses plan interventions to target and ameliorate the painful, frightening, harmful, and/or dysfunctional phenomena their clients are experiencing. Specific phenomena can include the following (ANA et al. 1994a, p. 8):

- Self-care limitations related to mental and emotional distress
- Crisis or emotional stress
- Self-concept changes
- Problems related to emotions such as anxiety, anger, sadness, loneliness, and grief
- Alterations in thinking and perceiving (hallucinations, delusions)
- Difficulty relating to others
- Self-violence (suicidal behaviors/thinking) or violence to others
- Difficulty relating to others

Refer to Box 1–1 for psychiatric mental health nursing's phenomena of concern.

BOX 1–1 PSYCHIATRIC MENTAL HEALTH NURSING'S PHENOMENA OF CONCERN

ACTUAL OR POTENTIAL MENTAL HEALTH PROBLEMS OF CLIENTS PERTAINING TO

- The maintenance of optimal health and well-being and the prevention of psychobiological illness.
- Self-care limitations or impaired functioning related to mental and emotional distress.
- Deficits in the functioning of significant biological, emotional, and cognitive systems.
- Emotional stress or crisis components of illness, pain, and disability.
- Self-concept changes, developmental issues, and life process changes.
- Problems related to emotions such as anxiety, anger, sadness, loneliness, and grief.
- Physical symptoms that occur along with altered psychological functioning.
- Alterations in thinking, perceiving, symbolizing, communicating, and decision making.
- Difficulties relating to others.
- Behaviors and mental states that indicate the client is a danger to self or others or has a severe disability.
- Interpersonal, systematic, sociocultural, spiritual, or environmental circumstances or events that affect the mental and emotional well-being of the individual, family, or community.
- Symptom management, side effects/toxicities associated with psychopharmacological intervention and other aspects of the treatment regimen.

From ANA, APNA, ACAPN, SERPN. (1994). *Statement on psychiatric–mental health clinical nursing practice and standards of psychiatric–mental health clinical nursing practice.* Washington, DC: American Nurses' Association.

TABLE 1–1 PSYCHIATRIC NURSING INTERVENTIONS AS DEFINED BY THE STANDARDS OF PSYCHIATRIC MENTAL HEALTH CLINICAL NURSES

LEVEL	INTERVENTION	DESCRIPTION
		Basic Level
Psychiatric Mental Health Nurse (RN, C)	A. Case management B. Counseling C. Health promotion and health maintenance D. Health teaching E. Milieu therapy F. Psychobiological intervention G. Self-care activities	In inpatient and outpatient settings: a. Coordinates health and human services b. Designs and evaluates the use of culturally appropriate services (refer to text) Use of communication skills and interviewing skills, problem-solving skills, crisis intervention, stress management, assertiveness training, and behavior modification. a. Conduct health assessments b. Targets at-risk situations c. Initials interventions: 1. Assertiveness training 2. Stress management 3. Parenting classes 4. Health teaching d. Targets potential complications related to symptoms or treatment Formal and informal information regarding coping, interpersonal relationships, mental health problems, mental disorders, treatments and their effects on daily living, developmental needs, and more. Information is given in gender, developmental, cultural, and educational appropriate levels. Provision of a therapeutic environment (hospital, community, home) focusing on a wide range of factors such as physical environment, social structures interactions, and cultural setting. Administering and monitoring responses to medications as well as emergency procedures, relaxation techniques, nutrition/diet regulations, exercise and rest schedules, and other somatic treatment.
		Advanced Practice
Certified specialist in Psychiatric Nursing (RN, CS)	All of the above plus: H. Consultation I. Prescription of pharmacological agents J. Psychotherapy	Encourage highest level of independent functioning in such areas as personal hygiene, feeding, recreational activities, practical skills (e.g., shopping, using public transportation) Provides consultation to health care providers and others as well as supervision to other mental health care providers and trainers. In accordance with the State Practice Act where the nurse works, the RN, CS Mental Health Nurse may prescribe pharmacological agents (medications) to treat symptoms of mental illness and improve functional health status. Performs individual, group, family, child, and adolescent psychotherapy and other therapeutic treatments in inclient, outclient, community mental health, and private practice settings.

Data from ANA, APNA, ACAPN, SERPN. (1994). *Statement on psychiatric–mental health clinical nursing practice and standards of psychiatric–mental health clinical nursing practice.* Washington, DC: American Nurses' Association.

PSYCHIATRIC NURSING: AN OVERVIEW

The Beginnings

1892–1950

The history of psychiatric nursing is slightly over a century old. Linda Richards, who studied under Florence Nightingale, was the first graduate nurse in the United States, as well as the first psychiatric nurse. Richards was graduated in 1873 from the New England Hospital for Women and Children, which had opened in 1872. Nine years later, Richards and a physician named Edward Cowles started the first formally organized training school for nurses at McLean Hospital for the mentally ill in Massachusetts. This marked the beginning of psychiatric nursing.

We identify important happenings and milestones by their dates, but history is also about the trends, patterns, and themes that categorize those happenings (Peplau 1994, p. 96). Peplau has written:

> The history of psychiatric nursing is about the struggles, choices, and progress that nurses have made over the many years of its development. It is the story of the continuities—the beginnings and the forward steps—that were taken by psychiatric nurses in the United States to get to their present position in nursing and society. The whole history of psychiatric nursing has not yet been told. It is a long story . . .
>
> There are always lessons to be learned from history. One such lesson comes from very courageous nurses, working in psychiatric hospitals, who were willing to take a stand on unpopular issues of their day. At the turn of the twentieth century and earlier, psychiatric nursing was an unpopular field of work. It shared the general stigma attached to mental illness and to the institutions that cared for psychiatric clients.
>
> Another lesson is that after World War II, when a change in attitude toward the mentally ill occurred, the nursing profession was able to rise to this challenge. It was able to pursue opportunities promised in the provisions of the National Mental Health Act of 1946. Nursing's readiness occurred not so much by design but rather as a consequence of the persistence of a few psychiatric nursing leaders. In earlier years, at the beginning of organized nursing, they had spoken out, persuaded, and therefore helped to shape the general direction taken by the nursing profession. Their perspective, eventually adopted by the profession, was to include psychiatric nursing as an important component of the whole of nursing.

The National Institute of Mental Health (NIMH), through the passage of the National Mental Health Act in 1946, provided funding for training mental health professionals. These funds played a significant role in the education of advanced practice psychiatric mental health nurses.

The 1950s

Psychiatric nursing began taking great strides beyond the giving of custodial care to the mentally ill in state hospitals. It was in the early 1950s that the first antipsychotic medications were introduced. These drugs produced profound behavior changes for many clients, lowering the need for restraints, straightjackets, and other constraints. Through the use of these new antipsychotic medications, more people became amenable to treatment and benefited from therapy. During the same period, Maxwell Jones of Great Britain wrote a book in 1953, *The therapeutic community*, that introduced the concept of the "therapeutic milieu" and the nurse's role in this therapy. The time was ripe for expanding the nurse's role in the ways Jones suggested. Although exposure to psychiatric clients was offered in many schools of nursing at the time, it was in 1953 that the National League for Nursing (NLN) adopted the position that all accredited nursing schools should give their students a psychiatric nursing experience.

In 1920 Harriet Bailey wrote the first psychiatric nursing textbook, *Nursing mental disease*. However, it was Hildegard Peplau in 1952 who formulated the first systematic theoretical framework in psychiatric nursing, presented in her groundbreaking work *Interpersonal relations in nursing*. Peplau emphasized that theoretical concepts and psychological techniques are essential to nursing practice and laid the foundation for the nurse-client relationship that is the cornerstone of psychiatric nursing (see Chapter 6).

June Mellow introduced the second theoretical approach to psychiatric nursing, calling it "nursing therapy." Mellow emphasized providing corrective emotional experience by focusing on psychosocial needs and the client's strengths. At a later date, Mellow would provide leadership for the first doctor of nursing science degree in psychiatric nursing, which was offered at the Boston University School of Nursing (Dumas 1994).

During this time, many other nursing leaders expanded the role of the psychiatric nurse and added to the theoretical base. The description of psychiatric nursing was evolving from caretaking duties to roles and subroles that nurses perform, including surrogate parent, teacher, resource person, counselor, and more.

In 1955 Rutgers University was the first to receive a federal grant for a graduate program for psychiatric clinical nurse specialists at the master's level. This was the first 2-year program to prepare nurses for individual, group, and family psychotherapy. It was during this time that nurse theoreticians began to differentiate between general practitioners, who were staff nurses working on a psychiatric unit, and psychiatric nurses, who were expert clinical practitioners with master's degrees.

The 1960s

In 1963 the Community Mental Health Center (CMHC) Act was passed, providing federal moneys to plan, construct, and staff mental health community centers. The original idea was to take clients out of the state mental hospitals and care for them in the community, in effect de-institutionalizing them. Five essential services were required in a federally funded CMHC. These services were to be provided through geographical areas called *catchment areas*. The services included (Hillard 1994)

- Inpatient services
- Outpatient services
- Emergency services
- Partial hospitalization
- Consultation and education

The CMHC Act of 1963 opened the way for the expansion of the nurse's role from the hospital into the community. Thus, the term *psychiatric nurse* evolved into *psychiatric mental health nurse*. Unfortunately, for many clients released from state institutions, de-institutionalization led to isolation, victimization, homelessness, and disintegration. Billings (1993) states that the failure during the 1960s and 1970s of the many efforts to improve access to mental health care and to develop new models of care were related to three factors:

1. Changed government spending policies
2. The system's failure to convert to the proposed new approaches
3. The pervasively negative public attitude surrounding the mentally ill and mental illness

Chapter 27 addresses more fully the needs of the severely and persistently mentally ill and the homeless populations.

Throughout the 1960s and 1970s, many other nurse leaders emphasized the importance of self-awareness and therapeutic use of self, nurse-client relationship therapy, and therapeutic communication. Peplau identified the main thrust of the psychiatric nurse's work with clients as that of counselor or psychotherapist (Peplau 1962). The nurses' theoretical base was expanding, and it was during this time that Peplau formulated the levels of anxiety and the steps in anxiety reduction used by all health care professionals today. In 1963 two journals specific to psychiatric nursing were first published: *Perspectives in Psychiatric Care* and what is today the *Journal of Psychosocial Nursing and Mental Health Services.*

The 1970s

In 1975 the federally funded CMHC added seven other residential services:

- Children's services
- Geriatric services
- Aftercare
- State hospital prescreening
- Drug abuse treatment
- Alcohol abuse treatment
- Transitional housing

During the 1970s the specialty of psychiatric nursing continued to develop. In 1973 the American Nurses' Association (ANA) established a certification program for nurses. In 1976 the ANA established two levels of professional nurse. Certification of psychiatric nurse generalists and specialists was established. The ANA's division on psychiatric and mental health nursing published the revised *Statement on psychiatric and mental health nursing practice.*

The 1980s

In 1980 the ANA published *Nursing: A social policy statement* with an emphasis on the nursing process. The definition of nursing in this publication represented a great shift from the roles nurses play (what do nurses *do*?) to "what *phenomena* do nurses fix, correct, ameliorate, relieve, or prevent by addressing nursing practices to them?" (Peplau 1994, p. 99). The *Standards of psychiatric–mental health nursing practice* was first published in 1982, delineating the scope of psychiatric nursing practice, and updated in 1994.

In the 1980s other nursing leaders were formulating theories of victimology and expanding crisis theory into nursing practice (see Appendix A). At the same time, nurse clinicians and theorists were carving out a classification system for psychiatric mental health nursing. A number of developments since the late 1980s were indicators of progress in the field of psychiatric nursing (McBride 1996):

- Debut of new journals (*Archives of Psychiatric Nursing, Journal of Child and Adolescent Psychiatric and Mental Health Nursing*, and *Capsules and Comments in Psychiatric Nursing)*
- Record-breaking attendance at annual professional meetings (see Appendix B for a list of psychiatric mental health nursing organizations)
- Acknowledgment of the specialty's interventions as being basic to nursing practice (e.g., music therapy, group psychotherapy, assertiveness training)
- Development of a classification system for psychiatric mental health nursing

This chapter does not permit a thorough overview of the historical trends, circumstances, happenings, and personalities that influenced the continually emerging role of the psychiatric nurse. However, it is a fascinating story, and you can find useful references at the end of the chapter if you want to explore the history of psychiatric nursing on your own. Also, Appendix A presents an overview of some of the trends and identifies some of the outstanding nursing leaders whose creativity, enthusiasm, strength of character, and hard work have influenced and helped to define the specialty of psychiatric nursing.

It is due to the efforts of outstanding leaders in the past who expanded the scope of nursing practice, as well as the knowledge base, through research and clinical observations that psychiatric nursing has developed into a profession in its own right.

The Present: Issues Affecting Nursing in the 1990s

The Decade of the Brain

The 1990s has been called the "decade of the brain." The advent of numerous imaging techniques opened up a new world of understanding the neurophysiology and neuroanatomy of the brain. Neurobiological changes can now be observed and categorized in people with mental disorders. This knowledge has led to a revolution in the understanding of mental health, providing evidence that many of the most serious mental disorders should be viewed as "diseases of the brain." Thus, there has been a major shift in the way to treat people with mental diseases, mainly through psychopharmacology.

In 1994 the ANA published a summary of the work of its psychopharmacology task force titled the *Psychiatric–mental health nursing psychopharmacology project.* The purpose of the project was to evaluate and advance the scope of psychiatric nursing practice with respect to psychopharmacology and related neuroscience for both certified and advanced practice nurses. The ANA advocates that undergraduate programs prepare their nurses with a solid foundation of neuroscience and psychopharmacology as they relate to mental illness. Graduate programs should include advanced learning, clinical application, and research inquiry in these essential fields. The ANA task force on psychopharmacology proposed that the future should include "a refinement of levels of psychopharmacology practiced by psychiatric mental health nurses, including appropriate credentials for psychiatric–mental health nurses in psychopharmacology" (ANA 1994b).

Each of the clinical chapters in this text presents the appropriate pharmacological treatment for specific mental health disorders. The discussion of medications appropriate for each clinical disorder includes the action, targeted symptoms, side effects, toxic effects, nursing implications, and medication teaching plans. Chapter 3 provides an overview of the psychotrophic drugs and how they affect the neurophysiology of the brain.

Many nursing leaders, while applauding the strides taken in the ameliorization of suffering for people with mental diseases, caution us not to lose sight of our identity and our unique strength as psychosocial and psychiatric nurses. A technician can be taught to be an expert in psychopharmacology; psychiatric nurses offer that expertise and a great deal more. Yes, we do need to educate ourselves and prepare future nurses to be competent regarding the growing body of information on the relationship among neuro-physio-anatomy, mental diseases, and psychopharmacology. Psychotropics are powerful chemicals. They are frequently prescribed, but nurses know that they do not always work (Schauer 1995). Clients are not always compliant with medications when the medications cause discomfort or embarrassing side effects. In these cases, compliance should not be expected until the issues around noncompliance are addressed. Nurses need to listen to the consumer (Schauer 1995).

Although the emphasis on psychopharmacology is not misplaced, Billings (1993) cautions that psychosocial nurses also need to continue to grow in their unique capacity to help people with the quality of their lives through psychoeducational approaches, clarification of verbal content, alteration of the environment stimuli, systems intervention within the family, or the classical application of a therapeutic nurse-client relationship.

Psychotropic drugs can have a profound and beneficial effect on cognition, mood, and behavior. However, they do not change the underlying process, which is often highly sensitive to intrapsychic and psychosocial stressors. Optimal benefits are achieved by simultaneously reducing symptoms and promoting the individual's capacity to adapt to the pressure and demands of life (Trubowitz 1994). Research substantiates that the combined treatment of psychopharmacology and psychotherapy for people with severe mental problems is superior to either treatment alone (ANA et al. 1994a).

> What medicine and I do is complementary, and our combined approach is invaluable in the restoration of a productive life for the client. If I simply narrow my focus to the medical perspective, then the client is deprived of the rich potential that additional or alternative views could have provided. Naming the "human response" with a nursing diagnosis sanctions my prescription and provides the basis for my nursing intervention. In our society, it is the diagnosis that justifies the prescription and codes the service for payment. In the future, it may be the only means by which we [nurses] will be compensated for our work. (Billings 1993, p. 176.)

The Changing Site of Practice: From Hospital to Community

The spiraling costs of health care, and diminished access to health care by large populations within our society, have contributed to the need for radical reform. The intense demands being made upon health care organizations and providers of care are increasingly complex and volatile (Hicks et al. 1993). Currently, the health care environment is in a state of chaos that is reverberating throughout the nation, with its future yet to be determined (Christensen and Bender 1994). In order to trim costs, hospitals cut down on the length of the clients' hospital stay and cut out available units and services (downsizing). The shortened length of stay is often guided by the use of **clinical** (sometimes called **critical**) **pathways.** A clinical pathway is a written plan, or map, that identifies predetermined times that specific nursing and medical interventions (e.g., diagnostic studies, treatments, activities, medications, client outcomes, discharge teaching) will be implemented. Clinical pathways are designed to allocate resources in the most effective and efficient manner. These pathways have been found to

- Target the focus of treatment for specific time periods
- Specify expected outcome criteria for each time period
- Improve the use of personalized client treatment strategies
- Streamline charting
- Enhance client/family teaching
- Enhance evaluation of client care activities and goal achievement

Clinical pathways have proved to be useful tools for teaching, for preventing complications, and for anticipating staffing needs (Redick et al. 1994). Other researchers found that the use of clinical pathways resulted in enhanced staff skills both in physical assessment and in communication with physicians (Milne and Pelletier 1994). Clinical pathways are used in many psychiatric health care centers across the United States. Although currently these pathways are not as widely used in psychiatric as in medical-surgical areas, their use in psychiatric health care is increasing. You will find more discussion of clinical/critical pathways in Chapter 8, and examples of specific clinical pathways for various psychiatric disorders are presented in some of the clinical chapters. Although clinical/critical pathways have their merits, there are also cautions with regard to their use. One of the nurses in the "A Nurse Speaks" section discusses the pros/cons of clinical/critical pathways.

The recent trend toward shorter hospital stays allows less time for tests, procedures, preparation for surgery, observation, client/family teaching, and discharge planning. This shortened length of stay means that many psychiatric clients are barely stabilized before they are released to home and/or the community. A shorter hospitalization period, coupled with downsizing of services, requires that the more acutely ill must continue to receive expert treatment in community settings. One result of the shorter hospital stay has been that emergency and outclient visits have greatly increased. CMHCs and emergency medical services are continuing to evolve toward providing for the increasing volume and variety of client needs. This rapid growth in emergency services has led to psychiatric emergency services taking on increasingly diversified functions, well beyond their initial role in diagnosis and referral (Hillard 1994). For example, some psychiatric emergency rooms are set up with beds for extended treatment where clients may stay for several days. Other emergency services offer outreach programs that send staff into the community to serve some clients. There is no question that nurses in general, and psychiatric nurses in particular, will increasingly work in a variety of community-based settings, both traditional and nontraditional.

It is not just that the locations where nurses work will undergo radical changes; there are changes in the types of agencies under which they will work. The reformed health care system will see more managed care facilities, and there will be much more emphasis on proving the cost effectiveness of provider services. More and more nurses will be working for corporations, in a move away from nonprofit or private hospital organizations. This will bring both obvious and subtle changes. One area of concern is that the values and philosophies of corporate medicine are not always compatible with those of nursing. We will turn to this issue again later in the chapter.

While hospitals were downsizing and reducing services, they were also laying off nurses throughout the country, and they eliminated many nursing positions, both administrative and clinical. Of great concern to the nursing community is the replacing of RNs with unlicensed staff. For example, community care facilities complain that psychiatric nurses are too expensive and say that two non-nurses can be hired to do the job of one registered nurse (Stuart 1994). This is happening in all areas of nursing practice.

Challenges and Emerging Roles for Nurses

Shorter hospital stays have increased the need for community-based support for people with both acute and long-term illnesses. The acutely ill who are discharged to the community continue to need expert professional care and intensive case management. These changes in the environment of health care practices have posed many challenges for nurses. At the same time, the breaking up of static and ineffective patterns of health care delivery has paved the way for many exciting opportunities.

Among the challenges, many nurses find that the job qualifications for positions they have traditionally held now demand that they acquire new skills or practice their skills in less traditional settings or at a different level of preparedness. As a result of the downsizing and subsequent layoffs of nursing staff in many areas of the country, jobs for nurses are not plentiful. Many new graduates are having difficulty finding work. Some argue, however, that the scarcity of jobs is more related to economic factors than to an overabundance of nurses (Christensen and Bender 1994). Many hospitals, in their quest to provide more cost-effective care, are hiring auxiliary personnel to provide nursing care. For example, instead of hiring one registered nurse, a hospital may hire two licensed practical nurses (LPNs), or one LPN and a nursing assistant or other unlicensed person. In some hospitals, RNs have been told that if they want to keep their jobs they will have to work at the level and pay scale of an LPN so that the hospital can save money. The ethical and legal implications, and the dangers, for an RN working at the level of an LPN are discussed in Chapter 4.

On the other hand, new opportunities are opening up for many nurses. One potential direction for APRNs is to provide primary and preventive care in community settings, including urban, rural, and school-based clinics (Christensen and Bender 1994). Nurses at the advanced practice level are prepared to provide safe, efficient, and cost-effective health care. As more nurses move into the community, they will need to possess astute assessment and evaluation skills as well as the ability to make independent decisions about client care (Christensen and Bender 1994).

A number of nursing care delivery models have evolved in an attempt to meet the challenges of maintaining high-quality care in a changing health care environment that places an emphasis on cost containment.

CASE MANAGEMENT. Case management is perhaps one of the most enduring of the many models of care that has emerged as a framework for quality client-centered nursing care. Many nurses are now finding that they need to redefine their primary function from providers of care to "managers of care." Case management is an extension of the primary care model. However, in case management there is more deliberation in planning resources needed by the client and more emphasis on interdisciplinary collaboration (McCloskey et al. 1994).

"Nurses who are case managers take on the responsibility for a client or group of clients, arrange assessment of need, formulate a comprehensive plan of care, arrange for delivery of suitable services to address the individual client's needs, and assess and monitor the services delivered" (Marshall et al. 1995). Case management is becoming the recommended method for the treatment of severely and persistently mentally ill clients. It allows for optimal community adjustment for individuals with long-term mental illness by providing a link between the clients and the support services they require (Forchuck et al. 1989).

Forchuck and associates have formulated a case management model incorporating Peplau's theory. The authors identify the essential component of case management as that of the one-to-one long-term therapeutic nurse-client relationship. Within this relationship, the case manager plays a variety of roles, as dictated by the client's needs. Roles include (Forchuck et al. 1989)

- Counselor or therapist
- Client advocate
- Teacher
- Community organizer
- Coordinator of services

Figure 1–1 portrays this case management model and helps to outline the overall goals of the case manager.

Nursing Informatics

Informatics refers to computer-based information systems and computer literacy. **Nursing informatics** is the study of information science applied to nursing and health care. Nursing informatics contains "building blocks" of knowledge that include basic computer literacy and accessing of information management systems (through the Internet or databases such as Medline).

Computer technology is gradually making an impact in the health care area. Computers affect the delivery of health care through diagnostic, treatment, monitoring, and documentation processes. Computers have been used since the mid-1980s in the continuing education of health care professionals, and now the use of computers for client teaching is emerging as an option (Chambers and Frisby 1995). Many nurses routinely use computers to access laboratory reports, client records, and administrative programs (Blythe et al. 1995). Nurse managers can access reports on everything from staffing to linen use (Kovner 1995). Some intensive care units have, or are planning for, the use of bedside computers (Colson et al. 1995). There are computer programs that offer standardized nursing care plans and protocols, and their use is becoming more common among nurses in hospital and community environments. Many nurses find the use of computers to devise nursing care plans to be very effective, ultimately leading to better plans, once they have mastered the technique.

The use of computers for education is also becoming commonplace. Since the early 1980s, educators in various schools of nursing have been adding computers to their array of teaching strategies. Many schools of nursing now have state-of-the-art computer laboratories in which students have easy access to computer-assisted instruction programs (CAIs) and multimedia video computer software, which can greatly enhance their learning experience. According to the literature, three variables can influence the learning experience for the students: the quality of the software programs, the environment of the computer, and the characteristics of the learner (Khoiny 1995). One way to classify learning styles is through brain hemisphere dominance. People with left-brain dominance are believed to learn best through auditory cues. Those with right-brain dominance are believed to be primarily visual learners. Khoiny cites a study by Benedict and Coffield (1989) that revealed that students with right-hemisphere dominance (visual learners) scored higher with CAI teaching strategies than those who were left-hemisphere dominant (auditory learners). Left-hemisphere learners did better in a lecture format.

Nurses who are interested in the specialty of nursing informatics and would like to work in this area can take the informatics nurse certification examination sponsored by the ANCC.

COMPUTERIZED RECORD-KEEPING SYSTEMS. Many hospitals have, or are in the process of establishing, computerized record-keeping systems. Since computerized information can be accessed more readily than going through charts or obtaining old records, the use of computers has great appeal. The more sophisti-

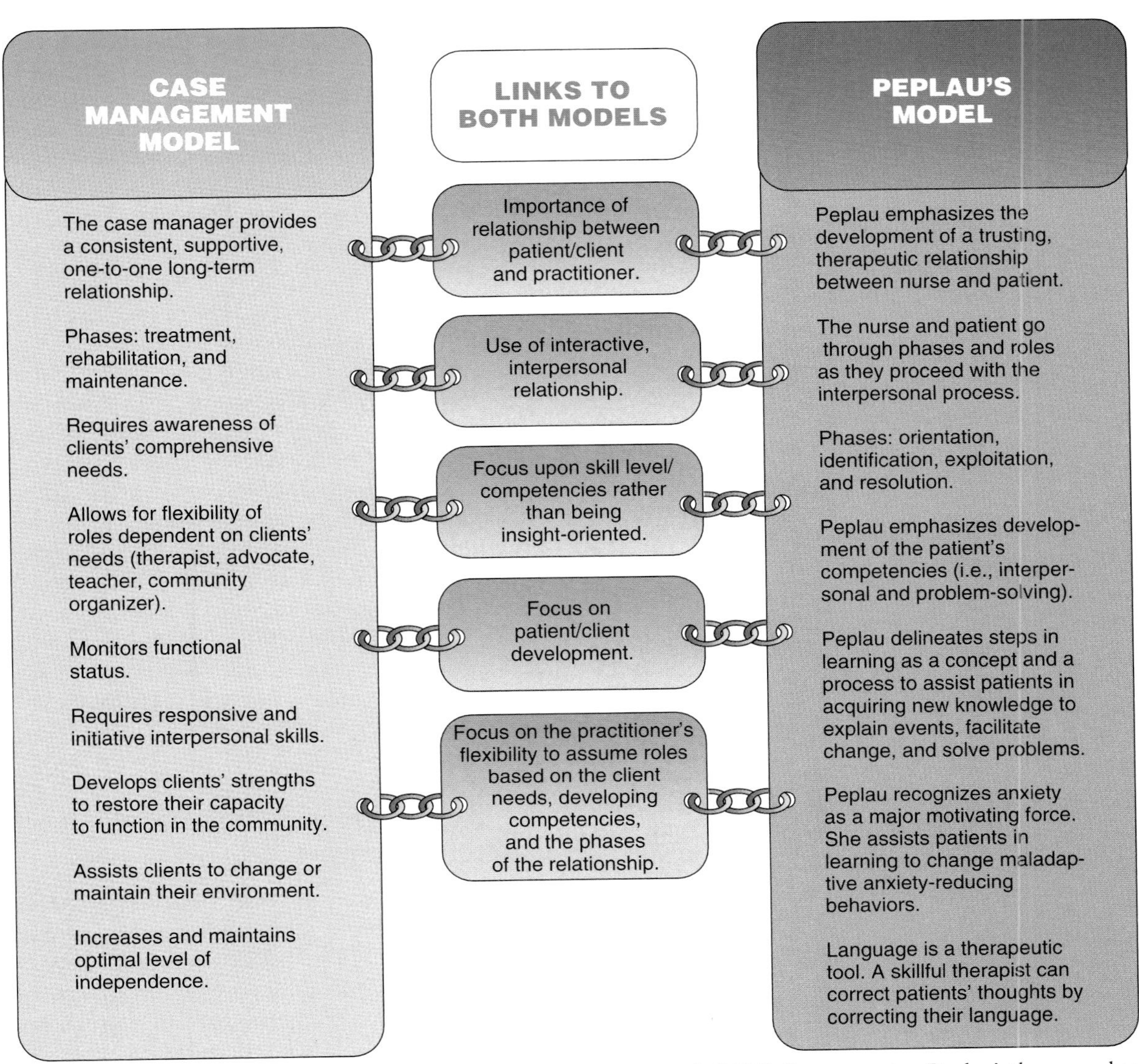

Figure 1–1 Case management model. (Adapted from Forchuck, C., et al. (1989). Incorporating Peplau's theory and case management. *Journal of Psychosocial Nursing*, 27(2):36.)

cated systems include "expert systems," which can provide checks on practice (e.g., screening for adverse drug interactions, therapeutic drug monitoring). Advanced systems would also make it possible to access large databases (e.g., Medline) to access literature on the most current nursing care (Kovner 1995). Some clinicians believe that clinical decisions can be better informed and nurses can more easily receive feedback on their practice through the use of a computerized record-keeping system (Modai and Rabinowitz 1993). For example, physicians or nurses in the hospital setting could access clinical records to monitor clients they send to community health care settings. In this way they could evaluate if their predictions of medication, client teaching, referrals, and supportive therapies were accurate and could use this information to improve planning for those with similar disorders and problems. Using this same computerized record-keeping system, visiting nurses would be able to access key components from the inpatient stay, as would nurses in any community-based health care service. Local physicians and mental health counselors would be able to access information about their client's earlier hospitalizations and recorded medical progress. Proponents of computerized client databased systems believe that such systems can greatly enhance the continuity of care for clients who may be shunted from one part of the health care system to another. The Institute of Medicine carried out a study to find likely indicators for the success of **computer-based client records (CPRs)** (Andrew and Richard 1995), which included

- Ever-increasing uses of, and legitimate demands for, client data
- Availability of more powerful and affordable technologies to support both CPRs and CPR systems
- An aging, mobile population

- A widely held belief that health care reform will not be achieved easily without routine use of CPRs and CPR systems

The question is, *should* health care personnel be able to access any individual's chart at any time? How available should data be, and to whom should it be available? You may recognize parallels in your own life concerning access by others to your credit records, reading preferences, and other personal information. There is great concern that, with the advent of computerized records, a break in security could lead to a breach in confidentiality. These concerns regarding security of information and confidentiality are areas of ongoing debate, and nurses need to be involved in these discussions (Kovner 1995).

NURSES ON-LINE. Nurses and other health care professionals are already on-line. They are beginning to use the information superhighway (Internet) to discuss, critique, evaluate, and solve health care problems or create nursing innovations by using electronic forums called discussions groups, newsgroups, and electronic mail (e-mail) (Tomaiuolo 1995). Nurses use the Internet to access databases all over the globe from their hospitals, offices, laboratories, clinics, classrooms, and homes. Downloaded images and data can be used for client care, client education, teaching, research, publications, and presentations (Tomaiuolo 1995). There are forums for nurses interested in almost all areas of nursing, including psychiatric mental health nursing. Nurses from all levels—students, graduates, baccalaureates, master-prepared, and PhDs—share information, resources, experiences, and most anything else regarding nursing concerns.

Some bulletin boards are free, while others require the user to be registered. See Table 1–2 for a brief list of search engines, bulletin boards, networks, and forums available on the Internet. Your instructor is a good source for further information on how you can become involved in dialoguing with colleagues and obtaining information from hundreds of databases in this country and around the world.

There is no doubt that in the future computers will become an integrated part of nursing practice for education, research, and client care. Health care personnel will be equipped with computers, video monitors, and computer telephone lines (modems); clients and families will also use computerized devices in the home. This will give health care staff a way of checking on the progress of many of their clients at home, and give clients and families opportunities for asking questions about medication, side effects, or symptoms and obtaining updated health care information. Providers of care will be able to respond readily by e-mail or voice mail in a timely fashion.

Christensen and Bender (1994) point out that studies show nurses spend more and more time with documentation and only 35% of their time with clients. Will computers allow more time with clients once the drudgery of charting is made easier, or will they lead to a more impersonal and mechanized approach to care? Kovner (1995) states that these are some of the many issues that nurses of the twenty-first century will continue to assess.

The Future: Into the Twenty-First Century

A change in nursing education is needed to prepare mental health nurse practitioners for the future. Owen and Sweeney (1995) state that the reliance on developing skills associated with problem removal should no longer be the focus for future practice. Current and future trends in mental health nursing education need to place greater emphasis on the development of skills to empower clients in diverse settings who have severe and persistent mental heath problems. A number of priorities in mental health services are evident. These priorities acknowledge the special needs of people from ethnic minority groups, people with severe and persistent mental health problems, people with problems associated with poverty, and people who are socially disadvantaged (Owen and Sweeney 1995).

The Changing Face of America: More Cultural Diversity

It is predicted that by the year 2020 the United States will have a very different ethnic and racial mix from that of today (Sills 1995) (Fig. 1–2). In addition, the U.S. population is growing older. There is an ever-increasing need for all who work in the health care arena to become comfortable with people who represent a diversity of life styles, have disabilities, are infected with human immunodeficiency virus (HIV), are afflicted with Alzheimer's disease, have addictions, or come from other stigmatized populations (Sills 1995).

Our whole concept of family life in America has gone through radical changes in the past few decades. The suburban, nuclear family of the 1950s is no longer the American way of life for most. For example, today 25% of American households consist of a single person, up from 8% in 1940 (Wright 1995, p. 53). The divorce rate has edged over 50%. One out of five children today lives in a single-parent home. Many gays and lesbians are choosing to live openly in "marriages," and many are adopting children. Other families may consist of a group of people who choose to live together, although unrelated genetically, and function as a family unit. "Mixed marriages" used to refer to people of different religions forming a married unit. Today many couples are marrying partners of different color or different culture. People are having children later in their lives, and many couples are opting not to have children at all. To provide respectful and relevant health care needs to this increasingly diverse population,

TABLE 1–2 SOME NURSING AND MEDICAL WEBSITES

NAME	ADDRESS	ABOUT AREA
American Journal of Nursing	http://www.ajn.org	Recent articles, information, nursing forum to talk to colleagues
The American Psychiatric Nurses Association	http://musc.edu/apna/	Journal articles, professional resources, links to many other nursing websites
Centers for Disease Control and Prevention (CDC)	http://www.cdc.gov	Link site for health information, data and statistics, travelers' health, and more
HyperDOC	http://www.nim.nih.gov	National Library of Medicine; includes access to all the library's database servers (some require accounts) and a great deal more
Internet Mental Health	http://www.mentalhealth.com/	Excellent site: disorders, diagnoses, medications, Internet links, and more
Mental Health Net	http://www.CMHC.com/	The largest mental health link site: self-help groups, professional resources, discussions, and more; over 6000 resources
National Institutes of Health (NIH)	http://www.nih.gov	Excellent link site for health information, grants, scientific resources, and more
National Institute of Nursing Research (NINR)	http://www.nih.gov/ninr/	Documents and publication, research and other links
The NetNurse	http://www.wp.com/NetNurse/	Great links to nursing journals, schools, student nurses, and other nursing related topics
Nursing/Medical Journals	http://www.nursingnet.com/jou.html	Articles from a variety of nursing journals
NursingNet	http://www.nursing.net.org	A marvelous website for students with numerous links to all nursing specialties
The Nursing Resource Home Page	http://www.nursingnet.com/	Professional points of interest pertaining to nursing; nice student section
Nurse Week Hot Links	http://www.nurseweek.com/alana.html	List of "hot" websites for information on nursing, allied health, and related topics
Nursing World	http://www.nursingworld.org/	Site sponsored by the American Nurses' Association; good site for visiting specialty nursing organizations, articles, and current information
University of Pennsylvania Multimedia Oncology Resource	http://cancer.med.upenn.edu	Offers cancer news, cancer searchers, and other updates
U.S. National Library of Medicine (NLM)	http://www.nlm.nih.gov	Databases (Medline), special information programs, research, grants, publications, and more
	Gopher Sites:	
MATERNAL AND CHILD HEALTH (gopher)	MCHNET.ICHP.UFT.EDU *Enter at prompt:* gophermchnet.ichp.ufl.edu	Infant topics, including breast feeding and working mothers
MEDICAL INFORMATION (1)	TJGOPHER.TJU.EDU *Enter at prompt:* gophertjgopher.tju.edu	Medical information by topic
NIGHTINGALE (gopher)	NIGHTINGALE.CON.UTK.EDU *Enter at prompt:* gopher nightingale.con.utk.edu	A nursing gopher, still under construction but currently contains some good resources

(1) Once at TJU's gopher, choose option 5 "medicine," then choose option 12 "client care," then choose option 1 "caring for clients," and finally choose option 8 "nursing care resources."

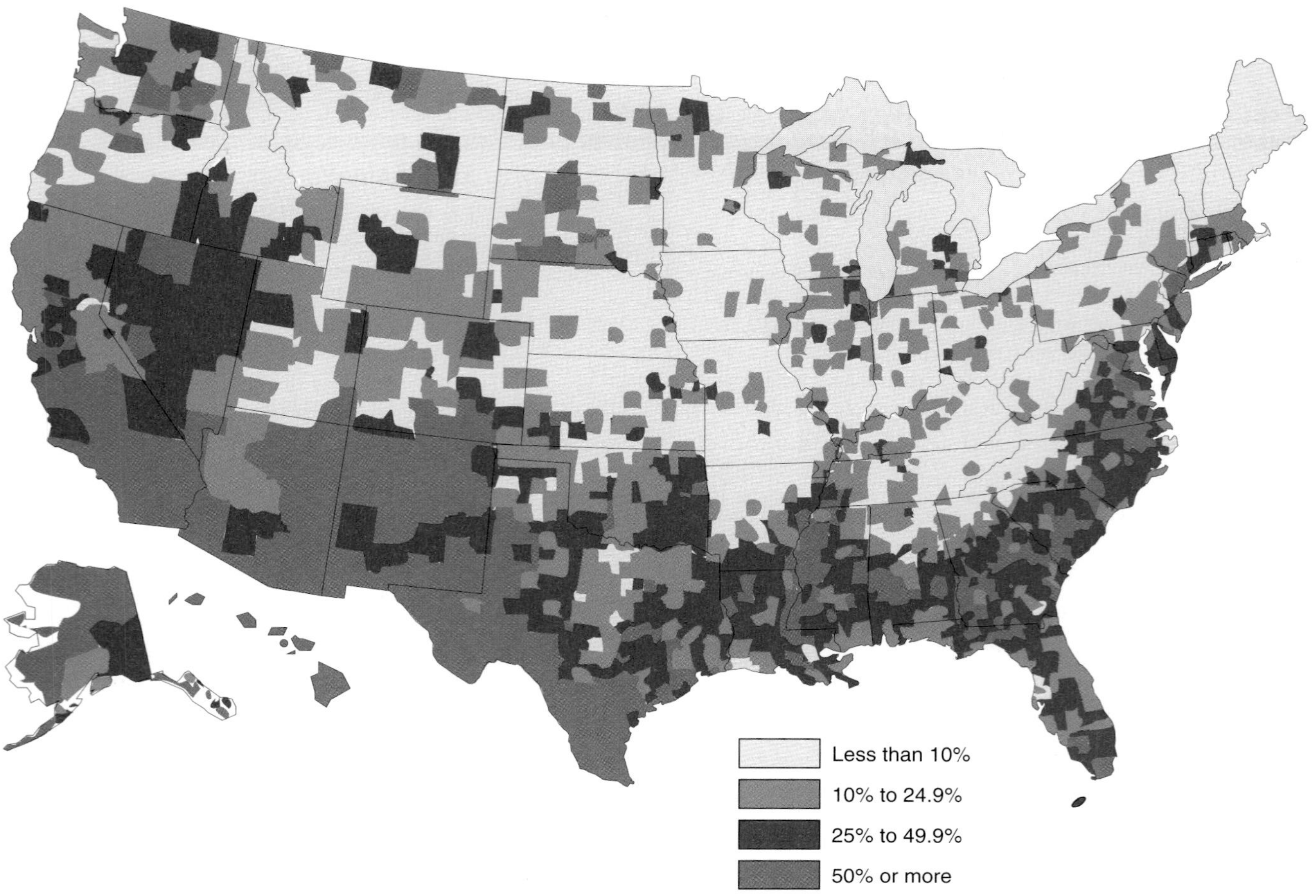

Figure 1–2 Projected percentages of the population, by county, that will be black, Asian, Native American, or Hispanic in the year 2020. (Rodger Doyle (c) 1995, for *U.S. News & World Report*, October 30, 1995.)

we must become more flexible and better informed; people need the preventive and sustaining mental and medical interventions that are culturally appropriate.

The health care workforce is also changing radically. The number of minorities joining this workforce continues to increase, bringing with them diverse cultural perspectives on health, illness, and health care. Lowenstein and Glanville (1995) point out that today's workforce has different experiences and looks, thinks, and acts differently from the workforce of the past. Men are joining the ranks of nursing, and increased numbers of older and nontraditional students are entering nursing programs (Lowenstein and Glanville 1995). The workforce of the present also does not hold the same values, or pursue the same needs and desires, as previous health care personnel. With cultural diversity issues affecting both the workplace and nursing practice, it would benefit nurses to become increasingly sensitive to the cultural nuances and issues, not only of their clients but also of their colleagues and subordinates (Lowenstein and Glanville 1995).

The rapid changes of the world we live in, especially in the health care arena where we choose to work, mandates that health care workers become more flexible, sensitive, and accepting of their clients, their co-workers, and themselves. Those who cannot do so may experience extreme stress and even burnout, and some may decide to leave the field.

Many nursing programs are making changes in their curriculum to focus on the care of "particular age groups (e.g., child, adolescent, and the elderly) or populations (e.g., survivors of violence, cocaine-addicted mothers, homeless families, and immigrants); psychiatric nurses are continuing to develop the in-depth knowledge, cultural sensitivity, and therapeutic skills necessary to build new models for care and to design relevant interventions" (ANA et al. 1994, p. 5).

Future Trends

The White (1991) study, which looked toward mental health nursing in the year 2000, identified areas for further expansion of the role of the mental health nurse. Three areas include

1. Expanding the advocacy role of the psychiatric mental health nurse
2. Supporting people with HIV and AIDS
3. Creating mental health nursing development units

EXPANDING THE ADVOCACY ROLE. Schauer (1995) states that nurses play a critical advocacy role in protecting the rights of clients, especially those with psychiatric disabilities. Nurses are also in a position to play an important role in identifying and reporting incidences of abuse and neglect. Five actions that pertain to the nurse's role of patient advocate are presented in Box 1–2.

Many nurses will be working as case managers in managed care settings (e.g., health maintenance organizations [HMOs]). Many of these managed care facilities will be corporately managed, with an eye to cost-effective care; therefore, nurses will increasingly practice in corporate settings. Nurses working in these settings will be affected by corporate goals and rules, which could lead to ethical dilemmas for nurses and threaten the appropriateness and quality of client care. Mohr (1995) points out that the role of client advocate may become increasingly difficult in the health care environment as nurses are becoming corporate employees, or even day laborers dispatched from agencies.

The nursing code of ethics defines the nurse's primary commitment as being to the client. "Nurses are employed by institutions, but their allegiance is to the client and his or her welfare, rather than to a group of shareholders" (Mohr 1995, p. 31). The mission, goals, and values of the corporate health care system are not always consistent with those of nursing. Mohr further warns nurses not to be placated by temporary guarantees of material concessions or to allow the fear of dismissal to push aside nursing's humanistic values of commitment to clients. The ANA published *Guidelines on reporting incompetent, unethical, or illegal practices.* All nurses should know about this publication and have a copy available for guidance, because these issues and concerns will follow us, and perhaps haunt us, into the next century. Sines (1994) states that the central concepts of nursing remain those of empowerment and advocacy, and the art of accurate empathy is a prerequisite for contemporary mental health care.

SUPPORTING PEOPLE WHO ARE HIV POSITIVE. AIDS has taken a heavy toll on the poor, urban, and minority populations in the United States. People who are HIV positive show a full range of psychiatric symptoms: mania, depression, psychosis, anxiety, and obsessive-compulsive disorders, and suicide is not uncommon. The mental health care community has an obligation to support and provide education and care for those health care workers and others who are directly involved in caring for HIV-positive persons. The challenges and rewards are both enormous.

CREATION OF MENTAL HEALTH NURSING UNITS. In the United States the community nursing center is not a new concept. One of the earliest nursing centers, the Henry Street Nurses Settlement, was founded by Lilian Wald in 1893 in New York City. In 1916 Margaret Sanger opened the first birth control clinic, also in New York City. Throughout the 1980s, a

BOX 1–2 THE NURSE'S ROLE OF PATIENT ADVOCATE *

1. **Nurses need to improve their observation, listening, and communications skills.** Patients complain that some nurses are "burned out," hide behind their desks, take the easy way out, and are quick to punish for infraction of rules rather than doing what is best for the patient. Nurses need to "ensure that a good nursing care plan exists, that activities of daily living and personal hygiene are addressed, and that bodily functions are monitored and assisted. . . . They need to be sensitive to assessing consumer's comfort levels regarding noise, temperature, lighting, and access to personal belongings." (p. 236.)
2. **Nurses need to develop and implement policies and procedures that affect the client quality of care.** These include the Patient's Bill of Rights; informed consent; policies addressing confidentiality, seclusion, and restraint; and policies for reporting and providing appropriate remedies for staff abuse. (To review the Patient's Bill of Rights, see Chapter 8.)
3. **Nurses need to know that unaddressed, ongoing abusive or neglectful behaviors may be brought to the attention of a Protection and Advocacy system (P&A) from any source, including nurses.** Examples of such behaviors include assault, failure to provide appropriate mental health or medical diagnostic evaluation or treatment, financial exploitation, and failure to provide discharge planning. The P&A is authorized to investigate incidents of abuse and neglect of mentally ill individuals. "Unfortunately, the P&A cannot protect nurses from retaliation from employers, but reports can be made anonymously and systemic problems can be identified." (p. 237.)
4. **Nurses can provide mental health consumers with the telephone number of the appropriate P&A System; it should be posted next to the patient's phone.**
5. **Nurses have a vital role in the administration of medication.** Mental health care consumers complain of being overmedicated, wrongly medicated, and poorly medicated. Nurses must take the responsibility for ensuring that the appropriate medication is administered, at a dose that makes sense, and that side effects are immediately noted, reported, and addressed. Nurses are responsible for seeing that patients are provided with understandable medication teaching plans. Patients are to be well informed of what medications they are getting, what side effects they might expect, any toxic effects, whom to contact when they suspect problems, and actions they can take to lessen side effects.

*Schauer 1995.

number of nurse-managed centers were opened, including those that were academically based, hospital based, freestanding, and agencies for home health care (Knauth 1994). **Community nursing centers (CNCs)**, or nurse-managed centers, are "organizations that provide direct access to professional nurses who offer holistic, client-centered health services for reimbursement" (Fehring et al. 1986, p. 63). Historically, CNCs provided care to the poor and underserved populations. Today, CNCs are expanding to provide care in both rural and urban settings (Walker 1994).

For community centers that work primarily with people with mental health diseases, current and future trends in mental health nursing should concentrate on and address the needs of those with severe and persistent mental health problems. In the community setting, nursing actions for this population need to focus appropriately on teaching skills to empower their clients and contribute to their ability to live up to their potential for independence, social assimilation, and work performance; in so doing, they provide the chance for clients to experience the optimal quality of life for themselves and their families.

The 1992 NLN study on community nursing centers clarified the characteristics that nursing centers had to meet to be included in the study:

- A nurse had to occupy the chief management position.
- Accountability and responsibility for client care and professional practice had to remain with the nursing staff.
- Clients had to have direct access to professional nurses as their primary providers.

At that time (1992), the NLN identified 250 nursing centers and found their cost effectiveness promising. These centers offered a range of health services such as physical examinations, screenings, immunizations, health teaching, case management, infusion therapy, home care, and respite care to children (Knauth 1994).

It is apparent that the growth and progress of nursing go hand in hand with the political and social developments of the time. For nursing to take a leading role in the reformed health care of the future, it is imperative that more nurses become involved with legislative and policy initiatives. Nursing research showing that nurse-managed health care agencies do indeed provide quality of care in a cost-effective manner can affect legislative decisions.

Trends in the profession of psychiatric mental health nursing are greatly influenced by trends in the social and political arenas. From this vantage point, we can try to predict how the present will affect the future. Nurses still have the time to influence the role they will play in the twenty-first century. Hildegard Peplau says it most eloquently:

> Nursing leaders and all other nurses are in one way or another participants in the drama of making nursing history. It is out of this ongoing history-making process that the present role of psychiatric nursing has emerged. Nurses who know the history of psychiatric nursing gain a sense of the cohesion and continuity that exists between the work of their nursing forebears and their own present-day work. The future of psychiatric nursing can be more clearly determined when its past is appreciated; that future lies in the hands of the present generation of nurses—especially those who care deeply about the needs of the mentally ill." (Peplau 1994, p. 96.)

Through the efforts of the many leaders who have gone before and of the nurses who are working diligently today, "psychiatric nurses are prepared to greet the future with a proud history, standards, credentials, advanced powers of observation, and communication skills" (McBride 1996, p. 3).

SUMMARY

All nurses need to know and be able to apply psychosocial concepts in order to give effective and competent care. However, some of you may go on to choose a career in psychiatric nursing. Psychiatric nurses work in a wide array of settings with people who have acute and long-term mental health problems. They work with homeless persons and families; with people in jails; with people who have survived abusive situations; with people who are HIV positive; with people in crisis; with children, adults, and the elderly.

Many staff nurses currently work in psychiatric units. However, specific criteria must be met by a nurse to be qualified as either a psychiatric mental health registered nurse (RN, C) or a psychiatric mental health advanced practice registered nurse (APRN) (RN, CS).

Psychiatric nurses are responsible for counseling clients, crisis intervention, managing the therapeutic environment, health and psychoeducational teaching, case management, administration and monitoring of psychobiological treatments, and much more. The "decade of the brain" has brought great strides in the relief of mental anguish for many people with mental health diseases, and great opportunities for nurses. Nurses on the advanced level are trained to prescribe pharmacological treatment according to their state's Nursing Practice Act, perform psychotherapy (individual, group, family, and other forms), and carry out consultation and supervision with other health care providers; some may also have admitting privileges to admit their clients into the hospital in times of crisis.

Psychiatric nursing has an important history that has grown out of the work of dedicated and gifted nurses who were innovators in their time. This history clearly reflects the social and political movements of the times. The advent of psychotropic drugs and the move to the community that resulted from the CMHC Act of 1963 were two trends that stimulated growth of the role of the psychiatric mental health nurse. These two trends provide exciting opportunities for psychiatric nursing that will continue into the twenty-first century.

Health care reform is focused on cutting costs while maintaining quality of care. Shorter hospital stays mean that some clients are going back into the community before they are stabilized, and are thus in greater need of supervision and community support. The shorter length of stay has opened the way to the use of critical (or clinical) pathways, which help focus daily medical and nursing care so that clients will have needed services while in the hospital, and discharge planning will be well outlined by the time they are discharged into the community. The requirement for orchestrating of support services to meet clients' needs once they are discharged has increased the importance of the role of case manager.

Computer-based patient records (CPRs) can enhance the quality of client care when health care workers from a variety of support services have access to a client's record. There are pros and cons of CPRs; one of the most serious concerns is that of maintaining client confidentiality. Computers are currently employed for student, staff, and client teaching, client hospital monitoring, and home supervision, research and more.

America is becoming ethnically, culturally, and racially more diverse. Nurses must become ever more sensitive and better informed if they are to give culturally appropriate nursing care. Nurses will also need to grow in their sensitivity and flexibility toward their colleagues, both their peers and those they supervise.

With the changes in the health care system and the growing role of managed care, nurses must become ever more diligent as client advocates. Nurses will be increasingly affected by corporate rules, and this will pose many new and challenging ethical dilemmas for members of our profession.

Today's trends will continue into the twenty-first century. A study by White (1991) identified areas for expansion and development of the role of the mental health nurse: (1) client advocacy, (2) support for people who are HIV positive or have other infectious and degenerative diseases, and (3) the creation of mental health nursing units.

REFERENCES

American Nurses' Association (ANA), American Psychiatric Nurses Association, Association of Child and Adolescent Psychiatric Nursing, Society for Education and Research in Psychiatric– Mental Health Nursing. (1994a). *A statement on psychiatric–mental health clinical nursing practice and standards of psychiatric–mental health clinical nursing practice.* Washington, DC: American Nurses' Association.

American Nurses' Association. (1994b). *Psychiatric–mental health nursing psychopharmacology project.* Washington, DC: American Nurses' Association.

American Psychiatric Nurses Association. (1995). Position statement: Prescriptive authority for advanced practice psychiatric nurses. September 15, 1995. Washington, DC: American Psychiatric Nurses Association.

Andrew, W. F., and Richard, D. S. (1995). Applied information technology: A clinical perspective feature focus: The computer-based client record (part 3). *Computers in Nursing,* 13:176–181.

Benedict, S. C., and Coffield, K. (1989). The effect of brain hemisphere dominance on learning by computer assisted instruction and the traditional lecture method. *Computers in Nursing,* 4, 152–156.

Billings, C. V. (1993). Psychiatric–mental health nursing professional progress notes. *Archives of Psychiatric Nursing,* 7(3):174–181.

Blythe, J., Royle, J. A., Oolup, P., et al. (1995). Linking the professional literature to nursing practice: challenges and opportunities. *AAOHN,* 42(6):342–345.

Chambers, J. K., and Frisby, A. J. (1995). Computer-based learning for ESRD client education: Current status and future directions. *Advances in Renal Replacement Therapy,* 2(3):234–245.

Christensen, P., and Bender, L. H. (1994). Models of nursing care in a changing environment: Current challenges and future directions. *Orthopedic Nursing,* 13(2):64–70.

Colson, A. R., Bounds, J. A., Alt-White, A. C., and McDermott, S. (1995). Preparing for an ICU bedside computer. *Nursing Management,* 26(5):48A–48B.

Dumas, R. G. (1994). Psychiatric nursing in an era of change. *Journal of Psychosocial Nursing,* 32(1):11–14.

Fehring, R., Riesch, S., and Schulte, J. (1986). Toward a definition of nurse managed centers. *Journal of Community Health Nursing,* 3(2):59–67.

Forchuck, C., et al. (1989). Incorporating Peplau's theory and case management. *Journal of Psychosocial Nursing,* 27(2):35–37.

Goldberg, R. J. (1995). *Practical guide to the care of the psychiatric client.* St. Louis, MO: Mosby–Year Book.

Hicks, L.L., Stallmeyer, J.M., and Coleman, J.R. (1993). *The role of the nurse in managed care.* Washington, DC: American Nurses Publishing.

Hillard, R. (1994). The past and future of psychiatric emergency services in the U.S. *Hospital and Community Psychiatry,* 45(6):541–543.

Khoiny, F. E. (1995). Factors that contribute to computer-assisted instruction effectiveness. *Computers in Nursing,* 13(4):165–168.

Knauth, D. G. (1994). Community nursing centers: Removing impediments to success. *Nursing Economics,* 12(3):140–145.

Kovner, C. (1995). Computers in nursing: From the pencil to the PC. *Journal of the New York State Nurses' Association,* 26(1):30–31.

Lowenstein, A. J., and Glanville, C. (1995). Cultural diversity and conflict in the health care workplace. *Nursing Economics,* 13(4):203–209.

Marshall, M., Lockwood, A., and Gath, D. (1995). Social services case management for long-term mental disorders: A randomized controlled trial. *Lancet,* 345(8947):409–412.

McBride, A. B. (1996). Psychiatric–mental health nursing in the twenty-first century. In A. B. McBride and J. K. Austin (Eds.), *Psychiatric–mental health nurse: integrating the behavioral and biological sciences* (pp. 1–10). Philadelphia: W. B. Saunders.

McCloskey, J.C., et al. (1994). Nursing management innovations: A need for systematic evaluation. *Nursing Economics,* 12(1):35–44.

Milne, C. T., and Pelletier, L. C. (1994). Enhancing staff skill. Developing critical pathways at a community hospital. *Journal of Nurse Staff Development,* 10(3):160–162.

Modai, I., and Rabinowitz, D. S. W. (1993). Why and how to establish a computerized system for psychiatric case records. *Hospital and Community Psychiatry,* 14(11):1091–1095.

Mohr, W. K. (1995). Values, ideologies, and dilemmas: Professional and occupational contradictions. *Journal of Psychosocial Nursing and Mental Health Services,* 33(1):29–34.

Owen, S., and Sweeney, J. (1995). The future role of the mental health nurse. *Nurse Education Today,* 15(1):17–21.

Peplau, H. E. (1994). Evolution of psychiatric nursing. In E. M. Varcarolis (Ed.), *Foundations of psychiatric mental health nursing* (pp 89–107) (2nd ed.). Philadelphia: W. B. Saunders.

Peplau, H. E. (1962). Interpersonal technique: The crux of psychiatric nursing. *American Journal of Nursing,* 62:53.

Redick, E. L., Stroud, A. R., and Kurack, T. B. (1994). Expanding the use of critical pathways in critical care. *Dimensions in Critical Care Nursing,* 13(6):316–321.

Schauer, C. (1995). Special report: Protection and advocacy: What nurses need to know. *Archives of Psychiatric Nursing,* 9(5):233–239.

Sills, G. M. (1995). Psychiatric nursing: Trends for clinicians. *Journal of the New York State Nurses' Association,* 26(1):42–43.

Sines, D. (1994). The arrogance of power: A reflection on contemporary mental health nursing practice. *Journal of Advanced Nursing,* 20(5):894–903.

Stuart, G. (1994). Vulnerable or valuable: Psychiatric nursing's future in health care reform. *Journal of Psychosocial Nursing,* 32(6):53–54.

Tomaiuolo, N. G. (1995). Assessing nursing resources on the internet. *Computers in Nursing,* 13(4):159–168.

Trubowitz, J. (1994). Personality theories and therapies. In E. Varcarolis (Ed.), *Foundations of psychiatric mental health nursing (2nd ed.).* Philadelphia: W. B. Saunders.

Walker, P. H. (1994). Dollars and sense in health reform: Interdisciplinary practice and community nursing centers. *Nursing Administration Quarterly,* 19(1):1–11.

White, E. (1991). *The future of psychiatric nursing by the year 2000. A Delphi study.* Department of Nursing, University of Manchester.

Wright, R. (1995). 20th century blues. *Time,* August 28th, 50–57.

SELF-STUDY AND CRITICAL THINKING

Multiple choice

1. A psychiatric nurse at the basic level
   - A. is a staff nurse
   - B. has a baccalaureate degree and has completed a certification examination
   - C. has at least a master's degree and has taken a national certification examination
   - D. is a baccalaureate nurse who works on a psychiatric unit

2. Psychiatric nurses work mainly in
   - A. the hospital
   - B. half-way houses
   - C. private practice
   - D. all kinds of community-based settings and in the hospital

Matching

3. Identify the areas that a basic level psychiatric mental health nurse (C) can perform and those that an advanced practice psychiatric mental health nurse (CS) can perform. When appropriate, you can check both.
   - A. ________ Counseling
   - B. ________ Consultation
   - C. ________ Self-care activities
   - D. ________ Case management
   - E. ________ Prescription of pharmacological agents
   - F. ________ Health teaching
   - G. ________ Health promotion and health maintenance
   - H. ________ Psychotherapy
   - I. ________ Milieu therapy
   - J. ________ Psychobiological interventions

4. Identify the five original services funded by the Community Mental Health Center Act of 1963 by putting an "O" next to the letter. Put an "L" next to those residential services that were funded later (in 1975).
   - A. __L__ Children's services
   - B. __O__ Outpatient service
   - C. __O__ Emergency service
   - D. __L__ Alcohol abuse treatment
   - E. __O__ Partial hospitalization
   - F. __L__ Geriatric services
   - G. __L__ Drug abuse treatment
   - H. __O__ Consultation and education
   - I. __O__ Inpatient services
   - J. __L__ Transitional housing

True or false

Correct any false statements; explain the true statements.

5. Clinical/critical pathways can

A. ___T___ Target the focus of treatment for specific time periods
B. ___T___ Improve the use of personalized client treatment strategies
C. ___T___ Enhance client teaching
D. ___T___ Enhance client goal achievement
E. ___T___ Save time and increase efficiency of charting
F. ___F___ Be specific only for nursing care
G. ___T___ Improve discharge planning

Critical thinking

6. Discuss what is meant by the "decade of the brain."

7. Refer to Box 1–1 on the phenomena that psychiatric nurses target for intervention. Explain at least five of the phenomena more fully. If you are not sure, look them up in the text.

8. Define for a friend the term *case manager*. Discuss what a case manager does. For a client you are following, identify the kinds of services this client needs and the role of the case manager in coordinating these services, either from hospital to community or within the community.
9. Discuss your experience with computers with a fellow student. Identify three ways the use of computer-assisted instruction (CAI) was helpful to you. Identify ways that you can envision computers as useful tools for client and family teaching.
10. In a small group (your study group would be ideal), share experiences you have had with others from unfamiliar cultural, ethnic, or racial backgrounds, and identify two positive learning experiences from these encounters.
11. What level of nursing do you think would be most appropriate for someone working in a nurse-managed community center? What would be some of the advantages for a nurse in such a setting? What are some of the concerns and questions you might have? What populations would be the best served? To a friend, describe a community-managed nursing center.
12. Identify from the list in Table 1–2 one computer on-line forum you would be interested in exploring and the kind of information that would be useful for you. Assess a nursing network on the Internet.

2

Mental Health: THEORIES AND THERAPIES

JULIUS TRUBOWITZ

OUTLINE

KEY TERMS AND CONCEPTS

The key terms and concepts listed here also appear in bold where they are defined or discussed in this chapter.

health maintenance organizations (HMOs)
DSM-IV
DSM-IV axis system
conscious
preconscious
subconscious
unconscious
id
ego
superego
defense mechanisms
selective inattention
psychoanalysis
dream analysis

KEY TERMS AND CONCEPTS

The key terms and concepts listed here also appear in bold where they are defined or discussed in this chapter.

transference
psychoanalytic psychotherapy
short-term psychodynamic therapy
rational emotive behavioral therapy (REBT)
cognitive therapy
pleasant events schedule
cognitive rehearsal
role playing
recording dysfunctional thoughts
behavioral therapy
modeling
operant conditioning
self-control therapy
systematic desensitization
aversion therapy
milieu therapy

OBJECTIVES

After studying this chapter, the reader will be able to

1. Assess his or her own mental health using the five signs of mental health identified in this chapter.
2. Analyze the pros and cons of the emerging health maintenance organization (HMO) concept of health care.
3. Explain in a small group how, by using the DSM-IV multiaxial system, a clinician is forced to consider a broad range of information before making a DSM diagnosis.
4. Give an example from your own culture of how consideration of norms and other cultural influences affect making a DSM-IV diagnosis.
5. Compare and contrast the developmental stages of Freud, Erikson, and Piaget.
6. Evaluate the premise behind the approaches to the various therapeutic models discussed in this chapter.
7. Choose the one therapeutic model you think would be most useful for you, if you had an issue you wanted to resolve. Which one would you recommend to a friend?

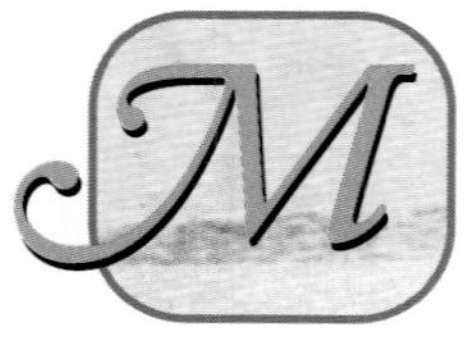

Mental health professionals are faced with a multitude of problems in defining mental illness and mental health. Agreement on the definitions has been elusive throughout history. Early definitions were based on statistical measures. The term *mental illness* was applied to behaviors, described as "strange" and "different," that occurred infrequently and deviated from an established norm. Such criteria are inadequate because they suggest that mental health is based on conformity. If such definitions were used, nonconformists and independent thinkers such as Abraham Lincoln, Mahatma Gandhi, and Socrates would be judged mentally ill. There is a further problem in viewing those people whose behavior is statistically infrequent as mentally ill. Simply stated, the sacrifices of a Mother Teresa and the dedication of a Martin Luther King, Jr., are uncommon, but none of us would consider these much-admired behaviors to be signs of mental illness.

This chapter discusses concepts of mental health and mental illness and how we currently categorize mental illness using the *Diagnostic and statistical manual of mental disorders (DSM-IV)*. You will review major theorists and their contributions, and are given an overview of major therapeutic modalities used today.

CONCEPTS OF MENTAL HEALTH AND ILLNESS

One approach to differentiating mental illness from mental health is based on what a particular culture regards as acceptable or unacceptable. In this view, the mentally ill are those who violate social norms and thus threaten (or make anxious) those who are observing them. This definition seems partly true. The callous psychopathic person fits the definition, as does the sometimes wild manic person and the schizophrenic person who is displaying strange antics. However, this definition explicitly makes mental illness a relative concept. Many forms of unusual behavior can be tolerated, depending on the prevailing cultural norms. People whose only problem is that they see things and hear things that no one else does may be put into a mental hospital, or they may be revered as visionaries, depending on the belief of their society (Leff 1981). The difficulty with defining mental illness through a particular behavior unacceptable to society is that it does not tell us what behavior a society should accept. Some totalitarian governments, to serve their own repressive goals, have classed all political dissidents as "mentally ill."

The field of mental illness is plagued by a host of myths and misconceptions. One myth is that to be mentally ill is to be different and odd. Another misconception is that to be healthy, a person must be logical and rational. All of us dream "irrational" dreams every night, and "irrational" emotions are not only universal human experiences but also essential to a fulfilling life. There are people who show extremely abnormal behavior and are characterized as mentally ill who are far more like than different from the rest of us. There is no obvious and consistent line between mental illness and mental health. In fact, all human behavior lies somewhere along a continuum of mental health and mental illness.

The following comments of a 40-year-old woman illustrate the continuum between illness and health as her condition changes from (1) deep depression to (2) mania to (3) health.

1. It was horror and hell. I was at the bottom of the deepest and darkest pit there ever was. I was worthless and unforgivable. I was as good as—no, worse than—dead.
2. I was incredibly alive. I could sense and feel everything. I was sure I could do anything, accomplish any task, create whatever I wanted, if only other people wouldn't get in my way.
3. Yes, I am sometimes sad and sometimes happy and excited, but nothing as extreme as before. I am much more calm. I realize now that, when I was manic, it was a pressure-cooker feeling. When I am happy now, or loving, it is more peaceful and real. I have to admit that I sometimes miss the intensity—the sense of power and creativity—of those manic times. I never miss anything about the depressed times, but of course the power and the creativity never bore fruit. Now I do get things done, some of the time, like most people. And people treat me much better now. I guess I must seem more real to them. I certainly seem more real to me. (Altrocchi 1980.)

Finally, many people think that mental illness is incurable. Translating this statement into "Abnormal behavior doesn't change" reveals its inaccuracy. Some abnormal behavior changes on its own; some can be changed after many weeks or months of effort; some stay the same despite time and effort; and a small fraction becomes progressively more abnormal no matter what we do.

A helpful approach in defining mental illness and mental health is based on evaluating individual behavior in two dimensions:

1. On a continuum from adaptive to maladaptive
2. On a continuum from constructive to destructive

Along the *adaptive-maladaptive continuum*, behaviors are assessed to the degree that they contribute to or are detrimental to the individual's psychological well-being. For example, does the behavior widen or restrict the range of possible responses to a problem of living? Does it raise or lower self-esteem? Does it create situations in which the individual or others are more likely to experience relief of tension or stress?

Maladaptive behavior allows a problem to continue and often generates new problems, interfering significantly—often over an extended period—with an individual's ability to function in such important areas of life as health, work, love, and interpersonal relationships. On the other hand, adaptive behavior solves problems in living and enhances an individual's life.

Regarding the second dimension, behavior along the *constructive-destructive continuum* often affects others as much as the individual. Destructive behavior not only results in failure to deal with a problem (and thus is maladaptive) but also undermines or destroys the psychological and biological well-being of the individual and others. Such behavior, whether it occurs once or repeatedly, may seriously undermine health, significantly increase chances of (or actually bring about) death, or drastically affect psychological functioning in the individual or others. On the other hand, constructive behavior contributes to psychological growth and biological well-being. It improves the health and positively influences the psychological functioning of the individual and others.

Table 2–1 identifies important aspects of mental health on a continuum. These aspects include degree of (1) happiness, (2) control over behavior, (3) appraisal of reality, (4) effectiveness in work, and (5) healthy self-concept.

DIRECTION OF MENTAL HEALTH NURSING

Community Mental Health Programs

Mental health advocates have supported community treatment programs designed to help people cope more effectively with their problems and thus achieve a better quality of life. Community-based programs for the mentally ill also provide rehabilitation and supportive therapy for those trying to cope with daily life outside of institutions.

The greatest single impetus to the community mental health movement was a practical one. In 1955, Congress authorized the Joint Commission on Mental Illness and Health to examine state mental hospitals. On the basis of a 6-year survey, the commission concluded that the care offered was largely custodial and that steps must be taken to provide effective treatment. Its 1961 report recommended that no additional large hospitals be built and that community mental health clinics be established instead. In 1963, President Kennedy sent a message to Congress calling for a "bold new approach" and proposing the Community Mental Health Centers Act to pro-

TABLE 2–1 MENTAL HEALTH VERSUS MENTAL ILLNESS

SIGNS OF MENTAL HEALTH	SIGNS OF MENTAL ILLNESS
Happiness	**Major Depressive Episode**
A. Finds life enjoyable B. Can see in objects, people, and activities their possibilities for meeting one's needs	A. Loss of interest or pleasure in all or almost all usual activities and pastimes B. Mood as described by person is depressed, sad, hopeless, discouraged, "down in the dumps"
Control Over Behavior	**Control Disorder, Undersocialized, Agressive**
A. Can recognize and act on cues to existing limits B. Can respond to the rules, routines, and customs of any group to which one belongs	A. A repetitive and persistent pattern of aggressive conduct in which the basic rights of others are violated
Appraisal of Reality	**Schizophrenic Disorder**
A. Accurate picture of what is happening around one B. Good sense of the consequences, both good and bad, that will follow one's acts C. Can see the difference between the "as if" and "for real" in situations	A. Bizarre delusions, such as delusions of being controlled B. Auditory hallucinations C. Delusions with persecutory or jealous content
Effectiveness in Work	**Adjustment Disorder with Work (or Academic Inhibition)**
A. Within limits set by abilities, can do well in tasks attempted B. When meeting mild failure, persists until determines whether or not one can do the job	A. Inhibition in work or academic functioning where previously there was adequate performance
A Healthy Self-Concept	**Dependent Personality Disorder**
A. Sees self as approaching one's ideals, as capable of meeting demands B. Reasonable degree of self-confidence helps in being resourceful under stress	A. Passively allows others to assume responsibility for major areas of life because of inability to function independently B. Lacks self-confidence, e. g., sees self as helpless, stupid

Data from Redl, F., and Wattenberg, W. (1959). *Mental hygiene in teaching* (pp. 198–201). New York: Harcourt, Brace & World, and American Psychiatric Association (1994). *Diagnostic and statistical manual of disorders* (DSM-IV) (4th ed.) Washington, DC: American Psychiatric Association.

vide comprehensive services in the community and to implement programs for the prevention and treatment of mental disturbances. The act was passed. For every 100,000 people, a mental health center was to provide outpatient therapy, short-term inpatient care, day hospitalization for those able to go home at night, 24-hour emergency services, and consultation with and education to other agencies in the community. Throughout the 1960s and 1970s, the government-funded program moved forward with the support of citizens' groups, unions, and mental health professionals and aided by the major policy attention given to it in 1977–1978 when President Carter established the President's Commission on Mental Health. However, by the 1980s the program had established fewer than 800 of the 2000 community mental health centers envisioned by Congress. Because of significant financial constraints, and because many aspects of the legislation resulting from the Carter Commission were reversed shortly after President Reagan took office, the community mental health center function has continued to be severely limited, and this program is considered by many to be ineffective (Kaplan and Sadock 1995).

Since the mid-1960s, the national trend of transferring responsibility for mental health services to local communities has led to a large and complex delivery system. Various kinds of organizations evolved to serve the mentally ill: halfway houses; board-and-care homes for clients discharged from a mental hospital; and more private, proprietary psychiatric hospitals. The community mental health movement and its available resources are covered in Chapter 9.

Health Maintenance Organizations (HMOs)

Since 1990, unprecedented changes have taken place within the administration, financing, and delivery of mental health programs and services. Among the most important of these changes is the rapid emergence of managed care strategies in the form of **health maintenance organizations (HMOs),** within which mental health providers in both public and private sectors are seeking to contain costs while maintaining access. Many of these managed care planning efforts are proceeding rapidly with inadequate experience to undergird them. In fact, HMOs are a burgeoning field, growing at the rate of 25% per year. By the year 2000, it is estimated that they will be the mainstream form of mental health services delivery in the United States (Boaz 1988). At present, millions of people participate in health plans that use managed care for their physical and mental health benefits. Currently, relatively little is known about how the financing, program design, and program delivery strategies will relate to existing local mental health programs.

Managed care programs attempt to provide care equal to or better in quality than the client has received in the past, for less cost, and with more accountability to the payer. Changes in the relationship between provider and consumer are at the core of what managed mental health seeks to accomplish. As part of an effort to conform systems, improve client outcomes, and control costs, health and mental health managers are implementing a number of strategies designed to monitor and assess treatment plans and outcomes that were, in the past, largely free from such oversight. These efforts have taken many forms, ranging from preadmission reviews to continuing treatment authorizations, concurrent reviews, and "screen" design (increasingly computerized) to determine the appropriateness of a treatment plan. With the growth of private HMOs and coverage by private insurance companies, the professional autonomy of providers has been significantly affected. Physicians and mental health personnel have been organized under strict treatment and financial guidelines. Changes have affected such key areas as provider income, system and client cost, provider control, and quality of care. The delivery of services has been centralized to flow through a primary care provider and thence to specialists of all types.

There has been a flood of criticism directed at HMOs to the effect that their entire philosophy of service is antithetical to the well-being of the client (often referred to as the "consumer"). Many observers have noted an explosion of complaints from psychologists who feel their clients are being shortchanged, and a conflict of interest in those who decide how much therapy is warranted (Goleman 1996; Korb 1996; Wolf 1996; Bush 1996). Contrary to reports by Seligman (1995), who showed that clients who are in psychotherapy for more than 6 months fare better than those whose treatment period is shorter, the practice of many managed care plans has been to cut back the number of sessions to 20, or even as few as 12. HMOs experience maximum profit when services are limited; the less they provide, the bigger is the profit. Thus, HMOs may exert a subtle pressure against treatment that is essential to the well-being of subscriber members. Similarly, financial incentives have been offered participating physicians to limit treatment or services; some HMOs award bonuses to physicians who use less than the allocated funds. This practice has come under review, because such incentives might influence primary providers to refer fewer clients to specialists. Clearly, primary providers may feel undue pressure when making a decision that is in the client's interest rather than in the economic interest of the HMO.

Another major concern with managed care has been communication and coordination between mental health and primary care providers. The primary care provider plays a vital role in identifying, supplying, and referring care for clients with mental difficulties, yet such problems frequently go unidentified by the primary health care system. Primary care providers face special problems in assessing mental health difficulties because they are often present in somatic forms. Consequently, people with mental health problems often fail to receive appropriate treatment, are subject to needless tests and procedures, and consume an undue proportion of the limited resources of the primary care system. The impact of managed care for the hospitalized client is discussed in Chapter 8. The impact of managed care on community services is discussed in Chapter 9.

Neglected Populations

Finally, as mental health care moves into the twenty-first century, it is confronted with populations that have been traditionally underserved and unserved (e.g., women, children, the elderly, and those in rural populations). Possibly 10% of the population is in need of mental health services at any one time, and only about one third of this group comes to the attention of any sort of mental health treatment facility. Women are still underserved, or even harmed, particularly when their problems run counter to societal stereotypes, as is the case with female alcoholics. Two of three seriously disturbed children in the United States are not receiving the mental health services they need. Generally, there are few mental health services in rural areas.

By the year 2000, one in every six Americans will be over 65 years of age. Never before have there been so many older people relative to the number of younger people, a situation presenting greater demands for mental health services. There is considerable evidence that older adults do not receive as much mental health care as would be desirable, and ethnic minority elders are even less well served. There are a number of reasons for this inadequate level of mental health services: (1) elders are reluctant to seek aid for emotional problems, (2) funding to community mental health centers does not provide effective outreach to older adults, (3) programs in some mental health professions (such as psychology) do not emphasize geriatric specialization, and (4) there are few financial incentives for private practitioners to seek out older clients who have only Medicare coverage.

CATEGORIZING MENTAL ILLNESS (DSM-IV)

To carry out their professional responsibilities, clinicians and researchers need clear and accurate guidelines for identifying and categorizing mental illness. Such guidelines help clinicians plan and evaluate treatment for their clients. Necessary elements for categorizing include agreement regarding which specific behaviors constitute mental illness.

The current DSM-IV (1994) incorporates the most recent changes: (1) moving away from any particular theoretical framework for understanding mental disorders; (2) increasing validity and reliability for each diagnostic category through a systematic and extensive review of relevant research results, clinical data, and field trials (APA 1994); and (3) establishing more specific criteria to identify disorders.

In **DSM-IV**, each of the mental disorders is conceptualized as a clinically significant behavioral or psychological syndrome or pattern that occurs in an individual and is associated with present *distress* (e.g., a painful symptom) or *disability* (e.g., impairment in one or more important areas of functioning) or with a significantly increased risk of suffering death, pain, disability, or an important loss of freedom. This syndrome or pattern must not be merely an expectable and culturally sanctioned response to a particular event, such as the death of a loved one. Whatever its original cause, it must currently be considered a manifestation of a behavioral, psychological, or biological dysfunction in the individual. Deviant behavior (e.g., political, religious, or sexual) and conflicts between the individual and society are not considered mental disorders unless the deviance or conflict is a symptom of a dysfunction in the individual.

A common misconception is that a classification of mental disorders classifies *people*. For this reason, the text of DSM-IV avoids the use of such expressions as "a schizophrenic" or "an alcoholic" and instead uses the more accurate "an individual with schizophrenia" or "an individual with alcohol dependence."

Since DSM-III appeared in 1980, the criteria for classification of mental disorders have been sufficiently detailed for clinical, teaching, and research purposes. See Box 2–1 for an example of how DSM-IV provides specific criteria for the diagnosis of generalized anxiety disorder.

DSM-III and DSM-III-R introduced a new multiaxial system of classification to allow for multiple complexities of people's lives. DSM-IV has continued individual evaluation on five dimensions as well as addressing ethnic and cultural considerations (Table 2–2).

BOX 2–1 DSM-IV CRITERIA FOR GENERALIZED ANXIETY DISORDER

A. Excessive anxiety and worry (apprehensive expectation), occurring more days than not for at least 6 months, about a number of events or activities (such as work or school performance)
B. The person finds it difficult to control the worry
C. The anxiety and worry are associated with three (or more) of the following six symptoms (with at least some symptoms present for more days than not for the past 6 months). Note: Only one item is required in children.
   (1) Restlessness or feeling keyed up or on edge
   (2) Being easily fatigued
   (3) Difficulty concentrating or mind going blank
   (4) Irritability
   (5) Muscle tension
   (6) Sleep disturbance (difficulty falling or staying asleep; or restless, unsatisfying sleep)
D. The focus of the anxiety and worry is not confined to features of an Axis I disorder; e.g., the anxiety or worry is not about having a panic attack (as in panic disorder), being embarrassed in public (as in social phobia), being contaminated (as in obsessive-compulsive disorder), being away from home or close relatives (as in separation anxiety disorder), gaining weight (as in anorexia nervosa), having multiple physical complaints (as in somatization disorder), or having a serious illness (as in hypochondriasis), and the anxiety and worry do not occur exclusively during posttraumatic stress disorder.
E. The anxiety, worry, or physical symptoms cause significant distress or impairment in social, occupational, or other important areas of functioning.
F. The disturbance is not due to the direct physiological effects of a substance (e.g., a drug of abuse, a medication) or a general medical condition (e.g., hyperthyroidism) and does not occur exclusively during a mood disorder, psychotic disorder, or pervasive developmental disorder.

Diagnostic criteria from American Psychiatric Association (1994). *Diagnostic and statistical manual of mental disorders (DSM-IV)* (4th ed.). Washington, DC: American Psychiatric Association. Reprinted with permission.

Special efforts have been made in DSM-IV to incorporate an awareness that the manual is used in culturally diverse populations in the United States and internationally. Clinicians evaluate individuals from numerous ethnic groups and cultural backgrounds (including many who are recent immigrants). Diagnostic assessment can be especially challenging when a clinician from one ethnic or cultural group uses the DSM-IV classification to evaluate an individual from a different ethnic or cultural group. For example, among some cultural groups, certain religious practices or beliefs (e.g., hearing or seeing a deceased

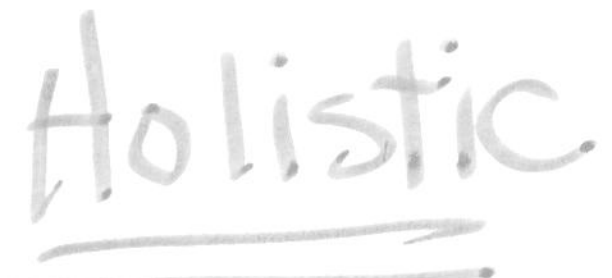

TABLE 2–2 DMS-IV MULTIAXIAL SYSTEM OF EVALUATION

Axis I	Clinical disorders Other conditions that may be a focus of clinical attention
Axis II	Personality disorders Mental retardation
Axis III	General medical conditions
Axis IV	Psychosocial and environmental problems
Axis V	Global assessment of functioning

From American Psychiatric Association (1994). *Diagnostic and statistical manual of disorders* (DSM-IV) (4th ed.) Washington, DC: American Psychiatric Association. Reprinted with permission. Copyright 1994 American Psychiatric Association.

relative during bereavement) may be misdiagnosed as manifestations of a psychotic disorder; furthermore, a syndrome often takes on different superficial forms in different cultures. Also, people from minority or migrant populations may have good reason to be distrustful, and it should not be assumed that these clients are suffering from paranoia or paranoid schizophrenia (Westmeyer 1986).

The **DSM-IV axis system,** by requiring judgments to be made on each of the five axes, forces the diagnostician to consider a broad range of information. Axis I refers to the collection of signs and symptoms that together constitute a particular disorder. Axis II refers to long-term patterns of behavior and mental retardation. Thus, axes I and II constitute the classification of abnormal behavior. Axes I and II were separated to ensure that the possible presence of long-term disturbance is considered when attention is directed to the current one. For example, a heroin addict would be diagnosed on axis I as having a substance-related disorder; this client might also have a long-standing antisocial personality disorder, which would be noted on axis II.

Although the remaining three axes are not needed to make the actual diagnosis, their inclusion in the DSM indicates recognition that factors other than a person's symptoms should be considered in an assessment. On axis III the clinician indicates any general medical conditions believed to be relevant to the mental disorder in question. In some individuals a physical disorder (e.g., a neurological dysfunction) may be the cause of the abnormal behavior, whereas in others it may be an important factor in their overall condition (e.g., diabetes in a child with a conduct disorder). Axis IV is for reporting psychosocial and environmental problems that may affect the diagnosis, treatment, and prognosis of a mental disorder. These may include occupational problems, economic problems, interpersonal difficulties with family members, and a variety of problems in other life areas. Finally, axis V, called global assessment of functioning (GAF), gives an indication of the person's best level of psychological, social, and occupational functioning during the preceding year, rated on a scale of 1 to 100 (from persistent danger of severely hurting oneself or others to superior functioning in a variety of activities) at the time of the evaluation, as well as the highest level of functioning for at least a few months during the past year. For children and adolescents, this should include at least 1 month during the school year. Ratings of current functioning generally reflect the current need for treatment or care. Ratings of the highest level of functioning during the past year frequently have prognostic significance because the goal of treatment is often to return the person to a previous level of functioning after an episode of illness. Table 2–3 illustrates how the multiaxial system of classification might be applied to a hypothetical case.

Caution needs to be exercised in diagnosing or labeling, whether a medical diagnosis or a nursing diagnosis is being formulated. The premise that every society has its own view of health and illness and its own classification of diseases has long been observed by anthropologists, historians, and other students of cross-cultural society (Klerman 1986). The process of psychiatric labeling can have harmful effects on an individual and family, especially if the diagnosis was made on insufficient evidence and proves faulty. A cross-national study of the diagnosis of mental disorders demonstrates, for example, a dramatic difference between British and American psychiatrists. The study revealed that London psychiatrists tend to "diagnose" people more frequently as having bipolar or character disorders, whereas New York psychiatrists use the diagnosis of schizophrenia much more readily (Rothblum et al. 1986).

An example of cultural and social bias influencing psychiatric diagnosis is that homosexuality was labeled a psychiatric disease in both DSM-I and DSM-II. All research consistently failed to demonstrate that people with a homosexual orientation were any more maladjusted than heterosexuals, but despite the research data, change occurred in the medical community only when gay rights activists advocated an end to discrimination against lesbians and gay men. No longer is homosexuality classified as a mental disorder. Other instances of bias may extend to many minority groups, including blacks, elderly persons, children, and women. These biases are often reflected in our power structures and political systems. A proposed category thought by many to reflect social bias was *self-defeating personality disorder*, found in the appendix to DSM-III-R (APA 1987). Most people who would come under this category are women. The American Psychological Association declared this new diagnosis potentially dangerous to women and without scientific basis, so the category was not adopted for DSM-IV. Awareness of the cultural bias and dangers in labeling carries enormous implications for nursing practice, especially in the field of mental health, because nurses often take their cues from the medical structure. Doctors diag-

TABLE 2–3 CLINICAL EXAMPLE DEMONSTRATING DSM-IV AXES

EVALUATION	DATA
	Axis I
Schizophrenic disorder, paranoid	For the past 9 months, Michael, a 33-year-old representative, has suffered delusions of grandeur and persecution. Believing himself to be a genius, he became convinced that another salesman in his firm was trying to kill him because the other man could not tolerate Michael's superiority. In the past 2 weeks, Michael has become certain that this other man has had a pale green gas pumped into his office through the air-conditioning ducts, but there is no objective evidence of such gas or any other malfunctioning of the air-conditioning system.
	Axis II
Paranoid traits, no personality disorder	Michael has always tended to be suspicious and distrustful of people. He looks constantly for evidence that others are trying to get the better of him or to harm him, and his manner is guarded. He has trouble relaxing, and others see him as cold and unemotional. He has no close friends and is considered a "loner." He was extremely jealous of his wife, from whom he is now separated, and often accused her, falsely, of having affairs with other men.
	Axis III
Colitis	Michael sees a flare-up of his colitis (inflammation of the colon) as evidence that the salesman is poisoning him, even though Michael has had the same symptoms many times before.
	Axis IV
Psychosocial and environmental problems a. Marital separation b. Loss of work responsibility Rated severe	Michael left his wife 10 months ago. Two months ago, the president of Michael's firm reassigned one of Michael's important accounts to the salesman Michael now suspects of hostile intent. Michael thinks this was maneuvered by the other salesman, but in fact the president acted because the quality of Michael's work was deteriorating. His work had slowed visibly, and co-workers complained that they could not perform their work properly when he was present.
	Axis V
Highest level of adaptive functioning in past year (GAF) Rated fair	Michael's functioning was adequate until he separated from his wife. At that point, he began to withdraw further from friends and acquaintances. He appeared to concentrate more on his job but actually spent his time checking and rechecking his work. When the firm's president reassigned his major account, Michael's work deteriorated further and Michael began to air some of his suspicions about the partner who took over the account. When his colitis flared up 2 weeks ago, he requested an appointment with the president and accused the partner openly. Michael was fired.

GAF, global assessment of functioning.
Adapted from Altrocchi, J. (1980). *Abnormal behavior.* New York: Harcourt Brace Jovanovich.

nose "diseases." Nurses diagnose "a perceived difficulty or need" (ANA 1994). The more objectively we as nurses observe, assess, and diagnose the individuals under our care, the more effectively we will administer our skills.

CULTURE AND MENTAL ILLNESS

▶ Over the past 4 months, George has struck and injured several dozen people. Most of them he hardly knew. Two of them had to be sent to the hospital. George expresses no guilt, no regrets. He says he would attack every one of them again if he got the chance.

What should society do with George?

1. Send him to jail?
2. Commit him to a mental hospital?
3. Give him an award for being the best defensive lineman in the league?

Before you can answer, you must know the context of George's behavior. Behavior that seems normal at a party might seem bizarre at a business meeting. Behavior that earns millions for a rock singer might earn a trip to the mental hospital for a college professor. Behavior that is perfectly routine in one culture might be considered criminal in another.

Even when we know the context of someone's behavior, we may wonder whether it is "normal." Suppose your Aunt Tillie starts to pass out $5 bills to strangers on the street and vows she will keep doing so until she has exhausted her entire fortune. Is she mentally ill? Should the court commit her to a mental hospital and turn her fortune over to you as her trustee?

A man claims to be Jesus Christ and asks permission to appear before the United Nations to announce God's message to the world. A psychiatrist is sure that he can relieve this man of his disordered thinking by giving him antipsychotic drugs, but the man refuses to take them and insists that his thinking is normal. Should we force him to take the drugs, just ignore him, or put his speech on the agenda of the United Nations?

In determining the mental health or mental illness of these individuals, we must consider the norms and influence of culture. Throughout history, people (including us) have interpreted health or sickness according to their current views. People in the Middle Ages, for example, regarded bizarre behavior as a sign that the disturbed person was possessed by a demon. To exorcise the demon, priests resorted to religious rituals. During the 1880s, when the "germ theory" of illness was popular, physicians interpreted bizarre behavior as stemming from biological causes. A striking example of how cultural change influences the interpretation of mental illness is the diagnosis of hysteria, which is much less common today than it was in the nineteenth century; according to some authors, this is because of a less restrictive family atmosphere and more permissive childrearing, especially in sexual areas (Chodoff 1954).

Cultures differ not only in their views of regarding mental illness but also in the types of behavior categorized as mental illness (Berry et al. 1992). For example, one form of mental illness recognized in parts of Southeast Asia is *running amok*, in which someone (usually a male) runs around engaging in furious, almost indiscriminate, violent behavior. *Pibloqtoq* is an uncontrollable desire to tear off one's clothing and expose oneself to severe weather; it is a recognized form of psychological disorder in parts of Greenland, Alaska, and the Arctic regions of Canada. In our own society, we recognize *anorexia nervosa* as a psychological disorder that entails voluntary starvation. That disorder is well known in Europe, North America, and Australia but unheard-of in many other parts of the world.

What is to be made of the fact that certain disorders occur in some cultures but are absent in other cultures? One interpretation is that the conditions necessary for causing a particular disorder occur in some places but are absent in other places. Another interpretation is that people learn certain kinds of abnormal behavior by imitation. However, the fact that some disorders may be culturally determined does not prove that all mental illnesses are so determined. The best evidence suggests that schizophrenia and bipolar affective disorders are found throughout the world. The symptom patterns of schizophrenia have been observed among indigenous Greenlanders and West African villager, as well as among our own Western culture. Refer to Chapter 5 for discussion of the differing ways people view the world and a review of discrete cultural syndromes.

MAJOR THEORIES OF PERSONALITY

All people go through a series of stages in their development from infancy to old age. Each stage has its own character and offers its own unique opportunities for growth. The meaning of particular events and relationships is deeply influenced by the stage in the life cycle in which they occur. Although each of us is unique, we all go through the same basic stages of growth. Each has its own special contribution to the individual as a whole. Hebrew, Chinese, and Greek writings dating back more than 2000 years attest to our interest in and observation of the "stages of man." Each ancient writing has identified similar stages in the human life cycle (Levison and Gooden 1985).

Nurses draw on relevant theories of personality and human development as a basis for assessment, nursing diagnosis, planning, intervention, and evaluation. Different theorists view the life cycle through their own disciplines and individual theories of personality development.

The contributions of Freud, Erikson, Sullivan, Piaget, Maslow, and Kohlberg form important theoretical foundations used in all medical and nursing practices, not just in the specialties of psychiatry or psychiatric nursing.

Freud

Sigmund Freud (1856–1939), an Austrian psychiatrist and the founder of psychoanalysis, developed a complex theoretical formulation of the nature of the human personality. The major components of his theory discussed here include levels of awareness, personality structure, the concept of anxiety and defense mechanisms, and psychosexual stages of development.

Levels of Awareness

Essentially, Freud's levels of awareness provide a mental typography that is divided into three parts: the conscious, the preconscious, and the unconscious.

CONSCIOUS. The **conscious** includes all experiences that are within a person's awareness at any given time. For example, all intellectual, emotional, and interpersonal aspects of a person's behavior that he or she is aware of and is able to control are within conscious awareness. All information that is easily remembered and immediately available to an individual is in the conscious mind. The conscious mind is logical and, according to Freud, regulated by the reality principle.

PRECONSCIOUS. The **preconscious** includes experiences, thoughts, feelings, or desires that might not be in immediate awareness but can be recalled to consciousness. The preconscious (sometimes called **subconscious)** can help screen out extraneous information and can enhance concentration. It can censor certain wishes and thoughts and helps repress unpleasant thoughts or feelings.

UNCONSCIOUS. Although Freud cannot be credited with discovering the unconscious, it was he who developed the concept of the unconscious in clear, rich, and original terms. Freud described the mind as an iceberg to convey the relationship between the conscious and the unconscious. The water's surface represents the boundary between conscious and unconscious, with nine tenths of the mind submerged (Fig. 2–1).

The **unconscious** refers to all memories, feelings, thoughts, or wishes that are not available to the conscious mind. Often these repressed memories, feelings, thoughts, or wishes could, if made prematurely conscious, trigger enormous anxiety. However, unconscious material often does become manifest in dreams, slips of the tongue, or jokes; or through the use of hypnosis, therapy, or certain drugs (e.g., sodium pentothal and hallucinogens).

The unconscious exists comfortably with extreme contradictions and ambivalence (love and hate toward the same object), intense emotions, and strong sexual urges. The unconscious is not logical, has no conception of time, and is governed by what Freud calls the pleasure principle.

Conscious, *preconscious*, and *unconscious* are not mental processes or systems. They are adjectives that describe the quality of psychological activity.

Personality Structure

Freud sought to describe what he called the "anatomy of the mental personality." He isolated three categories of experience—the id, the ego, and the superego—that represent a method of looking at the way an individual functions. They are not separate entities or sections of the mind. Very roughly, they may be identified as biologically driven energy (id), ways of coping with reality (ego), and conscience (superego). The way the three interact, the conflicts they produce, and their blending provide a comprehensive picture of the behavior of the individual.

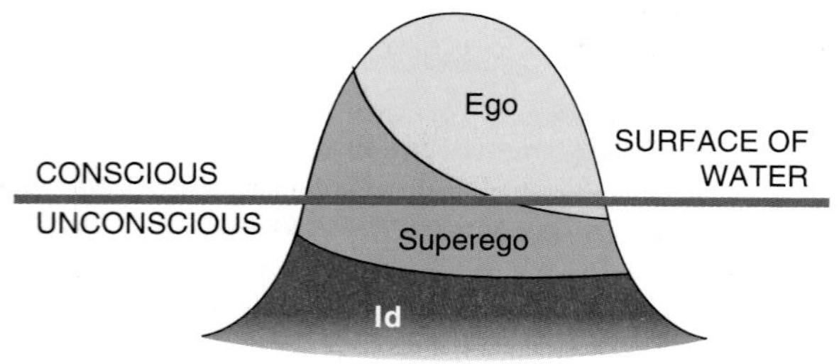

Figure 2–1 The mind as an iceberg.

THE ID. The **id** is the "core of our being." It is the source of all drives and the reservoir of instincts. The id is the oldest and the first original function of the personality, and it is the basis out of which the ego and the superego develop. The id includes all our genetic inheritance, our reflexes, and our capacities to respond, including the instincts, basic drives, needs, and wishes that motivate us. It is the reservoir of psychic energy and furnishes all the power for the operation of the other two systems. It is with us at birth.

The id operates according to the pleasure principle and uses primary processes. The *pleasure principle* refers to the seeking of immediate tension reduction. The id cannot tolerate increases in libido, or tension, which are experienced as uncomfortable states. Therefore, the id seeks to discharge the tension and return to a more comfortable, constant level of energy. To avoid painful tension and obtain pleasure, the id acts immediately in an impulsive, irrational way. It pays no attention to the consequences of actions and therefore often behaves in ways harmful to self and others.

Freud makes a distinction between primary and secondary process thinking. *Primary process* is a psychological activity in which the id attempts to reduce tension by hallucinating or forming an image of the object that will satisfy its needs and remove the tension. For example, the primary process provides the hungry individual with a mental picture of food. Picturing a hamburger momentarily reduces hunger pangs. This hallucinatory experience in which the desired object is present in the form of a memory image is called *wish fulfillment.* This activity is present in the mental functioning of newborns, in nocturnal dreams, and in the hallucinations of psychotics. Picturing a bottle or the breast partly pacifies the hungry infant, but it does not satisfy the need. The primary process by itself is not capable of reducing tension. The hungry infant cannot eat mental images of food. A new, or secondary, psychological process must develop if the individual is to survive. When this occurs, the structure of the second system of the personality, the ego, begins to take form.

THE EGO. The **ego** emerges because the needs, wishes, and demands of the id require appropriate exchanges with the outside world of reality. Hungry people have to be able to seek, find, and eat food in order to meet their needs and survive. The ego emerges out of the id and acts as an intermediary between the id and the external world. The ego is said to begin its development during the fourth or fifth month of life. The ego distinguishes between things in the mind and things in the external world, whereas the id knows only the subjective reality of the mind. Reality testing is one function of the ego.

The ego follows the *reality principle* and operates by means of the *secondary process* (i.e., realistic thinking). The aim of the reality principle is to satisfy the id's impulses in the external world with a suitable object. The reality principle determines whether an experience is true or false and whether it has external existence or not. Whereas the id employs fantasies and wishes of the primary process to satisfy a need, the ego uses the realistic thinking characteristic of the secondary process. Using the secondary process, the ego devises a plan and then tests it, usually by some kind of action, to see whether it will work. Problem solving, then, is another function of the ego. For example, the hungry person figures out where to find food and then proceeds to look for it in that place.

The ego has been called the executive of the personality. The ego becomes the mediator between the organism and the outer world. Through the use of mental functions of judgment and intelligence, the ego selects the parts of the environment to which it will respond and decides which instincts will be satisfied, and in what fashion. Carrying out its executive function is not an easy task for the ego. The ego has to try to integrate the often-conflicting demands of its "three harsh masters": external reality, the id, and the superego.

THE SUPEREGO. The third and last system of personality to be developed is the **superego,** the internal representative of the values, ideals, and moral standards of society. It comes from the interactions with one's parents during the extended period of childhood dependency. From a system of rewards and punishments originally imposed on the child from without, the child internalizes the moral standards of parents and society. The superego is the moral arm of personality. It strives for perfection rather than pleasure and represents the ideal rather than the real.

The development of the superego is a necessary part of socialization because young children's egos are too weak to control their impulses. Parental "thou shalt nots" are needed for a time. However, a harsh superego can be uncompromising and may lead to blocking of necessary and reasonable satisfactions. Furthermore, a rigid superego can create feelings of inferiority (expressed as "I'm a bad person") when the individual fails to meet parental dictates. The superego is said to have its development between 3 and 5 years of age.

The three systems of the personality—the id, the ego, and the superego—are names for the psychological processes that follow different operating principles. In a mature and well-adjusted personality, they work together as a team under the administrative leadership of the ego. However, development does not always proceed smoothly. Too powerful an id or a superego may gain control, and imbalance and maladjustment may be the result.

Let's take a look at a hypothetical situation and consider the roles of the id, ego, and superego. A young person is out on a date with an attractive member of the opposite sex with whom there may be a wish to have a sexual relationship. The id would declare, "I want, I want!" while the superego might assert "Thou shalt not!" The ego would be faced with the problem of meeting the id's demands within the limitations and standards of society. A solution might involve the young person's waiting until better acquainted with the other individual or until some other social norm is met.

Defense Mechanisms and Anxiety

Freud believed that anxiety was an inevitable part of living. The environment, physical and social, presents dangers and insecurities, threats and satisfactions. It can produce pain and increase tension or produce pleasure and decrease tension. Everyone must cope with anxiety. The ego develops defenses, or **defense mechanisms,** to ward off anxiety by preventing conscious awareness of threatening feelings. Without defense mechanisms, anxiety might overwhelm and paralyze us and interfere with daily living.

Defense mechanisms share two common features: (1) they operate on an unconscious level (except suppression), so that we are not aware of their operation; and (2) they deny, falsify, or distort reality to make it less threatening. We cannot survive without defense mechanisms. However, if they become too extreme in distorting reality, interference with healthy adjustment and personal growth may occur. It is useful to become familiar with the common defense mechanisms. Table 2–4 includes an overview of some of these and a brief description of their characteristics, with examples from daily living. A fuller discussion of defense mechanisms is found in Chapter 13.

Psychosexual Stages of Development

Freud believed that human development proceeds through a series of stages from infancy to adulthood. Each stage is characterized by the inborn tendency of all individuals to reduce tension and seek pleasure. During the first 5 years of life, each stage is defined by and named for the erogenous zone that produces the main source of gratification during that stage. Each stage is associated with a particular conflict that must be resolved before the child can move successfully to the next stage. Freud believed that the experiences during the early stages determine an individual's adjustment patterns and the personality traits that he or she has as an adult. In fact, Freud thought that personality was rather well formed by the time the child entered school, and that subsequent growth consisted of elaborating this basic structure.

The three early stages, collectively called the *pregenital stage,* are the oral, anal, and phallic stages. The child then enters a prolonged *latency period,* the quiet years in which the dynamics become more or less stabilized. With the arrival of adolescence, there is a burst of libidinal forces, primitive impulses from the id, which upsets the stabilization of the latency period and gradually comes under

TABLE 2–4 COMMON DEFENSE MECHANISMS

DEFENSE MECHANISMS	CHARACTERISTICS	EXAMPLE
Repression	Blocking a wish or desire from conscious expression	You forget the name of someone for whom you have intense negative feelings
Projection	Attributing an unconscious impulse, attitude, or behavior to someone else (blaming or scapegoating)	A man who is attracted to his friend's wife on an unconscious level accuses his wife of flirting with his friend
Reaction-formation	An intense feeling regarding an object, person, or feeling is out of awareness and is unknowingly acted out consciously in an opposite manner	You treat someone whom you unconsciously dislike intensely in an overly friendly manner
Regression	Returning to an earlier level of adaptation when severly threatened	A child resumes bed-wetting after having long since stopped when his baby brother is born and fussed over at home
Rationalization	Unconsciously falsifying an experience by giving a contrived, socially acceptable and logical explanation to justify an unpleasant experience or questionable behavior	A student who did not study for an examination blames his failure on the teacher's poor lecture material and the unfairness of the examination
Identification	Modeling behavior after someone else	A 6-year-old girl dresses up in her mother's dress and high-heeled shoes
Displacement	Discharging intense feelings for one person onto another object or person who is less threatening, thereby satisfying an impulse with a substitute object	A child who has been scolded by her mother hits her doll with a hairbrush
Sublimation	Rechanneling an impulse into a more socially desirable object	A student satisfies sexual curiosity by conducting sophisticated research into sexual behaviors

control as the adolescent moves into adulthood. The final developmental stage of adolescence and adulthood is the *genital stage.* Table 2–5 summarizes Freud's psychosexual stages of development and can be used to follow the narrative here.

ORAL STAGE (0 TO 1 YEAR). The first stage is the oral stage, which lasts from birth to 1 year of age. The baby is "all mouth," getting most of his or her gratification from sucking. The erogenous zones are the lips and mouth, through which the infant receives nourishment, has the closest contact with the mother (in breast-feeding), and discovers information about the world.

During this stage, which Freud called *primary narcissism,* the infant is concerned only with gratification of self. The infant is all id, operating on the pleasure principle and striving for immediate gratification of needs. The ego begins to emerge during this time (fourth or fifth month of life), as the infant begins to see the self as separate from the mother; this is the beginning of the development of a "sense of self." When the infant experiences gratification of basic needs, a sense of trust and security begins.

THE ANAL STAGE (1 TO 3 YEARS). Freud's second psychosexual stage is the anal stage, which is experienced in the second year of life. Generally, toilet training occurs during this period. According to Freud, the child gains pleasure both from the elimination of feces and from their retention. Toilet training involves converting an involuntary activity, the elimination of bodily wastes, into a voluntary one. Until this time, the infant has experienced few demands from others, but now there appear to be direct attempts by the parents to interfere with the pleasure obtained from the excretory functions. Thus, the conflict of this stage is between those demands from society in the persons of the parents and the sensations of pleasure associated with the anus.

According to Freud, parents' reactions during this stage may have far-reaching effects on the formation of specific traits and values. If the mother is very strict and repressive in her methods, the child may hold back the feces in defiance and become constipated. If this mode of reaction generalizes to other forms of behavior, the child will develop a retentive character (i.e., the child will become stubborn and stingy, unwilling to give). Alternatively, under the pressure of coercive measures in toilet training, the child may vent rage by expelling the feces at the most inappropriate times. This can become the original model for all kinds of expulsive traits, including cruelty, malicious destructiveness, temper tantrums, and messy disorderliness. On the other hand, according to Freudian theorists, if the mother is warm and sensitive in her urging and extravagantly praises the child in toilet activity, the child will acquire the notion that the whole activity of producing feces is extremely important.

TABLE 2–5 FREUD'S PSYCHOSEXUAL STAGE OF DEVELOPMENT

STAGE (AGE)	SOURCE OF SATISFACTION	PRIMARY CONFLICT	TASKS	DESIRED OUTCOME	OTHER POSSIBLE PERSONALITY TRAITS
Oral (0–1 yr)	Mouth (sucking, biting, chewing)	Weaning	Mastery of gratification of oral needs; beginning of ego development (4–5 mos)	Trust in the environment develops with the realization that needs can be met	Fixation at the oral stage is associated with passivity, gullibility and dependence, the use of sarcasm, and the development of orally focused habits (e.g., smoking, nail-biting)
Anal (1–3 yrs)	Anal region (expulsion and retention of feces)	Toilet training	Beginning to gain a sense of control over instinctual drives; learns to delay immediate gratification to gain a future goal	Control over impulses	Fixation associated with anal retentiveness (stinginess, rigid thought patterns, obsessive-compulsive disorder) or anal expulsive character (messiness, destructiveness, cruelty)
Phallic (oedipal) (3–6 yrs)	Genitals (masturbation)	Oedipus and Electra complexes	Sexual identity with parent of same sex; beginning of superego development	Identification with parent of the same sex	Unresolved outcomes may result in difficulties with sexual identity and difficulties with authority figures
Latency (6–12 yrs)	—	—	Growth of ego functions (social, intellectual, mechanical) and the ability to care about and relate to others outside the home (peers of the same sex)	The development of skills needed to cope with the environment	Fixations can result in difficulty in identifying with others and in developing social skills, resulting in a sense of inadequacy and inferiority
Genital (12 yrs and beyond	Genitals (sexual intercourse)	—	Developing satisfying sexual and emotional relationships with members of the opposite sex; emancipation from parents—planning life goals and gaining a strong sense of personal identity	The ability to be creative and find pleasure in "love and work"	Inability to negotiate this stage could result in difficulties in becoming emotionally and financially independent, lack of strong personal identity and future goals, and inability to form satisfying intimate relationships

Data from Gleitman, H. (1981). *Psychology*. New York: W. W. Norton.

According to Freud, this idea may be the basis for creativity and productivity. The child learns to delay immediate gratification (expelling feces) to obtain a future goal (parental approval).

THE PHALLIC STAGE (3 TO 6 YEARS). The phallic stage (or oedipal phase) of development occurs between the ages of 3 and 6 years. The child experiences both pleasurable and conflicting feelings associated with genital organs. At this time, children devote much energy to examining their genitalia, masturbating, and expressing interest in sexual matters. Children are curious about everything, including anatomical differences between the sexes and the origin of babies. They create unconscious fantasies about the sexual act itself and about the birth process. Their ideas are frequently inaccurate and unrealistic, such as believing that a pregnant woman has swallowed her baby or that a baby is expelled through the mouth or the anus.

The pleasures of masturbation and the fantasy life of children set the stage for the oedipus complex, the concept of which Freud considered to be one of his greatest contributions to the study of personality development. Freud's concept was suggested by the Greek tragedy of Sophocles in which King Oedipus unwittingly murdered his father and married his mother. To Freud, the Greek myth symbolized the unconscious psychological conflict that each child faces: the child's unconscious sexual attraction to, and wish to possess, the parent of the opposite sex; and the hostility toward, and desire to remove, the parent of the same sex; as well as subsequent guilt for these wishes. The conflict is resolved when the child identifies with the parent of the same sex.

According to Freud, the emergence of the superego is both the solution to, and the result of, these intense forbidden impulses. Because these intense erotic and murderous impulses have no prospect of succeeding, children channel this emotional energy through the defense mechanisms of identification and introjection. As a result, children not only identify with the parent of the same sex but also incorporate into their own belief system the values and social standards of their parents and those of their culture and subculture.

THE LATENCY PERIOD (6 TO 12 YEARS). After the phallic stage, the child enters school and begins what Freud termed *latency*. This period, encompassing approximately 6 years between the phallic and genital stages, is marked by a tapering off of conscious biological and sexual urges. The sexual impulses, which are unacceptable in their direct expression, are channeled and elevated into more culturally accepted levels of activity, such as sports, intellectual interests, and peer relations. Freud was relatively silent about the latency period. He did not consider it a genuine psychosexual stage, but viewed it rather as a period of transition and comparative sexual quiescence.

Today, Freud's view of latency has been questioned by most critics, who consider a more accurate observation is that during this period children learn to hide their sexuality from disapproving adults.

THE GENITAL STAGE (12 YEARS AND BEYOND). Freud's final stage is termed the *genital stage*, which emerges as adolescence with the onset of puberty, when the genital organs mature. The impulses of the pregenital period are narcissistic in character: i.e., the individual gains gratification from his or her own body. The child values other people because they satisfy his or her narcissistic pleasures. During adolescence, some of this self-love (narcissism) becomes redirected toward gratification involving genuine interaction with other people. Sexual attraction, socialization, group activities, vocational planning, and preparation for marrying and rearing a family begin to manifest themselves. By the end of adolescence, the person becomes transformed from what was originally a pleasure-seeking individual to a more reality-oriented, socialized adult.

According to Freud, a mature individual is one who has reached conventional genital sexuality; one who satisfies his or her needs in socially approved ways; and one who is able, in Freud's words, "to love and to work."

Although Freud differentiated five stages of personality growth, he did not assume that there were any sharp breaks or abrupt transitions in proceeding from one stage into another. The final organization of personality represents contributions from all stages.

Long-Term Effects of Freud's Psychosexual Stages

Freudian theorists contend that the effects of Freud's psychosexual stages can be seen in various adult character types or traits. They believe that children who have been either unduly frustrated or overindulged may become fixated on a particular stage. *Fixation* refers to growth arrestment in which excessive needs, characteristics of an earlier stage, are recreated.

For example, practitioners from a psychoanalytic school may believe that a child who persists in thumbsucking well beyond the preschool years may be showing evidence of being fixated at the oral stage. These theorists believe that the child has an inability to satisfy oral needs in an age-appropriate manner. The example of a chain-smoking adult who persists in smoking despite all health warnings also suggests to Freudians a fixation on oral needs. The character traits of an orally fixated person include being dependent on and easily influenced by others.

Likewise, adults who experienced frustration or overindulgence at the anal stage, according to Freudian thought, may be described as having anal personalities. They may be orderly, parsimonious, and stubborn, or the opposite: disorganized, explosive, and uncontrolled. Most of us do not reflect a pure type, but these personality types and their opposites are thought to have their origin in the various psychosexual stages.

Maddi (1972) summarized the various character traits described by Freud as bipolar dimensions. These traits may be seen as attitudes that developed during the various psychosexual stages. Consider each of the traits in Table 2–6. Do you recognize them as characteristics of yourself or of someone you know?

Erikson's Psychosocial Stages of Development

Erik Erikson (1902–1994), an American psychoanalyst who was initially a follower of Freud, broadened Freud's theory of human development. First, Erikson stressed the role of the ego, or the rational part of the personality, whereas Freud had concentrated largely on the nonrational, instinctual parts of the personality (the id). Second, Erikson viewed the growing individual within the larger social setting of the family and its cultural heritage rather than in the more restricted triangle of mother-child-father. Third, Erikson's stages span the full life cycle, in contrast to Freudian theory, which views basic personality as established by 5 years of age. Fourth, Erikson differed from Freud in that he studied healthy personali-

TABLE 2–6 FREUD'S PSYCHOSEXUAL TRAITS AS BIPOLAR DIMENSIONS

ORAL TRAITS	
Optimism	Pessimism
Gullibility	Suspiciousness
Manipulativeness	Passivity
Admiration	Envy
Cockiness	Self-belittlement
ANAL TRAITS	
Stinginess	Overgenerosity
Constrictedness	Expansiveness
Stubbornness	Acquiescence
Orderliness	Messiness
Rigid punctuality	Tardiness
Meticulousness	Dirtiness
Precision	Vagueness
PHALLIC TRAITS	
Vanity	Self-hatred
Pride	Humility
Blind courage	Timidity
Brashness	Bashfulness
Gregariousness	Isolation
Stylishness	Plainness
Flirtatiousness	Avoidance of heterosexuality
Chastity	Promiscuity
Gaiety	Sadness

Adapted with permission from Engler, B. O. (1979). *Personality theories: An introduction* (p. 55). Boston: Houghton Mifflin. Copyright © 1979 by Houghton Mifflin Company. Maddi, S. R. (1972). *Personality theories: A comparative analysis* (pp. 271–276). Holmwood, IL: Dorsey Press.

ties to arrive at his theory, rather than analyzing neurotic clients, as Freud had done.

In summary, Erikson remolded Freud's psychosexual stages of development into psycho*social* stages, emphasizing the growth of individuals as they establish new ways of understanding and relating to themselves and to their changing social world throughout the whole life cycle.

Erikson's recognition that humans continue to develop throughout the life span resulted in a developmental scheme of eight stages extending from infancy to old age. Erikson states that at each stage individuals are faced with a particular crisis or conflict, which can have a positive or negative outcome.

The stages listed in Table 2–7 are the major stages in the life cycle as described by Erikson. They clearly build on Freud's psychosexual stages, but they emphasize the social determinants of personality development. The conflicts are not simply caused by frustration or instinctual drives early in one's life; they take into account the roles that society and the individual play throughout life in the formation of the personality. Furthermore, Erikson's view of the individual is an optimistic one, for he demonstrates that each phase of growth has its strengths as well as its weaknesses, and that failures at one stage of development can be rectified by successes at later stages.

Sullivan's Interpersonal Theory

Harry Stack Sullivan (1892–1949), an American-born theorist in interpersonal psychiatry, used the Freudian framework early in his career. Later he developed a new concept of personality. Sullivan stopped trying to deal with what he considered unseen and private mental processes within the individual (Freud's intrapsychic processes) and began to focus on interpersonal processes that could be observed in a social framework. The basis of Sullivan's theory was the contention that personality can be observed and studied only when a person is actually behaving in relation to one or more other individuals. Thus, he defines personality as "the group of characteristic ways in which an individual relates to others" (Sullivan 1953). According to Sullivan, personality consists of behavior that can be observed.

Sullivan believes that individuals are motivated by two sets of purposes or goals: (1) the pursuit of satisfactions and (2) the pursuit of security. *Satisfactions* refer to biological needs, including sleep and rest, sexual fulfillment, food and drink, and physical closeness to other human beings. *Security* was used by Sullivan to refer to a state of well-being, belonging, and being accepted.

Anxiety and the Self-System

Anxiety is a key concept in Sullivan's interpersonal psychiatry that refers to any painful feeling or emotion. It comes from tension that arises from social insecurity or blocks to satisfaction (organic needs). According to Sullivan, there are a number of characteristics of anxiety. First, it is interpersonal in origin. For example, a mother's anxious feelings can be transmitted to a child. Second, anxiety can be described, and behaviors stemming from anxiety can be observed. The anxious person can tell how he or she feels, and behavior resulting from anxiety can be observed and studied. Third, individuals strive to reduce anxiety. For example, children learn that they can avoid anxiety that comes from punishment and the threat to their security by conforming to their parents' wishes.

Sullivan used the term *security operations* to describe those measures that the individual employs to reduce anxiety and enhance security. There are many parallels between Sullivan's notion of security operations and Freud's concept of defense mechanisms. Both are processes of which we are unaware, and both are ways in which we reduce anxiety. Although at times the concepts overlap, the major difference between security operations and defense mechanisms is Sullivan's emphasis on what is observable. For example, Freud's defense mechanism of repression is an *intrapsychic* activity, whereas Sullivan's security operations are *interpersonal* relationship activities that can be observed. Some examples of the observable manifestations of security operations are sublimation, selective inattention, and dissociation.

TABLE 2–7 ERIKSON'S EIGHT STAGES OF DEVELOPMENT 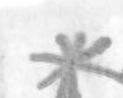

Approximate Age	Developmental Task	Psychosocial Crisis	Successful Resolution of Crisis	Unsuccessful Resolution of Crisis
Infancy (0–1½ yr)	Attachment to mother, which lays foundations for later trust in others	Trust vs. mistrust	Sound basis for relating to other people; trust in people; faith and hope about environment and future	General difficulties relating to people effectively; suspicion; trust-fear conflict; fear of future
Early childhood (1½–3 yr)	Gaining some basic control of self and environment (e.g., toilet training, exploration)	Autonomy vs. shame and doubt	Sense of self-control and adequacy; will power	Independence-fear conflict; severe feelings of self-doubt
Late childhood (3–6 yr)	Becoming purposeful and directive	Initiative vs. guilt	Ability to initiate one's own activities; sense of purpose	Aggression-fear conflict; sense of inadequacy or guilt
School age (6–12 yrs)	Developing social, physical, and school skills	Industry vs. inferiority	Competence; ability to learn and work	Sense of inferiority; difficulty learning and working
Adolescence (12–20 yr)	Making transition from childhood to adulthood; developing sense of identity	Identify vs. role confusion	Sense of personal identity; fidelity	Confusion about who one is; identity submerged in relationships or group memberships
Early adulthood (20–35 yr)	Establishing intimate bonds of love and friendship	Intimacy vs. isolation	Ability to love deeply and commit oneself	Emotional isolation; egocentricity
Middle adulthood (35–65 yr)	Fulfilling life goals that involve family, career, and society; developing concerns that embrace future generations	Generativity vs. self-absorption	Ability to give and care for others	Self-absorption; inability to grow as a person
Later years (65 yr to death)	Looking back over one's life and accepting its meaning	Integrity vs. despair	Sense of integrity and fulfillment; willingness to face death; wisdom	Dissatisfaction with life; denial of or despair over prospect of death

Data from Erikson, E. H. (1963). *Childhood and society.* New York: W. W. Norton and Altrocchi, J. (1980). *Abnormal psychology* (p. 196). New York: Harcourt Brace Jovanovich.

SUBLIMATION. When a child's behavior brings disapproval, the child experiences anxiety and threats to self-esteem. He or she learns to reduce the anxiety by behaving in a more acceptable manner. For example, the child learns to express anger verbally instead of biting, hitting, or kicking the person who is the object of the anger. This expression of unacceptable drives as more acceptable behaviors is called *sublimation.*

SELECTIVE INATTENTION. Sullivan (1953) states that **selective inattention** refers to an individual who "doesn't happen to notice an almost infinite series of more-or-less meaningful details of one's living" that might cause anxiety. For example, a husband may not notice his wife's seductive behavior toward other men because it threatens his own self-esteem.

DISSOCIATION. Some things are so threatening to the security of the self that they cannot be faced by the individual. For example, abused children—needy, helpless, and dependent on the abusing parent—block out or dissociate themselves from the experience of hate or anger toward the parent. Such feelings are excluded from conscious awareness before they are able to trigger overwhelming and intolerable anxiety. Thus, *dissociation* is similar to the defense Freud referred to as repression.

Interpersonal Theory and Psychiatric Nursing Practice

Sullivan's interpersonal theory has had a great impact on the direction of nursing practice. Hildegard Peplau, influenced by the work of Sullivan and learning theory, developed the first systematic theoretical framework for psychiatric nursing in her groundbreaking book *Interpersonal relations in nursing* (1952). Peplau laid the foundation for the professional practice of psychiatric nursing and has continued to enrich psychiatric nursing theory and the advancement of nursing practice. The discussions in Chapters 6 and 7 of the one-to-one nurse-client relationship and the clinical interview illustrate how Peplau's theoretical framework has become a cornerstone for the practice of psychiatric nursing, and consequently for all nursing practice that incorporates psychosocial principles.

Piaget

Jean Piaget (1896–1980), after earning a doctorate in zoology in his homeland of Switzerland, went on to explore the field of psychology. Piaget believed that, just as other living organisms adapt to their environment biologically, so humans adapt to their environment *psychologically*. He considered cognitive acts as ways in which the mind organizes and adapts to its environment. Piaget used the word *schema* to refer to the child's cognitive structure or framework of thought. Schemata are categories that people form in their minds to organize and understand the world. At the beginning, the young child has only a few schemata with which to understand the world. Gradually, these are increased. Adults use a wide variety of schemata to comprehend the world.

Two complementary processes of adaptation help in the development of schemata: assimilation and accommodation. *Assimilation* refers to the ability to incorporate new ideas, objects, and experiences into the framework of one's thoughts. Through assimilation, the growing child will perceive and give meaning to new information according to what is already known and understood. Assimilation is conservative, in that its main function is to make the unfamiliar familiar, to reduce the new to the old. In contrast, *accommodation* refers to the ability to change a schema in order to introduce new ideas, objects, or experiences. Whereas the process of assimilation molds the object or event to fit the child's existing frame of reference, accommodation changes the mental structure in order that new experiences may be added. These two processes are constantly working together to produce changes in the growing child's understanding of the world.

The acquisition of knowledge is an active process that depends on interaction between the child and the environment. Children do not passively receive stimulation from the environment; they learn about the world through active encounters with it. The development of the child's thinking relies on changes made in the mental structure of the child as he or she interacts with the environment. The true measure of a child's intellectual growth depends on the ability to change old ways of thinking to solve new problems.

Piaget's Stages of Cognitive Development

The development of children's thinking progresses through a sequence of four major stages, each very different from the others: (1) the sensorimotor period (0 to 2 years), (2) the preoperational period (2 to 7 years), (3) the period of concrete operations (7 to 11 years), and (4) the period of formal operations (11 years to adulthood) (Table 2–8).

The sequence of these four stages and of the substages they comprise never varies; no stage is ever skipped, because each one further develops the preceding stage and lays the groundwork for the next. The stages are somewhat related to chronological age. As with all development, however, each individual reaches each stage according to his or her own timetable. For this reason—and also because there is considerable overlapping between the stages of retention, and some characteristics from preceding stages occur in those that follow—all age norms must be considered approximate.

Maslow

Abraham Maslow (1908–1970), one of the founders of humanistic psychology, introduced the concept of a "self-actualized personality," a better-than-merely-normal personality, associated with high productivity and enjoyment of life (Maslow 1970). His unique contribution to a humanistic sociopsychological viewpoint lies in his focus on healthy people rather than sick ones, and his insistence that studies of these two groups generate different types of theory. He believed that psychology has been too concerned with humanity's frailties, and not enough with its strengths—that in the process of exploring our sins we had neglected our virtues. Where is the psychology, Maslow asks, that takes into account such experiences as love, compassion, gaiety, exhilaration, and well-being to the same extent that it deals with hate, pain, misery, guilt, and conflict? Maslow has undertaken to supply the other half of the picture, the brighter, better half, and to round out a portrait of the whole person.

Maslow offers a theory of human motivation that assumes people to have a hierarchy of needs. He proposes that each person has five *basic needs*, which are arranged in hierarchical order. Maslow describes basic needs as physiological (food, drink) and psychological (security, love, esteem), and *metaneeds* as higher-level needs (desire to know, the appreciation of truth and beauty, and the tendency toward growth and fulfillment—qualities that define *self-actualization*).

The basic needs are labeled *deficiency needs* because, when they are not satisfied, we try to remedy what we lack. For example, hunger represents a deficiency that can be satisfied by eating. Similarly, the metaneeds are termed *growth needs* because activities that relate to them do not fulfill a lack but instead lead to growth.

TABLE 2–8 PIAGET'S STAGES OF COGNITIVE DEVELOPMENT

PERIOD	CHARACTERISTIC OF THE PERIOD	MAJOR CHANGE OF THE PERIOD
Sensorimotor (0–2 yr)	—	
Stage 1 (0–1 mo)	Reflex activity only; no differentiation	Development proceeds from reflex activity to representation and sensorimotor solutions to problems
Stage 2 (1–4 mos)	Hand-mouth coordination; differentiation via sucking reflex	
Stage 3 (4–8 mos)	Hand-eye coordination; repeats unusual events	
Stage 4 (8–12 mo)	Coordination of two schemata; object performance attained	
Stage 5 (12–18 mo)	New means through experimentation—follows sequential displacements	
Stage 6 (18–24 mo)	Internal representation; new means through mental combinations	
Preoperational (2–7 yrs)	Problems solved through representation; language development (2–4 yr); thought and language both egocentric; cannot solve conservation problems	Development proceeds from sensorimotor representation to prelogical thought and solutions to problems
Concrete operational (7–11 yr)	Reversibility attained; can solve conservation problems—logical operations developed and applied to concrete problems; cannot solve complex verbal problems	Development proceeds from prelogical thought to logical solutions to concrete problems
Formal operational (11 yr to adulthood)	Logically solves all types of problems—thinks scientifically; solves complex verbal problems; cognitive structures mature	Development proceeds from logical solutions to concrete problems to logical solutions to all classes of problems

From *Piaget's theory of cognitive and affective development* by Barry J. Wadsworth. Copyright © 1989 by Longman Publishers. Reprinted with permission.

Our needs are hierarchically arranged, says Maslow, in the sense that the metaneeds will not be attended to unless the basic needs have been reasonably well satisfied; that is, we pay attention to beauty, truth, and the development of our potential when we are no longer hungry or feel unloved.

In order to study what makes healthy people healthy, or great people great, or extraordinary people extraordinary, Maslow has made intensive clinical investigations of people who are, or were, in the truest sense of the word, self-actualizing; that is, they move in the direction of achieving and reaching their highest potentials. People of this sort are rare, as Maslow discovered when he was selecting his group. Some were historical figures (Lincoln, Jefferson, Harriet Tubman, Walt Whitman, Beethoven, William James, F. D. Roosevelt), while others were living at the time they were studied (Einstein, Eleanor Roosevelt, Albert Schweitzer, along with some personal acquaintances of the investigator). Upon studying healthy, self-actualizing individuals, Maslow was able to sort out some basic personality characteristics that distinguished them from what might be called "ordinary" people. This is not to suggest that each person he studied reflected all of these characteristics, but each did exhibit a greater number of these characteristics and in more different ways than might be expected in a less "self-actualized" person. Maslow (1962, 1970) described the features as follows:

1. They are realistically oriented.
2. They accept themselves, other people, and the natural world for what they are.
3. They are spontaneous in thought, emotions, and behavior.
4. They are problem centered rather than self centered.
5. They are autonomous, independent, and able to remain true to themselves in the face of rejection or unpopularity.
6. They have a continual freshness of appreciation and the capacity to stand in awe again and again of the basic goods of life (a sunset, a flower, a baby, a melody, a person).
7. Their intimate relationships with a few specially loved people tend to be profound and deeply emotional rather than superficial.
8. They have unhostile senses of humor, which are expressed in their capacity to make common human foibles, pretensions, and foolishness the subject of laughter, rather than sadism, smut, or hatred of authority.
9. They have a great fund of creativeness.
10. They resist total conformity to culture.

Critics have attacked Maslow's description on the grounds that it is based on his own choice of subjects and that it reflects the characteristics he himself admired. In any case, Maslow set a precedent for other attempts to define a healthy personality as something more than personality without disorder.

Kohlberg

The provocative view of moral development in recent years was crafted by Lawrence Kohlberg (1958, 1976, 1986). Kohlberg's theory of moral development is deeply rooted in Piaget's work. His unique contribution was to apply to the study of moral development the concept of a progression of stages that Piaget worked out in relation to cognitive development (Table 2–9). Kohlberg arrived at his view after about 20 years of using a unique interview with children. In the interview, children are presented with a series of stories in which characters face moral dilemmas. The following is the most popular of the Kohlberg dilemmas:

> In Europe a woman was near death from a special kind of cancer. There was one drug that the doctors thought might save her. It was a form of radium that a druggist was charging ten times what the drug cost him to make. He paid $200 for the radium and charged $2000 for a small dose of the drug. The sick woman's husband, Heinz, went to everyone he knew to borrow the money, but he could only get together $1000, which is half of what it cost. He told the druggist that his wife was dying and asked him to sell it cheaper or let him pay later. But the druggist said, "No, I discovered the drug, and I am going to make money from it." So Heinz got desperate and broke into the man's store to steal the drug for his wife. (Kohlberg 1969, p. 379)

The story is one of 11 Kohlberg devised to investigate the nature of moral thought. After reading the story, interviewees answer a series of questions about the moral dilemma. Should Heinz have stolen the drug? Was stealing it right or wrong? Why? Is it a husband's duty to steal the drug for his wife if he can get it no other way? Would a good husband steal? Did the druggist have the right to charge that much when there was no law setting a limit on the price? Why?

On the basis of the answers interviewees gave for this and other moral dilemmas, Kohlberg concluded that three levels of moral development exist, each of which is characterized by two stages. A key concept in understanding moral development, especially for Kohlberg's theory, is *internalization*, the developmental change from behavior that is externally controlled to behavior that is controlled by internal, self-generated standards and principles. As children develop, their moral thoughts become more internalized.

Kohlberg believed that children's moral orientation unfolds as a consequence of their cognitive development. Children construct their moral thoughts as they pass from one stage to the next, rather than passively accepting a cultural norm of morality. He believed that peer interaction is a critical part of the social stimulation that challenges children to change their moral orientation. Whereas adults characteristically impose rules and regulations on children, the mutual give-and-take in peer interaction provides children with an opportunity to take the perspective of another person and to generate rules democratically.

Kohlberg stressed that perspective-taking opportunities can, in principle, be engendered by any peer group encounter. Although he believed that such perspective-taking opportunities are ideal for moral development, he also believed that certain types of parent-child experiences can induce the child to think at more advanced levels of moral thinking. In particular, parents who allow or encourage conversation about value-laden issues promote more advanced moral thought in their children; however, many parents do not systematically provide their children with such perspective-taking opportunities. Nonetheless, in one study, children's moral development was related to their parents' discussion style, which involved questioning and supportive interaction (Walker and Taylor 1991). There is an increasing emphasis on the role of parenting in moral development (Eisenberg and Murphy 1995).

Kohlberg's provocative theory of moral development has not gone unchallenged (Kurtines and Gewirtz 1991; Lapsley 1992; Puka 1991). The criticisms involve the link between moral thought and moral behavior, the quality of the research, inadequate consideration of culture's role in moral development, and underestimation of the care perspective.

Kohlberg's theory has been criticized for placing too much emphasis on moral thought and not enough on moral behavior. Moral reasons can sometimes be a shelter for immoral behavior. For example, bank embezzlers and presidents may endorse the loftiest of moral virtues when commenting about moral dilemmas, but their own behavior may be immoral. No one wants a nation of cheaters and thieves who can reason at the postconventional level. The cheaters and thieves may know what is right, yet still do what is wrong.

Some developmentalists fault the quality of Kohlberg's research and believe that more attention should be paid to the way moral development is assessed (Boyes et al. 1993). For example, James Rest (1976, 1983, 1986) argued that alternative methods should be used to collect information about moral thinking instead of relying on a single method that requires individuals to reason about hypothetical moral dilemmas. Researchers have also found that the hypothetical moral dilemmas posed in Kohlberg's stories do not match the moral dilemmas many children and adults face in their everyday lives (Walker et al. 1987; Yussen 1977). Most of Kohlberg's stories focus on the family and authority. However, when one researcher invited adolescents to write stories about their own moral dilemmas, they generated dilemmas that were broader in scope, focusing on friends, acquaintances, and other issues, as well as family and authority (Yussen 1977).

Yet another criticism of Kohlberg's view is that it is culturally biased (Banks 1993; Jensen 1995; Miller 1991).

TABLE 2–9 KOHLBERG'S SIX STAGES OF MORAL REASONING

LEVELS	STAGES OF REASONING	TYPICAL ANSWERS TO HEINZ'S DILEMMA
Level I: Preconventional (ages 4–10) Emphasis in this level is on external control. The standards are those of others, and they are observed either to avoid punishment or to reap rewards.	*Stage 1: Orientation toward punishment and obedience.* "What will happen to me?" Children obey the rules of others to avoid punishment. They ignore the motives of an act and focus on its physical form (such as the size of a lie) or its consequences (e.g., the amount of physical damage).	*Pro:* "He should steal the drug. It isn't really bad to take it. It isn't as if he hadn't asked to pay for it first. The drug he'd take is worth only $200; he's not really taking a $2000 drug." *Con:* "He shouldn't steal the drug. It's a big crime. He didn't get permission; he used force and broke and entered. He did a lot of damage, stealing a very expensive drug and breaking into the store, too."
	Stage 2: Instrumental purpose and exchange. "You scratch my back, I'll scratch yours." Children conform to rules out of self-interest and consideration for what others can do for them in return. They look at an act in terms of the human needs it meets, and differentiate this value from the act's physical form and consequences.	*Pro:* "It's all right to steal the drug because his wife needs it and he wants her to live. It isn't that we want to steal, but that's what he has to do to get the drug to save her." *Con:* "He shouldn't steal it. The druggist isn't wrong or bad; he just wants to make a profit. That's what you're in business for—to make money."
Level II: Morality of conventional role conformity (ages 10–13) Children now want to please other people. They still observe the standards of others, but they have internalized these standards to some extent. Now they want to be considered "good" by those persons whose opinions are important to them. They are now able to take the roles of authority figures well enough to decide whether an action is good by their standards.	*Stage 3: Maintaining mutual relations, approval of others, the golden rule.* "Am I a good boy or girl?" Children want to please and help others, can judge the intentions of others, and develop their own ideas of what a good person is. They evaluate an act according to the motive behind it or the person performing it, and they can take circumstances into account.	*Pro:* "He should steal the drug. He is only doing something that is natural for a good husband to do. You can't blame him for doing something out of love for his wife. You'd blame him if he didn't love his wife enough to save her." *Con:* "He shouldn't steal. If his wife dies, he can't be blamed. It isn't because he's heartless or that he doesn't love her enough to do everything that he legally can. The druggist is the selfish or heartless one."
	Stage 4: Social concern and conscience. "What if everybody did it?" People are concerned with doing their duty, showing respect for high authority, and maintaining the social order. They consider an act always wrong, regardless of motive or circumstances, if it violates a rule and harms others.	*Pro:* "You should steal the drug. If you did nothing, you'd be letting your wife die. It's your responsibility if she dies. You have to take it with the idea of paying the druggist." *Con:* "It's a natural thing for Heinz to want to save his wife, but it's still always wrong to steal. He knows that he is stealing and taking a valuable drug from the man who made it."
Level III: Morality of autonomous moral principles (age 13, or not until young adulthood, or never) This level marks the attainment of true morality. For the first time, the person acknowledges the possibility of conflict between two socially accepted standards and tries to decide between them. The control of conduct is now internal, both in the standards observed and in the reasoning about right and wrong. Stages 5 and 6 may be alternative methods of the highest level of moral reasoning.	*Stage 5: Morality of contract, of individual rights, and of democratically accepted law.* People think in rational terms, valuing the will of the majority and the welfare of society. They generally see these values best supported by adherence to the law. While they recognize that there are times when human need and the law conflict, they believe that it is better for society in the long run if they obey the law.	*Pro:* "The law wasn't set up for these circumstances. Taking the drug in this situation isn't really a right, but it's justified." *Con:* "You can't completely blame someone for stealing, but extreme circumstances don't really justify taking the law into your own hands. You can't have people stealing whenever they are desperate. The end may be good, but the ends don't justify the means."

TABLE 2–9 KOHLBERG'S SIX STAGES OF MORAL REASONING *(Continued)*

LEVELS	STAGES OF REASONING	TYPICAL ANSWERS TO HEINZ'S DILEMMA
	Stage 6: Morality of universal ethical principles. People do what they as individuals think is right, regardless of legal restrictions or the opinions of others. They act in accordance with internalized standards, knowing that they would condemn themselves if they did not.	*Pro:* "This is a situation that forces him to choose between stealing and letting his wife die. In a situation where the choice must be made, it is morally right to steal. He has to act in terms of the principle of preserving and respecting life." *Con:* "Heinz is faced with a decision of whether to consider the other people who need the drug just as badly as his wife. Heinz ought to act not according to his particular feelings toward his wife, but considering the value of all the lives involved."

Adapted from Kohlberg, 1969, 1976.

A review of research on moral development in 27 countries concluded that moral reasoning is more culture specific than Kohlberg envisioned, and that Kohlberg's scoring system does not recognize higher-level moral reasoning in certain cultural groups (Snarey 1987). Examples of higher-level moral reasoning that would not be scored as such by Kohlberg's system are values related to communal equity and collective happiness in Israel, the unity and sacredness of all life forms in India, and the relation of the individual to the community in New Guinea. These examples of moral reasoning would not be scored at the highest level in Kohlberg's system because they do not emphasize the individual's rights or abstract principles of justice.

Another critique of Kohlberg's theory of development comes from Gilligan (1982, 1990, 1991, 1992), who believes that this theory does not adequately reflect relationships and concern for others. The justice perspective is a moral perspective that focuses on the rights of the individual; individuals stand alone and independently make moral decisions. Kohlberg's theory is a *justice perspective.* By contrast, the *care perspective* is a moral perspective that views people in terms of their connectedness with others and emphasizes interpersonal communication, relationships with others, and concern for others. Gilligan's theory is a care perspective. According to Gilligan, Kohlberg greatly underplayed the care perspective in moral development. She believes that this may have happened because he was a male, because most of his research was with males rather than females, and because he used male responses as a model for his theory.

In extensive interviews with girls 6 to 18 years of age, Gilligan and her colleagues found that girls consistently interpret moral dilemmas in terms of human relationships and base these interpretations on listening and watching other people (Gilligan 1990, 1992). According to Gilligan, girls have the ability to sensitively pick up different rhythms in relationships and can often follow the pathways of feelings. She believes that girls reach a critical juncture in their development when they reach adolescence. Usually around 11 to 12 years of age, girls become aware that their intense interest in intimacy is not prized by the male-dominated culture, even though society values women as caring and altruistic. The dilemma is that girls are presented with a choice that makes them look either selfish or selfless. Gilligan believes that, as adolescent girls experience this dilemma, they increasingly silence their "distinctive voice."

SOME CURRENT THERAPEUTIC APPROACHES

Classical Psychoanalysis

Classical psychoanalysis is perhaps the least prevalent approach to therapy today, for many reasons. It is extremely expensive, it takes years and years, and Freud's original premise that all mental illness is caused by early intrapsychic conflict is no longer thought to be valid by most clinicians.

The term **psychoanalysis** describes the school and the system of therapy based on Freud's theory of personality and developed from Freud's treatment methods with neurotic clients in Vienna at the beginning of the twentieth century. In psychoanalytic treatment a number of techniques are employed by the analyst to uncover unconscious feelings and thoughts that interfere with the client's living a fuller life. One such technique is called *free association.* This refers to a technique in which the client is permitted to verbalize whatever comes to mind, no matter how insignificant, trivial, or even unpleasant the idea, thought, or picture might seem. Free association is based on the premise that no idea that occurs to the client is arbitrary and insignificant.

Another method of uncovering unconscious material is through **dream analysis.** For Freud, the dream is the royal road to the unconscious. Dreams provide a particular wealth of information because in dreams a person is more relaxed than during the waking state, and may be caught off guard (without resistance). Dreams express unsatisfied wishes, but because many of these wishes have become unacceptable to the self-concept, the dream undergoes a disguise.

In classical analysis the client lies on a couch while the analyst sits behind the client and out of view. The client is instructed to verbalize whatever comes to mind, that is, to free associate. The client obtains relief just by being able to unburden the self to a sympathetic listener. A positive **transference** is developed, even though the work of analysis has barely begun; there are undisclosed feelings that the client has not yet explored. The analyst gently assists the client in exploring these emotion-loaded areas by pointing out and interpreting the resistance in an effort to weaken the client's defenses and bring repressed conflicts into the open. Through the development of the transference, the client experiences the analyst as if the latter were a significant person in his or her life and *transfers* feelings for other persons onto the analyst. The client re-experiences crucial episodes from childhood, including both insufficiently resolved traumatic events and (more important) inadequately resolved interpersonal relationships. The analyst's stance enables the client to "work through" these situations to a more satisfactory conclusion. Finally, the analyst assists the client in converting newly won insights into everyday existence and behavior. This emotional re-education enables the new insights to become a permanent part of the client's personality.

In its traditional form, analysis is a very protracted and expensive procedure. The client meets with the analyst an average of four or five times a week for 45- or 50-minute sessions over a period of several years. The procedure requires a considerable commitment in terms of time, emotional effort, and money (Box 2–2).

Psychoanalytic Psychotherapy

The **psychoanalytic model of psychotherapy** uses many of the tools of psychoanalysis, such as free association, dream analysis, and transference, but the therapist is much more involved and interacts with the client more freely. Clinical nurse specialists, psychiatric social workers, and psychologists with special training at the master's level or above may undertake psychotherapy with clients in private practice. The therapist works with the client to uncover unconscious material that appears in the form of symptoms or unsatisfactory life patterns. This is done through an intimate professional relationship between the therapist and the client over a period of months to years. The process proceeds through stages—introductory, working, termination—that are described with examples in Chapter 6.

Short-Term Dynamic Psychotherapy

Although many people assume that clients usually spend many months, even years, in psychotherapy, most dynamic therapies last fewer than ten sessions (Garfield 1978). One of many reasons for the short duration of therapy is that relatively few people are interested in the personality overhaul that was the goal of classical analytic treatment. Another factor, both in shortening treatment and in encouraging therapists to adapt analytic ideas to time-limited psychotherapy *(brief therapy)*, is the growing reluctance of insurance companies to cover more than perhaps 25 psychotherapy sessions in a given calendar year, along with their limits on the amount of reimbursement provided. The emergence of cognitive and behavioral therapies over the past 20 to 30 years has also played a role; these approaches focus on discrete problems and avoid long-term therapy.

Another strand in the history of **short-term psychodynamic therapy** grew out of the need to provide short-term treatment for the posttraumatic stress disorder of returning veterans from World War II and Vietnam.

The best candidate for brief psychotherapy is the relatively healthy and well-functioning individual, with a clearly circumscribed area of difficulty, who is intelligent, psychologically minded, and well motivated for change. Psychotic, severely depressed, and borderline clients, as well as individuals with severe character disorders, are excluded from this type of treatment. Supportive therapies are useful for these clients, however, and you will be introduced to a variety of supportive therapies in chapters about specific disorders (Chapters 18, 19, 20, 21, and 22).

Although many of the tools employed in traditional psychotherapy are used in brief therapy (e.g., uncovering unconscious processes through transference and dream interpretation), other methods, such as free association, are discouraged. At the start of treatment, client and therapist agree both on what the focus will be and to concentrate their work on the area of focus. Sessions are held weekly, and the total number of sessions to be held (anywhere from 12 to 40) is determined at the outset of therapy. There is a rapid, back-and-forth pattern between client and therapist, both participating actively. The therapist intervenes constantly to keep the therapy on track, either by redirecting the client's attention or by interpreting deviations from the focus to the client.

BOX 2–2 EXAMPLE OF PSYCHOANALYSIS

In psychoanalysis, through the development of the transference, the client transfers feelings toward significant figures from the past toward the analyst. Inadequately resolved interpersonal relationships are reexperienced in the relationship with the analyst. The analyst helps the client deal with these feelings and conflicts in a more satisfactory way. The following is the case of a 28-year-old woman suffering from severe depression. She had a history of sexual molestation and she reported a series of stormy, painful adult relationships. After 1 year of analysis she entered a relationship with a man (Bob) who was gentle, warm, and loving.

The client begins the session by glaring at the therapist.

CLIENT: I'm in a dangerous mood.
THERAPIST: (Waits for her to continue, but she just sits silently.)
CLIENT: I'm tired of always regretting everything I do. I can't control my outbursts of temper at Bob, then I feel ashamed.
THERAPIST: (Remains silent, but feels that the client is having a temper outburst at him.)
CLIENT: I'm a failure. Nothing goes right.
THERAPIST: Are you angry with me?
CLIENT: No I'm not angry at you—it's myself I hate. I can't continue going through life like this. I have to get a handle on myself.
THERAPIST: (Waits.)
CLIENT: (Yelling) I'm really pissed at you. Why am I still so fat! Why am I still blowing up! You know what's wrong with me! You just won't tell me! I have to do everything for myself! You just sit there and don't do anything!

The therapist's withdrawal scared the client, and she became anxious and ashamed and began putting herself down.

CLIENT: I shouldn't get so upset. I shouldn't complain. I should be nice. I should be appreciative.
THERAPIST: By putting yourself down first, you protect yourself from the criticism that you expect from me.
CLIENT: You don't care! It doesn't make any difference to you.
THERAPIST: You feel that I'm indifferent.
CLIENT: Yes, I'm so ugly and you don't even care.
THERAPIST: Have I indicated in any way that I saw you as ugly?
CLIENT: No, but you wouldn't tell me if you did.
THERAPIST: But you expect that I'm put off by you, that I'm not pleased that you're able to be more assertive with me and speak up for yourself. It's a struggle for you to talk about your feelings of anger and disappointment, your fear of hurting people and driving them away. But you seem to be learning to express angry feelings in here with me.
CLIENT: I would rather be angry with you than with Bob.
THERAPIST: It's hard when you anticipate that the other person will be put off or hurt.

This session illustrates how the client uses the analyst in her effort to recover from the effects of early abuse. Through the transference the client expresses her hurt, fear of abandonment, and rage.

From Shapiro, S. (1995). *Talking with patients: A self psychological view of creative intuition and analytic discipline* (pp. 139–142). Northvale, NJ: Jason Aronson.

Brief therapies share the following common elements (Flegenheimer 1982):

1. Assessment tends to be rapid and early.
2. It is made clear right away to the client that therapy will be limited and that improvement is expected within a small number of sessions.
3. Goals are concrete and focused on the amelioration of the client's worst symptoms, on helping the client understand what is going on in his or her life, and on enabling the client to cope better in the future.
4. Interpretations are directed toward present life circumstances and client behavior rather than on the historical significance of feelings.
5. Some positive transference to the therapist is fostered in an effort to encourage the client to follow the therapist's suggestions and advice.
6. There is a general understanding that psychotherapy does not cure, but that it can help troubled individuals learn to deal better with life's inevitable stressors.

Refer to Box 2–3 for an example of short-term dynamic psychotherapy.

Rational Emotive Behavioral Therapy

Albert Ellis (b. 1913), founder of **rational emotive behavioral therapy (REBT),** was trained in the classical psychoanalytic model, but found that over time it was disappointingly ineffective "even though my clients liked it and thought they had significantly improved" (Bernard 1991). He did notice that his clients improved when he

BOX 2–3 EXAMPLE OF SHORT-TERM DYNAMIC PSYCHOTHERAPY

One of the chief techniques that is most distinctive of short-term psychotherapy is the use of anxiety-provoking confrontation. The most common example is the direct attack on the client's defenses rather than attempts at interpreting the meaning or function of the defenses. Other aspects of the client's productions or behavior may be challenged directly, sometimes in what seems to be a mocking or sarcastic manner. Behavioral manifestations of resistance such as lateness or missed appointments may be dealt with in a similar fashion.

The following is an example of the use of anxiety-provoking techniques with a 40-year-old man. Note how the therapist circumvents the client's defense of sadness and goes directly to the client's wish to be given something. Note also that at the end of this exchange the therapist helps to raise the client's self-esteem by pointing out the client's strengths.

CLIENT: I am not feeling very well today, as I have told you already. I feel sick. I want you to do the talking for a while. I want something soothing today. After all, it's partly your fault that I'm feeling the way I do today. I'm achy, I have . . .

THERAPIST: (interrupting) And why is it my fault?

CLIENT: Because you did not make an offer to give me another appointment after you canceled the one last week.

THERAPIST: We discussed all this before.

CLIENT: Yes, I know, but you never offered to make up the time.

THERAPIST: If you wanted another appointment, why didn't you ask for one?

CLIENT: You canceled it, so it was up to you to give me another one.

THERAPIST: What's going on today?

CLIENT: I told you I wanted to be soothed.

THERAPIST: I'm not going to soothe you, and you know better than that. Now stop feeling sorry for yourself and let's get back to work.

CLIENT: (sarcastic) I don't feel like being self-inquisitive today.

THERAPIST: So, you are self-destructive today. Having had no hour last week, which you blame on me, now you are determined to waste this hour so as to be even with me. Now, what about all this appointment controversy?

CLIENT: I told you that I wanted you to offer me another appointment.

THERAPIST: I know that. I also said that you could have asked for one if you wanted to. You are entitled to ask for what you want, in a mature way, but you are not entitled to act like a spoiled child in here, because this is what we are trying to help you understand and overcome. Now let me clarify something that I am sure you know only too well. I deal with you as a grown-up person, not as a child, and furthermore I am not here to play soothing games. Now, are you going to settle down and get to work, which you are perfectly capable of performing, as you have already demonstrated, or not?

From Sifneos, P. (1979). *Short-term dynamic psychotherapy* (pp. 120–121). New York: Plenum.

used a more active role, offering advice and giving direct interpretations. Ellis realized, after a number of years of careful observations, that much of people's dysfunctional behavior and emotional responses was a direct result of their irrational thinking. He found that if people could accept with conviction a more rational approach to another person or situation, it would greatly influence how they felt and how they behaved in a more positive and functional manner. He was greatly influenced throughout his life by the philosophies of Epictetus, Marcus Aurelius, Spinoza, and Bertrand Russell. In 1955, Ellis combined philosophical and rational thinking with behavioral therapy and started rational emotive therapy (RET), later called rational emotive behavioral therapy (REBT); thus, he became the forefather of the cognitive-behavioral therapy (CBT) movement.

THE ABC MODEL. Ellis uses a simple ABC model to illustrate the role that the thinking process plays in emotional disturbance. **A** stands for the *activating event* (person, circumstance) surrounding a client's distress (e.g., "He doesn't love me anymore"). **B** stands for the *belief system* regarding the **A** event. The **B** can be either a rational or an irrational belief. A *rational belief* **(rB)** to "He doesn't love me anymore" might be "I feel so disappointed because I really loved him and I was hoping this would work out. I will be sad and lonely for a while, but I will live through it and there will be others, even though it's hard to think about that now."

However, it is usually the *irrational beliefs* **(iBs)** which lead to emotional turmoil and self-defeating behaviors. An **iB** regarding "He doesn't love me anymore" might take the form of "I'm unlovable, no one will ever love me, and I'll be alone all my life. I need to be loved and I couldn't stand living alone all my life."

C stands for the emotional and behavioral *consequence* that people experience as a result of their belief. Ellis believes that it is not the **A** that causes our unhappiness and self-defeating behaviors, but rather the beliefs we hold about the activating event. For example, for the same **A,** "He doesn't love me anymore," the following demonstrates the belief system and possible resultant emotional reactions.

Belief	**Consequences**
Irrational Belief (iB) I'm unlovable, no one will ever love me, and I'll be alone all my life. I need to be loved and and I couldn't stand living alone all my life.	Depressed and hopeless
Rational Belief (rB) I feel so disappointed for I was hoping this would work out. I will be sad and lonely for a while, and this will be a hard time, but I will live through it and there will be others, even though it's hard to think about that now.	Sad and disappointed

Table 2–10 identifies common **iBs,** or thoughts that can lead to emotional distress, and gives the corresponding **rBs** that can foster emotional self-control.

The crux of REBT is *disputing* **(D)** clients' irrational beliefs, while supporting the rational beliefs. The therapist identifies the activating event **(A)** and the emotional and behavioral consequence, **C,** then elicits the irrational beliefs **(iBs)** clients have that they are using to make themselves miserable. In the example above, one person who had a more rational belief **(rB)** might look upon the loss of a love affair as sad and unfortunate, and an experience that will take time getting over. Another person who holds more irrational beliefs **(iBs)** might see the end of a love affair as proof that no one would ever love them and that they would end up alone all their life, and that they wouldn't be able to stand that. Since the definition of *irrational* is that there are no bases in fact for such beliefs, the therapist actively disputes with clients their irrational beliefs. The aim is not to have the client feel "good" about the event, but rather to respond appropriately to the activating event **(A)** and not remain self-defeating or irrationally angry, depressed, or anxious. Using the example above, you might rarely feel "good" about the end of a love affair that held promise for you, but it **is** self-defeating and self-downing to feel worthless, hopeless, and depressed when more rationally you could feel sad, temporarily lonely, and regretful and then get on with your life.

Although the **ABCDs** of REBT looks simple, it isn't necessarily an easy task to change years of an ingrained self-defeating belief system. Often the irrational beliefs are peppered with either overt or implied shoulds or musts: "I should be happy," "I should love my job," "I must be loved," "I must do well." When these should and musts aren't working, people become anxious, depressed, and angry. Therefore, therapists who use the REBT model give both cognitive and behavioral homework that clients can work on between sessions to strengthen their ability to replace their irrational beliefs with more rational beliefs. Homework might take the form of articles, tapes, writing a log, disputing throughout the week specific irrational beliefs identified in the most recent session, attending a lecture or a group, relaxation training, or some other activity. Refer to Box 2–4 for an example of rational emotive behavioral therapy.

TABLE 2–10 RATIONAL VS. IRRATIONAL THOUGHTS

Irrational Thoughts That Cause Disturbance	**Rational Thoughts That Promote Emotional Self-Control**
1. How *awful.*	This is disappointing.
2. I can't stand it.	I can put up with what I don't like.
3. I'm stupid.	What I *did* was stupid.
4. He stinks!	He's not perfect, either.
5. This *shouldn't* have happened.	This should have happened because it did!
6. I am to be blamed.	I am at fault but am not to be blamed.
7. He has no right.	He has every right to follow his own mind though I wish he hadn't exercised that right!
8. I *need* him to do that.	I want/desire/prefer him to do that, but I don't have to have what I want.
9. Things *always* go wrong.	Sometimes—if not frequently—things will go wrong.
10. *Every time* I try I fail.	Sometimes—even often—I may fail.
11. Things *never* work out.	More often than I would like, things don't work out.
12. This is bigger than life.	This is an important part of my life.
13. This *should* be easier.	I wish this was easier, but often things that are good for me aren't—no gain without pain. Tough, too bad!
14. I *should* have done better.	I would have *preferred* to do better, but I did what I could at the time.
15. I am a failure.	I'm a person who sometimes fails.

From Bernard, M. E., and Wolfe, J. L. (Eds.). (1993). *The RET resource book for practitioners.* New York: Institute for Rational-Emotive Therapy.

BOX 2–4 EXAMPLE OF RATIONAL EMOTIVE BEHAVIOR THERAPY

Rational emotive behavior therapy (REBT) seeks to identify assumptions and modify consequent self-defeating behaviors. In this case, the therapist actively questions the client to uncover the individual's basic stance toward self and the belief system that supports it. The REBT therapist is direct, challenging, and often contronting. The following is the case of a 25-year-old single woman who complains of being depressed all the time. The therapist begins by reading from the biographical information that the clients at the Albert Ellis Institute for Rational Emotive Behavior in New York City fill out before their first session: "Inability to control emotions: tremendous feelings of guilt, unworthiness, insecurity; constant depression; conflict between inner and outer self; overeating; drinking; diet pills."

THERAPIST: All right, what would you like to start on first?

CLIENT: I don't know. I'm petrified at the moment.

THERAPIST: You're petrified—of what?

CLIENT: Of you!

THERAPIST: No, surely not of me—perhaps of yourself!

CLIENT: (laughs nervously)

THERAPIST: Because of what I am going to do to you?

CLIENT: Right! Because you are threatening me, I guess.

THERAPIST: But how? What am I doing? Obviously, I'm not going to take a knife and stab you. Now in what way am I threatening you?

CLIENT: I guess I'm afraid, perhaps, of what I'm going to find out about me.

THERAPIST: Well, let's suppose you find out something dreadful about you—that you're thinking foolishly, or something. Now why would that be so awful?

CLIENT: Because I guess I'm the most important thing to me at the moment.

THERAPIST: No, I don't think that's the answer. I believe it's the opposite! You're really the least important thing to you. You are prepared to beat yourself over the head if I tell you that you're acting foolishly. If you were not a self-blamer, then you wouldn't care what I said. It would be unimportant to you—but you'd just go around correcting it. But if I tell you something really negative about you, you're going to beat yourself mercilessly. Aren't you?

CLIENT: Yes, I generally do.

THERAPIST: All right. So perhaps that's what you're really afraid of. You're not afraid of me. You're afraid of your own self-criticism.

CLIENT: (sighs) All right.

THERAPIST: So why do you have to criticize yourself? Suppose I find you're the worst person I ever met? Let's just suppose that. All right, now why would you have to criticize yourself?

CLIENT: I'd have to. I don't know any other behavior pattern. I guess in this point of time, I always do. I guess I just think I'm a shit.

THERAPIST: Yeah. But that, that isn't so. If you don't know how to ski or swim, you could learn. You could also learn not to condemn yourself, no matter what you do.

CLIENT: I don't know.

THERAPIST: Well, the answer is: you don't know how.

CLIENT: Perhaps.

THERAPIST: I get the impression you're saying, "I have to berate myself if I do something wrong." Because isn't that where your depression comes from?

CLIENT: Yes, I guess so. (Silence for a while.)

THERAPIST: Now what are you mainly putting yourself down for right now?

CLIENT: I don't seem quite able, in this point in time, to break it down very neatly. This form gave me a great deal of trouble. Because my tendency is to say everything. I want to change everything; I'm depressed about everything.

THERAPIST: Give me a couple of things, for example.

CLIENT: What am I depressed about. I, uh, don't know that I have any purpose in life. I don't know what I—what I am. And I don't know in what direction I am going.

THERAPIST: Yeah. But that's—so you're saying "I'm ignorant!" (Client nods.) Well, what's so awful about being ignorant? It's too bad you're ignorant. It would be nicer if you weren't—if you had a purpose and knew where you were going. But let's just suppose the worst: for the rest of your life you didn't have a purpose, and you stayed this way. Let's suppose that. Now why would you be so bad?

CLIENT: Because everyone should have a purpose?

THERAPIST: Where did you get this "should"?

CLIENT: 'Cause it's what I believe in. (Silence for a while.)

THERAPIST: I know. But think about it for a minute. You're obviously a bright woman; now where did that "should" come from?

From Ellis, A. (1978). Rational emotive therapy. In R. Corsini (Ed.), *Current psychotherapies* (2nd ed.). Itasca, IL: F. E. Peacock. Reproduced by permission of the publisher, F. E. Peacock Publishers Inc.

Cognitive Therapy

Aaron Beck's (Beck et al. 1979) approach to therapy for people suffering from depression illustrates the major components of **cognitive therapy.** This is an active, directive, time-limited, structured approach used to treat a variety of psychiatric disorders (e.g., depression, anxiety, phobias, pain problems). It is based on an underlying theoretical rationale that individuals' affect and behavior are largely determined by the way in which they structure the world (Beck 1967, 1976). Their cognitions (verbal or pictorial "events" in their stream of consciousness) are based on attitudes or assumptions (schemata) developed from previous experiences. For example, if a person interprets all experiences in terms of whether he or she is competent and adequate, thinking may be dominated by the schema "Unless I do everything perfectly, I'm a failure." Consequently, the person reacts to situations in terms of adequacy even when they are unrelated to whether he or she is personally competent.

The therapeutic techniques of the cognitive therapist are designed to identify, reality-test, and correct distorted conceptualizations and the dysfunctional beliefs (schemata) underlying these cognitions. Clients learn to master problems and situations they previously considered insuperable by reevaluating and correcting their thinking. The cognitive therapist helps clients to think and act more realistically and adaptively about their psychological problems, and thus to reduce symptoms.

A variety of cognitive and behavioral strategies are utilized in cognitive therapy. Cognitive therapies are aimed at delineating and testing clients' specific misconceptions and maladaptive assumptions. This approach consists of highly specific learning experiences designed to teach clients the following operations:

1. To monitor their negative, automatic thoughts (cognitions)
2. To recognize the connections between cognition, affect, and behavior
3. To examine the evidence for and against their distorted automatic thoughts
4. To substitute more reality-oriented interpretations for these biased cognitions
5. To learn to identify and alter the dysfunctional beliefs that predispose them to distort their experiences

For example, the depressed people's tendency to feel responsible for negative outcomes while consistently failing to take credit for their own success is identified and discussed. The therapy focuses on specific "target symptoms" (e.g., suicidal impulses). The cognitions supporting these symptoms are identified ("My life is worthless and I can't change it") and then subjected to logical and empirical investigation.

In cognitive therapy the client begins to incorporate many of the therapeutic techniques of the therapist. For example, clients frequently find themselves spontaneously assuming the role of the therapist in questioning some of their conclusions or predictions. Some examples of self-questioning are: What is the evidence for my conclusion? Are there other explanations? How serious is the loss? How much does it actually subtract from my life? What is the degree of harm to me if a stranger thinks badly of me? What will I lose if I try to be more assertive? Such self-questioning plays a major role in the generalization of cognitive techniques from the interview to external situations. Without such questioning, the depressed individual is pretty much bound by stereotyped automatic patterns, a phenomenon labeled "thoughtless thinking."

In contrast to those employing more traditional psychotherapies such as psychoanalytic therapy, the therapist applying cognitive therapy is continuously active and deliberately interacting with clients, exploring their psychological experiences, setting up schedules of activities, and making homework assignments. Unlike psychoanalytic therapy, the content of cognitive therapy is focused on "here and now" problems. Little attention is paid to childhood recollections except to clarify present observations. The major thrust is toward investigating clients' thinking and feeling during the therapy session and between the sessions. Interpretations of unconscious factors are not made.

Cognitive therapy contrasts with behavioral therapy in its greater emphasis on clients' internal (mental) experiences such as thoughts, feelings, wishes, daydreams, and attitudes. The overall strategy of cognitive therapy may be differentiated from the other schools of therapy by its emphasis on the empirical investigation of clients' automatic thoughts, inferences, conclusions, and assumptions. Clients' dysfunctional ideas and beliefs about themselves, their experience, and their future are formulated into hypotheses, and an attempt is made to test the validity of these hypotheses in a systematic way. Thus, almost every experience may provoke an opportunity for an experiment relevant to clients' negative views or beliefs. If clients believe, for example, that everybody they meet turns away from them in disgust, they are helped to set up a system for judging other people's reactions, and are motivated to make objective assignments of the facial expression and bodily movements of other people. Alternatively, for example, if clients believe that they are incapable of carrying out simple hygienic procedures, the therapist may jointly with the client devise a checklist or graph that clients can use to record the degree of success in carrying out these activities.

Cognitive therapists may use the following behavioral techniques:

1. *Pleasant events schedule* (MacPhillamy and Lewinsohn 1971). The therapist may assign the client the task of undertaking a particular pleasurable activity for a specified number of minutes each day and request that

the client note changes in mood or reduction of depressive ruminations associated with the activity on a **pleasant events schedule.**

2. *Cognitive rehearsal.* Effective with depressed clients who have problems in carrying out well-learned tasks, **cognitive rehearsal** refers to the technique of asking the client to imagine each successive step in the sequence leading to the completion of a task, and helps to identify potential "road blocks" (cognitive, behavioral, or environmental) that might impede the achievement of the assignment. The central plan of the therapist is to identify and develop solutions for such problems before they produce an unwanted failure experience.
3. *Assertiveness and role playing.* **Role playing** involves the adoption of a role by the client, therapist, or both, and the subsequent social interaction based on the assumed role. As with other techniques that have a behavioral focus, the therapist attempts to clarify self-defeating or interfering cognitions. Role playing may also be employed to demonstrate an alternative viewpoint to the client or to further elucidate the factors that interfere with appropriate emotional expression.
4. *Recording dysfunctional thoughts.* **Recording dysfunctional thoughts,** with cognitions and responses in parallel columns, is a way to begin examining, evaluating, and modifying the cognitions. The written assignment may include columns for describing the client's affect and behavior and the specific description of the situation or event preceding a cognition.

The therapist's major task is to help the client think of reasonable responses to negative cognitions. The therapist's goal is to increase the client's objectivity about cognitions, unpleasant affect, and unproductive behavior and (most important) to differentiate between a realistic accounting of events and an accounting distorted by idiosyncratic meanings. The following is an example of this behavioral technique.

A 24-year-old nurse recently discharged from the hospital for severe depression presented this record (Beck et al. 1979):

EVENT	FEELING	COGNITIONS	OTHER POSSIBLE INTERPRETATIONS
While at a party, Jim asked me "How are you feeling?" shortly after I was discharged from the hospital.	Anxious	Jim thinks I am a basket case. I must really look bad for him to be concerned.	He really cares about me. He noticed that I look better than before I went into the hospital and wants to know if I feel better too.

Refer to Box 2–5 for an example of cognitive therapy.

Behavioral Therapy and Behavior Modification

Behavioral therapists work on the assumption that changes in maladapted behavior can occur without insight into the underlying cause. Behavioral therapy is based on learning theory. This theory works best when it is directed at specific problems and the goals are well defined. Behavioral therapy is effective in people with agoraphobia (graded exposure and flooding) and other phobias (desensitization), alcoholism (aversion therapy), schizophrenia (token economy), and many other conditions. Refer to Chapter 17 for an explanation of these and other behaviorist treatments of anxiety disorders.

The many types of **behavioral therapy** can be grouped into five categories: (1) modeling, (2) operant conditioning, (3) self-control therapy, (4) systematic desensitization, and (5) aversion therapy.

MODELING. In **modeling** the therapist provides a role model for specific identified behaviors, and the client learns through imitation. The therapist may do the modeling, provide another person to model the behaviors, or present a video for the purpose. Bandura and colleagues (1969) were able to help people reduce their phobias about nonpoisonous snakes by having them view both live and filmed close and successful confrontations between people and snakes. In an analogous fashion, some behavior therapists use role playing in the consulting room. They demonstrate to clients patterns of behaving that might prove more effective than those the clients usually engage in, and then have the clients practice them. Lazarus (1971), in his *behavior rehearsal* procedures, demonstrates exemplary ways of handling a situation and then encourages clients to imitate them during the therapy session. For example, a student who does not know how to ask a professor for an extension on a term paper would watch the therapist portray a potentially effective way of making the request. The clinician would then help the student practice the new skill in a similar role-playing situation. Modeling is frequently used in conjunction with other behavioral therapy, as well as with other therapeutic approaches.

OPERANT CONDITIONING. Operant conditioning entails rewarding a person for desired behaviors and is the basis for *behavior modification.* In behavior modification, someone sets a specific behavior goal and then systematically reinforces the subject's successive approximations to it. Called *positive reinforcement,* it is thought to be one of the best ways to increase desired behaviors. For example, when desired goals are achieved or behaviors are performed, clients are rewarded with "tokens." These tokens can be exchanged for food, small luxuries, or privileges. This reward system is known as "token economy."

BOX 2-5 EXAMPLE OF COGNITIVE THERAPY

The client was an attractive woman in her early twenties. Her depression of 18 months' duration was precipitated by her boyfriend's leaving her. She had numerous automatic thoughts that she was ugly and undesirable. These automatic thoughts were handled in the following manner.

THERAPIST: Other than your subjective opinion, what evidence do you have that you are ugly?

CLIENT: Well, my sister always said I was ugly.

THERAPIST: Was she always right in these matters?

CLIENT: No. Actually, she had her own reasons for telling me this. But the real reason I know I'm ugly is that men don't ask me out. If I weren't ugly, I'd be dating now.

THERAPIST: That is a possible reason why you're not dating. But there's an alternative explanation. You told me that you work in an office by yourself all day and spend your nights alone at home. It doesn't seem like you're giving yourself opportunities to meet men.

CLIENT: I can see what you're saying, but still, if I weren't ugly, men would ask me out.

THERAPIST: I suggest we run an experiment: that is, for you to become more socially active, stop turning down invitations to parties and social events, and see what happens.

After the client became more active and had more opportunities to meet men, she started to date. At this point, she no longer believed she was ugly.

Therapy then focused on her basic assumption that one's worth is determined by one's appearance. She readily agreed this didn't make sense. She also saw the falseness of the assumption that one must be beautiful in order to attract men or be loved. This discussion led to her basic assumption that she could not be happy without love (or attention from men). The latter part of treatment focused on helping her to change this belief.

THERAPIST: On what do you base this belief that you can't be happy without a man?

CLIENT: I was really depressed for a year and a half when I didn't have a man.

THERAPIST: Is there another reason why you were depressed?

CLIENT: As we discussed, I was looking at everything in a distorted way. But I still don't know if I could be happy if no one was interested in me.

THERAPIST: I don't know either. Is there a way we could find out?

CLIENT: Well, as an experiment I could not go out on dates for a while and see how I feel.

THERAPIST: I think that's a good idea. Although it has its flaws, the experimental method is still the best way currently available to discover the facts. You're fortunate in being able to run this type of experiment. Now, for the first time in your adult life you aren't attached to a man. If you find you can be happy without a man, this will greatly strengthen you and also make your future relationships all the better.

In this case, the client was able to stick to a "cold turkey" regimen. After a brief period of dysphoria, she was delighted to find that her well-being was not dependent on another person.

There were similarities between both of these interventions. In both, the distorted conclusion or assumption was delineated and the client was asked for evidence to support it. An experiment to gather data was also suggested in both instances. However, in order to achieve the results, a contrasting version of the same experimental situation was required.

From Beck, A., et al. (1979). *Cognitive theory of depression.* New York: Guilford Press.

Operant conditioning has been useful in improving verbal behaviors of mute, autistic, and developmentally disabled children. In hospitalized clients with severe and persistent mental illness, behavior modification has helped to increase levels of self-care, social behavior, attendance in group activities, and more.

We use positive reinforcement all the time in everyday life, whether we know it or not. Reinforcers can increase, decrease, or maintain a behavior. Here is an example of three ways in which behavior can be reinforced (Aldinger 1992). A mother takes her son to the market. The child starts acting out, wanting this and that, nagging, crying, and yelling.

ACTION	RESULT
1. The mother gives the child what he wants.	The child continues to use this behavior. This is positive reinforcement of negative behavior.
2. The mother scolds the child.	Acting out may continue because the child gets what he or she really wants—attention. This positively rewards negative behavior.
3. The mother ignores the acting out but gives attention to the child when he is acting appropriately.	The child gets a positive reward for appropriate behavior.

SELF-CONTROL THERAPY. Self-control therapy is a combination of cognitive and behavioral approaches. A basic theme is that the "talking to ourselves" in which we all indulge can be altered to help us direct and control our actions more effectively. Stress is one area in which self-control therapy can be useful. For example, the therapist would teach clients to say to themselves when they feel stress affecting their bodies, "All right, my chest is starting to feel tight. Take it easy. Sit down, and breathe deeply. There, I'm feeling calmer." One advantage of this technique is that change is likely to last in many cases, and it is easily applied to new situations in the future.

SYSTEMATIC DESENSITIZATION. Systematic desensitization is another form of behavior modification therapy. For example, a client who has a fear of a particular situation or object (a phobia) will be introduced to short periods of exposure to the phobic object or situation while in a relaxed state. Gradually, over a period of time, exposure is increased until the anxiety about or fear of the object or situation has ceased. This is a common treatment for a variety of phobias (e.g., school phobia, fear of flying, fear of closed spaces).

AVERSION THERAPY. Aversive conditioning, or *negative reinforcement*, is another technique used to change behavior. In aversive conditioning, a stimulus attractive to the client is paired with an unpleasant event, such as shock to the fingertips, in hopes of endowing it with negative properties. One example of the use of **aversion therapy** is with people who have drinking problems. Each time the person takes a drink, he or she is given a mild electric shock or an emetic. Over time, it is hoped that the taking of a drink will be associated with an unpleasant experience, which will eventually override the desire for a drink. Disulfiram (Antabuse), a medication, works on the same principle (see Chapter 25). Aversive therapy has also been used with people who have *paraphilias*, a condition in which the sources of sexual gratification are unconventional (e.g., exhibitionism, voyeurism, sadism, masochism). For example, an electric shock or other noxious stimulus is applied at the time of the paraphiliac impulse. Refer to Box 2–6 for an example of behavior therapy.

Milieu Therapy

The roots of milieu therapy can be found at the end of the eighteenth century when a new humanitarianism, exemplified by Philippe Pinel, led to a new way of helping clients in mental hospitals. Pinel helped to put an end to some barbaric ways of dealing with clients and to institute humane forms of treatment for the mentally troubled.

In 1948, Bruno Bettelheim coined the term **milieu therapy** to describe his use of the total environment to treat disturbed children. Bettelheim created a comfortable, secure environment (or milieu) in which psychotic children were helped to form a new world. Staff members were trained to provide 24-hour support and understanding for each child on an individual basis. It was Bettelheim's goal "to create for (each child) a world that is totally different from the one he abandoned in despair, and moreover a world he can enter right now" (Bettelheim 1967). In 1953, Maxwell Jones wrote a book in Great Britain, *The therapeutic community*, that laid the groundwork for the movement in the United States toward a therapeutic milieu and the nurse's role in this therapy.

There are certain basic characteristics of milieu therapy, whether the setting involves psychotic children, clients in a psychiatric hospital, drug abusers in a residential treatment center, or psychiatric clients in a day hospital. Milieu therapy, or "therapeutic community," has as its locus a living, learning, or working environment. Such therapy may be based on any number of therapeutic modalities, from structured behavioral therapy to spontaneous, humanistically oriented approaches. However, most programs encompass the following (Liberman and Mueser 1989):

1. An emphasis on group and social interaction
2. Rules and expectations mediated by peer pressure
3. Blurring of the client's role through viewing of clients as responsible human beings
4. An emphasis on clients' rights through involvement in setting goals
5. Freedom of movement and informality of relationships with staff
6. An emphasis on interdisciplinary participation
7. Goal-oriented, clear communication

Community meetings, activity groups, social skills groups, and physical exercise programs are some of the ways that milieu management is achieved. Treatment units that set clearly defined and time-limited goals with clients, and units that organize and schedule prosocial activities for most waking hours, are thought to be the most effective.

Milieu therapy consists of the establishment of an environment that is adapted to the individual client's needs but that also provides greater comfort and freedom of expression than had been experienced in the past. The environment is staffed by persons trained to provide support and understanding and give individual attention. All members of the environment contribute to the planning and functioning of the setting. The power hierarchy is diminished, since all members are viewed as significant and valuable members of the community.

Hospital Settings

There have been efforts to apply milieu therapy as a treatment in present-day mental hospitals in which the entire hospital becomes a "therapeutic community" (Jones 1953). All of the hospital's ongoing activities and all of its personnel become part of the treatment pro-

BOX 2-6 EXAMPLE OF BEHAVIOR THERAPY

A 30-year-old married woman, mother of three boys, presented a complaint of anxiety and depression as a chronic state for several years. She became disheveled, hair and clothes in disarray, her walk a shuffling pace—all overt signs of psychomotor retardation.

An attempt was made to get details about the things that were disturbing her. She felt inadequate as a mother, and situations that involved making decisions concerning her three boys, ages 6, 5, and 2½, were distressing to her. In addition, she felt that her husband, to whom she had been married for 9 years, gave her no emotional support, constantly criticized her, and never gave her any positive advice, although he was quick to tell her about the things she did wrong.

The first interview was productive primarily as an opportunity for her to unburden herself about the things she had not been able to talk about with anyone before, and it was felt by the therapist that an excellent working relationship had been established. It was possible to get some idea about the things that were distressing her, but more details were needed, since she reported being distressed all the time. So far, it was impossible to tell what situations made her feel either worse or better, so she was asked to do some homework: to keep records about any upsetting events that occurred during the ensuing week. In addition, she was asked to fill out and bring in a Fear Survey Schedule.

When she came back the next time, she brought in her homework assignment. She said "I went to a movie and I became very upset." Only upon closer questioning about what specifically was happening at the time she became distressed did it become apparent that the disturbing scene was one in which people were drinking. The second thing she noted was that her husband would withdraw when they were talking about emotionally laden things, when what she really needed was for him to put his arms around her and give her some comfort. The third event she noted was that she was very sensitive to the fact that her husband had asked her to make an appointment with the dentist that he had not kept. She felt as though the dentist wouldn't think her trustworthy. In some way, she felt she would be seen by the dentist as being less of a person; he would be critical of her. The fourth area that she brought up was that anytime her children were engaged in fighting, or disagreement, she became upset. The fifth observation was that sudden noises distressed her.

In subsequent sessions the therapist went over each of these situations with the client to further clarify them. Assertive training was begun using a hierarchical approach, by giving her the instruction that between that session and the next session she was to go up and greet anyone that she knew even slightly. A list of people from whom she feared criticism was obtained; these were graded in terms of how distressing each might be to her.

Relaxation training was begun at this point to prepare for systematic desensitization in the areas of criticism and rejection. In subsequent sessions the assignments in assertive training were continued, as she was carrying them out effectively.

At termination, the client no longer looked depressed. A 1-year follow-up indicated that she was continuing to function fully, no longer experiencing depression, and on the whole enjoying life.

From Goldstein, A.. (1978). Behavior therapy. In R. Corsini (Ed.), *Current psychotherapies* (2nd ed.) (pp. 239–245). Itasca, IL: F. E. Peacock. Reproduced by permission of the publisher, F. E. Peacock Publishers Inc.

gram. Social interaction and group activities are encouraged, so that through group pressure the clients are directed toward normal functioning. Clients are expected to participate in their own readjustment as well as that of their fellow clients. Both individually and as a group, clients are expected to act responsibly and to participate in discussions about how the ward is to function. In general, they are treated more as normal individuals than as incompetent mental clients. Open wards allow them considerable freedom. Staff members impress on the residents their positive expectations and praise them for doing well. When they behave symptomatically, staff members stay with them, making clear the expectation that they would soon behave more appropriately.

Studies have provided some evidence for the efficacy of milieu therapy (Fairweather 1964; Greenblatt et al. 1965), the most convincing from a milestone project by Paul and Lentz (1977). In this ambitious study, Paul and Lentz demonstrated encouraging improvement in severely and persistently ill schizophrenic clients living in a state institution through both milieu and social-learning therapy. Before the program began the staff was carefully trained to adhere to detailed instructions in therapy manuals; regular observations confirmed that they were implementing the principles of a milieu therapy program. Over the 4½ years of hospitalization, and the 1½ years of follow-up, the clients were carefully evaluated at regular 6-month intervals by structured interviews and by meticulous, direct behavioral observations. The milieu therapy helped to reduce both positive and negative symptoms. The residents also acquired self-care, housekeeping, social, and vocational skills. The behavior of the clients in milieu therapy was found to be superior to that of the residents of a routine hospital ward. By the end of treatment, more of the severely ill clients in the milieu therapy program than those clients in a routine hospital ward were stable enough to be discharged. An interesting finding emerged on medication usage. Over time, such usage among the routine hospital management group increased, while in the milieu therapy group the percentage of clients on drugs dropped dramatically.

Community Settings

The concept of milieu therapy has also been extended to halfway houses. Because some people function too well to remain in a mental hospital, and yet are unable to function independently enough to live on their own or even within their own families, halfway houses have been established. These are protected living units, typically located in large, formerly private residences. Here, clients discharged from a mental hospital live, take their meals, and gradually return to ordinary community life by holding a part-time job or going to school. Living arrangements may be relatively unstructured; some houses set up money-making enterprises that help to train and support the residents. Depending on how well funded the halfway house is, the staff may include psychiatrists or clinical psychologists. The most important staff members are paraprofessionals, often graduate students in clinical psychology or social work who live in the house and act both as administrators and as friends to the residents. Group meetings, at which residents talk out their frustrations and learn to relate to others in honest and constructive ways, are often part of the routine. Encouraging findings have been reported on the application of such milieu therapy community programs in nonhospital residential settings (Mosher and Butti 1989; Mosher et al. 1986). The clients were young adults experiencing their first psychotic episodes. Had they been in the hospital, treatment would have relied heavily on psychotropic drugs, whereas in the alternative setting employing the principles of Jones' (1953) therapeutic community, clients showed marked improvement. The positive outcomes for such community-based programs indicate that hospitalization may not even be necessary for some acutely disturbed clients. Each clinical chapter discusses the types of milieu therapy useful for a variety of disorders.

SUMMARY

Definition of mental illness or recognition of mental health may change with the culture, the time in history, the political system and power, and the person or group doing the defining. There is no question that mental health and mental illness do exist on a continuum. One continuum is called *adaptive-maladaptive;* another is termed *constructive-destructive.* General indications of a mentally healthy person can be assessed by the degree of (1) happiness, (2) control over behavior, (3) appraisal of reality, (4) effectiveness in work, and (5) self-concept.

Vast changes in the health care setting dictate that more and more people will be cared for in a community setting, not a hospital setting. The trend going into the twenty-first century is the proliferation of health maintenance organizations (HMOs). There are controversial aspects of HMOs: neglected populations remain, and the needs of these people remain unmet.

Mental disorders are categorized by the *Diagnostic and statistical manual of mental disorders.* DSM-IV provides specific behavioral criteria for each diagnostic category of mental disorders and includes five axes to incorporate other data relevant for best diagnosing and planning appropriate care. DSM-IV increases the validity and reliability of each diagnostic category through extensive use of research results, and stresses cultural influences.

However, caution in adopting labels is advised, and some problems in applying information from DSM-IV were identified (e.g., the diagnostician's potential or actual bias toward specific minority groups, and the need to incorporate cultural norms when making a diagnosis). Awareness of these biases and caution in adopting and promoting labeling have enormous implications for nurses.

Sigmund Freud advanced the first theory of personality development, which still influences the thinking of many mental health workers today. He articulated levels of awareness (unconscious, preconscious, conscious) and demonstrated the influence of our unconscious behavior on everyday life, as evidenced by the use of defense mechanisms. Freud identified three psychological processes of personality (id, ego, superego) and described how they operate and develop. He proposed one of the first modern developmental theories of personality based on five psychosexual stages of human growth from infancy to adulthood.

Erik Erikson viewed the growth of the individual in terms of social setting (family, community, and culture). He expanded on Freud's developmental stages to include middle age through old age. Erikson called his stages *psychosocial* and emphasized the social aspect of personality development.

Harry Stack Sullivan proposed the interpersonal theory of personality development, which focuses on interpersonal processes that can be observed in a social framework. Anxiety is a key concept in Sullivan's theory, and he described certain *security operations* people use to decrease anxiety (e.g., sublimation, selective inattention, and dissociation). Hildegard Peplau was influenced by Sullivan's interpersonal theory. Peplau's theoretical framework in psychiatric nursing has become the foundation of psychiatric nursing practice.

Jean Piaget added to the understanding of personality development by identifying four cognitive stages in an individual's development: (1) the sensorimotor period, (2) the preoperational period, (3) the period of concrete operations, and (4) the period of formal operations. All stages follow this sequence, and each stage lays the groundwork for the next stage. Lawrence Kohlberg applied Piaget's concept of stage development to the study of moral development.

Abraham Maslow, the founder of humanistic psychology, offered the theory of human motivation that is basic to all nursing education today. He also described the features of a "self-actualized person" that can be used as another yardstick to measure mental health.

Kohlberg's view of moral development is important for bringing another dimension to growth and development; however, there is some criticism on his need for cultural consideration and emphasis on thought, not behavior.

Finally, six basic therapy approaches have been discussed. The four in greatest use today are psychoanalytic psychotherapy, short-term dynamic therapy, cognitive-behavioral therapy, and behavior modification.

REFERENCES

Aldinger, B. (1992). Personal communication.

Altrocchi, J. (1980). *Abnormal behavior.* New York: Harcourt Brace Jovanovich.

American Nurses' Association (1994). *Nursing: A social policy statement.* Kansas City, MO: American Nurses' Association.

American Psychiatric Association (1987). *Diagnostic and statistical manual of mental disorders (DSM-III-R)* (3rd ed., revised). Washington, DC: American Psychiatric Association.

American Psychiatric Association (1994). *Diagnostic and statistical manual of mental disorders (DSM-IV)* (4th ed.) Washington, DC: American Psychiatric Association.

Bandura, A., Balanchard, E. B., and Ritter, B. (1969). Relative efficacy of desensitization and modeling approaches for inducing behavioral, affective, and attitudinal changes. *Journal of Personality and Social Psychology,* 13:173–199.

Banks, E. C. (1993, March). Moral education curriculum in a multicultural context: The Malaysian primary curriculum. Paper presented at the biennial meeting of the Society for Research in Child Development, New Orleans.

Beck, A. T. (1967). *Depression: Clinical, experimental and theoretical aspects.* New York: Harper & Row.

Beck, A. T. (1976). *Cognitive therapy and the emotional disorders.* New York: New American Library.

Beck, A. T., Rush, A. J., Shaw, B. F., and Emery, G. (1979). *Cognitive theory of depression.* New York: Guilford Press.

Bernard, M. E. (1991). *Using rational-emotive therapy effectively: A practitioner's guide.* New York: Plenum Press.

Bernard, M. E., and Wolfe, J. L. (Eds.) (1993). *The RET resource book for practitioners.* New York: Institute for Rational Emotive Therapy.

Berry, J. W., Pourtinga, Y. H., Segal, H., and Dasen, P. R. (1992). *Cross-cultural psychology.* Cambridge, England: Cambridge University Press.

Bettelheim, B. (1967). *The empty fortress.* New York: Free Press.

Boaz, J. T. (1988). *Delivering mental health care: A guide for HMOs.* Chicago: Pluritus Press.

Boyes, M. C., Giordano, R., and Galperyn, K. (1993, March). Moral interpretation and interpretive contexts of moral deliberation. Paper presented at the biennial meeting of the Society for Research in Child Development, New Orleans.

Bush, J. W. (1996). Long-term therapy may not survive managed-care model (letter to the editor). *New York Times,* January 26, p. A26.

Chodoff, P. (1954). A reexamination of some aspects of conversion hysteria. *Psychiatry,* 17:75–81.

Eisenberg, N., and Murphy, B. (1995). Parenting and children's moral development. In M. H. Bornstein (Ed.), *Children and parenting* (Vol. 4). Hillsdale, NJ: Erlbaum.

Ellis, A. (1978). Rational emotive therapy. In R. Corsini (Ed.), *Current psychotherapies* (2nd ed.). Itasca, IL: F. E. Peacock.

Fairweather, G. W. (Ed.). (1964). *Social psychology in treating mental illness: An experimental approach.* New York: John Wiley.

Flegenheimer, W. V. (1982). *Techniques of brief psychotherapy.* New York: Jason Aronson.

Garfield, S. L. (1978). Research on client variables in psychotherapy. In S. L. Garfield and A. E. Bergin (Eds.), *Handbook of psychotherapy and behavior change* (2nd ed.). New York: John Wiley.

Gilligan, C. (1982). *In a different voice.* Cambridge, MA: Harvard University Press.

Gilligan, C. (1990). Teaching Shakespeare's sister. In C. Gilligan, N. Lyons and T. Hammer (Eds.), *Making connections: The relational worlds of adolescent girls at Emma Willard School.* Cambridge, MA: Harvard University Press.

Gilligan, C. (1991, April). How should "we" talk about development? Paper presented at the biennial meeting of the Society for Research in Child Development, Seattle.

Gilligan, C. (1992, May). Joining the resistance: Girls' development in adolescence. Paper presented at the Symposium on Development and Vulnerability in Close Relationships, Montreal.

Goldstein, A. (1978). Behavior therapy. In R. Corsini (Ed.), *Current psychotherapies.* Itasca, IL: F. E. Peacock.

Goleman, D. (1996). Critics say managed-care savings are eroding mental care. *New York Times,* January 24, p. C9.

Greenblatt, M., Solomon, M. H., Evans, A. S., and Brooks, G. W. (Eds.). (1965). *Drugs and social therapy in chronic schizophrenia.* Springfield, IL: Charles C Thomas.

Jensen, L. A. (1995, March). The moral reasoning of orthodox and progressive Indians and Americans. Paper presented at the meeting of the Society for Research in Child Development, Indianapolis.

Jones, M. (1953). *The therapeutic community.* New York: Basic Books.

Kaplan, H. I., and Sadock, B. I. (Eds.). (1995). *Comprehensive textbook of psychiatry-VI* (6th ed.) (Vol. 2). Baltimore: Williams & Wilkins.

Klerman, G. L. (1986). *Contemporary directions in psychopathology: Toward the DSM IV.* New York: Guilford Press.

Kohlberg, L. (1958). The development of modes of moral thinking and choice in the years 10 to 16. Unpublished doctoral dissertation, University of Chicago.

Kohlberg, L. (1976). Moral stages and moralization: The cognitive developmental approach. In T. Lickona (Ed.), *Moral development and behavior.* New York: Holt, Rinehart & Winston.

Kohlberg, L. (1986). A current statement on some theoretical issues. In S. Modgil and C. Modgil (Eds.), *Lawrence Kohlberg.* Philadelphia: Palmer.

Kohlberg, L. (1969). Stage and sequence: The cognitive-developmental approach to socialization. In D. A. Guslin (Ed.), *Handbook of socialization theory and research.* Chicago: Rand McNally.

Korb, L. J. (1996). Long-term therapy may not survive managed-care model (letter to the editor). *New York Times,* January 26, p. A26.

Kurtines, W. M. and Gewirtz, J. (Eds.). (1991). *Moral behavior and development: Advances in theory, research, and application.* Hillsdale, NJ: Erlbaum.

Lapsley, D. K. (1992, April). Moral psychology after Kohlberg. Paper presented at the meeting of the Midwestern Psychological Association, Chicago.

Lazarus, A. A. (1971). *Behavior therapy and beyond.* New York: McGraw-Hill.

Leff, J. (1981). *Psychiatry around the globe.* New York: Marcel Dekker.

Levison, D. I., and Gooden, W. E. (1985). Theoretical trends in psychiatry. In H. I. Kaplan and B. I. Sadock (Eds.), *Comprehensive textbook of psychiatry* (4th ed.). Baltimore: Williams & Wilkins.

Liberman, R. P., and Mueser, K. T. (1989). Schizophrenia: Psychosocial treatment. In Kaplan, H. I. and Sadock, B. I. (Eds.), *Comprehensive textbook of psychiatry* (4th ed.). Baltimore: Williams & Wilkins.

MacPhillamy, D. S., and Lewinsohn, P. M. (1971). Pleasant events schedule. Unpublished manuscript, University of Oregon.

Maddi, S. R. (1972). *Personality theories: A comparative analysis* (revised). Homewood, IL: Dorsey Press.

Maslow, A. H. (1970). *Motivation and personality* (2nd ed.). New York: Harper & Row.

Maslow, A. H. (1962). *Toward a psychology of living.* Princeton, NJ: Van Nostrand.

Miller, J. G. (1991). A cultural perspective on the morality of beneficence and interpersonal responsibility. In S. Ting-Toomey and F. Korzenny (Eds.), *International and intercultural communication annual* (Vol. 15). Newbury Park, CA: Sage.

Mosher, L. R., and Butti, L. (1989). *Community mental health principles and practice.* New York: Norton.

Mosher, L. R., Kresky-Wolff, M., Mathews, S., and Menn, S. (1986). Milieu therapy in the 1980s: A comparison of two residential alternatives to hospitalization. *Bulletin of the Menninger Clinic,* 50:257–268.

Paul, G. L., and Lentz, R. J. (1977). *Psychosocial treatment of chronic mental patients: Milieu versus social learning programs.* Cambridge, MA: Harvard University Press.

Peplau, H. E. (1952). *Interpersonal relations in nursing.* New York: G. P. Putnam's Sons.

Puka, B. (1991). Toward the redevelopment of Kohlberg's theory: Preserving essential structure, removing controversial content. In W. M. Kurtines and J. Gewirtz (Eds.), *Moral behavior and development: Advances in theory, research, and application.* Hillsdale, NJ: Erlbaum.

Rest, J. R. (1976). New approaches in the assessment of moral judgment. In T. Lickona (Ed.), *Moral development and behavior.* New York: Holt, Rinehart & Winston.

Rest, J. R. (1983). Morality. In P. H. Mussen (Ed.), *Handbook of child psychology* (4th ed., Vol. 3). New York: John Wiley.

Rest, J. R. (1986). *Moral development: Advances in theory and research.* New York: Praeger.

Rothblum, E. D., Solomon, L. I., and Albee, G. W. (1986), A sociological perspective of the DSM-III. In T. Millon and G. L. Klerman (Eds.), *Contemporary directions in psychopathology towards the DSM-IV.* New York: Guilford Press.

Seligman, M. E. P. (1995). The effectiveness of psychotherapy: The consumer reports study. *American Psychologist,* 50:965–974.

Shapiro, S. (1995). *Talking with patients: A self psychological view of creative intuition and analytic discipline* (pp. 139–142). Northvale, NJ: Jason Aronson.

Sifneos, P. (1979). *Short term dynamic psychotherapy* (pp. 120–121). New York: Plenum.

Snarey, J. (1987). A question of morality. *Psychology Today,* June:6–8.

Sullivan, H. S. (1953). *The interpersonal theory of psychiatry.* New York: W. Norton.

Walker, L. J., de Vries, B., and Trevethan, S. D. (1987). Moral stages and moral orientation in real-life and hypothetical dilemmas. *Child Development,* 58:842–858.

Walker, L. J., and Taylor, J. H. (1991). Family interaction and the development of moral reasoning. *Child Development*, 62:264–283.

Westmeyer, J. (1986). Cross cultural diagnosis. *Harvard Medical School Mental Health Letter*, 2(12):4.

Wolf, P. F. (1996). Long-term therapy may not survive managed-care model (letter to the editor). *New York Times*, January 26, p. A26.

Yussen, S. R. (1977). Characteristics of moral dilemmas written by adolescents. *Developmental Psychology*, 12:162–163.

SELF-STUDY AND CRITICAL THINKING

Mark true or false; correct the false statements.

1. __T__ Happiness, control of behavior, sound reality testing, ability to work effectively, and good self-concept are measures of mental health.
2. __T__ Behaviors that allow problems to continue and that interfere with an individual's health and ability to function in work, love, or interpersonal relationships are deemed maladaptive behaviors.
3. __T__ Destructive behaviors undermine or destroy the psychological or physical well-being of a person or others around the person.
4. __T__ DSM-IV provides specific diagnostic criteria as guides for diagnosis of mental disorders.
5. __F__ DSM-IV is free of cultural, social, and political bias and always provides accurate labels.

Match the stage of psychosocial development (Erikson) with the correct age group.

6. __C__	Initiative versus guilt	A. Infancy (birth to 18 months)
7. __E__	Identity versus role confusion	B. 18 months to 3 years
8. __H__	Generativity versus stagnation	C. 3 to 6 years
9. __G__	Integrity versus despair	D. School age (sixth year to puberty)
10. __B__	Autonomy versus shame	E. Adolescence (12 to 20 years)
11. __F__	Intimacy versus isolation	F. Early adulthood (20 to 35 years)
12. __A__	Trust versus mistrust	G. Middle adulthood (35 to 65 years)
13. __D__	Industry versus inferiority	H. Later years (65 to death)

Complete the statements by filling in the appropriate missing information.

14. Receiving a reward for a desired behavior is a form of __Behavioral__ therapy.
15. Lying on a couch, free-associating to a neutral analyst on whom transference feelings are directed, is part of __classical psychoanalytic__.
16. Therapy is limited in time, and although certain tools (e.g., transference and dream interpretation) are used, the therapist often influences the direction of the content. This is called __psycoanalytic psychotherapy__.
17. The therapist interacts actively with the client within the context of an intimate professional relationship to change symptoms or uncover unsatisfactory life patterns. This is called __short-term Dynamic psychotherapy__.

Multiple choice

Choose the answer that most accurately completes the statement.

18. The psychoanalytic theory of Freud placed major emphasis on

    A. Sex instincts
    B. Unconscious motivation
    C. Fixation in psychosexual stages
    D. All of the above

19. Freud called the structure of personality that represents our basic drives, needs, and wishes the

    A. Id
    B. Ego
    C. Superego
    D. Unconscious

20. According to Freud, the ego

    A. Is totally conscious
    B. Obeys the pleasure principle
    C. Follows the reality principle
    D. Is in control of the personality

21. The order in which Freud's three personality components appear as a result of the division of psychic energy is

    A. Ego, id, superego
    B. Superego, ego, id
    C. Id, ego, superego
    D. Ego, superego, id

22. Defense mechanisms

    A. Ward off anxiety
    B. Occur on an unconscious level
    C. Deny or distort reality
    D. All of the above

23. According to Freud, anxiety

    A. Is an inevitable aspect of the human condition
    B. Is a cultural and social product
    C. Has its source in the birth trauma
    D. Invariably leads to severe neurosis

24. A child identifies with the parent of the same sex and starts to take in the values and standards of his or parents (superego) during the

    A. Oral stage
    B. Anal stage
    C. Phallic (oedipal) stage
    D. Genital stage

25. The stage that is *not* one of the four major stages of cognitive development according to Piaget is the

    A. Sensorimotor period (0 to 2 years)
    B. Preoperational period (2 to 7 years)
    C. Period of concrete operations (7 to 11 years)
    D. Period of adolescence (11 to 21 years)

26. According to Piaget's theory, children progress from one stage to another

    A. In an orderly and invariant sequence
    B. Totally on the basis of chronological age
    C. And occasionally may skip a stage
    D. Only when their behavior is consistent with the final stage

27. Sullivan believed that anxiety

    A. Usually leads to ineffective relationships
    B. Results from failure to satisfy physiological needs
    C. Is interpersonal in origin
    D. Enhances an individual's self-esteem

28. The security operation in which one fails to observe some factor in interpersonal relations that might cause anxiety is termed

    A. Sublimation
    B. Selective inattention
    C. "As if"
    D. Suppression

29. Rational emotive behavioral therapy (REBT) theorists of personality emphasize

    A. Unconscious modes of perception and awareness
    B. Motivational factors in personality development
    C. Behavioral responses to the environment
    D. Processes of knowing and understanding the world

Critical thinking

30. Using Table 2–2, evaluate yourself and one of your clients in terms of mental health.
31. In groups of four (two for and two against), debate the pros and cons of the health maintenance organization (HMO) system of health care. Then switch and argue the opposite.
32. Using all DSM-IV axes, discuss (in small peer groups) your client in as much detail as you can. Encourage others to ask questions. **Remember this information is confidential and should not be discussed outside the study group.**
33. Choose two of the therapy models discussed in this chapter and explain to a classmate the premise of how they work. Have your classmate explain two additional therapy modalities to you.
34. If you were to choose a therapeutic model for yourself, explain to a classmate why you think that particular model would be best for you.

3

Psychobiology of Mental Disorders

JOHN RAYNOR

OUTLINE

KEY TERMS AND CONCEPTS

The key terms and concepts listed here also appear in bold where they are defined or discussed in this chapter.

circadian rhythms
neurons
dendrite
axon
neurotransmitters
synapse
reuptake
receptors
reticular activating system (RAS)
limbic system
basal ganglia
antagonists
therapeutic index

OBJECTIVES

After studying this chapter, the reader will be able to

1. Discuss at least eight functions of the brain and how these functions can be altered by psychotropic drugs.
2. Describe how a neurotransmitter functions as a neuromessenger.
3. Draw the three major areas of the brain and identify at least three functions of each.
4. Apply to a medication teaching plan the knowledge gained from this chapter that the blockage of dopamine at the receptor site can result in motor abnormalities and hyperprolactinemia.
5. Demonstrate the administration of the Abnormal Involuntary Movement Scale (AIMS).

6. **Describe the result of blockage to the muscarinic receptors and the $alpha_1$ receptors by the standard neuroleptics.**
7. **Contrast and compare the side-effect profile of the standard antipsychotics with those of (a) clozapine and (b) risperidone.**
8. **Briefly identify the main neurotransmitters that are affected by the following psychotropic drugs:**
   (a) standard (first-generation) antipsychotics
   (b) tricyclic antidepressants (TCAs)
   (c) selective serotonin reuptake inhibitors (SSRIs)
   (d) monoamine oxidase inhibitors (MAOIs)
   (e) antianxiety agents (benzodiazepines, buspirone)
9. **Apply knowledge of why a person on an MAOI would have special dietary and drug restrictions to a medications teaching plan.**

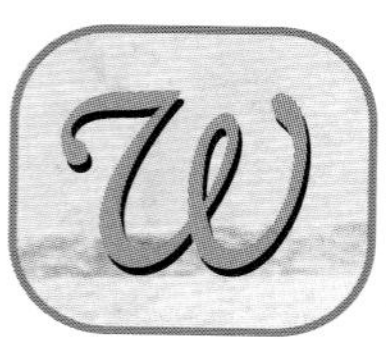

hether conscious or unconscious, focused on the logical or filled with fantasy, the locus of all mental activity is the brain. This implies that a primary goal of psychiatry is to understand both normal and abnormal mental processes in terms of brain function. Ultimately, we would like to be able to apply this understanding to the treatment of mental disease and the alleviation of mental suffering. Approached in terms of brain function, psychiatric problems are explained and treated in the same way as any other biological problems.

Implied in the biological approach to psychiatric illness is the idea that, while the origin of a psychiatric illness may involve any of a number of factors (genetics, drugs, infection, psychosocial experience), there will eventually be an alteration in cerebral function that accounts for the disturbances in the client's behavior and mental experiences. These physiological alterations are the targets of the psychotropic drugs used to treat mental disease.

The goal of this chapter is to relate psychiatric disturbances, and the psychotropic drugs used to treat these disturbances, to normal brain structure and function. We will first look at the normal functions of the brain and how these functions are carried out from an anatomical and physiological perspective. We will then review current theories of the neurophysiological basis of various types of emotional and physiological dysfunctions. As will be seen, these theories focus primarily on neurotransmitters and their receptors. Finally, we will attempt to relate both the beneficial and the untoward effects of psychiatric drugs to their proposed physiological actions.

This information is becoming increasingly important for nurses to understand. It is particularly crucial for advanced practice psychiatric nurses who, in many states, have prescriptive authority. This chapter includes an overview of the major drugs used to treat mental disorders and explains how they work, to help the reader understand why specific side effects are experienced by individual clients. Additional and detailed information regarding the side and toxic effects, dosage, nursing implications, and teaching tools are covered in the appropriate clinical chapters.

FUNCTIONS OF THE BRAIN

In addition to its role in regulating behavior and mental processes, the brain has a large number of other responsibilities; these are summarized in Box 3–1. Since all of these brain functions are carried out by similar mechanisms (interactions of neurons), and often in similar locations, it is not surprising that mental disturbances are often associated with alterations in other brain functions and that the drugs used to treat mental disturbances can also interfere with other activities of the brain.

The brain serves as the coordinator and director of the body's response to both internal and external changes. Appropriate responses require a constant monitoring of the environment, interpretation and integration of the incoming information, and control over the appropriate organs of response. The goal of these responses is to maintain homeostasis and thus to maintain life. Information about the external world is relayed from various senses to the brain by the peripheral nerves. This information, which is at first received as gross sensation (light, sound, touch), must ultimately be interpreted (a key, a train whistle, a hand on the back). Interestingly, a component of major psychiatric disturbance (e.g., schizophrenia) is an alteration of sensory experience. Thus, the client may experience a sensation that does not originate in the external world. People with schizophrenia may

BOX 3–1 FUNCTIONS OF THE BRAIN

1. Monitor changes in the external world
2. Monitor the composition of the body fluids
3. Regulate the contractions of the skeletal muscles
4. Regulate the internal organs
5. Initiate and regulate the basic drives: hunger, thirst, sex, aggressive self-protection
6. Conscious sensation
7. Memory
8. Mood (affect)
9. Thought
10. Regulate sleep cycle
11. Language

hear voices talking to them (auditory hallucination) or they may misinterpret incoming information that does originate in the external world—for instance, thinking that a broom is a rifle (illusion).

The brain not only monitors the external world but also keeps a close watch on the internal one. Thus, information about blood pressure, body temperature, blood gases, and the chemical composition of the body fluids is continuously received by the brain so that it can direct the appropriate responses required to maintain homeostasis.

To respond to external change, the brain must and does have control over the skeletal muscles. This control involves not only the ability to initiate contraction (e.g., to contract the biceps and flex the arm) but also the ability to fine-tune and coordinate contraction so that a person can guide his fingers to the correct keys on the piano. Unfortunately, both psychiatric disease and the treatment of psychiatric disease with psychotropic drugs are associated with disturbances of movement.

It is important to remember that the skeletal muscles controlled by the brain include the diaphragm, which is essential for breathing, and the muscles of the throat, tongue, and mouth, which are essential for speech. Thus, drugs that affect brain function can stimulate or depress respiration or lead to slurred speech.

Adjustments to changes within the body require that the brain exert control over the various internal organs. For example, if blood pressure drops, the brain must direct the heart to pump more blood and the smooth muscles of the arterioles to constrict. This increase in cardiac output and vasoconstriction allows the body to return blood pressure to its normal level.

The autonomic nervous system and the endocrine system serve as the communication links between the brain and the cardiac muscle, smooth muscle, and glands of which the internal organs are composed (Fig. 3–1). Thus, if the brain needs to stimulate the heart, it must activate the sympathetic nerves to the sinoatrial node and the ventricular myocardium, and if it needs to bring about vasoconstriction, it must activate the sympathetic nerves to the smooth muscles of the arterioles.

The linkage between the brain and the internal organs that allows for the maintenance of homeostasis may also serve to translate mental disturbances, such as anxiety, into alterations of internal function. For example, anxiety in some people can cause activation of parasympathetic nerves to the digestive tract, leading to hypermotility and diarrhea. Likewise, anxiety can activate the sympathetic nerves to the arterioles, leading to vasoconstriction and hypertension.

In attempting to understand the neurobiological basis of mental disease and its treatment, it is helpful to distinguish between the various types of brain activities that serve as the basis of mental experience and of behavior.

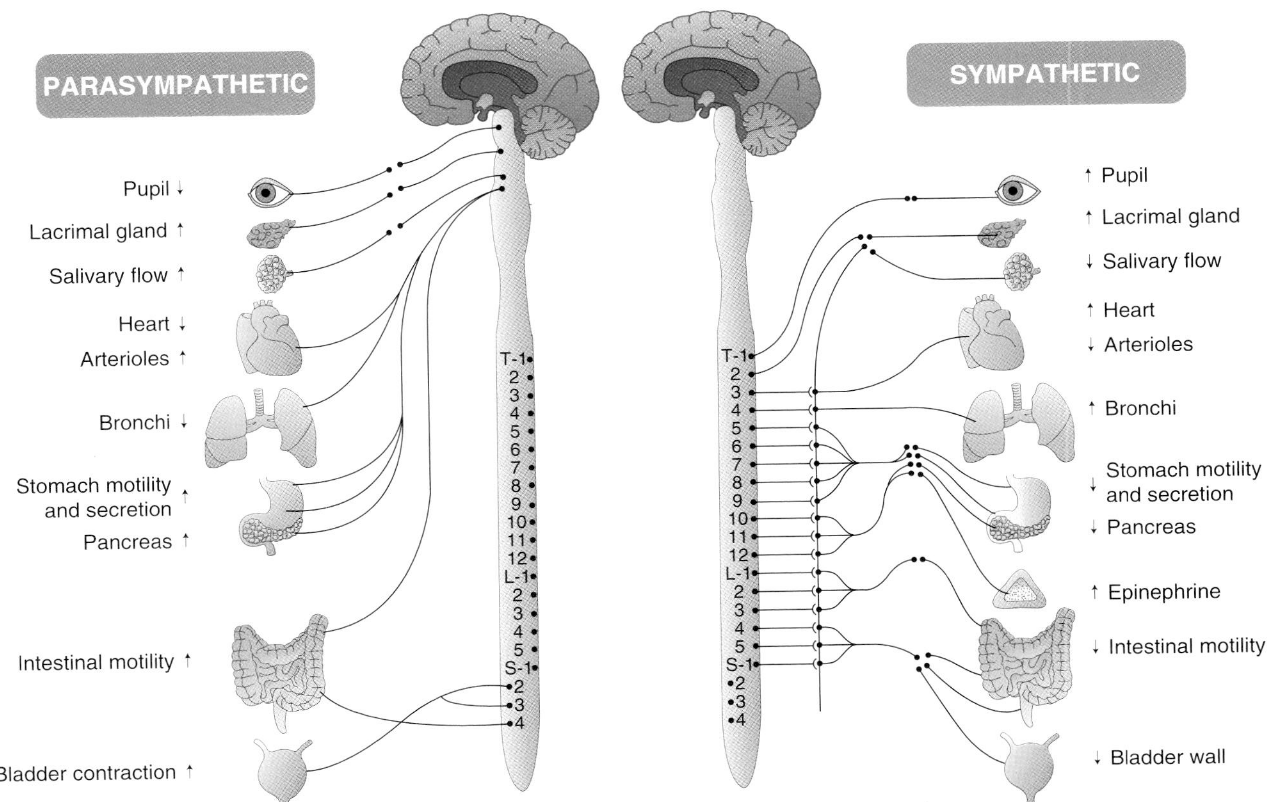

Figure 3–1 The autonomic nervous system has two divisions: the sympathetic and parasympathetic. The sympathetic division is dominant in stress situations, such as fear and anger—known as the fight or flight response.

An understanding of these activities focuses attention on where to look for disturbed function and what to hope for in treatment.

The brain, for example, is responsible for the basic drives, such as sex and hunger, that play a strong role in molding behavior. Disturbances of these drives (e.g., over- or under-eating, loss of sexual interest) can be an indication of an underlying psychological disease such as depression.

The entire cycle of sleep and wakefulness, as well as the intensity of alertness while the person is awake, is regulated and coordinated by various regions of the brain. Although we are far from a full understanding of the true homeostatic function of sleep, there is no question that it is essential for both physiological and psychological well-being. Sleep disturbances are often a symptom of psychological distress, and an assessment of sleep patterns is part of what is required to determine a psychiatric diagnosis.

When a person is awake, the degree of alertness and the ability to focus attention are regulated in complex ways by the brain. Disturbances in alertness and focus—hypervigilence in a person with paranoid schizophrenia or inability to concentrate in a person who is depressed—can be indications of mental disturbance.

Unfortunately, many of the drugs used to treat psychiatric problems interfere with the normal regulation of sleep and alertness. Drugs with a sedative-hypnotic effect can blunt the degree to which the client feels alert and can focus attention, and can make the client feel drowsy and fall asleep. A sedative-hypnotic effect demands caution in using these drugs while engaging in activities that require a great deal of attention, such as driving a car or operating farm machinery. One way of minimizing the danger is to give such drugs at night just before the client goes to sleep.

The cycle of sleep and wakefulness is only one aspect of what we call **circadian rhythms,** the fluctuation of various physiological and behavioral parameters over a 24-hour cycle. Other variations include changes in body temperature, the secretion of hormones such as adrenocorticotropic hormone and cortisol, and the secretion of neurotransmitters such as norepinephrine and serotonin. Both norepinephrine and serotonin are thought to be involved in mood (affect), whether normal or abnormal; thus, daily fluctuations of mood may be related in part to circadian variations in these transmitters. There is some evidence that the circadian rhythm of neurotransmitter secretion is altered in psychological disease, particularly in disorders that involve alteration of mood.

All aspects of conscious mental experience and sense of self must ultimately result from the neurophysiological activity of the brain. The most basic type of conscious mental activity is probably the loose, meandering stream of consciousness that can jump back and forth between thoughts of future responsibilities, past experiences, fantasized activities, interpersonal grievances, and so on. Conscious mental activity must, of course, become much more organized when it is applied to problem solving and the interpretation of the external world. Both the random stream of consciousness and the ability to interpret the environment can become extremely distorted in psychiatric illness. Thus, a person with schizophrenia can present with chaotic and seemingly incoherent speech and thought patterns (a jumble of unrelated words known as *word salad,* unconnected phrases and topics known as *looseness of association*) and delusional interpretations of personal interactions, such as beliefs about people or events that are not supported by data or reality.

An extremely important component of mental activity is memory, the ability to retain and recall past experience. From both an anatomical and physiological perspective, it is thought that there is a major difference in the processing of short- and long-term memory. Clinically, this can be seen dramatically in some forms of cognitive mental disorders such as dementia, in which a person has no recall of the events of the previous 8 minutes but may have vivid recall of events that occurred 80 years ago.

Another important component of mental experience, and therefore of brain function, is the feeling or emotion that exists along with the thought process. Although we might argue theoretically about the role of emotion in homeostasis and survival, there is no question that, for individuals, emotion is at the core of their sense of well-being. Attempts to understand the biological basis of emotional status are a major focus of psychiatric research.

One major way in which the human brain differs from that of other animals is seen in the ability to add language to mental experience and then communicate that experience to others. It seems that the addition of language occurs in anatomically distinct areas of the brain (e.g., the frontal and temporal lobes) and by physiologically distinct processes. Thus, in various types of aphasias (loss of language ability), a person may know that a key is used to open a door, but not be able to name the object a *key.*

NEURONS

Nerve cells are called **neurons** or nerve fibers. Each neuron has a cell body containing the nucleus and its surrounding cytoplasm, a **dendrite** that transmits impulses *toward* the cell body, and an **axon** that conveys electrical impulses *away from* the cell body. All the functions of the brain, from regulation of blood pressure to the conscious sense of self, must result from the actions of individual neurons and the interconnections between neurons. Although neurons come in a great variety of shapes and sizes, all carry out the same three types of physiological actions: (1) they respond to stimuli, (2) they conduct electric impulses, and (3) they release chemicals called neurotransmitters.

An essential feature of neurons is their ability to conduct an electrical impulse from one end of the cell to the other. This electrical impulse consists of a self-propagating change in membrane permeability that first allows the inward flow of sodium ions and then the outward flow of potassium ions. The inward flow of sodium ions changes the polarity of the membrane from positive on the outside to positive on the inside. Movement of potassium ions out of the cell returns the positive charge to the outside of the cell. Since these electrical charges are self-propagating, a change at one end of the cell is conducted along the membrane until it reaches the other end of the cell (Fig. 3–2). The functional significance of this propagation is that the electrical impulse serves as a means of communication between one part of the body and another.

Once an electrical impulse reaches the end of a neuron, a chemical called a neurotransmitter is released. A **neurotransmitter** is a chemical substance that functions as a neuromessenger. Neurotransmitters are released from the axon terminal at the *presynaptic* neuron on excitation. This transmitter then diffuses across a narrow space, or **synapse,** to an adjacent *postsynaptic* neuron, where it attaches to specialized receptors on the cell surface and either inhibits or excites the postsynaptic neuron. It is the interaction between transmitter and receptor that allows the activity of one neuron to influence the activity of other neurons. Depending on the chemical structure of the transmitter and the specific type of receptor to which it attaches, the postsynaptic cell will be rendered either more or less likely to have an electrical impulse. As we shall see, it is the interaction between transmitter and receptor that is a major target of the drugs used to treat psychiatric disease. Table 3–1 lists some of the most important neurotransmitters and the types of receptors to which they attach.

After attaching to a receptor and exerting its influence on the postsynaptic cell, the transmitter separates from the receptor and is destroyed. The process of transmitter destruction is illustrated in Box 3–2. As can be seen, there are two basic mechanisms by which transmitters are destroyed. Some transmitters (e.g., acetylcholine) are destroyed by specific enzymes at the postsynaptic cell. The specific enzyme that destroys acetylcholine is called *acetylcholinesterase.* Other transmitters (e.g., norepinephrine are taken back into the presynaptic cell from which they were originally released by a process called cellular **reuptake.** Upon their return to these cells, the transmitters are either reused or destroyed by intracellular enzymes. In the case of the monoamine transmitters, the destructive enzyme is called *monoamine oxidase (MAO).*

As a means of regulating the concentration of transmitters at the postsynaptic receptors, many of the transmitters exert a feedback inhibition of their own release. This inhibition is accomplished by the attachment of transmitters to what are called presynaptic **receptors,** as illustrated in Figure 3–3 for the transmitter norepinephrine. As can be seen, norepinephrine not only attaches to receptors on the postsynaptic cell but also attaches to receptors on the cell from which it was released. This interaction informs the presynaptic cell that there is already sufficient norepinephrine at the synapse, and acts to inhibit the release of further transmitters.

ORGANIZATION OF THE NERVOUS SYSTEM

Structurally, the nervous system consists of the brain and spinal cord (the central nervous system [CNS]) and the peripheral nerves that link these structures with the rest of the body. These peripheral nerves, sensory and motor, allow the CNS to monitor both the inside of the body and the external world and to alter body function as necessary.

The brain is divided into three major areas: brainstem, cerebellum, and cerebrum. Although each of these areas has distinct responsibilities, they are interconnected by a vast network of neurons so that they work in a coordinated fashion.

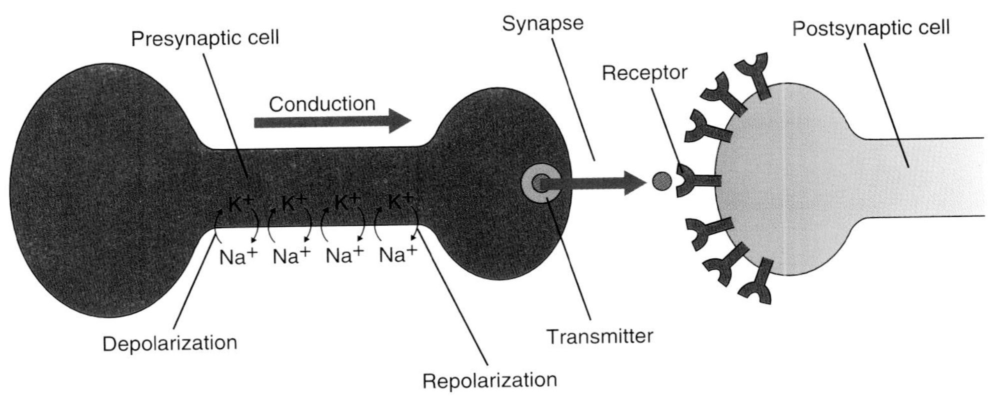

Figure 3–2 Activities of neurons. Conduction along a neuron involves the inward movement of sodium (Na^+) followed by the outward movement of potassium (K^+). When the current reaches the end of the cell, a neurotransmitter is released. The transmitter crosses the synapse and attaches to a receptor on the postsynaptic cell. The attachment of transmitter to receptor either stimulates or inhibits the postsynaptic cell.

TABLE 3–1 TRANSMITTERS/RECEPTORS

TRANSMITTERS	RECEPTORS	EFFECTS/COMMENTS	WHERE SECRETED
		Bioamines	
Dopamine (DA)	D_1, D_2, D_3, D_4, D_5	▶ Fine muscle movement ▶ Integration of emotions and thoughts ▶ Involved with decision making ▶ Stimulates hypothalamus to release hormones (sex, thyroid, adrenals)	Limbic system; cerebral system; basal ganglia; hypothalamus
Norepinephrine (NE)	Alpha$_1$, alpha$_2$, beta$_1$, beta$_2$	▶ Level in brain affects mood ▶ Stimulates sympathetic branch of ANS for "fight or flight"	Autonomic system; reticular activating system; other areas of brain and spinal cord
Serotonin (5-HT)	5-HT, 5-HT$_2$, 5-HT$_3$, 5-HT$_4$	▶ Plays a role in sleep regulation, hunger, mood states, and pain perception ▶ Plays a role in aggression and sexual behavior	Limbic system; hypothalamus; cerebellum; spinal cord
		Amino Acids	
Gama-aminobutyric Acid (GABA)	GABA$_A$, GABA$_B$	▶ Plays a role in inhibition; reduces aggression, excitation, and anxiety ▶ May play a role in pain perception ▶ Anticonvulsant and muscle-relaxing properties	Cerebral cortex; cerebellum; spinal cord
		Cholinergics	
Acetylcholine (ACH)	Nicotinic Muscarinic (M_1, M_2, M_3)	▶ Plays a role in learning, memory ▶ Mood regulator: manic, sexual aggression ▶ Affects sexual and aggressive behavior ▶ Stimulates parasympathetic nervous system	Muscle-nerve junctions; autonomic system; parts of brain
		Neuropeptides	
Histamine	H_1, H_2	▶ Alertness ▶ Inflammatory response ▶ Stimulates gastric secretion	Brain; throughout body; stomach

ANS-Autonomic Nervous System

The Brainstem

The central core of the brainstem regulates the internal organs and is responsible for such vital functions as the regulation of blood gases and the maintenance of blood pressure. The brainstem also serves as an initial processing center for sensory information that is then sent on to the cerebral cortex. Through projections of what is called the **reticular activating system** *(RAS)*, the brainstem regulates the entire cycle of sleep and wakefulness and the ability of the cerebrum to carry out conscious mental activity.

The influence of the brainstem on consciousness extends beyond a simple on-off control of the sleep cycle. Neurons extending from the brainstem to the cerebrum influence those areas of cerebrum, collectively referred to

BOX 3–2 DESTRUCTION OF NEUROTRANSMITTERS

A full explanation of the various ways in which psychotropic drugs alter neuronal activity requires a brief review of the manner in which neurotransmitters are destroyed after attaching to the receptors. As a means of avoiding continuous and prolonged action on the postsynaptic cell, the neurotransmitter is released shortly after attaching to the postsynaptic receptor. Once released, the transmitter is destroyed in one of two ways. *One* is the immediate inactivation of the transmitter at the postsynaptic membrane.

An example of this method of destruction is the action of the enzyme acetylcholinesterase on the neurotransmitter acetylcholine. Acetylcholinesterase is present at the postsynaptic membrane and destroys acetylcholine shortly after it attaches to nicotinic or muscarinic receptors on the postsynaptic cell.

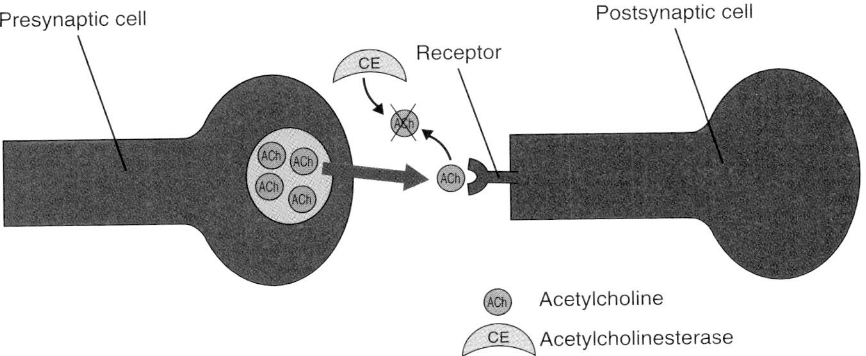

A *second* method of neurotransmitter inactivation is a little more complex. After interacting with the postsynaptic receptor, the transmitter is released and taken back into the presynaptic cell, the cell from which it was released. The process, referred to as the reuptake of neurotransmitter, is a common target for drug action. Once inside the presynaptic cell, the transmitter is either recycled or inactivated by an enzyme within the cell. The monoamine transmitters norepinephrine, dopamine, and serotonin are all inactivated in this manner by the enzyme monoamine oxidase.

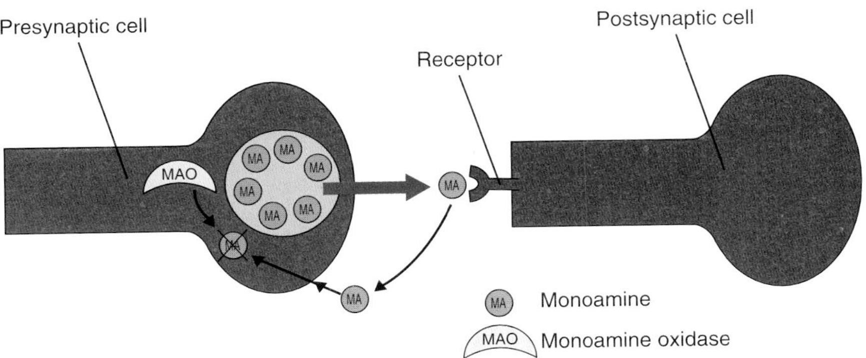

Looking at this second method, you might naturally ask what prevents the enzyme from destroying the transmitter before its release. The answer is that before release the transmitter is stored within a membrane and is thus protected from the degradative enzyme. After release and reuptake, the transmitter is either destroyed by the enzyme or reenters the membrane to be used once again.

as the **limbic system,** that play a crucial role in emotional status and psychological function. Figure 3–4 helps you visualize the network of neurons. These neurons, which use the monoamines norepinephrine, dopamine, and serotonin as their transmitters, are prime suspects as a cause of psychic distress and are prime targets for the psychotropic drugs used to treat it. Table 3–2 identifies the function and location of components of the limbic system.

The Cerebellum

Located posteriorly to the brainstem, the cerebellum (Fig. 3–5) is primarily involved in the regulation of skeletal muscle coordination and contraction and the maintenance of equilibrium. It plays a crucial role in coordinating contractions so that movement is accomplished in a smooth and directed manner.

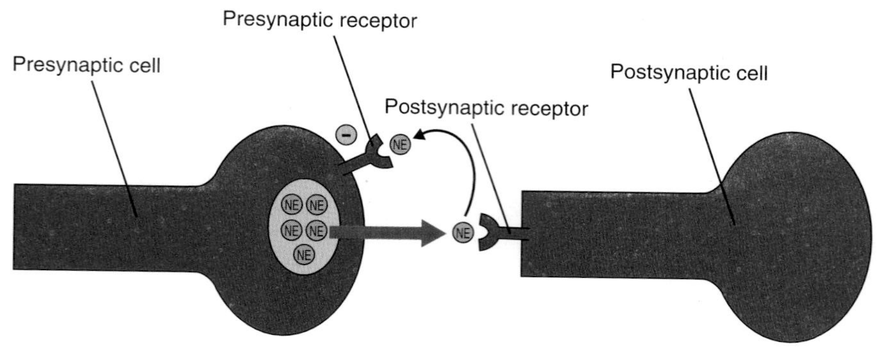

Figure 3–3 Presynaptic inhibition, showing feedback inhibition of transmitter release by attachment of norepinephrine to presynaptic receptors.

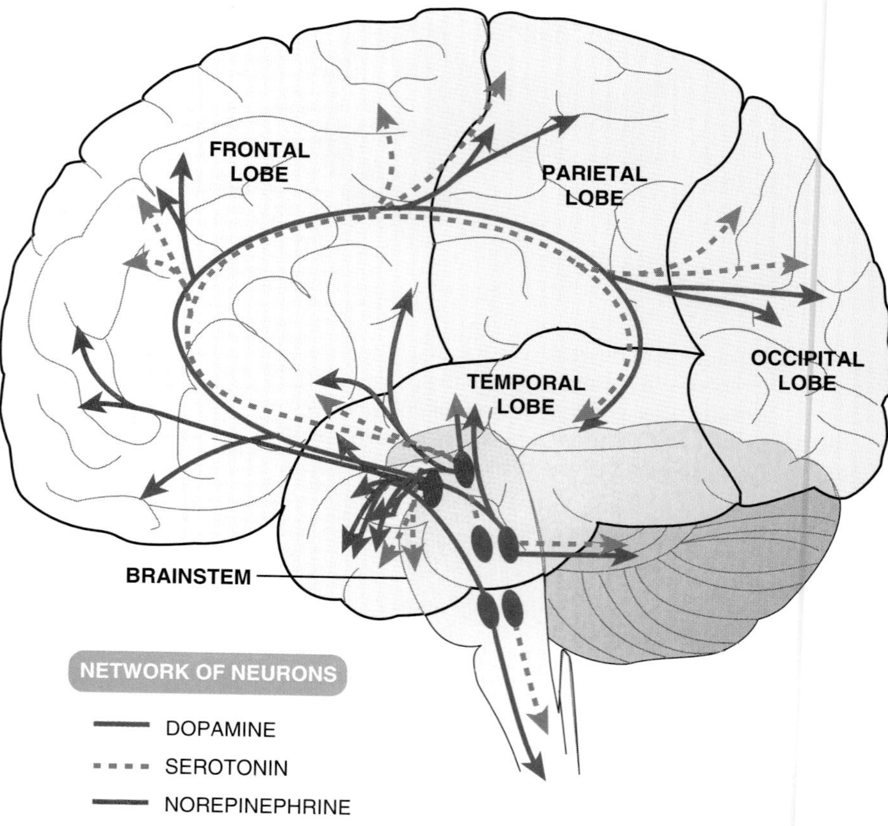

Figure 3–4 The brain: cerebrum (comprised of the frontal, parietal, occipital, and temporal lobes), brainstem, and cerebellum. The network of neurons extending from the brainstem, collectively called the limbic system, is crucial to regulation of emotional status.

TABLE 3–2 THE LIMBIC SYSTEM

LIMBIC STRUCTURE	FUNCTION	LOCATION
Amygdala	Controls behavior for each social occasion	Deep inside anterior end of each temporal lobe
Hippocampus	Determines which sensory information will be committed to memory	Medial border of each cerebral hemisphere
Mamillary body	Perhaps helps to determine mood and degree of wakefulness	Posterior to hypothalamus
Septum pellucidum	Perhaps helps to control temper and autonomic nervous system	Midline of cerebrum anterior and superior to hypothalamus
Limbic cortex: Cingulate gyrus, cingulum, insula, parahippocampal gyrus	Conscious components in control of behavior	Ring of cerebral cortex in medial part of cerebrum around deeper limbic structures

From Guyton, A. C. (1991). *Basic neuroscience anatomy and physiology* (2nd ed.) (p. 20). Philadelphia: W. B. Saunders.

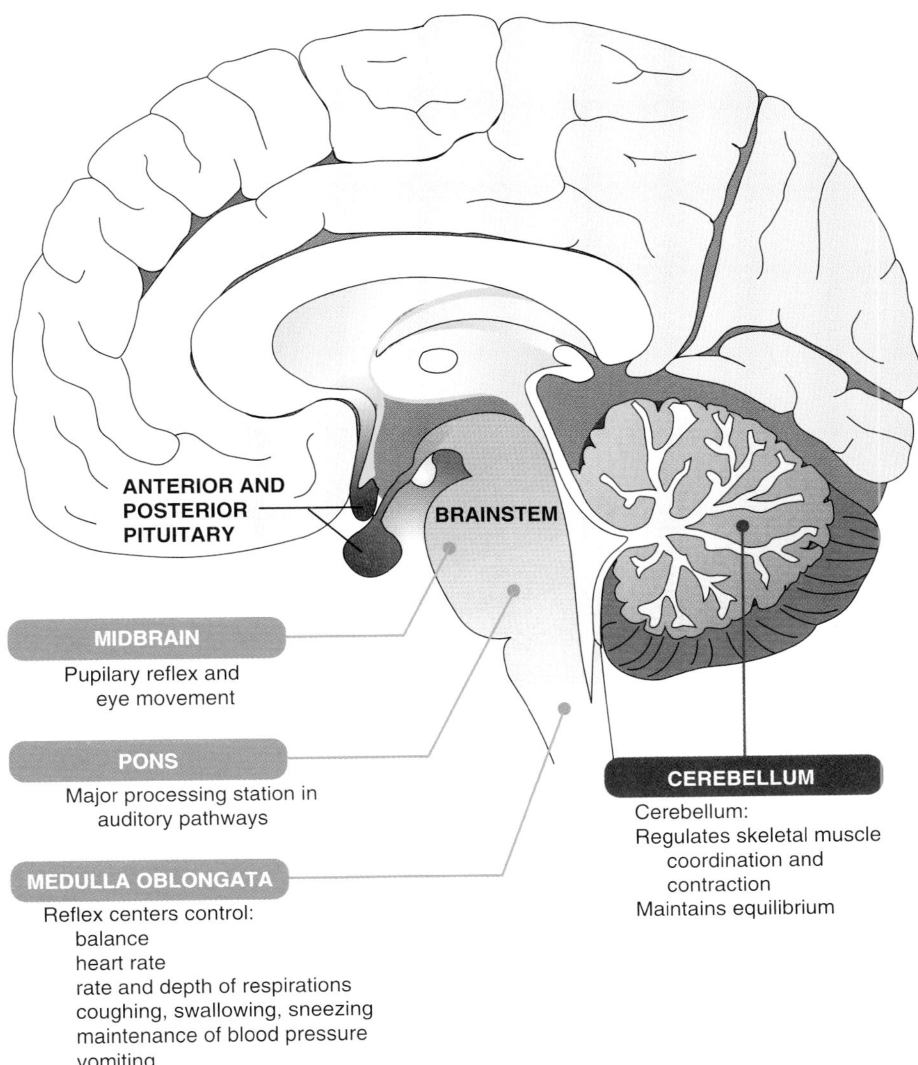

Figure 3–5 The functions of the brainstem and cerebellum.

The Cerebrum

The brainstem and cerebellum of the human brain are similar in both structure and function to these same structures in the brains of other mammals. The development of a much larger and more elaborate cerebrum is what distinguishes human beings from the rest of the animal kingdom.

The cerebrum, situated on top of and surrounding the brainstem, is responsible for mental activities and a conscious sense of being. Thus, the cerebrum is responsible for our conscious perception of the external world and of our own body, for emotional status, for memory, and for the control of the skeletal muscles that allow the willful direction of movement. The cerebrum is also responsible for language and the ability to communicate.

Anatomically, the cerebrum consists of surface and deep areas of integrating gray matter, of the cerebral cortex and basal ganglia, and of the connecting tracts of white matter that link these areas with each other and with the rest of the nervous system. The cerebral cortex, which forms the outer layer of the brain, is responsible for conscious sensation and the initiation of movement. It is organized in such a way that specific areas of the cortex are responsible for specific sensations: the parietal cortex is responsible for touch, the temporal cortex for sound, the occipital cortex for vision, and so on. Likewise, the initiation of skeletal muscle contraction is controlled by a specific area of the frontal cortex. Of course, all the areas of the cortex are interconnected so that an integral picture of the world can be formed and, if necessary, linked to an appropriate response (Fig. 3–6).

Specialized areas of the cerebral cortex are responsible for language in both its sensory and motor aspects. Sensory language functions include the ability to read, to understand spoken language, and to know the names of objects that are perceived by the senses, whereas motor functions involve the ability to use muscles properly for speech and writing. In both neurological and psychological dysfunction, the use of language may become com-

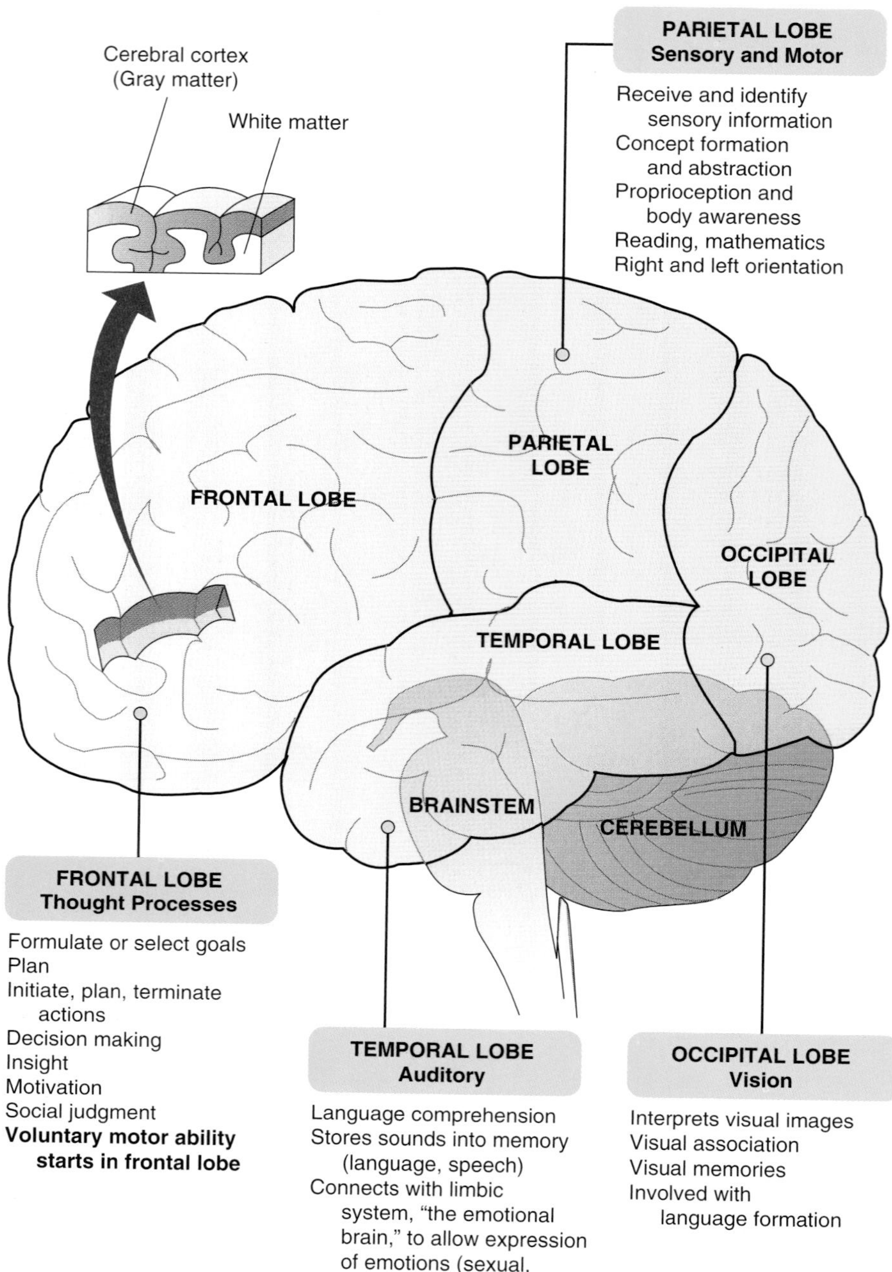

Figure 3–6 The functions of the cerebral lobes; frontal, parietal, temporal, and occipital.

promised or distorted. The change in linguistic ability may be a factor in determining a diagnosis.

In addition to forming the surface of the cerebrum, there are pockets of integrating gray matter deep within the cerebrum. These areas are referred to collectively as **basal ganglia.** Some areas of the basal ganglia are involved in the regulation of movement; others are involved in the emotions and basic drives. Significantly, there is an overlap of these various areas both anatomically and in the types of neurotransmitters employed. One consequence of this is that drugs used to treat emotional disturbances may cause movement disorders and that drugs used to treat movement disorders may cause emotional changes.

A variety of noninvasive imaging techniques are used to visualize brain structure, functions, and metabolic activity in clients experiencing various mental disorders. Positron-emission tomography (PET) scans are particularly useful in identifying physiological and biochemical changes as they occur in live tissue. Usually a radioactive "tag" is used to trace compounds, such as glucose, in the brain. Glucose is related to functional activity in certain areas of the brain. For example, in clients with schizophrenia, PET scans may show a decreased use of glucose in the frontal lobes of unmedicated individuals. Figure 3–7 shows reduced brain activity in the frontal lobe of a twin diagnosed with schizophrenia as compared with the

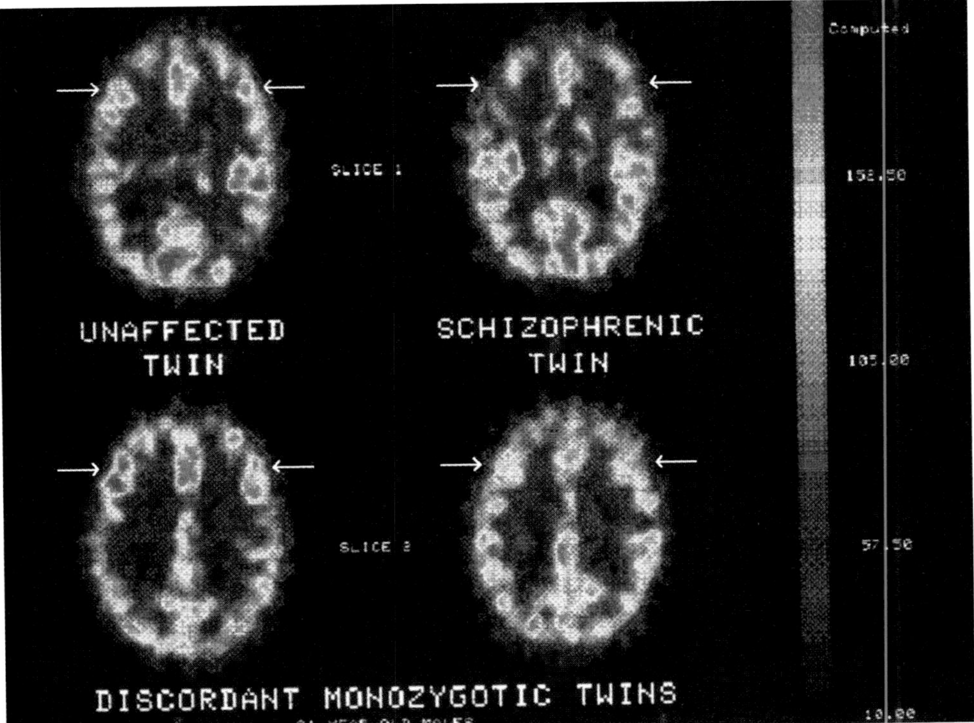

Figure 3–7 Positron-emission tomography (PET) scans of blood flow in identical twins, one of whom has schizophrenia, illustrate that individuals with this illness have reduced brain activity in their frontal lobes when asked to perform a reasoning task that requires activation of this area. Schizophrenic clients also perform poorly on the task. This suggests a site of functional impairments in schizophrenia. (From Karen Berman, MD, courtesy of National Institute of Mental Health, Clinical Brain Disorders Branch.)

twin who does not have schizophrenia. The area affected in the frontal cortex of the schizophrenic twin is an area associated with reasoning skills, which are greatly impaired in people with schizophrenia. Scans such as these suggest a location in the frontal cortex as the site of functional impairment in people with schizophrenia.

Increased brain metabolism shows up in PET scans in certain areas of the frontal cortex in people with obsessive-compulsive disorder (OCD). Figure 3–8 shows increased brain metabolism as compared with a normal control, suggesting altered brain function in people with OCD.

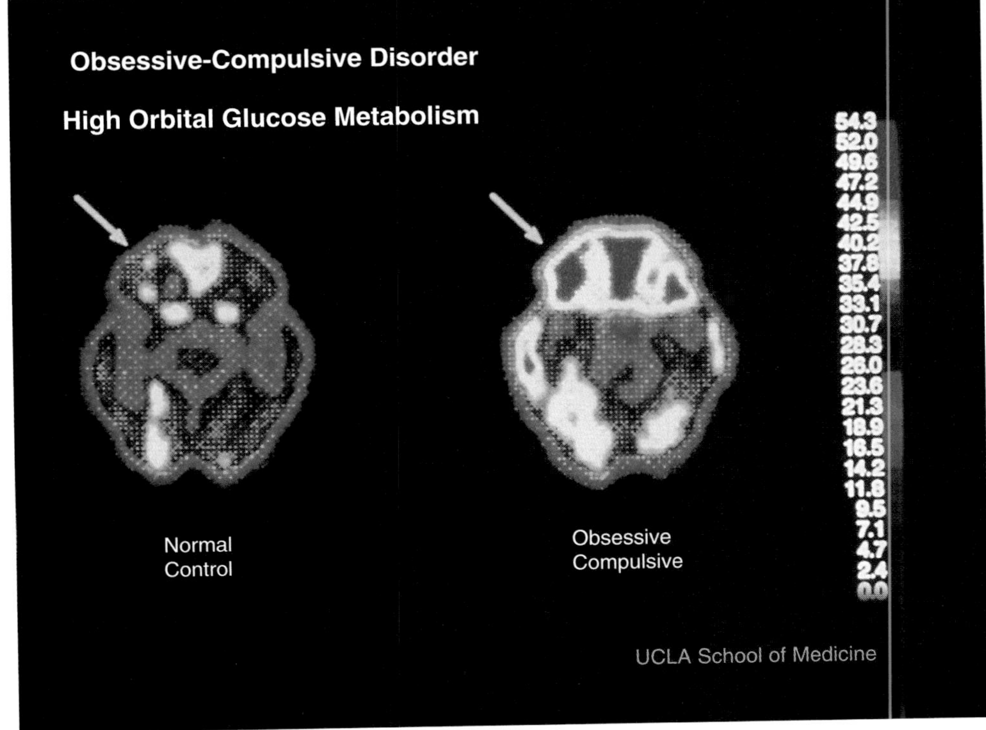

Figure 3–8 PET scans show increased brain metabolism *(brighter colors)*, particularly in the frontal cortex, in an obsessive-compulsive disorder (OCD) client, compared with a normal control. This suggests altered brain function in OCD. (From Lewis Baxter, MD, University of Alabama, courtesy of National Institute of Mental Health.)

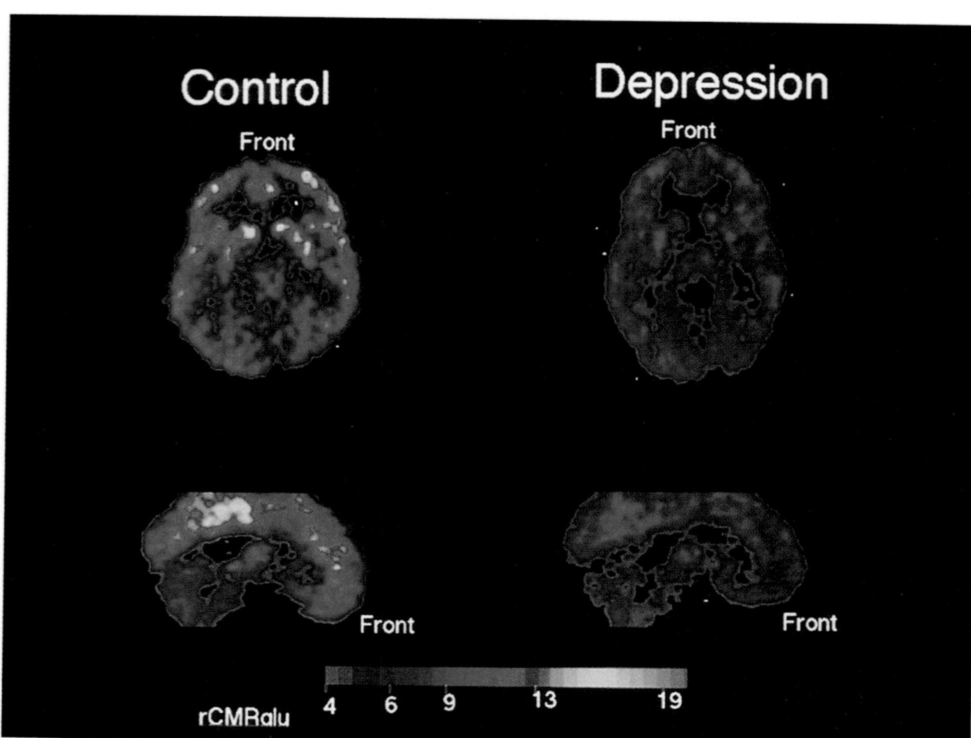

Figure 3–9 PET scans of a normal subject *(left)* and a depressed client *(right)* reveal reduced brain activity *(darker colors)* during depression, especially in the prefrontal cortex. A form of radioactively tagged glucose was used as a tracer to visualize levels of brain activity. (From Mark George, MD, courtesy of National Institute of Mental Health, Biological Psychiatry Branch.)

Decreased brain activity may be seen on PET scans in the prefrontal cortex of many depressed individuals. Figure 3–9 shows the results of a PET scan taken after a form of radioactively tagged glucose was used as a tracer to visualize levels of brain activity. The depressed client shows reduced brain activity as compared with a nondepressed control.

From a psychiatric perspective, we would like to be able to understand where in the brain the various components of psychological activity take place, and what are the types of neurotransmitters and receptors that underlie this activity physiologically. Currently, our understanding of both these questions is far from complete. However, it is thought that the limbic system—a group of structures that include parts of the frontal cortex, the basal ganglia, and the brainstem—is a major locus of psychological activity. Within these areas the monoamine transmitters (norepinephrine, dopamine, and serotonin), as well as the transmitters acetylcholine and gamma-aminobutyric acid (GABA), play a major role.

DISTURBANCES OF MENTAL FUNCTION

Although in a limited number of clients the cause of mental dysfunction is known, most occurrences are of unknown origin. Among known causes are drugs (lysergic acid diethylamide [LSD], long-term use of prednisone), excess levels of hormones (thyroxine, cortisol), infection (encephalitis, AIDS), and physical trauma. However, even when the etiology is known, the link between the causative factor and the mental disruption is far from understood.

Results from numerous studies seem to indicate that there is at least in part a genetic component to psychological dysfunction. The incidence of both thought and mood disorders is higher in relatives of people with these diseases than in the general population. There is also a strong concordance, although certainly not 100%, among identical twins even when they are raised apart. Psychosocial stress, either in the family of origin or in contacts with society at large, increases the likelihood of mental problems, as does physical disease. Genetics and environment are linked in complex ways so that some people are better able to cope with stress than others.

Researchers want ultimately to be able to understand mental changes in terms of altered activity of neurons in specific areas of the brain; the hope is that such understanding could lead to better treatments and possible prevention of mental disorders. Current interest is focused on certain neurotransmitters and their receptors, particularly in the limbic system linking the frontal cortex, basal ganglia, and upper brainstem. As mentioned, the transmitters that have been most consistently linked to mental activity are norepinephrine, dopamine, serotonin, and GABA.

Although the underlying physiology is complex, in simple terms it is thought that a deficiency of norepinephrine and/or serotonin serves as the biological basis of depression. Figure 3–10 shows that an insufficient degree of

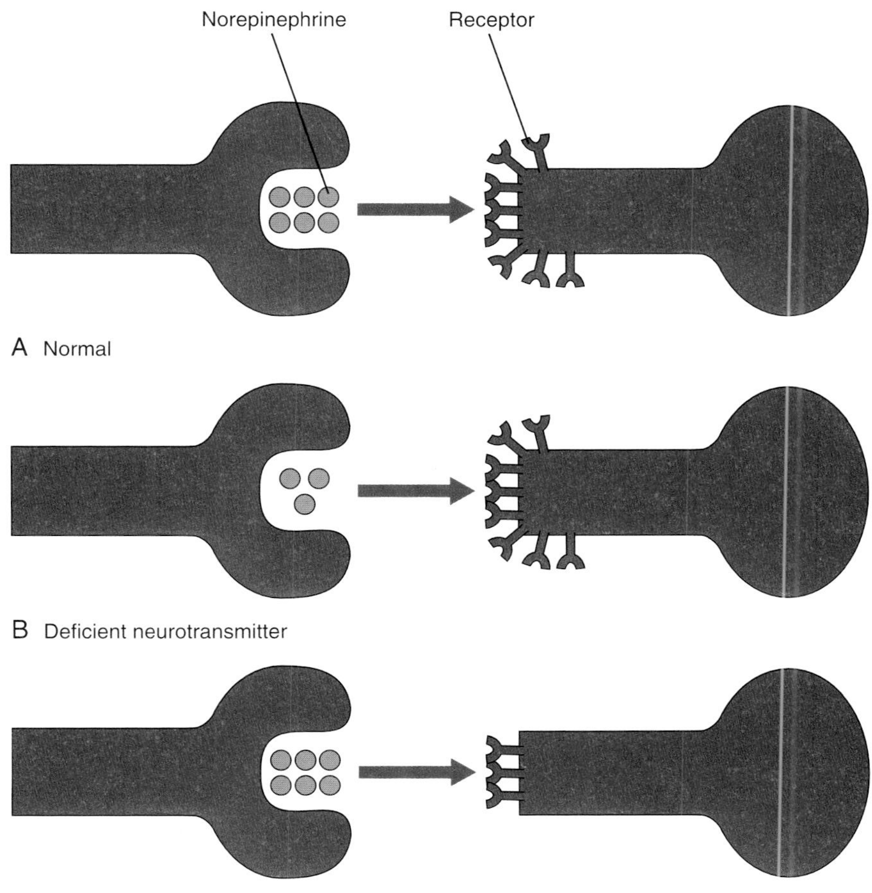

Figure 3–10 Normal transmission of neurotransmitters *(A)*. Deficiency in transmission may be due to deficient release of transmitter, as shown in *(B)*, or by reduction in receptors, as shown in *(C)*.

transmission may be due to a deficient release of the transmitters by the presynaptic cell or to a loss of the ability of postsynaptic receptors to respond to the transmitters.

Thought disorders such as schizophrenia are associated physiologically with excess transmission of the neurotransmitter dopamine. As illustrated in Figure 3–11, this may be due either to excess release of transmitter or to increased receptor responsiveness.

The neurotransmitter GABA seems to play a role in modulating neuronal excitability and anxiety. Not surprisingly, most antianxiety (anxiolytic) drugs act by increasing the effectiveness of this transmitter. This is accomplished primarily by increasing receptor responsiveness.

It is important to keep in mind that the various areas of the brain are interconnected structurally and functionally by a vast network of neurons. This network serves to integrate the many and varied activities of the brain. A limited number of neurotransmitters are used in the brain, and thus a particular transmitter is often used by different neurons to carry out quite different activities. For example, dopamine is used not only by neurons involved in thought processes but also by neurons involved in the regulation of movement.

As a result of the use of the same transmitter by different types of neurons, alterations in transmitter activity, either as the causative factor of a mental disturbance or brought about by the drugs used to treat the disturbance, can affect more than one area of brain activity. In other words, alterations in mental status, whether arising from disease or from medication, are often accompanied by changes in basic drives, sleep patterns, body movement, and autonomic function.

PSYCHOTROPIC DRUGS

An ideal psychiatric drug would relieve the mental disturbance of the client without inducing untoward cerebral (mental) or somatic (physical) effects. Unfortunately, in psychiatry, as in most other areas of pharmacology, there are no drugs that are both fully effective and at the same time free of undesired complications. Researchers work toward achieving the ideal.

Since all the activities of the brain involve the actions of neurons, neurotransmitters, and receptors, these are the targets of pharmacological intervention. Most psychotropic drugs act by either increasing or decreasing the activity of certain transmitter-receptor systems. It is generally agreed that different transmitter-receptor systems

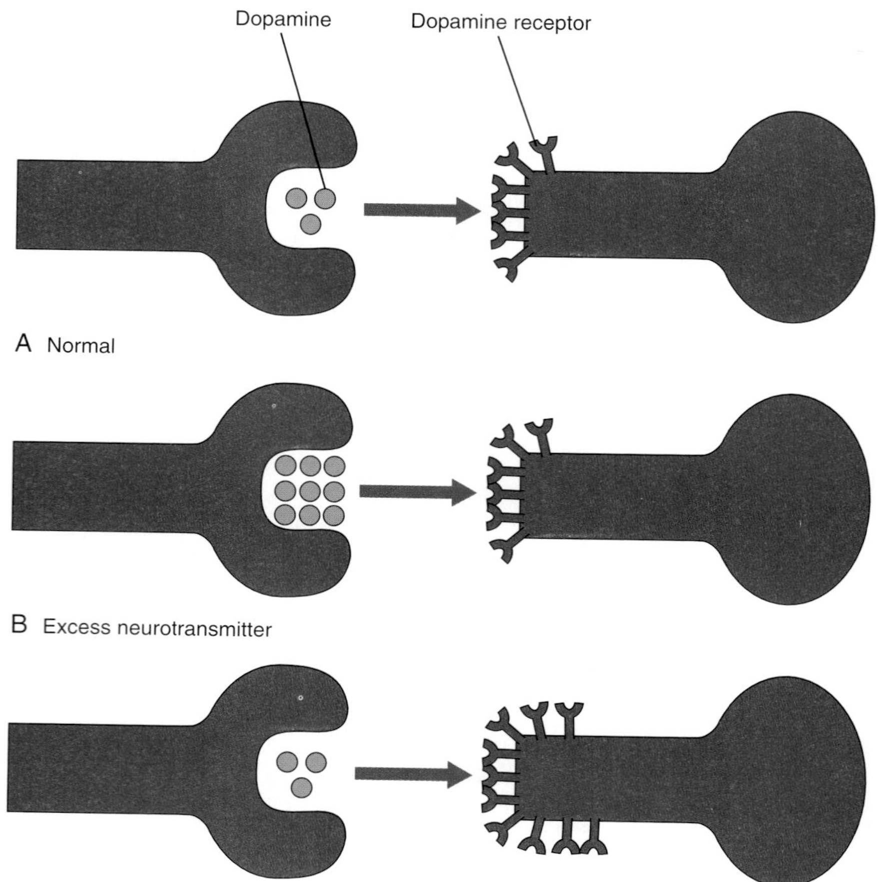

Figure 3–11 Causes of excessive transmission of neurotransmitters. Excess in transmission may be due to excess release of transmitter, as shown in *(B)*, or by excess responsiveness of receptors, as shown in *(C)*.

are dysfunctional in different psychiatric conditions. These differences offer more specific targets for drug action. In fact, much of what is known about the relationship between specific transmitters and specific disturbances has been derived from a knowledge of the pharmacology of the drugs used to treat these conditions. For example, it was found that most agents that were effective in reducing the delusions and hallucinations of schizophrenia block the D_2 receptors for dopamine. From this information, it was concluded that delusions and hallucinations result from overactivity of dopamine at these receptors.

Antipsychotic Drugs

Standard Antipsychotics

Box 3–3 illustrates the proposed mechanism of action of the standard (first-generation) antipsychotic drugs: the phenothiazines, thioxanthenes, butyrophenones, and pharmacologically related agents. These drugs are strong antagonists of the D_2 receptors for dopamine. By attaching to these receptors and blocking the attachment of dopamine, they reduce dopaminergic transmission. It has been postulated that an overactivity of the dopamine system in certain areas of the limbic system may be responsible for at least some of the symptoms of schizophrenia; thus, blockage of dopamine may reduce these symptoms. This is thought to be particularly true of the "positive" symptoms of schizophrenia, such as delusions (e.g., paranoid and grandiose ideas) and hallucinations (e.g., hearing or seeing things not present in reality) (refer to Chapter 22).

These drugs, however, are also to varying degrees **antagonists** (blocking the action) at muscarinic receptors for acetylcholine and $alpha_1$ receptors for norepinephrine. Although it is unclear if this antagonism plays a role in the beneficial effects of the drugs, it is certain that antagonism is responsible for some of the major side effects.

As summarized in Box 3–4, many of the untoward side effects of these drugs can be understood as a logical extension of their receptor-blocking activity. Thus, since dopamine in the basal ganglia plays a major role in the regulation of movement, it is not surprising that dopamine blockage can lead to motor abnormalities such as parkinsonism, akinesia, akathisia, and tardive dyskinesia. Nurses and physicians often monitor clients for evidence of involuntary motor movement after administration of the standard antipsychotic agents. One popular scale is called the Abnormal Involuntary Movement Scale

BOX 3–3 HOW THE STANDARD (FIRST-GENERATION) ANTIPSYCHOTIC DRUGS WORK

It is thought that at least some of the symptoms of psychosis are due to an excess of the neurotransmitter dopamine in those areas of the brain involved in thought and in emotions. Most antipsychotic drugs (phenothiazines and related compounds) seem to produce many of their beneficial effects as well as some of their undesired side effects by blocking dopamine receptors and thus reducing dopamine-induced responses in the brain.

When a patient takes an antipsychotic medication, even though excess dopamine may be released by presynaptic cells in the brain, it will not cause a corresponding response in the postsynaptic cells because the receptors to which dopamine must attach are blocked by the medication. Because dopamine is used as a neurotransmitter in many areas of the brain in addition to those involved in thought and emotion, blocking of these receptors can also lead to serious untoward effects. Specifically, dopamine is a neurotransmitter in the basal ganglia, where it is involved in modulating and fine-tuning motor activity. Blocking of dopamine receptors in this area of the brain probably accounts for the disorders of movement (known as extrapyramidal effects), such as parkinsonian symptoms, that can result from the use of antipsychotic drugs. In fact, Parkinson's disease is thought to result from a deficiency of dopamine in the basal ganglia.

Dopamine also plays a normal physiological role as an inhibitor of prolactin release. Blocking of dopamine receptors by the antipsychotic drugs can therefore lead to elevated levels of prolactin in the blood. This abnormally high level of prolactin may induce disturbances such as galactorrhea in women and gynecomastia in men.

To understand more fully the pharmacology of the antipsychotic drugs, it is necessary to recognize that these agents block other types of receptors in addition to those for dopamine. In particular, they can block the muscarinic receptors for acetylcholine and the alpha$_1$ receptors for norepinephrine. The degree to which individual drugs block these receptors varies to a considerable extent.

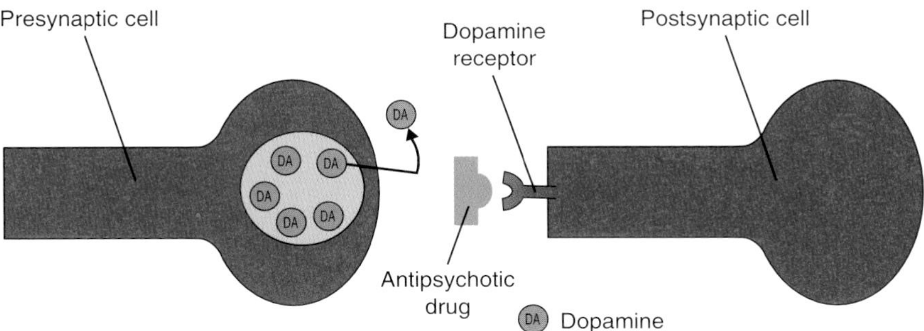

BLOCKING OF MUSCARINIC RECEPTORS

Because it is the attachment of acetylcholine to muscarinic receptors on smooth muscle, cardiac muscle, and exocrine gland cells that is responsible for the actions of the parasympathetic nervous system, it follows that blockage of these receptors will have antiparasympathetic effects. Included in these effects are blurred vision, tachycardia, constipation, and urinary retention.

BLOCKING OF ALPHA$_1$ RECEPTORS

Stimulation of alpha$_1$ receptors by norepinephrine is normally responsible for the vasoconstriction necessary to maintain blood pressure when a person is in the upright position. Therefore, the consequence of alpha$_1$-receptor blocking is often orthostatic hypotension.

(AIMS). See Box 3–5 and practice with a classmate the administration of AIMS. These disturbances and others are discussed in Chapter 22, which details the clinical use of the antipsychotic drugs along with specific nursing interventions and client teaching strategies.

An important physiological function of dopamine is that it acts as the hypothalamic factor that inhibits the release of prolactin from the anterior pituitary gland; thus, blockage of dopamine transmission can lead to increased pituitary secretion of prolactin. In women this hyperprolactinemia can result in amenorrhea (absence of the menses) or galactorrhea (milk flow), and in men it can lead to gynecomastia (development of the male mammary glands).

Acetylcholine is the neurotransmitter released by the postganglionic neurons of the parasympathetic nervous system; through its attachment to muscarinic receptors on internal organs, it serves to help regulate internal function. Blockage of the muscarinic receptors by phenothiazines and a wide variety of other psychiatric drugs can lead to a constellation of untoward effects predictable from a knowledge of the normal physiology of the

BOX 3–4 UNTOWARD EFFECTS OF DOPAMINE, MUSCARINIC, AND ALPHA$_1$ ANTAGONISM

DOPAMINE BLOCKAGE

Movement defects
- Parkinsonian symptoms
- Akinesia
- Akathisia
- Tardive dyskinesia

Decreased prolactin
- Gynecomastia in men
- Galactorrhea-amenorrhea in women

MUSCARININC BLOCKAGE

Blurred vision
Dry mouth
Constipation
Urinary difficulty

ALPHA$_1$ ANTAGONISM

Orthostatic hypotension
Failure to ejaculate

parasympathetic nervous system. These side effects typically involve blurred vision, dry mouth, constipation, and urinary hesitancy.

In addition to blocking dopamine and muscarinic receptors, many of the first-generation antipsychotic drugs act as antagonists at the alpha$_1$ receptors for norepinephrine. These receptors are found on smooth muscle cells that contract in response to norepinephrine from sympathetic nerves. For example, the ability of sympathetic nerves to constrict blood vessels is dependent on the attachment of norepinephrine to alpha$_1$ receptors; thus, blockage of these receptors can bring about vasodilation and a consequent drop in blood pressure. Sympathetic mediated vasoconstriction is particularly essential for maintaining normal blood pressure in the upright position; blockage of the alpha$_1$ receptors can lead to orthostatic hypotension.

Alpha$_1$ receptors are also found on the vas deferens and are responsible for the propulsive contractions leading to ejaculation. Blockage of these receptors can lead to a failure to ejaculate.

Atypical Antipsychotics

The atypical antipsychotic agents have few or no extrapyramidal symptoms and also target the negative and the positive symptoms of schizophrenia, as discussed in Chapter 22.

CLOZAPINE. Clozapine (Clozaril) is an antipsychotic drug that is relatively free of the untoward motor effects of the phenothiazines and other first-generation antipsychotics. It is thought that clozapine preferentially blocks the dopamine receptors in the limbic system rather than those in the neostriatal area of the basal ganglia. This allows this agent to exert an antipsychotic action without leading to difficulties with movement.

Clozapine can have a possibly fatal side effect in about 1% of clients. This is due to its potential to suppress bone marrow and induce agranulocytosis. Any deficiency in white blood cells renders a person prone to serious infection. For this reason, regular weekly measurement of white blood cell count is mandatory for any client taking clozapine.

Clozapine also has the potential for inducing convulsions in a small percentage (3%) of clients. This means that all clients taking the drug must be monitored closely.

The most common side effects are drowsiness and sedation (40%), hypersalivation (30%), tachycardia (25%), and dizziness (20%).

RISPERIDONE. Risperidone (Risperdal) is an antipsychotic drug that shares with clozapine the ability to treat psychotic symptoms of delusions and hallucinations without frequently inducing motor abnormalities, as many of the older drugs did. Unlike clozapine, it does not seem to have the potential for inducing agranulocytosis or convulsions. These advantages are offset, however, by the fact that at doses of risperidone only slightly higher than those that are effective, clients taking this drug may begin to experience motor difficulties. Because risperidone blocks alpha$_1$ and histamine-1 (H_1) receptors, it can cause orthostatic hypotension and sedation. Keep in mind that orthostatic hypotension can lead to falls, which are a serious problem among the elderly.

OLANZAPINE. Olanzapine (Zyprexa) is a more recent antipsychotic that appears to have the efficacy of clozapine, but without the dangerous side effects.

Chapter 22 discusses thought disorders and the treatments and nursing care for them, giving detailed information about action, dosage, nursing implications, and teaching strategies for both the standard and atypical antipsychotic medications.

SERTINDOLE. At this writing, sertindole has not yet been released. Preliminary studies support sertindole's efficacy with the positive symptoms of schizophrenia and at higher doses (e.g., 20 mg or higher) with the negative symptoms of schizophrenia.

Mood Stabilizers

Antimanic Drugs

LITHIUM. Although the efficacy of lithium as a mood-stabilizing drug in bipolar (manic-depressive) clients has been established for many years, its mechanism of action is still far from understood. As a positively charged ion, similar in structure to sodium and potassium, it may well act by affecting electrical conductivity in neurons.

BOX 3-5 ABNORMAL INVOLUNTARY MOVEMENT SCALE

DEPARTMENT OF HUMAN SERVICES
PUBLIC HEALTH SERVICE
Alcohol, Drug Abuse, and Mental Health Administration
NIMH Treatment Strategies in Schizophrenia Study

ABNORMAL INVOLUNTARY MOVEMENT SCALE (AIMS)

PATINET NUMBER	DATA GROUP	EVALUATION DATE
— — — —	aims	— — — — — — M M D D Y Y

PATIENT NAME

RATER NAME

RATER NUMBER — — —

EVALUATION TYPE (*Circle*)

1 Baseline	4 Start double-blind	7 Start open meds	10 Early termination
2 2-week minor	5 Major evaluation	8 During open meds	11 Study completion
3	6 Other	9 Stop open meds	

INSTRUCTIONS: Complete Examination Procedure (reverse side) before making ratings.
MOVEMENT RATINGS: Rate highest severity observed.

Code: 1 = None; 2 = Minimal, may be extreme normal; 3 = Mild; 4 = Moderate; 5 = Severe

		(Circle One)				
FACIAL AND ORAL MOVEMENTS:	**1. Muscles of facial expression** e.g., movements of forehead, eyebrows, periorbital area, cheeks; include frowning, blinking, smiling, grimacing	1	2	3	4	5
	2. Lips and perioral area e.g., puckering, pouting, smacking	1	2	3	4	5
	3. Jaw e.g., biting, clenching, chewing, mouth opening, lateral movement	1	2	3	4	5
	4. Tongue Rate only increase in movement both in and out of mouth, NOT inability to sustain movement	1	2	3	4	5
EXTREMITY MOVEMENTS:	**5. Upper** (*arms, wrists, hands, fingers*) Include choreic movements (rapid, objectively purposeless, irregular, spontaneous), athetoid movements (slow, irregular, complex, serpentine). Do NOT include tremor (repetitive, regular, rhythmic)	1	2	3	4	5
	6. Lower (*legs, knees, ankles, toes*) e.g., lateral knee movement, foot tapping, heel dropping, foot squirming, inversion and eversion of foot	1	2	3	4	5
TRUNK MOVEMENTS:	**7. Neck, shoulders, hips** e.g., rocking, twisting, squirming, pelvic gyrations	1	2	3	4	5

GLOBAL JUDGMENTS:	**8. Severity of abnormal movements**	None, minimal	1
		Minimal	2
		Mild	3
		Moderate	4
		Severe	5
	9. Incapacitation due to abnormal movements	None, minimal	1
		Minimal	2
		Mild	3
		Moderate	4
		Severe	5
	10. Patient's awareness of abnormal movements Rate only patient's report	No awareness	1
		Aware, no distress	2
		Aware, mild distress	3
		Aware, moderate distress	4
		Aware, severe distress	5
DENTAL STATUS:	**11. Current problem with teeth and/or dentures?**	No	1
		Yes	2
	12. Does patient usually wear dentures?	No	1
		Yes	2

Continued

BOX 3–5 ABNORMAL INVOLUNTARY MOVEMENT SCALE *(Continued)*

EXAMINATION PROCEDURE

Either before or after completing the examination procedure, observe the patient unobtrusively, at rest (e.g., in waiting room).

The chair to be used in this examination should be a hard, firm one without arms.

1. Ask patient to remove shoes and socks.
2. Ask patient whether there is anything in his/her mouth (i.e., gum candy, etc.) and if there is, to remove it.
3. Ask patient about current condition of his/her teeth. Ask patient if he/she wears dentures. Do teeth or dentures bother the patient *now?*
4. Ask patient whether he/she notices any movements in mouth, face, hands, or feet. If yes, ask to describe and to what extent they *currently* bother patient or interfere with his/her activities.
5. Have patient sit in chair with hands on knees, legs slightly apart, and feet flat on floor. (Look at entire body movements while in this position.)
6. Ask patient to sit with hands hanging unsupported: if male, between legs; if female and wearing a dress, hanging over knees. (Observe hands and other body areas.)
7. Ask patient to open mouth. (Observe tongue at rest within mouth.) Do this twice.
8. Ask patient to protrude tongue. (Observe abnormalities of tongue movement.) Do this twice.
9. Ask patient to tap thumb, with each finger, as rapidly as possible for 10 to 15 seconds: separately with right hand, then with left hand. (Observe each facial and leg movement.)
10. Flex and extend patient's left and right arms (one at a time). (Note any rigidity.)
11. Ask patient to stand up. (Observe in profile. Observe all body areas again, hips included.)
12. Ask patient to extend both arms outstretched in front with palms down. (Observe trunk, legs, and mouth).
13. Have patient walk a few paces, turn, and walk back to chair. (Observe hands and gait.) Do this twice.

As we saw in Figure 3–2, an electrical impulse consists of the inward, depolarizing flow of sodium followed by an outward, repolarizing of potassium. These electrical charges are propagated along the neuron so that if they are initiated at one end of the neuron they will pass to the other end. Once they reach the end of a neuron, a transmitter is released.

It may be that an overexcitement of neurons in some parts of the brain underlies bipolar disorders, and that lithium interacts in some complex way with sodium and potassium at the cell membrane to stabilize electrical activity. Even if not responsible for its beneficial effects, an alteration in electrical conductivity certainly explains some of the untoward effects and toxicity of lithium.

By altering electrical conductivity, lithium represents a potential threat to all body functions that are regulated by electrical currents. Foremost among these functions, of course, is cardiac contraction, so that lithium can induce cardiac dysrhythmias. Extreme alteration of cerebral conductivity can lead to convulsions. Alteration in nerve and muscle conduction can lead to tremor or more extreme motor dysfunction.

The fact that sodium and potassium play a strong role in regulating fluid balance and the distribution of fluid in various body compartments explains the disturbances in fluid balance that can be caused by lithium. These include polyuria (the output of large volumes of urine), polydipsia (the intake of large volumes of water), and edema (the accumulation of fluid in the interstitial space). There seems to be some evidence that long-term use of lithium increases the risk of kidney and thyroid disease.

Primarily because of its effects on electrical conductivity, lithium has the lowest therapeutic index of all psychiatric drugs. The **therapeutic index** represents the ratio of the lethal dose to the effective dose, and thus the safety of a drug. A low therapeutic index means that the blood level of a drug that can cause death is not far removed from the blood level required for drug effectiveness. This means that the blood level of lithium needs to be monitored on a regular basis to be sure that the drug is not accumulating and rising to dangerous levels. Table 3–3 lists some of the untoward effects of lithium.

CARBAMAZEPINE AND CLONAZEPAM. Carbamazepine and clonazepam were originally introduced as anticonvulsant agents but are now being used to treat a variety of psychiatric conditions. Their anticonvulsant properties derive from the fact that they alter electrical conductivity in membranes; in particular, they reduce the firing rate of very-high-frequency neurons in the brain. It is possible that this membrane-stabilizing effect accounts for the ability of these drugs to reduce the mood swings that occur in bipolar clients. The drugs are particularly effective in reducing the excitement of the manic phase of this disease; thus, they are sometimes used to calm a manic client before long-term stabilization with lithium. When the client cannot tolerate lithium, carbamazepine or clonazepam may be used for long-term maintenance therapy.

Carbamazepine (Tegretol) is structurally similar to the tricyclic antidepressants (TCAs) (see below), although it is not clear if it shares the ability of these drugs to treat unipolar depression. Carbamazepine does, however, share the ability of TCAs to serve as a neurological analgesic. It is particularly effective in conditions such as trigeminal neuralgia that involve paroxysms (bursts) of severe pain. The efficacy of carbamazepine as an analgesic may be related to its ability to reduce the firing rate of overexcited neurons as well as to its ability to calm the accompanying psychological agitation associated with the pain.

Clonazepam (Klonopin) is structurally a benzodiazepine, a type of antianxiety drug discussed later in this chapter. These drugs have strong sedating properties, which may in part account for the ability of clonazepam to calm a client rapidly in the manic phase of a bipolar disorder. Clonazepam is also increasingly being used as part of a multiple-drug regimen to treat clients who show a mixture of anxious and depressive symptoms concomitantly; these individuals are sometimes given both antidepressants and antianxiety agents.

The dosage, side effects, nursing implications, and client teaching strategies for the antimanic drugs are covered in Chapter 21.

TABLE 3–3 UNTOWARD EFFECTS OF LITHIUM

SYSTEM	UNTOWARD EFFECTS
Nervous system and muscle	Tremor, ataxia, confusion, convulsions
Digestive	Nausea, vomiting, diarrhea
Cardiac	Arrhythmias
Fluid and electrolyte	Polyuria, polydipsia, edema
Endocrine	Goiter and hyperthyroidism

Antidepressant Drugs

Our understanding of the neurophysiological basis of mood disorders is far from complete. However, a great deal of evidence seems to indicate that the neurotransmitters norepinephrine and serotonin play a major role in regulating mood. It is thought that a transmission deficiency of one or both of these monoamines within the limbic system underlies depression. One of the lines of evidence pointing in this direction is that all the drugs that show efficacy in the treatment of depression increase the synaptic level of one or both of these transmitters. Figure 3–12 illustrates the normal release, reuptake, and destruction of the monoamine transmitters. A grasp of this underlying physiology is essential for understanding the mechanisms by which the antidepressant drugs are thought to act.

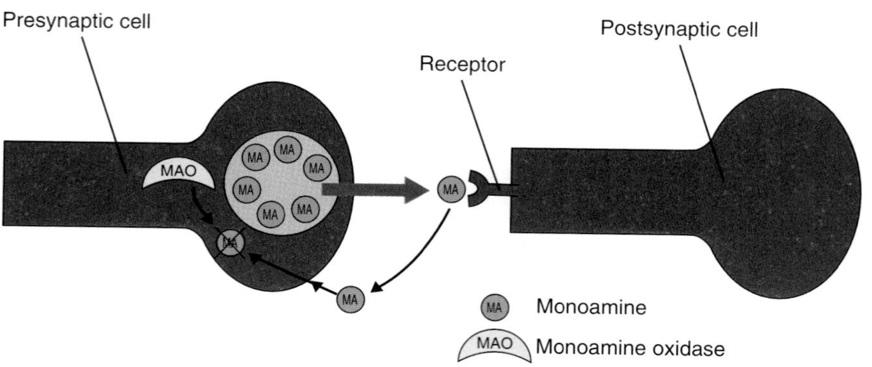

Figure 3–12 Normal release, reuptake, and destruction of the monoamine transmitters.

Box 3–6 HOW THE TRICYCLIC ANTIDEPRESSANT DRUGS WORK

Whether the original cause of depression is biological, psychological, or social, its symptomatic expression seems to be associated with a deficiency of either or both of the monoamine neurotransmitters norepinephrine and serotonin. The most commonly used pharmacological interventions for the treatment of depression are directed at increasing the activity of these transmitters. Tricyclic antidepressant drugs accomplish this task by blocking the reuptake of norepinephrine and, to a lesser degree, of serotonin into the presynaptic cell, as illustrated.

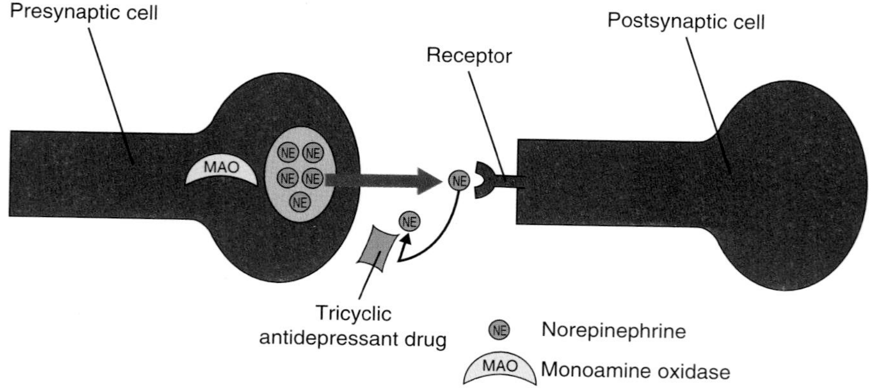

Blocking norepinephrine reentry into the presynaptic cell increases the concentration of this transmitter in the synaptic space and, presumably, its action on the postsynaptic cell. This explanation of the beneficial actions of tricyclic drugs is called into question somewhat by the fact that the blockage of transmitter reuptake occurs immediately, whereas the alleviation of depressive symptoms by these drugs usually takes 2 or 3 weeks. Although a number of theories attempt to explain this discrepancy, a proved and agreed explanation is not available at present.

The pharmacological actions of the tricyclic antidepressants are not limited to the blockade of monoamine reuptake and destruction. As is the case with the phenothiazines, these drugs can block muscarinic and alpha$_1$-adrenergic receptors. Many of these agents have quite strong muscarinic blocking ability and can produce the predictable antiparasympathetic responses of blurred vision, constipation, tachycardia, and urinary retention. Alpha$_1$ antagonism blocks the pressor response necessary to avoid orthostatic hypotension.

Although an antidepressant drug might be thought to be somewhat of a stimulant, this is not the case for the tricyclic drugs. In fact, many of these drugs have strong sedating properties. The sedating actions of tricyclic drugs are believed to be due to their ability to block histamine receptors in the brain.

In addition to those untoward effects attributable to known mechanisms of action, most drugs can also have undesirable actions for which there is no clear-cut explanation at present. The most serious toxic and life-threatening effects of tricyclic drugs at high doses are convulsions and the depression of cardiac conductivity and contractility. The therapeutic index (ratio of toxic dose to safe dose) of tricyclic drugs is low, and they are potential agents of accidental and deliberate death.

TRICYCLIC ANTIDEPRESSANTS. The TCAs, such as amitriptyline (Elavil), imipramine (Tofranil), and nortriptyline (Pamelor), are thought to act primarily by blocking the reuptake of norepinephrine and, to a lesser degree, serotonin. As described in Box 3–6, this blocking prevents norepinephrine from coming into contact with its degrading enzyme, MAO, and thus increases the level of norepinephrine at the synapse. Similarly, the TCAs block the reuptake and destruction of serotonin and also increase the synaptic level of this type of transmitter. Exactly how the increased level of these transmitters alleviates depression is far from clear; however, many controlled scientific studies attest to the efficacy of these drugs.

To varying degrees, many of the tricyclic drugs also block the muscarinic receptors that normally bind acetylcholine. As discussed in the previous section, this blockage leads to typical anticholinergic effects such as blurred vision, dry mouth, tachycardia, and constipation. These untoward effects can be troubling to clients and can limit their compliance with the regimen.

Again to varying degrees, depending on the individual drug, the drugs can block H_1 receptors in the brain. Blockage of these receptors by any drug causes sedation and drowsiness, an unwelcome symptom in daily use.

SELECTIVE SEROTONIN REUPTAKE INHIBITORS. As the name implies, the selective serotonin reuptake inhibitors (SSRIs), such as fluoxetine (Prozac), sertraline (Zoloft), and paroxetine (Paxil), preferentially block the reuptake and thus the destruction of serotonin, with little or no effect on the other monoamine transmitters. These drugs, as a group, also have less ability to block the muscarinic and H_1 receptors than do the tricyclic agents. As a result of their more selective action, they seem to show comparable efficacy while not presenting the anticholinergic and sedating side effects that limit client compliance (Box 3–7).

MONOAMINE OXIDASE INHIBITORS. These are a group of antidepressant drugs that illustrate the principle that drugs can have a desired, beneficial effect in the brain, while at the same time having possibly dangerous effects elsewhere in the body. To understand the action of these drugs, keep in mind the following definitions:

- Monoamines: a type of organic compound; includes the neurotransmitters norepinephrine, epinephrine, dopamine, and serotonin as well as many different food substances and drugs
- Monoamine oxidase (MAO): an enzyme that destroys monoamines
- Monoamine oxidase inhibitors (MAOIs): drugs that prevent the destruction of monoamines by inhibiting the action of MAO

The monoamine neurotransmitters, as well as any monamine food substance or drugs, are degraded (destroyed) by the enzyme MAO, which is located in neu-

BOX 3–7 HOW THE INHIBITORS OF SEROTONIN REUPTAKE (SSRIs) WORK

Fluoxetine, sertraline, paroxetine, and related selective serotonin reuptake inhibitors (SSRIs) specifically block the reuptake of serotonin (5-hydroxytryptamine) into the presynaptic cell from which it was originally released. As a result of this blockage, in a fashion analogous to the action of tricyclic antidepressants on norepinephrine, the destruction of the transmitter is reduced and its concentration at the postsynaptic cell increased. Because these drugs are specific to serotonin and have little or no ability to block muscarinic and other receptors, they tend to have fewer untoward autonomic effects than the tricyclic drugs. In addition, they do not cause as much sedation or have cardiac toxicity. However, to the degree that depression involves norepinephrine deficiency and presents with symptoms of agitation, the serotonin blockers may have less efficacy than the tricyclic antidepressants. Major untoward effects of the serotonin blockers include excessive stimulation and anorexia among susceptible patients.

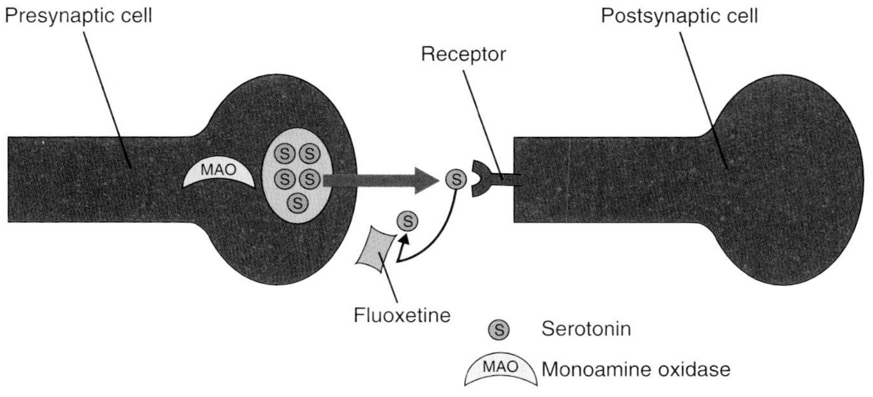

rons and in the liver. Antidepressant drugs such as phenelzine (Nardil) and tranylcypromine (Parnate) are MAOIs; that is, they act by inhibiting the enzyme and interfering with the destruction of the monoamine neurotransmitters. This in turn increases the synaptic level of the transmitters (Box 3–8) and makes possible the antidepressant effects of these drugs.

The use of MAO-inhibiting drugs is complicated by the fact that the enzyme is also present in the liver and is responsible for degrading monoamine substances that enter the body via food or drugs. Of particular importance is the monoamine tyramine, which is present in many food substances such as aged cheeses, pickled or smoked fish, and wine. Tyramine poses a threat of hypertensive crises because it can produce intense vasoconstriction, and thus an elevation in blood pressure, if allowed to circulate freely in the blood. Normally, this does not happen, because tyramine is destroyed by MAO as it passes through the liver before entering the general blood circulation. However, in the presence of MAOIs, tyramine is not destroyed by the liver and can cause serious, even life-threatening, hypertension.

A substantial number of drugs are chemically monoamines. The dosage of these drugs is determined by the rate at which they are destroyed by MAO in the liver. In a client on MAOIs, the blood level of monoamine drugs can reach high levels and present serious toxicity.

Because of the dangers that result from destruction of

BOX 3–8 HOW THE MONOAMINE OXIDASE INHIBITORS WORK

As illustrated, inhibitors of the enzyme monoamine oxidase (MAO) act by interfering with the ability of this enzyme to destroy the monoamines norepinephrine, dopamine, and serotonin (5-hydroxytryptamine). Enzyme inhibition eventually leads to an increase in the presynaptic, synaptic, and postsynaptic concentrations of these neurotransmitters. Increased postsynaptic activity of one or more of these transmitters would then account for the beneficial effects of these drugs in certain forms of depression. As with the tricyclic drugs, this explanation still leaves unsolved the problem of the 2- to 3-week time lag between enzyme inactivation and clinical improvement.

MAO is present in liver cells, as well as in monoamine-releasing neurons. In the liver, this enzyme has the function of destroying circulating endogenous monoamines (e.g., the hormone epinephrine) and exogenous monoamines (e.g., tyramine), which are present in many foods and readily absorbed from the digestive tract. Inactivation of hepatic MAO by MAO-inhibiting drugs can lead to a potentially fatal interaction between these drugs and foods such as aged cheeses, which contain significant amounts of tyramine. This is because tyramine can trigger the release of norepinephrine from sympathetic nerve endings. Norepinephrine is a potent vasoconstrictor, and the sudden release of large amounts of norepinephrine in response to tyramine can produce a life-threatening hypertensive crisis. In the absence of MAO-inhibiting drugs, tyramine does not present a problem because it is destroyed by MAO when the absorbed food is brought to the liver by the blood passing through the hepatic portal system. To avoid the possibility of a hypertensive crisis, patients are given a list of proscribed foods that contain large amounts of tyramine.

A large number of pharmacological agents, particularly sympathomimetic drugs, are monoamines and are broken down by hepatic MAO. The plasma level of such drugs resulting from a given dose may be vastly increased in the presence of MAO-inhibiting drugs. Thus, these drugs must be used with great care, if at all, in a patient who is also taking MAO inhibitors. Because many of the monoamine drugs are sold over the counter, patients taking MAO inhibitors must be given a list of drugs as well as foods to be avoided.

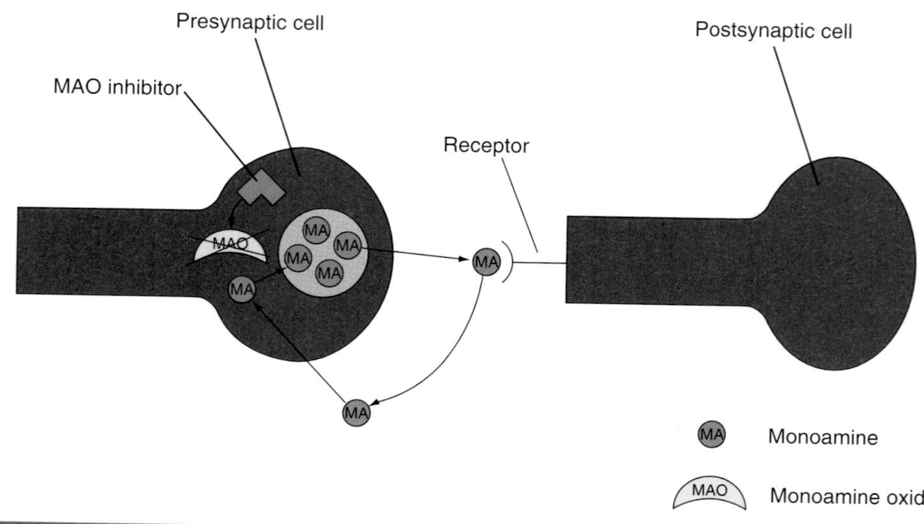

hepatic MAO, clients on MAO-inhibiting drugs must be given a list of food and drugs high in tyramine that need to be avoided. Chapter 20 discusses the treatment of depression and contains a list of forbidden foods and foods to be taken in moderation, along with nursing measures and instructions for client teaching.

ATYPICAL ANTIDEPRESSANTS. A number of drugs that seem to work by mechanisms less clearly defined than those of the TCAs, SSRIs, and MAOIs are sometimes grouped together under the heading of atypical antidepressants. Of these, we will briefly discuss three: trazodone, nefazodone, and venlafaxine.

Trazodone and nefazodone are chemically related compounds that affect the reuptake of serotonin and, to a lesser degree, norepinephrine. They differ from the TCAs and SSRIs in that they and their metabolites (chemicals formed from the drugs by the liver) can act directly on the 5-hydroxytryptamine (5-HT) postsynaptic receptors for serotonin. The complexity of relating the biological actions of a drug to its clinical effects is well illustrated by these agents, in that the drugs themselves can antagonize the receptors while their metabolites act as receptor agents. Thus, we have drugs that increase the concentration of serotonin at the synapse by blocking its reuptake, that mimic serotonin at the receptor, and that form chemicals that block serotonin at the receptor. We are left with a question as to the overall physiological results of these drugs and how they stack up to their proved efficacy in reducing depression.

Trazodone (Desyrel) is a very weak antagonist of muscarinic receptors that was originally introduced as an alternative to the TCAs, which have strong anticholinergic actions. It does, however, block $alpha_1$ and H_1 receptors and thus can cause orthostatic hypotension and sedation. These are very serious problems in the elderly, since they can increase the likelihood of falls and broken bones. Trazodone has also been associated with priapism in males; this is a painful, continuous erectile state unrelated to sexual desires or activity.

Nefazodone (Serzone), a newer relative of trazodone, does not block $alpha_1$ and H_1 receptors, so it does not lead to orthostatic hypotension and sedation, but it has proved to be an effective antidepressant agent.

Venlafaxine (Effexor) is a newer antidepressant that blocks the reuptake of both norepinephrine and serotonin. Since it does not block muscarinic, $alpha_1$, or H_1 receptors, it is relatively free of the untoward effects that occur when these receptors are inhibited. It has been found particularly useful in the treatment of severely depressed and melancholic clients. For reasons not currently understood, it can cause some clients to feel heightened anxiety and the very uncomfortable sensations of nausea, vomiting, and dizziness. It has also been associated with abnormal ejaculation and impotence in males. Refer to Chapter 20 for the nursing implications, dosages, side effects, and toxic effects of each group of antidepressants, as well as teaching tools.

Antianxiety/Anxiolytic Drugs

As illustrated in Figure 3–13, the neurotransmitter GABA seems to exert an inhibitory effect on neurons in many parts of the brain. Drugs that can enhance this effect exert a sedative-hypnotic action on brain function. Many drugs with this type of effect tend to reduce anxiety and some are actually used as antianxiety agents. The most commonly used drugs of this group are the benzodiazepines.

BENZODIAZEPINES. Figure 3–14 shows that benzodiazepines—e.g., diazepam (Valium), clonazepam (Klonopin), and alprazolam (Xanax)—bind to specific receptors adjacent to the GABA receptors. Because of their ability to bind benzodiazepines, these receptors are called benzodiazepine receptors. Binding of benzodiazepines to these receptors strengthens the action of GABA; that is, binding of benzodiazepines at the same time as GABA allows GABA to inhibit more forcefully than it would if binding alone. The fact that benzodiazepines do not inhibit neurons in the absence of GABA limits the potential toxicity of these drugs.

Of the various benzodiazepines, some, such as flurazepam (Dalmane) and triazolam (Halcion), have a predominantly hypnotic (sleep-inducing) effect, whereas others, such as lorazepam (Ativan) and alprazolam (Xanax), reduce anxiety without being as soporific (sleep producing). Currently, there is no clear explanation for the differential effects of the various benzodiazepines. There seems to be some evidence that there are subtypes of the benzodiazepine receptors in different areas of the brain, and these subtypes differ in their ability to bind the different drugs.

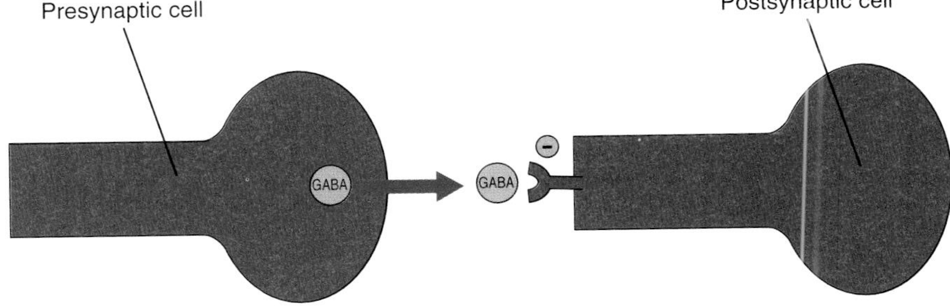

Figure 3–13 Action of gamma-aminorbutyric acid (GABA). GABA has primarily inhibitory effects on postsynaptic cells; it renders them less likely to have electrical impulses.

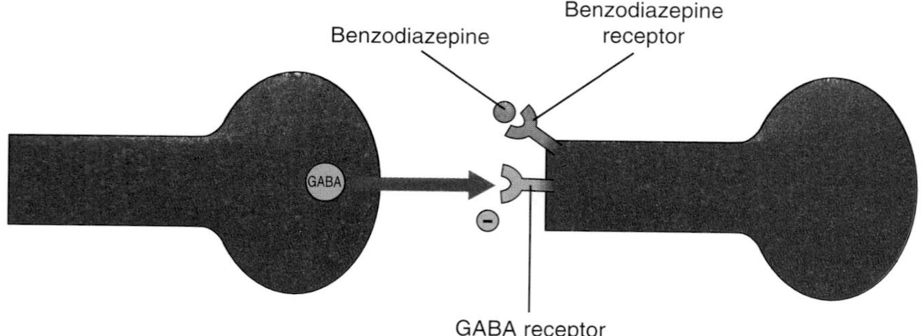

Figure 3–14 Action of benzodiazepines. The group of drugs called benzodiazepines attach to receptors adjacent to the receptors for the neurotransmitter GABA. Drug attachment to receptors results in a strengthening of the inhibitory effects of GABA. In the absence of GABA, there is no inhibitory effect of benzodiazepines.

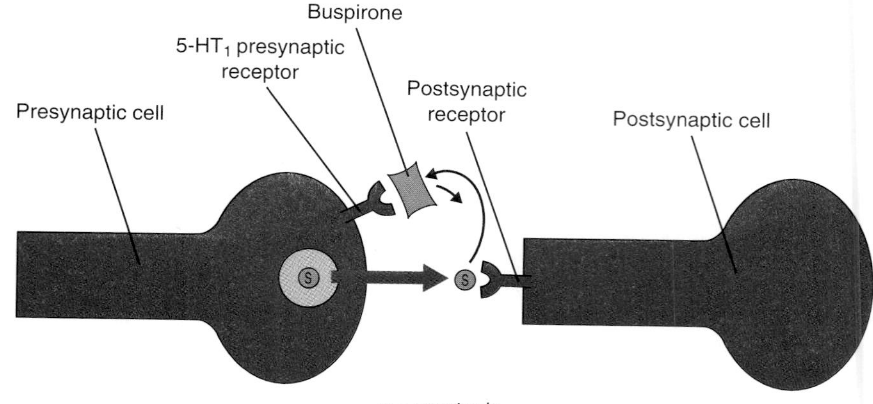

Figure 3–15 Action of buspirone. A proposed mechanism of action for buspirone is that it blocks feedback inhibition by serotonin. This leads to increased release of serotonin by the presynaptic cell.

The fact that the benzodiazepines potentate the ability of GABA to inhibit neurons probably accounts for their efficacy as anticonvulsants and for their ability to reduce the neuronal overexcitement of alcohol withdrawal. When used alone, even at high doses, these drugs rarely inhibit the brain to the degree of respiratory depression, coma, and death. However, when combined with other CNS depressants, such as alcohol, opiates, or TCAs, the inhibitory actions of the benzodiazepines can lead to life-threatening respiratory depression.

Any drug that inhibits electrical activity in the brain can interfere with motor ability, attention, and judgment; a client taking benzodiazepines must be cautioned about activities that could be dangerous if reflexes and attention are impaired. This includes specialized activities such as working in construction on a tall building and more common activities such as driving a car. In the elderly, the use of benzodiazepines may contribute to falls and broken bones. Chapter 17 discusses the nursing considerations, indications, side and toxic effects, and teaching strategies for clients taking benzodiazepines.

BUSPIRONE. Buspirone (BuSpar) is a drug that reduces anxiety, without having strong sedative-hypnotic properties. Since this agent does not leave the client sleepy or sluggish, it is often much better tolerated than the benzodiazepines. It is also not a CNS depressant and thus does not represent as great a danger of interaction with other CNS depressants such as alcohol, nor is there the potential for addiction that exists with benzodiazepines.

Although at present the mechanism of action of buspirone is not clearly understood, one possibility is illustrated in Figure 3–15. Buspirone seems to act as an antagonist at presynaptic 5-HT_1 receptors. The normal function of these receptors is to monitor the synaptic level of serotonin; that is, serotonin released by the neurons binds not only to postsynaptic receptors to exert its effects on adjacent neurons but also to presynaptic receptors on the neuron from which it is released. Once bound to the presynaptic receptor, serotonin inhibits the further release of this transmitter; this release serves as negative feedback. Buspirone, by blocking these presynaptic receptors, prevents the negative feedback and allows more transmitter to be released. The end result is an increased synaptic level of serotonin that presumably accounts for the beneficial action of this drug.

SUMMARY

The brain is responsible for directing appropriate responses to change in both the external and internal environments. To carry out this responsibility, the brain must receive information from sensory structures, process the information, and then direct appropriate responses. It is guided in its responses by basic drives, emotional status, memory, and thought processes. For interpersonal responses, language must also be employed.

All these responsibilities must be carried out physiologically through the interactions of nerve cells. These interactions involve impulse conduction, transmitter release, and receptor response. Alterations in these basic processes can lead to mental disturbances and physical manifestations.

In particular, it seems that excess activity of dopamine is involved in the thought disturbances of schizophrenia, and that deficiencies of norepinephrine and/or serotonin underlie the mood disturbances of depression. Insufficient activity of GABA seems to play a role in anxiety.

Pharmacological treatment of mental disturbances is directed at the suspected transmitter-receptor problem. Thus, antipsychotic drugs block dopamine receptors, antidepressant drugs increase synaptic levels of norepinephrine and/or serotonin, and antianxiety drugs increase the effectiveness of GABA.

Unfortunately, as is the case for almost all pharmacological agents, the agents used to treat mental disease can also cause various undesired effects. Prominent among these can be sedation or excitement, motor disturbances, muscarinic blockage, and alpha antagonism. There is a continuing effort on the part of pharmacologists to develop new drugs that are effective as well as safe and comfortable for people suffering from emotional disorders.

FURTHER READING

American College of Neuropsychopharmacology. (1992). Suicidal behavior and psychotropic medication (consensus statement). *Neuropsychopharmacology*, 8:177.

Andersen, P. H., et al. (1990). Dopamine receptor subtypes. *Trends in Pharmacological Science*, 11:231.

Baldessarini, R. J., et al. (1991). Clozapine—a novel antipsychotic agent. *New England Journal of Medicine*, 324:746.

Ballenger, J. C. (1995). Benzodiazepines. In A. F. Schatzberg and C. B. Nemeroff (Eds.), *Textbook of psychopharmacology*. Washington, DC: American Psychiatric Press.

Beare, R. G., and Myers, J. L. (1994). *Principles and practices of adult health nursing* (2nd ed.) (p. 1167). St. Louis: Mosby–Year Book.

Blier, P., et al. (1990). A role for the serotonin system in the mechanism of action of antidepressants. *Journal of Clinical Psychiatry*, 51(Suppl. 4):14.

Boyer, W. E., and Feighner, J. P. (1991). The efficacy of selective serotonin uptake inhibitors in depression. In Feighner and W. E. Boyer (Eds.), *Selective serotonin uptake inhibitors*. Chichester, England: John Wiley.

Briley, M., and Chopin, P. (1991). Serotonin in anxiety: Evidence from animal models. In M. T. Sandler et al. (Eds.), *5-Hydroxytryptamine in psychiatry*. New York: Oxford Medical Publications.

Charney, D. S., et al. (1991). Current hypotheses of the mechanism of antidepressant treatment: Implications for the treatment of refractory depression. In J. D. Amsterdam (Ed.), *Advances in neuropsychiatry and psychopharmacology* (Vol. 2). New York: Raven Press.

Cole, J. O., and Yonkers, K. A. (1995). Nonbenzodiazepine anxiolytics. In A. F. Schatzberg and C. B. Nemeroff (Eds.), *Textbook of psychopharmacology*. Washington, DC: American Psychiatric Press.

Cooper, J. R., Bloom, F. E., and Roth, R. H. (1992). *The biochemical basis of neuropharmacology* (6th ed.). New York: Oxford University Press.

Dechant, K. L., and Cissold, S. P. (1991). Paroxetine. *Drugs*, 41:225.

Dunner, D. L., and Rosenbaum, J. F. (1997). *Psychiatric Clients of North America*, 4:00. Annual of drug therapy.

Fitton, A, and Heel, R. C. (1990). Clozapine—a review of pharmacological properties and therapeutic use in schizophrenia. *Drugs*, 40:722.

Gerlach, J. (1991). New antipsychotics classification, efficacy and adverse effects. *Schizophrenia Bulletin*, 17(2):289.

Goodwin, F. K., and Jamison, K. R. (1990). *Manic-depressive illness*. New York: Oxford University Press.

Hollister, L. E. (1995). Antipsychotic agents and lithium. In G. G. Katzung (Ed.), *Basic and clinical pharmacology*. Norwalk: Appleton & Lange.

Kasper, S., et al. (1992). Comparative efficacy of antidepressants. *Drugs*, 43(Suppl. 2):11.

Knable, M. B., et al. (1995). Neurobiology of schizophrenia. In A. F. Schatzberg and C. B. Nemeroff (Eds.), *Textbook of psychopharmacology*. Washington, DC: American Psychiatric Press.

Krishnan, K. R. (1995). Monoamine oxidase inhibitors. In A. F. Schatzberg and C. B. Nemeroff (Eds.), *Textbook of psychopharmacology*. Washington, DC: American Psychiatric Press.

Lavin, M. R., and Rifkin, A. (1992). Neuroleptic induced parkinsonianism. In J. M. Kane and J. A. Lieberman (Eds.), *Adverse effects of psychotropic drugs*. New York: Guilford Press.

Lenox, R. H., and Manji, H. K. (1995). Lithium. In A. F. Schatzberg and C. B. Nemeroff (Eds.), *Textbook of psychopharmacology*. Washington, DC: American Psychiatric Press.

Manji, H. K., et al. (1991). Mechanisms of action of lithium. *Archives of General Psychiatry*, 48:505.

Mansour, A., et al. (1995). Biochemical anatomy: Insights into the cell biology and pharmacology of neurotransmitter systems in the brain. In A. F. Schatzberg and C. B. Nemeroff (Eds.), *Textbook of psychopharmacology*. Washington, DC: American Psychiatric Press.

Marder, S. R., and Van Patten, T. (1995). Antipsychotic medications. In A. F. Schatzberg and C. B. Nemeroff (Eds.), *Textbook of psychopharmacology*. Washington, DC: American Psychiatric Press.

Marder, S. R., et al. (1991). Drug treatment of schizophrenia: Overview of recent research. *Schizophrenia Research*, 4:81.

Nathan, K. I., et al. (1995). Biology of mood disorders. In A. F. Schatzberg and C. B. Nemeroff (Eds.), *Textbook of psychopharmacology*. Washington, DC: American Psychiatric Press.

Owens, M. J., and Risch, S. L. (1995). Atypical antipsychotics. In A. F. Schatzberg and C. B. Nemeroff (Eds.), *Textbook of psychopharmacology*. Washington, DC: American Psychiatric Press.

Paykel, E. S. (1989). Treatment of depression: The relevance of research for clinical practice. *British Journal of Psychiatry*, 155:754.

Pickar, D., et. al. (1992). Clinical and biologic response to clozapine in patients with schizophrenia. *Archives of General Psychiatry*, 49:345.

Potter, W. Z., et al. (1995). Tricyclics and tetracyclics. In A. F. Schatzberg and C. B. Nemeroff (Eds.), *Textbook of psychopharmacology*. Washington, DC: American Psychiatric Press.

Potter, W. Z., et al. (1991). The pharmacological treatment of depression: An update. *New England Journal of Medicine*, 523:633.

Ray, W. A. (1992). Psychotropic drugs and injuries among the elderly: A review. *Journal of Clinical Psychopharmacology*, 12:386.. Norwalk: Appleton & Lange.

Risby, E. D., et al. (1991). The mechanisms of action of lithium. *Archives of General Psychiatry*, 48:513.

Rudorfer, M. S. (1994). Comparative tolerability profiles of the newer versus the older antidepressants. *Drug Safety*, 10:18.

Snyder, S. H. (1990). The dopamine connection. Nature, 247:121.

Siever, L. J., et al. (1991). Critical issues in defining the role of serotonin in psychiatric disorders. *Pharmacological Reviews*, 43:509.Snyder, S. H. (1990). The dopamine connection. *Nature*, 247:121.

Stein, M. B., and Uhde, T. W. (1995) Biology of anxiety disorders. In A. F. Schatzberg and C. B. Nemeroff (Eds.), *Textbook of psychopharmacology*. Washington, DC: American Psychiatric Press.

Tollefson, G. D. (1995). Selective serotonin reuptake inhibitors. In A. F. Schatzberg and C. B. Nemeroff (Eds.), *Textbook of psychopharmacology*. Washington, DC: American Psychiatric Press.

Trevor, A. J., and Way, W. L. (1995). Sedative-hypnotics. In G. G. Katzung (Ed.), *Basic and clinical pharmacology*. Norwalk: Appleton & Lange.

Wilcox, R. E., and Gonzales, R. A. (1995). Introduction to neurotransmitters, receptors, signal transaction, and second messengers. In A. F. Schatzberg and C. B. Nemeroff (Eds.), *Textbook of psychopharmacology*. Washington, DC: American Psychiatric Press.

Wyatt, R. J. (1991). Neuroleptics and the natural cause of schizophrenia. *Schizophrenia Bulletin*, 17:325.

SELF-STUDY AND CRITICAL THINKING

Circle the correct answer.

1. Where are the basal ganglia located?

   A. cerebrum
   B. cerebellum
   C. brainstem
   D. spinal cord

2. Which of the following neurotransmitters is *not* destroyed by monoamine oxidase?

   A. dopamine
   B. acetycholine
   C. serotonin
   D. norepinephrine

3. Which of the following neurotransmitters is thought to be overactive in schizophrenia?

   A. dopamine
   B. acetylcholine
   C. serotonin
   D. norepinephrine

4. A drug that blocked a *presynaptic* receptor would lead to ________________ transmitter at the synapse.

   A. more
   B. less
   C. no change in

5. Which of the following does *not* result from blocking muscarinic receptors?

   A. tachycardia
   B. constipation
   C. hypotension
   D. blurred vision

6. Benzodiazepines potentiate the neurotransmitter

   A. dopamine
   B. acetycholine
   C. GABA
   D. serotonin

7. Fluoxetine blocks the reuptake of

   A. dopamine
   B. acetylcholine
   C. GABA
   D. serotonin

8. Which of the following is most likely to interfere with fluid balance?

   A. clozapine
   B. lithium
   C. phenothiazines
   D. anxiety

9. Buspirone is a drug used to treat

   A. schizophrenia
   B. depression
   C. manic-depression
   D. anxiety

10. Which of the following can cause parkinsonian movement disorders?

    A. serotonin reuptake inhibitors
    B. tricyclic antidepressants
    C. phenothiazines
    D. benzodiazepines

Write a short answer to the following:

11. Name at least eight functions of the brain.
12. Name at least five neurotransmitters in the brain.
13. What type of untoward effects would be expected from a drug that blocked muscarinic receptors?
14. Explain the destruction of norepinephrine and of acetylcholine.
15. Explain the function of presynaptic receptors.
16. What is the life-threatening aspect of clozapine?
17. What are some of the major untoward effects of lithium?

Critical thinking

18. Describe the ionic movements across the cell membrane during an electrical impulse.
19. What factors might influence a person not to take prescribed psychotropic drugs?
20. Why do phenothiazines cause motor problems?

4

Legal and Ethical Aspects of Mental Health Care

PENNY S. BROOKE

OUTLINE

ETHICAL CONCEPTS
- American Nurses' Association (ANA) Code of Ethics
- Mental Illness and the Social Norm
- Responsibilities of the Therapeutic Relationship

MENTAL HEALTH LAWS
- Civil Rights and Other Client's Rights
  - *The Patient's Bill of Rights*
  - *Due Process in Civil Commitment*
  - *The Right to Treatment*
  - *The Right to Refuse Treatment*
  - *Informed Consent*
  - *Restraint and Seclusion*

TORT LAW APPLIED TO PSYCHIATRIC SETTINGS
- Common Liability Issues
- Intentional Torts
  - *Assault and Battery*
  - *False Imprisonment*
  - *Punitive Damages*
- Violence
- Negligence

DETERMINING A STANDARD OF CARE
- Guidelines for Students Who Suspect Negligence

THE DUTY TO INTERVENE AND THE DUTY TO REPORT

DOCUMENTATION OF CARE
- Purpose
- Facility Use of Medical Records
- The Medical Record as Evidence
- Nursing Guidelines for Charting

MAINTAINING CLIENT CONFIDENTIALITY
- Ethical Considerations: ANA Code for Nurses
- Legal Considerations
- Exceptions to the Rule
  - *Duty to Warn Third Parties*
  - *Nursing Implications*
- Child and Elder Abuse Reporting Statutes

KEY TERMS AND CONCEPTS

The key terms and concepts listed here also appear in bold where they are defined or discussed in this chapter.

ethical dilemma
ethics
bioethics
beneficence
autonomy
justice
fidelity
nonmaleficence
social norms
civil rights
confidentiality
parens patriae

state's police power
least restrictive alternative
voluntary admission
involuntary admission
commitment
conditional release
discharge
right to treatment
right to refuse treatment
informed consent
implied consent
torts
intentional tort
defamation of character
assault
battery
false imprisonment
punitive damages
negligence
right to privacy
duty to warn
child abuse reporting statutes
elder abuse reporting statutes

OBJECTIVES

After studying this chapter, the reader will be able to

1. Define the following terms: (a) ethics and bioethics, (b) torts, (c) battery, (d) assault, (e) false imprisonment, and (f) negligence.
2. Analyze the relationship between social norms, ethics, and mental deviation.
3. Compare and contrast (a) voluntary admission with two types of involuntary admission (civil commitment) and (b) conditional release with discharge.
4. Apply knowledge of what is meant by a client's civil rights to a client situation in his or her clinical setting.
5. Discuss a client's civil rights and how they pertain to restraint and seclusion.
6. Discuss the standards of care for psychiatric nursing practice.
7. Develop an awareness of the balance between the client's rights and the rights of society with respect to these legal concepts relevant in nursing and psychiatric nursing: (a) duty to intervene, (b) documentation and charting, (c) confidentiality, (d) right to treatment, (e) right to refuse treatment, and (f) informed consent.

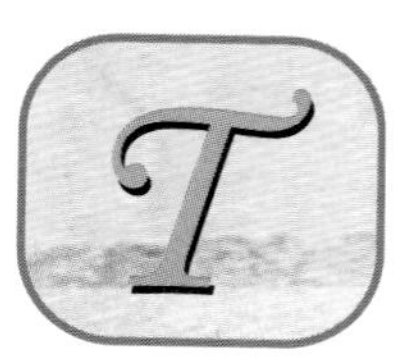

The underlying premise of this chapter is that the client's rights and the nurse's responsibilities are necessarily intertwined. Knowledge of the Nurse Practice Act is merely a starting point; numerous statutes, regulations, and court decisions may affect the way a nurse practices. This is particularly true in the area of psychiatric nursing, because every state has enacted mental health laws regarding the care and treatment of the mentally ill.

Through licensure, a state confers on the registered nurse the privilege of practicing the profession of nursing in that state. Nursing practice is regulated through licensure. As noted in Chapter 1, a growing number of states specifically license psychiatric nurse specialists as advanced practice nurses. Prescriptive authority licenses are also granted in some states to psychiatric nurse specialists (RN, CS). Implicit in this right to practice psychiatric nursing is the responsibility to practice safely and competently and in a manner consistent with state laws and regulations. Each state has a licensing agency, a state board of nursing composed of experts in nursing, that is charged with the implementation of the nurse practice act in that state. The state law sets forth the legal parameters of the practice of nursing, minimal qualifications for practicing nursing, and actionable offenses for disciplinary purposes. Each board establishes rules and regulations that specifically define the nurse practice act of its state. The board also serves as the hearing panel in disciplinary matters.

Nurses who work for the federal government in facilities such as Veterans Administration hospitals must also be aware of the policies and procedures of these institutions, as well as of the federal statutes that apply to these settings.

This chapter introduces you to current legal and ethical issues that may be encountered in the practice of psychiatric nursing. Because the law is dynamic and evolving, it does not always lend itself to clear answers. Accordingly, in situations where the law is not clearly stated by statute, regulation, or court decision, the nurse often encounters an **ethical dilemma** (a situation that requires a choice between morally conflicting alternatives).

The fundamental concept in any legal or ethical issue confronting the nurse in a psychiatric setting is striking the balance between the rights of the individual client and the rights of society at large. This chapter is designed to assist you in identifying competing ethical or legal interests involved in various nursing interventions and to help you consider their impact on decision making.

Although the New York and California statutes and cases cited in this chapter may differ from those of your state, these statutes are representative of modern mental health law in the United States. A variety of state cases are cited to demonstrate different principles of law. *You are encouraged to be aware of the mental health statutes in your own state.* These state codes are available in law school libraries and other state agencies that must evaluate laws.

ETHICAL CONCEPTS

Ethics is the study of philosophical beliefs about what is considered right or wrong in a society. Discussions of ethical practice in nursing involve the topics of morals and values. Whenever morals and values are being debated, there is no right or wrong answer. Ethical beliefs are generally very personal beliefs that arise from your own experiences in society. Judgments made about the ethical beliefs of another are often unfounded. It is important for all nurses to be consciously aware of their own ethical beliefs. Nurses who are not aware of how they feel about ethical dilemmas are more likely to impose their beliefs on clients; it is important to allow clients to act autonomously according to their own beliefs. The term *bioethics* is used in relation to ethical dilemmas surrounding client care. **Bioethics** in psychiatric nursing is the application of ethical principles within the scope of the psychiatric nursing practice setting.

The four principles of bioethics are (1) beneficence, (2) autonomy, (3) justice, and (4) fidelity (nonmaleficence). **Beneficence** is the duty to benefit or promote the good of others; for example, the decision to remain by the bedside of an extremely anxious client in order to be supportive, even if the shift has ended, until a replacement can be found. **Autonomy** is the right to make one's own decisions and respect the rights of others to make their own decisions; for example, acknowledging the client's right to make decisions that do not conform with the recommendation of the staff. **Justice** is the treating of others fairly and equally. **Fidelity (nonmaleficence)** is the observance of loyalty and commitment to the client and "doing no wrong" to the client; for example, the commitment of the nurse to clinical expertise through participation in continuing education.

Everyone has an inner set of standards that results from the influences of family, culture, and teachers, as well as from life's experiences. The development of a value system is a dynamic process, and exposure to different values provides an opportunity for reordering and incorporating new values. Self-exploration to identify your own belief system through reading, questioning, and discussing ethical issues (i.e., clarifying your value system) is an essential element in the process of becoming a professional. Knowledge of your own value system helps in formulating a sturdy foundation for professional development. Without this knowledge, you may feel vulnerable and become confused when confronted with work situations that present a different set of values. However, flexibility in allowing your values to grow, change, and evolve is necessary to professional development. See Chapter 6 for a discussion of, and exercise in, values clarification.

When the psychiatric nurse is presented with an ethical dilemma or a difficult decision that has no response that would apply to all clients, it is often helpful to discuss possible solutions with others. Through small-group discussions, the nurse is able to clarify the facts of the situation and the real ethical decisions to be made. Input from several persons, including members of the health team and the client's family, may be most productive in clarifying these issues and in protecting the client's autonomy and right to decide. There are no easy answers to ethical dilemmas, but having input from several persons will help you arrive at a reasonable solution. Nurses need to study ethical decision making through continuing education programs after graduation. New ethical issues continue to develop. Ethical dilemmas typically result in final decisions that do not please everyone.

Ethical decisions involve morals and values that may differ widely among decision makers. Therefore, it is important to respect and protect the client's autonomy and the client's right to be the ultimate decision maker about decisions that affect his or her life. The nurse must avoid trying to impose personal values on the client. The nurse's life experiences may be dramatically different from those of the client, and part of becoming a professional is developing the ability to recognize and accept the client's right to have an opinion that differs from your own.

Furthermore, a nurse's values may be in conflict with the value system of the institution. This situation further complicates the decision-making process and necessitates careful consideration of the client's desires. For example, the nurse may experience a conflict in a setting in which there is abundant use of tranquilizers for the treatment of an elderly or a depressed client. Whenever one's value system is challenged, increased stress results.

Ethical standards, although lacking the clarity and power of law, do serve as a field guide for decision making. As each generation advances in both knowledge and technology, society inherits increased options. Choices exist today that were nonexistent just 10 years ago. Such dynamic progress promotes more questions than answers. In such a society, the most limited, and thus the most dangerous, way of proceeding is to assume with moral certitude that there is only one "right" or "correct" thing to do. The nurse's role as a client advocate is a prime example of the need to be able to view a situation from another vantage point: through the eyes of the client.

American Nurses' Association (ANA) Code of Ethics

The ANA code (Box 4–1) provides helpful general guidelines for nurses dealing with ethical dilemmas. The distinction between legal and ethical issues is often vague. However, there is an important distinction when the nurse relies on ethical guiding principles instead of on the guiding principles of law. The nurse is bound to comply with the laws, and even though the nurse may feel morally obligated to follow ethical guidelines, these guiding principles should not override laws. For example, if the nurse is aware of a statute, or of a specific rule or regulation created by the state board of nursing, that prohibits certain behavior (e.g., restraining clients against their will) and the nurse feels an ethical obligation to protect the client by using restraints, the nurse would be wise to follow the law. Laws override ethical principles, which do not have the same legal strength. However, ethical dilemmas can influence laws when society is concerned enough to take specific ethical issues to the courts or to the legislature.

Ethical issues become legal issues through court case decisions or when the legislature has heard from many people that a law is needed to protect certain rights. Laws are specific, and they address only what is wrong in a particular society. It is not always possible or desirable to translate an ethical principle into law. Laws protect people's rights and freedoms, but they also infringe on other rights and freedoms. Laws are fluid: they change from time to time and from place to place. Laws reflect a community's standards, which is the reason nurses must become aware of the specific laws of the community in which they are practicing. The law is narrow and deals with a system of compliance in a given society.

Laws are developed to protect the population as a whole, or at least a segment of the population. Specific laws are written to protect psychiatric clients and persons who are not competent to protect their own rights. Ethical principles are much broader and express more universal concepts than do laws. Ethical values address what is wrong or right or what are the nurse's duties and obligations to the client. Ethical choices are based on the individual's attitudes, values, and beliefs. Although it is important to follow one's ethical beliefs, they cannot be relied on as guiding principles when they contradict a law.

Box 4–1 AMERICAN NURSES' ASSOCIATION (ANA) CODE FOR NURSES

1. The nurse provides services with respect for human dignity and the uniqueness of the client unrestricted by considerations of social or economic status, personal attributes, or the nature of health problems.
2. The nurse safeguards the client's rights to privacy by judiciously protecting information of a confidential nature.
3. The nurse acts to safeguard the client and the public when health care and safety are affected by the incompetent, unethical, or illegal practice of any person.
4. The nurse assumes responsibility and accountability for individual nursing judgments and actions.
5. The nurse maintains competence in nursing.
6. The nurse exercises informed judgment and uses individual competence and qualifications as criteria in seeking consultation, accepting responsibilities, and delegating nursing activities to others.
7. The nurse participates in activities that contribute to the ongoing development of the profession's body of knowledge.
8. The nurse participates in the profession's efforts to implement and improve standards of nursing.
9. The nurse participates in the profession's efforts to establish and maintain conditions of employment conducive to high-quality nursing care.
10. The nurse participates in the profession's effort to protect the public from misinformation and misrepresentation and to maintain the integrity of nursing.
11. The nurse collaborates with members of the health professions and other citizens in promoting community and national efforts to meet the health needs of the public.

Mental Illness and the Social Norm

Social norms are known to every society, and most members of society conform to these norms. However, some members of society do not conform. What happens to them? Must all people conform? Does society need the nonconformist (the artist, the scientist, the inventor)? Does the majority have the right to impose its will on the individual?

What about the freedom of individuals to do what they want to do when they want to do it? When is the right of the individual curtailed for the benefit of society? Take, for example, the street lady who for years has been unobtrusively pilfering from trash containers every evening. This behavior, although not desirable, is acceptable. Eventually, she starts rummaging after midnight, and as the noise level escalates, the community responds by notifying authorities of the violation of the peace. What was once tolerable behavior becomes unacceptable.

What constitutes desirable or acceptable behavior of the individual is decided by the group (society) that establishes the norms. Methods of changing human behavior include behavior modification techniques and psychotherapy. Psychotropic drugs can also dramatically alter behavior and must therefore be prescribed carefully. Freedom of expression is a fundamental value of our society, a right embodied in the Constitution. Some hold the view that many psychiatric treatment modalities alter the individual's thought processes and thus challenge our fundamental societal values.

Responsibilities of the Therapeutic Relationship

The psychotherapeutic relationship carries with it serious ethical and legal obligations to the client. The psychotherapist becomes extremely important to the client and must assume this role conscientiously. Termination of the psychotherapeutic relationship can be traumatic to the client if the break is not handled skillfully. (Refer to Chapter 6 regarding the termination phase.) The psychotherapist also has a legal and ethical obligation to the client and to society not to abuse the power that can exist when a client relies on a therapist.

Protection of the client when he or she is in a vulnerable state of mind must be considered. Sadly, many therapeutic relationships are in the news because of sexual abuse of clients by therapists. This misuse of the therapeutic relationship constitutes grounds for losing a license and violates the ethical duty of fidelity to the client. Protection of the confidentiality and privacy of the client's disclosures during therapeutic communication is also vitally important. Because of the complexity of human behavior, therapeutic relations may be long-lasting and very complicated. Skilled psychotherapists must have great insight into their own behavior as well as the client's behavior. Without self-awareness, therapists risk imposing their own value system upon the client.

In summary, essential to an understanding of ethical questions and issues is a knowledge of your own personal value system, the professional code of ethics, and societal values. Laws reflect society's values. In the area of mental health and psychiatric nursing, it is further necessary to understand the mental health laws at both the state and federal levels. Nurses must also be educated regarding models for ethical decision making.

MENTAL HEALTH LAWS

A fundamental component of psychiatric nursing care is understanding the legal framework for the delivery and provision of mental health services in the particular state in which you practice.

Laws have been enacted in each state to regulate the care and treatment of the mentally ill. Many of these laws have undergone major revision in the years since 1963, reflecting a shift in emphasis from state institutional care of the mentally ill to community-based care. This was heralded by the enactment of the Community Mental Health Center Act of 1963 under President Kennedy. Along with this shift in emphasis has come the more widespread use of psychotropic drugs in the treatment of mental illness—enabling many people to integrate more readily into the larger community—and an increasing awareness of the need to provide the mentally ill with humane care that respects their civil rights.

Included in a client's right to remain protected are the issues of inappropriate and indefinite involuntary commitment of mentally disordered persons, developmentally disordered persons, and persons with chronic alcoholism. The timeliness and appropriateness of the evaluation and treatment of persons with serious mental disorders or chronic alcoholism are also issues of concern. An emphasis is now placed not only on protecting public safety but also on safeguarding the individual rights of persons through judicial review. Conservatorships for gravely disabled persons and better use of public funds for social service agencies are being established by legislation at the state and federal levels. There can be competing interests between protection of the individual client's rights and protection of the public safety. Public safety and health issues are generally legislated at the state level.

Civil Rights and Other Clients' Rights

Nowhere is the conflict between the client's expressed interests and the nurse's judgment of the client's best interest more apparent than in the hospital psychiatric setting. As mentioned in Chapter 1, the nurse's role of client advocate can be difficult to exercise in the psychiatric setting, given this inherent conflict. Questioning your ability to be an effective advocate and separating your clinical judgment from the client's expressed desires are both essential.

Facilities may employ a designated institution-based client advocate to mediate such conflicts. This is an attempt to equalize the power of the individual and that of the institution. Some states, recognizing the inability of mentally ill clients to assert their own rights effectively in the psychiatric setting, have developed ombudsman programs for these clients. State law in California mandates an independent client advocate, and New York provides for mental health legal services. Both programs ensure that clients' constitutional rights are protected and that their expressed interests are represented.

The single most important action a nurse can take to protect client's rights is to be familiar with state laws regarding the care and treatment of mentally ill clients and any rights specified by the state. If state law mandates legal services for mental clients or a clients' rights advocate program, client concerns regarding confinement, treatment, change in status, release, medication, and any other treatment modality can be referred to the appropriate offices.

Nurses also need to be familiar with their own hospital's policies regarding admission, change in status, release, medications, informed consent, and use of restraints. The following paragraphs discuss clients' rights in depth. (One version of the Patient's Bill of Rights can be found in Chapter 8.) These rights are prominently displayed on all hospital inpatient units.

Persons with mental illness are guaranteed the same rights under federal and state laws as any other citizen. Included in these are the right to treatment provided by the least restrictive means; the right to prompt medical care and treatment; the right to be free from hazardous procedures; and the right to dignity, privacy, and humane care.

The Patient's Bill Of Rights

CIVIL RIGHTS. Most states specifically prohibit any person from depriving a recipient of mental health services of his or her **civil rights,** including the right to vote; the right to civil service ranking; rights related to granting, forfeit, or denial of license; and the right to make purchases and to enter contractual relationships (unless the client has lost legal capacity by being adjudicated incompetent). The psychiatric client's rights include the right to humane care and treatment. The medical, dental, and psychiatric needs of the client must be met in accordance with the prevailing standards accepted in these professions. The mentally ill in prisons and jails are afforded the same protections.

The right to religious freedom and practice, the right to social interaction, and the right to exercise and recreational opportunities are also protected.

CLIENT CONSENT. Proper orders for specific therapies and treatments are required and must be documented in the client's charts. Consent for surgery, electroconvulsive treatment, or the use of experimental drugs or procedures must be obtained. Clients have the right to refuse participation in experimental treatments or research, and the right to voice grievances and recommend changes in policies or services offered by the facility, without fear of punishment or reprisal.

COMMUNICATION. Clients have the right to communicate fully and privately with those outside the facility. They have a right to have visitors, to have reasonable access to phones and mail, and to send as well as receive unopened correspondence. Clients may seek, at their own expense, consultation with other mental health professionals or attorneys. Clients may not be forced to work for the hospital, with the exception of being assigned routine duties that are developed to enhance their living abilities outside the agency. The rules and regulations of the hospital need to be explained to the client, and the client needs to have reasonable access for communicating with persons outside the hospital.

FREEDOM FROM HARM. Most state laws also provide for the right to be free from harm, which includes freedom from unnecessary or excessive physical restraint, isolation, medication, abuse, or neglect. Use of medications for staff convenience, as a punishment, or as a substitute for treatment programs is explicitly prohibited.

DIGNITY AND RESPECT. Clients in psychiatric hospitals have the right to be treated with dignity and respect. These rights are not only ethically important but also legally protected. Clients have the right to be free from discrimination on the basis of ethnic origin, gender, age, handicap, or religion.

CONFIDENTIALITY. Confidentiality of care and treatment is also an important right for all clients, in particular psychiatric clients. The client's records must be treated as confidential by the staff. Photographs may not be taken without the client's written consent. The client's privacy is protected along with the confidentiality of the treatment. Any discussion or consultation involving a client should be conducted discreetly and only with individuals who have a need and a right to know this privileged information. *Discussions about a client in public places such as elevators and the cafeteria, even when the client's name is not mentioned, can lead to disclosures of confidential information and liabilities for the nurse and the hospital.*

The client's permission must be given to share information with persons who are not directly involved in his or her care. These protections also apply to the client's medical record, which should be read only by individuals directly involved in the client's treatment or in monitoring the quality of care given. Clients must issue a written authorization to allow others to read their medical record. They have a right to expect that all communications and other records relating to treatment are treated as confidential. Institutions that use computerized records must safeguard against intrusion into their client record systems. This issue of client confidentiality is discussed in more detail later in the chapter.

PARTICIPATION IN THEIR PLAN OF CARE. Additional rights the psychiatric client enjoys include a written individualized treatment plan that is reviewed regularly and that involves the client in the planning decisions. Clients are also entitled to a discharge plan that includes follow-up care or continuing care requirements. The treatment plan needs to include the least restrictive treatment environment that is appropriate. Reasonable safety is an expectation of this environment. If the client is unable to make these decisions, the person legally authorized to act on the client's behalf must be consulted.

Clients have the right to be informed by their physician of the benefits, risks, and side effects of all medications and treatment procedures used. They cannot be subjected to any procedure or treatment without their consent, or a battery will have occurred. (*Assault* is the threat of harm or putting a person in a state of apprehension; *battery* is the actual contact with the person. These principles are discussed in greater detail later in this chapter.)

Due Process in Civil Commitment

The courts have recognized that involuntary civil commitment to a mental hospital is a "massive curtailment of liberty" (*Humphrey v. Cady* 1972, p. 509) requiring due process protections in the civil commitment procedure. This right derives from the Fifth Amendment of the U.S. Constitution, which states that "no person shall . . . be deprived of life, liberty or property without due process of law." The Fourteenth Amendment explicitly prohibits states from depriving citizens of life, liberty, and property without due process of law. State civil commitment statutes, if challenged in the courts on constitutional grounds, will have to afford minimal due process protections to pass the court's scrutiny.

A state's power in enacting a civil commitment procedure is based either on the *parens patriae* power or on state police power. ***Parens patriae*** is the power of the state to act for the care, treatment, or protection of an individual or class of individuals who are unable to act on their own behalf in their own best interests.

For example, in an 1845 Massachusetts case, *In re Oakes,* the court found justification for depriving a person of liberty for his own safety and that of others when such restraint might be beneficial to him. Mr. Oakes, an elderly widower, was confined when he became engaged to a woman of questionable character and involved in speculative financial ventures after the death of his wife. This case is an example of early judicial application of the *parens patriae* doctrine to civil commitment of the mentally ill.

In contrast, a **state's police power** is a plenary power to make laws and regulations to protect the public health, safety, and welfare. Civil commitment statutes are enacted to protect societal interests and have their basis in the police power.

The privilege of the writ of habeas corpus and the least restrictive alternative doctrine are two other important concepts applicable to civil commitment cases. A writ of habeas corpus is the procedural mechanism, guaranteed by Article I, Section 9 of the U.S. Constitution, used to challenge unlawful detention by the government. The doctrine of the **least restrictive alternative** mandates that the least drastic means be taken to achieve a specific purpose.

ADMISSIONS TO THE HOSPITAL. *All students are encouraged to become familiar with the important provisions of the laws in their own states regarding admissions, discharges, client rights, and informed consent,* because a state-by-state review of the law is beyond the scope of this chapter. Admissions to mental institutions are governed by statutes that vary from state to state. Admissions are either voluntary or involuntary, and this categorization affects a client's rights with regard to release, notice of rights, and treatment.

A medical standard or justification for admission should exist. A well-defined psychiatric problem must be established, based on current DSM-IV illness classifications. The presenting illness should also be of such a nature that other less restrictive alternatives are inadequate or unavailable, or cause an immediate crisis situation. There should also be a reasonable expectation that the hospitalization will improve the presenting problems.

Voluntary Hospitalization. Generally, **voluntary admission** is sought by the client or the client's guardian through a written application to the facility. Voluntary clients have the right to demand and obtain release. If the client is a minor, the release may be contingent on the consent of the parents or guardian. However, few states require voluntary clients to be notified of the rights associated with their status. In addition, many states require that a client submit a written release notice to the facility staff, who reevaluate the client's condition for possible conversion to involuntary status according to criteria established by the state law.

A few states have statutes that provide for a less restricted form of voluntary admission called *informal admission.* Informal admission permits a client to make a verbal application for admission, similar to that made for hospital admission for medical treatment.

Involuntary Hospitalization. Involuntary admission is made without the client's consent. Although criteria vary from state to state, there are two common threads found in states that justify involuntary admissions that may result in the client being committed to the institution. Involuntary admission is necessary when a person is a danger to self or others or is in need of psychiatric treatment or physical care. Three different commitment procedures are commonly available—judicial determination, administrative determination, and agency determination. Additionally, a specified number of physicians must certify that a person's mental health justifies detention and treatment.

Involuntary hospitalization can be further categorized by the nature and purpose of the involuntary admission. It may be emergency, observational or temporary, or indeterminate or extended.

Emergency Involuntary Hospitalization. Most states provide for emergency involuntary hospitalization or civil **commitment** for a specified period (1 to 10 days on average) to prevent dangerous behavior that is likely to cause harm to self or others. Police officers, physicians, and mental health professionals may be designated by statute to authorize the detention of mentally ill persons who are dangers to themselves or others.

Observational or Temporary Involuntary Hospitalization. Civil commitment for observational or temporary involuntary hospitalization is of longer duration than emergency hospitalization. The primary purpose of this type of hospitalization is observation, diagnosis, and treatment of persons who suffer from mental illness or pose a danger to themselves or others. The length of time is specified by statute and varies markedly from state to state. Application for this type of admission can be made by a guardian, family member, physician, or other public health officer. Some states permit any citizen to make an application for aid to another. States vary as to their procedural requirements for this type of involuntary admission. Medical certification by two or more physicians that a person is mentally ill and in need of treatment or a judicial or administrative review and order are often required for involuntary admission.

Indeterminate or Extended Involuntary Hospitalization. Indeterminate or extended commitment for involuntary hospitalization has as its primary purpose extended care and treatment of the mentally ill. Like clients who undergo observational involuntary hospitalization, those who undergo extended involuntary hospitalization are committed solely through judicial or administrative action or medical certification. States that do not require a judicial hearing before commitment often provide the client with an opportunity for a judicial review after commitment procedures. This type of involuntary hospitalization generally lasts 60 to 180 days, but it may be for an indeterminate length of time.

Clients who are involuntarily committed do not lose their right of informed consent. Clients must be considered legally competent until they have been declared incompetent through a legal proceeding. Competency is related to the capacity to understand the consequences of one's decisions. If the psychiatric nurse believes a client lacks this ability, action should be initiated to have a legal guardian appointed by the court.

RELEASE FROM THE HOSPITAL. Release from hospitalization depends on the client's admission status. Clients who sought informal or voluntary admission, as previously discussed, have the right to demand and receive release. Some states, however, do provide for conditional release of voluntary clients, which enables the treating physician or administrator to order continued treatment on an outpatient basis if the clinical needs of the client warrant further care.

Conditional Release. Conditional release usually requires outpatient treatment for a specified period to determine the client's compliance with medication protocols, ability to meet basic needs, and ability to reintegrate into the community. Generally, a voluntary client who is conditionally released cannot be reinstitutionalized without consent unless the institution complies with the procedures for involuntary hospitalization. However, an involuntary client who is conditionally released may be reinstitutionalized while the commitment is still in effect without recommencement of formal admission procedures.

Discharge. Discharge, or unconditional release, is the termination of a client-institution relationship. This release may be court ordered or administratively ordered by the institution's officials. Generally, the administrative officer of an institution has the discretion to discharge clients. In most states a client can institute a court proceeding to seek a judicial discharge. This is referred to as a writ of habeas corpus, meaning "free the person." Follow-up care is critical to these clients. Discharge planning is important for the continued well-being of the psychiatric client. Aftercare case managers are needed to facilitate the client's adaptation back into the community and to provide early referral if the treatment plan is not being followed (see Chapter 8). Nursing measures and protocols are discussed in Chapter 12 (Angry and Aggressive Clients) and Chapter 21 (The Bipolar Client).

The Right to Treatment

With the enactment of the Hospitalization of the Mentally Ill Act in 1964, the federal statutory right to psychiatric treatment in public hospitals was created. The statute requires that "a person hospitalized in a public hospital for a mental illness shall, during his hospitalization, be entitled to medical and psychiatric care and treatment."

Although state courts and lower federal courts have decided that there may be a federal constitutional right to treatment, the U.S. Supreme Court has never firmly grounded the **right to treatment** in a constitutional principle. The evolution of these cases in the courts provides an interesting history of the development and shortcomings of our mental health delivery system.

The initial cases presenting the psychiatric client's right to treatment arose in the criminal justice system. In *Rouse v. Cameron* (1966) the petitioner filed a writ of habeas corpus alleging that he was unlawfully detained and without psychiatric treatment after 4 years in a maximum security pavilion of the hospital. Mr. Rouse had pleaded not guilty by reason of insanity to a misdemeanor charge, which carried a 1-year maximum sentence, for having a dangerous weapon in his possession. The court concluded, on the basis of state law as well as a federal statutory right, that without treatment the petitioner would be deprived of liberty. The ruling also indicated that there might also be a constitutional basis for the right to treatment.

The next significant right-to-treatment case served as a sorry indictment of mental health hospitals in Alabama. The central issue in *Wyatt v. Stickney* (1971) was the absence of adequate treatment for the involuntarily committed clients. Five thousand clients were cared for by a professional staff of 17 doctors, 21 registered nurses, 12 psychologists, and 13 social workers and a nonprofessional staff of 12 activity workers and 850 psychiatric aides.

The court found that the state hospitals lacked individualized client treatment plans, adequate qualified professional staff to administer treatment, and a humane physical and psychological environment. In fashioning a remedy, the court issued several standards, including minimal staffing requirements, treatment in the least restrictive setting required by the individual, and development of a human rights committee in each institution. The court stated that "when clients are so committed for treatment purposes, they unquestionably have a right to receive such individualized treatment as will give each of them a realistic opportunity to be cured or improve his or her mental condition" (*Wyatt v. Stickney* 1971, p. 784).

The U.S. Supreme Court first considered the right-to-treatment issue in *O'Connor v. Donaldson* (1975) (Box 4–2).

The U.S. Supreme Court, in declining to affirm the lower court's finding of damages and a broad constitutional right to treatment, narrowly defined the issue for consideration: whether or not a finding of mental illness alone can justify the state's indefinite custodial confinement of a mentally ill person against his or her will. The Supreme Court held that a "state cannot constitutionally confine a nondangerous individual who is capable of surviving safely in freedom by himself or with the help of willing and responsible family members or friends" (*O'Connor v. Donaldson* 1975, p. 576).

BOX 4–2 RIGHT TO TREATMENT: *O'CONNOR V. DONALDSON*

In 1957, Mr. Donaldson was involuntarily committed, on his father's initiation, to a Florida state hospital for care, treatment, and maintenance. For 14 years before his commitment, he was gainfully employed. Despite the fact that Mr. Donaldson posed no danger to himself or others, his requests for ground privileges, occupational training, and an opportunity to discuss his case with the superintendent, Dr. O'Connor, or others were denied. During his 15 years of confinement, he was not provided with any treatment.

Mr. Donaldson frequently requested his release, which the superintendent was authorized to grant even though Mr. Donaldson was lawfully confined, because even if he continued to be mentally ill, he posed no danger to himself or others. Between 1964 and 1968, Mr. Donaldson's friend requested on four separate occasions that he be released into his custody. These requests, and requests made by a halfway house on Mr. Donaldson's behalf, were all denied by Dr. O'Connor, who believed that Mr. Donaldson should be released into his parents' custody. Dr. O'Connor further believed that Mr. Donaldson's parents were too old and infirm to care for him adequately.

The court found that Mr. Donaldson's care was merely custodial because he received no treatment. He was not dangerous, community alternatives were available for him, and the doctor's refusal to release him was "malicious." The Federal Court of Appeals ruled that Mr. Donaldson had a constitutional right to treatment and awarded him $38,000 in damages.

In 1982 the Supreme Court again considered an aspect of the right-to-treatment issue in *Youngberg v. Romeo*. The issue before the Supreme Court was whether or not involuntarily committed mentally retarded clients have a constitutionally protected interest in safety, freedom from undue restraint, and minimally adequate or reasonable training. Although the court affirmed these rights, it further noted that the substantive liberty interests established in the case were not absolute and that the client's interests in liberty must be balanced against the state's reasons for restraint.

Although not specifically dealing with the rights of psychiatric clients, *Youngberg v. Romeo* has had an impact on cases regarding the psychiatric client's right to refuse treatment. Federal regulations enacted on the use of restraints would override these case precedents.

The Right to Refuse Treatment

A corollary to the right to consent to treatment is the right to withhold consent. A client may also withdraw consent at any time. Retraction of consent previously given must be honored, whether it is a verbal or written retraction. However, the mentally ill client's **right to refuse treatment** with psychotropic drugs has been debated in the courts, turning in part on the issue of mental clients' competency to give or withhold consent to treatment and their status under the civil commitment statutes. These cases, initiated by state hospital clients, consider principles of constitutional law, balancing competing state interests and societal interests against the client's interest in autonomy and self-determination, in the face of the often permanent and disfiguring side effects of psychotropic drugs. The analyses in these cases included medical, legal, and ethical considerations, such as basic treatment problems, the doctrine of informed consent, and the bioethical principle of autonomy.

In *Rogers v. Okin* (1979) the district court ruled that clients involuntarily committed are not incompetent and have constitutionally protected liberty and privacy interests in making treatment decisions for themselves. Without consent by the client or the client's guardian, this right could not be overridden except in an emergency. Forcible administration of medication is justified when the "need to prevent violence outweighs the possibility of harm to the medicated individual" and when reasonable alternatives to medication have been ruled out (*Rogers v. Okin* 1979, p. 1365).

The court of appeals (*Rogers v. Okin* 1980) affirmed the lower court's ruling that mental clients have the constitutionally protected right to make treatment decisions and refuse treatment. The court of appeals ruled that the police power provides the hospital staff with substantial discretion in an emergency, and that the *parens patriae* doctrine justifies forcible administration of psychotropic medication to competent clients only when necessary to prevent further deterioration of their mental health. The court of appeals reversed the lower court's conclusion that a guardian may make psychotropic drug treatment decisions for incompetent clients in nonemergency situations; instead, it decided that the client's rights must be protected by a judicial determination of incompetency and application of the "substituted judgment rule." With a competent client, then, treatment with antipsychotic medication is justified only if he or she has voluntarily accepted treatment. For a summary of the evolution of the cases regarding the client's right to refuse treatment, see Table 4–1.

The precedent for the Rogers decision, summarized in Table 4–1, was set in the case of *In re guardianship of Roe* (1981), which held that noninstitutionalized mental clients who are adjudicated incompetent have a right to refuse treatment with antipsychotic drugs by the use of a substituted judgment rule. The court enunciated general standards for courts to use in applying substituted judgment.

The factors underlying the court's decision that guardians do not have inherent authority to consent to antipsychotic drug treatment for their wards are (1) the intrusiveness of the treatment, (2) the potential for side effects, (3) the absence of an emergency, (4) the nature and extent of poor judicial involvement, and (5) the likelihood of conflicting interests.

In discussing the intrusiveness of the treatment and the possibility of adverse side effects, the court stated that there are "few . . . medical procedures which are more intrusive than forcible injection of antipsychotic medication because it affects the person's thought processes and personality." It further noted that the very significant side effects are frequently devastating and often irreversible (In *re guardianship of Roe* 1981, p. 52).

After concluding that previous court approval was necessary in a substituted judgment, the court identified six relevant factors in applying this standard:

- The person's expressed preferences regarding treatment when competent
- The person's religious belief
- The effect of treatment, or lack of it, on the person's family
- The probability of an adverse side effect
- The risks involved in the refusal of the treatment
- The prognosis with treatment

In instances in which forcible medication is sought to prevent violence to third persons, to prevent suicide, or to preserve security, the court noted that the medication is being used as a "chemical restraint," and the justification for medication thus changes from individual treatment to public protection. Accordingly, the infringement on a person's liberty is at least equal to that with involuntary commitment. In this circumstance, the noninstitutionalized, incompetent, mentally ill client has the right, through substituted judgment, to determine whether to be involuntarily committed or to be medicated.

In New Jersey, involuntarily committed psychiatric clients also brought a suit in federal court alleging violation of their constitutional rights through forcible administration of antipsychotic drugs. See Table 4–2 for a

TABLE 4–1 RIGHT TO REFUSE TREATMENT: EVOLUTION OF MASSACHUSETTS CASE LAW TO PRESENT LAW

CASE	COURT	DECISION
Rogers v. Okin, 478 F Supp 1342 (D Mass 1979)	Federal District Court	Involuntary mental patients are competent and have the right to make treatment decisions. Forcible administration of medication is justified in an emergency if needed to prevent violence and if other alternatives have been ruled out. A guardian may make treatment decisions for an incompetent client.
Rogers v. Okin, 634 F2nd 650 (1st Cir 1980)	Federal Court of Appeals	Affirmed that involuntary mental patients are competent and have the right to make treatment decisions. The staff has substantial discretion in an emergency. Forcible medication is also justified to prevent the client's deterioration. A client's rights must be protected by judicial determination of incompetency.
Mills v. Rogers, 457 US 291 (1982)	U.S. Supreme Court	Set aside the judgment of the court of appeals with instructions to consider the effect of an intervening state court case.
Rogers v. Commissioner of the Department of Mental Health, 458 NE 2d 308 (Mass 1983)	Massachusetts Supreme Judicial Court answering questions certified by Federal Court of Appeals	Involuntary clients are competent and have the right to make treatment decisions unless they are judicially determined to be incompetent.

TABLE 4–2 RIGHT TO REFUSE TREATMENT: EVOLUTION OF NEW JERSEY CASE LAW TO PRESENT LAW

CASE	COURT	DECISION
Rennie v. Klein, 476 F Supp 1294 (D NJ 1979)	Federal District Court	Involuntary mental patients have a qualified constitutional right to refuse treatment with antipsychotic drugs. Voluntary clients have an absolute right to refuse treatment with antipsychotic drugs under New Jersey law.
Rennie v. Klein, 653 F2d 836 (3rd Cir 1981)	Federal Court of Appeals	Involuntary mental patients have a constitutional right to refuse antipsychotic drug treatment. The state may override a client's right when the client poses a danger to self or others. Due process protections are required before forcible medication of clients in nonemergency situations.
Rennie v. Klein, 454 US 1078 (1982)	U.S. Supreme Court	Set aside the judgment of the court of appeals with instructions to consider the case in light of the U.S. Supreme Court decision in *Youngberg v. Romeo.*
Rennie v. Klein, 720 F2d 266 (3rd Cir 1983)	Federal Court of Appeals	Involuntary mental patients have the right to refuse treatment with antipsychotic medication. Decisions to forcibly medicate must be based on "accepted professional judgment" and must comply with due process requirements of the New Jersey regulations.

summary of the evolution of the *Rennie v. Klein* (1979) case.

Cases involving the right to refuse psychotropic drug treatment are still evolving. Without clear direction from the Supreme Court, there will be different case outcomes in different jurisdictions. In the 1989 case of *State of Washington v. Harper,* the Supreme Court addressed the issue of whether mentally ill prisoners' refusal of medication can be overridden by administrative procedures or whether a full judicial hearing is required. The court held that the State of Washington Department of Corrections policy provided adequate due process protections and that prisoners were not entitled to a separate judicial hearing on the right to refuse medication. The court did not address the rights of involuntarily committed mentally ill clients.

The relationship between these cases on the right to refuse psychotropic drug treatment and cases on the right to terminate life support presents compelling ethical, legal, and philosophical questions. The Massachusetts courts, using a substituted judgment rule, and the New York courts, basing their rulings on common law, have honored incompetent medical clients' previously expressed desires, made while they were competent, to terminate life support. Other states, such as California, have enacted statutes that permit persons to designate a health care representative to consent to treatment should they become incompetent, with instructions delineating the client's treatment wishes.

These court cases and statutes are based on the individual's right to self-determination. The fundamental issue is whether there is a difference between medical and mental illness that justifies a distinction between the rights afforded to persons in making treatment decisions. The cases on the right to refuse medication have illustrated the complex and difficult task of translating social policy concerns into a clearly articulated legal standard.

On December 1, 1991, a federal law entitled the Patient Self-Determination Act became effective. This advance-directive law requires that all persons 18 years of age and older who are admitted to a hospital or to a Medicaid-participating organization (e.g., home health agencies, prepaid health maintenance organizations, hospice programs, or skilled nursing facilities) must be asked if they have an advance directive to clarify their wishes and philosophy regarding life, death, and medical care. The act does not require every person to have prepared a living will or special directive, but it is hoped that the inquiry will encourage clients to record their wishes.

The act also requires that the agency provide written information regarding clients' rights under state law to accept or reject medical treatment, and that the agency inform clients about durable powers of attorney (e.g., appointing a surrogate decision maker if the client is unable to make decisions). The agency must document in the client's record whether he or she has completed a directive. Agencies that do not comply with this law will lose their eligibility for federal funding reimbursement. Refer to Chapter 31, "The Elderly," for more discussions on this issue.

Informed Consent

The principle of **informed consent** is based on a person's right to self-determination, as enunciated in the landmark case *Canterbury v. Spence* (1972, p. 780):

> The root premise is the concept, fundamental in American jurisprudence, that every human being of adult years and sound mind has a right to determine what shall be done with his own body . . . true consent to what happens to one's self is the informed exercise of choice, and that entails an opportunity to evaluate knowledgeably the options available and the risks attendant on each.

For consent to be effective legally, it must be informed. Generally, the informed consent of the client must be obtained by the physician or other health professional to perform the treatment or procedure. Clients must be informed of the nature of their problem or condition, the nature and purpose of a proposed treatment, the risks and benefits of that treatment, alternative treatment options, the probability that the proposed treatment will be successful, and the risks of not consenting to treatment.

Because psychiatric nursing procedures are generally noninvasive and are commonly understood by the client, the need for the nurse to obtain informed consent does not occur as frequently as in medical treatment. Many procedures that nurses perform have an element of implied consent attached. For example, if the nurse approaches the client with a medication in hand and the client indicates a willingness to receive the medication, **implied consent** has occurred. A general rule for the nurse to follow is that the more intrusive or risky the procedure, the higher is the likelihood that informed consent must be obtained. The fact that the nurse may not have a legal duty to be the person to inform the client of the associated risks and benefits of a particular medical procedure does not excuse the nurse from explaining the procedure to the client and obtaining his or her expressed or implied consent. *Client teaching is a recognized legal duty of nurses.*

Restraint and Seclusion

Legally, behavioral restraint and seclusion are authorized as an intervention

1. When behavior is physically harmful to the client or a third party
2. When the disruptive behavior presents a danger to the facility
3. When alternative or less restrictive measures are insufficient in protecting the client or others from harm
4. When the client anticipates that a controlled environment would be helpful and requests seclusion.

As indicated, most state laws prohibit the use of unnecessary physical restraint or isolation. The use of seclusion and restraint is permitted only on the written order of a physician, which must be reviewed and renewed every 24 hours and which also must specify the type of restraint to be used. "As necessary" orders are prohibited.

Only in an emergency may the charge nurse place a client in seclusion or restraint and obtain a written or verbal order as soon as possible thereafter. Federal laws require the consent of the client unless an emergency situation exists in which an immediate risk of harm to the client or others can be documented. The client must be removed from restraints when safer and quieter behavior is observed. While in restraints, the client must be protected from all sources of harm. The nurse documents the behavior leading to restraint or seclusion and the time the client is placed in and released from restraint. The client in restraint must be assessed at regular and frequent intervals (e.g., every 15 to 30 minutes) for physical needs (food, toileting), safety, and comfort, and these observations are also documented (every 15 to 30 minutes).

Restraint and seclusion should never be used as punishment or for the convenience of the staff. For example, if the unit is short-staffed, restraining a client to protect him or her while the nurse passes medications is an inappropriate use of restraints. The least restrictive means of restraint for the shortest duration is always the general rule. Verbal interventions are the first approach; restraints are used only to prevent harm or to provide benefit to the client. Chemical restraints are more subtle than physical restraints but can have a greater impact on the client's ability to relate to the environment. The psychiatric nurse must be aware of the severe and powerful impact of chemical restraints on psychiatric clients. The client's personality and ability to relate to others is greatly controlled by chemical restraints. The practice of secluding a client is comparable with the practice of sedating a client until the client is secluded within himself or herself. An example of the misuse of chemical restraints is a case in which a verbally abusive or pacing client is deeply sedated and placed in his or her room in order to control the unit's environment. The nurse must always be able to document professional judgment regarding the use of physical or chemical restraint, as well as for the use of seclusion. With recent changes in the law regarding the use of restraint and seclusion that require a client's consent to be restrained, agencies have revised their policies and procedures, greatly limiting these practices of the past. Most agencies have found no negative impact associated with the reduced use of restraints and seclusion. Alternative methods of therapy and cooperation with the client have been successful.

TORT LAW APPLIED TO PSYCHIATRIC SETTINGS

Torts are civil wrongs for which money damages are collected by the injured party (the plaintiff) from the wrongdoer (the defendant). The injury can be to persons, property, or reputations. Because tort law has general applicability to nursing practice, this section may contain a review of material previously covered elsewhere in your nursing curriculum.

In a psychiatric setting, nurses are more likely to encounter provocative, threatening, or violent behavior. Such behavior may require the use of restraint or seclusion until a client demonstrates quieter and safer behavior. Accordingly, the nurse in the psychiatric setting should understand the **intentional torts** of battery, assault, and false imprisonment.

Common Liability Issues

Legal issues common in psychiatric nursing relate to the failure to protect the safety of clients. If a suicidal client is left alone with the means to harm himself or herself, the nurse who has a duty to protect the client will be held responsible for the resultant injuries. Leaving a suicidal client alone in a room on the sixth floor with an open window is an example of unreasonable judgment on the part of the nurse. Precautions must be taken whenever a client is restrained to prevent harm. Miscommunications and medication errors are common in all areas of nursing, including psychiatric care. A common area of liability in psychiatry revolves around abuse of the therapist-client relationship. Issues of sexual misconduct during the therapeutic relationship have become a source of concern among the psychiatric community. Misdiagnosis is also frequently charged in legal suits.

Charges of **defamation of character,** either written (libel) or oral (slander), can be brought if confidential information regarding clients is divulged that harms their reputation. The privacy protections afforded all clients by the law are especially protective of the rights of psychiatric clients.

Supervisory liability may be incurred if nursing duties are delegated to persons who cannot safely perform these duties. The nurse who does not verify that the assistive personnel can safely and appropriately provide the care being delegated will be held vicariously liable for any harm or injury the client suffers. Supervision of assistive personnel is essential. Supervisors are no longer protected under the National Labor Relations Act because of a ruling that held they were closely aligned with employers in these roles and therefore fell outside the bargaining units of organized unions. This ruling makes it even more important that nurses who delegate tasks to others clarify whether or not they will be considered supervisors and therefore outside the protections of the employee bargaining unit.

Short-staffing issues have raised concerns about client safety as well as of delegation to assistive personnel. If the nurse believes that a staffing pattern is not allowing appropriate and reasonable care, a written appeal to the nurse's supervisor and the institution will document the nurse's concerns. Nurses should not perform tasks for which they are not prepared, including the assumption of responsibility for the safety and care of an unreasonable number of clients. If the institution is unwilling to correct an unsafe situation, the nurse must determine whether he or she wishes to remain employed and incur possible liability if a client is injured for whom the nurse is ultimately responsible. Proper channels of appeal must be followed to avoid charges of insubordination and possible firing. Institutional policies should outline the correct procedure for voicing a reasonable grievance.

There are constant changes in the health care system and in those who use it. One area of concern is that in many parts of the United States nurses are often asked to work outside the scope of their license because of decreased hiring of RNs and an increase in hiring of unlicensed personnel and LPNs. It is important for nurses to keep in mind that they must not work outside the scope of their license. In many states an LPN license is forfeited when the nurse becomes an RN. If the nurse is hired in an LPN position, even though an RN license is held, it is likely that the nurse will be held to the standards of care of an RN. This situation may place nurses in the position of working beyond the scope of their present employment. This is a conflict that must be resolved by the nurse, the State Board of Nursing, and the employer on a state-by-state basis.

Legal issues involving care of clients who are human immunodeficiency virus (HIV) positive are another area of concern for nurses in all areas of the health care system. This is especially true for psychiatric mental health nurses. Refer to Table 4–3 for some legal issues involved HIV and psychiatric mental health nursing.

Some guidelines for avoiding liability include the following:

1. Always put the client's rights and welfare first.
2. Observe the hospital's or agency's policy manual.
3. Practice within the scope of the nurse practice act.
4. Maintain current understanding and knowledge of established practice standards.

Intentional Torts

Torts are a category of civil law that commonly applies to health care practice. Some torts can also carry criminal penalties. *An intentional tort requires a voluntary act and an intent to bring about a physical consequence.* In the most basic terms, a voluntary act is a voluntary movement of the body. The requirement for intent is met when the defendant acts purposefully to achieve a result or is substantially certain that the result will occur. If the injured party consents to participate in an act, there can be no intentional tort. Likewise, self-defense and defense of others are privileges that can be used to defend successfully against a court action for intentional torts. Reckless behavior may be classified as intentional or negligent. Mal-

TABLE 4–3 LEGAL ISSUES INVOLVING HUMAN IMMUNODEFICIENCY VIRUS (HIV) AND PSYCHIATRIC MENTAL HEALTH NURSING

ISSUE	THE LAW
1. Involuntary HIV testing of psychiatric patients	1. Consent from the psychiatric patient must be sought to test blood for HIV. Substitute decision making applies only to children age 13 or younger and to involuntarily committed adult psychiatric patients (Lo, 1989).
2. Involuntary confinement of a psychiatric patient who is HIV positive and having sex with other patients.	2. Knowing transmission of HIV through sexual contact is prohibited by law. The institution has the legal means to prohibit such contact. The Illinois Supreme Court held that a statute prohibiting a person from knowingly transmitting HIV was constitutional (*Illinois v. Russel,* 1994).
3. Duty to warn the partner of a psychiatric patient who is HIV positive	3. In 1988, New York and California enacted laws permitting notification of contacts of HIV persons. These laws require that the informant persuade the patient to allow notification without disclosing the identity of the patient. Alternatively, public health officials may be asked to notify contacts. Recent statutes, however, do not require notification, encouraging voluntary notification (Lo, 1989).
4. Disclosure of a psychiatric patient's HIV status by the nurse to an unauthorized person	4. The Arkansas Supreme Court held that a nurse who disclosed information about a man's HIV test to an unauthorized third party did not constitute medical malpractice (*Wyatt v. St. Paul Fire & Marine Insurance Co.,* 1994).
5. Psychiatric nurses' refusal to care for an HIV-positive psychiatric patient	5. In general, nurses have no legal duty to care for HIV-positive psychiatric patients. However, moral obligation, employment contracts, and professional and ethical standards may impose some authority to obligate the nurse to care for HIV-positive patients.
6. Psychiatric nurses' duty to inform employer of HIV status	6. While HIV-positive psychiatric nurses have a moral obligation to inform their employer of their HIV status, their right to privacy should be balanced with the risk of infection to co-workers or patients who come under their care.
7. Nurses' claims for emotional distress caused by exposure to AIDS or needlestick	7. In *Tischler v. Dimenna* (1994), a New York court recognized claims for emotional distress caused by exposure to AIDS. Moreover, the Montana Supreme Court held that the State Worker's Compensation Act provided the exclusive remedy for a former employee who developed a fear of AIDS after being punctured by a needle (*Blythe v. Radiometer America, Inc.,* 1993).

From Constantino, R., E., B. (1996) Legal issues in psychiatric-mental health nursing. In S. Lego (2nd ed.). *Psychiatric nursing: A comprehensive reference,* Philadelphia: J. B. Lippincott.

practice actions typically result from negligent behavior. For example, the foreseeability that a suicidal client will harm himself or herself if left alone with sharp objects or an open window is great enough for negligence to be found on the part of the nurse, who has a duty to protect the client. If the nurse left the client alone, knowing of the likelihood of self-harm, an intentional decision could be argued. It would not be a wise nursing judgment to test the suicidal client's ability to be left alone with dangers in the immediate environment.

Assault and Battery

An **assault** is an act resulting in a person's apprehension of an immediate harmful or offensive touching (battery). In an assault, there is no physical contact. The aggressor's act must amount to a threat to use force, although threatening words alone are not enough. The aggressor must also have the opportunity and the ability to carry out the threatened act immediately. A **battery** is a harmful or offensive touching of another's person. For example, the nurse approaches the client with a restraint in hand. The client fearfully pleads not to be restrained. If the nurse proceeds to apply the restraints, both an assault and a battery may be charged against the nurse.

False Imprisonment

False imprisonment is an act with the intent to confine a person to a specific area. The use of seclusion or restraint that is not defensible as being necessary and in the client's best interest may result in false imprisonment of the client and liability for the nurse. As another example, if a psychiatric client wants to leave the hospital and the nurse prohibits the client from leaving, the nurse may have falsely imprisoned the client if the client was voluntarily admitted and if there are no agency or legal policies for detaining the client. On the other hand, if the client was involuntarily admitted or had agreed to an evaluation before discharge, the nurse's actions would be reasonable.

Punitive Damages

Punitive damages may be recoverable by an injured party in an intentional tort action. Because these damages are designed to punish and make an example, punitive damage awards can be very large. Often, the plaintiff's actual damages are insignificant, and nominal damages may be awarded in the sum of 1 dollar. However, intentional acts are not covered by malpractice insurance, which makes intentional torts a less attractive theory of liability for injured clients to pursue against health professionals and hospitals. The case *Plumadore v. State of New York* (1980) (Box 4–3) illustrates the use of intentional tort in the psychiatric setting.

Violence

Violent behavior is not acceptable in our society. Nurses must protect themselves in both institutional and community settings. Employers are not typically held responsible for employee injuries due to violent client behavior. Nurses have placed themselves knowingly in the range of danger by agreeing to care for unpredictable clients. It is therefore important for nurses to protect themselves by participating in setting policies that create a safe environment. Good judgment means not placing oneself in a potentially violent situation. Nurses, as citizens, have the same rights as clients not to be threatened or harmed. Appropriate security support should be readily available to the nurse practicing in an institution. Nurses who work in community settings must avoid placing themselves unnecessarily in dangerous settings, especially when alone at night. Common sense should be used and the support of local law enforcement officers enlisted when needed. A violent client is not being abandoned if placed safely in the hands of the authorities.

BOX 4–3 FALSE IMPRISONMENT AND NEGLIGENCE: *PLUMADORE V. STATE OF NEW YORK*

Mrs. Plumadore was admitted to Saranac Lake General Hospital for a gallbladder condition. Her medical work-up revealed emotional problems stemming from marital difficulties, which had resulted in suicide attempts several years before her admission. After a series of consultations and tests, she was advised by the attending surgeon that she was scheduled to have gallbladder surgery later that day. After the surgeon's visit, a consulting psychiatrist who examined her directed her to dress and pack her belongings because he had arranged to have her admitted to a state hospital at Ogdensburg.

Subsequently, two uniformed state troopers handcuffed her and strapped her into the back seat of a patrol car. She was also accompanied by a female hospital employee and was transported to the state hospital. On arrival, the admitting psychiatrist recognized that the referring psychiatrist lacked the requisite authority to order her involuntary commitment. He therefore requested that she sign a voluntary admission form, which she refused to do. Despite Mrs. Plumadore's protests regarding her admission to the state hospital, the psychiatrist assigned her to a ward without physical or psychiatric examination and without the opportunity to contact her family or her medical doctor. The record of her admission to the state hospital noted an "informed admission," which is the patient-initiated voluntary admission in New York.

The court awarded $40,000 to Mrs. Plumadore for false imprisonment, negligence, and malpractice.

Negligence

Negligence is an act or an omission to act that breaches the duty of due care and results in or is responsible for a person's injuries. The five elements required to prove negligence are (1) duty, (2) breach of duty, (3) cause in fact, (4) proximate cause, and (5) damages. Foreseeability of harm is also evaluated.

Duty is measured by a standard of care. When nurses represent themselves as being capable of caring for psychiatric clients and accept employment, a duty of care has been assumed. The duty is owed to psychiatric clients to understand the theory and medications used in the specialty care of these clients. Persons who represent themselves as possessing superior knowledge and skill, such as psychiatric nurse specialists in nursing, are held to a higher standard of care in the practice of their profession. The staff nurse who is assigned to a psychiatric unit must be knowledgeable enough to assume a reasonable or safe duty of care to the clients.

If the nurse is not capable of providing the standard of care that other nurses would be expected to supply under similar circumstances, the nurse has breached the duty of care. *Breach of duty* is the conduct that exposes the client to an unreasonable risk of harm, through either commission or omission of acts on the part of the nurse. If a nurse does not have the required education and experience to provide certain interventions, the nurse has breached the duty by neglecting or omitting to provide necessary care. The nurse can also act in such a way that the client is harmed and can thus be guilty of negligence through acts of commission.

Cause in fact may be evaluated by questioning: but for what the nurse did, would this injury have occurred? *Proximate cause*, or legal cause, may be evaluated by determining whether there have been any intervening actions or persons that were, in fact, the causes of harm to the client. *Damages* include actual damages (e.g., loss of earnings, medical expenses, and property damage) as well as pain and suffering.

DETERMINING A STANDARD OF CARE

Professional standards of practice determined by professional associations differ from the minimal qualifications set forth by state licensure for entry into the profession of nursing. The ANA has established standards for psychiatric nursing practice and credentialing of clinical psychiatric nurse specialists (ANA 1994).

Standards for psychiatric nursing practice differ markedly from minimal state requirements because the primary purposes for setting these two types of qualifications are different. The state's qualifications for practice provide consumer protection by ensuring that all practicing nurses have successfully completed an approved nursing program and passed the national licensing examination. The professional association's primary focus is to elevate the practice of its members by setting standards of excellence. The ANA Standards of Psychiatric and Mental Health Nursing Practice are provided inside the front cover of this book.

Nurses are held to the standard of care exercised by other nurses possessing the same degree of skill or knowledge in the same or similar circumstances. In the past, community standards existed for urban and rural agencies. However, with greater mobility and expanded means of communication, national standards have evolved. Psychiatric clients have the right to receive the standard of care recognized by professional bodies governing nursing, whether they are in a large or a small, a rural or an urban, facility. Nurses must participate in continuing education courses to stay current with existing standards of care.

The most common method of establishing a standard of care in a court case is to use an expert witness. Expert witnesses testify about their opinions and conclusions, usually on the basis of a hypothetical fact pattern that is presented by counsel and that resembles the fact pattern of the actual case. The testimony of expert witnesses differs from that of other witnesses. Other witnesses can testify as to facts only. The expert's testimony carries no greater weight, except for credibility, than the testimony of any other witness.

In a professional negligence case or a disciplinary action, the expert witness testifying should not only be a member of the profession about which he or she is testifying but should also practice in the specialty area concerned in the case. The witness is qualified as an expert by reason of education, clinical practice, and research. An expert's opinion should not be bought: the integrity of the expert's opinion must be protected by the nurse acting as an expert.

Hospital policies and procedures set up institutional criteria for care, and these criteria, such as the frequency of rounds on clients in seclusion, may be introduced to prove a standard that the nurse met or failed to meet. The shortcoming of this method is that the hospital's policy may be substandard. For example, the state licensing laws for institutions might set a minimal requirement for staffing or frequency of rounds on certain clients, and the hospital policy might fall below that minimum. Substandard institutional policies do not absolve the individual nurse of responsibility to practice on the basis of professional standards of nursing care.

Like hospital policy and procedures, custom can be used as evidence of a standard of care. For example, in the absence of a written policy on the use of restraint, testimony might be offered regarding the customary use of restraint in emergency situations in which the combative, violent, or confused client poses a threat of harm to self or others. Using custom to establish a standard of care may result in the same defect as in using hospital policies and procedures: custom may not comply with the laws, accrediting body recommendations, or other recognized standards of care. Custom must be carefully and regularly evaluated to ensure that substandard routines have not developed. Substandard customs will not protect the nurse when a psychiatric client charges that a right has been violated or that harm has been caused by the staff's common practices.

Guidelines for Students Who Suspect Negligence

It is not unusual for a student or practicing nurse to suspect negligence on the part of a peer. In most states, nurses have a legal duty to report such risks of harm to the client. It is also very important that the nurse document clear and accurate evidence before making serious accusations against a peer. If the nurse questions a physician's orders or actions, or those of a fellow nurse, it is wise to communicate these concerns directly to the person involved. If the risky behavior continues, the nurse has an obligation to communicate these concerns to a supervisor, who should then intervene to ensure that the client's rights and well-being are protected. If a nurse suspects a peer of being chemically impaired or of practicing irresponsibly, the nurse has an obligation to protect not only the rights of the peer but also the rights of all clients who could be harmed by this impaired peer. If, after the nurse has reported suspected behavior of concern to a supervisor, the danger persists, the nurse has a duty to report the concern to someone at the next level of authority. It is important to follow the channels of communication in an organization, but it is also important to protect the safety of the clients. If the supervisor's actions or inactions do not rectify the dangerous situation, the nurse has a continuing duty to report the behavior of concern to the appropriate authority, such as the state board of nursing.

THE DUTY TO INTERVENE AND THE DUTY TO REPORT

The psychiatric nurse has a duty to intervene when the safety or well-being of the client or another person is obviously at risk. A nurse who follows an order that is known to be incorrect or that the nurse believes will harm the client is responsible for the harm that results to the client. If the nurse has information that leads her or him to believe that the doctor's orders need to be clarified or changed, it is the nurse's duty to intervene and protect the client. It is important that the nurse communicate with the physician who has ordered the treatment to explain the concern. If the treating physician does not appear willing to consider the nurse's concerns, the nurse should carry out the duty to intervene through other appropriate channels.

It is important for the nurse to express concerns to the supervisor in order to allow the supervisor to communicate with the appropriate medical staff for intervention in the physician's treatment plan. The nurse, as the client's advocate, has a duty to intervene to protect the client; at the same time, the nurse does not have the right to interfere with the physician-client relationship.

It is very important to follow agency policies and procedures for communicating differences of opinion. If the nurse fails to intervene and the client is injured, the nurse may be partly liable for the injuries that result because of the nurse's failure to use safe nursing practice and good professional judgment. The legal concept of abandonment may also arise when a nurse does not leave a client safely back in the hands of another health professional before discontinuing treatment. Abandonment issues arise when accurate, timely, and thorough reporting has not occurred or when follow-through of client care, on which the client is relying, has not occurred. The same principles apply for the psychiatric nurse who is working in a community setting. For example, if a suicidal client refuses to come to the hospital for treatment, the nurse cannot abandon the client but must take the necessary steps to ensure the client's safety. These actions may include enlisting the assistance of the law in temporarily involuntarily committing the client.

The duty to intervene on the client's behalf poses many legal and ethical dilemmas for the nurse in the workplace. Institutions that have a chain-of-command policy or other reporting mechanisms offer some assurance that the proper authorities in the administration are notified. Most client care issues regarding physician's orders or treatments can be settled fairly early in the process by nurses' discussing their concerns with the physician. If further intervention by the nurse is required to protect the client, the next step in the chain of command can be initiated. Generally, the nurse then notifies the immediate nursing supervisor; the supervisor thereupon discusses the problem with the physician, and then with the chief of staff of a particular service, until a resolution is reached. If there is no time to resolve the issue through the normal process because of the life-threatening nature of the situation, the nurse must act to protect the client's life.

The issues become more complex when a professional colleague's conduct, including a student nurse's, is criminally unlawful. Specific examples include the diversion of drugs from the hospital, or sexual misconduct with clients. Increasing media attention and the recognition of substance abuse as an occupational hazard for health professionals have led to substance abuse programs for health care workers in many states. These programs provide appropriate treatment for impaired professionals in order to protect the public from harm and to rehabilitate the professional.

The problem previously discussed, of reporting impaired colleagues, becomes a very difficult one, particularly when no direct harm has occurred to the client. Concern for professional reputations, damaged careers, and personal privacy rather than public protection has generated a code of silence regarding substance abuse among health professionals. Several states now require reporting of impaired or incompetent colleagues to the professional licensing boards. Without this legal mandate, the questions of whether to report and to whom to report become ethical ones. Chapter 25 deals more fully with issues related to the chemically impaired nurse.

The duty to intervene includes the duty to report known abusive behavior. Most states have enacted statutes to protect children and the elderly from abuse and neglect. Psychiatric nurses working in the community may be mandated by the law to report unsafe relationships they discover.

DOCUMENTATION OF CARE

Purpose

The purpose of the medical record is to provide accurate and complete information about the care and treatment of clients and to give health care personnel responsible for that care a means of communicating with each other. The medical record allows for continuity of care. A record's usefulness is determined by evaluating, when the record is read at a later date, how accurately and completely it portrays the client's behavioral status at the time it was written.

Timeliness in recording nursing actions and observations is as important as the accuracy of the information shared. Clients' safety is compromised when their high-risk behavior or statements are not immediately communicated. Miscommunications and delays in sharing pertinent information are major causes of legal liability. If a member of the health care team relies on old information because the nurse has not recently charted new data, and the client is harmed, the nurse shares the responsibility for the resultant injury. For example, if a psychiatric client describes to a nurse a plan to harm either self or another, and the nurse fails to document the information, including the need to protect the client or the identified victim, the information will be lost when the nurse leaves work and the client's plan may be carried out. The harm caused could be linked directly to the nurse's failure to communicate this important information. Even though documentation takes time away from the client, the importance of communicating and preserving the nurse's memory through the medical record cannot be overemphasized.

Accrediting agencies, such as the Joint Commission on Accreditation of Healthcare Organizations (JCAHO) and state regulatory agencies, require health care facilities to maintain records on clients' care and treatment. Noncompliance with record-keeping responsibilities may result in fines, loss of accreditation, or both.

Facility Use of Medical Records

The medical record has many other uses aside from providing information on the course of the client's care and treatment to health care professionals. A retrospective chart review can provide valuable information to the facility on the quality of care provided and on ways to improve that care. A facility may conduct reviews for risk management purposes, to determine areas of potential liability for the facility, and to evaluate methods used to reduce the facility's exposure to liability. For example, documentation of the use of restraints and seclusion for psychiatric clients may be reviewed by risk managers. Accordingly, the chart may be used to evaluate care for quality assurance or peer review. Utilization review analysts review the chart to determine appropriate use of hospital and staff resources consistent with reimbursement schedules. Insurance companies and other reimbursement agencies rely on the medical record in determining payments they will make on the client's behalf.

The Medical Record As Evidence

From a legal perspective, the chart is a recording of data and opinions made in the normal course of the client's hospital care. It is deemed to be good evidence because it is presumed to be true, honest, and untainted by memory lapses. Accordingly, the medical record finds its way into a variety of legal cases for a variety of reasons. Some examples of its use include determining (1) the extent of the client's damages and pain and suffering in personal injury cases, such as when a psychiatric client attempts suicide while under the protective care of a hospital; (2) the nature and extent of injuries in child abuse or elder abuse cases; (3) the nature and extent of physical or mental disability in disability cases; and (4) the nature and extent of injury and rehabilitative potential in workers' compensation cases.

Medical records may also be used in police investigations, civil conservatorship proceedings, competency hearings, and commitment procedures. In states that mandate a mental health legal services or clients' rights advocacy program, audits may be performed to determine the facility's compliance with state laws or violation of clients' rights. Finally, medical records may be used in professional and hospital negligence cases.

During the discovery phase of litigation, the medical record is a pivotal source of information for attorneys in determining whether a cause of action exists in a professional negligence or hospital negligence case. Evidence of the nursing care rendered will be reflected in what the nurse charted at the time. Incomplete or poor notes will raise suspicion about the quality of care delivered.

Nursing Guidelines For Charting

Accurate, descriptive, and legible nursing notes serve the best interests of the client, the nurse, and the institution. As computerized charting becomes more widely available, it will also be important for psychiatric nurses to understand how to protect the confidentiality of these records. Institutions must also protect against intrusions into the privacy of the client record systems.

The nurse's charting should reflect factual observations and not contain generalized opinions. For example, if the notation is made that the client "had a good night," does this indicate merely that the nurse was not bothered by the client during the night? More appropriate notations would indicate the time(s) that the client was checked on and what, specifically, the nurse observed.

The various systems utilized will allow specific time frames within which the nurse must make any necessary corrections if a charting error is made. The information charted will assist those on the following shift to understand the client's current status. Information on whether the psychiatric client slept through the night or continued to pace the hallway has significant treatment implications. It is important never to obliterate or erase previous charting. A presumption of fraud will be made if it appears that an error is being hidden. Instead, a line drawn through the error with correct information provided in the next available space will maintain the integrity of the record.

Integrated charting systems encourage all members of the health team to read each other's documentation of care. Any charting method that improves communication between care providers should be encouraged. Courts assume that nurses and physicians read each other's notes on client progress. Many courts reflect the attitude that if care is not documented, it did not occur. The nurse's charting also serves as a valuable memory refresher if the client sues years after the care is provided. In providing complete and timely information on the care and treatment of clients, the medical record enhances communication among health professionals. Internal, institutional audits of the record can improve the quality of care rendered. The nurse's charting will be improved by following the guidelines in Box 4–4. Chapter 8 identifies four common charting forms and gives examples as well as the pros and cons of each.

MAINTAINING CLIENT CONFIDENTIALITY

Ethical Considerations: ANA Code for Nurses

The ANA Code for Nurses states that "the nurse safeguards the client's right to privacy by judiciously protecting information of a confidential nature" (ANA 1985).

BOX 4–4 DO'S AND DON'TS OF CHARTING

DO'S

- Chart in a timely manner all pertinent and factual information.
- Be familiar with the nursing documentation policy in your facility and make your charting conform to this standard. The policy will generally state the method of charting, the frequency, pertinent assessments, interventions, and outcomes. If your agency's policies and procedures do not encourage or allow for quality documentation, bring the need for change to the administration's attention. (Refer to Chapter 8 for four charting methods.)
- Chart legibly in ink.
- Chart facts fully, descriptively, and accurately.
- Chart what you see, hear, feel, and smell.
- Chart a total patient assessment on admission, discharge, and transfer, and in between when pertinent.
- Chart pertinent observations: psychosocial observations, physical symptoms pertinent to the medical diagnosis, and behaviors pertinent to the nursing diagnosis.
- Chart follow-up care provided when a problem has been identified in earlier documentation. For example, if a patient falls and injures a leg, describe how the wound is healing.
- Chart fully the facts surrounding unusual occurrences and incidents, *but do not note in the chart that an incident report was filed.* This form is generally a privileged communication between the hospital and the hospital's attorney. Charting it may destroy the privileged nature of the communication.
- Chart *all* nursing interventions, treatments, and outcomes, including teaching efforts and patient responses, and safety and patient protection interventions.
- Chart the patient's expressed subjective feelings.
- Chart each time you notify a physician, the reason for notification, what was communicated, the accurate time, the physician's instructions or orders, and the follow-up activity.
- Chart doctor visits and treatments.
- Chart discharge medications and instructions given for use, as well as all discharge teaching performed and which family members were included in the process.

DON'TS

- Do *not* chart opinions that are not supported by the facts.
- Do *not* defame clients by calling them names or by making derogatory statements about them (e.g., "an unlikable client/person who is demanding unnecessary attention").
- Do *not* chart before an event occurs.
- Do *not* chart generalizations, suppositions, or "pat phrases" (e.g., "client in good spirits").
- Do *not* obliterate, erase, alter, or destroy a record. If an error is made, draw one line through the error, write "mistaken entry" or "error," and initial. Follow your agency's guidelines closely.
- Do *not* leave blank spaces for chronological notes. If you must chart out of sequence, chart "late entry." Identify the time and date of the entry and the time and date of the occurrence.

The applicable interpretive statement provides further explanation for maintaining client confidentiality and recognizes the distinction between legal and ethical obligations. The interpretive statement follows:

> The right of privacy is an inalienable right of all persons, and the nurse has a clear obligation to safeguard any confidential information about the client acquired from any source. The nurse-client relationship is built on trust. This relationship could be destroyed and the client's welfare and reputation jeopardized by injudicious disclosing of information provided in confidence. Since the concept of confidentiality has legal as well as ethical implications, an inappropriate breach of confidentiality may also expose the nurse to liability.

Legal Considerations

The psychiatric client's right to have treatment and medical records kept confidential is legally protected. The fundamental principle underlying the ANA code on confidentiality is a person's constitutional **right to privacy.** Generally, the nurse's legal duty to maintain confidentiality is to act to protect the client's right to privacy. Therefore, the nurse may not, without the client's consent, disclose information obtained from the client or information in the medical record to anyone except those necessary for implementation of a client's treatment plan.

For example, the nurse's release of information to the client's employer about the client's condition, without the client's consent, is a breach of confidentiality that subjects the nurse to liability for the tort of invasion of privacy. On the other hand, discussion of clients' history with other staff members to ascertain a consistent treatment approach is not a breach of confidentiality.

Many states have enacted privileged communication statutes that prohibit specified health professionals from disclosing client information unless the client has either consented to the disclosure or waived the privilege of consent. These state statutes differ markedly.

Generally, to create a situation in which information is privileged, a client-health professional relationship must exist, and the information must relate to the care and treatment of the client. The health professional may refuse to disclose information in order to protect the client's privacy. However, the right to privacy is the client's right, and health professionals cannot involve confidentiality for their own defense or benefit. A person's reputation can be damaged even after death. It is therefore important not to divulge information after a person's death that could not have been legally shared before the death. The Dead Man's Statute protects confidential information about people when they are not alive to speak for themselves.

A legal privilege of confidentiality is enacted legislatively and exists to protect the confidentiality of professional communications (e.g., nurse-client, physician-client, attorney-client). The theory behind such privileged communications is that clients will not be comfortable or willing to disclose personal information about themselves if they fear that the nurse will repeat their confidential conversations. In some states in which the legal privilege of confidentiality has not been legislated for nurses, the nurse must respond to a court's inquiries regarding the client's disclosures even if this information implicates the client in a crime. In these states, the confidentiality of communications cannot be guaranteed. If a duty to report exists, the nurse may be required to divulge private information shared by the client. For example, some states have enacted mandatory or permissive statutes that direct health care providers to warn a spouse if a partner is HIV positive (Table 4–3). Nurses must understand the laws in their jurisdiction of practice regarding privileged communications and warnings of infectious disease exposure.

Exceptions To The Rule

Duty To Warn Third Parties

The California Supreme Court, in its 1976 landmark decision *Tarasoff v. Regents of University of California*, ruled that a psychotherapist has a **duty to warn** the client's potential victim of potential harm. This decision created much controversy and confusion in the psychiatric and medical communities over breach of client confidentiality and its impact on the therapeutic relationship in psychiatric care and on the ability of the psychotherapist to predict when a client is truly dangerous. This trend continues as other jurisdictions have adopted or modified the California rule despite the psychiatric community's objections. These jurisdictions view public safety to be more important than privacy in narrowly defined circumstances.

The *Tarasoff* case acknowledged that generally there is no common-law duty to aid third persons. An exception is when special relationships exist, and the court found the client-therapist relationship sufficient to create a duty of the therapist to aid Ms. Tarasoff, the victim. The duty to protect the intended victim from danger arises when the therapist determines—or, pursuant to professional standards, should have determined—that the client presents a serious danger to another. Any action reasonably necessary under the circumstances, including notification of the potential victim, the victim's family, and the police, discharges the therapist's duty to the potential victim.

Arguing that predictions of future violence are inaccurate at best and speculative at worst, the psychiatric community raised concerns over the use of a professional standard to determine when a therapist should have known of the client's future violence toward another, as required by *Tarasoff.* The courts and other legal commentators have recognized the therapist's difficulty in forecasting violence but have also noted that therapists' assessment for predicting violence are used in civil commitment procedures to determine whether a client poses a threat to others.

The psychologist's diagnostic function, a professional service rendered within the legal scope of practice, was central to the California Supreme Court's ruling in *Hedlum v. Superior Court of Orange County* (1983). The court stated that the duty to warn was composed of two elements: (1) the duty to diagnose and predict the client's danger of violence and (2) the duty to take appropriate action to protect the identified victim. The court stated that "a negligent failure to diagnose dangerousness in a *Tarasoff* action is as much a basis for liability as is a negligent failure to warn a known victim once such a diagnosis has been made."

A limited duty to investigate the client's history was enunciated in *Jablonski v. United States* (1983). Mr. Jablonski had attempted to rape his girlfriend's mother. He agreed to undergo psychiatric treatment. The police notified the chief psychiatrist that Mr. Jablonski had a criminal record that included threatening others, and recommended that he be treated on an inpatient basis. The chief psychiatrist failed to communicate this information to the treating psychiatrist. The treating physician noted the client's potential violence, learned of his criminal rape record, and noted his past psychiatric treatment during the initial interview. However, the treating psychiatrist did not attempt to locate the previous medical records and did not believe that the client met the civil commitment criteria. While being treated on an outpatient basis, Mr. Jablonski killed his girlfriend.

The court found that the psychiatrist's failure to obtain the client's records and the failure to record and communicate the telephone contact by the police were negligent acts. Although no specific threats were made toward the girlfriend, Mr. Jablonski's previous history indicated that his violence would probably be directed toward her.

In *Thomas v. County of Alameda* (1980), a juvenile with dangerous and violent propensities toward young children was released from the custody of the county to the custody of his mother for a home visit. While home, he killed a neighborhood child. The deceased child's parents sued the county for wrongful death, alleging that the county had a duty to warn the police, the juvenile's mother, and other local parents. The court held that there was no duty to warn because the victim was a "member of a large amorphous public group of potential targets and not a known, identifiable victim." This is distinguishable from the *Jablonski* case, in which sufficient information existed to identify the victim.

Nursing Implications

As this trend toward making it the therapist's duty to warn third persons of potential harm continues to gain wider acceptance, it is important for students and nurses to understand its implications for nursing practice. Although none of these cases to date has dealt with nurses, it is fair to assume that, in jurisdictions that have adopted the *Tarasoff* doctrine, the duty to warn third persons will be applied to clinical psychiatric nurse specialists in private practice who engage in individual therapy.

It is unlikely that a duty to warn potential victims will be extended to staff psychiatric nurses working in the institutional setting, because nurses at present do not have primary case management responsibilities. However, if a staff psychiatric nurse who is a member of a team of psychiatrists, psychologists, psychiatric social workers, and other psychiatric nurses does not report client threats of harm against specified victims or classes of victims to the team of the client's management psychotherapist for assessment and evaluation, this failure is likely to be considered substandard nursing care.

So, too, the failure to communicate and record relevant information from police, relatives, or the client's old records might also be deemed negligent. Breach of client-nurse confidentiality should not pose ethical or legal dilemmas for nurses in these situations, because a team approach to the delivery of psychiatric care presumes communication of pertinent information to other staff members in order to develop a treatment plan in the client's best interest.

Child and Elder Abuse Reporting Statutes

Because of their interest in protecting children, all 50 states and the District of Columbia have enacted **child abuse reporting statutes.** Although these statutes differ from state to state, they generally include a definition of child abuse, a list of persons required or encouraged to report, and the governmental agency designated to receive and investigate the reports. Most statutes include civil penalties for failure to report. Many states specifically require nurses to report cases of suspected abuse.

There is a conflict between federal and state laws with respect to child abuse reporting when the health care professional discovers child abuse or neglect during the suspected abuser's alcohol or drug treatment. Federal laws and regulations governing confidentiality of client records, which apply to almost all drug abuse and alcohol treatment providers, prohibit any disclosure without a court order. In this case, federal law supersedes state reporting laws, although compliance with the state law may be maintained (1) if a court order is obtained, pursuant to the regulations; (2) if a report can be made without identifying the abuser as a client in an alcohol or drug treatment program; or (3) if the report is made anonymously. Some states, to protect the rights of the accused, do not allow anonymous reporting.

As reported incidents of abuse to other persons in society surface, states may require health professionals to report other kinds of abuse. A growing number of states are enacting **elder abuse reporting statutes,** which require registered nurses and others to report cases of abuse of the elderly. The elderly are defined as adults 65 years of age and older. These laws also apply to dependent adults—that is, adults between 18 and 64 years of age whose physical or mental limitations restrict their ability to carry out normal activities or protect themselves—when the registered nurse has actual knowledge that the person has been the victim of physical abuse. The nurse may also report knowledge of, or "reasonable suspicion" of, mental abuse or suffering. Both dependent adults and elders are protected by the law from purposeful physical or fiduciary neglect or abandonment. *Because state laws vary, students are encouraged to become conversant with the requirements of their state.*

SUMMARY

The states' power to enact laws for public health and safety and for the care of those unable to care for themselves often pits the rights of society against the rights of the individual. The complexities of these relationships can manifest as legal and ethical dilemmas in the psychiatric setting. Increasingly, the nurse encounters problems requiring ethical choices. The nurse's privilege to practice nursing carries with it responsibility to practice safely, competently, and in a manner consistent with state and federal laws. Knowledge of the law, the ANA Code for Nurses, and the Standards of Psychiatric and Mental Health Nursing Practice will enhance the nurse's ability to provide safe, effective psychiatric nursing care and will serve as a framework for decision making when the nurse is presented with complex problems involving competing interests.

ACKNOWLEDGMENTS

The author wishes to recognize and thank Lorenza M. Valvo and Mary Ursula Guthormsen for their contribution to the first edition.

REFERENCES

American Nurses' Association (1994). *A statement on psychiatric-mental health clinical nursing practice and standards of psychiatric and mental health nursing practice.* Washington, DC: American Nurses' Publishing.

American Nurses' Association (1985). *Code for nurses.* Kansas City, MO: American Nurses' Association.

Blythe v. Radiometer America, Inc. 866 P.2d 218 (Mont. Sup. Ct. 1993).

Canterbury v. Spence, 464 F2d 722 (DC Cir 1972), quoting *Schloendorf v. Society of NY Hosp,* 211 NY 125 105 NE2d 92, 93 (1914).

Hedlum v. Superior Court of Orange County, 34 C3d 695 (1983).

Humphrey v. Cady, 405 US 504 (1972).

Illinois vs. Russel, 630 NE2nd 794 (Ill. Sup. Ct. 1994).

In re guardianship of Roe, 421 NE2d 40 (Mass 1981).

In re Oakes, 8 Law Rep 122 (Mass 1845).

Jablonski v. United States, 712 F2d 391 (9th Cir 1983).

L., B. (1989). Clinical ethics and HIV-related illnesses: Issues in treatment and health services. In W. Le Vee (ed.), New Perspectives on HIV-Related Illnesses: Progress in Health Services Research (pp. 170–179). Washington, DC: U. S. Dept. of Health and Human Services.

Mills v. Rogers, 457 US 291 (1982).

O'Connor v. Donaldson, 422 US 563 (1975).

Pisel v. Stamford Hospital, 430 A2d 1 (Cone 1980).

Plumadore v. State of New York, 427 NYS2d 90 (1980).

Rennie v. Klein, 476 F Supp 1294 (DNJ 1979).

Rennie v. Klein, 653 F2d 836 (3rd Cir 1981).

Rennie v. Klein, 454 US 1078 (1982).

Rennie v. Klein, 720 F2d 266 (3rd Cir 1983).

Rogers v. Commissioner of the Department of Mental Health, 458 NE2d 308 (Mass 1983).

Rogers v. Okin, 478 F Supp 1342 (D Mass 1979).

Rogers v. Okin, 634 F2d 650 (1st Cir 1980).

Rouse v. Cameron, 373 F2d 451 (DC Cir 1966).

State of Washington v. Harper, 489 US 1064 (1989).

Tarasoff v. Regents of University of California, 17 C3d 425 (1976).

Thomas v. County of Alameda, 27 C3d 741 (1980).

Wyatt v. Stickney, 325 F Supp 781 (MD Ala 1971).

Wyatt v St. Paul Tire & Marine Ins. Co., 868 S. W. 2d 505 (Ark. Sup. Ct. 1994).

Youngberg v. Romeo, 457 US 307 (1982).

Further Reading

Beck, J. C. (1987). The psychotherapists' duty to protect third parties from harm. *Mental Health and Physical Disability Law Reporter,* 2, 2 (Mar-Apr).

Bellah v. Greenson, 81 CA 3rd 614 (1978).

Brakel, S. J., Parry, J. Weiner, B. A. (1985). *Mentally disabled and the law* (2nd ed.). Chicago: American Bar Foundation.

Brennan, J. (1973). *Ethics and morals.* New York: Harper & Row.

California Department of Mental Health (1985). *Patients' rights advocacy manual.* Sacramento, CA: California Department of Mental Health.

Chalmers-Frances v. Nelson, 6 C2d 402 (1936).

Cole, R. (1981). Patients' rights to refuse antipsychotic drugs. *Law, Medicine and Health Care,* 9(4):1, 1981.

Darling v. Charleston Community Memorial Hospital, 211 NE2d 253 (Ill. 1965).

Feuntz, S. A. (1987). Preventative legal maintenance. *Journal of Nursing Administration,* 17(1):8–10.

Garritson, S. (1983). Degrees of restrictions in psychosocial nursing. *Journal of Psychosocial Nursing,* 21(12):9.

Goldstein, A. S., Perdew, S., and Pruitt, S. S. (1989). *The nurse's legal advisor: Your guide to legally safe practice.* Philadelphia: J. B. Lippincott.

Miller, R., and Fiddleman, P. (1984). Outpatient commitment: Treatment in the least restrictive environment? *Hospital and Community Psychiatry,* 35(2):147.

Rhoden, N. (1985). The presumption for treatment: Has it been justified? *Law, Medicine and Health Care,* 13(2):65.

Saunders, J., and DuPlessis, D. (1985). A historical view of right to treatment. *Journal of Psychosocial Nursing,* 23(9):12.

Schmid, D., Applebaum, P., Roth, L., and Lidz, C. (1983). Confidentiality in psychiatry: A study of the patients' view. *Hospital and Community Psychiatry,* 34(4):353.

Vitek v. Jones, 445 US 480 (1980).

Wyatt v. Aderholt, 503 F2d 1305 (5th Cir 1974).

SELF-STUDY AND CRITICAL THINKING

Match the word with the correct definition.

1. ________ Civil wrongs for which money damages are collected by the injured party.
2. ________ Harmful or offensive touching of another's person.
3. ________ The act or omission to act that breaches the duty or care and is the actual or proximate cause of a person's injuries.
4. ________ Based on the principle of a person's right to self-determination.
5. ________ Verbal or written retraction of consent previously given must be honored.

A. Negligence
B. Assault
C. Battery
D. Torts
E. Informed consent
F. Right to refuse treatment

True or false

6. ________ Voluntarily admitted clients have the right to demand and obtain release.
7. ________ In many states, common criteria for involuntary admission to mental health facilities include need for psychiatric treatment and danger to self and others.

For discussion:

8. Discuss what is meant by *client's civil rights,* and give examples.
9. Discuss some of the legal responsibilities of the nurse in the care and discharge of a client in seclusion or restraints, as identified in this chapter.
10. Discuss guidelines for nurses who suspect negligence.
11. Define what is meant by confidentiality and the right to privacy. Discuss two exceptions to the rule.

Critical thinking

The distinction between minimal entry practice standards and professional practice standards is important in a discussion of standards of care for psychiatric nurses. Consider the legal and ethical issues posed by the following situations.

12. Nurse A has worked in a psychiatric setting for 5 years, since she was licensed by the state. She arrives at work on her unit and is informed that the nursing office has requested a nurse from the psychiatric unit to assist the intensive care unit staff in caring for an agitated car accident victim with a history of schizophrenia. Nurse A works with Nurse B in caring for the client. While the client is sleeping, Nurse B leaves the unit for a coffee break. Nurse A, unfamiliar with the telemetry equipment, fails to recognize an arrhythmia, and the client has a cardiopulmonary arrest. The client is successfully resuscitated after 6 minutes but suffers permanent brain damage.
    - Can Nurse A legally practice? (That is, does her license permit her to practice in the intensive care unit?)

- Does the ability to practice legally in an area differ from the ability to practice competently in that area?
- Did Nurse A have any legal or ethical grounds to refuse the assignment to the intensive care unit?
- What are the risks in accepting an assignment to an area of specialty practice in which you are professionally unprepared to practice?
- What are the risks in refusing an assignment to an area of specialty practice in which you are professionally unprepared to practice?
- Would there have been any way for Nurse A to minimize the risk of action for insubordination by the employer had she refused the assignment?
- What action could Nurse A have taken to protect the client and herself when Nurse B left the unit for a coffee break?
- If Nurse A is negligent, is the hospital liable for any harm to the client caused by Nurse A?

13. A 40-year-old man who is admitted to the emergency room for a severe nosebleed has both nares packed. Because of his history of alcoholism and the probability of ensuing delirium tremens, the client is transferred to the psychiatric unit. He is admitted to a private room, placed in restraints, and checked by a nurse every hour per physician order. While unattended, the client suffocates, apparently by inhaling the nasal packing, which had become dislodged from the nares. On the next 1-hour check, the nurse finds the client without pulse or respiration.

    A state statute requires that a restrained client on a psychiatric unit be assessed by a nurse every hour for safety, comfort, and physical needs.

    - If standards are not otherwise specified, do statutory requirements set forth minimal or maximal standards?
    - Does the nurse's compliance with the state statute relieve her of liability in the client's death?
    - Does the nurse's compliance with the physician's order relieve her of liability in the client's death?
    - Was the order for the restraint appropriate for this type of client?
    - What factors did you consider in making your determination?
    - Was the frequency of rounds for assessment of client needs appropriate in this situation?
    - Did the nurse's conduct meet the standard of care for psychiatric nurses? Why or why not?
    - What nursing action should the nurse have taken to protect the client from harm?

Assume that there are no mandatory reporting laws for impaired or incompetent colleagues in the following clinical situations.

14. Jane Smith, 45 years of age, is admitted to the surgical unit for a biopsy of the thyroid gland. Her admitting physician has recommended a psychiatric consultation because Mrs. Smith has had a history of pronounced mood swings for the past 3 months, after the break-up of her marriage of 20 years. The nurse introduces the client to the psychiatrist and is called away because of a new admission. Within the hour, the nurse is summoned to Mrs. Smith's room and finds the client alone, agitated and crying. The nurse encourages Mrs. Smith to share her concerns, and the client then states that the doctor touched her "private areas" while talking with her and exposed himself to her. She states that she pushed him away as he advanced toward her. She tells the nurse that she feels violated and humiliated. What action, if any, can the nurse take?

    - Should the nurse chart the incident?
    - Should the nurse inform the admitting physician?
    - Should the nurse inform the nursing supervisor?
    - Should the nurse talk with the consulting psychiatrist about the client's allegations?

- Should the nurse inform the chief of staff of psychiatry of the incident reported by the client?
- Should the nurse report the incident to the chairperson of the peer review committee of the hospital?
- If the nurse initiates the reporting mechanism in her facility, must she take any further action?
- Should the nurse report the psychiatrist to the medical board?
- Should the nurse notify the police?

15. Two nurses, Joe and Beth, have worked on the psychiatric unit for 2 years. During the past 6 months, Beth has confided to Joe that she has been going through a particularly difficult marital situation. Joe has noticed that for 6 months Beth has become increasingly irritable and difficult to work with. He notices that minor tranquilizers are frequently missing from the unit dose cart on the evening shift. He complains to the pharmacy and is informed that the drugs were stocked as ordered. Several clients state that they have not been receiving their usual drugs. Joe finds that Beth has recorded that the drugs have been given as ordered. He also notices that Beth is diverting the drugs. What action, if any, should Joe take?
    - Should Joe confront Beth with his suspicions?
    - If Beth admits that she has been diverting the drugs, should Joe's next step be to report Beth to the supervisor or to the board of nursing?
    - Should Joe make his concern known to the nursing supervisor directly by identifying Beth or should he state his concerns in general terms?
    - Legally, must Joe report his suspicions to the board of nursing?
    - Does the fact that harm to the clients is limited to increased agitation affect your responses?

16. A 23-year-old woman in an agitated state is admitted to a psychiatric unit and placed in a seclusion room without furniture, per physician order. Four days after her admission, a bed frame inexplicably arrives in the room. On the ninth day of hospitalization, her psychosis becomes more acute, and the staff intensify their care. The following day, the client reports to the staff that she heard voices telling her to hurt herself. The client is sedated and locked in her room. Four hours later, the room is unlocked and the client is found unconscious, with her head wedged between the bed frame and the side rails. She suffers neurological damage. The following day, the director of the nurses orders the staff to remove the original charting, rewrite their notes, and place the falsified notes in the chart.*
    - Which acts or omission by the staff breach the staff's duty to provide the client with a safe environment?
    - What nursing action should the staff have taken after sedating the client to protect her from harm?
    - Discuss the legal and ethical ramifications of the staff's falsification of the client's record on the order of the director of nurses.

17. In a private psychiatric unit in California, a 15-year-old boy is admitted voluntarily at the request of his parents because of violent, explosive behavior that seems to stem from his father's recent remarriage after his parents' divorce. A few days after admission, while in group therapy, he has an explosive reaction to a discussion about weekend passes for Mother's Day. He screams that he has been abandoned and that nobody cares about him. Several weeks later, on the day before his discharge, he elicits from the nurse a promise to keep his plan to kill his mother confidential.

---

*This clinical situation was taken from the facts in a Connecticut case. In Pisel v. Stamford Hospital (1980), the falsification of the record was not disclosed until after a lawsuit had been filed. The Connecticut Supreme Court, in upholding a $3.6 million award for the client, decided that the jury was entitled to consider the falsified record as evidence that the hospital was conscious of its negligence.

Consider the ANA code of ethics on client confidentiality, the principles of psychiatric nursing, statutes on privileged communications, and the duty to warn third parties in answering the following questions:

- Did the nurse use appropriate judgment in promising confidentiality?
- Does the nurse have a legal duty to warn the client's mother of her son's threat?
- Is the duty owed to the client's father and stepmother?
- Would a change in the admission status from voluntary to involuntary protect the client's mother without violating the client's confidentiality?
- Would your response be different depending on the state where the incident occurred? Why or why not?
- What nursing action, if any, should the nurse take after the disclosure by the client?

18. How would your responses to the concepts in the previous question differ in relation to the changes in the following clinical situation?

    A 25-year-old woman is attending a federally funded outpatient rehabilitative center for alcoholism after successfully completing the inpatient program. The client's husband comments to the nurse that he believes his wife is showing improvement because she no longer beats their 3-year-old son. A few weeks later, the son is admitted to the hospital with a fractured arm and several bruises and contusions over his body.

5

Framework for Culturally Relevant Psychiatric Nursing

DENISE SAINT ARNAULT

OUTLINE

KEY TERMS AND CONCEPTS

The key terms and concepts listed here also appear in bold where they are defined or discussed in this chapter.

cultural ideology
world view
ethnocentrism
cultural relativism
independent world view
interdependent world view
culture-bound syndromes
explanatory models (EMs)

OBJECTIVES

After studying this chapter, the reader should be able to

1. Analyze the relationship between dominant American cultural values and Western psychological theory and practice.
2. Compare and contrast conceptions of the self within the Western world view and within other major world views.
3. Evaluate the psychiatric nursing implications of using culture in planning care.
4. Apply the concepts of culture to psychiatric mental health nursing assessment and practice.

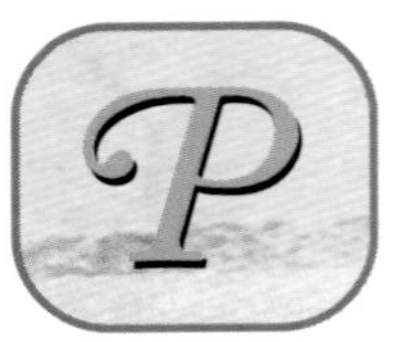

sychiatric mental health nurses are often required to provide skilled assessment and intervention for people very different from themselves. Standard practice around the world has been to utilize psychological theories derived from the Western tradition. However, non-Western practitioners are beginning to question whether Western theories can be applied universally (Box 5–1). As the people of many nations have increased their access to advanced education and high technology, they are not as likely to accept Western thinking as authoritative, choosing instead to work from their own models of understanding the world and the human condition. These views can differ substantially from those of Western theory.

The challenge to contemporary nurses is to recognize that there are vast differences among the world's peoples, and that these differences profoundly affect our assessment of psychiatric nursing phenomena (e.g., family functioning, expression of feelings, appropriate behavioral modes). This chapter explores Western and non-Western conceptions of the self and of relationships and suggests some strategies for intervention that arise from these differences.

RELEVANCE OF CULTURE IN PSYCHIATRIC NURSING

In recent years there has been growing attention to the relationship between the white, English-speaking, middle class that dominates American society and the rest of the diverse U.S. population. While there is some debate about whether we can talk about *one* culture in referring to such a multicultural mix of peoples, many scholars agree that there *is* an American culture, and that this culture has its roots in Western tradition (Sahlins 1996; Markus and Katayama 1991).

There has also been growing concern about the limited understanding most Americans have about the differences in customs, languages, and traditions of both nonwhite Americans and non-Western peoples worldwide. Many attempts have been made in nursing to describe the infinite varieties of traditions held by the peoples with whom nurses may encounter in the health care setting, and to begin to catalog the ways that peoples around the world understand and treat illness and disease.

Within psychology and psychiatry, there have been similar calls for compassion about the variety of ways in which the world's peoples understand and treat mental and emotional problems. These efforts in psychological anthropology, cognitive anthropology, and cultural psychology have called into question the psychological theories derived from Western tradition about the nature of the personality. These theories have also been challenged regarding the limited attention paid to the influence of cultural processes on personality development. Practitioners working in all the mental health fields have found that the study of the personality must include an understanding of how culture shapes personality characteristics such as emotional expression, ego boundaries, and inter- and intrapersonal perceptions.

One of the roles of culture is to define what is good, what is right, and what is normal. Therefore, it is through the culture that our individual self is molded, our relationships with others are prescribed, and our own thoughts and feelings are defined and reinforced.

An American television commercial depicts a 2- to 3-year-old toddler in a high chair. The announcer describes that this child is at the point in her life where she is learning to make choices. The video shows the mother offering the toddler a choice of two different juices to drink. The commercial then shows her making a choice, depicting at some length her pleasure in drinking the juice that she selected.

This illustrates that it is a value within American society to determine our desires, needs, and preferences. We value exploring our inner selves to get a clear sense of who we are and what we need. In the commercial, the toddler is being taught the values held *within her culture*—that this ability to choose is an important ability to have. It also conveys to the mother that this is an important skill to provide for her child. The mother is being instructed, by the media as an agent of culture, that choice making is an ideal behavior in a child. The mother in American society learns that it is her task to assist the child in the full development of this ability if her child is to become a competent member of American society.

Box 5–1 DEFINING WESTERN AND NON-WESTERN

There are a number of ways to categorize the variety of the world's peoples. In American culture there has been a tendency to focus on skin color. This has had mixed results. For example, it has confused the issue of genetic differences with cultural differences, focusing on racial differences rather than on cultural understanding. However, many diverse cultural groups have used the term *people of color* as a unifying term, pointing up the gap in understanding between peoples who were colonized and the nations that were historically involved in colonization: Britain, France, Germany, The Netherlands, Spain, Portugal, and the United States. Throughout this chapter, the term *Western* is used to refer to the nations of Europe and North America, predominantly white, who tend to hold a common world view, who share substantial economic and social power, and who have generally dominated people of color worldwide.

However, these kinds of intrapersonal awareness, self-directed behavior, and interpersonal autonomy are not the only preferred way.

> [In a day care center in Japan] each item of the menu is served on a separate plate or bowl for each child . . . Each teacher brings food for her children on several trays from the kitchen to her classroom. For the younger children (ages 1 to 4), teachers set the table for the children. However, among the oldest children, a boy and a girl are assigned this duty each day. These children are called *toban*. They serve the plates and bowls, which are already filled with food, from the trays to each child. Meanwhile the other children are supposed to sit quietly. When the children on duty finish serving, they stand in front of everyone and say *itadakimasu* (I will gratefully receive this food) and the others follow . . . every child has an equal opportunity to be a toban . . . [and] each child knows when his or her turn comes next . . . each one takes pride in being responsible and also in being able to do the task as well as the other children do. (Fujita and Sano 1988, p. 82.)

This vignette demonstrates another set of cultural values. This time, the values lie in doing well in other's eyes and fulfilling responsibilities and obligations with pride. The children are excited about the opportunity to be "in charge," but the role of being in charge carries with it a responsibility to do your best and to do well for the others who are dependent upon you. At another time, the children will practice being attended to, and the gratefulness that they should show for a job well done.

The beliefs and values held by a culture about what is good, right, and normal are referred to as their **cultural ideology,** or **world view.** The ideology or world view of a culture refers to the available symbols, meanings, and values about what is important and what behaviors are right and correct. This is the link between the larger world view of a culture and the individual psychological functioning of any given person. Mental health is the degree to which a person is able to fulfill the cultural expectations of his or her society (Markus and Katayama 1991). Mental health is defined by the culture, and deviance from cultural expectations is considered to be a problem.

The culture defines what types of differences are still within the range of normal (mentally healthy) and which ones are outside the range of normal (mentally ill). In the examples given above, there is a range within which the American toddler would be considered mentally healthy. For example, it is still considered normal for her to want her mother to choose, or to resist choice altogether and refuse to eat (the so-called "terrible two's"). However, it might be considered mentally unhealthy for the child to have tantrums at every mealtime, or for her to be unable to initiate any action on her own. In the Japanese example, it might be considered normal for a child to take excessive pride in being the *toban*, or to be very shy in front of others, or to be afraid of making a mistake. It might be considered mentally unhealthy for the child to refuse to help, or to be selfish or ungrateful. It might also be unhealthy for a Japanese child to focus on self-needs to the exclusion of those of others, or to be unable to allow others to do for them (Johnson 1995).

In a discussion of the role of culture in the socialization of children, and the misapplication of Western-derived psychological theory across cultures, Turkish researcher Kagitcibasi writes:

> To illustrate the point, I shall refer to the maternal regulation strategies of the Japanese mother. . . . Here is the contrast between two meaning systems that render the same pattern normal or abnormal. The Japanese mother's message to the child, "I am one with you, and we can be of the same mind," . . . is exactly the definition of a "symbiotic" relationship, an expression of pathological "enmeshment" in the Western family, as interpreted by Western psychology. (Kagitcibasi 1989, p. 155.)

WORLD VIEW IN THE WESTERN TRADITION

Nurses learning about mental health, psychology, and psychiatry throughout the world are generally schooled in the classic personality and developmental theories of Freud, Erikson, Maslow, Piaget, and other Europeans and Americans. While these theories may be applicable to people who share their world view, they have been challenged as being unable to explain or predict behavior and mental health across diverse populations (Johnson 1995; Gergen 1992; Markus and Kitayama 1991). It is important for psychiatric nurses to understand the beliefs and values embedded in these theories before attempting to provide culturally relevant psychiatric nursing care.

The values of a given culture are the framework or context within which a health care system (as well as a legal and educational system) is developed. The health care system embraces and upholds the values of its culture. In the case of cultural ideals about what is right or good, the health care system defines these and prescribes the treatment for deviations from them. For example, in a culture that values behavioral and emotional self-control, vigorous outward expressions of emotions, or a perceived lack of emotional self-control, may be deemed by the health care system as deviant and abnormal. For a cross-cultural view of mental health, see Box 5–2.

As stated above, a culture defines for its people what is important and what is true and real in the world. It defines for us what we should pay attention to, and what we should overlook. It helps us understand the relationships between one thing and another. In American society, we also hold ideals and values about what is right, wrong, true, important, and normal. These values are based on traditions within our Western European cultural, philosophical, and historical roots (Gergen 1992; Levan 1992; Markus and Katayama 1991). Table 5–1 presents a brief look at the relationship between our Western roots and

BOX 5–2 A CROSS-CULTURAL VIEW OF POSITIVE MENTAL HEALTH

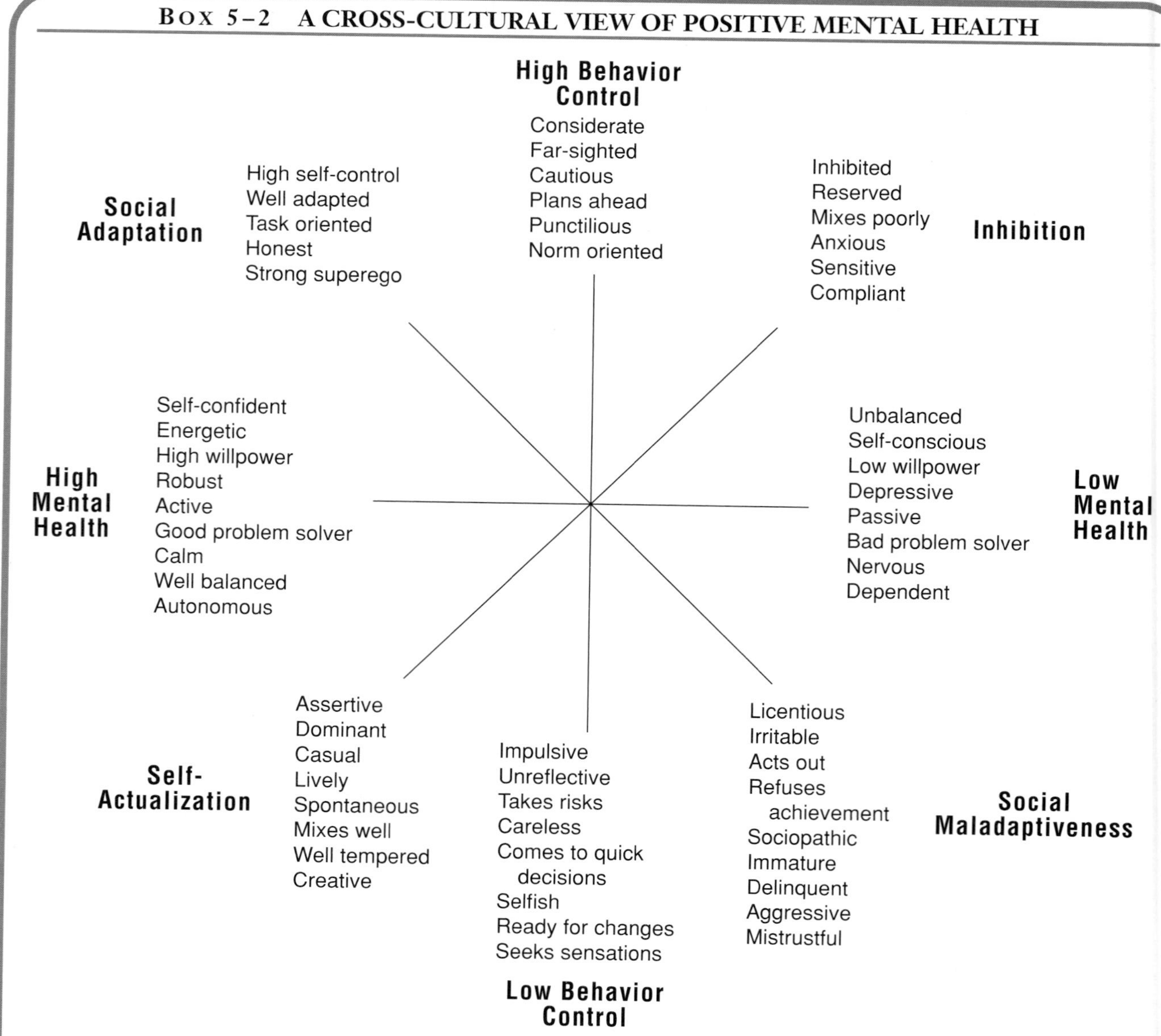

Student teachers, working teachers, and retired teachers (N = 595) from four countries (France, Germany, Greece, United States) completed a questionnaire containing 186 items in Likert format with instructions to describe the mentally healthy person. Principal component analyses of item responses showed two cross-culturally invariant orthogonal factors, which were interpreted as high versus low mental health and high versus low behavior control. Factor loadings revealed a circumplex structure similar to that repeatedly found by Becker in studies of self-description of personality. Four scales were constructed representing the two main axes and the two diagonals of the circumplex structure. The scales were named mental health, behavior control, social adaptation versus social maladaptiveness, and self-actualization versus inhibition. Analyses of variance showed cultural and age differences, which were interpreted as reflecting different degrees of permissiveness, varying self-concepts, and differences in economic wealth of the countries studied.

From Becker, P., Korchin, S. J., and Minsel, B. (1991). A cross-cultural view of positive mental health, Two orthogonal main factors replicable in four countries. *Journal of Cross-Cultural Psychology,* 22:157–181. © 1991 Western Washington University.

our modern expressions of them. Like people all around the world, we believe not only that the ideas we hold are true and right but also that other ideas and values are wrong or bad. This process of believing that one's own culture is generally right or best is called **ethnocentrism,** and it occurs in every culture.

Even though ethnocentrism is common, there are many ways in which it is a problem for health care

TABLE 5–1 THE UNDERPINNINGS OF WESTERN PHILOSOPHY IN MODERN PSYCHOLOGY

WESTERN PHILOSOPHICAL TRADITION	PSYCHOLOGICAL COROLLARY	AMERICAN CULTURE
Reason and abstraction are superior to emotion and passion	The ego must master the id to achieve developmental maturity	"Think before you act"—the belief that the mark of a healthy person is one who is "in control"
The spirit or soul does not perform in predictable ways—therefore it is unscientific—science is the search for universal law and order	What is real is that which can be observed, measured, and predicted—mental processes are essentially hign-order biological processes that operate in predictable ways	Belief that spiritual or faith healing is unreal, magical, and superstitious—real healing comes when biological causes are discovered and corrected
There is an essential separation between the self as the subject and the environment, which is the object of the self	The idea of the bounded self—the self as separate from context—agency, self-control, and an intact identity are the marks of developmental maturity	Value of independence of thought and action—"Be all that you can be," "Be your own man," "Follow your dreams," "Think for yourself"

providers. It is often the basis for fear of other ways of understanding the world and the basis for value judgments about people with other views.

> On an urban psychiatric unit, several African American male clients and an African American male staff member are playing cards in the day room. The game involves bluffing, with challenges to the bluffs, and counterbluffs. The staff and the clients are having a good game, and there are lots of bluffs and counters, accompanied by laughter. The nurses assigned to the unit are Filipina immigrants. They are becoming increasingly frightened by the noises in the day room, and discuss with each other how to handle what they perceive as clients becoming "out of control."

In this vignette, each group has expectations about what is right and normal. In the urban African American culture, verbal banter and vocality are important cultural traditions. Here, the group was showing cohesiveness and trust by talking simultaneously and teasing and challenging each other. From the Filipina perspective, talking loudly and outward challenges are a sign of a loss of control and a breakdown in trust. Trust and togetherness for the Filipinas are demonstrated by harmonious and peace-seeking behaviors. There is a value placed on behaviors that foster harmony, such as quietness and polite forgiveness of another's mistakes. Ethnocentricity leads each group to see their own perspective as right and good, and fosters poor relationships, mistrust, and potentially disastrous misunderstandings between the groups.

It is essential that the nurse working with people with diverse cultural beliefs and values recognize that each group has its own cultural definitions and perceptions. Nurse managers must help each staff team to communicate these values and arrive at a mutually agreed upon set of behavioral expectations that reflects all members of the team. In a multicultural milieu, behavioral expectations and care plans should be reviewed to avoid ethnocentric biases.

Ethnocentrism is like a blinder to an understanding of other ways of thinking or knowing. When blinded by ethnocentrism, health care personnel may unwittingly abuse their power. Problems in a multicultural society (e.g., discrimination and prejudice) are based on ethnocentric attitudes of superiority. Ethnocentrism is only one of the "isms" that can get in the way of harmonious relationships (Box 5–3). From an anthropological point of view, these phenomena can be understood as the dominant ideology of the culture's shaping the social relations of its members. In this way, the values and beliefs of the dominant Western culture have shaped social policy and all the major institutions in the United States, including medicine and nursing. In psychiatric nursing, then, our practices and assessments have reflected our Western world view. (For further discussion of these ideas, see Bellah et al. 1985; Geertz 1975; Hsu 1983; Johnson 1985; Sampson 1988; Shweder and Borne 1984; Spindler and Spindler 1987.)

To avoid the problems posed by ethnocentricity, the nurse needs to cultivate multicultural understanding actively (Box 5–4). These activities can dispel myths, help the nurse gather realistic knowledge, and create a stance that is open to new cultural understandings. In a health care encounter, it is helpful to assume that you have only partial understanding of the client's values, and thus to enter into the assessment with broad questions and an open mind about the client's values and beliefs.

Kavanaugh (1995) suggests the following general strategies when entering into a cultural encounter:

- *Promote a feeling of acceptance* by providing clients with adequate time and space to present their situation fully, including the social and cultural components, and hearing their symptoms in the context of their life.
- *Anticipate diversity* by eliciting cultural information and challenging stereotypes and generalizations, using respect for differences and similarities, and emphasizing strengths.
- *Affirm diversity* by assessing the knowledge and skills of each interested party—the nurse, the client, and the community— regarding the care of the client.

BOX 5–3 THE "ISMS"

Egocentrism: The assumption that one is superior to others. An example of this involves someone who has never been diagnosed as mentally ill (a staff member, for instance) who thinks he or she is better than those who are diagnosed as ill.

Ethnocentrism: The assumption that one's own cultural or ethnic group is superior to that of others. Ethnicity refers to cultural differences and should not be confused with race. Ethnocentrism occurs, for example, when everyone is expected to speak English and to know the rules (many of which are implicit) for living in this society.

Sociocentrism: The assumption that one society's way of knowing or doing is superior to others. It may be assumed, for instance, that biomedicine is effective and folk medicines are not. Actually, there is much evidence that this is not always the case. Many traditional societies have highly effective, community-oriented ways of treating those clients that modern Western medicine calls "psychiatric."

Racism: The assumption that members of one race are superior to those of another (*race* refers to presumed biological differences).

Sexism: The assumption that members of one sex are superior to those of the other. For example, women have historically been viewed as less rational and more emotional and subject to mental illness than men.

Heterosexism: The assumption that everyone is or should be heterosexual and that heterosexuality is superior and expectable. It is relatively recently that homosexuality was redefined as a life style rather than a disease.

Ageism: The assumption that members of one age group are superior to those of others. Young clients and staff may not be taken seriously as those who are older.

Adultism: The assumption that adults are superior to youths and can or should control, direct, reprimand, or reward them or deprive them of respect. For example, children in American society are often interrupted and ignored by adults. They may not be given choices that allow them to learn how to cope with specific situations.

Sizism: The assumption that people of one body size are superior to or better than those of other shapes and sizes. Positions involving interaction with the public, for example, may be denied to individuals who are very heavy or who otherwise fail to meet the standards of ideal appearance.

Classism/elitism: The assumption that certain people are superior because of their social and economic status or position in a group or organization. This often assumes that those with more money or education are superior. A poorly dressed high school drop-out, for example, may not be given the same treatment options offered to a well-dressed college graduate.

"Ableism": The assumption that the able-bodied and sound of mind are physically or developmentally superior to those who are disabled, retarded, or otherwise different. An example of "ableism" is not offering a chronically ill client choices owing to the assumption that he or she does not want to or cannot make decisions.

From Kavanaugh, K. (1995). Transcultural perspectives in mental health. In M. Andrews and J. Boyle (Eds.), *Transcultural concepts in nursing care* (2nd ed.) (p. 263.) Philadelphia: J. B. Lippincott.

- *Learn what it means to be the client* by assessing health beliefs, including the roles of the client and family; health, illness and hygiene; the causes and care of illnesses.
- *Understand the client's goals and expectations* by assessing what the client (and the family and community) expect from the nurse and the client. (Kavanaugh 1995, p. 279.)

These Western cultural ideals have become the standard for the mental health of the people in American society. Individuals may be considered emotionally and developmentally immature if the Western culturally valued abilities of autonomy, individuation, and clear self-control are lacking (see the classic works of Erikson 1968; S. Freud 1923; A. Freud 1936; Kernberg 1976; Mahler et al. 1975; Rapaport 1960).

The ethnocentric bias described above has been criticized as being one of the underlying causes for institutionalized sexism and racism within American medicine and psychology. Many of the diverse groups in American society value cultural patterns such as interdependence, sensitivity to the needs of others, or suspending one's own needs in favor of external obligations or responsibilities. Yet, within the dominant medical and psychological systems, these behaviors have been viewed as the mark of developmental immaturity—*those* people have not met the expected level of autonomy, self-control, ego integrity, or independence, and they may be labeled as developmentally immature. Symptoms of mental illness in these individuals may be attributed to their perceived psychological deficits, and treatment has traditionally been directed toward correcting these perceived deficits.

With this new awareness of such cultural diversity in psychological functioning, some critics of the American health care system and the Western model of psychology have called for a culturally relative model of mental health (Table 5–2) (for a discussion of this debate, see Gergen 1992). **Cultural relativism** is the practice of using culturally derived definitions of mental health, illness,

BOX 5-4 PROMOTING MULTICULTURALISM

1. Take the opportunity to learn about the history and culture of African, Native, Latin, and Asian people. Read literary works and historical perspectives written by people of color; attend ethnic plays and films; listen to ethnic music. Spend time with people culturally different from yourself. Are you and your family comfortable interacting with ethnic people? Multicultural people have diversity reflected in their home and in social circles.
2. Do not assume an authoritarian role in understanding and dealing with discrimination, stereotyping, and racism if you have not experienced it directly. European Americans need to be willing to put themselves in the role of learner, taking direction from ethnic people as opposed to only listening to other members of the dominant group, who tend to view issues of racism from an "outsider's" perspective.
3. Learn about your ethnic heritage to enhance your understanding of culture in general. It is impossible to embrace multiculturalism without self-knowledge of your own cultural roots. Recognizing strengths and weaknesses inherent in *all* cultures is a part of the multicultural learning process.
4. Do not assume that ethnic people can speak only on ethnic issues. Recognize that all people are well rounded and talented and can speak on varied subjects. Remember to include ethnic people to serve on committees or groups that do not pertain to diversity.
5. Encourage and support culturally self-defining structures such as task forces, advocacy groups, cultural committees, and other bodies established by and for ethnic people rather than viewing these efforts as attempts to segregate.
6. Do not assume that anyone who has claims of discrimination is overreacting or misreading a situation, especially if as a member of the dominant group you have not experienced discrimination based on your skin color.
7. Recognize that if you are in the dominant group, you have a unique role in educating others on multiculturalism, as most European Americans will consider your opinions to be more objective and credible. Take advantage of formal and informal teaching opportunities that most ethnic people are not privileged to receive.
8. Do not be offended by such terms as *European American* or *dominant group*. These terms illustrate the power and privilege that many people of European descent receive just by virtue of their skin color and cultural preparation.
9. Recognize that multiculturalism benefits everyone and is not just an issue of concern only to ethnic people. Be a well-informed social activist working *with* rather than *on behalf of* those who are oppressed.
10. Do not assume that oppression is a thing of the past and that your community and/or workplace is culturally sensitive. If your surroundings are composed primarily of European Americans and/or if there is a high degree of turnover of ethnic people, evaluate and analyze the environment. When possible, talk to ethnic people (in a sensitive manner) to get a more accurate perspective on how multicultural your work/home community is.
11. Educate yourself on language and culture so that others are not offended by your use of anachronistic or racist terminology such as "wetbacks," "squaw," or "colored." Learn why these terms are offensive. In many instances there is no such thing as *the correct* term; nonetheless, it is valuable to understand the context within which various words and phrases are used.
12. Continue attending multicultural trainings, lectures, and programs; however, understand that becoming multicultural is a lifelong learning process that must include interacting on a regular basis with people culturally different from yourself.

From: Moody, M. (1994). Unpublished manuscript. Used with permission.

and treatment; discussing the change in contemporary urban Egyptian women, Rugh (1985) describes the term:

> As a cultural relativist sees it, every society develops a unique set of shared understandings, modes of action it considers appropriate, and a specific world view. Seen together as a system, these parts mesh with reasonable internal consistency . . . each culture reserves for its members the potential to act directly, without the hesitation that unlimited choice would require. To begin to understand what motivates people's behavior, one needs to look not only at individual needs but the rationales and the desired ends the society sets for its members. People seek the social rewards that accompany accepted behaviors. They feel guilty when they behave in a way that is socially unacceptable. (Rugh 1985, p. 276.)

Critics of the use of the cultural relativist model for understanding mental health argue that this approach leaves scientific questions about the nature of mental health and illness to the common beliefs of the culture, and therefore definitions of mental health, illness, and treatment include all types of folk beliefs, understandings of supernatural phenomena, and poorly tested remedies (Gergen 1992; Kleinman 1980).

Whatever the outcome of this debate, psychiatric nurses, as members of an eclectic and humanistic profession, must leave room for indigenous cultural perspectives about behavior, and should have a clear view of what clients within that culture want from the health encounter. A goal for culturally competent psychiatric nurses is to recognize the cultural origins of their own

TABLE 5–2 CULTURALLY RELATIVE PHENOMENA IN PSYCHIATRIC NURSING

PHENOMENA	COMMENTS	GUIDELINES
Perception of reality	The inability to perceive the consensual reality of others may indicate a focus on internal perceptions and experiences. These perceptions may be 1. culturally prescribed. 2. spiritually induced in a traditional healing system. 3. otherwise sanctioned by cultural group.	Representatives from those cultures must assist in the understanding of the "psychotic" state before a diagnosis is made.
Needs, feelings, thoughts of others and self	The ability to attend to the needs, feelings, and thoughts of the self and others, whether they are internal or external to the patient, demonstrates interpersonal awareness and the development of this awareness. Conforming to and fulfilling culturally and socially prescribed obligations and expectations are not the mark of mental illness or emotional immaturity.	The concern for psychiatric nurses is whether this is in concert with expectations and culturally defined values and ideals for that culture.
Decision making	The ability to make decisions within a socially and culturally prescribed arena should be separated from the delegation of certain decisions to another. Families and cultures designate decision makers, which may include health care decisions.	Asking for direction from the health care provider (who may be the culturally defined decision maker) or another family member is not necessarily the mark of an inability to decide for oneself but may be an indication that the person is operating within a culturally defined set of relationships.

beliefs and health care practices, and to constantly and vigilantly act as an advocate for their clients (Table 5–3). This requires that we define a culture- and gender-sensitive model of mental health, one that recognizes culturally derived differences and separates them from pathological deviations in mental functioning (Table 5–4). It is also important to recognize that ethical decisions about how to define essential human rights, and how and when to act as an advocate for our clients to ensure that our clients' culturally derived values, beliefs, and needs are respected.

Variations in Self-Understandings

The self is conceptualized in many different ways across the cultures of the world (Fig. 5–1). Traditional psychoanalytic theory conceptualized the self as the ego (see Chapter 2). The ego is the psychological structure that moderates the conflict between the *biological* drives of the individual and the internalized *social* mandates for conformity and self-restraint (S. Freud 1923; A. Freud 1936; Rapaport 1960; Levan 1992). The ego is where individuals define who they are in relation to others.

TABLE 5–3 COMMON VALUE ORIENTATIONS IN THE UNITED STATES

VALUE ORIENTATION	DESCRIPTION
Active, agentic	Determination, competition, solve problems through direct confrontation, "just do it," "actions speak louder than words"
Future orientation	Progress and goal oriented, self-development, trying to make things better for the children, "be all that you can be"
Individualistic	Accessing thoughts and feelings is valued, able to articulate needs and desires clearly, emphasis on getting what one needs, self-reliance
Universalistic morality	Laws based on universal truths rather than particular situations; context-independent thinking is encouraged
Multiple group membership	Groups form on basis of singular characteristics or needs rather than family, clan, or other traditional characteristics; emphasize similarities rather than hierarchy whenever possible

TABLE 5–4 CROSS-CULTURAL EXAMPLES OF CULTURAL PHENOMENA AFFECTING NURSING CARE

Nations of Origin	Communication	Space	Time Orientation	Social Organization	Environmental Control	Biological Variations
Asian China Hawaii Philippines Korea Japan Southeast Asia (Laos, Cambodia, Vietnam)	National language preference Dialects, written characters Use of silence Nonverbal and contextual cueing	Noncontact people	Present	Family: hierarchical structure, loyalty Devotion to tradition Many religions, including Taoism, Buddhism, Islam, and Christianity Community social organizations	Traditional health and illness beliefs Use of traditional medicines Traditional practitioners: Chinese doctors and herbalists	Liver cancer Stomach cancer Coccidioidomycosis Hypertension Lactose intolerance
African West Coast (as slaves) Many African countries West Indian Islands Dominican Republic Haiti Jamaica	National languages Dialect: Pidgin, Creole, Spanish, French	Close personal space	Present over future	Family: Many female, single parent Large, extended family networks Strong church affiliation within community Community social organizations	Traditional health and illness beliefs Folk medicine tradition Traditional healer: rootworker	Sickle cell anemia Hypertension Cancer of esophagus Stomach cancer Coccidioidomycosis Lactose intolerance
Europe Germany Great Britain Italy Ireland Other European countries	National languages Many learn English immediately	Noncontact people Aloof Distant Southern countries: closer contact and touch	Future over present	Nuclear families Extended families Judeo-Christian religions Community social organizations	Primary reliance on modern health care system Traditional health and illness beliefs Some remaining folk medicine traditions	Breast cancer Heart disease Diabetes mellitus Thalassemia
Native American 170 Native American tribes Aleuts Eskimos	Tribal languages Use of silence and body language	Space very important and has no boundaries	Present	Extremely family oriented Biological and extended families Children taught to respect traditions Community social organizations	Traditional health and illness beliefs Folk medicine tradition Traditional healer: medicine man	Accidents Heart disease Cirrhosis of liver Diabetes mellitus
Hispanic countries Spain Cuba Mexico Central and South America	Spanish or Portuguese primary language	Tactile relationships Touch Handshakes Embracing Value physical presence	Present	Nuclear family Extended family *Compadrazgo:* Godparents Community social organizations	Traditional health and illness beliefs Folk medicine tradition Traditional healers: *Curandero, Espiritista, Partera, Senora*	Diabetes mellitus Parasites Coccidioidomycosis Lactose intolerance

From Specter, R. (1993). In P. A. Potter and A. G. Perry (Eds.). *Fundamentals of nursing: Concepts, process and practice* (3rd ed.). St. Louis: Mosby–Year Book.

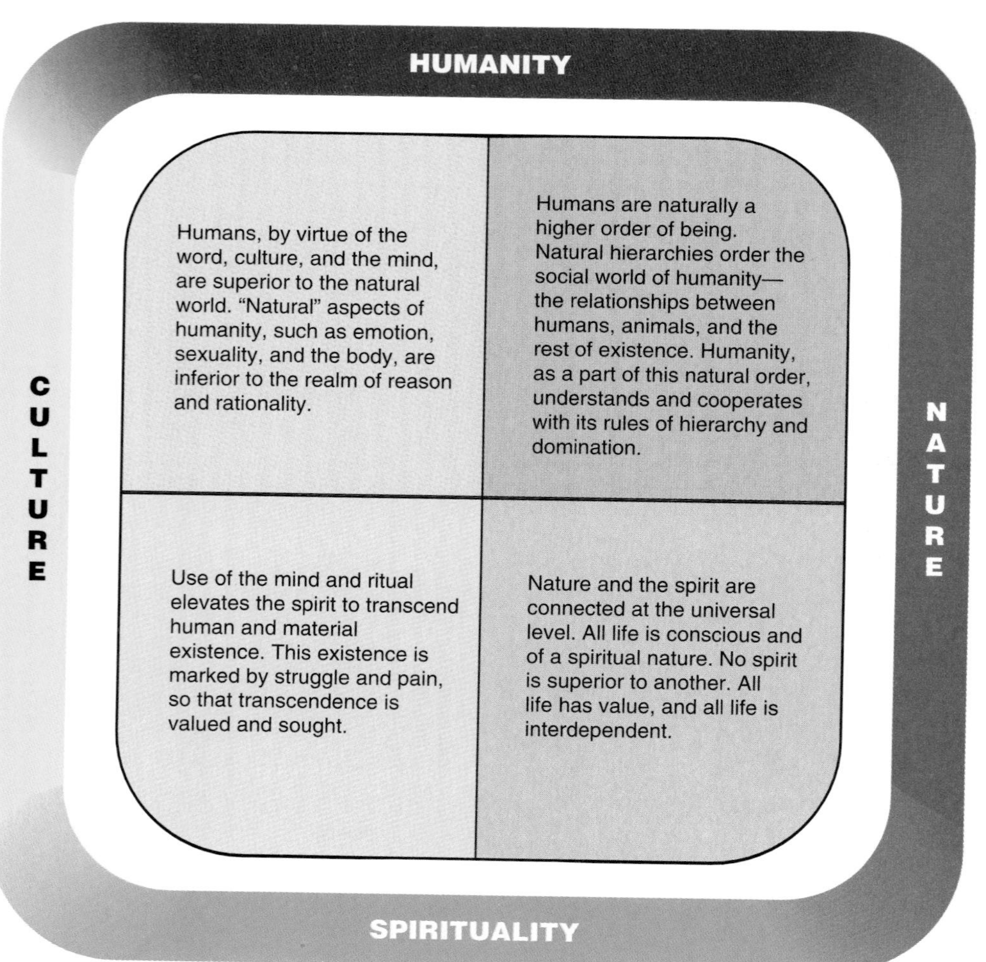

Figure 5–1 The self across cultures: major world views along experiential dimensions. (Inspired by Lebra, T.S., 1992.) Because of natural and forced migration, colonization, and human expansion, cultures around the world have historically exchanged language and traditions. Any culture represents a hybrid of lifeways and—to a much less extent—world views. For example, Mesoamerican and South American cultures represent a blend of indigenous nature-based/spiritual world views with the humanity/culture world view imposed by Spanish colonization in the early 1400s. Similarly, the culture/spirit world view is represented by Hindu and Buddhist traditions in India and the surrounding nations. However, Buddhism has been exported to, and is widely practiced in, China, Japan, and other Asian countries. Moreover, in Japan these world views are superimposed on the nature-based ideology of the Shinto religion, which might more clearly fit with the spirit/nature quadrant of this grid.

In many of the world's non-Western cultures, however, the ego self is articulated in terms of roles and obligations, and defined in terms of similarities to others in the social sphere (Triandis et al. 1988). Indeed, research within American society has shown that definitions of the self differ from male to female; for example, white women in the dominant society are more likely than white men to see themselves as part of a social system and operating in relation to the social context. (For more about the self and gender, see Lyons 1983; Lykes 1985; Gilligan 1986; Gergen and Gergen 1988; Gergen 1992.) The self, from this perspective, is inseparable from the social context in which it emerges. Indeed, perception may be guided by gender (Markus and Oyserman 1989; Cross and Markus 1993) and by a culturally formed world view (Triandis et al. 1988). Some authors in cultural and gender psychology have focused on how the different socialization and acculturation experiences of people could theoretically account for variations in the organization or content of the ego or self (Chodorow 1978; Stoller 1985).

WORLD VIEW FROM MAJOR NON-WESTERN TRADITIONS

As stated earlier, the ideal of the self-determined, emancipated individual is rooted in European and American values (Gergen 1992; Kleinman 1988). This **independent world view** has also been described as *individualistic* or *ideocentric* and has been broadly differentiated from cultures that have an **interdependent world view** (that are *collectivist, sociocentric*) (Triandis et al. 1988; Kagitcibasi 1989; Markus and Katayama 1991).

People from cultures different from our own experience life as part of an interdependent web of relationships and expectations. Their concept of the self is better described in terms of roles, responsibilities, and relationships. Personal feelings and desires, while certainly present, are a much less relevant piece of information in understanding behavior. Authority, group needs, and family obligations carry more weight (Espin 1985; Kleinman 1988; Shweder and Miller 1991; Roland 1991; Dien 1992; Johnson 1995).

People within these *sociocentric* cultures have personality styles and behavioral norms very unlike those in the West. The generalizations that follow are for the purposes of a broad understanding of differences among the world's major philosophical and cultural ideologies, and may not necessarily fit any particular group (Table 5–5). Differences between groups evolve throughout time, because of intercultural contact, economic and material conditions, and both immigration and migration into vastly different ecological regions.

An example of cultural change can be seen in the forced migration of thousands of Native Americans from North Carolina and Tennessee to Oklahoma over the infamous "Trail of Tears" (Brown 1982). Hundreds died and hundreds more were unable to adapt to the social, ecological, and biological changes demanded of them. Moreover, Native American nations with vastly different traditions and ways of life were thrown together in an unfamiliar milieu. Some new traditions emerged; some old traditions were retained.

In addition to cultural changes, Native Americans across the continent were forced to adapt to or incorporate aspects of the dominant European world view, including the Christian religion, although the indigenous people had practiced a nature-based spiritual life and a cooperative social life. The concept of a pure culture becomes meaningless when one considers these and other economic forces of change.

It is important for the nurse to be aware of the forces of change that exist within any given social group. Dominant views may arise from the upper socioeconomic levels of society because members control such institutions as education and the law. Other socioeconomic groups may hold competing cultural views and behaviors, which can result in conflict, struggle, and resistance to the status quo. Consider what happened in the United States during the 1960s. Although the dominant ideology included values such as hard work and striving for financial or professional success, radical subcultures embraced living in the moment, living in harmony, and lack of material possessions. Cultures are constantly in flux, and economic factors are central to this process (Johnston and Klandermans 1995).

When trying to develop a general understanding of cultural psychology, it is not helpful to talk about specific values of a people in a given time and place. Rather, it is necessary to try to understand how world view affects the way a person from any culture understands self as a member of that culture. In other words, we do not understand the psychology of a people by looking at their dietary preferences or clothing styles, or even their religious beliefs. We need to look at the world view of the person as a member of a culture, and acknowledge that his or her self is molded by the culture, in order to help the person operate in ways that fit the broad beliefs and values about what is good, right, and normal. Assessment would include people's conception of the cultural values and beliefs from their upbringing, including how they have subscribed to or resisted them.

For our purposes, the major world views can be grouped broadly into Asian, indigenous, Arabic/Islamic, African, and Western European traditions. Within any major tradition, however, there can be significant variations among national, ethnic, religious, and socioeconomic groups. For example, within the Asian tradition, there are Chinese, Japanese, Korean, Vietnamese, and Asian Indian variations, and more. Similarly, cultures from northern Africa may share many of the beliefs and values with the Islamic tradition. Finally, cultures from Central and South America may represent a blending of the Western traditions of Spain and those of the indigenous people living at the time of the Spanish conquest. So we see that these major traditions represent only starting points in understanding the ways that the world view of a culture shapes and defines mental health, psychological functioning, and self-development of its people.

The Asian Tradition

Within the broad framework of the Asian world view, a primary concern is interpersonal relationships. In the Korean culture, for example, there is a concept of We-ness, in which each person is not seen as an isolated personality, but is first and foremost part of a group (Choi and Choi 1990). The person is a part of an interdependent network, and role obligations carry a heavy significance in individual lives. Duty and obligation are generally considered more important than individual needs.

The Asian cultures share a concern for harmony and balance within relationships and between the individual and the natural world. The world is seen as composed of complementary forces, opposite in nature and always seeking a balance. These forces can be identified as hot/cold, female/male, or light/dark, but they are not viewed as being in conflict; rather, the forces of nature are understood to be constantly changing and seeking a balance.

Kleinman (1980, 1988) has documented that the experience of depression in Taiwan Chinese tends to take the form of somatic illness. This illness experience is seen not as an individual problem but as the result of disharmonious interrelationships, whether with spirits, the person and the environment, or the person in his or her relationship with others.

Asian Indian culture shares characteristics of both the Western and the Asian world views. For example, interpersonal relationships, obligation, and duty play a central role in social relationships, but there appears to be a cultural recognition of the self as separate from society. There is a religious and cultural striving for transcendence from the personal and the interpersonal within the

TABLE 5–5 SELF AND CULTURE

DOMAIN	EUROPEAN AMERICAN	ASIAN	NATIVE AMERICAN	ARABIC OR ISLAMIC	AFRICAN OR AFRICAN AMERICAN
Socially constructed self	Individualization and articulation of ideas, desires, and needs; progress and goal oriented	Individual is incomplete, needs to give and receive to be complete; part of cooperative, hierarchical group of insiders with common needs, goals, concerns	Spiritual nature of all beings is linked; humans are part of an interdependent web of life	One is part of a corporate group, which includes a lineage; one's value is derived from these social units; honor is for and among members of the social group	Self includes one's ancestors, nature, and community; the authentic self is emotionally vital and interactive
Roles and obligations	To be true to oneself; to develop the self fully and clearly separate one's needs from those of others; to strive to make life better for the children	To give fully and receive gratefully; to meet the expectations held by others fully to save face or the honor of the group	Right action in relation to humans and nonhumans; to give generously; to care for those in one's charge, which includes the rest of life and the earth	To maintain honor for those dependent on you; to behave in honorable, modest, and appropriate ways to protect and preserve the honor of the corporate group	To keep alive the presence of the truth, the history of the ancestors; to assist those within the community through active and engaged support
Maturity	Bounded and highly articulated ego or self; motivation and future orientation; independence and ability and willingness to compete; emotional self-control and self-restraint; verbal expression of feeling instead of action	High receptivity to the needs and emotions of others; reliance on others to meet person needs; interdependence and corporation with others to meet group needs; clear recognition of hierarchical and reciprocal relationships	Truthfulness; respect for all needs in a given situation or group such as group consensus building and negotiation skills; noncompetitiveness and cooperation; nonpossessiveness; self-responsibility	Assertiveness within one's ascribed, hierarchical social place; powerfulness and unwillingness to allow another to dominate; self-restraint; adherence to social customs	Facility with oral and vocal expression of emotional and authentic self; recognition of and resistance to oppression through renewal and community support
Psychiatric nursing implications	Nondirective, empathy-based, verbal psychotherapy; assertiveness and identity therapy; self-esteem and intrapsychic therapy; individual focus	Recognition of and differentiation between inner thoughts and needs and group needs; development of spontaneous and authentic self outside hierarchical system; foster ability to give and receive fully in reciprocal relationship	Return to indigenous spirituality; combat the isolation and estrangement of dominant society with reaffirmation of essential values of interconnection with all life, respect, and nonpossessiveness	Recognition of corporate needs and individual responsibility to retain honor; recognition of strength and power within a hierarchical system	Value the spontaneous vocal and oral traditions; assist with authentic and emotional self-expression; recognize the healing power of the community

East Indian culture (Derne 1992; Kakar 1978; Triandis et al 1988).

Much has been written about the psychological make-up of the Japanese people. Interest in the self-structure of the Japanese personality was discussed as early as the World War II years, and these studies have been central in comparative psychology texts. The findings of these studies highlight the importance of the primacy of the group in the development of the self. Interdependency is a central aspect of Japanese social relationships and, therefore, the Japanese personality (Doi 1984; Johnson 1995; Roland 1991). The concept that the Japanese use to describe this characteristic is *amae* (noun form); the term means "to depend or presume upon another's benevolence." The hierarchical social system in this culture creates a world in which any individual is both dependent on, and depended on by, others. Therefore, the skills necessary to relate successfully through *amearu* (verb form) are valued and supported in the development of personality. These skills include a sensitivity to the needs, thoughts, wishes, and emotions of others, and the ability to provide nurturance, support, and assistance. Moreover, individuals within this society learn that to give, and to receive gratefully, are characteristics of primary value. When one views these cultural characteristics as psychologically healthy, it is possible to expand ideas about the ways a healthy self can develop.

The interdependence within this social world leaves open the question of whether the ego or the self is bounded, divided, or separated. Roland (1991) theorized that the Japanese have ego boundaries despite the intensely interpersonal nature of their personality structures, but that it is important to think of these boundaries in layers: one type of ego boundary is between the individual and others; another is between the person and his or her personal thoughts and feelings. Roland suggested that the Japanese have a relatively permeable "outer ego boundary" that enables them to be successful in their social life. He notes that they develop a strong "inner ego boundary" that takes the form of a "private self." This allows the individual to retain a kind of personal integrity in the face of a collectivist societal structure. He also notes that this inner ego boundary is somewhat rigid, and that the Japanese clients he has treated have little access to their own thoughts and feelings.

Indigenous Peoples of the Americas

The indigenous people of the Americas have survived hundreds of years of cultural contact that included forced migration, governmental attempts at cultural extermination, religious oppression, and forced separation of families (Brown 1982). This cultural imposition has left a painful legacy of suicide, substance abuse, family violence, alienation, powerlessness, and depression. Despite this, many cultural values and beliefs held by Native Americans survived and grew stronger.

The interconnection of all life is an essential and inescapable element of existence for indigenous peoples around the world. Humans, animals—indeed, all living beings—are held to share a spirit or quality that is precious. Hierarchies among living beings and between the living and the nonliving are irrelevant because every entity has an interdependent relationship with every other. Human beings, capable of willful and thoughtful action, are charged with caring for those with less control, will, and power. Therefore, humans have a responsibility to protect and ensure that their actions do not injure or impair the lives of others (Hollowell 1963).

Power is an important concept for this world view and is only partly attributed to willful or thoughtful action. Instead, it is seen as an integral part of spiritual life that can be harnessed and directed; spiritual power is both respected and honored. The acquisition of power carries with it obligations to share with others and to avoid waste and greed. Nature is taken as a model for ethical behavior and is seen as abundant, generous, conservative in that it is not wasteful, and noncompetitive. Therefore, humans should also adopt a position of sharing, generosity, nonpossessiveness, and noncompetitiveness (Hollowell 1963; Kaplan and Johnson 1964; Brown 1982).

Attitudes and behavior that do not foster the correct relationships between humans, other animals, and nature are offensive. Deference to that which is more powerful, protection of available resources, and honesty are valued characteristics. Indigenous people honor group needs, in that consensus and the longevity of the group over time is important. Individual needs and positions are also deemed important. Everyone must have a voice and be treated with respect, and compromise and collective decision making are important interpersonal skills. Each person is expected to behave responsibly. Confession of disrespectful, possessive, or competitive desires is expected, for this fosters overall harmony within the group (Kaplan and Johnson 1964; La Barre 1964; Dinges et al. 1991).

The native peoples of Central and South America have been influenced by a different set of cultural forces from those experienced by natives of North America. It has been 500 years since their conquest by the Spanish culture, and the resultant tradition, commonly referred to as Hispanic, shares features of both the indigenous and European world views. In understanding Hispanic peoples, the model presented above is useful, with some slight modifications. Balance in relationships was of primary importance to the pre-Columbian peoples of Central America. This balance is achieved through moderation, obedience, and a sense of duty (Ortiz de Montellano 1990). Moderation and equilibrium must be maintained between people and the deities, within the community, and within the physical body. Sharing, moderate consumption, and egalitarian social relationships serve to promote balance and harmony. Imbalance in any of these domains creates a vulnerability to illness, and health is restored when harmony and balance are restored.

The Arabic Tradition

The Middle East exhibits cultural traditions and religious beliefs that are seen to share characteristics of both East and West. Some authors have suggested that the Arabic world view has features in common with, and perhaps originated from, the Greek and Roman philosophies that also undergird the Western traditions described above (Abu-Lughod 1986). The Arabic world view sees personal existence in the context of an intensely social world in which aloneness is feared and tolerance of it demonstrates courage and strength. The identity of an Arabic person is defined in terms of a collective—a family genealogy that can be traced for generations. A person's worth is tied to the distinction of his or her male lineage. The Arabic world view embraces a moral code of honor that values moral excellence, honor (strength to master temptations and personal desires), sincerity and honesty, and generosity. Fearlessness and courage are also important attributes (Rugh 1985; Abu-Lughod 1986).

One way that moral superiority and strength of character are demonstrated in the culture is through strict rules about sexual segregation. Sexual "purity" is held in very high esteem by both men and women, and failure to practice it is a sign of inferiority, weakness, and lack of honor. Shame and modesty are highly valued signs of character; immodesty is a sign of inferiority. This culture embraces hierarchy and allows closeness, affiliation, and sentimentality to those who have earned it, either through an honored patrilineage, demonstrated strength of character, or closeness based on proximity (such as a long-standing neighbor, wife, or friend). Trust is conferred only on those who have earned it.

This culture places supreme value on strength, that is, being free of weakness and shamefulness coupled with being responsible for dependents. Those who are weaker, such as women, servants, and children, are always under the protection of another. The protector has an obligation to protect their honor by being honorable himself. This independence is also an independence against the possibility of being dominated by another.

Those who are in dependent positions in relationship to the men (i.e., women and servants) also hold the ideals of autonomy and honor, although their social position does not allow them access to these higher positions. For them, the honor they achieve is the honor of the dependent. People in this social position show honor by deferring to the earned authority of another—this means to accept another's authority willingly when it is earned and just. To accept another's rule who is unworthy or because one has no choice is to show a lack of honor and earn pity, not respect.

Women are expected to maintain a code of modesty that includes the ability to maintain self-control, which is seen as strength of character. "Having shame" is to recognize the need for honor, self-restraint, and appropriate social behavior. It also refers to the woman's recognition of her social place, just as a younger man would know his place relative to an older man—it is a deference to an authority that is earned. However, women are expected to be strong, energetic, industrious, and tough. Boys and girls are taught not to allow others to dominate or intimidate them—they are both to demonstrate power, personal courage, and strength and to challenge dominance.

> An older man was sitting with his younger brother. His youngest daughter, a charming and much-loved toddler, wandered in and went to cuddle with her father. Her uncle teased her, threatening to kill her (using the same word used to talk about slaughtering sheep). Her father coached her to throw back the challenge, asking rhetorically "*Yagdar*?" which implied both "Is he capable?" and "Does he dare?" This interchange was repeated several times as the little girl, standing close to her father for support, challenged her uncle with emphatic "no's" every time he threatened. (Abu-Lughod 1986 p. 88.)

The attributes of assertiveness, power, and willfulness are respected and admired in women as an expression of their honor and courage, even as women are expected to know their place, behave modestly, and have shame.

The African Tradition

African Americans have to some degree retained the cultural beliefs, values, and world view of their African heritage throughout their centuries in the United States. Authors have documented a cultural ideology that is radically different from the Eurocentric one outlined above (Forde 1954; Levine 1977; Mbiti 1970) and have termed this ideology *Afrocentric* (Asante 1987, 1988). The term *Afrocentric* is not synonymous with African American; it simply refers to making African cultural values central to one's life. African peoples do share commonalities of value and belief, and many African American communities have been strengthened and empowered by the world view originating from Africa; however, African Americans vary widely in the degree to which they incorporate these values.

This Afrocentric world view is characterized by interdependence, interrelatedness, and connectedness with others (Burlew et al. 1992; Asante 1987, 1988). This cultural value of engagement and connection suggests that people interact in a dialogue with one another. The speaker is in direct connection with the listener, and the listener's behavior influences the speaker. There is a cultural value placed on the exchange between people, an exchange considered best when it is marked by realness and authenticity. *Realness* refers, in part, to the emotional vitality and expressiveness of the exchange. An exchange between people is honest when it is emotionally full and truthful, conveying affect as well as thoughts. A related cultural value is an emphasis on direct or lived experience. People are real and honest if they are expressing something that is real and true *for them*.

Afrocentricity suggests a philosophical understanding of the connection between the person, environment, ancestry, and responsibility to those not yet born. Culturally, this value is demonstrated in the oral tradition where a person is connected to the present and remains alive within the spoken word. The connection with history is also played out in the verbal exchange. This exchange may be between the elders and children, or between the minister and the congregation, but the spoken word keeps the past alive and each person connected with each other and their shared history. Recognition of shared history includes sharing joys and struggles, and reminding one another that the past has been filled with both triumphs and shared oppression. Keeping the experienced miseries of life alive is not meant to focus on the negative aspects of life and history but is intended to acknowledge triumph and shared struggle; it strengthens the connection with those who have gone before. An important part of keeping connection throughout the generations is to remember and share these joys, sorrows, and strengths.

Related to this memory of this shared history and interconnection is a feeling of distrust for those who have proved themselves to be dishonest and ingenuine. For many African Americans, this includes their history with white Americans. Oppression and racism continue to be a daily reality, to be faced and shared honestly. A person who denies the truth of this, whether a fellow African American or another, is dishonest and suspect.

In an urban African American church, people living with HIV and AIDS gather each week to have dinner, share stories and information about their lives, and provide each other support and strength. The sharing is eager, affectionate, and vocal. Missing members are noted, illness and death are acknowledged with praise for the person in life, and even small triumphs receive significant recognition. After gratefully acknowledging the cooks for dinner, the group gathers to discuss issues related to the HIV. Consistently, the speakers move from their personal struggles to the shared nature of their problems, and then to the small and big successes each have had—to be at the meetings, to be providing each other support, and to be alive in the face of this disease. Members talk about all of the blessings they have, and reframe the threat of death into a triumph of living and celebration.

CULTURALLY RELEVANT PSYCHIATRIC NURSING PRACTICE

As the above discussion indicates, psychiatric nurses cannot apply a standard model of assessment, diagnosis, and intervention to all clients with equal confidence. Using only the Western-derived model creates the possibility that inter- and intrapersonal characteristics may be poorly assessed and misdiagnosed, leading to culturally irrelevant interventions. The United States is an amalgam of cultural values that presents a special challenge to caregivers (Table 5–6). Complete understanding of all the possible self-structures, world views, and understandings about health and illness is impossible.

People do come to the therapeutic arena with differing adherences to traditional world views, and with differing acceptance and practice of the Western world view. Abstract ethnographic data about the traditions of various cultures and subcultures provide only limited information about any individual, family, or community. Assessment of the client's beliefs, values, and goals, along with ethnographic data about the person's primary group affiliation, is more helpful in providing culturally relevant

TABLE 5–6 CULTURAL VALUES, CARE MEANINGS, AND ACTION MODES

VALUES	CARE MEANINGS AND ACTION MODES
Anglo-American Culture (mainly U.S. middle and upper classes)	
1. Individualism—focus on a self-reliant person 2. Independence and freedom 3. Competition and achievement 4. Materialism (things and money) 5. Technology dependent 6. Instant time and actions 7. Youth and beauty 8. Equal sex rights 9. Leisure time highly valued 10. Reliance on scientific facts and numbers 11. Less respect for authority and the elderly 12. Generosity in time of crisis	1. Stress alleviation by ▸ Physical means ▸ Emotional means 2. Personalized acts ▸ Doing special things ▸ Individual attention 3. Self-reliance (individualism) by ▸ Reliance on self ▸ Reliance on self (self-care) ▸ Becoming independent ▸ Reliance on technology 4. Health instruction ▸ Teach us how "to do" this care for self ▸ Give us the "medical" facts

Continued

TABLE 5–6 CULTURAL VALUES, CARE MEANINGS, AND ACTION MODES *(Continued)*

VALUES	CARE MEANINGS AND ACTION MODES
Mexican American Culture*	
1. Extended family valued 2. Interdependence with kin and social activities 3. Patriarchal (machismo) 4. Exact time less valued 5. High respect for authority and the elderly 6. Religion valued (many Roman Catholics) 7. Native foods for well-being 8. Traditional folk-care healers for folk illnesses 9. Belief in hot-cold theory	1. Succor (direct family aid) 2. Involvement with extended family ("other care") 3. Filial love/loving 4. Respect for authority 5. Mother as care decision maker 6. Protective (external) male care 7. Acceptance of God's will 8. Use of folk-care practices 9. Healing with foods 10. Touching
Haitian American Culture†	
1. Extended family as support system 2. Religion—God's will must prevail 3. Reliance on folk foods and treatments 4. Belief in hot-cold theory 5. Male decision maker and direct caregivers 6. Reliance on native language	1. Involve family for support (other care) 2. Respect 3. Trust 4. Succor 5. Touching (body closeness) 6. Reassurance 7. Spiritual healing 8. Use of folk food, care rituals 9. Avoid evil eye and witches 10. Speak the language
African American Culture‡	
1. Extended family networks 2. Religion valued (many are Baptists) 3. Interdependence with "blacks" 4. Daily survival 5. Technology valued, e.g., radio, car 6. Folk (soul) foods 7. Folk-healing modes 8. Music and physical activities	1. Concern for my "brothers and sisters" 2. Being involved 3. Giving presence 4. Family support and "get-togethers" 5. Touching appropriately 6. Reliance on home folk remedies 7. Rely on "Jesus to save us" with prayers and songs
North American Indian Culture§	
1. Harmony between land, people, and environment 2. Reciprocity with "Mother Earth" 3. Spiritual inspiration (spirit guidance) 4. Folk healers (shamans) (the circle and four directions) 5. Practice culture rituals and taboos 6. Rhythmicity of life with nature 7. Authority of tribal elders 8. Pride in cultural heritage and "nations" 9. Respect and value for children	1. Establish harmony between people and environment with reciprocity 2. Actively listening 3. Using periods of silence ("Great Spirit" guidance) 4. Rhythmic timing (nature, land, people) in harmony 5. Respect for native folk healers, carers, and curers (use of circle) 6. Maintaining reciprocity (replenish what is taken from Mother Earth) 7. Preserving cultural rituals and taboos 8. Respect for elders and children

*These findings were from the author's transcultural nurse studies (1970, 1984) and other transcultural nurse studies in the United States.
†These data were from Haitians living in the United States (1981–1991).
‡These findings were from the author's study of two southern U.S. villages (1980–1981) and from a study of one large northern urban city (1982–1991) along with other studies by transcultural nurses.
§These findings were collected by the author and other contributors in the United States and Canada.
Cultural variations among all nations exist, and so these data are some general commonalities about values, care meanings, and actions.
From Andrews, M., and Boyle, J. (1995) *Transcultural concepts in nursing care* (2nd ed.) (pp. 63–64). Philadelphia: J. B. Lippincott. Leininger, M. M. (1991). *Culture care diversity and universality: A theory of nursing* (pp. 355–357). New York: National League for Nursing Press.

nursing care. Box 5–4 introduces a number of ideas for becoming fluent across cultures.

A model of cultural assessment presented by Giger and Davidhizar (1995) evaluates six cultural dimensions: communication, space, social orientation, time, environmental control, and biological variations (Fig. 5–2). While not specific to psychiatric nursing, the data gathered from this assessment tool provide general information about ways in which different cultural groups organize their activities and relationships. This general information will also help you understand how to organize a psychosocial interview (Table 5–7). A general assessment guide is included in Appendix D.

Illness and disease occur within a cultural and social context. Culture provides the framework within which the meaning of the illness, and the necessary care or cure, are determined. The types of mental illness seen within a given culture reflect the way that culture understands the self and its relationship to society; the way people within the culture understand themselves in the world; and the way they express grief, fear, anxiety, and depression (Table 5–8). Syndromes that seem to express certain cultural ideologies, and are not shared across cultures, are referred to as **culture-bound syndromes** (Table 5–9). For example, the preoccupation with feminine beauty, self-control, and sexuality in the United States is sometimes expressed in anorexia nervosa, a disorder unknown in many other parts of the world. Similarly, conflicts between the Japanese role expectations of the housewife and her desires for emotional fulfillment outside the home have come to be manifested in the "kitchen syndrome" (Lock 1987).

In summarizing the impact of culture on the expression of mental illness, Kleinman (1980) contrasted the experience of depression in the Western client and that of neurasthenia in the Chinese client. He encouraged health care providers to understand the cultural meaning of the illness experience; the roles of the client, family, and community regarding the illness; and the expectations the client and family have in the health care encounter. Kleinman referred to these as **explanatory models (EMs).** These models are the way that cultures understand the factors that cause and cure illnesses and shape

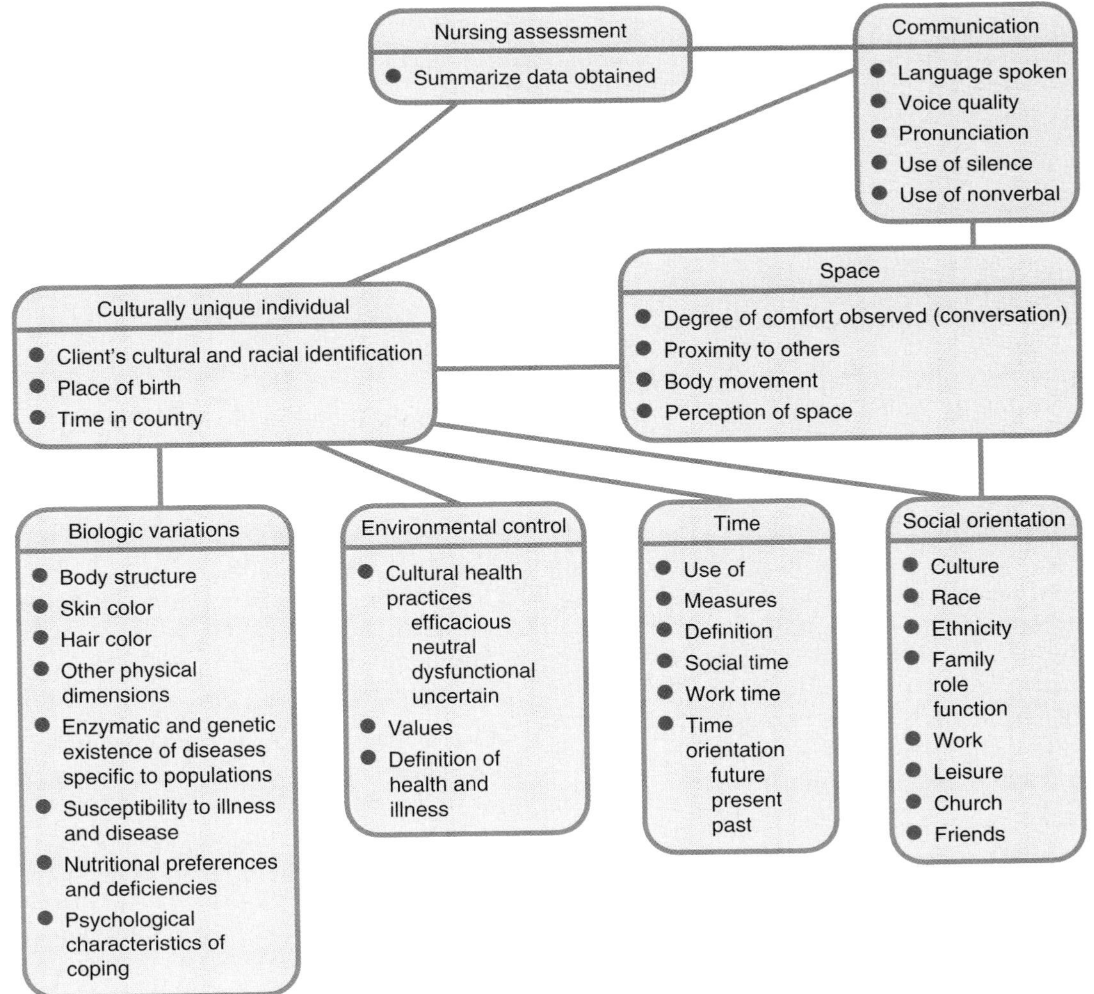

Figure 5–2 Giger and Davidhizar's transcultural assessment model. (From Giger, J. and Davidhizar, R. (1995). *Transcultural nursing: Assessment and intervention.* St. Louis: Mosby–Year Book.)

TABLE 5–7 CULTURAL ASSESSMENT IN PSYCHIATRIC NURSING

I. Relationships with Others

a. "What kinds of behavior do people in your culture believe are good or right?"
b. "How should people behave—What's the right way to be with others?"
c. "How should one deal with their personal needs?"
d. "What needs take high priority? Who takes care of whose needs?"
e. "If there is a conflict about needs, how is it resolved?"
f. "What are the most important things to pay attention to in your family/culture/social group?"

II. Modes of Expressing/Understanding Emotions

a. "How do people in your culture solve problems between each other?"
b. "What kinds of behaviors that people do are problems in your culture—what kinds of things that people do cause conflict or trouble?"
c. "What do people in your culture do when they are upset—when they have strong emotions or feelings? (Men? Women?)"

III. Understanding the Self and the World

a. "What's important in your culture to learn about yourself—others—life—what kinds of lessons are good to learn?"
b. "When you were learning about your place in the world, what kinds of things were you told? What do you think and feel about this?"
c. "When you were learning about yourself and the world as a child, how were you taught—told stories, shown, told, provided experiences?"

IV. Developmental Maturity

a. "What does it mean to be a good man or woman in your culture?"
b. "What does it mean in your culture if your life is going according to plan—What would you be like or be doing?"

V. Conceptions of Mental Health and Illness

a. "What has your family or community said about the problems you've been having?"
b. "Have you ever heard of someone in your culture who has had problems like you're having? What did people say the causes of these problems were? What kinds of help did they get—from the church—others in the community—healers? What helped?"

the expectations that the community, family, and client have for the health care encounter (Fig. 5–3).

Psychiatric nursing care is a culturally derived set of interventions designed to promote verbalization of feelings, teach individually focused coping skills, and assist clients with behavioral and emotional self-control consistent with Western cultural ideals. However, consideration should be given to providing psychiatric nursing care that is not bound to specific cultural ideologies but aimed at general mental health goals. Kleinman (1988) conducted an analysis of the curative factors of traditional healing worldwide and developed a list of factors that these healing systems have in common:

1. Healing needs to integrate the physical symptoms with the symbolic system of the culture.
2. The explanatory models of the client and the healer are congruent.
3. The healer has characteristics of charisma and confidence.
4. The illness is conceptualized by both the healer and the client in cultural terms.
5. There are elements of confession, or moral witnessing, especially in an emotionally charged or cathartic way.
6. There is emotional arousal and faith in the healing method, both within the client and within the community.
7. Social persuasion is used by the healer, the family, and the community.
8. Healing techniques use rhetorical devices such as irony and paradox

Consideration of these commonalities suggests that the psychiatric nurse should facilitate extensive involvement of the family and the community when delivering education and making treatment plans. For example, it is within the community that understanding of the cultural meaning of the disease is formed and the illness itself is dealt with. Family members and the community are primary factors in the success of a treatment plan based on whether they agree with the diagnosis and whether they support compliance with the treatment (Kleinman 1980).

It is also necessary that the goals of treatment be cul-

TABLE 5–8 CULTURAL DATA OF MAJOR WORLD VIEWS

CULTURAL PHENOMENON	EUROPEAN AMERICAN	ASIAN	PAN-AMERICAN INDIAN	ARABIC OR ISLAMIC*	AFRICAN
Communication	Verbally oriented; use of eye contact more common in men than in women; women tend to facilitate communication with questions; men tend to be more direct and declarative	Use of silence and nonverbal cueing; non–eye contact; communication based on contextual cues, sex, and social position; formal communication with those outside intimate circle	Use of tribal languages increasing; also Spanish and English; use of silence, nonverbal cues; limited eye contact; respectful silence; reserved manner and "small talk" until rapport established; tact and diplomacy	Personal; verbal with same sex; close eye contact (staring); communication is easier with peers, more reserved when there is a gap in social status	Oral and verbal orientation; use of verbal rhythms, feedback from listener; truth is expected; facial and hand gesturing and intonations create emphasis and emotive expression
Space	Consider close proximity and touch a sign of intimacy; use of touch more common between women; displays of affection between men and women and kissing in media and in public	Close personal space tolerated for long periods without social engagement; use of touch and space have subtle and distinct communication aspects and varies based on intimacy; touch among those of same sex and parent-child but not between opposite sex	Group orientation and touch among intimates; spaces carry social and religious/symbolic significance—each space may have appropriate uses or behavioral expectations	Close personal space; touch between parent and child and same sexes, limited between opposite sexes; hand-holding or arm in arm same sex only	Close personal space in company of familiars; may be guarded and reserved until rapport is established; touch may signify familiarity
Time orientation	Monochronic—see time in linear, segmented way; task oriented, concerned with punctuality; future oriented; consider concerns about the past old-fashioned	Polychronic—sees time as flowing with several simultaneous tasks; future orientation in work and technology; present orientation in social situations	Highly present oriented; relationships and present interactions must be handled well to achieve harmony and balance; past time orientation with regard to ancestry and tradition	Highly present oriented; no social regard for appointments—oriented to interaction at hand; social expectation that they will be tended to when someone is available; expectation of trustworthiness	Polychronic; orientation depends on adoption of dominant world view; continuity from past to future; may tend toward present orientation

Continued

TABLE 5–8 CULTURAL DATA OF MAJOR WORLD VIEWS *(Continued)*

CULTURAL PHENOMENON	EUROPEAN AMERICAN	ASIAN	PAN-AMERICAN INDIAN	ARABIC OR ISLAMIC*	AFRICAN
Social organization	Nuclear families; Judeo-Christian religion is hierarchical; organize relationships and groups around similarities	Hierarchical—obligations and duties to those a bove and below; filial-piety—loyalty and duty to male house head, superior; hierarchy based on sex and age; devotion to tradition varies by generation	Family oriented; nuclear family with extended kinships ties; hierarchy based on age and sex; family pride and honor regulate behavior	Organize by group affiliation, especially political/religious groups, also by lineage and tribe; born into established social status; affiliations are generally lifetime; hierarchical by age, sex, lineage, and social status	Social pattern greatly affected by history of discrimination; family oriented, with family extended to nonkin dependents and community members; emphasis on community
Environmental control	Value science and technology; action oriented; tendency to attempt to manipulate environment to adapt to human needs	Adjust to physical and social world; order is predetermined and acceptance of what is valued; individuals are expected to recognize consequences of actions and adjust behavior accordingly	Being oriented; focus on harmony with forces outside of person, including community, nature, and spirits or deities; concern for balance and moderation in relations with nature and others	Limited emphasis on personal control; control and authority are attained from those with established power and wealth; expectation that those in power and control over you have the obligation to care for their dependents; rely on benevolence of others	Interrelationship between person and external world is focus; proper relationships, nutrition, religious observances, and respect for those who came before affect health and well-being; history of social injustice may affect view of ability to alter social environment
Biological variations	Dominant focus in medicine is heart and lungs; fast-paced life style promotes stress-related diseases such as hypertension, migraines, ulcers, cancers	Dominant focus is chest and abdomen; "belly" is seat of soul or mind; somatic expression of mental distress in forms of dizziness, shoulder pain, stomach distress; diseases of industrialization; tropical diseases vary by region	Forced migration and reservation residence altered healthy traditional habits; currently plagued by diseases of poverty—alcohol abuse, STDs, TB, depression, and suicide; may be genetically predisposed to diabetes and alcohol addiction	Oriented to abdomen and chest area; may express feelings nonverbally through abdominal pain or joint and muscle pain	Discrimination and unemployment have created disease of poverty—substance abuse, STDs, TB, malnutrition; urbanization of poverty has created increased susceptibility to urban problems—violence, asthma; cultural meanings of blood—hypertension and HIV

*Kulwicki, A. (1996). Personal communication.
STDs, sexually transmitted diseases; TB, tuberculosis; HIV, human immunodeficiency virus.

TABLE 5–9 SELECTED CULTURE-BOUND SYNDROMES

GROUP	DISORDER	SYMPTOMS
Whites	Anorexia nervosa	Excessive preoccupation with thinness; self-imposed starvation
	Bulimia	Gross overeating and then vomiting or fasting
African American/ Haitians	Blackout	Collapse, dizziness, inability to move
	Low blood	Not enough blood or weakness of blood that is often treated with diet
	High blood	Blood that is too rich in certain things owing to ingestion of too much red meat or rich foods
	Thin blood	Occurs in women, children, and old people; renders individual more susceptible to illness in general
	Diseases of hex, witchcraft, conjuring	Sense of being doomed by spell; gastrointestinal symptoms, e.g., vomiting; hallucinations; part of voodoo beliefs
Chinese/S.E. Asians	Koro	Intense anxiety that penis is retracting into body
Greeks	Hysteria	Bizarre complaints and behavior because uterus leaves pelvis for another part of the body
Hispanics	Empacho	Food forms into a ball and clings to stomach or intestine, causing pain and cramping
	Fatigue	Asthma-like symptoms
	Mal ojo, "evil eye"	Fitful sleep, crying, diarrhea in children caused by a stranger's attention; sudden onset
	Pasmo	Paralysis-like symptoms of face of limbs; prevented or relieved by massage
	Susto	Anxiety, trembling, phobias from sudden fright
Native Americans	Ghost	Terror, hallucinations, sense of danger
North Indians	Ghost	Death from fever and illness in children; convulsions, delirious speech (or incessant crying in infants); choking, difficulty breathing; based on Hindu religious beliefs and curing practices
Japanese	Wagamama	Apathetic childish behavior with emotional outbursts
Korean	Hwa-byung	Multiple somatic and psychological symptoms; "pushing-up" sensation of chest; palpitations, flushing, headache, "epigastic mass," dysphoria, anxiety, irritability, and difficulty concentrating; mostly afflicts married women
	Amok	An acute reaction resulting from morbid hostility; our vernacular term "running amok" comes from the frenzied lashing out associated with this syndrome
	Malignant anxiety	Acute anxiety states with panic and varying degrees of egodisorganization that have been associated with criminality and loss of stable culture owing to colonialism
Polar Eskimos	Pibloktog	"Arctic hysteria"—accounts are of bizarre, overdramatized behavior, such as running naked through snow
Latin Americans	Susto	Traumatic, anxiety-depressive state with psychophysiological changes; "fright sickness" that results from such stimuli as a fall, a thunderclap, meeting some threat, or other frightening experiences; susto causes anxiety, insomnia, listlessness, loss of appetite, and social withdrawal
Native Americans	Trance dissociation	Possession syndromes occurring in various parts of world with varying degrees of social sanction; this differs from primary schizophrenic reactions and is believed to be caused by disease, the loss of one's soul, or the invasion of a benign or evil spirit; in some circumstances, it is viewed as a mystical state
	Voodoo death	"Magical" or sociocultural death that has been explained as result of flight-or-fight response, belief in power of threat and suggestion, and acceptance of hopelessness

Adapted from Giger, J., and Davidhizar, R. (1995). *Transcultural nursing: Assessment and intervention* (p. 80). St. Louis: Mosby–Year Book. Kavanaugh, K. (1995). Transcultural perspectives in mental health. In M. Andrews and J. Boyle (Eds.), *Transcultural concepts in nursing care* (2nd ed.) (p. 258). Philadelphia: J. B. Lippincott.

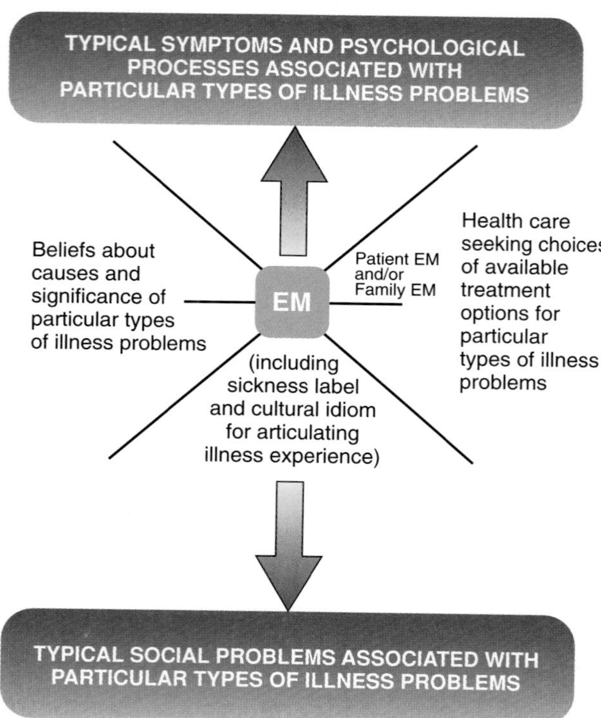

Figure 5–3 Popular explanatory models (EMs), semantic networks, and health care seeking. (From Kleinman, A. (1980). *Patients and healers in the context of culture.* Berkeley, CA: University of California Press.)

turally relevant and appropriate. For example, nurses who have the culturally derived belief that feelings should be expressed verbally might plan to engage the client in exercises and counseling that promote such expression. However, in cultures that do not support such a clear focus on the self and do not encourage the person to express such feelings verbally, this treatment is irrelevant and inappropriate. Techniques such as art therapy, journal writing, and experiential learning may be more appropriate. Understanding the client's goals will also help the treatment process. For example, a person may have a goal of coping quietly without verbal expression of feelings; thus, problem solving and other constructive strategies may be most effective for that client.

SUMMARY

All nursing care needs to accommodate cultural diversity; however, psychiatric mental health nursing has the special challenge of defining mental health and providing behavioral control. Western ideas of normalcy have been applied universally to quite different cultures, and little research was done historically about the role of culture in shaping psychological functioning. Recent research is only beginning to delineate these differences, and culturally relevant psychological care is still at the experimental stage. However, authors agree that the current model of Western psychotherapy must be used cautiously, and our definition of mental health must be expanded to include a broader range of behaviors.

Before making any cross-cultural encounter, nurses must be aware of personal values and beliefs, expose themselves to cultural diversity, challenge their own ethnocentrism, and dispel cultural myths. Understanding world views can help the nurse categorize and understand assessment data and promote critical thinking about culture and mental health.

While forming a therapeutic relationship with a client, family, or community of another culture, the nurse should conduct a relevant cultural assessment. General assessment data about cultural aspects of mental health include beliefs, values, and behaviors around the relationship between the self and others; modes of emotional expression; understanding the self and the world; developmental maturity; and conceptions of mental health and illness. Finally, cultural psychology data to date suggest that interdependent cultural models stress roles, relationships, interpersonal harmony, and authority. These values can inform nursing practice when the nurse incorporates the sociocultural factors into the plan of care. Curiosity, negotiation, compromise, and flexibility are attributes that can help the nurse provide culturally relevant care.

Future research is needed to test psychiatric nursing assessment tools. International psychiatric nursing models need to be developed that focus on general mental health goals along a continuum of normalcy. Finally, psychiatric nursing must develop and test goals and interventions that assist all clients to achieve culturally relevant outcomes.

REFERENCES

Abu-Lughod, L. (1986). *Veiled sentiments*. Berkeley, CA: University of California Press.

Andrews, M., and Boyle, J. (1995). *Transcultural concepts in nursing care* (2nd ed.) (pp. 153–285). Philadelphia: J. B. Lippincott.

Asante, M. K. (1987). *The Afrocentric idea*. Philadelphia: Temple University Press.

Asante, M. K. (1988). *Afrocentricity*. Trenton, NJ: Africa World Press.

Bellah, R. N., et al. (1985). *Habits of the heart: Individualism and commitment in American life*. Berkeley, CA: University of California Press.

Brown, J. E. (1982). *The spiritual legacy of the American Indian*. New York: Crossroads Publishing.

Burlew, A., Banks, W., McDoo, H., and Azibo, D. (1992). *African American psychology: Theory, research and practice*. Newbury Park, CA: Sage Publications.

Chodorow, N. (1978). *The reproduction of mothering: Psychoanalysis and the sociology of mothering*. Berkeley, CA: University of California Press.

Choi, S. C., and Choi, S. H. (1990, July). *We-ness: a Korean discourse of collectivism*. Paper prepared for the First International Conference on Individualism and Collectivism: Psychocultural Perspectives for East and West, Seoul, Korea.

Cross, S. E., and Markus, H. R. (1993). Gender in thought, belief and action: A cognitive approach. In A. E. Beall and J. Sternberg (Eds.), *The psychology of gender* (pp. 55–98). New York: Guilford Press.

Derne, S. (1992). Beyond institutional and impulsive conceptions of the self: Family structure and the socially anchored real self. *Ethos*, 20(3):259–288.

Dien, D. S. (1992). Gender and individuation: China and the west. *Psychoanalytic Review*, 79(1):105–119.

Dinges, N., Trimble, J., Manson, S., and Pasquale, F. (1991). Counseling and psychotherapy with American Indians and Alaska Natives. In A. Marsella and P. Pedersen (Eds.), *Cross-cultural counseling and psychotherapy* (pp. 243–276). New York: Pergamon Press.

Doi, L. T. (1984). *Amae*: A key for understanding Japanese personality structure. In H.P. Varley (Ed.), *Japanese culture* (3rd ed.) (pp. 132–139). Honolulu: University of Hawaii Press.

Erikson, E. H. (1968). *Identity, youth and crisis*. New York: Norton.

Espin, O. M. (1985). Psychotherapy with Hispanic women: Some considerations. In P. B. Pedersen (Ed.), *Handbook of cross-cultural counseling and therapy* (pp. 165–171). Westport, CT: Greenwood Press.

Forde, D. (1954). *African worlds: Studies in the cosmological ideas and social values of African peoples*. London: Oxford University Press.

Freud, A. (1936). *The ego and mechanisms of defense*. New York: International Universities Press, 1946.

Freud, S. (1923). *The ego and the id*. London: Hogarth, 1948.

Fujita, M., and Sano, T. (1988). Children in American and Japanese day care centers: Ethnograph and reflective cross-cultural interviewing. In H. T. Trueba and C. Delgado-Gaitan (Eds.), *School and society: Learning through culture*. New York: Praeger.

Geertz, C. (1975). On the nature of anthropological understanding. *American Scientist*, 63:47–53.

Gergen, K. J. (1992). *Psychology in the postmodern era*. Unpublished manuscript.

Gergen, K. J., and Gergen, M. M. (1988). Narrative and the self as relationship. In L. Berkowitz (Ed.), *Advances in experimental social psychology*, vol. 21. New York: Academic Press.

Giger, J., and Davidhizar, R. (1995). *Transcultural nursing: Assessment and intervention*. St. Louis: Mosby–Year Book.

Gilligan, C. (1986). Remapping the moral domain: New images of the self in relationship. In T. C. Heller, M. Sosna and D. E. Wellbery (Eds.), *Reconstructing individualism: Autonomy, individuality, and the self in Western thought* (pp. 237–252). Stanford, CA: Stanford University Press.

Hollowell, A. I. (1963). Ojibwa world view and disease. In I. Galdston (Ed.), *Man's image in medicine and anthropology* (pp. 258–315). New York: International Universities Press.

Hsu, F. L. K. (1983). *Rugged individualism reconsidered*. Knoxville: University of Tennessee Press.

Johnson, F. (1985). The Western of self. In A. Marsella, G. De Vos and F. Hsu (Eds.), *Culture and self*. London: Tavistock.

Johnson, F. (1995). *Dependency and Japanese socialization*. New York: New York University Press.

Johnston, H., and Klandermans, B. (Eds.) (1995). *Social movements and culture*. Minnesota: University of Minnesota Press.

Kagitcibasi, C. (1989). Family and socialization in cross cultural perspectives: A model of change. In J. Berman (Ed.), *Nebraska Symposium on Motivation* (vol 37). Lincoln, NB: University of Nebraska Press.

Kakar, S. (1978). *The inner world: A psychoanalytic study of childhood and society in India*. Delhi, India: Oxford University Press.

Kaplan, B., and Johnson, D. (1964). The social meaning of Navaho psychopathology and psychotherapy. In A. Kiev (Ed.), *Magic, faith and healing* (pp. 203–227). New York: Free Press.

Kavanaugh, K. (1995). Transcultural perspectives in mental health. In M. Andrews and J. Boyle (Eds.), *Transcultural concepts in nursing care* (2nd ed.) (pp. 153–285). Philadelphia: J. B. Lippincott.

Kernberg, O. (1976). *Object relations theory and clinical psychoanalysis*. New York: Jacob Aronson.

Kleinman, A. (1980). *Patients and healers in the context of culture*. Berkeley, CA: University of California Press.

Kleinman, A. (1988). *Rethinking psychiatry*. New York: Free Press.

Kolwicki, A. (1996). Personal communication.

La Barre, W. (1964). Confession as cathartic therapy in American Indian tribes. In A. Kiev (Ed.), *Magic, faith and healing* (pp. 36–49). New York: Free Press.

Lebra, T. S. (1992, June). Culture, self and communication. Paper presented at the University of Michigan, Ann Arbor.

Levan, J. D. (1992). *Theories of the self*. Washington, DC: Taylor & Frances.

Levine, L. (1977). *Black culture and black consciousness*. New York: Oxford University Press.

Lock, M. (1987). Protests of a good wife and wise mother. In M. Lock and E. Norbeck (Eds.), *Health, illness and medical care in Japan* (pp. 130–157). Honolulu: University of Hawaii Press.

Lykes, M. B. (1985). Gender and individualistic vs. collectivist notions about the self. In A. J. Stewart and M. B. Lykes (Eds.), *Gender and personality: Current perspectives on theory and research* (pp. 269-295). Durham, NC: Duke University Press.

Lyons, N. P. (1983). Two perspectives: On self, relationships and morality. *Harvard Educational Review*, 53(2):125–145.

Mahler, M., Pine, F., and Bergman, A. (1975). *The psychological birth of the human infant: Symbiosis and individuation*. New York: Basic Books.

Markus, H., and Katayama, S. (1991). Culture and the self: Implications for cognition, emotion and motivation. *Psychological Review*, 98(2):224–253.

Markus, H., and Oyserman, D. (1989). Gender and thought: The role of the self-concept. In M. Crawford and M. Gentry (Eds.), *Gender and thought: Psychological perspectives* (pp. 100–127). New York: Springer-Verlag.

Mbiti, J. (1970). *African religions and philosophy*. Garden City, NY: Doubleday.

Moody, M. (1994). *For racial harmony*. Unpublished manuscript.

Ortiz de Montellano, B. (1990). *Aztec medicine, health and nutrition*. New Brunswick, NJ: Rutgers University Press.

Rapaport, D. (1960). On the psychoanalytic theory of motivation. In *Nebraska Symposium on Motivation* (pp. 173–247). Lincoln: University of Nebraska Press.

Roland, A. (1991). Psychoanalysis in India and Japan: Toward a comparative psychoanalysis. *American Journal of Psychoanalysis*, 51(1):1–10.

Rugh, A. B. (1985). *Family in contemporary Egypt*. Cairo, Egypt: American University Press.

Sahlins, M. (1996). Personal communication.

Sampson, E. E. (1988). The debate of individualism: Indigenous psychologies of the individuals and their role in personal and social functioning. *American Psychologist*, 43:15–22.

Shweder, R. A., and Borne, E. J. (1984). Does the concept of person vary cross-culturally? In R. A. Shweder and R. A. LeVine (Eds.), *Culture theory: Essays on mind, self and emotion* (pp. 158–199). Cambridge, England: Cambridge University Press.

Shweder, R. A., and Miller, J. G. (1991). The social construction of the person: How is it possible? In R. A. Shweder (Ed.), *Thinking through cultures: Expeditions in cultural psychology* (pp. 156–185). Cambridge, MA: Harvard University Press.

Spindler, G., and Spindler, L. (1987). *Interpretive ethnography of education at home and abroad*. Hillsdale, NJ: Lawrence Erlbaum Associates.

Stoller, R. (1985). *Presentations of gender*. New Haven, CT: Yale University Press.

Triandis, H., et al. (1988). Individualism and collectivism: Cross-cultural perspectives on self-ingroup relationships. *Journal of Personality and Social Psychology*, 54:323–338.

SELF-STUDY AND CRITICAL THINKING

Multiple choice

1. Understanding the relevance of culture to mental health nurses requires a nurse to do all the following *except:*

   A. Expose self to a variety of cultural ideals, values, and beliefs about relationships and the world.
   B. Study specific traditional ways of life of a variety of cultures (e.g., diet, religious practices, manner of dress).
   C. Carefully assess the goals of development, roles and responsibilities, and self-definitions of any given clients and their family.
   D. Understand the values and beliefs embedded within one's own culture and medical practices.

2. Which of the following behaviors should the psychiatric nurse carry out in the preintroductory phase of a cultural encounter?

   A. Gather relevant cultural data.
   B. Dispel myths and understand own cultural beliefs.
   C. Facilitate communication with appropriate use of touch and space.
   D. Interact with the family and community leaders.

For discussion:

3. Define the term "explanatory models of health and illness" and discuss how this affects therapeutic goals and interventions.
4. "Women from Arabic cultures are passive in relationship to men." Discuss why this statement is untrue and give an example.
5. Describe the African American cultural values of emotional honesty and interpersonal connection. Use these ideas to dispel myths and stereotypes.
6. Differentiate between the self-structure of the individualist and collectivist societies. Relate this to psychiatric nursing practice.
7. The suicide rate in the American Indian population is very high. Compare and contrast the conflict between traditional and European American values, and discuss why native counseling centers stress traditional values as a way to prevent suicide.

Critical thinking

8. A Chinese woman has recently moved to America from Taiwan. She is a wife and the mother of two small children, and lives in a tight-knit Chinese community with her husband's parents. She comes to an emergency room with complaints of fatigue, headache, and stomach pain. Diagnostic tests are unrevealing. Inquiry by the nurse reveals that the woman wants to be more like an American woman, and has been trying to "speak her mind" to her husband's parents. She has received increasing pressure from her husband and the family to "be a good wife."

   A. What are the symbolic or cultural meanings of her symptoms?
   B. What are the cultural expectations for this client and the possible cultural explanations for her suffering?

C. What might the family and her community recommend for her, and how does this contrast with the typical psychiatric nursing approach to her problems?
D. How might a culturally relevant approach modify these? What can a culturally competent psychiatric nurse do for this client?

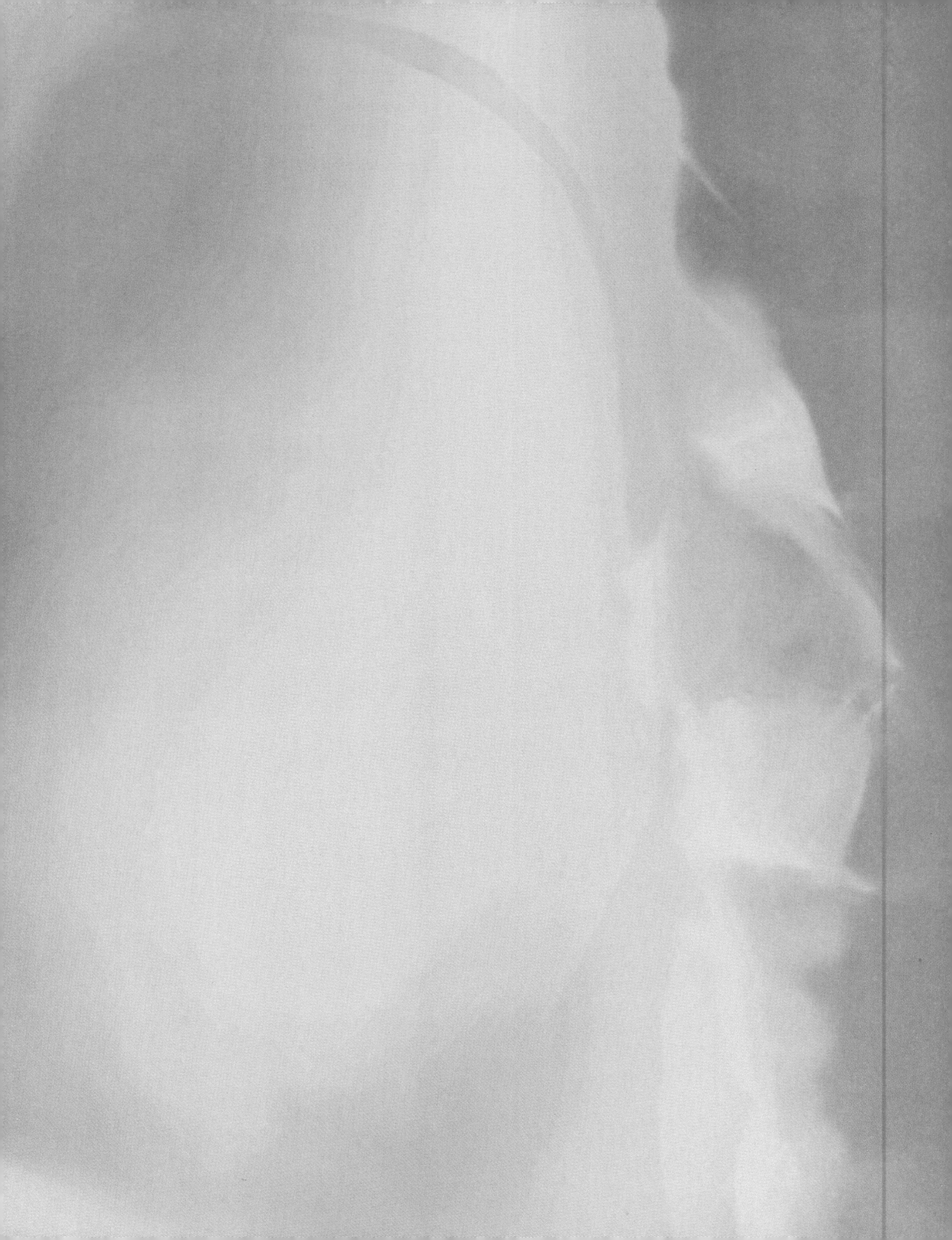

Unit Two

Basic Concepts in Psychiatric Nursing

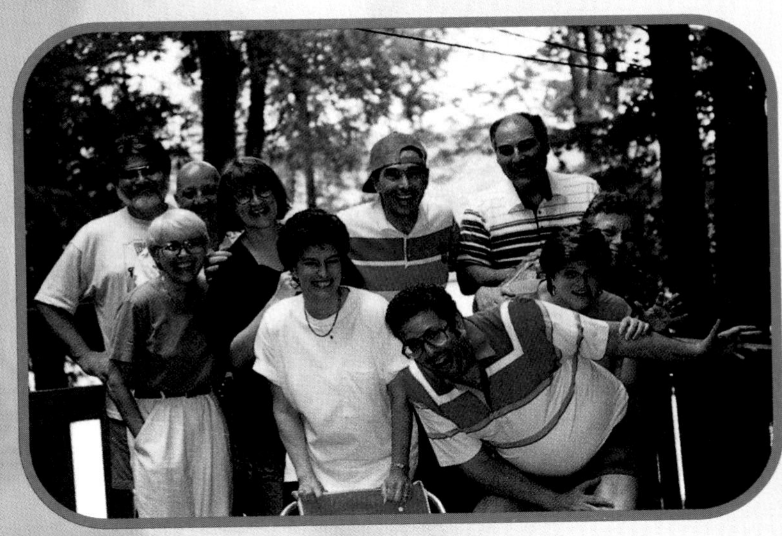

Against the assault of laughter, nothing can stand.

MARK TWAIN, THE MYSTERIOUS STRANGER

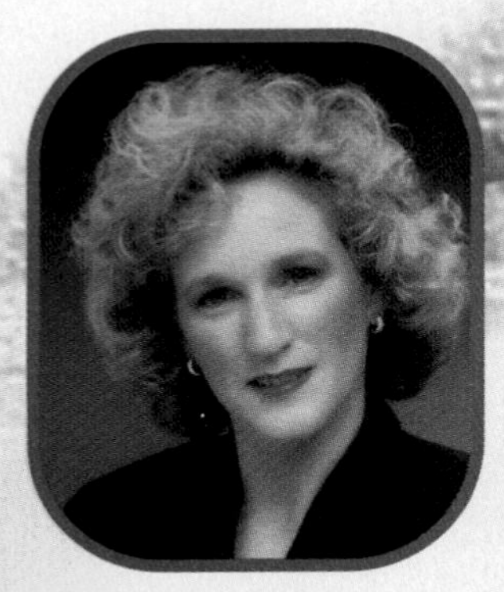

A Nurse Speaks

Constance Kolva Taylor

As client acuity has risen, lengths of stay have diminished, the number of professional nurses relative to the number of clients on a unit has decreased, and the locus of care moves rapidly to the community, nurses have needed an alternative to the tried and true way of doing nursing care planning. Nurses have also realized that the scope of practice and the scope of care of nursing are limited not only from a regulatory perspective, but because of the nature of basic nursing education and other social, political, and economic factors. This limitation creates a situation in which nursing can be imparting high-quality care but cannot achieve the quality outcomes because of not having the power to admit and discharge or having limited, if any, prescriptive authority. Thus, the interdisciplinary plan of care came into being. It was sanctioned by the Joint Commission on Accreditation of Healthcare Organizations (JCAHO) and had always been the intent of the Health Care Financing Administration (HCFA) regulations pertaining to treatment planning.

Clinical pathways are interdisciplinary plans of care that specify only those major care events that are to occur during the client's stay. They are diagnostically driven and intended to communicate expectations about the client's care to the client, the family, the payer, the provider, and the clinicians. As such, they describe the major care activities that are to occur and the time frame within which those activities are to occur. They are applied prospectively—that is, they are prescriptive and the same for all people with a given diagnosis, e.g., schizophrenia. They define the care to be delivered before its delivery and are anchored by time-based benchmarks. In essence, they are a way to assure payers that no more care than is absolutely necessary will be delivered, and that the client will be at the most expensive level of care for the shortest time possible. This translates into an assurance that the client's care will cost the least possible amount because of adherence to the pathway.

However, hospital administrators are trying to keep their facilities in the running for managed care contracts, and clinical pathways are perceived as a primary tool to engage the managed care entities into discussions and contract negotiations. The net result may be the arbitrary imposition of pathways with little choice by the clinician about their implementation or evaluation.

The elements of clinical pathways are to be appropriate and applied for at least 70% of those seeking treatment for a particular diagnosis. Unfortunately, no one knows for which clients the pathway will be appropriate and for which the pathway is inappropriate or at variance. Technically, the key to variance management is individualized care that is justified and substantiated by the clinical reasonings of the pracitioners and relative to the resources available. This begins to sound a lot like individualized care planning, which is where it all began.

When one takes into consideration the unique way in which each individual manifests an illness and the family and support system responds to the same and applies all of this to mental health care, it would seem that the odds are that variance is more likely to occur than compliance, especially when one considers the prevalence of comorbidity (two or more diagnoses) within the mental health treatment population. Additionally, the way in which the outcomes are defined must be scrutinized. As the pathways are diagnostically based, staff oriented, and time driven, it would follow that the outcomes will be time-based descriptions of what the staff accomplished. While the net result of the care delivered vis-à-vis the pathway is described by all as "clinical outcomes," there are some pathways that fail to define the outcome(s). Some describe mental health care outcomes as specific changes in psychometric scores. Others rely on broad descriptions of changes in behavior and/or verbalizations, such as "Client verbalizes understanding why he is violent" or "Client copes better with illness." It is curious that just a few years ago, such broad, non-measurable outcome statements were unsatisfactory to surveyors from JCAHO and HCFA alike!

It is important that nurses understand the origins of clinical pathways and their current purpose, scope, and intent. Issues relating to patient acuity, staff mix, and score of practice and care must be considered when using clinical pathways as guides for care. The lines of accountability must be defined and adhered to when using pathways so that the nurse is not, once again, the whipping child of the organization. Finally, one must cautiously use the pathways and rely primarily on sound clinical judgment by applying the most judicious care relative to the individual client circumstances and manifestations. It may be that the greatest value clinical pathways have to offer is when they are applied retrospectively to a group of patients over a predefined period. It is in this historical analysis that major systems issues that impede quality care can be identified and total quality management (TQM) methods applied to their remedy—all for the benefit of the client, first and foremost.

6

The Nurse-Client Relationship and the Nursing Process

ELIZABETH M. VARCAROLIS

OUTLINE

KEY TERMS AND CONCEPTS

The key terms and concepts listed here also appear in bold where they are defined or discussed in this chapter.

social relationship
intimate relationship
therapeutic relationship
congruence
empathy
transference
countertransference
values
values clarification
therapeutic encounter
orientation phase
contract
confidentiality
working phase
termination phase
assessment
outcome criteria
counseling
health teaching
self-care activities
milieu therapy

OBJECTIVES

After studying this chapter, the reader will be able to

1. Contrast and compare the purpose, focus, communication styles, and goals for (a) a social relationship, (b) an intimate relationship, and (c) a therapeutic relationship.
2. Define and discuss the role of empathy, genuineness, and positive regard on the part of the nurse in a nurse-client relationship.
3. Identify two attitudes and four actions that may reflect the nurse's positive regard toward a client.
4. Analyze what is meant by boundaries and the influence of transference and countertransference on boundary blurring.
5. Act out four common nonhelpful nurse responses and state the ways the nurse can minimize each one.
6. Assess five of your most important values using a values clarification exercise.
7. Contrast and compare the three phases of the nurse-client relationship.
8. Discuss the four areas of concern you will address during your first interview with a client.
9. Identify four testing behaviors a client may demonstrate and discuss possible nursing interventions for each behavior.
10. Perform a mental health assessment on a client agreed upon with your instructor.
11. Explain three principles the nurse follows in planning nursing actions to meet the client's goals.
12. Identify three advanced practice interventions.

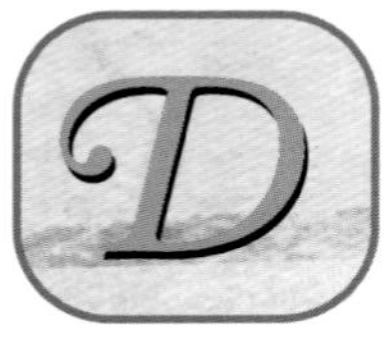

Does helping help? The answer is yes, no, and sometimes. When helping is done by skilled and socially intelligent people, it can do a great deal of good (Egan 1994). However, helping is a powerful process that can be mismanaged. Egan goes on to state that "helping is not neutral; it is for better or worse." In reviewing the process of human change, Mahoney (1991) suggested three fundamental questions:

1. Can humans change?
2. Can humans help humans change?
3. Are some forms of helping better than others?

Mahoney answered yes to all three questions.

So we see that helping can be, and often is, useful; unfortunately, sometimes it is not. Helping a person with a medical or emotional problem is rarely a straightforward proposition, and assisting a person to gain or regain physiological and functional normality can be a difficult goal to reach (Parsons and Wicks 1994). How can we become effective helpers? Some of the issues that need to be addressed before learning specific helping skills were outlined by Egan (1994):

- What specific stages and steps make up the helping process?
- What techniques aid the process?

- What communication skills are needed to interact with clients?
- How are these skills and techniques acquired?
- What do clients need to do to collaborate in the helping process and to manage their problems and [further] develop their opportunities?
- How do we evaluate [our] own and [our] client's efforts?

This chapter, along with Chapter 7 on communication techniques, offers guidelines for answering these queries. Elaboration on these issues—specific techniques, communication and evaluation strategies, and tools for specific diagnostic disorders—are interwoven throughout the text, especially in the clinical chapters (Chapters 11 to 26). Now we will take a look at the attributes of a helpful relationship.

THE HELPFUL NURSE-CLIENT RELATIONSHIP

Types of Relationships

The nurse-client relationship is often loosely defined, but a therapeutic relationship incorporating principles of mental health nursing is more clearly defined and differs from other relationships. A helpful (or therapeutic) nurse-client relationship has specific goals and functions. Goals in a therapeutic relationship include

- Facilitating communication of distressing thoughts and feelings.
- Assisting a client with problem solving to help facilitate activities of daily living.
- Helping clients examine self-defeating behaviors and test alternatives.
- Promoting self-care and independence.

Look again at Chapter 1 for a discussion of the roles and goals of psychiatric mental health nurses and a reminder that the nurse-client relationship develops over time and goes through specific stages. Chapter 1 also noted that *specific phenomena occur during the process of the relationship*. We are going to explore these phenomena here.

A relationship is an interpersonal process that involves two or more people. Throughout life, we meet people in a variety of settings and share a variety of experiences. With some individuals we develop long-term relationships; with others the relationship lasts only a short time. Naturally, the kinds of relationships we enter into vary from person to person. Generally, they may be defined as (1) social, (2) intimate, or (3) therapeutic in nature.

Social Relationships

A **social relationship** can be defined as a relationship that is primarily initiated for the purpose of friendship, socialization, enjoyment, or accomplishing a task. Mutual needs are met during social interaction (e.g., participants share ideas, feelings, and experiences). Communication skills used in this type of relationship include giving advice and (sometimes) meeting basic dependency needs, such as lending money and helping with jobs. Often the content of the communication remains superficial. During social interactions, roles may shift. Within a social relationship, there is little emphasis on the evaluation of the interaction.

Staff nurses as well as students may struggle with requests by clients to "be my friend." When this occurs, the nurse should make it clear that the relationship is a therapeutic (helping) one. This does *not* mean that the nurse is not "friendly" toward the client at times. It does mean, however, that the nurse follows the stated guidelines regarding a therapeutic relationship; essentially, the focus is on the client, and the relationship is not designed to meet the nurse's needs. The client's problems and concerns are explored and potential solutions are discussed by both client and nurse, and solutions are implemented by the client.

Intimate Relationships

An **intimate relationship** occurs between two individuals who have an emotional commitment to each other. Those in an intimate relationship usually react naturally to each other. Often the relationship is a partnership wherein each member cares about the other's needs for growth and satisfaction. Within the relationship, mutual needs are met and intimate desires and fantasies shared. Short- and long-range goals are usually mutual. Information shared between these individuals may be personal and intimate. People may want an intimate relationship for many reasons, such as procreation, sexual or emotional satisfaction, economic security, social belonging, and reduced loneliness. Depending on the style, level of maturity, and awareness of both parties, evaluation of the interactions may or may not be ongoing.

Therapeutic Relationships

The **therapeutic relationship** between nurse and client differs from both a social and an intimate relationship in that the nurse maximizes inner communication skills, understanding of human behaviors, and personal strengths in order to enhance the client's growth. The focus of the relationship is on the client's ideas, experiences, and feelings (Smitherman 1982). Inherent in a therapeutic (helping) relationship is the nurse's focus on significant personal issues introduced by the client during the clinical interview. The nurse and the client identify areas that need exploration and periodically evaluate the degree of change in the client. *Although the nurse may assume a variety of roles* (e.g., teacher, counselor, socializing agent, liaison), *the relationship is consistently focused on the client's problem and needs.* Health care workers do well to get their needs met outside the relationship. When nurses begin to want the client to "like them," "do as they suggest," "be nice to them," or "give them recognition," the needs of the client cannot be adequately met and the interaction could be detrimental to the client. Working under supervision is an excellent way to keep the focus and boundaries clear. Communication skills and knowledge of the stages and phenomena occurring in a therapeutic relationship are crucial tools in the formation and maintenance of that relationship. Within the context of a helping relationship:

1. The needs of the client are identified and explored.
2. Alternate problem-solving approaches are taken.
3. New coping skills may develop.
4. Behavioral change is encouraged.

Factors That Enhance Growth in Others

Rogers (1967) identified three personal characteristics that help promote change and growth in clients: (1) genuineness, (2) empathy, and (3) positive regard (Rogers and Truax 1967). These personal characteristics continue to be regarded as crucial ingredients in effective helpers.

Genuineness

Rogers uses the word **congruence** to signify genuineness, or an awareness of one's own feelings as they arise within the relationship, and the ability to communicate them when appropriate. Essentially, congruence is the ability to meet "person to person" in a therapeutic relationship. It is conveyed by such actions as not hiding behind the role of nurse, listening to and communicating with others without distorting their messages, and being clear and concrete in communications with clients. Congruence connotes the ability to use therapeutic communication tools in an appropriately spontaneous manner, rather than rigidly or in a parrot-like fashion.

Genuine helpers do not take refuge in the role of nurse or therapeutic counselor. "People who are genuine are at home with themselves, and therefore can comfortably be themselves in all their interactions" (Egan 1994, p. 55).

Empathy

Empathy is the ability to see things from the other person's perspective and to communicate this understanding to the other person. Empathy denotes understanding and acceptance of the client and his or her situation. Myrick and Erney (1984) state that the word *empathy* is often used as a substitute for the word *understanding*. Empathy means that one understands the ideas expressed, as well as the feelings that are present in the other person. La-Monica (1980), a nurse researcher who developed a valid empathy instrument, defines empathy:

> Empathy signifies a central focus and feeling with and in the client's world. It involves (1) accurate perception of the client's world by the helper, (2) communication of this understanding to the client, and (3) the client's perception of the helper's understanding.

People often confuse the term *empathy* with *sympathy*. Being empathetic and being sympathetic are two different things. Egan (1994) states that sympathy has more to do with feelings of compassion, pity, and commiseration. Although these are human traits, they may not be particularly useful in a counseling situation. When people express sympathy, they express agreement with another, which may in some situations discourage further exploration of a client's thoughts and feelings. Sympathy is the actual sharing of another's feelings, and consequently experiencing the need to reduce one's own personal distress. When a helping person is "feeling sympathy" with another, objectivity is lost, and the ability to assist the client in solving a personal problem ceases. For example, a friend tells you her mother was just diagnosed with inoperable cancer. Your friend then begins to cry and pounds the table with her fist.

- *Sympathetic response:* "I know exactly how you feel. My mother was hospitalized last year and it was awful. I was so depressed. I still get upset just thinking about it."

You go on to tell your friend about the incident. Sometimes, when nurses try to be sympathetic, they are in danger of projecting their own feelings onto the client's, thus limiting the client's range of responses (Morse et al. 1992). A more useful response might be as follows:

- *Empathetic response:* "How upsetting this must be for you. Something similar happened to my mother last year. What thoughts and feelings have you had?"

You continue to stay with your friend and listen to his or her thoughts and feelings.

In the practice of psychotherapy or counseling, it is believed by many that empathy is an essential ingredient both for the better-functioning client and for the client who functions at a more primitive level (Book 1988). However, if a nurse feels empathetic toward a client and his or her situation, is therapeutic empathy *always* an effective or helpful response? Morse and associates (1992) question the use of therapeutic empathy in *all* nurse-client relationships. Although therapeutic empathy may be appropriate in community, psychiatric, and rehabilitation settings or with long-term clients, it might not be so in all nursing situations or settings. One example might be the case of acute and sudden illness. During this crisis phase, clients and families are learning to cope with discomfort and learning to accept their radically changed reality. This is a phase that must be "experienced before reaching the phases in which adaptation and change (personal growth) are important, relevant or possible" (Morse et al. 1992, p. 277). The authors go on to say that responses that facilitate clients' and families' acceptance of their crisis situations are perhaps more appropriate and useful. Such facilitating responses include sympathy, compassion, pity, consolation, and commiseration.

Morse and associates (1992) argue that the essence of the nurse-client relationship is the engagement, the identification of the nurse with the client, and the identification with the human experience of the other person. These authors propose a theory of engagement in the nurse-client relationship where pity and sympathy and other "devalued responses" play an acknowledged part in some nurse-client relationships, to the benefit of both nurse and client. Readers are encouraged to review this model (Morse et al. 1992).

Positive Regard

Positive regard implies respect. It is the ability to view another person as being worthy of caring about and as someone who has strengths and achievement potential. Respect is usually communicated not directly in words but indirectly by actions.

ATTITUDES. One attitude through which a nurse might convey respect is willingness to work with the client. That is, the nurse takes the client and the relationship seriously. The experience is viewed not as "a job," "part of a course," or "time spent talking," but as an opportunity to work with people to help them develop their own resources and actualize more of their potential in living.

ACTIONS. Some actions that manifest an attitude of respect are attending, suspending value judgments, and helping clients develop their own resources.

Attending. This refers to an intensity of presence, or being with the client (Egan 1994). At times, simply being with another person during a painful time can make a difference. Some nonverbal behaviors that reflect the degree of attending are the nurse's body posture (leaning forward toward the client, arms comfortably at sides), degree of eye contact, degree of relaxation during the interaction, and evaluating the client's response to such nurse behaviors.

Suspending Value Judgments. Nurses are more effective when they guard against using their own value systems to judge a client's thoughts, feelings, or behaviors. For example, if a client is taking drugs or is sexually promiscuous, the nurse might recognize that these behaviors are hindering the client from living a more satisfying life or from developing satisfying relationships. However, labeling these activities "bad" or "good" is not useful. Rather, the nurse focuses on exploring the behavior of the client and works toward identifying the thoughts and feelings that influence this behavior. Judgmental behavior on the part of the nurse will most likely interfere with further exploration.

The first steps in eliminating judgmental thinking and behaviors are to (1) identify its presence, (2) identify how or where the nurse learned these responses to the client's behavior, and (3) reconstruct alternative ways to view the client's thinking and behavior. Just denying judgmental thinking will only compound the problem. Egan (1994, p. 53) cites the following example:

Client: I am really sexually promiscuous. I give in to sexual tendencies whenever they arise and whenever I can find a partner. This has been going on for at least 3 years.

Judgmental response:

Nurse A: Immature sex hasn't been the answer, has it? It's just another way of making yourself miserable. These days it's just asking for AIDS.

A more helpful response would be:

Nurse B: So, letting yourself go sexually is part of the picture also. You sound as if you're not happy about this.

In this example, Nurse B focuses on the client's behaviors and the possible meaning they might have to the client. Nurse B does not introduce personal value statements or prejudices regarding promiscuous behaviors as does Nurse A.

Helping Clients Develop Resources

The nurse becomes aware of clients' strengths and encourages them to work at their optimal level of functioning. The nurse does not act for clients unless absolutely necessary, and then only as a step toward helping them act on their own.

Client: This medication makes me so dry. Could you get me something to drink?

Nurse: There is juice in the refrigerator. I'll wait here for you until you get back.

or

I'll walk with you while you get some juice from the refrigerator.

Client: Could you ask the doctor to let me have a pass for the weekend?

Nurse: Your doctor will be on the unit this afternoon. I'll let her know that you want to speak with her.

Consistently encouraging clients to use their own resources helps to minimize the clients' feelings of helplessness and dependency and also validates their potential for change.

Establishing Boundaries

The nurse's role in the therapeutic relationship is rather well defined. The client's needs are separated from the nurse's needs, and the client's role is different from that of the nurse. Therefore, the boundaries of the relationship seem to be well stated. In reality, boundaries are at risk for blurring, and a shift in the nurse-client relationship may lead to nontherapeutic dynamics. Philette and associates (1995) describe two common behaviors that may occur and blur boundaries:

1. When the relationship slips into a social context
2. When the nurse's behavior reflects getting the self's needs met at the expense of the client's needs

Resultant actions by the nurse may be manifested in specific groups of behaviors (Philette et al. 1995), although these violations are mostly unwitting, subtle, and unconscious. These behaviors include

- *Overhelping:* going beyond the wishes or needs of the client.
- *Controlling:* asserting authority and assuming control of clients "for their own good."
- *Narcissism:* having to find weakness, helplessness, and/or disease in clients in order to feel helpful. This is at the expense of recognizing and supporting the client's healthier, stronger, and more competent features.

Role blurring (Philette et al. 1995) may take the form of

- What is too helpful?
- What is not helpful enough?

Table 6–1 points out certain behaviors that identify role boundary blurring when nursing behaviors reflect being "too helpful" and "not helpful enough." When situations such as these arise, the relationship has ceased to be a helpful one and the phenomenon of control becomes an issue. Role blurring is often a result of unrecognized *transference* or *countertransference.*

Transference

Transference is a phenomenon originally identified by Sigmund Freud when using psychoanalysis to treat clients. **Transference** is the process whereby a person unconsciously and inappropriately displaces (transfers) onto individuals in his or her current life those patterns of behavior and emotional reactions that originated with significant figures from childhood. Although the transference phenomenon occurs in all relationships, transference seems to be intensified in relationships of authority. Because the process of transference is accelerated toward a person in authority, physicians, nurses, and social workers are all potential objects of transference. It is important to realize that the client may experience thoughts, feelings, and reactions toward a health care worker that are realistic and appropriate; these are *not* transference phenomena.

Common forms of transference include the desire for affection or respect and the gratification of dependency needs. Other transferential feelings the client might experience are hostility, jealousy, competitiveness, and love. Requests for special favors (e.g., cigarettes, water, extra time in the session) are concrete examples of transference phenomena.

Countertransference

Countertransference refers to the tendency of the therapist to displace onto the client feelings caused by people in the therapist's past. Frequently, the client's transference to the nurse will evoke countertransference feelings in the nurse. For example, it is normal to feel angry when attacked persistently, annoyed when frustrated unreasonably, or flattered when idealized. A nurse might also feel omnipotent or very important when depended on exclusively by a client (Bonnivien 1992).

TABLE 6–1 EVIDENCE OF BLURRED BOUNDARIES

CLIENT'S AND NURSE'S BEHAVIORS THAT ARE	
Too Helpful	**Not Helpful Enough**
▸ Increased requests for assistance that cause increased dependency on the nurse ▸ Inability of the client to perform tasks of which he or she is known to be capable prior to the nurse's help, which causes regression ▸ Unwillingness on the part of the client to maintain performance or progress in the nurse's absence ▸ Expressions of anger by other staff who do not agree with the nurse's interventions or perceptions of the client ▸ The nurse keeping secrets about the nurse-patient relationship	▸ The client's increased verbal or physical expression of isolation (depression) ▸ Lack of mutually agreed goals ▸ Lack of progress toward goals ▸ Avoiding spending time with the client ▸ The nurse not following through on agreed interventions

Data from Philette, P.C., et al. (1995). Therapeutic management of helping boundaries. *Journal of Psychosocial Nursing and Mental Health Services,* 33(1):40–47.

If the nurse feels either a very strong positive or negative reaction to a client, the feeling may signal a countertransferential process in the nurse. A common sign of countertransference in the nurse is overidentification with the client. In this situation the nurse may have difficulty recognizing or understanding problems the client has that are similar to the nurse's own. For example, a nurse who is struggling with an alcoholic family member may feel disinterested, cold, or disgusted toward an alcoholic client. Other indications of countertransference occur when the nurse gets involved in power struggles, competition, or arguing with the client. Table 6–2 identifies some common reactions and gives some suggestions for self-intervention.

This identification, and working through, of various transference and countertransference issues is crucial for the nurse's professional and clinical growth and for positive change in the client. These issues are best dealt with by the use of supervision, either by a more experienced professional or by a peer. Regularly scheduled supervision sessions provide the nurse with the opportunity to increase self-awareness, clinical skills, and growth, as well as allowing for progression of growth in the client. Look at Chapter 7 for more on clinical supervision.

Understanding Self and Others

Values

More and more we are working, living, and caring for people from diverse cultures and subcultures whose life experiences and life values may be very different from our own. Refer back to Chapter 5. **Values** are abstract standards and represent an ideal, either positive or negative. For example, in the United States, to create a social order in which people can live peaceably together and feel secure in their persons and property, two of society's values are a respect for one another's liberty and working cooperatively for the common goal. Not all the nation's people live up to these ideals all the time, and there may exist for some a dichotomy between theory and practice. For example, some people may pay lip service to the values of authority or the culture, while their behavior contradicts these values. For example, they may stress honesty and respect for the law, yet cheat on their taxes and in their business practices. They may "love" their neighbors on Sunday, and demean or downgrade them for the rest of the week. They may declare themselves patriots, yet deny freedom of speech to any dissenters whose concept of patriotism is different from theirs.

A person's value system greatly influences both everyday and long-range choices. Values and beliefs provide a framework for the life goals people develop and for what they want their life to include. Our values are usually culturally oriented and influenced in a variety of ways through our parents, teachers, religious institutions, workplaces, peers, and political leaders and through Hollywood and the media. All these influences attempt to instill their values and to form and influence ours (Simon et al. 1995).

We also form our values through the example of others. *Modeling* is perhaps one of the most potent means of value education because it presents a vivid example of values in action (Simon et al. 1995). We all need role models to guide us in negotiating life's many choices. Young people in particular are hungry for role models and will find them among adults or their peers, for better or worse. As nurses, parents, bosses, co-workers, friends, lovers, teachers, spouses, singles, or whatever, we are constantly (in either a positive or negative manner) providing a role model to others.

One of the steps in the nursing process is represented by the planning outcome criteria (long- and short-range goals). We stress that the client and the nurse identify realistic and measurable goals together. What happens when the nurse's beliefs and values are very different from those of a client? For example, the client wants an abortion, which is against the nurse's values (or vice versa). The client is sexually promiscuous, and that is against the nurse's values. The client puts material gain and objects way ahead of loyalty to friends and family, in direct contrast to a nurse's values. The client's life style includes the taking of illicit drugs, and substance abuse is against the nurse's values. The client is deeply religious, and the nurse is a nonbeliever who shuns organized religion. Can a nurse develop a working relationship and help a client solve a problem when the values and the goals of the client are so different from his or her own?

As nurses, it is useful for us to understand that our values and beliefs are not necessarily "right," and certainly not right for everyone. It is helpful for us to realize that our values (1) reflect our own culture, (2) are derived from a whole range of choices, and (3) are those we have *chosen* for ourselves from a variety of influences and role models. These chosen values guide us in making decisions and taking the actions we hope will make our lives meaningful, rewarding, and full. Personal values may change over time; indeed, personal values may change many times over the course of a lifetime. Self-awareness requires that we understand what we value and those beliefs that guide our behavior. It is critical that as nurses we not only understand and accept our own values but also are sensitive to and accepting of the unique and different values of others.

Values Clarification

Values clarification is a process that helps people to understand and build their value system, addressing some questions in the process. For example, "Where do we learn whether to stick to the old moral and value standards or try new ones? How do we learn to relate to people whose values differ from our own? What do we do

TABLE 6–2 COMMON COUNTERTRANSFERENCE REACTIONS

As a nurse, you'll sometimes experience countertransference feelings. Once you're aware of them, use them for self-analysis to understand those feelings that may inhibit productive nurse-client communication.

NURSE'S REACTION TO CLIENT	CHARACTERISTIC NURSE BEHAVIOR	SELF-ANALYSIS	SOLUTION
Boredom (indifference)	▶ Inattention ▶ Frequently asking client to repeat statements ▶ Inappropriate responses	▶ Is the content of what the client presents uninteresting? Or is the style of communication? Does the client exhibit an offensive style of communication? ▶ Have you anything else on your mind that may be distracting you from the client's needs? ▶ Is the client discussing an issue that makes you anxious?	▶ Redirect client if he provides more information than you need or goes "off the track." ▶ Clarify information with client. ▶ Confront ineffective modes of communication.
Rescue	▶ Reaching for unattainable goals ▶ Resisting peer feedback and supervisory recommendations	▶ What behavior stimulates your perceived need to rescue the client? ▶ Has anyone evoked such feelings in you in the past? Who? ▶ What are your fears or fantasies about failing to meet the client's needs?	▶ Avoid secret alliances. ▶ Develop realistic goals. ▶ Do not alter meeting schedule. ▶ Let client guide interaction.
Overinvolvement	▶ Coming to work early, leaving late ▶ Ignoring peer suggestions, resisting assistance ▶ Buying the client clothes or other gifts ▶ Behaving judgmentally at family interventions ▶ Keeping secrets ▶ Calling client when off-duty	▶ What particular client characteristics are attractive? ▶ Does the client remind you of someone? Who? ▶ Does your current behavior differ from your treatment of similar clients in the past?	▶ Establish firm treatment boundaries, goals, and nursing expectations. ▶ Avoid self-disclosure. ▶ Avoid calling client when off-duty.
Overidentification	▶ Special agendas, secrets ▶ Increased self-disclosure ▶ Feelings of omnipotence ▶ Physical attraction	▶ With which of the client's physical, emotional cognitive, or situational characteristics do you identify? ▶ Recall similar circumstances in your own life. How did you deal with the issues now being created by the client?	▶ Allow client to direct issues. ▶ Encourage a problem-solving approach from client's perspective. ▶ Avoid self-disclosure.
Misuse of honesty	▶ Withholding information ▶ Lying	▶ Why are you protecting the client? ▶ What are your fears about the client's learning the truth?	▶ Be clear in your responses and aware of your hesitation; do not "hedge." ▶ If you cannot provide information, tell client and give your rationale. ▶ Avoid keeping secrets. ▶ Reinforce client about interdisciplinary nature of treatment.
Anger	▶ Withdrawal ▶ Speaking loudly ▶ Using profanity ▶ Asking to be taken off case	▶ What client behaviors are offensive to you? ▶ What dynamic from your past may this client be recreating?	▶ Determine origin of anger (nurse, client, or both). ▶ Explore roots of client anger. ▶ Avoid contact with client if anger is not understood.

Continued

TABLE 6–2 COMMON COUNTERTRANSFERENCE REACTIONS *(Continued)*

NURSE'S REACTION TO CLIENT	CHARACTERISTIC NURSE BEHAVIOR	SELF-ANALYSIS	SOLUTION
Helplessness or hopelessness	▶ Sadness	▶ Which client behaviors evoke these feelings in you? ▶ Has anyone evoked similar feelings in the past? Who? ▶ What past expectations were placed on you (verbally and nonverbally) by this person?	▶ Maintain therapeutic involvement. ▶ Explore and focus on client's experience rather than on your own.

Data from Aromando, L. (1995). *Mental health and psychiatric nursing* (2nd ed.). Springhouse, PA: Springhouse. Used with permission.

when two important values are in conflict?" (Simon et al. 1995).

A popular approach to values clarification has been formulated by Louis Raths (1966). In his framework, a value has three components: emotional, cognitive, and behavioral. We do not just hold our values, we *feel* deeply about them and will stand up for them and affirm them when appropriate. We *choose* our values from a variety of choices after weighing the pros and cons, including the consequences of these choices and positions. And, ultimately, we *act* upon our values. Our values determine how we live our lives. Values, according to Raths (1966), are composed of seven subprocesses:

PRIZING one's beliefs and behaviors (emotional):

1. Prizing and cherishing
2. Publicly affirming, when appropriate

CHOOSING one's beliefs and behaviors (cognitive):

3. Choosing from alternatives
4. Choosing after consideration of consequences
5. Choosing freely

ACTING on one's beliefs (behavioral):

6. Acting
7. Acting with a pattern, consistency, and repetition

Simon and associates (1995) have added that part of the values-clarification process should be to attend to the needs and rights of others. They suggest such questions as "What affect will this choice have on others around me? What is the ethical thing to do? If everyone followed my example, what kind of world would this become?" Box 6–1 is a values clarification exercise that you can use to identify and prioritize those things that are important to you; you might also find this useful when counseling clients. There are many values clarification exercises that can help clients, individuals, partners, friends, and groups identify important values in their lives, and compare values with others in a friendship, partnership, or group situation.

Phases of the Nurse-Client Relationship

The ability of the nurse to engage in interpersonal interactions in a goal-directed manner for the purpose of assisting clients with their emotional or physical health needs is the foundation of nursing practice (Hagerty 1984).

The nurse-client relationship is synonymous with a professional helping relationship. Behaviors that have relevance to health care workers, including nurses, are as follows:

1. *Accountability.* The nurse assumes responsibility for the conduct and consequences of the assignment and nurses' actions.
2. *Focus on client needs.* The interest of the client, not that of other health care workers or of the institution, is given first consideration. The nurse's role is that of client advocate.
3. *Clinical competence.* The criteria on which the nurse bases his or her conduct are principles of knowledge and appropriateness to the specific situation. This involves awareness and incorporation of the latest knowledge made available from research.
4. *Supervision.* Validation of performance quality is through regularly scheduled supervisory sessions. Supervision is conducted either by a more experienced clinician or through discussion with the nurse's peers in professionally conducted supervisory sessions. (Refer to Chapter 7.)

Nurses interact with clients in a variety of settings, such as emergency rooms, medical-surgical units, maternity and pediatric units, clinics, community settings, schools, and clients' homes. Nurses who are sensitive to the client's needs and have effective assessment and communication skills can significantly help the client confront current problems and anticipate future choices.

Sometimes, the type of relationship that occurs may be informal and not extensive, such as when the nurse and client meet for only a few sessions. However, even

BOX 6–1 VALUES CLARIFICATION

YOUR VALUES ARE YOUR IDEAS ABOUT WHAT IS MOST IMPORTANT TO YOU IN YOUR LIFE—WHAT YOU WANT TO LIVE BY AND LIVE FOR. THEY ARE THE SILENT FORCES BEHIND MANY OF YOUR ACTIONS AND DECISIONS. THE GOAL OF "VALUES CLARIFICATION" IS FOR THEIR INFLUENCE TO BECOME FULLY CONSCIOUS, FOR YOU TO EXPLORE AND HONESTLY ACKNOWLEDGE WHAT YOU TRULY VALUE AT THIS TIME IN YOUR LIFE. YOU CAN BE MORE SELF-DIRECTED AND EFFECTIVE WHEN YOU KNOW WHICH VALUES YOU REALLY CHOOSE TO KEEP AND LIVE BY AS AN ADULT, AND WHICH ONES WILL GET PRIORITY OVER OTHERS. IDENTIFY YOUR VALUES FIRST, AND THEN RANK YOUR TOP THREE OR FIVE.

- ☐ Being with people
- ☐ Being loved
- ☐ Being married
- ☐ Having a special partner
- ☐ Having companionship
- ☐ Loving someone
- ☐ Taking care of others
- ☐ Having someone's help
- ☐ Having a close family
- ☐ Having good friends
- ☐ Being liked
- ☐ Being popular
- ☐ Getting someone's approval
- ☐ Being appreciated
- ☐ Being treated fairly
- ☐ Being admired
- ☐ Being independent
- ☐ Being courageous
- ☐ Having things in control
- ☐ Having self-control
- ☐ Being emotionally stable
- ☐ Having self-acceptance
- ☐ Having pride or dignity
- ☐ Being well organized
- ☐ Being competent
- ☐ Learning and knowing a lot
- ☐ Achieving highly
- ☐ Being productively busy
- ☐ Having enjoyable work
- ☐ Having an important position
- ☐ Making money
- ☐ Striving for perfection
- ☐ Making a contribution to the world
- ☐ Fighting injustice
- ☐ Living ethically
- ☐ Being a good parent (or child)
- ☐ Being a spiritual person
- ☐ Having a relationship with God
- ☐ Having peace and quiet
- ☐ Making a home
- ☐ Preserving your roots
- ☐ Having financial security
- ☐ Holding on to what you have
- ☐ Being safe physically
- ☐ Being free from pain
- ☐ Not getting taken advantage of
- ☐ Having it easy
- ☐ Being comfortable
- ☐ Avoiding boredom
- ☐ Having fun
- ☐ Enjoying sensual pleasures
- ☐ Looking good
- ☐ Being physically fit
- ☐ Being healthy
- ☐ Having prized possessions
- ☐ Being a creative person
- ☐ Having deep feelings
- ☐ Growing as a person
- ☐ Living fully
- ☐ "Smelling the flowers"
- ☐ Having a purpose

From Bernard, M.E., and Wolfe, J.L. (Eds.) (1993). *The RET resource book for practitioners.* New York: Institute for Rational-Emotive Therapy.

though it is brief, the relationship may be substantial, useful, and important for the client. This limited relationship is often referred to as a **therapeutic encounter.**

At other times, the encounters may be of longer duration and more formal, such as in inpatient settings, mental health units, crisis centers, and mental health centers. This longer time span allows the development of a therapeutic nurse-client relationship, which is the medium through which the nursing process is implemented (Hagerty 1984).

Three distinctive phases of the nurse-client relationship are generally recognized: (1) the orientation phase, (2) the working phase, and (3) the termination phase. Although various phenomena and goals are identified for each phase, they often overlap from phase to phase. However, even beforehand, the nurse may have many thoughts and feelings related to the first clinical session. This is sometimes referred to as the preorientation phase.

Preorientation Phase

Beginning health care professionals who are new to the psychiatric setting usually have many concerns and experience a mild to moderate degree of anxiety on their first clinical day. One common concern involves fear of physical harm or violence. Your instructor will discuss this common concern in your first pre-conference. There are unit protocols for intervening with clients who have poor impulse control, and staff and unit safeguards should be constantly in place to help clients gain self-control. Although such disruptions are not common, the concern is valid. Most unit staff are trained and practice interventions for clients who are having difficulty with impulse control. Hospital security is readily available to give the staff support. Chapter 12 describes communicating with angry and aggressive clients.

Some of you may be concerned with "saying the wrong thing," using the client as a guinea pig, feeling inadequate about new and developing communication skills, feeling vulnerable without the uniform as a clear indicator of who is the nurse and who is the client, and feeling vulnerable as you relate to your own earlier personal experiences or crises. These are universal and valid feelings; if they were not discussed in class, they will be brought up on the first clinical day, either by you or by your instructor. Chapter 7 deals with a variety of clinical concerns student nurses have when beginning their psychiatric nursing rotation (e.g., what to do if clients do not want to talk, if they ask the nurse to keep a secret, if they cry). Usually after the first clinical day your anxiety will be much lower and you will focus on clinical issues more easily with the support of your instructor and classmates.

Orientation Phase

The **orientation phase** can last for a few meetings or can extend over a longer period. This first phase may be prolonged in the case of severely and persistently ill mental health clients. Forchuk's study (1992) found that lengthy hospitalization patterns were related to a lengthy orientation phase. In this study the length of the orientation phase ranged from 1 to 23 months.

The first time the nurse and the client meet, they are strangers to each other. When strangers meet, whether or not they know anything about each other, they interact according to their own backgrounds, standards, values, and experiences. This fact—that each person has a unique frame of reference—underlies the need for self-awareness on the part of the nurse.

As the relationship evolves through an ongoing series of reactions, each participant may elicit in the other a wide range of positive and negative emotional reactions (Bonnivien 1992). Remember that the stirring up of feelings in the client by the nurse is referred to as *transference*, and the stirring up of feelings in the nurse or therapist by the client is referred to as *countertransference*. As we discussed earlier, the nurse is responsible for identifying these two phenomena and maintaining appropriate boundaries.

ESTABLISHING TRUST. A major emphasis during the first few encounters with the client is upon providing an atmosphere in which trust can grow. As in any relationship, trust is nurtured by demonstrating genuineness (congruence) and empathy, developing positive regard, showing consistency, and offering assistance in alleviating the client's emotional pain or problems. This may take only a short time, but in many instances it may take a long time before a client feels free to discuss painful personal experiences and private thoughts.

During the orientation phase, four important issues need to be addressed:

1. The parameters of the relationship
2. The formal or informal contract
3. Confidentiality
4. Termination.

The Parameters of the Relationship. The client needs to know about the nurse (who the nurse is and what his or her background is) and the purpose of the meetings. For example, a student might furnish the following information:

Student: Hello, Mrs. James. I am Nancy Rivera from Orange Community College. I am in my psychiatric rotation, and I will be coming to York Hospital for the next six Thursdays. I would like to spend time with you each Thursday if you are still here. I'm here to be a support person for you as you work on your treatment goals.

The Formal or Informal Contract. A contract emphasizes the client's participation and responsibility because it shows that the nurse does something *with* the client rather than *for* the client (Collins 1983). The **contract**, either stated or written, contains the place, time, date, and duration of the meetings. During the orientation phase, the client may begin to express thoughts and feelings, identify problems, and discuss realistic goals. Therefore, the mutual agreement on goals is also part of the contract. If the goals are met, the client's level of functioning will return to a previous level, or at least improve from the present level. If fees are to be paid, the client is told how much they will be and when the payment is due.

Student: Mrs. James, we will meet at 10 AM each Thursday in the consultation room at the clinic for 45 minutes, from September 15th to October 27th. We can use that time for further discussion of your feelings of loneliness and anger with your husband and to explore some things you could do to make things better for yourself.

Confidentiality. The client has a right to know who else will know about the information being shared with the nurse. He or she needs to know that the information may be shared with specific people, such as a clinical supervisor, the physician, the staff, or other students in conference. The client also needs to know that the information will *not* be shared with his or her relatives, friends, or others outside the treatment team, except in extreme situations. Extreme situations include (1) information that may be harmful to the client or others, (2) when the client threatens self-harm, and (3) when the client does not intend to follow through with the treatment plan. If information must be given to others, this is usually done by the physician, according to legal guidelines (refer to Chapter 4). The nurse must be aware of the client's right to **confidentiality** and must not violate that right.

Student: Mrs. James, I will be sharing some of what we discuss with my nursing instructor, and at times I may discuss certain concerns with my peers in conference or with the staff. However, I will *not* be sharing this information with your husband or any other members of your family without your permission.

Termination. Termination begins in the orientation phase. It may also be mentioned when appropriate during the working phase if the nature of the relationship is time limited (e.g., six or ten sessions). The date of the termination phase should be clear from the beginning. In some situations the nurse-client contract may be renegotiated when the termination date has been reached. In other situations, when the therapeutic nurse-client relationship is an open-ended one, the termination date is not known.

Student: Mrs. James, as I mentioned earlier, our last meeting will be on October 27th. We will have three more meetings after today.

During the orientation phase and later, clients often unconsciously employ "testing behaviors" that may be used to test the nurse. The client wants to know if the nurse will

- Be able to set limits when the client needs them.
- Still show concern if the client acts angry, babyish, unlikable, or dependent.
- Still be there if the client is late, leaves early, refuses to speak, or is angry.

Table 6–3 identifies some testing behaviors and possible responses by nurses.

In summary, the initial interview includes the following:

1. The nurse's role is clarified and the responsibilities of both the client and the nurse are defined.
2. The contract containing the time, place, date, and duration of the meetings is discussed.
3. Confidentiality is discussed and assumed.
4. The terms of termination are introduced.

Throughout the orientation phase and beyond:

5. The nurse becomes aware of transference and countertransference issues and discusses them in conference/supervision.
6. An atmosphere where trust can grow is established.
7. Articulation of client problems and mutually agreed goals are established.

Working Phase

Moore and Hartman (1988) identify specific tasks of the **working phase** of the nurse-client relationship:

1. Maintain the relationship.
2. Gather further data.
3. Promote the client's problem-solving skills, self-esteem, and use of language.
4. Facilitate behavioral change.
5. Overcome resistance behaviors.
6. Evaluate problems and goals and redefine them as necessary.
7. Practice and express alternative adaptive behaviors.

During the working phase, the nurse and client together identify and explore areas in the client's life that are causing problems. Often, the client's present ways of handling situations stem from earlier ways of coping devised in order to survive in a chaotic and dysfunctional family environment. Although certain coping methods may have worked for the client at an earlier age, they now interfere with the client's interpersonal relationships and prevent him or her from attaining current goals. The client's dysfunctional behaviors and basic assumptions about the world are often defensive in nature and the client is usually unable to change the dysfunctional behavior at will. Therefore, most of the problem behaviors or thoughts continue because of unconscious motivations and needs that are out of the client's awareness.

The nurse can work with the client to identify these unconscious motivations and assumptions that keep the client from finding satisfaction and reaching potential. Describing, and often reexperiencing, old conflicts generally awakens high levels of anxiety in the client. Clients may use various defenses against anxiety and displace their feelings onto the nurse. Therefore, during the working phase, intense emotions such as anxiety, anger, self-hate, hopelessness, and helplessness may surface. Behaviors such as acting out anger inappropriately, withdrawing, intellectualizing, manipulating, and denying are to be expected.

During the working phase, strong transferential feelings may appear. The emotional responses and behaviors in the client may also awaken strong countertransferential feelings in the nurse. *The nurse's awareness of personal feelings and reactions to the client is vital for effective interaction with the client.* Common transferential feelings, the reactions that nurses experience in response to different behaviors and situations, are discussed in the planning component of each of the clinical chapters.

The development of a strong working relationship can allow the client to experience increased levels of anxiety and demonstrate dysfunctional behaviors in a safe setting, and to try out new and more adaptive coping behaviors.

Termination Phase

Termination is discussed during the first interview. During the working stage, the fact of eventual termination may also be raised at appropriate times. Reasons for terminating the nurse-client relationship include

1. Symptom relief
2. Improved social functioning
3. Greater sense of identity
4. More adaptive behaviors in place
5. Accomplishment of the client's goals
6. An impasse in therapy that the nurse is unable to resolve

In addition, forced termination may occur, such as when the student completes the course objectives or a nurse leaves the hospital or clinical setting and there is a change of staff. Forchuk (1992) points out that, for the long-term mentally ill client, sudden termination with

TABLE 6–3 TESTING BEHAVIORS USED BY CLIENTS

CLIENT BEHAVIOR	CLIENT EXAMPLE	NURSE RESPONSE	RATIONALE
Shifts focus of interview *to* the nurse, *off* the client.	"Do you have any children?" or "Are you married?"	"This time is for you." If appropriate, the nurse should add: 1. "Do you have any children?" or "What about your children?" 2. "Are you married?" or "What about your relationships?"	The nurse refocuses back to the client and client's concerns. The nurse sticks to the contract.
Tries to get the nurse to take care of him or her.	"Could you tell my doctor"	"I'll leave a message with the ward clerk that you want to see him" or "You know best what you want him to know. I'll be interested in what he has to say."	1. The nurse validates that the client is able to do many things for him- or herself. This aids in increasing self-esteem.
	"Should I take this job"	"What do you see as the pros and cons of this job?"	2. The nurse always encourages the person to function at the highest level, even if he or she doesn't want to.
Makes sexual advances toward the nurse, e.g., touching the nurse's arm, wanting to hold hands or kiss nurse.	"Would you go out with me? . . . Why not?" or "Can I kiss you? . . . Why not?"	"I am not comfortable having you touch (kiss) me." The nurse briefly reiterates the nurse's role: "This time is for you to focus on your problems and concerns." If the client stops: "I wonder what this is all about?" 1. Is the client afraid the nurse won't like him or her? 2. Is the client trying to take the focus off problems? If the client continues: "If you can't cease this behavior, I'll have to leave. I'll be back at (time) to spend time with you then."	1. The nurse needs to set clear limits on expected behavior. 2. Frequently restating the nurse's role throughout the relationship can help maintain boundaries. 3. Whenever possible, the meaning of the client's behavior should be explored. 4. Leaving gives the client time to gain control. The nurse returns at the stated time.
Continues to arrive late for meetings.	"I'm a little late because (excuse)."	The nurse arrives on time and leaves at the scheduled time. (The nurse does not let the client manipulate him or her or bargain for more time.) After a couple of times, the nurse can explore behavior, e.g.: "I wonder if there is something going on you don't want to deal with?" or "I wonder what these latenesses mean to you?"	1. The nurse keeps the contract. Clients feel more secure when "promises" are kept, even though clients may try to manipulate the nurse through anger, helplessness, and so forth. 2. The nurse doesn't tell the client what to do, but nurse and client need to explore what the behavior is all about.

the nurse the client has been working with may trigger a return to the orientation phase with a new nurse or counselor. The **termination phase** is the final phase of the nurse-client relationship. Important reasons for the student/nurse counselor to address the termination phase are as follows:

1. Termination is an integral phase of the therapeutic nurse-client relationship, and without it the relationship remains incomplete.
2. Feelings are aroused in both the client and the nurse with regard to the experience they have had; when these feelings are recognized and shared, clients learn

that it is acceptable to feel sadness and loss when someone they care about leaves.
3. The client is a partner in the relationship and has a right to see the nurse's needs and feelings about their time together and the ensuing separation.
4. Termination can be a learning experience; clients can learn that they are important to at least one person.
5. By sharing the termination experience with the client, the nurse demonstrates caring for the client.
6. This may be the first successful termination experience for the client.

Termination often awakens strong feelings in both nurse and client. Termination of the relationship between the nurse and the client signifies a loss for both, although the intensity and meaning of termination may be different for each. If a client has unresolved feelings of abandonment or loneliness, or feelings of not being wanted or of being rejected by others, they may be reawakened during the termination process. This process can be an opportunity for the client to express these feelings, perhaps for the first time.

It is not unusual to see a variety of client behaviors that indicate defensive maneuvers against the anxiety of separation and loss. For example, a client may withdraw from the nurse and not want to meet for the final session or may become outwardly hostile and sarcastic—for instance, accusing the student of using the client for personal gains ("like a guinea pig") as a way of deflecting the awakening of anger and pain that is rooted in past separations. Often, a client will deny that the relationship had any impact or deny that ending the relationship evokes any emotions whatsoever. Regression is another behavioral manifestation; it may be seen in increased dependency on the nurse or a return of earlier symptoms.

It is important for the nurse to work with the client to bring into awareness any feelings and reactions the client may be experiencing related to separations. If a client denies that the termination is having an effect (assuming the nurse-client relationship was strong), the nurse may say something like "Goodbyes are difficult for people. Often they remind us of other goodbyes. Tell me about another separation in the past." If the client appears to be displacing anger, either by withdrawing or by being overtly angry at the nurse, the nurse may use generalized statements such as "People may experience anger when saying goodbye. Sometimes they are angry with the person who is leaving. Tell me how you feel about me leaving." New practitioners and students new to the psychiatric setting need to give thought to their last clinical experience with their client and to work with their supervisor or instructor to facilitate communication during this time.

Summarizing the goals and objectives achieved in the relationship is part of the termination process. Reviewing situations that occurred during the time spent together and exchanging memories can help validate the experience for both nurse and client and facilitate closure of that relationship.

A common response of beginning practitioners is feeling guilty about terminating the relationship. These feelings may be manifested in students' giving the client their telephone number, making plans to get together for coffee after the client is discharged, continuing to see the client afterward, or exchanging letters. Beginning practitioners need to understand that such actions may be motivated by their own sense of guilt or by misplaced feelings of responsibility, not by concern for the client. Indeed, part of the termination process may be to explore, after discussion with the client's case manager, the client's plans for the future: where to go for help in the future, which agencies to contact, and which specific resource persons may be available.

During the student affiliation, the nurse-client relationship exists for the duration of the clinical course only. The termination phase is just that. Thoughts and feelings the student may have about continuing the relationship are best discussed with the instructor or shared in conference with peers, because these are common reactions to the student's experience.

PSYCHIATRIC MENTAL HEALTH NURSING THROUGH THE NURSING PROCESS

The nursing process continues to be the basic framework for nursing practice and has been used as a basis for the following:

1. Criteria for certification
2. Legal definition of nursing, as reflected in many states' nurse practice acts
3. The National Council of State Boards of Nursing licensure examination (NCLEX-RN) format

The nurse uses the nursing process when evaluating the client at any point on the health-illness continuum. A client may be an individual, a family, a group, or a community. Assessment is made on many levels: physical, social, emotional, intellectual, spiritual, and cultural. Psychiatric and mental health nursing practice bases nursing judgments and behaviors on an accepted theoretical framework. The importance of a theoretical framework has been supported by the Standards of Psychiatric and Mental Health Nursing, developed by the ANA (1994 revised) (see inside front cover). Figure 6–1 depicts psychiatric mental health nursing through the nursing process.

Assessment

Although high levels of anxiety and maladaptive behaviors are commonly seen by psychiatric nursing practitioners, these phenomena are encountered in all areas in the health care setting. Depression, suicidal thoughts,

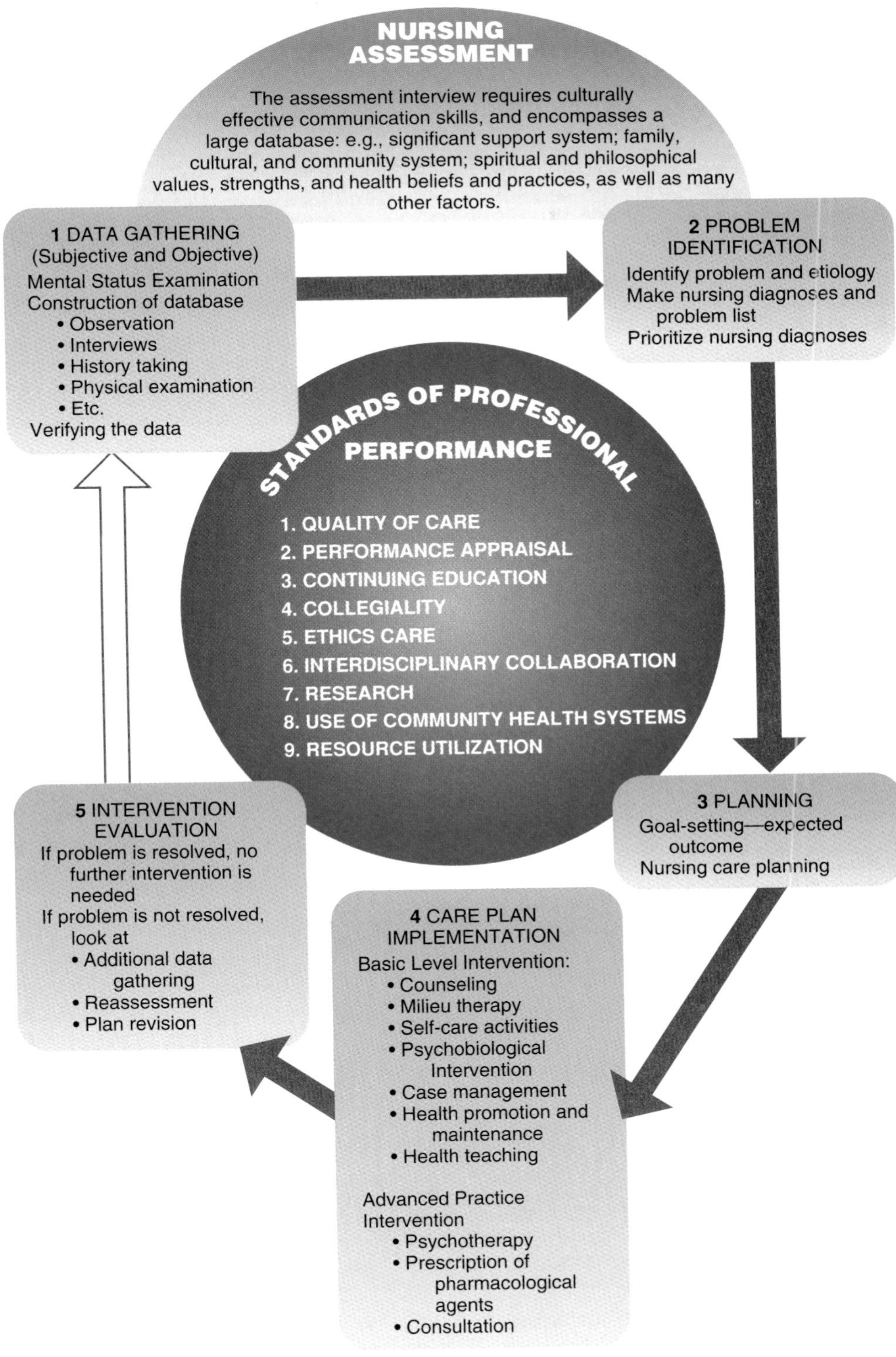

Figure 6–1 The nursing process in psychiatric mental health nursing.

anger, disorientation, delusions, and hallucinations may be encountered in medical-surgical wards, obstetrical and intensive care units, outpatient settings, extended care facilities, emergency departments, clinics, and pediatric settings. The **assessment** of the client's psychosocial status is a part of any nursing assessment, along with assessment of the client's physical health.

The nursing process is a cyclical one. Assessment is ongoing and continues throughout the planning, intervention, and evaluation phases. The initial assessment often clarifies the client's immediate needs. As the nurse works further with the client, the database is enlarged and other problems may become evident.

Psychiatric nursing assessment is done within the

framework of the psychiatric interview. The assessment interview or intake interview is often conducted in the psychiatric inpatient setting, but it may take place in many other settings such as emergency rooms, medical-surgical units, intensive care units, crisis units, community mental health centers, private practice, homes, and schools. The time given for the interview varies, depending on the clinical setting and the circumstances of the client. During emergencies, immediate intervention is often based on a minimal amount of data. A scheduled psychiatric interview and psychosocial assessment in a structured setting allows more time for an elaborate assessment. At times, completing the assessment process may involve many interviews.

The purpose of the psychiatric assessment (Hagerty 1984) is to

- Assess a person's current level of psychological functioning.
- Establish a trusting rapport.
- Understand how previous modes of coping contributed to the person's psychosocial development.
- Formulate a plan of care.

Although the nurse may obtain a lot of needed data from the physician's assessment, the nurse's primary source for data collection is the client; however, there may be times when the client is unable to assist with the assessment. For example, if the client is severely delusional, mute, comatose, or extremely confused, secondary sources should be used. Such sources include members of the family, friends, neighbors, police, other members of the health team, medical records, and laboratory results. Both primary and secondary sources need to be used during assessment.

Process of the Psychiatric Nursing Assessment

If the nursing process is the framework for nursing practice, *the therapeutic relationship is the medium through which the nursing process is implemented.* Although the client is the focus, the nurse and the client work together to reduce anxiety, relieve pain, satisfy unmet needs, and promote optimal functioning. Assisting a person toward optimal functioning is accomplished through three levels of nursing intervention:

- Preventive (primary intervention)
- Restorative (secondary intervention)
- Rehabilitative (tertiary intervention)

Underlying these three levels of nursing intervention are certain premises (Bower 1982):

- Individuals have the right to decide their destiny and to be involved in decisions that affect them.
- Nursing intervention is designed to assist individuals to meet their own needs or to solve their own problems.
- The ultimate goal of all nursing action is to assist individuals to maximize their independent level of functioning.

The development of the therapeutic relationship is a crucial factor in the implementation of the nursing process.

When assessment occurs during the initial interview, the nurse and the client are essentially strangers. Both experience anxiety, as in any other meeting between strangers. The interviewer's anxiety may stem from the client's perception of the interviewer's ability (or inability) to help the client. If the interviewer is a nursing student, anxiety regarding the instructor's evaluation becomes an added dimension. Clients' anxiety centers on their problems, the nurse's view of them, and what is ahead for them in treatment.

Both client and nurse bring to their relationship their total background experiences. These experiences include cultural beliefs and biases, religious attitudes, educational background, and occupational and life experiences, as well as attitudes regarding sexual roles. These attitudes, beliefs, and values influence the nurse's interactions with clients. As emphasized earlier in this chapter, it is important for nurses, through examining their personal beliefs and clarifying their values, to be aware of their biases and values and not feel compelled to impose their personal beliefs on others. Look again at Chapter 5 to review how clients from various cultural backgrounds and with differing belief systems experience their roles and hold their views of mental health and illness. Although the nurse shares perceptions and alternatives with the client, the goal is to work with the client so that decisions and actions taken are the right ones for the client. Theoretically, this sounds easy, but often it is not. When beginning practitioners share their perceptions and thoughts with a more experienced nurse, unrecognized biases and value judgments often become evident. Countertransference issues may also play a role in the beginning practitioner's perceptions. *Experience and supervision help a nurse separate what is important to the client from any bias that might impede mutually agreed goals.*

Although the purpose of the psychiatric assessment is to gather data that will help clarify the client's situation and problem, this is best done in an atmosphere of minimal anxiety. Therefore, if an individual becomes upset, defensive, or embarrassed regarding any topic, the topic should be abandoned. The nurse can acknowledge that this is a subject that makes the client uncomfortable and can suggest that it would best be discussed when the client feels more comfortable. It is important that the nurse not probe, pry, or push for information that is difficult for the client to discuss. However, recognize that increased anxiety about any subject is "data" in itself. The nurse can note this in the assessment without obtaining any further information. The purpose of an assessment is to gather data pertaining to the client's problem, *not* to collect a lot of data.

Content of the Psychiatric Nursing Assessment

The actual assessment consists of (1) gathering and (2) verifying the data.

GATHERING DATA. The use of a standardized nursing assessment tool facilitates the assessment process. Many assessment forms are available. Most health care systems and schools of nursing have their own assessment tool; however, even though an assessment tool is used, it is best to gather information from the client in an informal fashion, with the nurse clarifying, focusing, and exploring pertinent data with the client. This method allows clients to state their perceptions in their own words and enables the nurse to observe a wide range of nonverbal behaviors. When the order and the questions on the assessment tool are too rigidly applied, spontaneity is reduced. Assessment is a skill that is learned over a period of time. The development of this skill is enhanced by practice, supervision, and patience. A personal style of interviewing congruent with the nurse's personality develops as comfort and experience increase.

The basic components of the psychiatric nursing assessment include the client's history and mental and emotional status. Box 6–2 is an example of a basic mental status examination. Appendix D contains a complete assessment tool with three defining tables. The sheets are perforated and can be torn out, copied, and used in the clinical area. Sometimes it is not possible to complete a full mental status examination. Folstein's Mini Mental State Examination (MMSE) is a good tool for evaluating cognitive states (Box 6–3).

The client's history is most often the *subjective* part of the assessment. The focus of the history is the client's perceptions and recollections in three broad areas: presenting problem, current life style, and life in general (family, friends, education, work experience). See Appendix D.

The mental and emotional status is the *objective* part of the assessment. The nurse observes the person's physical behavior and nonverbal communication, appearance, speech patterns, thought content, and cognitive ability. Objective data are measurable.

The assessment covers the social, physical, emotional, cultural, cognitive, and spiritual aspects of an individual. It elicits information about the systems in which a person operates. To conduct such an assessment, the nurse should have fundamental knowledge of growth and development and of basic cultural and religious practices, as well as pathophysiology, psychopathology, and pharmacology.

After the nurse has concluded the assessment, it is use-

BOX 6–2 MENTAL STATUS EXAMINATION/BASIC

1. Behavior and general appearance
   a. Dress (overly neat, sloppy, bizarre . . .)
   b. Posture
   c. Gait
   d. Motor activity level (e.g., retarded)
   e. Attitude (cooperative, hostile . . .)
   f. Behavioral mannerism (tics, pacing . . .)
   g. Speech (monotonous, pressured, unusual aspects, aphasia, stuttering, slurring, relevance, pitch, level . . .)
2. Affect and emotional state
   a. As reported by client
   b. As client appears to interviewer
   c. Duration, intensity, appropriateness, anxieties, swings . . .)
   d. How emotionalism is handled
3. Sensorium
   a. Attention and alertness (understanding, responsiveness . . .)
   b. Orientation
      (1) Time
      (2) Place
      (3) Identity
   c. Memory
      (1) Recent: President's name, address, experience last few days
      (2) Remote: Date of marriage, children's birthdays, where grew up
4. Intelligence, insight, and general information
   a. General fund of information
   b. Insight
      (1) Awareness of illness
      (2) Ability to report etiological, supporting, and personal factors involved in development and continuance of illness
5. Cognitions and cognitive processes
   a. Speed
   b. Associative abilities (neologisms, word salad . . .)
   c. Organization
   d. Content
      (1) Disturbances: perceptual (hallucinations, illusions . . .) and thought (referential ideas, delusions . . .)
      (2) Productivity
      (3) Concerns (physical, environmental, obsessions, compulsions, antisocial, sexual . . .)
   e. Abstract thinking
   f. Judgment
      (1) Social convention
      (2) Planning, problem-solving abilities
6. Summary of findings
7. Diagnostic and prognostic impressions
8. Management and treatment recommendations

BOX 6–3 FOLSTEIN'S MINI MENTAL STATE EXAMINATION (MMSE)

Patient's Name: ______________________ Social Sec. #: ______________________

Examiner's Name: ______________________ Date Administered: ______________________

Assess the patient's level of consciousness along this continuum

Alert Drowsy Stupor Coma

Maximum Score	**Patient Score (Score one point for each correct response)**		
		Orientation	
5	________	What is the (year) (season) (date) (day) (month)?	
5	________	Where are we (state) (county) (town) (hospital) (floor)?	
		Registration	
3	________	Remember these three words: cup pencil airplane Ask the patient to say all three. If the patient fails to say one or more of the words, repeat all three again up to a maximum of six repetitions. Number of repetitions ________	
		Attention and Calculation	
5	________	I want you to count backwards from 100 by sevens. Stop after five subtractions (93, 86, 79, 72, 65). Score one point for each correctly placed number. **If the patient refuses or will not attempt serial sevens,** ask the patient to spell the word "WORLD" backwards (D-L-R-O-W).	
		Recall	
3	________	Please tell me the three words I gave you earlier.	
		Language	
2	________	*Naming*	Point to a pencil and a watch. Have the patient name them as you point.
1	________	*Repetition*	Ask the patient to repeat the following: "No ifs ands or buts"
3	________	*Three-Stage Command*	Place a piece of paper in front of the patient and say: (1) "Take the paper in your right hand, (2) fold it in half, (3) and put it on the table."
1	________	*Reading*	Write the following in large letters.

"CLOSE YOUR EYES"

			Ask the patient to read and obey the command.
1	________	*Writing*	Ask the patient to write a sentence. Score one point if the sentence has a subject, an object, and a verb.
1	________	*Copying*	Ask the patient to copy the intersecting five-angle designs and give one point if all sides and angles are preserved and if the intersecting sides form a quadrangle.

Continued

BOX 6–3 FOLSTEIN'S MINI MENTAL STATE EXAMINATION (MMSE) *(Continued)*

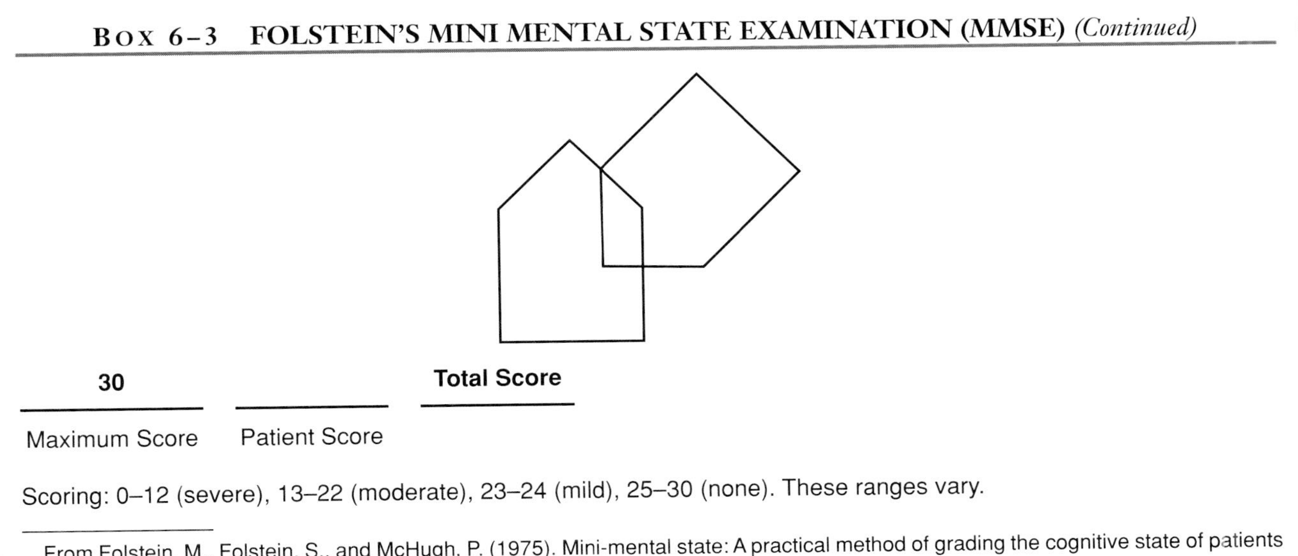

30		**Total Score**
Maximum Score	Patient Score	

Scoring: 0–12 (severe), 13–22 (moderate), 23–24 (mild), 25–30 (none). These ranges vary.

From Folstein, M., Folstein, S., and McHugh, P. (1975). Mini-mental state: A practical method of grading the cognitive state of patients for the clinician. *Journal of Psychiatric Research,* 12:189.

ful to summarize pertinent data with the client. This summary provides clients with reassurance that they have been heard and it allows them the opportunity to clarify any misinformation. They should be told what will happen next. For example, if the initial assessment takes place in the hospital, the nurse should tell the client who else the client will be seeing. If the initial assessment was conducted by a psychiatric nurse in a mental health clinic, the nurse will let the client know when and how often they will meet to work on the client's problems. If the nurse feels a referral is necessary (e.g., to a psychiatrist, social worker, or physician), he or she will discuss this with the client.

VERIFYING DATA. It is necessary that the nurse validate data obtained from the client with secondary sources. Whenever possible, family members should be a part of the assessment. Is there anything going on in the family that is affecting the family? How does the family define the problem? How do the client's problems affect the family?

Family, friends, and neighbors may verify or contradict the client's self-perception and actions or may add information.

Often, police officers are the ones who bring clients into the psychiatric emergency rooms. It is important for the nurse to know as much as possible about what the client was doing that warranted police intervention.

Other members of the health team are important sources of information and data verification. Many members of the health team will have contact with the client on admission to the hospital. The psychiatrist or psychologist, social worker, psychiatric nurse, recreation therapist, therapy aides, and student nurses can add to the nurse's database.

Old charts and medical records can help validate information the nurse already has or add new information. In some communities, client records may have been computerized. Medical history can aid in assessing physical losses and stress and can alert the staff to potential medical problems. If the client has been admitted to a psychiatric unit in the past, information about the client's previous level of functioning and behavior gives the nurse a baseline for making clinical judgments.

Laboratory reports can provide useful information. When the body's chemistry is abnormal, personality changes and violent behaviors can result. For example, abnormal liver enzymes can explain irritability, depression, and lethargy. People who have chronic renal disease often suffer from the same symptoms when their blood urea nitrogen and electrolyte levels are abnormal. People with endocrine diseases such as diabetes can have changes in mood and level of consciousness related to sugar and insulin levels. A toxicology screen for the presence of either prescription or illegal drugs may also provide useful information.

Nursing Diagnosis

Nursing diagnoses provide the basis for selection of nursing interventions to achieve outcomes for which the nurse is responsible (Box 6–4) (Gordon 1997).

Because nurses are increasingly faced with caring for culturally diverse populations, there is increasing need for nursing diagnoses and subsequent care to be planned around unique cultural health care beliefs, values, and practices. Awareness of individual cultural beliefs and health care practices can help nurses minimize "labeling" of clients (see Chapter 5).

BOX 6-4 NURSING DIAGNOSTIC CATEGORIES

BOLDFACE TYPE INDICATES DIAGNOSES CURRENTLY ACCEPTED BY THE NORTH AMERICAN NURSING DIAGNOSIS ASSOCIATION (NANDA). OTHERS ARE EITHER DIAGNOSES RECEIVED BY NANDA FOR DEVELOPMENT OR NOT ACCEPTED BY NANDA, BUT ARE FOUND USEFUL IN CLINICAL PRACTICE.

HEALTH PERCEPTION–HEALTH MANAGEMENT

Health-Seeking Behaviors (Specify)
Altered Health Maintenance (Specify)
Ineffective Management of Therapeutic Regimen (Specify Area)
Risk for Ineffective Management of Therapeutic Regimen (Specify Area)
Effective Management of Therapeutic Regimen
Ineffective Family Management of Therapeutic Regimen
Ineffective Community Management of Therapeutic Regimen
Health-Management Deficit (Specify Area)
Risk for Health-Management Deficit (Specify Area)
Noncompliance (Specify Area)
Risk for Noncompliance (Specify Area)
Risk for Infection (Specify Type/Area)
Risk for Injury (Trauma)
Risk for Perioperative Positioning Injury
Risk for Poisoning
Risk for Suffocation
Altered Protection (Specify)
Energy Field Disturbance

NUTRITIONAL-METABOLIC PATTERN

Altered Nutrition: More Than Body Requirements or Exogenous Obesity
Altered Nutrition: More Than Body Requirements or Risk for Obesity
Altered Nutrition: Less Than Body Requirements or Nutritional Deficit (Specify Type)
Ineffective Breastfeeding
Interrupted Breastfeeding
Effective Breastfeeding
Ineffective Infant Feeding Program
Impaired Swallowing (Uncompensated)
Risk for Aspiration
Altered Oral Mucous Membrane (Specify Alteration)
Fluid Volume Deficit
Risk for Fluid Volume Deficit
Fluid Volume Excess
Risk for Impaired Skin Integrity or Risk for Skin Breakdown
Impaired Skin Integrity
Pressure Ulcer (Specify Stage)
Impaired Tissue Integrity (Specify Type)
Risk for Altered Body Temperature
Ineffective Thermoregulation
Hyperthermia
Hypothermia

ELIMINATION PATTERN

Colonic Constipation
Perceived Constipation
Intermittent Constipation Pattern
Diarrhea
Bowel Incontinence
Altered Urinary Elimination Pattern
Functional Incontinence
Reflex Incontinence
Stress Incontinence
Urge Incontinence
Total Incontinence
Urinary Retention

ACTIVITY EXERCISE PATTERN

Activity Intolerance (Specify Level)
Risk for Activity Intolerance
Fatigue
Impaired Physical Mobility (Specify Level)
Impaired Bed Mobility
Transfer Deficit
Impaired Locomotion
Impaired Ambulation
Risk for Disuse Syndrome
Risk for Joint Contractures
Total Self-Care Deficit (Specify Level)
Self-Bathing–Hygiene Deficit (Specify Level)
Self-Dressing–Grooming Deficit (Specify Level)
Self-Toileting Deficit (Specify Level)
Altered Growth and Development: Self-Care Skills (Specify Level)
Diversional Activity Deficit
Impaired Home Maintenance Management (Mild, Moderate, Severe, Potential, Chronic)
Dysfunctional Ventilatory Weaning Response (DVWR)
Inability to Sustain Spontaneous Ventilation
Ineffective Airway Clearance
Ineffective Breathing Pattern
Impaired Gas Exchange
Decreased Cardiac Output
Altered Tissue Perfusion (Specify)
Dysreflexia
Disorganized Infant Behavior
Risk for Disorganized Infant Behavior
Potential for Enhanced Organized Infant Behavior
Risk for Peripheral Neurovascular Dysfunction
Altered Growth and Development

Continued

BOX 6–4 NURSING DIAGNOSTIC CATEGORIES *(Continued)*

SLEEP-REST PATTERN

Sleep-Pattern Disturbance
Delayed Sleep Onset
Sleep Pattern Reversal
Sleep Deprivation

COGNITIVE-PERCEPTUAL PATTERN

Pain (Specify Type and Location)
Chronic Pain (Specify Type and Location)
Pain Self-Management Deficit (Acute, Chronic)
Uncompensated Sensory Loss (Specify Type/Degree)
Sensory Overload (Sensory-Perceptual Alteration)
Unilateral Neglect
Sensory Deprivation (Sensory-Perceptual Alteration)
Knowledge Deficit (Specify Area)
Altered Thought Processes (Specify)
Attention-Concentration Deficit
Acute Confusion
Chronic Confusion
Impaired Environmental Interpretation Syndrome
Uncompensated Memory Loss
Impaired Memory
Risk for Cognitive Impairment
Decisional Conflict (Specify)
Decreased Intracranial Adaptive Capacity

SELF-PERCEPTION–SELF-CONCEPT PATTERN

Fear (Specify Focus)
Anxiety
Mild Anxiety
Moderate Anxiety
Severe Anxiety (Panic)
Anticipatory Anxiety (Mild, Moderate, Severe)
Reactive Situational Depression (Specify Situation)
Risk for Loneliness
Hopelessness
Powerlessness (Severe, Moderate, Low)
Low Self-Esteem
Chronic Low Self-Esteem
Situational Low Self-Esteem
Body Image Disturbance
Risk for Self-Mutilation
Personal Identity Disturbance

ROLE-RELATIONSHIP PATTERN

Anticipatory Grieving
Dysfunctional Grieving
Altered Role Performance (Specify)
Unresolved Independence-Dependence Conflict
Social Isolation or Social Rejection
Social Isolation
Impaired Social Interaction
Altered Growth and Development: Social Skills (Specify)
Relocation Stress Syndrome
Altered Family Processes (Specify)
Altered Family Process: Alcoholism
Altered Parenting (Specify Alteration)
Risk for Altered Parenting (Specify Alteration)
Parental Role Conflict
Weak Parent-Infant Attachment
Risk for Altered Parent-Infant/Child Attachment
Parent-Infant Separation
Caregiver Role Strain
Risk for Caregiver Role Strain
Support System Deficit
Impaired Verbal Communication
Altered Growth and Development: Communication Skills (Specify Type)
Risk for Violence

SEXUALITY-REPRODUCTIVE PATTERN

Altered Sexuality Patterns
Sexual Dysfunction
Rape Trauma Syndrome
Rape Trauma Syndrome: Compound Reaction
Rape Trauma Syndrome: Silent Reaction

COPING—STRESS-TOLERANCE PATTERN

Ineffective Coping (Individual)
Avoidance Coping
Defensive Coping
Ineffective Denial or Denial
Impaired Adjustment
Post-Trauma Response
Family Coping: Potential for Growth
Compromised Family Coping
Disabling Family Coping
Ineffective Community Coping
Potential for Enhanced Community Coping

VALUE-BELIEF PATTERN

Spiritual Distress (Distress of Human Spirit)
Potential for Enhanced Spiritual Well-Being

From Gordon, M. (1997). *Manual of nursing diagnosis 1997–1998.* St. Louis: Mosby–Year Book.

A nursing diagnosis has three structural components:

1. Problem (unmet need)
2. Etiology (probable cause)
3. Supporting data (signs and symptoms)

The *problem,* or unmet need, describes the state of the client at present. Problems that are within the nurse's domain to prescribe and treat are termed *nursing diagnoses.* The nursing diagnostic title states what should change. For example: *Hopelessness.*

Etiology, or probable cause, is linked to the diagnostic title with the words *related to. Stating the etiology or probable cause tells what needs to be done to effect the change and identifies causes that the nurse can treat through nursing interventions.*

Hopelessness: *related to long-term stress*

Supporting data, or signs and symptoms, state what the condition is like at present.

Altered thought processes: related to psychological conflicts

Supporting data (defining characteristics) that validate diagnosis:

- Client states "It's no use, nothing will change."
- Lack of involvement with family and friends.
- Lack of motivation to care for self or environment.

Refer to Figure 6–1 to follow Mr. Saltzberg through the steps in the nursing process.

- Mr. Saltzberg is a 47-year-old married man, the father of two boys 7 and 9 years of age. He is admitted to the hospital because of depression and potential for suicide. Two months ago his business failed. Mr. Saltzberg states "I built that business up from nothing; now I am left with nothing." He states he has been feeling depressed and "I just want to be alone."
- He has been anorexic and has lost 12 pounds in the past 2 months. He weighs 140 pounds and is 10 pounds under his range for normal body weight (150 to 165 pounds). He has no interest in sex or any other activity. Family history reveals that his father suffered from depression and attempted suicide at age 60.
- Mr. Saltzberg appears unkempt—his clothes are wrinkled and he has not shaved for 3 days. He sits slumped in the chair with his head down, facing the interviewer but seldom making eye contact. His speech is slow and his mood depressed. His thinking has slowed and he says "I can't think."
- He admits that the idea of suicide has occurred to him. His wife says that he just sits and stares into space all day, keeping to himself. She states that this is the first time she has ever known him to react like this, and that his behavior is a constant concern for the whole family. Mrs. Saltzberg says she feels overwhelmed without his help and support. The children are confused and miss doing things with their father. The family has not gone to temple, the movies, or sports activities—all of which are important events for this family—for 2 months.
- Mr. Saltzberg was seen by the psychiatrist on the unit and was given the DSM-IV diagnosis of *major depression.*
- The nurse meets with Mr. Saltzberg and makes an initial assessment. She speaks with Mrs. Saltzberg, verifies her assessment, and adds it to the database. The nurse also shares information with other staff and members of the health team in conference.

Nursing Diagnosis

After the nurse assesses Mr. Saltzberg, the data are organized into problems and placed in order of priority.

Three major problem areas are identified:

1. Risk of suicide
2. Inadequate nutrition
3. Disrupted family functioning

From these problem areas, three nursing diagnoses are formulated:

Risk for self-directed violence: possible suicidal behavior related to multiple losses

Supporting data that validate diagnosis:

- Business failing.
- The client says "I have nothing left to live for."
- Difficulty with activities of daily living (ADLs) and lowering of mood lasting 2 months.
- Father attempted suicide at age 60.
- Client states he has had vague thoughts of killing himself.

Altered nutrition: less than body requirements, related to apathy and poor self-concept

Supporting data that validate diagnosis:

- Client has sustained a 12-pound weight loss in 2 months.
- He is 10 pounds under his recommended weight range.
- He refuses to eat prepared meals.
- He says he has no appetite.

Altered family process: related to an ill family member

Supporting data that validate diagnosis:

- Since client's illness, the family has not participated in usual family activities.
- Wife and husband have not shared usual activities involving companionship or sex since the onset of illness.
- Wife says she feels overwhelmed without the husband's help and support.
- Children are upset and confused over father's behavior.

Outcome Criteria

Determining the Desired Outcomes

The first part of planning involves identifying **outcome criteria.** For each nursing diagnosis, these are established. Outcome criteria are the behaviors or situations hoped for after the implementation of nursing interventions designed to remedy or lessen the problem identified in the nursing diagnosis. Outcome criteria or *long-term goals* are the hoped-for outcomes that reflect the maximal level of client health that can realistically be reached by nursing interventions. *Short-term goals* are the intermediate goals that assist the client in achieving the long-term goals.

Goals should be realistic and acceptable to both client and nurse. An appropriate goal meets the following criteria:

- It is stated in observable or measurable terms.
- It indicates client outcomes.
- It sets a specific time goal for achievement.
- It is short and specific.
- It is written in positive terms.

Referring to the nursing diagnoses formulated for Mr. Saltzberg, the nurse sets outcome criteria and short-term goals. The goals for the second nursing diagnosis are provided here as an example.

Nursing diagnosis: Altered nutrition: less than body requirements, related to apathy and poor self-concept

OUTCOME CRITERION	SHORT-TERM GOAL
1. Client will gain 2 pounds per week until low normal weight is achieved. Present weight (date) is 140 pounds.	1. Client will eat at least one half to three fourths of his three meals a day, plus one snack at bedtime.

Identifying Interventions To Help Clients Achieve Goals

The second part of planning consists of identifying nursing interventions that will help meet the outcome criteria and are appropriate to the client's level of functioning. The nurse writes a set of interventions appropriate for reaching each goal. Each stated goal should include nursing interventions, which should be seen as instructions for all people working with the client. These written plans aid in the continuity of care for the client and are points of information for all members of the health team. More and more units, both inpatient and community-based facilities, use standardized care plans or clinical pathways for clients with specific diagnoses (see Chapters 1 and 8). Other units are devising individual plans of care.

Even though many inpatient and outpatient units have adopted critical pathways, it is important for you, the student, to understand the process of planning care and evaluating that care. The critical pathways identify the tasks of each interdisciplinary team member; however, the nursing care plans spell out specific steps in the tasks that are part of the nurse's role. An understanding of how to formulate specific long- and short-term outcome criteria, and how to identify appropriate nursing interventions, is essential for the beginning practitioner and student. Therefore, each clinical chapter of this textbook has nursing interventions and rationales spelled out in nursing care plans. Many of the clinical chapters also have an example of a critical/clinical pathway identifying the tasks of other members of the health team along a time line. Refer to Chapter 8 for an example of a critical/clinical pathway. These clinical pathways identify each health care member's role (psychiatrist, psychiatric nurse, social worker, nutritionist, psychologist) in the caregiver's specific time frames for care to be given.

When the short-term goals are reached and charted, a picture of the client's progress is evident. You will note in your practice that computerized clinical documentation is the common trend in health care practice today. The nurse considers specific principles when planning care. Nursing interventions planned for meeting a specific goal need to be

1. *Safe.* They must be safe for the client as well as for other clients, staff, and family.
2. *Appropriate.* They must be compatible with other therapies and with the client's personal goals and cultural values, as well as with institutional rules.
3. *Effective.* They should be based on scientific principles.
4. *Individualized nursing care.* They should be realistic: (1) be within the capabilities of the client's age, physical strength, condition, and willingness to change; (2) be based on the number of staff available; (3) reflect actual available community resources; and (d) be within the student's or nurses' capabilities.

The nurse plans the interventions to meet the goals set for Mr. Saltzberg. The development of one goal follows:

Nursing diagnosis: Risk for self-directed violence: suicide related to multiple losses

Outcome criterion: **By discharge, client will state he wants to live.**

SHORT TERM GOAL	NURSING INTERVENTION
1. Client will remain safe while in the hospital, with the aid of staff.	1a. Remove all items that could potentially be used as weapons (e.g., belts, ties, shoelaces, razors, plastic bags).
	1b. Assess immediate degree of suicidal risk, and ask client if he is thinking of killing himself.
	1c. Check client every 15 minutes and keep him in view at all times.
	1d. Make a "no suicide contract" with the client stating he will not harm himself. (See Chapter 24 for specifics.)
	1e. Spend time with client for 15 minutes, three times a day.
	1f. Encourage client to express thoughts and feelings.
	1g. Encourage client to engage in unit activities even though he may resist and be withdrawn.
	1h. Document all assessments, interactions, and interventions.

Implementation

The *Standards of psychiatric-mental health clinical nursing practice* (ANA 1994) identify ten areas for intervention as discussed in Chapter 1. Seven of these areas of intervention are at the basic level. Recent graduates and practitioners new to the psychiatric setting will participate in many of these activities with the guidance and support of more experienced health care professionals. Interventions at the basic level include

- Counseling
- Milieu therapy
- Self-care activities
- Psychobiological interventions
- Health teaching
- Case management
- Health promotion and health maintenance

Three other areas are specific for the advanced level. The psychiatric mental health advanced practice registered nurse is prepared at the master's level or beyond. Advanced practice interventions include

- Psychotherapy
- Prescription of pharmacological agents
- Consultations

Many nurses who contribute to the practice of psychiatric mental health nursing and care for mentally ill clients are either entry-level RNs or RNs new to the specialty of psychiatric nursing; they are responsible for adhering to the specialty practice standards as designated by the profession (ANA 1994) (refer to Chapter 1).

The care for Mr. Saltzberg involved the following interventions at the basic level.

Counseling

Counseling is usually carried out by a nurse minimally prepared at the basic level in psychiatric mental health nursing. The nurse is skilled in basic techniques of therapeutic communication. Some of the interventions include reinforcing healthy patterns of behavior; employing problem-solving, interviewing, and communication skills; crisis intervention; stress management; relaxation techniques; conflict resolution; and behavior modification. The dialogue in Box 6–5 illustrates the use of communication and counseling skills during a nurse-client interaction with Mr. Saltzberg.

Health Teaching

Health teaching includes identifying health education needs of the client and teaching basic principles of physical and mental health, such as giving information about coping, mental health problems, mental disorders and treatments, and their effects on daily living. The following vignette illustrates health teaching.

- While working with Mr. Saltzberg on creating alternatives to his present solution, the nurse notes that family communications seem to break down when the client is faced with an issue that threatens his self-image. Mr. Saltzberg says that the family is usually able to talk about personal concerns. However, when the business started to falter, Mr. Saltzberg began to think of himself as a failure. He felt ashamed and impotent, and he isolated himself from his family emotionally, hiding his feelings. Thus, he increased his feelings of isolation and helplessness. As anxiety increases, the ability to solve problems decreases. Eventually, Mr. Saltzberg felt overwhelmed and defeated.

- The nurse intervenes to suggest alternative interpersonal communication skills Mr. Saltzberg can use within the family to minimize feelings of hopelessness and helplessness when problems arise. The nurse suggests to Mr. Saltzberg that the family and nurse meet together so that he can "practice" sharing personal feelings. Illness or problems of one family member usually affect all family members. By having the family meet together and work on important issues with some degree of safety and guidance, problems can be minimized. For example, the family may decide to encourage Mr. Saltzberg to talk things out when he seems preoccupied or upset. Discussing problem situations as a family can help put situations into a realistic perspective, provide a variety of alternative actions, and decrease feelings of isolation and helplessness. The family may also identify outside resources that could prove helpful; for example, religious counseling and sympathetic relatives and friends.

Self-Care Activities

Self-care activities assist the client in assuming personal responsibility for ADLs and are aimed at improving the client's functional status when appropriate.

The nursing interventions aimed at increasing Mr. Saltzberg's physical care center on nutrition.

Short-Term Goal

- Mr. Saltzberg will eat at least three quarters of his three meals a day, plus one snack.

- Getting an anorexic person to eat takes creative thinking and patience. In implementing the plan of care for Mr. Saltzberg, the nurse first finds out whether there are any religious or medical dietary restrictions. Mr. Saltzberg states that he eats only kosher foods and that he does have food preferences. These preferences are special dishes his wife makes for him at home.

BOX 6–5 COMMUNICATION AND COUNSELING INTERVENTION

SHORT-TERM GOAL: CLIENT WILL NAME THREE PERSONAL STRENGTHS THAT HAVE WORKED FOR HIM IN THE PAST.

INTERACTION	RATIONALE
NURSE: You mentioned everything coming down on you when your business began to fail.	Placing the event in time and sequence, validating the precipitating event.
CLIENT: Yes . . . everything I had worked for was lost. That business was my whole life. Everything I did was for my business. It was my baby.	
NURSE: You lost a great deal. You said it was like your baby?	Reflecting and showing empathy. Restating
CLIENT: Yeah, well, I had dreamed of it for years. My brother lent me some money, but it was my idea, and I did most of the work to get it going.	
NURSE: It seems to me that building up a business from scratch takes a lot of work and know-how.	Pointing out realities and assisting to clarify strengths.
CLIENT: Oh yes, I was never afraid of hard work. I used to be good at figuring my way out of a tight spot. Now . . . I don't know . . . Ever since that automated shop came in, I couldn't keep up with those prices. Everything caved in . . . It doesn't seem to matter anymore.	
NURSE: What doesn't seem to matter?	Clarifying.
CLIENT: Me . . . being a success . . . being somebody. I guess now I'll never be anybody.	
NURSE: Are you saying that you equate what happens in business with your personal worth?	Validating the client's perception.
CLIENT: Yes . . . I mean . . . no, I just felt so awful when everything caved in . . . I felt so responsible.	
NURSE: Responsible?	Restating.
CLIENT: Yeah . . . responsible to my family.	
NURSE: How did your family react?	Giving broad openings.
CLIENT: Well . . . I really didn't say too much to them. I didn't want to worry them . . . I guess I was afraid.	
NURSE: Afraid?	Restating.
CLIENT: Yeah. That they would think I was no longer a success now that the business was failing.	
NURSE: You were afraid they would see you as a failure if the business ran into trouble?	Reflecting.
CLIENT: I don't know . . . the business was such a great success in the beginning.	
NURSE: What do you think made the shop so successful in the beginning?	Encouraging the client to realistically appraise his strengths.
CLIENT: Well, I worked very hard . . . and I am good at knowing what people want. Everyone says I have a unique way of marketing and advertising.	
NURSE: You are conscientious, observant of others, and creative.	Restating what the client has said. At this point the client can agree or clarify what he meant.
CLIENT: Well . . . yes, but what does that matter now?	
NURSE: In what other ways could you use these qualities?	Encourage the client to problem-solve.
CLIENT: Huh . . . I hadn't thought about other ways . . . *Silence* Sam Cohn . . . well . . . Sam, he always wanted me to come in with him. I always wanted my own place though.	
NURSE: Well, that is one possibility. We talked this morning about some of your strengths and maybe this afternoon we can talk some more about other ways you can use these strengths in the future.	Summarizing and encouraging collaboration
CLIENT: Yeah . . . some other possibilities.	

▶ By working with Mr. Saltzberg and contacting other members of the health team and family, the nurse sets up optimal conditions for increasing his weight. The doctor is first contacted to approve Mrs. Saltzberg's bringing foods from home. The dietitian is contacted to visit Mr. Saltzberg. Kosher foods are requested and food preferences are listed. Mrs. Saltzberg is contacted and agrees to make foods her husband especially likes and that she feels will tempt him to eat.

▶ The importance of follow-up care, community resources, and suicide prevention centers is also a vital part of Mr. Saltzberg's total care. The nurse in charge of case management is involved in Mr. Saltzberg's discharge planning.

Psychobiological Interventions

One of the nurse's functions is the administration of medications to clients. Nurses are responsible for observing the therapeutic, as well as any untoward, effects of the drug. They are expected to know the intended action, therapeutic dose, and blood levels and to monitor these when appropriate (e.g., blood levels with lithium). The nurse is expected to discuss with the client and family both drug action and side effects and to provide time for questions.

▶ Mr. Saltzberg is taking the antidepressant paroxetine hydrochloride (Paxil). The nurse discusses the purpose of the drug with him and potential side effects that he might experience at home. Mr. Saltzberg will have written instructions about potential side effects, toxic effects, and whom to contact in case of difficulty once he is discharged to the community.

Milieu Therapy

Milieu therapy is an extremely important consideration for the nurse working with a client. The client should feel comfortable and safe and be assured that help is available. Milieu management includes reteaching activities that meet the client's physical and mental health needs. In the hospital setting and day-hospital setting, recreational, occupational, and dance therapists are often available to create appropriate activities for clients and give structure to their day. At times, milieu management might mean setting limits (restraints, seclusion, time out). In Mr. Saltzberg's case, milieu management includes certain environmental restrictions that can protect him from self-destructive behavior.

A safe environment for Mr. Saltzberg is the highest priority when he is first admitted to the unit. A person who is feeling overwhelmed and who is in a great deal of emotional pain often has difficulty figuring out ways to solve problems. Sometimes suicide appears to be the only solution. Mr. Saltzberg has suffered a great loss, is a male, and is over 45 years old; his father had attempted suicide at age 60; Mr. Saltzberg is clinically depressed. He has also disengaged himself from the support of his family and friends, and is not attending to ADLs (eating, dressing, appearance). All these factors place him at risk for suicide. (See Chapter 24 for assessing a person's suicide risk.)

A safe environment is arranged by providing Mr. Saltzberg with close observation and by setting limits. All potential weapons are removed and he is put on suicide precautions, which entail checking the client every 15 minutes and keeping him in view at all times. He is also observed for any behaviors that might indicate thoughts of suicide, such as a sudden sense of well-being, giving away possessions, or making out a will.

These nursing interventions occur within the framework of building a relationship with Mr. Saltzberg. The nurse sets aside at least 15 minutes three times a day for him. The content includes sitting, talking, walking, planning, and engaging him in recreational activities—whatever seems the most useful to Mr. Saltzberg at the time. The process is providing the presence of a person who is interested in the client's situation, is willing to work on issues in a nonjudgmental and nonthreatening manner, and is able to provide important resources when needed.

Continuing Data Collection

Data collection is an ongoing process throughout all the phases of the nursing process. While observing Mr. Saltzberg, one nurse noted that he had difficulty sharing problems with his family when his self-esteem was threatened. During these times, family communications broke down, and family members became confused and isolated. The added data directed future nursing intervention.

Evaluation

Evaluation is often the most neglected part of the nursing process. Ideally, evaluation should be part of each phase in the process.

Evaluating Outcome Criteria

There are three possible outcomes when goals are evaluated: goal met, goal not met, goal partially met. The nurse develops the statement of evaluation and documents the client's behavior to determine whether the goal has been met. Diagrammatically, evaluation of goal achievement appears as follows:

EVALUATION:
Goal met
Goal not met
Goal partially met

Whether the goal is met or only partially met, actual client behaviors should be added as evidence. For example, evaluation of the goals set by the nurse for Mr. Saltzberg's third nursing diagnosis might be as follows:

Nursing diagnosis: Altered family process related to an ill family member
Long-term goal: **By discharge, client and family will discuss and identify three outside supports available to them all.**

SHORT-TERM GOAL	EVALUATION
1. By 6/11, client will meet with family and discuss feelings each member is experiencing related to client's illness.	1. 6/11—Goal met. Family was able to share with client and each other their own experiences. Client stated he felt very supported and cared for. Wife and children said they felt relieved to talk about things together again like a family.
2. By 6/15, client will participate with family in planning two family activities they wish to resume.	2. 6/15—Goal met. Client suggested that he and his wife go to the movies once a week, as they had in the past. Client agreed to go with his sons to Little League practice at least three times a month.
3. By 6/18, family will discuss resources and supports they feel are important to the family unit.	3. 6/18—Goal partially met. Family states that going to temple and talking to their family rabbi was special to them. They mentioned certain family friends in whom they could confide and two relatives who were especially close to the family. At this time, Mr. Saltzberg resisted being followed up in the mental health clinic, although he would see the doctor once a month for medication supervision. Emergency number for clinic is given to client in case he has problems or decides he would like to see a counselor in the future.

▶ Mr. Saltzberg was discharged 9 days after he was admitted. By the third day he was taken off suicide precaution and stated, "I really do want to live. I feel a little better knowing there are some options." He was still feeling depressed but no longer hopeless. He understood that the medication might take up to 3 weeks to work. He also understood that, if this medication failed to work, or if the side effects interfered too much in his life, there were other types of medication to try. He had gained 2 pounds and his appetite had improved. Communication with his family was greatly improved and he was looking forward to going home at discharge. He readily agreed to be followed up in the clinic for medication monitoring, but told the caseworker that his rabbi was the person he would rather go to for guidance.

SUMMARY

The nurse-client relationship is well defined, and the role of the nurse and the client must be clearly stated. It is important that the nurse be aware of the differences between a therapeutic relationship and a social or intimate relationship. In a therapeutic nurse-client relationship, the focus is on the client's needs, thoughts, feelings, and goals. The nurse is expected to get personal needs met outside this relationship, in other professional, social, or intimate arenas.

Genuineness, positive regard, and empathy are personal strengths in the helping person that foster growth and change in others.

Even though the boundaries of the nurse-client relationship are clearly defined, the blurring of these boundaries can be insidious and may occur on an unconscious level. Usually, transference and countertransference phenomena are operating when boundaries are blurred. An indication of blurred boundaries might be identified when the nurse is too helpful or not helpful enough. It is important to have a grasp of common countertransferential feelings and behaviors, along with the nursing actions to counteract these phenomena.

The importance of supervision cannot be overemphasized. Supervision aids in the professional growth of the nurse, as well as safeguarding the integrity of the nurse-client relationship. It enhances the progression of the nurse-client relationship, allowing the client's goals to be worked on and met.

The phases of the nurse-client relationship include the orientation, working, and termination phases. At the first interaction of the orientation phase, certain issues need to be brought up: (1) setting the parameters of the relationship—who the nurse is and the purpose of the meetings; (2) the contract—who, what, where, when, and for how long; (3) the issues of confidentiality; and (4) the date of termination, if known. During the orientation phase (and at times throughout the relationship) a number of common client testing behaviors may arise that will require specific nursing interventions.

The nursing process is an adaptation of the problem-solving process used by many professions. The *primary source* of assessment is the client. The psychiatric nursing assessment is done within the psychiatric interview. *Secondary sources* of information include the family, neighbors, friends, police, and other members of the health team. The *process component* of the interview—use of communication skills and the therapeutic use of self—have a great impact on the resulting relationship. Both the nurse's and the client's anxiety levels need to be acknowledged, as do personal biases and value judgments. The content of the interview includes gathering subjective data (client history) and objective data (mental or emotional status). An assessment tool is provided, and charts defining motor behaviors and thought content are included in Appendix D. The student is urged to practice taking a client history using this assessment guide. Assessment tools are useful and can help the nurse focus the interview. When the nurse develops skill and becomes more comfortable in this role, the interview becomes less formal without sacrificing important data.

The nursing diagnosis is a crucial phase in the nursing process. It performs a number of functions: it defines the practice of nursing, improves communication between staff, assists in accountability for care, differentiates nursing from medicine, and so forth. A nursing diagnosis consists of (1) an unmet need or problem, (2) an etiology or probable cause, and (3) supporting data.

Planning nursing care involves (1) determining desired outcomes and goals and (2) planning nursing actions to reach those goals. A goal should be measurable, indicate the desired outcome, have a set time for achievement, and be short and specific. Goals identify the direction for nursing care. Planning nursing action to achieve the goals includes the use of specific principles: the plan should be (1) safe, (2) based on scientific rationale, (3) realistic, and (4) compatible with other therapies.

Practice in psychiatric nursing encompasses seven basic level interventions: counseling, milieu therapy, self-care activities, psychobiological interventions, health teaching, case management, and health promotion and management.

Advanced practice skills are carried out by a nurse who is educated at the master's level and above. Nurses certified for advanced practice psychiatric mental health nursing can practice psychotherapy, prescribe certain medications, and do consulting work.

The evaluation of care must include a look at goal achievement. The nurse judges the goal to be met, not met, or partially met. Supporting data are included to clarify the evaluation. If the goals have not been met, the nurse decides whether priorities in diagnosis need changing, new diagnoses need to be added, new interventions are required to meet goals—and whether diagnosis, goals, interventions, and plans are currently appropriate.

REFERENCES

American Nurses' Association (1994). *A statement on psychiatric-mental health clinical nursing practice and standards of psychiatric-mental health clinical nursing practice.* Washington, DC: American Nurses' Association.
Aromando, L. (1995). *Mental health and psychiatric nursing* (2nd ed.). Springhouse, PA: Springhouse.
Bernard, M. E., and Wolfe, J. L. (Eds.) (1993). *The RET resource book for practitioners.* New York: Institute for Rational-Emotive Therapy.
Bonnivien, J. F. (1992). A peer supervision group: Put countertransference to work. *Journal of Psychosocial Nursing,* 30(5):5.
Book, H. E. (1988). Empathy: Misconceptions and misuses in psychotherapy. *Journal of American Psychiatry,* 145(4):420–424.
Bower, F. L. (1982). *The process of planning nursing care.* St. Louis: C. V. Mosby.
Collins, M. (1983). *Communication in health care: The human connection in the life cycle* (2nd ed.). St. Louis: C. V. Mosby, 1983.
Egan, E. (1994). *The skilled helper: A problem-management approach* (5th ed.). Pacific Grove, CA: Brooks/Cole.
Forchuk, C. (1992). The orientation phase of the nurse-client relationship: How long does it take? *Perspectives in Psychiatric Care,* 28(4):7–10.
Gordon, M. (1997). *Manual of nursing diagnosis 1997–1998.* St. Louis: Mosby–Year Book.
Hagerty, B. K. (1984). *Psychiatric-mental health assessment.* St. Louis: C. V. Mosby.
LaMonica, E. (1980). Validity of empathy instruments. *Health, Education and Welfare Research Project Grant No. 5R01 NU00640* (December 1, 1977 to February 29, 1980).
Mahoney, M. J. (1991). *Human change processes.* New York: Basic Books.
Moore, J. C., and Hartman, C. R. (1988). Developing a therapeutic relationship. In C. K. Beck, R. P. Rawlins and S. R. Williams (Eds.), *Mental health-psychiatric nursing.* St. Louis: C. V. Mosby.
Morse, J. M., et al. (1992). Beyond empathy: Expanding expressions of caring. *Journal of Advanced Nursing,* (17):809–821.
Myrick, R. D., and Erney, T. (1984). *Caring and sharing.* Minneapolis: Educational Media.
Parsons, R. D., and Wicks, R. J. (1994). *Counseling strategies and intervention techniques for human services* (4th ed.). Needham Heights, MA: Allyn & Bacon.
Philette, P. C., et al. (1995). Therapeutic management of helping boundaries. *Journal of Psychosocial Nursing and Mental Health Services,* 33(1):40–47.
Rogers, C. R. (Ed.) (1967). *The therapeutic relationship and its impact.* Madison: University of Wisconsin Press.
Rogers, C. R., and Truax, C. B. (1967). The therapeutic conditions antecedent to change: A theoretical view. In C. R. Rogers (Ed.), *The therapeutic relationship and its impact.* Madison: University of Wisconsin Press.
Simon, S. B., Howe, L. W., and Kirschenbaum, H. (1995). *Values clarification.* New York: Warner Books.
Smitherman, C. (1982). *Nursing action for health promotion.* Philadelphia: F. A. Davis.

SELF-STUDY AND CRITICAL THINKING

Place an S (social), an I (intimate) or a T (therapeutic) next to the corresponding behaviors.

1. __________ The relationship is initiated primarily for socialization, enjoyment, and friendship.

2. ________ The relationship is initiated between two people who have an emotional commitment to each other.

3. ________ Sharing ideas, feelings, and experiences is part of the relationship.

4. ________ The focus of the relationship is on the ideas, experiences, and feelings of just one party in the relationship.

5. ________ The content may be superficial; giving advice or meeting certain dependency needs may be appropriate.

6. ________ Evaluation of specific stated goals is ongoing within the life of the relationship.

7. ________ Mutual fantasies and goals that meet mutual needs are an integral part of the relationship.

8. ________ The relationship is equal (on the same level).

True or false

9. ________ Transference is the attribution (projection) of feelings, wishes, and attitudes originally thought and felt regarding significant others in the client's life to the nurse.

10. ________ It is important for the nurse to be tuned in to personal feelings when the nurse works with a client and to use these feelings to understand the client's experience better.

Place an O (orientation), a W (working), or a T (termination) next to the appropriate phase of the nurse-client relationship. Discuss your rationale for each answer.

11. ________ Some regression and mourning may occur, although the client has reached a point of satisfaction, security, and competence in life.

12. ________ The nurse assesses the client's level of psychological functioning, and both begin to identify problems and set realistic goals.

13. ________ The client begins to seek connections between actions, thoughts, and feelings; takes a more active role in problem solving; and tries out alternative coping behaviors.

14. ________ The nurse summarizes the objectives achieved in the relationship.

Multiple choice

15. Juan Morales, RN, C, has been working with a young man with drug dependence. Juan has put in a great deal of time listening to his client, bringing in articles from the outside at his request, and even offering to go with him to the eye doctor in the client's old neighborhood in order to "keep him from temptation." In peer supervision with Juan, you would focus on

A. Juan's countertransference reaction toward his client.
B. Not going to the eye clinic with Juan.
C. Who the client may remind Juan of and what to Juan is attractive about this client.
D. Juan's altruistic (unselfish) caring and concern for a young man who needs his attention.

16. You are in the first interview with a client and it is extremely warm in the room. The client seems very concerned about your welfare, and a few minutes after you start the interview your client tells you he wants a glass of water and asks if he can get you one. You would best respond by saying

    A. Yes that is thoughtful of you . . . I am thirsty.
    B. I am fine, do as you like.
    C. If you are thirsty, I'll get the water for you.
    D. Yes, I am thirsty but I will get my own water.

17. A nurse has been working with a client in a community center for over 6 months. The client has reached her goal of increased understanding and improved communication with her son, who has long-term mental disorder. It has been an intense 6 months and the nurse and client have established a strong therapeutic alliance. Therefore, the nurse is surprised when the client comes to the last session seemingly carefree, says little, and just looks at her watch. A useful response for the nurse would be to

    A. Say "Well, I see that you are ready to get on with your life now. I am happy for you."
    B. Say very little, since the nurse doesn't want to bring up any new issues now.
    C. Say "You know . . . sometimes goodbyes are hard. We have spent a lot of time together dealing with painful issues. I am wondering how you feel about ending our sessions."
    D. Wonder aloud about the appropriateness of the lack of feelings and the client's use of denial, which could indicate there is still more work to be done.

Write a short answer to the questions that follow:

18. You are spending time with a young woman who is depressed. She tells you she wants to kill herself. How would you feel initially? What are some actions you could take? What are some rationales for supervision at this time?
19. You approach a middle-aged man, introduce yourself, and tell him your purpose and where you are from. When you mention to him that you would like to spend time with him, he looks down and does not respond. You become anxious. Name three actions you can take.

Critical thinking

Ms. Jamison is a 25-year-old woman who came to the hospital because voices told her to kill herself, and she became very frightened. She appears tense. Her posture is rigid, her respiration is rapid, and she says she has not eaten for 3 days. When asked what she usually does when she gets upset, she says that she used to talk to her mother, but her mother died a year ago. Since then, she has been extremely lonely. She tells the nurse she does not have any friends and works part-time as a temporary secretary. She says her voices started a week after her mother died. "They used to be friendly voices, but now they want me to die." She has an aunt and a brother but is hesitant to contact them. She states "They really don't need my problems . . . they have busy lives." She says she is frightened about the voices and is afraid she might obey them. She asks the nurse to help her.

Questions 20 to 23 refer to the above situation. They are organized according to the steps of the nursing process.

20. There are a number of diagnoses the nurse could choose. Formulate one nursing diagnosis for Ms. Jamison. Include the problem statement, probable etiology, and supporting data.

A. The diagnostic title: What should change? ____________________
B. The etiology or possible cause related to ____________________
C. Supporting data to validate diagnosis:

-
-
-

21. State one outcome criterion (long-term goal) and two short-term goals for the diagnosis in question 20, using all four criteria.

A. *Outcome criteria (long-term goal):* ____________________
B. *Short-term goal:* ____________________
C. *Short-term goal:* ____________________

22. When planning nursing care for Ms. Jamison, list four principles you would consider.

A. ____________________
B. ____________________
C. ____________________
D. ____________________

Ms. Jamison is to be discharged tomorrow. She tells the nurse that the voices no longer tell her to kill herself and do not seem as threatening. She says she would like to continue seeing the nurse therapist in the clinic and plans to continue visiting her brother on weekends, but she does not feel up to trying any other activity at this time, although she completes her self-care. As to her medication, she is able to explain to the nurse the dose and time of the medications and possible side effects.

23. For the following goals, state whether the goal was met, not met, or partially met, and give the supporting data.

Outcome criterion: By discharge, client will state she no longer hears threatening or frightening voices.

A. Goal: ____________________ Supporting data: ____________________
____

Short-term goal: Within 2 weeks, client will be able to name three sources of support (church, community health center, women's groups, relatives, neighbors) that she is comfortable using.

B. Goal: ____________________ Supporting data: ____________________
____

Short-term goal: Client will complete self-care while in the hospital, with the aid of medication and a daily therapy session with the nurse.

C. Goal: ____________________ Supporting data: ____________________
____

24. You have just introduced yourself to your client and attempted to establish an initial contact. The client responds that he doesn't think he wants to talk to you. What are some actions that you might take at this time? Generate a list of three or four possibilities, decide which you would attempt first, and give a rationale for your choice.

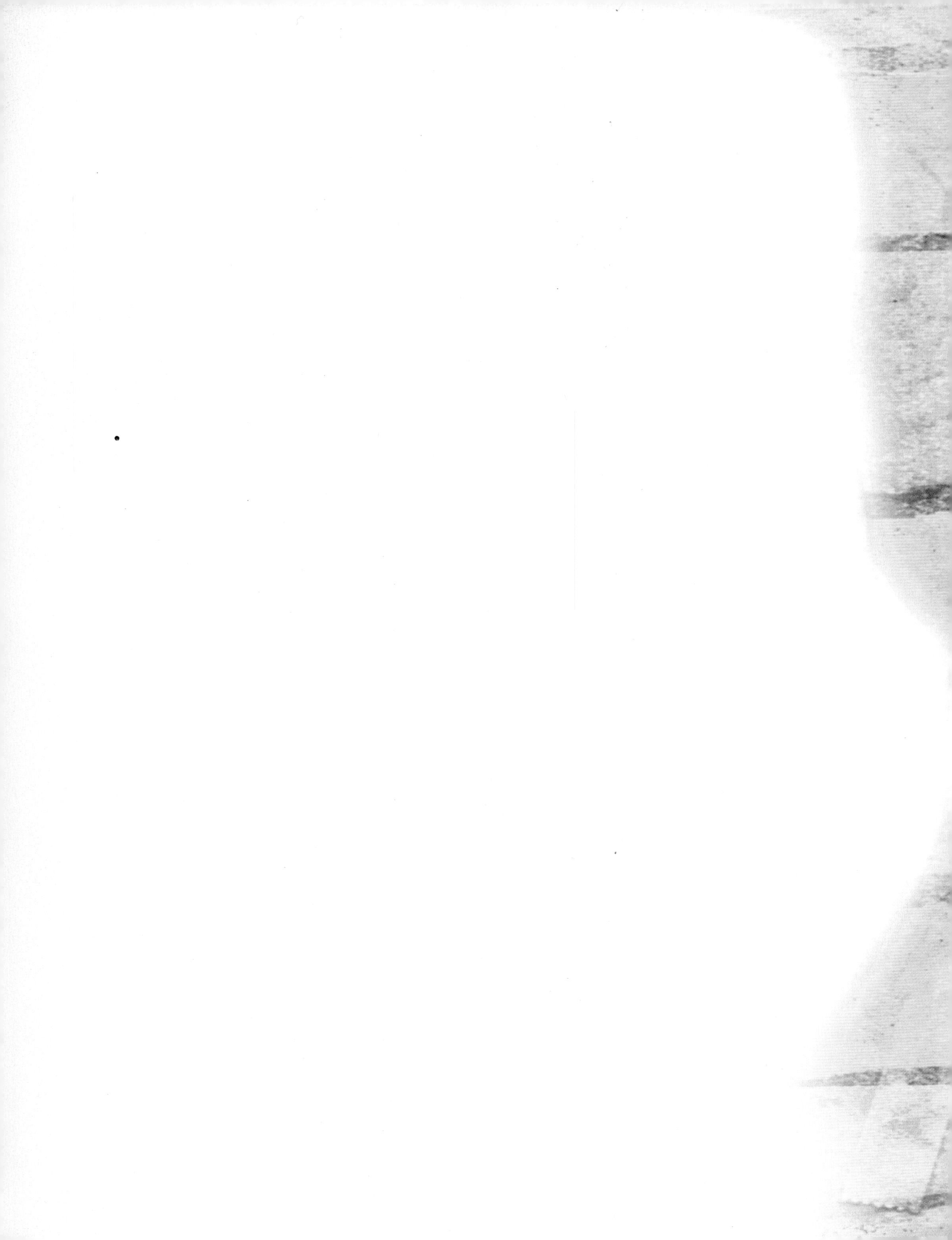

7

Communication and the Clinical Interview

ELIZABETH M. VARCAROLIS

OUTLINE

KEY TERMS AND CONCEPTS

The key terms and concepts listed here also appear in bold where they are defined or discussed in this chapter.

- communication model (Berlo's)
- feedback
- verbal communication
- nonverbal behaviors
- nonverbal communication
- therapeutic (helpful) techniques
- nontherapeutic (nonhelpful) techniques
- clarifying techniques
- paraphrasing
- restating
- reflecting
- exploring
- use of silence
- active listening
- cultural filters
- giving approval

giving advice
"why" questions

clinical supervision
process recordings

OBJECTIVES

After studying this chapter, the reader will be able to

1. Define the five components in Berlo's communication model.
2. Identify three personal factors that can impede accurate communication.
3. Identify two environmental factors that can impede accurate communication.
4. Discuss the differences between verbal and nonverbal communication and identify five areas of nonverbal communication.
5. Identify potential problems that can arise when nurses are insensitive to cultural differences in clients' communication styles.
6. Compare and contrast the range of nonverbal and verbal behaviors of different cultural groups in the areas of (a) communication style, (b) eye contact, and (c) touch. Give examples.
7. Identify four techniques that enhance communication, and discuss what makes them effective.
8. Identify four techniques that hinder communication, and discuss what makes them ineffective.
9. Identify and give rationales for suggested (a) setting, (b) seating, and (c) beginning of the nurse-client interaction.
10. Explain to a classmate the importance of clinical supervision and how it works.
11. Identify four client behaviors a nurse can anticipate, and discuss possible nursing interventions for each behavior.

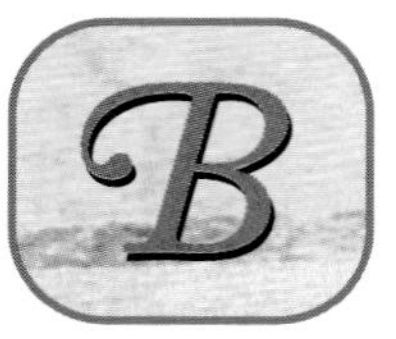

Beginning practitioners who are new to a psychiatric setting are often concerned that they may say "the wrong thing," especially when initially learning to apply therapeutic techniques. *Will* you say "the wrong thing"? The answer is, yes, you probably will. That is how we all learn to find more useful and effective ways of helping clients reach their goals. Will saying "the wrong thing" be harmful to the client? This is doubtful, especially if your intent is honest, your approach is respectful, and you have a genuine concern for the client. We know that special skills (e.g., communications skills) and methods have been identified through scientific investigations that can aid people to become more effective helpers. However, knowledge of skills and techniques is not enough. Being an effective communicator, whether in nursing or in any other area of life, is not just a matter of knowing what techniques to use. The very idea of using techniques is "sometimes met with skepticism because it can imply that someone is deliberately and consciously trying to manipulate someone else" (Myrick and Erney 1984). Mechanical or forced use of communication skills is not helpful. However, when such skills are a genuine part of the helping process, applied with concern and respect for the other person, communication techniques can be a dynamic tool in working effectively with people, in any setting. As you continue to practice and evaluate the use of these techniques, you will develop your own style and rhythm, and eventually they will become a part of the way you communicate with others.

Effective communication is an important foundation for a therapeutic nurse-client relationship. Communication is the medium through which the nursing process is realized. In this chapter, we review the basics of communication and give an introduction to a special form of communication—the clinical interview.

Portions of this chapter first appeared in Collins, M. (1983). *Communication in health care: The human connection in the life cycle* (2nd ed.). St. Louis: C. V. Mosby. We thank Dr. Mattie Collins for generously sharing her insights and ideas.

COMMUNICATION

Simply put, communication is the process of sending a message to one or more persons. One way of thinking about the process of communication is a **communication model,** which identifies the parts of an interaction. One such is **Berlo's** model, which has five parts: stimulus (referent), sender, message, medium (channel), and receiver (Berlo 1960).

The *stimulus* begins communication. For example, the stimulus can be a need for information, comfort, or advice. A stimulus in a nurse might be the perception that the client is feeling discomfort or confusion. A stimulus in a client could be the experience of anxiety, despair, or pain.

The *sender* initiates interpersonal contact. The *message* is the information sent or expressed to another. The clearest are those that are well organized and expressed in a manner familiar to the receiver. The message can be sent through a variety of *mediums*. A message can be sent through an auditory (hearing), a visual (seeing), or a tactile (touch) medium. For example, a person may send a very clear message through silence, body language, or a hug, as well as through the stated word.

The *receiver* receives and interprets the message. Often the message from the sender may act as a stimulus to the receiver. The receiver may then respond to the sender by giving feedback to the sender. The nature of the **feedback** often indicates whether the meaning of the message sent by the sender has been correctly interpreted by the receiver. Validating the accuracy of the sender message is extremely important. An accuracy check may be obtained by simply asking the sender "Is this what you mean?" or "It seems you are saying . . ." (Parsons and Wicks 1994). Feedback in a counseling situation may entail pointing out certain observed behaviors and giving your impression or reaction. "I notice you turn away when we talk about your going back to college. Is there a conflict there?" When the receiver gives feedback to the sender, communication becomes reciprocal. Communication is most effective when the message sent is the same as the message received.

Figure 7–1 shows this simple model of communication. However, communication is a complex process involving a variety of personal and environmental factors that can distort both the sending and the receiving of messages.

Personal factors that can impede accurate transmission or interpretation of messages include emotional factors

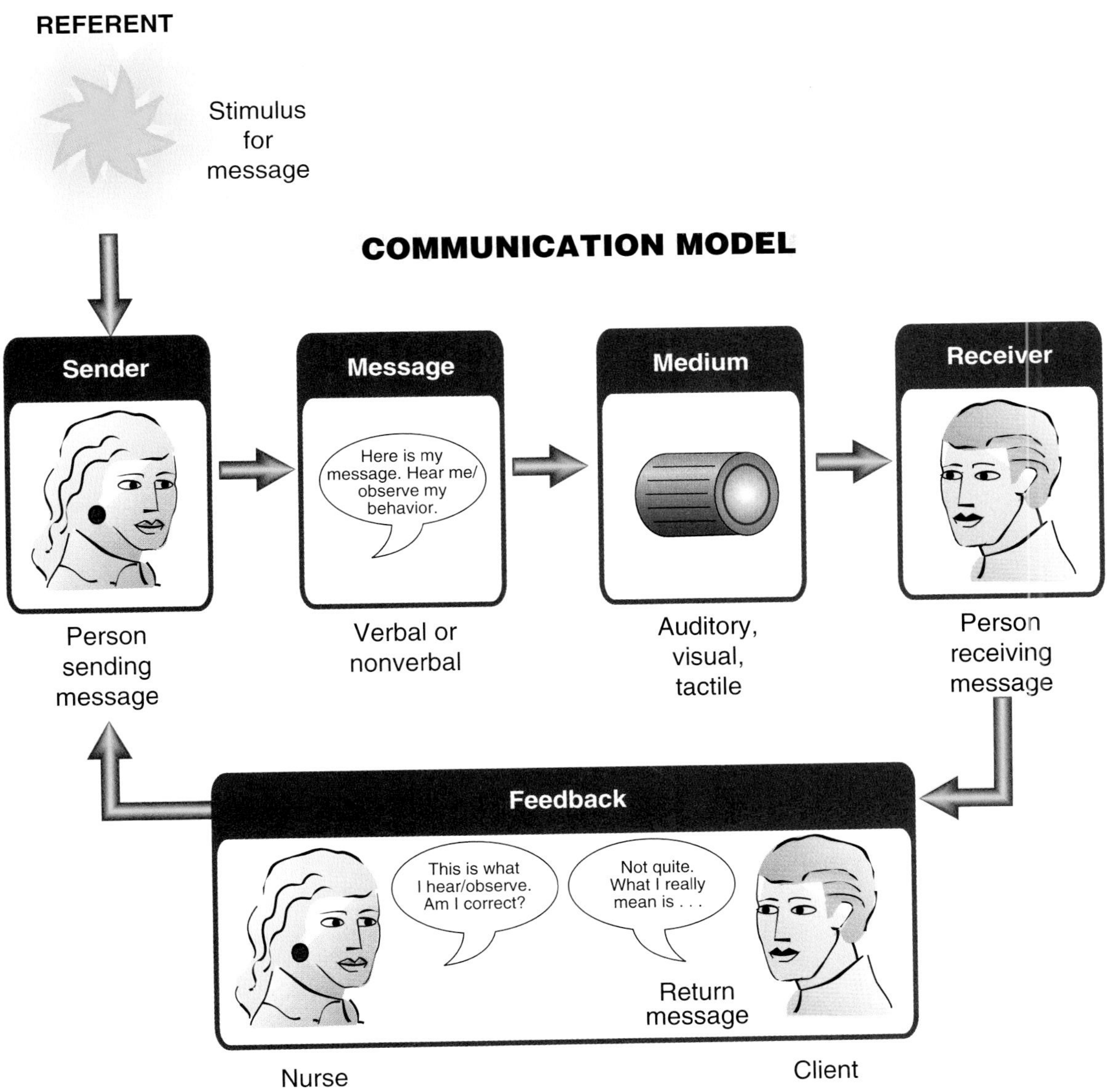

Figure 7–1 The reciprocal process of communication.

(e.g., mood, knowledge levels, language use) and social factors (e.g., previous experience, differences in culture, language).

Environmental factors include physical factors (e.g., background noise, lack of privacy, uncomfortable accommodations) and societal factors (e.g, the presence of others, the expectations of others).

Effective communication in helping relationships depends on nurses' knowing what they are trying to convey (the purpose of the message), communicating what is really meant to the client, and comprehending the meaning of what the client is intentionally or unintentionally conveying (Collins 1983). The success of such an interdependent activity can be evaluated by the degree to which each person understands what was communicated and can show the other person that the message was understood. Peplau (1952, p. 290) identified two main principles that can guide the communication process during the nurse-client interview: (1) *clarity*, wherein the meaning of the message is accurately understood by both parties "as the result of joint and sustained effort of all parties concerned"; and (2) *continuity*, which promotes connections among ideas "and the feelings, events, or themes conveyed in those ideas."

Communication consists of verbal and nonverbal elements. Shea (1988) states that communication is roughly 10% verbal and 90% nonverbal. Therefore, learning to be an effective communicator means using both verbal and nonverbal cues.

Verbal Communication

Verbal communication consists of all words a person speaks. We live in a society of symbols, and our supreme social symbol is words. Talking is our most common activity, our public link with one another, the primary instrument of instruction, a need, an art, and one of the most personal aspects of our private life. When we speak, we

- Communicate our beliefs and values.
- Communicate perceptions and meanings.
- Convey interest and understanding *or* insult and judgment.
- Convey messages clearly *or* convey conflicting or implied messages.
- Convey clear, honest feelings *or* disguised, distorted feelings.

Even if the nurse and client have the same cultural background, the mental image they have of a word may not be exactly the same. Although they believe they are talking about the same thing, the nurse and client may actually be talking about two quite different things. Words are the symbols for emotions as well as for mental images. For example, the word *trip* shows the manner in which differences in mental images can produce misunderstanding. If a nurse says to a client "I heard you had some trip!" the client will define *trip* according to the images that he or she has formed of the word from speaking, reading, writing, and listening. Depending on the client's life experience, the nurse's statement could convey interest or insult. Did the nurse think that the client stumbled and fell? Traveled to another city? Experimented with a drug? Reflecting the rapid and widespread changes in our society, words often change meanings and are therefore best interpreted in accordance with the company they keep (Collins 1983).

Conversation between persons of different cultures can be confusing if one statement simultaneously conveys different messages. One message is the *explicit* message (i.e., the precise or literal meaning of the sentence); the other is the *implicit* message (i.e., the meaning that the speaker wishes to convey at the moment). In some cultures the question, "Why don't you drop in sometime?" is not a request for a visit. If it were a true invitation, a specific date and hour would be set. However, someone from a different background may take the speaker at his or her word and create an embarrassing situation for all concerned. That a person can say one thing and at the same time mean another may be baffling to someone unfamiliar with the way a particular culture uses words. Many remarks are no more than social phrases: "Nice day, isn't it?" or "Hi, how are you?" These remarks are made in passing, and the speaker neither expects to discuss the weather seriously nor really wants to know how someone is. More information must be communicated, either verbally or nonverbally, to make the statement personally relevant (Collins 1983).

Nonverbal Communication

Nonverbal behaviors are the behaviors displayed by an individual, in contrast to the actual content of speech. Tone of voice and the manner in which a person paces speech are examples of **nonverbal communication.** Other common examples of nonverbal communication (often called *cues*) are facial expressions, body posture, amount of eye contact, eye cast (emotion expressed in the eyes), hand gestures, sighs, fidgeting, and yawning. Table 7–1 identifies key components of nonverbal behaviors. Nonverbal behaviors need to be observed and interpreted in light of a person's culture, class, gender, age, sexual orientation, and spiritual norms.

Interaction of Verbal and Nonverbal Communication

Communication thus involves two radically different but interdependent kinds of symbols: the deliberate impressions that you *give* and the less deliberate impressions that you *create*. The first type involves the *spoken word*, which represents our public selves. Verbal assertions can be skillfully used to distort, conceal, deny, and generally

TABLE 7–1 NONVERBAL BEHAVIORS

POSSIBLE BEHAVIORS	EXAMPLE
Body Behaviors	
Posture, body movements, gestures, gait	The client is slumped in a chair, puts her face in her hands, and occasionally taps her right foot.
Facial Expressions	
Frowns, smiles, grimaces, raised eyebrows, pursed lips, licking lips, tongue movements	The client grimaces when speaking to the nurse; when alone, he smiles and giggles to himself.
Eye Cast	
Angry, suspicious, and accusatory looks	The client's eyes harden with suspicion.
Voice-Related Behaviors	
Tone, pitch, level, intensity, inflection, stuttering, pauses, silences, fluency	The client talks in a loud, sing-song voice.
Observable Autonomic Physiological Responses	
Increase in respirations, diaphoresis, pupil dilation, blushing, paleness	When the client mentions discharge, she becomes pale, her respirations increase, and her face becomes diaphoretic.
General Appearance	
Grooming, dress, hygiene	The client is dressed in a wrinkled shirt and his pants are stained; his socks are dirty and he wears no shoes.
Physical Characteristics	
Height, weight, physique, complexion	The client appears grossly overweight and his muscle tone appears flabby.

disguise true feelings. The second type, *nonverbal behaviors*, covers a wide range of human activities, from body movements to responses to the messages of others. How a person listens and uses silence and sense of touch may also convey very important information about the private self that is not available from conversation alone, especially when viewed through a cultural perspective.

Some nonverbal communication, such as facial expressions, seems to be inborn and is similar across cultures (Table 7–1). Dee (1991) cited studies that found a high degree of agreement in spontaneous facial expressions or emotions across ten different cultures. In public, however, some cultural groups (e.g., the Japanese) may control their facial expressions when observers are present. Other types of nonverbal behaviors, such as how close people stand to each other when speaking, depend on cultural conventions. Some nonverbal communication is formalized and has very specific meanings (e.g., the military salute, the Japanese bow).

Therefore, an interaction consists of both verbal and nonverbal messages. Often, people have more conscious awareness of their verbal messages and less awareness of their nonverbal behaviors. The verbal message is sometimes referred to as the *content* of the message, and the nonverbal behavior is called the *process* of the message. When the content (verbal message) is congruent with (agrees with) the process (nonverbal behavior), the communication is more clearly understood and is considered healthy. For example, if a student says that it is important to earn high grades and proceeds to buy the text, read the notes, and study systematically, the content message is consistent with the process, or the nonverbal behaviors.

If, however, the verbal message is not reinforced or is in fact contradicted by the nonverbal behavior, the message is confusing. If the student who stated that it was important to earn high grades did not obtain a copy of the text, did not clarify questions from the notes, and did not study, the student would be sending out two different messages. Conflicting messages are known as double, or mixed, messages. Dee (1991) suggests that one way a nurse can respond to verbal and nonverbal incongruity is to reflect and validate the client's feelings. "You say you are upset that you did not pass this semester, but I notice that you look more relaxed and less conflicted than you have all semester. Do you want to share with me some of the pros and cons of not passing the course this semester?"

With experience, nurses become increasingly aware of a client's verbal and nonverbal communication. Nurses can compare the clients' dialogue with their nonverbal communication to gain important clues about the real message. What persons do may either express and reinforce, or contradict, what they say. As in the saying "actions speak louder than words," actions often reveal the true meaning of a person's intent, whether it is conscious or unconscious. The meaning of the nonverbal cues depends on the context of the situation, the client and his or her cultural orientation, each person's experience, and the total pattern of both nonverbal and verbal behavior. The cues need to be considered together to form an accurate interpretation. The greater the cultural distance between the nurse and the client, the greater is the possibility of miscommunication (Collins 1983).

Culturally Speaking

Ethnic minorities are the most rapidly growing segment of the American population. Health care professionals are gradually becoming aware of the need to become more familiar with the verbal and nonverbal communications of the diverse multicultural populations using the health care system. (Refer to Chapter 2 for a discussion of the *Diagnostic and statistical manual of mental disorders* [DSM-IV]'s emphasis on assessment within the cultural context of the client's symptoms, and look again at Chapter 5 on cultural experience.) The nurse's awareness of the cultural meaning of certain verbal and nonverbal communications in initial face-to-face encounters with a client can lead to the formation of positive therapeutic alliances with culturally diverse populations (Siantz 1991).

Unacknowledged differences between aspects of the cultural identities of client and nurse can result in assessment and interventions that are not optimally respectful of the client and can be inadvertently biased or prejudiced (Lu et al. 1995). Lu and colleagues further stress that health care workers not only need to have knowledge of various clients' cultures, but also need awareness of their own cultural identity. Especially important are nurses' attitudes and beliefs toward ethnic minorities, because these will affect their relationships with clients. Siantz (1991) identifies three areas that may prove problematic for the nurse interpreting specific verbal and nonverbal messages of the client: communication styles, the use of eye contact, and the perception of touch.

Communication Styles

People from some ethnic backgrounds may communicate in an intense and highly emotional manner. For example, Hispanic Americans may appear to use dramatic body language when describing their emotional problems, from the perspective of a non-Hispanic person. For clinicians from a non-Hispanic background, such behavior may be perceived as out of control, and thus viewed as having a degree of pathology that is not actually present. However, from within the Hispanic culture, intensely emotional styles of communication are culturally appropriate and are to be expected (Siantz 1991). French and Italian Americans also demonstrate animated facial expressions and expressive hand gestures during communication that can be mistakenly interpreted by others.

Conversely, in other cultures, a calm facade may mask severe distress. For example, in Asian cultures, expression of either positive or negative emotions is a very private affair, and open expression of emotions is considered to be in bad taste and possibly a weakness. A quiet smile by an Asian American may express joy, an apology, stoicism in the face of difficulty, or even anger (Poole et al. 1995). German and British Americans highly value the concept of self-control and may show little facial emotion in the presence of great distress or emotional turmoil.

Ingram (1991) and others believe it is important to understand an ethnic minority in light of the historical context from which it evolved and its relationship to the dominant culture. For example, the African American, whose historical background in the United States is one of slavery and oppression, is likely to be aware of a basic need for survival. As a result of their experience, many African Americans have become highly selective and guarded in their communication with those outside their cultural group. Therefore, a tendency toward guarded and selective communication among black clients may represent a healthy cultural paranoia and is a black norm (Ingram 1991; Grier and Cobbs 1968).

Eye Contact

Culture also dictates a person's comfort or lack of comfort with direct eye contact. Some cultures consider direct eye contact disrespectful and improper. For example, Hispanics have traditionally been taught to avoid eye contact with authority figures such as nurses, physicians, or other health care professionals. Avoidance of direct eye contact is seen as a sign of respect to those in authority. To nurses or other health care workers from non-Hispanic backgrounds, this lack of eye contact may be wrongly interpreted as disinterest in the interview, or even taken as a lack of respect. Conversely, the nurse is expected to look directly at the client when conducting the interview (Siantz 1991). Similarly, in Asian cultures, respect is shown by avoiding eye contact. For example, in Japan, direct eye contact is considered a lack of respect and a personal affront; preference is for shifting or downcast eyes. With many Chinese, gazing around and looking to one side when listening to another is considered polite. However, when speaking to the elderly, direct eye contact is used (Geissler 1993). Philippine Americans may try to avoid eye contact; however, once it is established, it is important to return and maintain eye contact. Many Native Americans also believe it is disrespectful to engage in direct eye contact, especially if the speaker is younger. Direct eye contact by members of the dominant culture in the health care system can and does cause discomfort for some clients (Poole et al. 1995).

Among German Americans, direct and sustained eye contact indicates that the person listens, trusts, is somewhat aggressive, or in some situations is sexually interested. Russians also find direct, sustained eye contact the norm for social interactions. In Haiti, it is customary to hold eye contact with everyone but the poor (Geissler 1993). French, British, and many African Americans maintain eye contact during conversation; avoidance of eye contact by another person may be interpreted as disinterest, not telling the truth, or avoiding the sharing of important information. In some Arab cultures, a woman making direct eye contact with a man may imply a sexual interest or even promiscuity. In Greece, staring in public is acceptable (Geissler 1993).

Touch

The therapeutic use of touch is a basic aspect of the nurse-client relationship and is normally perceived as a gesture of warmth and friendship. However, touch can be perceived as an invasion of privacy or an invitation to intimacy by some clients (Dee 1991). The response to touch is often culturally defined. For example, many Hispanic Americans are accustomed to frequent physical contact. For some Hispanics, holding the client's hand in response to a distressing situation or giving the client a reassuring pat on the shoulder may be experienced as supportive, and thus help facilitate openness early in the therapeutic relationship (Ramirez 1989). However, the degree and extent of comfort conveyed by touch in the nurse-client relationship is dependent on the country of origin. People from Italian and French cultural backgrounds may also be accustomed to frequent touching during conversation (Geissler 1993). In the Russian culture, touch is also an important part of nonverbal communication. In other cultures, personal touch within the context of an interview might be experienced as patronizing, intrusive, aggressive, or sexually inviting. For example, among German, Swedish, and British Americans, touch practices are infrequent, although a handshake may be common at the beginning and end of an interaction. In India, men may shake hands with other men, but not with women; an Asian Indian man may greet a woman by nodding and holding the palms of his hands together, but not touching. In Japan, handshakes are acceptable; however, a pat on the back is not. Chinese Americans do not like to be touched by strangers. Some Native Americans extend their hand and lightly touch the hand of the person they are greeting, rather than shake hands (Geissler 1993). Even among people of the same culture, the use of touch has clear interpretations and rules between people of different genders and class.

So we see that there are numerous ways to interpret verbal and nonverbal communications for each cultural and subcultural group. Even if a nurse is aware of how a specific cultural group responds to, say, touch, the nurse could still be in error when dealing with an individual within that cultural group. Ingram (1991, p. 40) proposes that a basic guiding principle when working with clients from various cultures is to recognize and use the client as the primary source of information:

> When approached from a posture of respect and compassion, clients of all cultures are the most accurate source of information about their own culturally specific behavior. Hence it is the task of nurses to identify and explore the meaning of nonverbal and verbal behavior with the clients with whom they interact.

Ingram (1991) offers some strategies that may increase the nurse's awareness of culturally specific verbal and nonverbal behavior:

- Engage in personal and professional workshops and training seminars that facilitate awareness of biases and prejudices toward people who are culturally different.
- Once trust has been established in a nurse-client relationship, share your observations with the client. Seek clarification and validate your perceptions with the client.
- Explore the meaning of the behavior with the client, being careful not to inject preconceived notions.
- Acquire knowledge outside your professional practice through participation in culturally diverse activities, and through nonprofessional contacts.
- Read history and literature written by members of the cultural group with whom you are working.
- Engage in discussion of racial issues when they emerge in the context of your interaction with clients, peers, and others outside your work setting.
- Gain an appreciation for how your own culture communicates and what you observe as different in others (e.g., foods, celebrations, issues of trust, expressions of joy or fear).

TECHNIQUES THAT ENHANCE OR HINDER COMMUNICATION

The goals of the nurse in the mental health setting are to help the client

- Identify and explore problems relating to others.
- Discover healthy ways of meeting emotional needs.
- Experience satisfying interpersonal relationships.
- Feel understood and comfortable.

Once specific needs and problems have been identified, the nurse can work with the client on increasing problem-solving skills, learning new coping behaviors, and experiencing more appropriate and satisfying ways of relating to others. To do this, nurses need to have a sound knowledge of communication skills. Therefore, nurses need to become more aware of their own interpersonal techniques, eliminating nonhelpful techniques and applying additional responses that maximize nurse-client interactions. Appropriate techniques are neither therapeutic nor nontherapeutic in themselves. They can, when used in the context of respect and genuine interest, greatly facilitate open communication.

Peplau's book *Interpersonal relations in nursing* (1952) and her groundbreaking article "Interpersonal techniques: The crux of psychiatric nursing" (1962) remain to this day the classic writings that defined nurses' understanding of the relationship between nurse and client.

Hays and Larson (1963) discussed and compiled from various sources and the works of various theorists examples of **therapeutic (helpful)** and **nontherapeutic (nonhelpful) techniques,** which are basic to communication skills used by mental health personnel today.

Techniques deemed nontherapeutic are often used in social relationships, but they may impede communications during a therapeutic relationship.

Table 7–2 identifies techniques that may enhance communication. In the description of the technique and

TABLE 7-2 TECHNIQUES THAT ENHANCE COMMUNICATION

DISCUSSION	EXAMPLE
Using Silence	
Gives the person time to collect thoughts or to think through a point.	Encouraging a person to talk by waiting for the answers.
Accepting	
Indicates that the person has been understood. The statement does not necessarily indicate agreement but is nonjudgmental. However, nurses do not imply they understand when they do not understand.	"Yes." "Uh-huh." "I follow what you say."
Giving Recognition	
Indicates awareness of change and personal efforts. Does not imply good or bad, or right or wrong.	"Good morning, Mr. James." "You've combed your hair today." "I notice that you shaved today."
Offering Self	
Offers presence, interest, and a desire to understand. Is not offered to get the person to talk or behave in a specific way.	"I would like to spend time with you." "I'll stay here and sit with you a while."
Offering General Leads	
Allows the other person to take direction in the discussion. Indicates that the nurse is interested in what comes next.	"Go on." "And then?" "Tell me about it."
Giving Broad Openings	
Clarifies that the lead is to be taken by the client. However, the nurse discourages pleasantries and small talk.	"Where would you like to begin?" "What are you thinking about?" "What would you like to discuss?"
Placing the Events in Time or Sequence	
Puts events and actions in better perspective. Notes cause-and-effect relationships and identifies patterns of interpersonal difficulties.	"What happened before?" "When did this happen?"
Making Observations	
The nurse calls attention to the person's behavior, e.g., trembling, biting nails, restless mannerisms. Encourages the person to notice the behavior in order to describe thoughts and feelings for mutual understanding. Helpful with mute and withdrawn persons.	"You appear tense." "I notice you're biting your lips." "You appear nervous whenever Mr. X enters the room."
Encouraging Description of Perception	
Increases the nurse's understanding of the client's perceptions. Talking about feelings and difficulties can lessen the need to act them out inappropriately.	"What do these voices seem to be saying?" "What is happening now?" "Tell me when you feel anxious."
Encouraging Comparison	
Brings out recurring themes in experiences or interpersonal relationships. Helps the person clarify similarities and differences.	"Has this ever happened before? "Is this how you felt when . . .?" "Was it something like . . .?"
Restating	
Repeats the main idea expressed. Gives the client an idea of what has been communicated. If the message has been misunderstood, the client can clarify it.	C: "I can't sleep. I stay awake all night." N: "You have difficulty sleeping?" C: "I don't know . . . he always has some excuse for not coming over or keeping our appointments." N: "You think he no longer wants to see you?"

Continued

TABLE 7–2 TECHNIQUES THAT ENHANCE COMMUNICATION *(Continued)*

DISCUSSION	EXAMPLE
Reflecting	
Directs questions, feelings, and ideas back to the client. Encourages clients to accept their own ideas and feelings. Acknowledges the right to have opinions and make decisions, and encourages clients to think of themselves as capable people.	C: "What should I do about my husband's affair?" N: "What do you think you should do?" C: "My brother spends all of my money and then has the nerve to ask for more." N: "This causes you to feel angry?"
Focusing	
Concentrates attention on a single point. It is especially useful when the client jumps from topic to topic. If a person is experiencing a severe or panic level of anxiety, the nurse should not persist until the anxiety lessens.	"This point you are making about leaving school seems worth looking at more closely." "You've mentioned many things. Let's go back to your thinking of 'ending it all'."
Exploring	
Examines certain ideas, experiences, or relationships more fully. If the client chooses not to elaborate, the nurse does not probe or pry. In such a case, the nurse respects the client's wishes.	"Tell me more about that." "Would you describe it more fully?"
Giving Information	
Makes available facts the person needs. Supplies knowledge from which decisions can be made or conclusions drawn. For example, the client needs to know the role of the nurse; the purpose of the nurse-client relationship; and the time, place, and duration of the meetings.	"My purpose for being here is . . ." "This medication is for . . ." "The test will determine . . ."
Seeking Clarification	
Helps clients clarify their own thoughts and maximizes mutual understanding between nurse and client.	"I am not sure I follow you." "What would you say is the main point of what you just said?" "Give me an example of one time you thought everyone hated you."
Presenting Reality	
Indicates what is real. The nurse does not argue or try to convince the client, just describes personal perceptions or facts in the situation.	"That was Dr. Todd, not a man from the Mafia." "That was the sound of a car backfiring." "Your mother is not here; I am a nurse."
Voicing Doubt	
Undermines the client's beliefs by not reinforcing the exaggerated or false perceptions.	"Isn't that unusual?" "Really?" "That's hard to believe."
Seeking Consensual Validation	
Clarifies that both the nurse and client share mutual understanding of communications. Helps clients become clearer about what they are thinking.	"Tell me whether my understanding agrees with yours." "Are you using this word to convey . . .?" "When you say 'terrible' do you mean . . .?"
Verbalizing the Implied	
Puts into concrete terms what the client implies, making the client's communication more explicit.	C: "I can't talk to you or anyone else. It's a waste of time." N: "Do you feel no one understands?"

Continued

TABLE 7–2 TECHNIQUES THAT ENHANCE COMMUNICATION *(Continued)*

DISCUSSION	EXAMPLE
Encouraging Evaluation	
Aids the client in considering people and events within his or her own set of values.	"How do you feel about . . .?" "What did it mean to you when he said he couldn't stay?"
Attempting to Translate into Feelings	
Responds to the feelings expressed, not just the content. Often termed "decoding."	C: "I am dead inside." N: "Are you saying that you feel lifeless? Does life seem meaningless to you?"
Suggesting Collaboration	
Emphasizes working with the client, not doing things for the client. Encourages the view that change is possible through collaboration.	"Perhaps you and I can discover what produces your anxiety." "Perhaps by working together we can come up with some ideas that might improve your communications with your spouse."
Summarizing	
Brings together important points of discussion to enhance understanding. Also allows the opportunity to clarify communications so that both nurse and client leave the interview with the same ideas in mind.	"Have I got this straight?" "You said that . . ." "During the past hour, you and I have discussed . . ."
Encouraging Formulation of a Plan of Action	
Allows clients to identify alternative actions for interpersonal situations they find disturbing, e.g., when anger or anxiety are provoked.	"What could you do to let anger out harmlessly?" "Next time this comes up, what might you do to handle it?" "What are some of the other ways you can approach your boss?"

From *Interacting with patients* by Joyce Samhammer Hays and Kenneth Larson. Copyright © 1963 Macmillan Publishing Company. Reprinted with permission from the Macmillan Publishing Company.

the examples given, you may recognize some techniques that you already use. Throughout this book, in case studies and in the text, you will find many examples of verbal communication. You can begin to identify various therapeutic techniques as you read, and in time learn to recognize and apply them in practice.

Table 7–3 provides examples of techniques that may get in the way of understanding between two people.

Even if you are new to a mental health setting, you can become aware of your own communication patterns, identify your responses, and increase your ability to alter responses and maximize open communication. Important therapeutic techniques discussed further in the next sections include (1) clarifying techniques, (2) the use of silence, and (3) active listening.

Clarifying Techniques

Understanding depends on clear communication, which is aided by verifying with a client the nurse's interpretation of the client's messages. The nurse must request feedback on the accuracy of the message received from both verbal and nonverbal cues. The use of **clarifying techniques** helps both participants to identify major differences in their frame of reference, giving them the opportunity to correct misperceptions before they cause any serious misunderstandings. The client who is asked to elaborate on or to clarify vague or ambiguous messages needs to know that the purpose is to promote mutual understanding.

Paraphrasing

For clarity, we might use **paraphrasing,** which means to restate in different (often fewer) words the basic content of a client's message. Using simple, precise, and culturally relevant terms, the nurse may readily confirm interpretation of the client's previous message before the interview proceeds. By prefacing statements with a phrase such as "I am not sure I understand" or "In other words, you seem to be saying . . .," the nurse helps the client form a clearer perception of what may be a bewildering mass of details. After paraphrasing, the nurse must validate the

TABLE 7–3 TECHNIQUES THAT HINDER COMMUNICATION

NONTHERAPEUTIC EXAMPLE	DISCUSSION	MORE HELPFUL RESPONSE
	Reassuring	
"I wouldn't worry about . . ." "Everything will be all right." "You're doing fine."	Underrates a person's feelings and belittles a person's concerns. May cause clients to stop sharing feelings if they think they will be ridiculed or not taken seriously.	"What specifically are you worried about?" "What do you think could go wrong?" "What are you concerned might happen?"
	Giving Approval	
"I'm glad you made the right decision." "You wrote such a good poem this AM."	Indicates that what the client is doing now is "good" and implies that not doing it is "bad." When praise is given, potential learning may be hindered because the client then seeks to gain the nurse's approval rather than to focus on the steps of learning.	"What factors led to the decision to leave that job?" "Your poem seemed to reflect a lot more of what you are feeling about your life."
	Rejecting	
"Talk to your doctor about this." "This topic is too painful."	May make the client feel rejected by the nurse because he or she is unable to express personal thoughts and feelings. Thus, the client avoids sharing thoughts or feelings to avoid the risk of further rejection.	"This sounds important—let's continue . . ." "This is a painful topic, this must have been painful for you . . . you were saying . . ."
	Disapproving	
"I'd rather you wouldn't talk incessantly in group meeting." "You really shouldn't yell at your roommate."	Is moralizing; implies the nurse has the right to judge the client's thoughts or actions. It further implies the client is expected to please the nurse. If the client's behavior is extreme or hurtful, the nurse should not label the behavior. Make an observation, e.g., "I notice that you are talking a lot even though you know it annoys others and pushes them away."	"I wonder what you're trying to prevent from happening with all your talking, or are you comfortable in group?" "Let's try to figure out what's going on between you and your roommate."
	Agreeing	
"That's right." "I agree."	Denies clients an opportunity to change their point of view.	"Tell me about your thinking in arriving at that conclusion." "That is one way of looking at the situation."
	Disagreeing	
"I disagree with that." "The FBI is not out to torture you for your secrets."	May make a person defensive. Defending one's ideas often tends to strengthen them. If a client has delusional thinking, defending such thinking prevents the exploration of feelings or refocusing energies into more productive activities or interactions.	"That is one point of view. I'd like to understand how you arrived at that conclusion." "I know nothing about the FBI. Do you feel frightened thinking people want to harm you?"
	Advising	
"I think you should get out of this situation immediately." "Why don't you go back to school?"	Conveys that the nurse knows best and that clients cannot think for themselves. Fosters dependency and inhibits the problem-solving process. Encourage clients' problem solving: "What have you thought about this situation?"	"What were some of the actions you thought you might take?" *or* "What are the pros and cons of your situation?" "What are some ways you have thought of to meet your goals?"

Continued

TABLE 7–3 TECHNIQUES THAT HINDER COMMUNICATION *(Continued)*

NONTHERAPEUTIC EXAMPLE	DISCUSSION	MORE HELPFUL RESPONSE
	Probing	
"Tell me about your dislike for your wife." "Tell me why you run around with other men."	May make clients feel used and valued only for the information they can give. Most people resent persistent personal questions, especially if they have not brought up the subject themselves.	"Tell me about you and your wife." "Tell me about important people in your life."
	Testing	
"What day is this?" "Do you know what kind of hospital this is?" "Do you remember . . .?"	Indicates that the nurse feels the client needs help, instead of asking questions such as "Can you remember?"	Unless the nurse is testing for T × P × P*, the nurse could say "Tell me what took place."
	Defending	
"No one around here would lie to you." "I am only trying to help you straighten out."	Implies that the client has no right to express his or her impressions, opinions, or feelings. Defending could also imply to the client that the nurse is taking the others' side against the client. It is better to explore the other person's perspective.	"It's important to have the correct information. What is it you want to know? I will try to get you the information." "Tell me what I did to upset you."
	Requesting an Explanation	
"Why did you stop taking your medication?" "Why did you do that?" "Why do you always start an argument when we start to talk about change?"	Implies criticism; the client may respond defensively. It is better to ask people to describe *what* is occurring rather than *why* it is occurring. Ask questions that focus on who, what, where, and when.	"Tell me some of the reasons that led to your not taking your medication." "I notice when we start to talk about change you get upset. What do you think will happen if you make some changes?"
	Minimizing Feelings	
C: "I wish I were dead." N: "Everyone gets down once in awhile." *or* N: "I know what you mean." *or* N: "I get that way sometimes."	Is evident when the nurse is unable to empathize or understand another point of view. When a nurse tells a client to "buck up" or "cheer up," the client's feelings or experiences are being belittled. This can cause a person to feel "small" or "insignificant."	C: "I wish I was dead." N: "You must be feeling very upset. Are you thinking of hurting yourself?"
	Making Stereotypical Comments	
"Things get worse before they get better." "It's for your own good." "Keep your chin up."	Lacks value in the nurse-client relationship. Encourages empty responses by the client and cuts off important areas of communication.	"It sounds like you're feeling overwhelmed. What about this is the most difficult to deal with?" "What about the medication bothers you the most?" "Things sound a bit confused right now. What would you say is the most distressing?"

*Time, place, and person.

Continued

TABLE 7–3 TECHNIQUES THAT HINDER COMMUNICATION *(Continued)*

NONTHERAPEUTIC EXAMPLE	DISCUSSION	MORE HELPFUL RESPONSE
	Using Denial	
C: "I am nothing." N: "Of course you're something. Everybody is something."	Blocks avenues of discussion. Clients are blocked from identifying and exploring their difficulties.	C: "I am nothing." N: "Give me an example of what you mean."
C: I'll never, never walk again." N: "Sure you will, a lot of people get better."		C: "I'll never, never walk again." N: "I don't know about that right now, but if that is true there are a number of options that can help you maintain your mobility. When we find what your situation is, you can discuss them with me and other members of the health team."
	Changing the Subject	
C: "I'd like to die." N: "Did you have any visitors this weekend?"	When the nurse changes the topic, he or she is usually threatened by an anxiety-provoking topic. It is important for the nurse to become aware of what precipitates these occurrences and to discuss them in peer counseling or with a supervisor.	C:"I'd like to die." N: "This sounds serious. Have you thought of harming yourself?"

Adapted from Hays, J.S., and Larson, K. (1963). *Interacting with patients.* New York: Macmillan.

accuracy of the restatement and its helpfulness to the discussion. The client may confirm or deny the perceptions through nonverbal cues or by directly responding to a question such as "Was I correct in saying . . . ?" As a result, the client is made aware that the interviewer is actively involved in the search for understanding.

Restating

With **restating,** the nurse mirrors the client's overt and covert messages; thus, this technique may be used to echo feeling as well as content. Restating differs from paraphrasing in that it involves repetition of the same key words the client has just spoken. If a client remarks "My life has been full of pain," additional information may be gained by restating, "Your life has been full of pain." The purpose of this technique is to explore more thoroughly subjects that may be significant. However, too frequent and indiscriminate use of restating might be interpreted by clients as inattention, disinterest, or worse. It is very easy to overuse this tool and become mechanical. Inappropriately parroting or mimicking what another has said may be perceived as poking fun at the person, making this nondirective approach a definite drawback to communication. To avoid overuse of restating, the nurse can combine restating with direct questions that encourage descriptions: "Tell me about how your life has been full of pain."

Reflecting

Reflection is a means of assisting people to better understand their own thoughts and feelings. **Reflecting** may take the form of a question or a simple statement that conveys the nurse's observations of the client when sensitive issues are being discussed (Parsons and Wicks 1994). The nurse might then describe briefly to the client the apparent meaning of the emotional tone of the client's verbal and nonverbal behavior. For example, to reflect a client's feelings about his or her life, a good beginning might be "You sound as if you have had many disappointments." Sharing *observations* with a client shows acceptance. The nurse helps make the client aware of inner feelings and encourages the client to own them. For example, the nurse may tell a client "You look sad." Perceiving the nurse's concern may allow a client spontaneously to share feelings. The use of a question in response to the client's question is another reflective technique (Parsons and Wicks 1994, p. 92). For example:

Client: Nurse, do you think I really need to be hospitalized?

Nurse: What do you think, Jane?

Client: I don't know, that's why I'm asking you.
Nurse: I'll be glad to share my impression with you at the end of this first session. However, you've probably thought about hospitalization and have some feelings about it. I wonder what they are.

Exploring

A technique that enables the nurse to examine important ideas, experiences, or relationships more fully is **exploring.** For example, if a client tells the nurse that he does not get along well with his wife, the nurse will want to further explore this area. Possible openers might include

- "*Tell me* more about your relationship with your wife."
- "*Describe* your relationship with your wife."
- "*Give me an example* of you and your wife not getting along."

Asking for an example can greatly clarify a vague or generic statement made by a client:

Mary: No one likes me.
Nurse: Give me an example of one person who doesn't like you.
Jim: Everything I do is wrong.
Nurse: Give me an example of *one* thing you do that you think is wrong.

Use of Silence

In many cultures in our society, and in nursing, there is an emphasis on action. In communication, we tend to expect a high level of verbal activity. Many students and practicing nurses find that when the flow of words stops, they become uncomfortable. The effective **use of silence,** however, is a useful communication technique.

Silence is not the absence of communication. Silence is a specific channel for transmitting and receiving messages. The practitioner needs to understand that silence is a significant means of influencing and being influenced by others.

In the initial interview the client may be reluctant to speak because of the newness of the situation, the strangeness of the nurse, self-consciousness, embarrassment, or shyness. Talking is highly individualized; some find the telephone a nuisance, whereas others believe they cannot live without it. The nurse must recognize and respect individual differences in styles and tempos of responding. How else can nurses learn of another's nature and their own but by courtesy, care, and time? People who are quiet, those who have a language barrier or speech impediment, the elderly, and those who lack confidence in their ability to express themselves may be communicating through their silences a need for support and encouragement in acts of self-expression (Collins 1983).

Although there is no universal rule concerning how much silence is too much, silence has been said to be worthwhile only as long as it is "serving some function and not frightening to the patient" (Schulman 1974). Knowing when to speak during the interview is largely dependent on the nurse's perception about what is being conveyed through the silence. Icy silence may be an expression of anger and hostility. Being ignored or "given the silent treatment" is recognized as an insult and is a particularly hurtful form of communication. Ingram (1991) points out that silence among some African American clients may relate to anger, insulted feelings, or acknowledgment of a nurse's lack of cultural sensitivity.

Silence may also indicate emotional blocking in some clients. A client who feels pressured to talk about a subject that is too painful or delicate may react by looking away in stony silence as a form of defiance or resistance. The nurse can intervene in a sure-footed manner against resistance only when the relationship has a reservoir of trust and intimacy that can help it withstand the strain. Timing is essential; the more positive experiences the participants have had together over time, the greater is the likelihood that the client will make painful disclosures. If the relationship has not reached the stage of mutual trust, more may be gained when the client's unreadiness is respected and the conversation is not pursued along the lines that evoked the initial reaction. Silence can communicate strength and support by allowing the client to regain composure and to continue the conversation at a more comfortable level. Thus, silence can show respect for the client's right to choose the nature, circumstances, and degree of openness in communication (Collins 1983).

Successful interviewing may be largely dependent on the nurse's "will to abstain"—that is, to refrain from talking more than necessary. Silence may provide meaningful moments of reflection for both participants. It gives each an opportunity to contemplate thoughtfully what has been said and felt, to weigh alternatives, to formulate new ideas, and to gain a new perspective of the matter under discussion. If the nurse waits to speak and allows the client to break the silence, the client may share thoughts and feelings that could otherwise have been withheld. Nurses who feel compelled to fill every void with words often do so because of their own anxiety, self-consciousness, and embarrassment. When this occurs, the nurse's need for comfort tends to take priority over the needs of the client.

On the other hand, prolonged and frequent silences by the nurse may hinder an interview that requires verbal articulation. Although the untalkative nurse may be comfortable with silence, this mode of communication may make the client feel like a fountain of information to be drained dry. Moreover, without feedback, clients have no way of knowing whether what they said was understood. The verbal patterns of nursing students have been demonstrated to correlate with communication competence (Johnson 1964). The appropriate use of verbal interviewing techniques helped the students to focus more directly on clients' needs and to elicit more emotional responses. Nurses who value silence highly may need to reassess the impact of nonverbal communication on the interviewing process. Without such a reassessment, there may be minimal use of the creative potential of mutuality, or working with the client toward goals (Collins 1983).

Active Listening

People want more than just physical presence in human communication. Most people are looking for the other person to be there for them psychologically, socially, and emotionally (Egan 1994). **Active listening** includes

- Observing the client's nonverbal behaviors.
- Listening to and understanding the client's verbal message.
- Listening to and understanding the person in the context of the social setting of his or her life.
- Listening for "false notes" (e.g., inconsistencies or things client says that need more clarification).

We have already noted that effective interviewers must become accustomed to silence. It is just as important, however, for effective interviewers to learn to become active listeners when the client is talking, as well as when the client becomes silent. During active listening, nurses carefully note what the client is saying verbally and nonverbally, as well as monitoring their own nonverbal responses (Parsons and Wicks 1994). Using silence effectively and learning to listen on a deeper, more significant level to both the client and your own thoughts and reactions are both key ingredients in effective communications. Both these skills take time, profit from guidance, and can be learned.

A word of caution about listening. It is important for all of us to recognize that it is impossible to listen to people in an unbiased way. In the process of socialization we develop **cultural filters** through which we listen to ourselves, others, and the world around us (Egan 1994). Cultural filters are a form of cultural bias or cultural prejudice.

> One of the functions of culture is to provide a highly selective screen between man and the outside world. In its many forms, culture therefore designates what we pay attention to and what we ignore. This screening provides structure for the world. (Hall 1977, p. 85.)

Egan (1994) states that we need these cultural filters to provide structure for ourselves and to help us interpret and interact with the world. However, unavoidably, these cultural filters also introduce various forms of bias in our listening, since they are bound to influence our personal, professional, familial, and sociological values and interpretations. Egan goes on to give an example of how strong cultural filters can influence the likelihood of bias with multicultural clients. For instance, he gives the example of a white, middle-class helper who would tend to use white, middle-class filters when listening. These cultural filters may not interfere with, and could even facilitate, working with someone from a white, middle-class background. However, if the awareness of our own cultural filters goes unacknowledged, the likelihood is great that they will distort our perceptions and interpretations of multiethnic clients. Therefore, the white, middle-class helper, if not cognizant of personal cultural biases, could easily introduce bias when working with, say, a well-to-do Asian client with high social status in the community; an African American mother from the urban ghetto; or a poor white subsistence farmer (Egan 1994). We all need a frame of reference to help us function in our world. The trick is to understand that people use many other frames of reference to help them function in their world. Acknowledging that others view the world quite differently, and trying to understand other people's ways of experiencing and living in the world, can go a long way toward minimizing our personal distortions in listening. Building acceptance and understanding of those culturally different from ourselves is a skill, too.

Active listening helps strengthen the client's ability to solve personal problems. By giving the client undivided attention, the nurse communicates that the client is not alone; rather, the nurse is working along with the client, seeking to understand and help. This kind of intervention enhances self-esteem and encourages the client to direct energy toward finding ways to deal with problems. Serving as a "sounding board," the nurse listens as the client tests thoughts by voicing them aloud. This form of interpersonal interaction often enables the client to clarify thinking, link ideas, and tentatively decide what should be done and how best to do it (Collins 1983).

Techniques to Monitor and Minimize

A number of techniques that can interfere with communication were listed in Table 7–3. Look these over and identify the ones you tend to use and want to modify. Although people frequently use these techniques in their daily lives, we will now look at how they can become problematic when one is working with clients who are under stress while attempting to cope with disruptions in their life.

Giving Approval

"You look great in that dress." "I am proud of the way you controlled your temper at lunch." "That's a great quilt you made." What could be bad about giving someone a pat on the back once in a while? Nothing, if it is done without involving a judgment (positive or negative) by the nurse. We often give our friends and family approval when they do something well. However, in a nurse-client situation, **giving approval** often becomes much more complex. A client may be feeling overwhelmed; experiencing low self-esteem; feeling unsure of where his or her life is going; and very needy of recognition, approval, and attention. Yet, when people are feeling vulnerable, a value comment might be misinterpreted. For example:

Nurse: "You did a great job in group telling John just what you thought about how rudely he treated you."

Implied in this message is that the nurse was pleased by the manner in which the client talked to John. The client then sees this response as a way to please the nurse, by doing "the right thing." In order to continue to please the nurse (and get approval), the client may continue the behavior. The behavior might be useful behavior for the client, but when a behavior is being done to please another person, it is not coming from the individual's own volition or conviction. Also, when the other person whom the client needs to please is not around, the motivation for the new behavior might not be there either. Thus, it really is not a change in behavior as much as a ploy to win approval and acceptance from another person. Giving approval also cuts off further communication. It is a statement of the observer's (nurse's) judgment on another person's (client's) behavior. A more useful response would be:

Nurse: "I noticed you spoke up to John in group yesterday about his rude behavior. How did it feel to be more assertive?"

This opens the way for finding out if the client was scared, was comfortable, wants to work more on assertiveness, or whatever. It also suggests that this was a self-choice the client made. The client is given recognition for the change in behavior, and the topic is also open for further discussion.

Advising

Although we ask for and give advice all the time in daily life, **giving advice** to a client is rarely helpful. Often, when we ask for advice, our real motive is to discover if we are thinking along the same lines as someone else or whether they would agree with us. When the nurse gives advice to clients who are having trouble assessing and problem-solving conflicted areas of their life, the nurse is interfering with their ability to make personal decisions. When we offer clients "solutions," they eventually begin to think that the nurse doesn't view them as capable of making effective decisions. People often feel inadequate when they are given no choices over decisions in their life. Giving advice to clients can foster dependency ("I'll have to ask the nurse what to do about . . .). Giving people advice can undermine their sense of competence and adequacy. It also keeps the nurse "in control" and feeling like the strong one, although this might be unconscious on the nurse's part. However, people do need information to make informed decisions. Often, the nurse can help the client define a problem and identify what information might be needed to come to an informed decision. A more useful approach would be "What do you see as some possible actions you can take?" It is much more constructive to encourage problem solving by the client. At times, the nurse can suggest several alternatives that a client might consider (e.g., "Have you ever thought of telling your friend about the incident?") Clients are then free to say yes or no and make their own decision from among the suggestions.

Requesting an Explanation: "Why" Questions

"Why did you come late?" "Why did you change your hair?" "Why didn't you study for the exam?" Very often a **"why" question** implies criticism. We may ask our friends or family such questions and, in the context of a solid relationship, the "why" may be more understood as "what happened?" With people we don't know—especially an anxious person who may be feeling overwhelmed—a "why" question from a person in authority (nurse, doctor, teacher) can be experienced as intrusive and judgmental, which only serves to make the person defensive. Most of the time we don't know why we do things, although when confronted by a "Why did you . . ." we may make up all sorts of responses on the spur of the moment.

It is much more useful to ask *what* is happening, rather than *why* it is happening. Questions that focus on who, what, where, and when often elicit important information that can facilitate problem solving and further the communication process.

THE CLINICAL INTERVIEW

The clinical interview is not a random meeting between nurse and client. It is a systematic attempt to understand those problems in clients' lives that interfere with meeting their goals, and to help them improve their skills or learn alternative ways of dealing effectively with their problems.

The clinical interview differs from the intake interview, or the assessment interview, which is described in Chapter 6 as part of the nursing process. In most cases, by the time a nurse meets a client for the first time, the intake interview has already been recorded. In the hospital setting the intake interview is often recorded in the chart by the physician or (in some places) a psychiatric nurse clinician. In the community setting the physician or nurse clinician is often the person doing the intake interview. However, during the clinical rotation, it is not uncommon for the student to obtain important data from the client that can be added to the client database.

The content and direction of the clinical interview are decided by the client. The client leads. The nurse employs communication skills and active listening (identifying what the client says as well as what the client does not say) to better understand the client's situation. The nurse also observes how congruent the content (what the client says) is with the process (what the client does). During the clinical interview, the nurse provides the opportunity for the client to reach goals mentioned earlier: (1) identify and explore problems relating to others, (2) discuss healthy ways of meeting emotional needs, (3) experience a satisfying interpersonal relationship, and (4) feel understood and comfortable.

Communication and interviewing techniques are acquired skills. Nurses learn to increase their ability to use communication and interviewing skills through practice and supervision by a more experienced clinician.

Health care practitioners new to the psychiatric setting often say they feel overwhelmed by the severity of some of the clients' problems and that they feel responsible for "doing something" to positively affect the emotional health of clients. It may help to know that numerous studies show the strength of the therapist-client relationship to be more important for a successful therapeutic outcome than a variety of other factors. Nicholi (1988) states that studies have borne out that the "therapist's ability to convey an intrinsic interest in the client has been found to be more important than . . . position, appearance, reputation, clinical experience, training, and technical or theoretical knowledge." This finding does not negate the importance of clinical training, skill, or experience. It does, however, emphasize the need for the nurse to convey genuine interest in another human being, without being patronizing or condescending.

Anxiety during the first interview is to be expected, as in any meeting between strangers. Clients may be anxious about their problems, about the nurse's reaction to them, or about their treatment. Students may be anxious about the client's reaction to them, their ability to provide help, what the instructor will think of them, and how they will do compared with their peers.

Students have many concerns when beginning their psychiatric experience. Two common concerns are (1) how to begin the interview and (2) what to do in response to specific client behaviors. The following section offers some basic guidelines for the first interview, identifies some common problems in clinical situations, and offers possible solutions.

How To Begin the Interview

Helping a person with an emotional or medical problem is rarely a straightforward task. The goal of assisting a client to regain psychological or physiological functional normality can be difficult to reach. Extremely important to any kind of counseling is permitting the client to set the pace of the interview, no matter how slow the progress happens to be (Parsons and Wicks 1994).

Setting

Effective communication can take place almost anywhere. However, because the quality of the interaction—whether in a clinic, a ward, an office, or the client's home—depends on the degree to which the nurse and client feel safe, establishing a setting that enhances feelings of security can be important to the helping relationship. A health care setting, a conference room, or a quiet part of the unit that has relative privacy but is within view of others is ideal. Home visits offer the nurse a valuable opportunity to assess the person in the context of everyday life.

Seating

In all settings, chairs need to be arranged so that conversation can take place in normal tones of voice and eye contact can be comfortably maintained, or avoided. For example, a nonthreatening physical environment for nurse and client would involve

- Assuming the same height—either both sitting or both standing.
- Avoiding a face-to-face stance when possible—a 90-degree angle or side by side may be less intense.
- Making sure that the door is easily accessible to both client and nurse.
- Avoiding a desk barrier between nurse and client.

Introductions

In the orientation phase, students tell the client who they are, the name of their school, the purpose of the meetings, and how long and at what time they will be meeting with the client. The issue of confidentiality is also covered at some point during the initial interview. The nurse can then ask the client how he or she would like to be addressed. This question accomplishes a number of tasks (Shea 1988), for example:

- It conveys respect.
- It gives the client direct control over an important ego issue. (Some clients do not like to be called by their last names; others dislike being called by their first names.)

How To Start

Once introductions have been made, the nurse can turn the interview over to the client by using one of a number of open-ended statements (Shea 1988; MacKinnon and Michels 1971):

- "Where should we start?"
- "Tell me a little about what has been going on with you."

- "What are some of the stresses you have been coping with recently?"
- "Tell me a little about what has been happening in the past couple of weeks."
- "Perhaps you can begin by letting me know what some of your concerns have been recently."
- "Tell me about your difficulties."

Communication can be facilitated by the appropriate use of offering leads (e.g., "Go on"), statements of acceptance (e.g., "Uh-huh"), or other conveyances of the nurse's interest.

Tactics To Avoid

The nurse needs to avoid some behaviors (Moscato 1988):

- Do not argue with, minimize, or challenge the client.
- Do not praise the client or give false reassurance.
- Do not interpret to the client or speculate on the dynamics of the client's problem.
- Do not question the client about sensitive areas.
- Do not try to "sell" the client on accepting treatment.
- Do not join in attacks the client launches on his or her mate, parents, friends, or associates.
- Do not participate in criticism of another nurse or any other staff member.

Helpful Guidelines

Some guidelines for conducting the initial interviews are offered by Meier and Davis (1989):

- Speak briefly.
- When you don't know what to say, say nothing.
- When in doubt, focus on feelings.
- Avoid advice.
- Avoid relying on questions.
- Pay attention to nonverbal cues.
- Keep the focus on the client.

Evaluation of Clinical Skills

After you have had some introductory clinical experience, you may find the facilitative skills checklist in Table 7–4 useful for evaluating your progress in interviewing skills. Note that some of the items might not be relevant with some of your clients (e.g., numbers 11 to 13 may not be possible with a person who is highly psychotic).

CLINICAL SUPERVISION AND PROCESS RECORDINGS

Communication and interviewing techniques are acquired skills. Nurses learn to increase their ability to use communication and interviewing skills through practice and through clinical supervision by a more experienced clinician. In **clinical supervision,** the focus is on the nurse's behavior in the nurse-client relationship. During clinical supervision, the nurse and the supervisor examine and analyze the nurse's feelings and reactions to the client, and how they affect the nurse-client relationship. Farkas-Cameron (1995, p. 34) states that "the nurse who does not engage in the clinical supervisory process stagnates both theoretically and clinically, while depriving him- or herself of the opportunity to advance professionally." She goes on to say that clinical supervision can be a therapeutic process for the nurse. During the process,

TABLE 7–4 FACILITATIVE SKILLS CHECKLIST

Instructions: Periodically during your clinical experience, use this checklist to identify areas needed for growth and progress made. Think of your clinical patient experiences. Indicate the extent of your agreement with each of the following statements by marking the scale: SA, strongly agree; A, agree; NS, not sure; D, disagree; SD, strongly disagree.

1. I maintain good eye contact.	SA	A	NS	D	SD
2. Most of my verbal comments follow the lead of the other person.	SA	A	NS	D	SD
3. I encourage others to talk about feelings.	SA	A	NS	D	SD
4. I am able to ask open-ended questions.	SA	A	NS	D	SD
5. I can restate and clarify a person's ideas.	SA	A	NS	D	SD
6. I can summarize in a few words the basic ideas of a long statement made by a person.	SA	A	NS	D	SD
7. I can make statements that reflect the person's feelings.	SA	A	NS	D	SD
8. I can share my feelings relevant to the discussion when appropriate to do so.	SA	A	NS	D	SD
9. I am able to give feedback.	SA	A	NS	D	SD
10. At least 75% or more of my responses help enhance and facilitate communication.	SA	A	NS	D	SD
11. I can assist the person to list some alternatives available.	SA	A	NS	D	SD
12. I can assist the person to identify some goals that are specific and observable.	SA	A	NS	D	SD
13. I can assist the person to specify at least one next step that might be taken toward the goal.	SA	A	NS	D	SD

Adapted from Myrick, D., and Erney, T. (1984). *Caring and sharing* (p. 154). Copyright © 1984 by Educational Media Corporation.

TABLE 7–5 SEGMENT OF A PROCESS NOTE

NURSE	CLIENT	COMMENTS	FEELINGS
"Good morning, Mr. L."		*Therapeutic.* Giving recognition. Acknowledging a client by name can enhance self-esteem and communicates that the client is viewed as an individual by the nurse.	
	"Who are you and where the devil am I?" *Looks around with a confused look on his face—quickly sits on the edge of the bed.*		
"I am Mrs. V. I am a student nurse from X college, and you are at Mt. Sinai Hospital. I would like to spend some time with you today."		*Therapeutic.* Giving information. Informing the client of facts needed to make decisions or come to realistic conclusions. *Therapeutic.* Offering self. Making oneself available to the client.	
	"What am I doing here? How did I get here?" *Spoken in a loud, demanding voice.*		
"You were brought in by your wife last night after swallowing a bottle of aspirin. You had to have your stomach pumped."		*Therapeutic.* Giving information. Giving needed facts so that the client can orient himself and better evaluate his situation.	
	"Oh . . . yeah." *Silence for two minutes. Shoulders slumped, Mr. L. stares at the floor and drops his head and eyes.*		
"You seem upset, Mr. L." "What are you thinking about?"		*Therapeutic.* Making observations. He looks sad. *Therapeutic.* Giving broad openings in an attempt to get at his feelings.	
	"Yeah, I just remembered . . . I wanted to kill myself." *Said in a low tone almost to himself.*		
"Oh Mr. L., you have so much to live for. You have such a loving family."		*Nontherapeutic.* Defending. *Nontherapeutic.* Introducing an unrelated topic.	I felt overwhelmed. I didn't know what to say—his talking about killing himself made me nervous. I could have said, "You must be very upset" (verbalizing the implied) or "Tell me more about this" (exploring).
	"What do you know about my life? You want to know about my family? . . . My wife is leaving me, that's what." *Faces the nurse with an angry expression on his face and speaks in loud tones.*		
"I didn't know. You must be terribly upset by her leaving."		*Therapeutic.* Reflective. Observing the angry tone and content of the client's message and reflecting back the client's feelings.	

TABLE 7–6 COMMON CLIENT BEHAVIORS AND NURSE RESPONSES

POSSIBLE REACTIONS BY NURSE	USEFUL RESPONSES BY NURSE
What To Do if the Client Cries	
The nurse may feel uncomfortable and experience increased anxiety or feel somehow responsible for making the person cry.	The nurse should stay with the client and reinforce that it is all right to cry. Often, it is at that time that feelings are closest to the surface and can be best identified. "You seem ready to cry." "You are still upset about your brother's death." "What are you thinking right now?" The nurse offers tissues when appropriate.
What To Do if the Client Asks the Nurse To Keep a Secret	
The nurse may feel conflict because the nurse wants the client to share important information but is unsure about making such a promise.	The nurse *cannot* make such a promise. The information may be important to the health or safety of the client or others. "I cannot make that promise. It might be important for me to share it with other staff." The client then decides whether to share the information or not.
What To Do if the Client Leaves Before the Session is Over	
The nurse may feel rejected, thinking it was something that he or she did. The nurse may experience increased anxiety or feel abandoned by the client.	Some clients are not able to relate for long periods of time without experiencing an increase in anxiety. On the other hand, the client may be testing the nurse. "I will wait for you here for 15 minutes, until our time is up." During this time, the nurse does not engage in conversation with any other client or even with the staff. When time is up, the nurse approaches the client, tells him or her the time is up, and restates the day and time he or she will see the client again.
What To Do if Another Client Interrupts During Time with Your Selected Client	
The nurse may feel a conflict. The nurse does not want to appear rude. Sometimes the nurse tries to engage both clients in conversation. 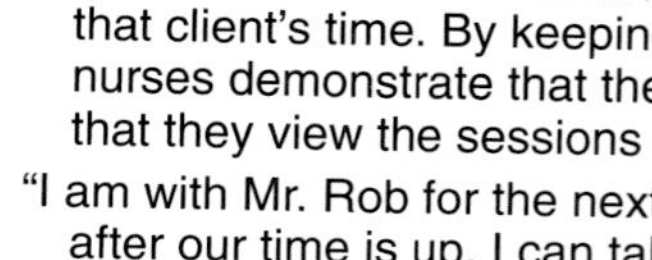	The time the nurse had contracted with a selected client is that client's time. By keeping their part of the contract, nurses demonstrate that they mean what they say and that they view the sessions as important. "I am with Mr. Rob for the next 20 minutes. At 10 AM, after our time is up, I can talk to you for 5 minutes."
What To Do if the Client Says He Wants to Kill Himself	
The nurse may feel overwhelmed or responsible to "talk the client out of it." The nurse may pick up some of the client's feelings of hopelessness. 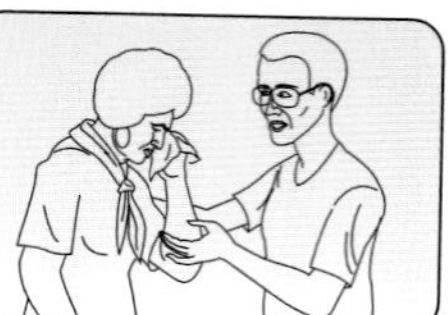	The nurse tells the client that this is serious, that he or she does not want harm to come to the client, and that this information needs to be shared with other staff. "This is very serious, Mr. Lamb. I do not want any harm to come to you. I will have to share this with the other staff." The nurse can then discuss with the client the feelings and circumstances that led up to this decision. (Refer to Chapter 24 for strategies in suicide intervention.)

Continued

TABLE 7–6 COMMON CLIENT BEHAVIORS AND NURSE RESPONSES *(Continued)*

POSSIBLE REACTIONS BY NURSE	USEFUL RESPONSES BY NURSE
What To Do if the Client Says She Does Not Want to Talk	
The nurse new to this situation may feel rejected or ineffectual. 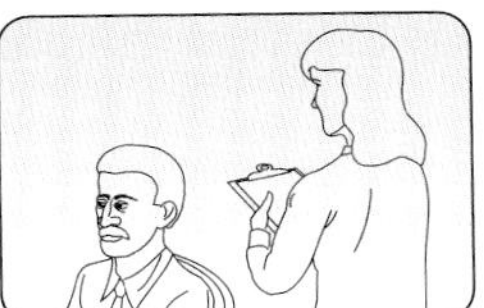	At first, the nurse might say something to this effect: "It's all right. I would like to spend time with you. We don't have to talk." The nurse might spend short, frequent periods (e.g., 5 minutes) with the client throughout the day. "Our 5 minutes is up. I'll be back at 10 AM and stay with you 5 more minutes." This gives the client the opportunity to understand that the nurse means what he or she says and is back on time consistently. It also gives the client time between visits to assess the nurse and perhaps feel less threatened.
What To Do if the Client Seeks to Prolong the Interview	
Sometimes, clients open up dynamic or "juicy" topics just before the interview time is up. This is often to test or manipulate the nurse. The nurse might feel tempted to extend scheduled time or might not want to hurt the client's feelings. 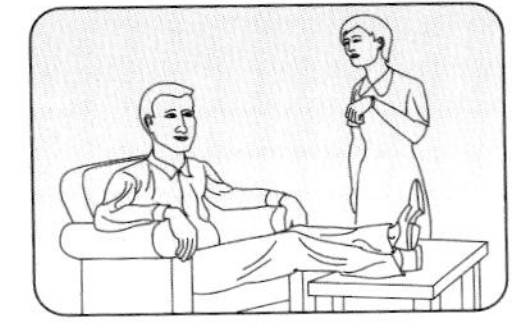	The nurse sets limits, and restates and reinforces the original contract. The nurse states that they will use the issues for the next session. "Our time is up now, Mr. Jones, This would be a good place to start at our next session, which is Wednesday at 10 AM."
What To Do if the Client Gives the Nurse a Present	
The nurse may feel uncomfortable when offered a gift. The meaning needs to be examined. Is the gift 1. A way of getting better care? 2. A way to maintain self-esteem? 3. A way of making the nurse feel guilty? 4. A sincere expression of thanks? 5. A cultural expectation? 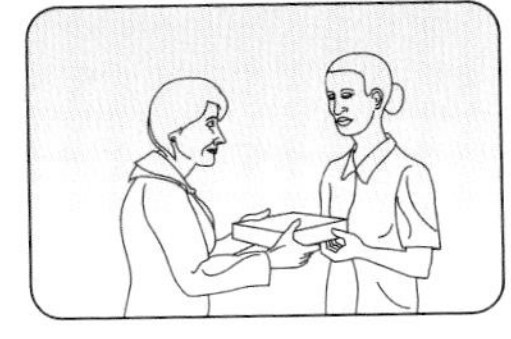	Possible guidelines: If the gift is expensive, the best policy is to perhaps graciously refuse. If it is inexpensive and 1. given *at the end* of hospitalization when a relationship has developed, graciously accept. 2. given *at the beginning* of hospitalization, graciously refuse and explore the meaning behind the present. "Thank you, but it is our job to care for our clients. Are you concerned that some aspect of your care will be overlooked?" If the gift is money, it may be best to graciously refuse.
What To Do if the Client Asks You a Personal Question	
The nurse may think that it is rude not to answer the client's question. *or* A new nurse might feel relieved to put off having to start the interview. *or* The nurse may feel put on the spot and want to leave the situation New nurses are often manipulated by a client to change roles. This keeps the focus off the client and prevents the building of a relationship. 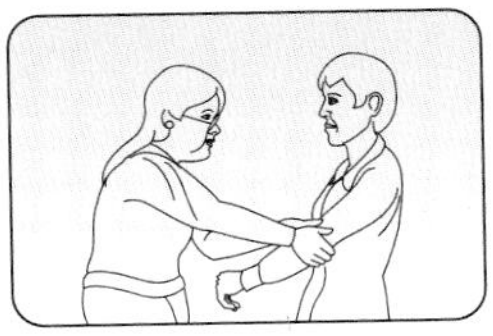	The nurse may or may not answer the client's query. If the nurse decides to answer a natural question, he or she answers in a word or two, then refocuses back on the client. P: Are you married? N: Yes, do you have a spouse? P: Do you have any children? N: This time is for you—tell me about yourself. P: You can just tell me if you any children. N: This is your time to focus on your concerns. Tell me something about your family.

feelings and concerns are ventilated as they relate to the developing nurse-client relationship. The opportunity to examine your interactions, obtain insights, and devise alternative strategies for dealing with various clinical issues enhances your clinical growth and minimizes frustration and burnout. Clinical supervision is a necessary professional activity that fosters professional growth and helps to minimize the development of nontherapeutic nurse-client relationships.

The best way to increase communication and interviewing skills is to review clinical interactions exactly as they occur. This process offers students the opportunity to identify themes and patterns in their own, as well as their client's, communication. The student also learns to deal with the variety of situations that arise in the clinical interview.

Perhaps the best way of reviewing nurse-client interactions is to view a videotape, which reveals the nonverbal as well as the verbal communications between both parties. The second-best method of capturing the interaction between nurse and client is through an audiotape recording. Unfortunately, these methods are often not possible. The most common form of evaluating the interactions in academic settings is through process recordings.

The use of process recordings is a popular way to identify patterns in the student's and the client's communication. **Process recordings** are written records of a segment from the nurse-client session that reflects as closely as possible the verbal and nonverbal behaviors of both client and nurse. Process recordings have some disadvantages because they rely on memory and are subject to distortions. However, they can be a useful tool for identifying communication patterns. It is usually best if the student can write notes verbatim (word for word) in a private area immediately after the interaction has taken place. Sometimes, a clinician takes notes during the interview. This practice also has disadvantages. One disadvantage is that it may be distracting for both interviewer and client; another is that some clients (especially those with a paranoid disorder) may resent or misunderstand the nurse's intent. Table 7–5 shows a segment of a process note. Nurses record their words and the client's words, identify whether the responses are therapeutic or not, and recall their emotions at the time.

WHAT TO DO IN RESPONSE TO SPECIFIC CLIENT BEHAVIORS

Often, students new to the mental health setting are concerned about being in situations that they may not know how to handle. These concerns are universal and often arise in the clinical setting. Table 7–6 identifies common client behaviors (e.g., crying, asking the nurse to keep a secret, threatening to commit suicide). The table gives an example of an appropriate response, the rationale for the response, and a possible verbal statement. Read the table, paying particular attention to the rationales for responses. The exact words will depend on the situation, but understanding the rationale will help you to apply the information later on.

SUMMARY

Communication is the foundation for any nurse-client relationship. When effective communication skills are a genuine part of the helping process and are applied with concern and respect for the other person, they can be a dynamic tool in working effectively with people. Berlo's model has five parts: stimulus, sender, message, medium, and receiver. Feedback is a vital component in the communication process for validating the accuracy of the sender's message.

A number of factors can minimize or enhance the communication process. For example, differences in culture, language, and knowledge levels; noise; lack of privacy; the presence of others; and the expectations of others can all influence communication.

There are verbal and nonverbal elements in communication; the nonverbal often plays the larger role in identifying a person's message. Verbal communication consists of all words a person speaks. Nonverbal communication consists of the behaviors displayed by an individual, in contrast to the actual content of speech.

Communication also has two levels. One is the content level (verbal) and the other the process level (nonverbal behavior). When content is congruent with process, the communication is said to be healthy. When the verbal message is not reinforced by the communicator's actions, the message is ambiguous; we call this a double (or mixed) message.

Cultural backgrounds (as well as individual differences) have a great deal to do with what nonverbal behavior means to different individuals. The degree of eye contact and the use of touch are two nonverbal behaviors that can be misunderstood across cultures.

There are a number of accepted therapeutic (messages that facilitate communication) and nontherapeutic (messages that impede communication) techniques. Some nurses are most effective when they can use nonthreatening and open-ended communication techniques with clients during everyday encounters.

Whether you are working in a psychiatric unit, in a clinic, or in the home, you will be confronted with an array of behaviors during your student experience. It is useful to be somewhat prepared for specific client behaviors (e.g., clients cry, ask you to keep a secret, or say they want to kill themselves). Effective communication is a skill that develops over time and is a crucial tool for all nurses in all settings all of the time.

REFERENCES

Berlo, D. K. (1960). *The process of communication*. San Francisco: Reinhart Press.
Collins, M. (1983). *Communication in health care: The human connection in the life cycle* (2nd ed.). St. Louis: C. V. Mosby.
Dee, V. (1991). How can we become more aware of culturally specific body language and use this awareness therapeutically? *Journal of Psychosocial Nursing*, 29(11):39–40.
Egan, G. (1994). *The skilled helper: A problem-management approach* (5th ed.). Pacific Grove, CA: Brooks/Cole.
Farkas-Cameron, M. M. (1995). Clinical supervision in psychiatric nursing. *Journal of Psychosocial Nursing and Mental Health Services*, 33(2):40–47.
Geissler, E. M. (1993). *Pocket guide to cultural assessment*. St. Louis: C. V. Mosby.
Grier, W. H., and Cobbs, P. M. (1968). *Black rage*. New York: Basic Books.
Hall, E. T. (1977). *Beyond culture*. Garden City, NJ: Anchor Press.
Hays, J. S., and Larson, K. H. (1963). *Interacting with patients*. New York: Macmillan.
Ingram, C. A. (1991). How can we become more aware of culturally specific body language and use this awareness therapeutically? *Journal of Psychosocial Nursing*, 29(11):40–41.
Johnson, B. (1964). The relationship between verbal patterns of nursing students and therapeutic effectiveness. *Nursing Research*, 13:339.
Lu, F. G., et al. (1995). Issues in the assessment and diagnosis of culturally diverse individuals. In J. M. Oldhan and M. B. Riba (Eds.), *Review of Psychiatry* (Vol. 14) (pp. 477–510). Washington, DC: American Psychiatric Press.
MacKinnon, R. A., and Michels, R. (1971). *The psychiatric interview in clinical practice*. Philadelphia: W. B. Saunders.
Meier, S. T., and Davis, S. R. (1989). *The elements of counseling* (2nd ed.). Pacific Grove, CA: Brooks/Cole.
Moscato, B. (1988). The one-to-one relationship. In H. S. Wilson and C. S. Kneisel (Eds.), *Psychiatric Nursing* (3rd ed.). Menlo Park, CA: Addison-Wesley.
Myrick, R. D., and Erney, T. (1984). *Caring and sharing*. Minneapolis: Educational Media Corporation.
Nicholi, A. M. (1988). The therapist-patient relationship. In A. M. Nicholi (Ed.), *The new Harvard guide to psychiatry*. Cambridge, MA: Belknap Press of Harvard University.
Parsons, R. D., and Wicks, R. J. (1994). *Counseling strategies and intervention techniques for human services* (4th ed.). Needham Heights, MA: Allyn & Bacon.
Peplau, H. E. (1952). *Interpersonal relations in nursing*. New York: G. P. Putnam & Sons.
Peplau, H. E. (1962). Interpersonal techniques: The crux of psychiatric nursing. *American Journal of Nursing*, 62:50.
Poole, V. C., et al (1995). Cultural aspects of psychiatric nursing. In N. L. Keltner, et al. (Eds.), *Psychiatric nursing* (2nd ed.) (pp. 185, 190).
Ramirez, D. (1989). Mexican American children and adolescents. In J. Gibbs et al. (Eds.), *Children of color: Psychological interventions with minority youth*. San Francisco: Jossey-Bass.
Schulman, E. D. (1974). *Intervention in human services*. St. Louis: C. V. Mosby.
Shea, S. C. (1988). *Psychiatric interviewing: The art of understanding*. Philadelphia: W. B. Saunders.
Siantz, M. L. (1991). How can we become more aware of culturally specific body language and use this awareness therapeutically? *Journal of Psychosocial Nursing*, 29(11):38–39.

SELF-STUDY AND CRITICAL THINKING

True or false

1. ______ A stimulant is the medium by which a message is sent.
2. ______ Feedback can indicate whether a message has been correctly interpreted.
3. ______ Communication is a reciprocal process.
4. ______ Emotional factors, intellectual factors, and social factors play no part in accurate transmission or interpretation of communications.
5. ______ Content expressed in the nurse-client interaction refers to what the client has already spoken.
6. ______ Process messages that are expressed in the nurse-client interaction refer to nonverbal communications.

Place a V (verbal) or an N (nonverbal) next to the appropriate communication.

7. ______ Hair is uncombed and stringy; clothes have food stains.
8. ______ The person states that his body feels heavy.
9. ______ The person licks her lips and grimaces while talking to the nurse.
10. ______ The person writes a note to the nurse before she leaves for the day.

Place a T (therapeutic) or an N (nontherapeutic) next to the appropriate communication and name the response.

11. ______ I know exactly how you feel. R __________
12. ______ I am not sure I understand what you mean. R __________

13. ________ I noticed you changed into a different dress this evening. R ____________

14. ________ You should call the doctor and tell him these pills make you dizzy. R ____________

15. ________ Tell me more about your bad dream. R ____________

16. ________ Student: I had to repeat Nursing I, and for a long time I felt like a failure. R ____________

Teacher: That must have been very painful for you. R ____________

17. ________ I observed several strengths that you bring to this difficult situation. R ____________

Choose the correct answer.

18. During your first visit with a restless young man, you notice that he does not make eye contact with you through most of the interview. You correctly assume that
    A. He is not to be trusted in what he says because he is avoiding honest communication.
    B. He is really feeling very sad inside and can't look you in the eye.
    C. You need more background data before making an assumption as to the meaning of his behavior.
    D. He is very shy and you have to be careful to go very slowly.

19. You are working with a young Asian woman who seems depressed. You try to cheer her up by being casual and humorous. You notice that at one point the woman smiles. You
    A. Have succeeded in reaching her and are on the way to cheering her up.
    B. Can now outline a plan of care that involves distraction and humor.
    C. Have identified an approach that would be useful in all situations.
    D. Need to seek supervision immediately since your approach is not acceptable.

20. When working with a woman for the first time who has just lost her son in a car accident, you feel so sorry for her that you instinctively reach out and touch her. Your response
    A. Is empathetic and will encourage the woman to continue to express her feelings.
    B. Will frighten her, and she may feel you are being intrusive and overstepping boundaries.
    C. Is perhaps premature until you understand how the use of touch might be interpreted by her both culturally and individually.
    D. Is threatening, and one never uses touch in a nurse-client relationship.

21. You are a white male nursing student talking to a black male client. When he says to you "How could you understand? You are white in a white world," your best response would be to
    A. Explain that we all go through the same experiences and that you do understand.
    B. Ask him to give you an example of one thing that he thinks you couldn't understand.
    C. Reassure him that you are being trained to deal with people from all cultures.
    D. Gently change the topic to one that is less emotionally laden.

22. You wish to use a clarifying technique with a client who is telling you that her mother is always putting her down. You would say

    A. "Uh huh . . . I hear what you are saying . . . go on."
    B. "Mothers and daughters have very complex relationships."
    C. "Your mother always puts you down . . . ?"
    D. "Tell me about one time that your mother put you down."

23. What is the most helpful response to a fellow classmate who tells you he is thinking of dropping out of nursing school because it is too stressful and he gets down sometimes?

    A. "Oh, John, I do know what you are going through. The stress is terrible."
    B. "You have two more semesters . . . just stick it out and you'll be glad you did."
    C. "Why would you drop out now when you only have two semesters to go?"
    D. "It is stressful. What do you find most stressful?"

24. You are talking to a young man and you have 5 minutes to go in your session with him. He has been silent and sullen most of the session, and has been staring at the floor for the last 15 minutes. A troubled young woman comes up to you and says she really wants to talk to you. You would

    A. End the session, since it is going badly, and spend time with the young woman, since she really needs you.
    B. Ask your instructor to give you another client, since this young man is really not interested in talking about his problems.
    C. Ask her to join you both. She might have problems similar to those of your young male client and perhaps this will get him to participate more readily.
    D. Tell the young woman that you have 5 more minutes with your client, and at XX time you can spend 5 (10) minutes with her.

Critical thinking

25. You are attempting to conduct a clinical interview with a very withdrawn client. You have tried silence and open-ended statements to engage the client, but all you get is one-word answers. What other actions could you take at this time?

26. You have been spending time with a client for 5 weeks, twice a week, at a community mental health center. Your client has been upset over the diagnosis that her son has AIDS, and you and she have been spending a lot of time discussing many of the painful issues she is presently dealing with. She is going away for 3 weeks to visit her son in Seattle, and she brings you a leather-covered notebook "to keep your client notes in." How would you handle this situation? If she had brought you the "present" during the first week, how would you have handled it?

27. Keep a log for one half-hour a day of your communication pattern (a tape recorder is ideal). Pick out four communication techniques that you notice you use frequently and that are identified as "nontherapeutic." In your log, rewrite those nontherapeutic techniques and replace them with statements that would better facilitate discussion of thoughts and feelings. Share your log and discuss the changes you are working on with one other classmate.

8

Psychiatric Nursing in the Acute Psychiatric Hospital Setting

THOMAS WENZKA

MARGARET SWISHER

OUTLINE

KEY TERMS AND CONCEPTS

The key terms and concepts listed here also appear in bold where they are defined or discussed in this chapter.

managed care

case manager

critical or clinical pathways (care MAPS)

elopement

codes

OBJECTIVES

After studying this chapter, the reader will be able to

1. Analyze the psychiatric hospital experience from the client's perspective.
2. Explain how the mental health team collaborates to plan and implement care for the hospitalized client.
3. Describe the role of the nurse as advocate and provider of care for the client.
4. Explain the interrelationships among the managed care system, interdisciplinary care MAPS (critical/clinical pathways), and the role of the nurse as case manager.
5. Discuss the managerial and coordinating roles of nursing on an inpatient acute care unit.
6. Document your nurse's notes using three of the four documentation formats described here.

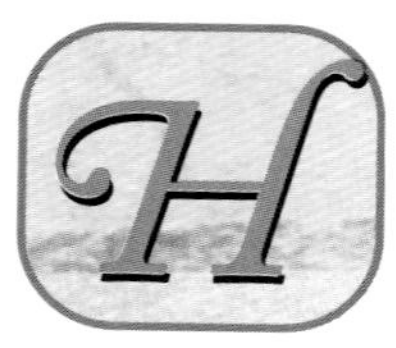

ospitalization is only one option for the treatment of mental disorders and emotional crises. It is now reserved for those conditions that cannot be safely treated in less restrictive and less costly settings. In the mid-1980s clients were admitted to inpatient care for initial evaluation, for intensive therapy, and even for respite from stressful situations. Changes in treatment today arise from the evolution of managed care, the principal model for delivery of health care services today.

Managed care is a generic term that refers to an organized system that integrates the issues of cost management and quality care. Health maintenance organizations (HMOs), preferred provider organizations (PPOs), and managed care options from government and private indemnity health insurance plans are the basic types of managed care organizations that represent this focus. In managed care, the insurer and the provider agree to a binding contract that delineates restrictions on the variables of treatment (e.g., length of stay, use of resources, admission and discharge criteria). Most psychiatric care providers negotiate an arrangement with multiple managed care insurers to provide services for a specific cost—usually a reduced or average cost. To provide care at this reduced cost, psychiatric hospitals must restructure their care delivery system to avoid unnecessary expenditures while striving to maintain standards of quality care and successful client outcomes. The provider also becomes a managed care organization, modifying its treatment system to deliver efficient, effective care within the guidelines established by the contractual agreement (Hicks et al. 1993). Thus, managed care also refers to the organization of a care process by any health care provider.

Hospitals that opt for a managed care approach to treatment assemble multidisciplinary teams that analyze the care process for similar client cases, usually diagnosis-related groups (DRGs). This analysis yields information about the patterns of care (e.g., lengths of stay, client outcomes, treatments and services utilized). The goals of a managed care initiative by the health care provider are to streamline the care process, eliminate obstacles to quality client outcomes, and avoid unnecessary costs (Abbot 1993; Etheredge 1989). Although psychiatric disorders are not included in the DRG classification, specific disorders, symptoms, or behaviors are frequently utilized to establish these patterns of resource consumption and reasonable outcomes. Today, health care providers must develop a managed care approach, since most reimbursement, whether or not it is from a managed care company, is set in advance. Providers who do not "manage care" may face financial losses and insolvency. Thus, in the present era of managed care, inpatient hospitalization must be justified by at least one of the following:

1. Clear risk of client danger to self or others
2. Dangerous decompensation of a client under long-term treatment
3. Failure of outpatient treatment with a clearly demonstrable need for more intensive and structured treatment to avoid harmful consequences
4. Medical need, either unassociated with psychiatric treatment (such as intractable pain experienced by a depressed person) or associated with treatment (such as serious adverse reactions to a psychotropic medication)

These criteria for acute care hospitalization are common to many third-party payers. Exceptions may occur with a few insurance companies or with clients who are paying for their own hospitalization. Currently, therefore, goals for acute psychiatric hospitalization tend to include

1. Prevention of self-harm to the client.
2. Prevention of harm to others by the client.
3. Stabilization of crisis (but only to the point where the client can manage with support from outpatient treatment sources).
4. Initiation or modification of a psychotropic medication regimen for clients requiring careful titration or observation.
5. Brief, specific problem solving designed to enable the client to gain or regain a state of compensation.
6. Rapid establishment of a plan for outpatient therapy.

The following two vignettes demonstrate the application of these criteria.

- Allen G., a 49-year-old computer programmer, has arrived at the emergency mental health center in tears, stating that he has had suicidal thoughts after losing his job during corporate restructuring. He has been divorced for the past 6 months. The clinical nurse specialist who interviews him determines that his risk of suicide is not high at this time. (Refer to Chapter 24 for assessment of suicide risk.) Allen responds to crisis counseling and agrees to an appointment for the next morning at an outpatient facility. The nurse assists Allen to identify supports and to begin to recognize coping skills that he has used to survive past crises. No hospitalization is required.
- Jordan S., age 31, arrives at the emergency mental health center in the company of a law enforcement officer. Jordan is nearly mute, so the officer explains to the clinical nurse specialist that Jordan was stopped from jumping off a bridge. After establishing a relationship with Jordan, the nurse determines that he has been treated for a severe and persistent mental disorder for the past 14 years and that his family has refused to support him in any way for the past 2 years. Jordan continually states that "God wants me to

liquidate myself." After consultation with the attending psychiatrist, the nurse specialist arranges for voluntary admission, and Jordan agrees.

RIGHTS OF THE HOSPITALIZED CLIENT

People, although hospitalized, retain their rights as citizens. The psychiatric team has an obligation to balance the client's needs for safety with his or her rights as a citizen. Nearly all mental health facilities provide a written statement of these rights, often with copies of applicable state laws attached. Students are also advised to become familiar with the client's handbook and the policy and procedure manual on the unit. Each student should be familiar with the unit's procedures for (1) suicide precautions, (2) seclusion and restraints, and (3) client elopement. (Refer again to Chapter 4 for a full account of clients' legal rights.) Box 8–1 gives an overview of a patient's rights. A listing of these should be displayed prominently on the unit. In addition, clients are frequently given a copy of their rights.

BOX 8–1 SAMPLE STATEMENT OF PATIENT'S RIGHTS

TYPICAL ITEMS INCLUDED IN HOSPITAL STATEMENT OF PATIENT'S RIGHTS

1. Right to be treated with dignity.
2. Right to be involved in treatment planning and decisions.
3. Right to refuse treatment, including medications.
4. Right to request to leave the hospital, even against medical advice.
5. Right to be protected against the possible impulse to harm oneself or others that might occur as a result of a mental disorder.
6. Right to the benefit of the legally prescribed process of an evaluation occurring over a limited period (in most states, 72 hours) in the event of a request for discharge against medical advice that may lead to harm to self or others.
7. Right to legal counsel.
8. Right to vote.
9. Right to communicate privately by telephone and in person.
10. Right to informed consent.
11. Right to confidentiality regarding one's disorder and treatment.
12. Right to choose or refuse visitors.
13. Right to be informed of research and to refuse to participate.
14. Right to the least restrictive means of treatment.
15. Right to send and receive mail and to be present during any inspection of packages received.
16. Right to keep personal belongings unless they are dangerous.
17. Right to lodge a complaint through a plainly publicized procedure.
18. Right to participate in religious worship.

- Helen Weaver, RN, C, is a certified psychiatric nurse. She has just heard the morning report, learning about the conditions of all the clients on the unit and about the status of the treatment community. Four clients have been assigned to her care during the coming shift. Upon hearing that Jordan is to be readmitted to her acute care unit, Ms. Weaver volunteers to conduct the admissions process, because Jordan had been one of her primary clients during his previous three hospital admissions.
- Ms. Weaver proceeds to interview Jordan. While her assessment priority is his risk for self-harm, she also gathers data regarding his biological, social, cognitive, and emotional status. The physician is contacted for orders based on these data. A plan of care is initiated.
- On the basis of her assessment of Jordan's current ability to understand, Ms. Weaver ensures that Jordan has freely consented to hospitalization and explains to him his rights as a hospitalized client. He is given a copy of the hospital's Patient's Bill of Rights and shown where it is displayed on the unit.
- Jordan is oriented to the unit and to the schedule of activities. With the assistance of a client who is designated the "host," Ms. Weaver introduces Jordan to a few of the other clients. Because of Jordan's risk for self-harm, Ms. Weaver maintains a distance of no more than an arm's length from him during these activities. After Jordan demonstrates some degree of comfort with his new situation, Ms. Weaver delegates responsibility for keeping Jordan under close watch to another staff member. Ms. Weaver then documents her assessment and plan. This initial plan will guide Jordan's care until the treatment team meets to consider his needs.

Refer to Chapter 24 for suicide precautions.

INTERDISCIPLINARY TEAMWORK AND CARE MANAGEMENT

The client's care is planned and implemented by a team composed of nurses, social workers, counselors, psychologists, occupational and activities therapists, psychiatrists, medical physicians, mental health workers, pharmacists, and other members of the hospital's health care team, according to the client's need.

Each discipline is responsible for gathering data and participating in the planning of care. For the newly admitted client, this can prove extremely stressful or threatening. The team, often upon the recommendation of the nurse, must consider the need for timing. These assessments should balance the urgency of the need for data against the client's ability to tolerate the assessments. Often, the assessments of the intake worker and the nurse provide the basis for initial care. In most settings the psychiatrist must assess and provide orders within a limited time frame. Medical problems are usually referred to a primary care physician or specialist, who assesses the client and consults with the unit physicians.

The various disciplines meet as soon as possible to formulate or select a plan of care that reflects the consensus of the team. The plan reflects nursing process or an interdisciplinary path-based approach to care. The latter approach, known also as a *clinical* or *critical pathway,* is a predetermined method for guiding care and measuring the client's progress based on the client's psychiatric diagnosis (Beyea 1996). The team either composes the plan of care or selects the clinical pathway, revising the plan or making clinical decisions if the client's progress differs from the expected outcomes. Many settings utilize a nursing case manager to monitor and facilitate the achievement of outcomes along the critical pathway. It is important for the student nurse to have an understanding of case management and critical pathways, since both are becoming common in health care settings.

Case management by nurses has evolved within the nursing profession to achieve managed care objectives, as discussed in Chapter 1. Insurance and rehabilitation companies employ case managers; hospitals may establish a case management department or develop a case management role to replace primary nursing as the practice model within their organization (Etheredge 1989). As we saw in Chapter 1, **case managers** are client advocates who interact with and assess clients and family members, coordinate services appropriate to the client, monitor the delivery of services, and evaluate the outcome for the client (Cohen and Cesta 1993). Cost-effective treatment leading to the best outcome for the client is the primary consideration. The American Nurses' Association (1988, p. 1) has described case management as encompassing the elements of "health assessment, planning, procurement, delivery, and coordination of services, and monitoring to assure that the multiple service needs of the client are met." The goal of case management is to facilitate comprehensive quality care from admission through discharge while meeting the fiscal objectives of the health care providers. Although social workers and counselors may be case managers, nurses are recognized as being "in a key position to implement case management and managed care by virtue of their clinical skills and the nature of their interactions with clients and other members of the health care team" (Etheredge 1989, p. 13).

Case management has been recognized as a useful approach for the severely and persistently mentally ill in a community setting (Forchuk et al. 1989; Intagliata 1982), since it fosters success outside the hospital. Recidivism by the client with long-term illness (the "revolving door" problem) refers to the frequent readmission of these clients to the acute care hospital. Case managers can establish enduring relationships with long-term clients, facilitate their involvement in outpatient settings, and help avoid the crises that result in readmission to the acute care hospital.

As described in Chapter 1, **critical or clinical pathways** and **care MAPS** provide a tool that assists the case manager as well as the multidisciplinary team in prospectively detailing the course of daily treatments and interventions for a particular psychiatric diagnosis or behavior problem. Beyea (1996, p. 3) defines critical pathways as "interdisciplinary client care plans that delineate assessments, interventions, treatments, and outcomes for specific health-related conditions across a designated time line." When the New England Medical Center Hospitals first developed the nursing case management model in 1985, critical pathways were described as "one-page, user-friendly tools . . . that focus primarily on the key tasks or technical aspects of care that must be completed within a specified time frame if cost-effective care is to be achieved" (Etheredge 1989, p. 76). Since that time, critical pathways have appeared in this format as well as in the more comprehensive format described by Beyea (1996), and are replacing traditional nursing care plans. Care MAPS, an acronym for multidisciplinary action plans (Del Togno-Armanasco et al. 1993), are conceptually identical to the expanded critical pathway and can also be found in psychiatric hospitals as a substitute for nursing care plans. Most hospitals customize their critical/clinical pathways, or care MAPS, to meet their individual needs, and may include a format to document completion of interventions and variances from the pathway on the critical/clinical pathway tool. See Box 8–2 for a sample interdisciplinary treatment plan. Many of the clinical chapters contain examples of actual clinical/critical pathways that are used by members of the health care team. We are moving fast in this age of managed care, and a cautious and thoughtful approach to critical pathways is advised. See Unit II, "a Nurse Speaks," for just such an analysis of pros and cons.

The use of clinical or critical pathways in case management is seen as efficient for the multidisciplinary team (Cohen and Cesta 1993). Nurses, as well as other clinical members of the team, participate as case managers, or as collaborators with the case manager. Because this approach allows for monitoring by means of computers, research into cost-effective treatment measures and containment of costs can more easily be carried out by providers and third-party payers.

In many inpatient settings, nurses convene and lead planning meetings. This nursing leadership reflects the holistic nature of nursing as well as the fact that nursing is the discipline that is present on the unit at all times. However, a variety of disciplines assume responsibility for implementing portions of the plan. See Box 8–3 for a brief description of the roles of other members of the health team.

BOX 8–2 SAMPLE INTERDISCIPLINARY TREATMENT PLAN

Date: 6/19/98 — INTERDISCIPLINARY TREATMENT PLAN — Page: A1

Axis: 1:	ICD No.	Axis IV Stressors
Maj. depr., sing. epis, severe, without psychotic feat.	*296.23*	*Conflictual relationships* *Family discord*
Axis II:	**ICD No.**	**Axis V**
Axis II deferred	0.00	**Current GAF:** *20*
Axis III Dx: *None*		**Highest GAF:** *50*

Assets	Problem	Date Active	Date Resolved
Domicile *Employment* *Good physical health* *Intelligence*	*Depressed mood* *Suicidal ideas/impulses*	*6/1/98* *6/1/98*	

Date	Legal Status	Expiration
6/5/98	*VOL*	*8/3/98*

Review Date	Participation
6/8/98	*Pt. unable to collaborate in treatment planning*

Problem: *Depressed mood*

Objective	Term	Date Achieved
Attends and participates in 2 activities daily (group therapy, movement group)	*Short term*	
Eats 3 balanced meals a day (1800 kcal)	*Short term*	
Mood will be free of depressive features in 2 weeks	*Short term*	
Sleeping 6–8 hours a night	*Short term*	
Will state 3 alternative strategies for managing stress	*Long term*	
Will state 3 feelings related to having a mental illness	*Long term*	
Will remain in outpatient treatment for 1 year	*Long term*	

Methods: *Activity therapy groups daily (AI)*
Fluoxetine 20mg PO qd (MD)
Group therapy 3 times a week (RN),
Individual therapy 3 times a week (CNS)

Problem: *Suicidal ideas/impulses*

Objective:	Term	Date Achieved
Absence of suicide attempts	*Short term*	
Cessation of suicidal impulses	*Short term*	
Will state 2 alternatives to inflicting harm to self	*Short term*	
Will immediately notify staff of suicidal thoughts or impulses	*Short term*	
Will state 3 plans for the future	*Long term*	

Methods: *Staff will assess patient at arm's length (RN)*
Staff will contract with patient not to hurt self (CNS, RN)
Primary RN will meet with patient every shift to discuss issues (RN)

Primary Nurse: *Fatima Ramos, RN, MS, CS*
Primary Therapist: *Susan L. Goldstein, MS, RN, C*
Social Worker: *Iris Gordon*
Activities Therapist: *Carol Gaffney*
Other:

From St. Barnabas Hospital, Bronx, NY and Ramas, F., and Gladstein, S.L. (1996). Documentation. In S. Lego, *Psychiatric nursing: A comprehensive reference* (p. 489). Philadelphia; JB Lippincott.

BOX 8–3 OTHER MEMBERS OF THE MENTAL HEALTH TEAM

Social workers	Basic social workers assist the client to prepare a support system that will promote mental health upon discharge from the hospital. This includes contacts with day treatment, employers, sources of financial aid, and landlords. Licensed clinical social workers are prepared in individual, family, and group therapies, often as primary care providers.
Counselors	Counselors, prepared in disciplines such as psychology, rehabilitation counseling, or addiction counseling, may augment the treatment plan by co-leading groups, providing basic supportive counseling, or assisting in psychoeducational and recreational activities.
Psychologists	According to their master or doctoral preparation, psychologists conduct psychological testing, provide consultation for the team, and offer direct services such as specialized individual, family, or marital therapies.
Occupational, recreational, art, music, and dance therapists	On the basis of their specialist preparations, these therapists assist the clients to gain skills that help them cope more effectively, to gain or retain employment, to use leisure time to the benefit of their mental health, and to express themselves in healthy ways.
Psychiatrists	Depending on their specialty of preparation, psychiatrists may provide in-depth psychotherapy, or medication therapy or head a team of mental health providers functioning as a private service based in the community. As physicians, psychiatrists may be employed by the hospital or may hold practice privileges in the facility. Owing to their legal power to prescribe and to write orders, psychiatrists often function as leaders of the team in terms of the patients assigned to the individual psychiatrist.
Medical physicians	These physicians provide, on a consultation basis, medical diagnosis and treatments. Occasionally, a physician prepared as an addictionologist may serve in a more direct role on the unit that offers treatment for addictive disease.
Mental health workers	Like nursing assistants, mental health workers function under the direction and supervision of registered nurses. They provide assistance to clients in meeting basic needs and also help the community to remain supportive, safe, and healthy.
Pharmacists	In view of the intricacies of prescribing, coordinating, and administering combinations of psychotropic and other medications, the consulting pharmacist can offer a valuable safeguard. Physicians and nurses collaborate with the pharmacist regarding new medications, which are proliferating at a steady rate.

- Jordan is approached by the nurse on the next shift as that nurse briefly assesses his well-being. He notices that once again he is being asked about thoughts of harming himself.
- So far he has spoken with the intake nurse, with his primary nurse Ms. Weaver, with his psychiatrist, with a counselor who conducts a group activity in conjunction with his nurse, and with a social worker who states that he will be meeting with Jordan tomorrow. He has been asked to take a medication that will "help you to think more clearly and to feel more secure."
- After Jordan's admission and assessments by the nurse and the psychiatrist, the treatment team meets to discuss several people under the care of that psychiatrist. Ms. Weaver introduces the team to the data and initial list of identified problems and needs. Priorities are set and agreements reached regarding what further data are needed and which members of the team will obtain these data.
- The team chooses a clinical pathway. They note that Jordan has already progressed in terms of a decreased risk for self-harm but has not yet met the expected criteria for a reduction in psychotic thinking.
- The team agrees upon use of prn medication, as ordered by the psychiatrist, and gentle guidance of Jordan's thought processes during one-to-one contacts with staff and during simple group activities to reduce psychotic thinking. It is agreed that the nurses will report on Jordan's progress in gaining clarity of thought at the next treatment planning meeting.

NURSING ON THE INPATIENT UNIT

Management

Nurses assume the bulk of the management of the daily functioning of the inpatient mental health unit. Organizationally, an arrangement of nursing management with a parallel "program" management or clinical coordinator may exist. The program staff may provide social services, activities, occupational therapy, and specialized counseling services, among others. On the other hand, these services may be managed by a nursing manager. Some healthy debate continues regarding the advantages of these and other creative systems of organization and management.

In either case, the nurse manager is responsible for an awareness of the safety of the unit, its effectiveness in the delivery of services, and how well the components of the health care team integrate their services. The nurse manager, either alone or in conjunction with the program manager or clinical coordinator, plans a schedule of therapeutic activities that is comprehensive but that can be reasonably carried out within the context of the hospital schedule, the constraints of the schedules of attending physicians, the availability of services, and the availability of adequately skilled staff members. In the event of problems in any of these areas, the nursing management must be able to campaign administratively to make corrections.

- Consistency and attentiveness are essential to Jordan's safety during the time that he poses a risk to his own safety. The system of staffing and shift-to-shift reporting on Ms. Weaver's unit provides for continuity of care by overlapping of shifts combined with both a tape-recorded report and an opportunity for face-to-face clarification by nurses and other staff members. (Refer to Chapter 24 for specific guidelines and suicide protocol.)
- By the end of the report, the staff knows its roles and responsibilities for the upcoming shift. While Jordan is at risk for self-harm, continuous one-to-one assignment of staff to his care is provided. A documentation sheet is maintained by the assigned staff member to indicate client status at frequent intervals.
- Two days after his admission, a neurologist arrives on the unit to examine Jordan because of neurologic symptoms that Helen Weaver has reported to the psychiatrist. Because the neurologist arrives during a group therapy session in which Jordan is participating, the charge nurse informs the neurologist that Jordan's chart may be reviewed, but that the physician must wait until the conclusion of group before Jordan can be examined. The neurologist accepts this restriction because of previous negotiations carried out by the nurse manager of the unit with the medical staff.

Therapeutic Strategies

Psychiatric nurses implement a major portion of the treatment plan. The plan is partly carried out in formal sessions with the client, but is carried out more frequently during informal contacts with individuals and with small groups of clients. Often, the effectiveness of the informal contacts can be viewed as more significant than the formal ones, because they occur during natural activities of daily and social living and are therefore based on reality.

Appropriate counseling skills are the basis for all nursing interventions. Nurses are prepared educationally with psychosocial skills to assist clients to feel heard and supported, to develop trust and increased feelings of safety, to receive feedback, and to learn more adaptive coping skills. Nurses who have furthered their formal education, participated in workshops, or gained recognition as certified psychiatric nurses or nurse specialists can carry out more intensive interpersonal or group therapies.

Nurses continue to carry out such therapeutic interventions as team members, sharing successes and difficulties with the team in order to provide for consistency of care and to gain feedback regarding timing and technique. Group work is typically co-led, with at least one of the co-leaders trained in such therapies. The co-leaders plan before sessions and examine the group process and their joint efforts afterward.

- Jordan continues to experience difficulty trusting and relating to others. The plan is to build trust gradually and to introduce Jordan to increasingly complex interpersonal and group challenges. Ms. Weaver and the other nurses approach Jordan cautiously in a nonthreatening way. They offer empathetic comments regarding his nonverbal messages of distrust and discomfort. As Jordan shows increasing comfort with such one-to-one interactions, the nurses invite him to join in simple social activities on the unit, such as eating and talking with other clients.
- Ms. Weaver and a social worker co-lead a structured group therapy session for clients whose goals include organizing their thought processes and socializing at a basic level. Jordan participates in this activity, gradually extending trust to several other clients and allowing himself to laugh and talk briefly about his immediate experiences and thoughts.
- After the most recent session, Ms. Weaver and the social worker discuss how Ms. Weaver's role with Jordan is purposely being reduced in order to encourage Jordan to interact more with others.

Milieu

Group Activities

Experienced mental health nurses conduct specific, structured activities involving the therapeutic community, special groups, or families on most mental health units. Examples of these activities include morning goal-setting meetings and evening goal-review meetings. Community meetings may be held daily or at other scheduled times of the week. At these meetings, new clients are greeted and departing clients given farewells, ideas for unit activities are discussed, community problems or successes are processed, and other business of the therapeutic community is conducted. Nurses also offer psychoeducational groups for clients and/or families on topics such as stress management, coping skills, grieving, management of medications, and communication skills. For a fuller discussion of unit groups run by nurses, refer to Chapter 10, "Communication Within Groups."

▶ Helen Weaver and another nurse are conducting a morning goal-setting meeting of the community. A thought for the day is chosen by the two nurses, taking into account some of the common concerns of a number of the clients. This is read from an inspirational book by a client who volunteers to do so, and Ms. Weaver encourages the clients to discuss the reading briefly. Clients and staff members then introduce themselves, and each states a goal that is specific and can realistically be accomplished that day. The two nurses assist community members to state realistic goals in measurable, concrete terms. They invite the other members of the community to offer words of encouragement. The meeting ends with the community's choice of another reading or with the ever-popular choice of the Serenity Prayer.

Management of the Milieu

On an inpatient unit, nursing is the discipline primarily responsible for maintenance of a therapeutic milieu. Each nurse, through the course of a workday, is constantly gathering data about the well-being of the therapeutic community. As noted above, reports from shift to shift attend to the status of the milieu.

To maintain an atmosphere in which healing and growth can take place, nurses strive to keep communications and interpersonal feedback open and constructively honest. Verbal messages must be clear or must be clarified as needed. Nonverbal messages must also be congruent with verbal messages. Ideally, staff and clients should be interacting often and be seen as sharing a number of community goals. Clients need to be involved in some decisions and given explanations for those decisions that must be left to the staff. Behavioral limits and rules should be plainly understood and consistently enforced by all staff. All clients and staff must be held responsible for their own behavior and for the well-being of the community.

The therapeutic milieu operates on the understanding that the community can serve as a real-life training ground for learning about self and for practicing communication and coping skills in preparation for a return to living outside the hospital. Even events that seemingly distract from the program of therapies can be turned into valuable learning opportunities for the members of the community.

▶ Sally K., age 34, is a client on the unit who is well known to both clients and staff. Her bright, intelligent, and outgoing manner has made her popular. Because of her leadership and knowledge, however, she has led a number of clients to begin to question the unit's rules, schedules, and therapies.

▶ One of the nurses, Bob Kay, notices that he has begun to feel uncomfortable among several clients with whom he formerly had good rapport. He thinks that they are avoiding him and withholding trust. He mentions this in his shift report. Ms. Weaver validates his feelings by noting that she had also experienced this but had assumed that it may have been her own personal reaction to being a member of a different sociocultural group.

▶ The nursing staff consults with the rest of the treatment team and decides to open the community meeting to questions regarding the unit's rules, schedules, and therapies. At the meeting, the airing of issues satisfies the client community. Several of the clients involved ask to speak privately with staff about their feelings of having been influenced by Sally. Sally herself speaks with her nurse about how she realizes that she was using the situation to avoid working on her own painful feelings and decisions.

Safety

The mental health nurse assumes a responsibility for ongoing vigilance regarding safety hazards. The nurse also carries out a variety of measures designed to reduce the risk of danger on a daily basis.

Nurses must be able to respond quickly to environmental threats such as fire. They have to be able to rapidly isolate or evacuate clients while remaining in control of cleints' whereabouts and minimizing their sense of threat.

The nurse must supervise the unit's systems for tracking which clients are on or off the unit, and for periodic or constant checks on those clients at risk of harm to self or others. The flow of visitors and objects being brought onto the unit must be managed. Procedures for the safe control of sharp objects must be implemented. Use of illegal drugs and alcohol must be prevented. Sexual activity between clients must be prevented. Violence and disruption must be minimized while retaining an atmosphere that promotes healthy and appropriate expression of anger and other feelings. **Elopement** (escape) of clients has to be prevented, but in a way that avoids an atmosphere of imprisonment. The routine concerns about slippery floors, client falls, and electrical hazards must be addressed, all on a unit where clients are more mobile and active than on medical or surgical units.

▶ Helen Weaver has woven concern for safety into her daily nursing practice. As she enters or leaves the unit, she is checking the functioning of the unit's locks. She is alert to any potential electrical or fire hazards. Her eyes routinely scan the unit for possible sharp objects. She tracks the locations of clients as she moves about the unit. If she is aware that staff have not been present in certain locations, she is sure to include those places in her rounds.

▶ Ms. Weaver informs new clients of rules regarding sharp objects, smoking, medications from home, visitors, leaving the unit, and behavioral restrictions. She clearly advises clients against the possession of alcohol and illicit drugs. She supervises inspection of clients' personal items and of any medications brought from home.

◗ She participates in community meetings where staff provide clarification of these rules. When visitors arrive, she teaches them the rules, and checks bags and other incoming items.

Documentation

Documentation of client progress is the responsibility of the entire mental health team. Although communication among team members and coordination of services are the primary goals when choosing a system for charting, practitioners in the inpatient setting must also consider professional standards, legal issues, requirements for reimbursement by insurers, and accreditation by regulatory agencies. Information must also be in a format that is retrievable for quality assurance monitoring, utilization management, peer review, and research. For nursing, documentation of the nursing process is a guiding concern and is reflected in different formats that are commonly found in psychiatric hospitals. See Table 8–1 for an overview of charting methods. As mentioned previously in Chapters 1 and 6, computerized clinical documentation is the common trend in inpatient settings today.

Psychobiological Responsibilities

Nurses are responsible for the safe administration and monitoring of medications on the inpatient acute care unit. Because of their active leadership during treatment planning, nurses often exert great influence regarding medication decisions on mental health units. Detailed knowledge of psychoactive medications and of the interactions and psychological side effects of other medications is expected of mental health nurses. Their observations of the expected and adverse effects of medication regimens provide data necessary for efficient and accurate medication decisions by the psychiatrist and treatment team. The issues of resistance to taking medication and of noncompliance are dealt with in the clinical chapters (e.g., see Chapters 4 and 22).

Medications may be administered according to various systems, but most of these can be categorized into one of two types: (1) medication by a nurse assigned to carry out the function of the "meds nurse" (team nursing) and (2) medication by the nurse assigned to the client on that shift (primary nursing). The former is simpler and efficient, but the latter provides for greater individualization of the medication regimen and for improved preparation of the client for self-care upon discharge. Medications are generally not brought to the client. Instead, clients are either called to a central location or are expected to arrive at a designated location and time to meet their nurses for medications.

Psychiatric nurses often have numerous decisions to make about prn medications. These decisions must be based on a combination of factors: the client's request, the team's plan, attempts to use alternative methods of coping, and the nurse's judgments regarding timing and the client's behavior. Nurses consult with team members when possible in order to make the best prn decision.

◗ Helen Weaver has provided the team with data leading to an accurate diagnosis and choice of medications for Jordan. This choice reflects Ms. Weaver's knowledge of how Jordan responded to medication regimens during previous hospitalizations. His current regimen includes orders for medications that reduce his disorganized thought processes and thereby reduce his risk for self-harm.

◗ On Ms. Weaver's day off, the nurse assigned to Jordan assesses that he hears voices "commanding me to cease living." The nurse refers to Jordan's chart. The plan directs the nurse to spend 15 minutes helping Jordan to recall that he has learned to understand that when he hears such voices, it is his mind's way of expressing his feeling of being overwhelmed. He is to use relaxation techniques, but if he does not obtain relief within 20 minutes, he may use his prn medication along with relaxation.

◗ The nurse notes that Jordan has received his oral dose of medication (same as the prn) only 10 minutes before her assessment. On the basis of her knowledge of the time needed for the onset of action of this medication, she follows the plan of care. The relaxation, along with the onset of action of Jordan's usual dose, leads to relief of his symptoms at this time.

Crisis Management

Nurses anticipate, prevent, and manage emergencies and crises on the unit. These crises may be of a medical or behavioral nature. Mental health units, whether situated in a general hospital or independently, must be able to stabilize the condition of a client who experiences a medical crisis. Mental health or addictive disease units that manage detoxification (withdrawal from alcohol or other drugs) must anticipate several common medical crises associated with that process. Mental health units therefore store "crash carts" containing the emergency medications used to treat shock and cardiorespiratory arrest. Nurses must maintain their cardiopulmonary resuscitation (CPR) skills and be able to use basic emergency equipment. In order to be effective and to practice at a high level of competency, nurses are advised to attend inservices and workshops designed to teach and maintain current skills. Nurses must be able to alert medical support systems quickly and mobilize transportation to the appropriate medical facilities.

◗ Lester D., age 55, has been started on a tricyclic antidepressant medication. Within 2 hours of his first

TABLE 8–1 CHARTING METHODS

	NARRATIVE	PROBLEM-ORIENTED CHARTING (SOAPIE)
Characteristics	A descriptive statement of client status written in chronological order throughout a shift. Used to support assessment finding from a flow sheet. In charting by exception, narrative notes are used to indicate significant symptoms, behaviors, or events that are exceptions to norms identified on an assessment flow sheet.	Developed in the 1960s for physicians to reduce inefficient documentation. Intended to be accompanied by a problem list. Originally SOAP, with IE added later. The emphasis is on problem identification, process, and outcome. S: Subjective data (patient statement). O: Objective data (nurse observations). A: Assessment (nurse interprets S and O and describes either a problem or a nursing diagnosis). P: Plan (proposed intervention). I: Interventions (nurse's response to problem). E: Evaluation (client outcome).
Example	Date/time/discipline Client was agitated in the morning and pacing in the hallway. Blinks eyes, muttering to self and looking off to the side. States he hears voices. Verbally hostile to another client. Offered 2 mg haloperidol (Haldol) prn and sat with staff in quiet area for 20 minutes. Client returned to community lounge and was able to sit and watch television.	Date/time/discipline S: "I'm so stupid. Get away, get away." "I hear the devil telling me bad things." O: Client pacing the hall, mumbling to self and looking off to the side. Shouted derogatory comments when approached by another client. Watching walls and ceiling closely. A: Client is having auditory hallucinations and increased agitation. P: Offer client Haldol prn. Redirect client to less stimulating environment I: Client received 2 mg Haldol PO prn; sat with client in quiet room for 20 minutes. E: Client calmer. Returned to community lounge, sat and watched television.
Advantages	Narrative writing is a common form of expression. Can address any event or behavior. Explains flow sheet findings. Multidisciplinary ease of use.	Structured. Consistent organization of data. Easy to retrieve data for quality assurance and utilization management Contains all elements of nursing process. Minimizes unnecessary data. Multidisciplinary ease of use.
Disadvantages	Unstructured. Organization of information may vary from note to note. Difficult format for retrieval of quality assurance and utilization management data. Elements of nursing process frequently omitted. Unnecessary and subjective information commonly included.	Time/effort to structure the information. Limits entries to problems. Data about progress may be lost. Not chronological. Negative connotation.

Data from Iyer and Camp (1995); Springhouse Corporation (1992).

dose, he complains of feeling faint. The nurse asks Lester to be seated and checks his vital signs, carefully listening to his apical pulse. Noting irregularities that were not observed upon previous assessments, the nurse stays with Lester while asking another nurse to notify the physician and to ready the crash cart. The portable electrocardiogram (ECG) monitor is attached and the nurse observes erratic, irregular heart beats. Transportation is arranged, and Lester is transferred after an intravenous line is started and ECG monitoring set up. The emergency is managed within 25 minutes of the client's first complaint.

Behavioral crises can lead to violence toward oneself or others. Crises are usually, but not always, observed to escalate through fairly predictable stages. Crisis prevention and management techniques are practiced by staff in most mental health facilities. Many psychiatric hospitals have special teams made up of nurses, psychiatric aides, and other professionals who respond to psychiatric emer-

TABLE 8–1 CHARTING METHODS *(Continued)*

	PROBLEM-ORIENTED CHARTING (*PIE OR APIE*)	FOCUS CHARTING (*DAR*)
Characteristics	Either APIE or PIE. Intended to parallel nursing process. Problem is described by nursing diagnosis. Assessment is either included in the progress note or referenced from an assessment flow sheet. A: Assessment P: Problems (nursing diagnosis) I: Interventions E: Evaluation	Uses key words to indicate the primary subject of the note. May be a symptom, event, behavior, or nursing diagnosis. Has replaced SOAP notes in many hospitals. D: Data (information pertinent to the focus). A: Action (intervention). R: Response (client outcome).
Example	Date/time A: Client at severe level of anxiety, muttering to self and looking off to the side. Making verbal threats, has psychomotor agitation, states he hears voices. P: Anxiety related to internal auditory stimulation. I: Client received 2 mg Haldol PO prn; sat with client in quiet room for 20 minutes. E: Client calmer. Returned to community lounge, sat and watched television.	Date/time/focus Agitated behavior D: Client pacing the hall, mumbling to self and looking off to the side; states he hears voices, verbal hostility. A: Given 2 mg Haldol PO prn; sat with client in quiet room for 20 minutes. E: Client calmer. Returned to community lounge, sat and watched television.
Advantages	Structured. Consistent organization of data. Easy to retrieve data for quality assurance and utilization management. Contains all elements of nursing process. Minimizes unnecessary data.	Structured. Consistent organization of data. Easy to retrieve data for quality assurance and utilization management. Fosters use of the nursing process. Not necessarily problem-oriented. Includes a variety of data on client status.
Disadvantages	Time/effort to structure the information. Specific for nursing. Limits entries to problems. Data about progress may be lost. Not chronological. Negative connotation.	Time/effort to structure the information. Not chronological.

gencies called **codes.** Each member of the team takes part in the team effort to defuse a crisis when it is in its early stages. If preventive measures fail, each member of the team participates in a rapid, organized movement designed to immobilize, medicate, or seclude a client. The nurse is most often this team's leader, not only organizing the plan but also timing the intervention and managing the concurrent use of prn medications. The nurse can initiate such an intervention in the absence of a physician in most states but must secure a physician's order for restraint or seclusion within a specified time. (Refer to Chapters 12 and 21 for further discussions and protocols on restraints and seclusions.)

The nurse also advocates for clients by ensuring that their legal rights are preserved, no matter how difficult their behaviors may be for the staff to manage.

Crises on the unit are upsetting and threatening to other clients in the therapeutic community. A staff member is usually reserved for the needs of the community. This person removes other clients from the area of crisis and helps them express their fears. Clients may be concerned for the involved client and may fear that they, too, might experience such a loss of behavioral control.

- Jordan appears upset as he approaches a mental health worker. Jordan reports that John, another client, is angrily throwing objects at the staff person assigned on a one-to-one basis to John. The mental health worker reports this to the charge nurse, who quickly assigns the worker to remove other clients from the area. The nurse organizes other staff and quickly checks John's prn orders. There is no order for restraints or seclusion. The team gathers at the far areas of the dayroom while the nurse and one other staff person use calm but limit-setting communication techniques: "John, you are not to hurt yourself or anyone here. If you are having trouble controlling your impulses, we will help you." Because John's behavior continues to escalate toward violence, the charge nurse directs another nurse to prepare John's prn medication while the rest of the staff prepares to direct John to the seclusion room. The staff uses its numbers as a "show of force" to convince John of the seriousness of this directive. John agrees and also reluctantly takes the prn medication. The staff remains prepared to intervene safely but decisively to take John to the seclusion room if he cannot agree to the directive.
- While the charge nurse telephones the physician to report the incident and to obtain orders for seclusion, another nurse gathers the community in the dayroom to allow for expression of feelings about the situation. The nurse is careful to avoid breaking John's confidentiality during this activity.
- Careful, accurate documentation in John's chart demonstrates the need for these measures and how the intervention was carried out. Once in seclusion, John will be monitored at frequent intervals by an assigned staff member.

Preparation for Discharge

As members of the multidisciplinary team, nurses assist clients and their families to prepare for independent or assisted living after hospitalization. This is especially important to the concept and practice of managed care, aiming toward the goal of decreased hospital stays by the client.

Given the current trend of brief hospitalizations, nurses focus on precipitants of the crisis that led to hospital admission. Clients are then assisted to learn coping skills and behaviors that will help them to avert future crises. Psychoeducational groups, individual exploration of options and supports, therapeutic leaves, and on-the-spot instruction (such as during medication administration) offer the client numerous opportunities. Nurses, during the 24-hour day experienced by the client, use the everyday experiences of the client as a testing ground for new, more adaptive behaviors.

The care plan or clinical pathway chosen for the client should reflect this discharge planning emphasis as early as the day of admission. The client is expected to begin to work toward achievement of self-care goals fairly early in the hospital stay and to show readiness for independence by the time of discharge. This readiness should include preparation by the client's support system for their role in enhancing the client's mental health.

- The unit's schedule reflects its commitment to discharge teaching. Once his condition permits, Jordan attends evening groups that present information about safe and consistent use of medications, availability and use of social activities in the outside community, communication skills, cognitive restructuring, self-esteem building, use of spiritual supports, and healthy interaction with one's family. Jordan uses role playing to learn more comfortable communication and assertiveness skills.
- A social worker learns that Jordan's boss at work has helped Jordan to remember to take his medications regularly. During a meeting attended by the boss, Jordan, the social worker, and Ms. Weaver, this support is strengthened, and the boss receives information and a back-up phone number to use if questions arise.
- In group, Jordan's peers encourage him to contact his family. He says one morning that his goal for the day is to phone his parents. The group helps him to decide how to communicate during the phone conversation and later encourages him to discuss the results.
- By the day of his discharge from the hospital, Jordan is arriving for his medications independently, has plans for his follow-up care, is ready to return to his job and apartment, and has been invited to lunch with his parents.

Policy Review and Revision

Mental health nurses are usually expected or invited to participate in decisions about the system of providing care and the working environment. Nurses may address such issues as problems of scheduling of activities, work schedules, assignments, opportunities to expand professional practice, and safety. Nurses may research novel approaches to these or other aspects of delivery of care. Committee work may offer the nurse the chance to participate in the management and future of the unit.

- Ms. Weaver has been collaborating with other nurses and program staff on development of a system for monitoring clinical outcomes. This system, based on the clinical pathways, will enable the staff to argue more persuasively for insurance payments for clients. It will also provide data useful for contracting with large regional employers to provide mental health services for their employees. Ms. Weaver describes her enthusiasm about participating in research and expanding beyond her customary nursing roles.

SUMMARY

Nursing on an inpatient acute care psychiatric unit calls for skills in management, communication, and collaboration with an interdisciplinary team. The mental health nurse assists the client to adjust to hospitalization and to benefit from the therapies available. The nurse provides direct services to the client, but also participates in the team effort to create a safe, supportive, and growth-enhancing environment for the client. With additional experience, education, and training, the nurse participates in advanced therapies. The nurse advocates for the client and ensures that the client's rights are protected.

The beginning practitioner needs to gather information about the functioning of this unique form of treatment from the clinical orientation, the unit's handbook for clients, policy and procedure books, and the patient's bill of rights. Students are advised to maintain open communication with staff, managers, and clinical instructors. Staff and clients often welcome an interest by students because of students' ability to provide clients with time and empathy, and because the students' fresh perspectives on the unit can offer the staff valuable feedback about the quality of its services.

Because of the sense of community of the inpatient unit, the student must be alert to the possibility of unwittingly becoming involved in divisive maneuvers initiated by some clients. Frequent verbal reporting to staff and seeking of evaluative comments from staff help to safeguard students from such pitfalls. Students are reminded to become familiar with plans of care or clinical pathways in order to join in the interdisciplinary team effort.

REFERENCES

Abbot, J. (1993). Making the commitment to managed care. *Nursing Management* 24(8):36–37.

American Nurses' Association (1988). *Nursing case management*. Publ. No. NS-32. Kansas City, MO: American Nurses' Association.

Beyea, S. C. (1996). *Critical pathways for collaborative nursing care*. Menlo Park, CA: Addison-Wesley Nursing.

Cohen, C. L., and Cesta, T. G. (1993). *Nursing case management: From concept to evaluation*. St. Louis: C. V. Mosby.

Del Togno-Armanasco, V., Hopkin, L., and Harter, S. (1993). *Collaborative nursing case management*. New York: Springer.

Etheredge, M. L. S. (Ed.) (1989). *Collaborative care, nursing case management*. Chicago: American Hospital Publishing.

Forchuk, C., et al. (1989). Incorporating Peplau's theory and case management. *Journal of Psychosocial Nursing*, 27(2):35–38.

Hicks, L. L., Stallmeyer, J. M., and Colemen, J. R.(1993). *Role of the nurse in managed care*. Washington, DC: American Nurses Publishing.

Intagliata, J. (1982). Improving the quality of community care for the chronically disabled: The role of case management. *Schizophrenic Bulletin*, 8(4):655–674.

Iyer, P., and Camp, N. (1995). *Nursing documentation. A nursing process approach* (2nd ed.). St. Louis: Mosby–Year Book.

Springhouse Corporation (1992). *Better documentation*. Springhouse, PA: Springhouse.

Further Reading

Etheredge, M. (1986). The maps for managed care. *Definition*, 1(3):1–3.

Ferguson, L. (1993). Steps to developing a critical pathway. *Nursing Administration Quarterly*, 17(3):58–62.

Joint Commission on the Accreditation of Healthcare Organizations (1995). *The accreditation manual for hospitals*. Oakbrook Terrace, IL: JCAHO.

Kolva, C. (1992). *Clinical nursing standards for inpatient psychiatric settings*. Joppa, MD: Publication Resources for Nurses.

SELF-STUDY AND CRITICAL THINKING

Multiple choice

1. When the mental health team meets to plan care for a client on the inpatient unit, the primary goal is

   A. Support for the psychiatrists
   B. Equal distribution of responsibility
   C. Coordinated multidisciplinary treatment
   D. Building team cohesion

2. The priority symptom to consider when evaluating a client for admission to an inpatient mental health unit is

   A. Suicidal thoughts
   B. Auditory hallucinations
   C. Anxiety
   D. Feelings of sadness

3. Which of the following always violates the rights of a client on the inpatient mental health unit?

   A. Searching the client's belongings
   B. Absence of a treatment plan
   C. Use of physical restraints
   D. Observing the client closely

4. The characteristics of a therapeutic milieu include

   A. Clear communication
   B. Few rules
   C. Conflict avoidance
   D. Staff control

5. When responding to a client who exhibits agitated behavior on the inpatient mental health unit, the first action by the nurse is to

   A. Offer prn medication
   B. Follow the team plan of care
   C. Place the client in seclusion
   D. Encourage angry outbursts

6. Which of the following goals must be met before the client is discharged from the inpatient mental health unit?

   A. The client can return to productive work.
   B. Family members are ready to accept the client.
   C. The client's mental illness is cured.
   D. The admissions crisis is resolved.

Critical thinking

7. State three arguments in favor of and three arguments in opposition to the use of hospitalization as part of treatment for mental disorders.
8. Compare mental disorders with medical or surgical disorders in terms of whether inpatient services are justified.
9. How does a nurse decide to place clients' safety needs before their right to make decisions for themselves?
10. If nurses function as fairly equal members of the multidisciplinary mental health team, what differentiates the nurse from the other members of the team?

9

Psychiatric Mental Health Nursing in Community Settings

SUSAN CAVERLY

SUSAN MEJO

OUTLINE

KEY TERMS AND CONCEPTS

The key terms and concepts listed here also appear in bold where they are defined or discussed in this chapter.

deinstitutionalization

transinstitutionalization

acculturation

ethical dilemma

OBJECTIVES

After studying this chapter, the reader will be able to

1. Explain the evolution of the community mental health movement.
2. Distinguish between the goals and interventions of mental health nursing care in the hospital and the community setting.
3. Compare and contrast the levels of education and the roles and functions of the community mental health nurse.
4. Give examples of the psychiatric nurse's role as a member of a multidisciplinary team.

5. **Summarize the role of the nurse and the goals of treatment for the following community resource facilities:**
   - **Community mental health center**
   - **Homeless shelter**
   - **Mobile health care units**
   - **Forensic setting**
   - **Private practice setting**
   - **Home psychiatric mental health care**
   - **Outpatient substance abuse treatment facility**
6. **Describe some of the ethical issues and conflicts a community mental health nurse might encounter.**
7. **Discuss how culture affects nurses and clients when formulating realistic and attainable health care goals in the community setting.**
8. **Assess how the future directions of health care in hospital and community settings could affect your career goals.**

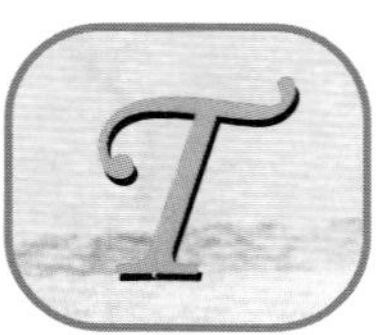

he first psychiatric nurses working in the community setting were community health nurses who developed a specialty practice in mental health. They were able to move within the community, were comfortable meeting with clients in the home or neighborhood center, were competent to act independently using professional judgment in sometimes unanticipated situations, and possessed knowledge of community resources. The heritage of these nurses began among European women who cared for the sick at home and American women who organized into religious and secular societies during the 1800s to visit the sick in their homes. By 1877, trained nurses worked as public health nurses visiting the homes of the poor in northeastern cities and generalist nurses engaged in community visits to rural areas for health promotion and care of the sick (Smith 1995).

THE CONTEXT FOR PSYCHIATRIC NURSING IN THE COMMUNITY

In 1963, President Kennedy signed into law the Community Mental Health Centers Act, thus solidifying the shift of mental health care from the institution to the community and heralding the era of **deinstitutionalization.** Media focus raising public awareness regarding the horrors of psychiatric institutions, the mental health care needs presented by returning servicemen, and the advent of psychopharmacologic agents all acted as catalysts for needed change in psychiatric treatment philosophy (Marcos 1990; Rochefort 1993).

The 1960s were also the time when federal entitlement programs proliferated: Social Security Disability, Supplemental Security Income, Medicaid, Medicare, housing assistance, and food stamps. These social programs provided the means for moving the mentally ill out of institutions and into the community. Talbott (1981) used the term **transinstitutionalization** to describe the process of providing institutional services in settings outside the institution. Policymakers of the time believed community care would be less expensive than the historic hospital-based care.

Caring for the severely and persistently mentally ill in the community is not without problems, and the community mental health system has been criticized for failing to serve those who are most severely ill. Funding is often inadequate to meet needs. Those who are most in need of psychiatric care are often the same clients who, for whatever reason, resist the use of available services. Despite these concerns, a second wave of deinstitutionalization took place in the 1980s after President Carter's Commission on Mental Health highlighted the needs of the underserved and unserved chronically mentally ill. Concepts of deinstitutionalization, rehabilitation, and long-term treatment of the severely and persistently mentally ill are embedded in the current mental health system and are the legacy of the Mental Health Services Act of 1980 (Bachrach 1994; Callahan 1994; Crosby 1987).

In recent years the sites in which psychiatric nursing is provided and the nursing specialties delivering this care have become more diverse (Scales et al. 1993; Kimball and Williams-Burgess 1995). Home health nurses often care for persons with undiagnosed mental or emotional disorders. Nurses working in the criminal justice system provide mental health nursing care by default, if not by specialty; the Los Angeles County Jail has been recognized as the largest mental health institution in the United States.

School-based clinics are becoming more common in all communities, and as a consequence nurses trained to work with children and adolescents are currently providing mental health care. The list of both traditional and nontraditional community mental health care settings

BOX 9–1 POSSIBLE COMMUNITY MENTAL HEALTH PRACTICE SITES (NONEXCLUSIVE LIST)

- Community mental health centers
- Youth centers
- Private practice office
- Crisis centers
- Shelters (homeless, battered women, adolescent)
- Correction facilities, local jails, courts
- Primary care offices
- Substance abuse program offices
- Client's home
- Schools and day care centers
- Nursing homes
- Day hospital facilities
- Group homes and adult foster homes or day care centers
- Work release housing
- Industry and business
- Emergency departments of community hospitals
- Outreach to multiple locations, including restaurants and shopping malls
- Churches, temples, synagogues, mosques
- Ethnic cultural centers
- Hospices and AIDS supportive living programs
- Client worksite

BOX 9–2 COMMUNITY PSYCHIATRIC MENTAL HEALTH NURSE ATTRIBUTES

- Awareness of self; personal and cultural values
- Nonjudgmental attitude
- Flexibility
- Problem-solving skills
- Ability to cross service systems (e.g., to work with schools, corrections, shelters, health care providers, employers)
- Knowledge of community resources
- Excellent psychosocial and health assessment skills
- Excellent communications skills
- Knowledge of psychopharmacology
- Ability to recognize need for consultation
- Calm external manner
- Ability to see strength and ability in even the severely ill
- Willingness to work with the family or significant others identified by the client as support people
- Understanding of the social, cultural, and political issues that affect mental health and illness
- Knowledge of political activism

continues to increase. It is a challenge for nurses to meet this community need and for educators to ensure that nurses possess the knowledge and skills required to provide community psychiatric mental health nursing care. Box 9–1 lists some of the possible sites in which nurses provide community psychiatric care.

ASPECTS OF COMMUNITY NURSING

Psychiatric nursing in the community setting differs markedly from its hospital counterpart. The community setting requires that the psychiatric nurse possess knowledge about a broad array of community resources and be flexible in approaching problems related to individual psychiatric symptoms, family and support systems, and basic living needs such as housing and financial support. The setting is the realm of the client rather than of the health care provider; the nurse is in essence a guest or a consultant to the client, the housing manager, or the corrections officer who requested or agreed to psychiatric nursing intervention (Sullivan and Cohen 1990).

Psychiatric nurses who have not previously worked in the community setting may find transition to this role difficult. It is an **acculturation** process, in which the nurse must revisit beliefs that there is a single definition of health or that professionals can or should control client behavior. A number of personal characteristics can ease the nurse's accommodation to the new role and enhance success at working in the community. Box 9–2 summarizes some of the attributes most helpful to the community psychiatric mental health nurse.

Community treatment hinges on enhancing client strengths in the same environment in which daily life must be maintained, thus making individually tailored psychiatric care imperative. The hospital represents a controlled setting and promotes stabilization, but strides made during hospitalization can be lost upon return home. Treatment in the community permits clients and those involved in their support to learn new ways of coping with symptoms or situational difficulties. The result can be one of empowerment and self-management, to the extent possible given the client's disability.

Psychiatric Nursing Assessment Strategies

Assessment of the biopsychosocial needs and capacities of clients living in the community requires expanding the general psychiatric nursing assessment. For the hospitalized client, the nurse must understand community living challenges and resources in order to assess presenting problems as well as to plan for discharge. The community psychiatric nurse must also develop a comprehensive understanding of the client's ability to cope with the demands of living in the community in order to be able to plan and implement effective treatment that will allow the client to stay in the community. Box 9–3 identifies the areas covered in a biopsychosocial assessment. Refer to Appendix D for a full assessment guide.

BOX 9–3 ELEMENTS OF BIO-PSYCHOSOCIAL NURSING ASSESSMENT

- Presenting problem and referring party
- Psychiatric history, including symptoms, treatments, medications, and most recent service utilization
- Health history, including illnesses, treatments, medications, and allergies
- Substance abuse: history and current use
- Family history, including health and mental health disorders and treatments
- Psychosocial history, including
  - Developmental history
  - School performance
  - Socialization
  - Vocational success or difficulty
  - Interpersonal skills or deficits
  - Income and source of income
  - Housing adequacy and stability
  - Family and support system
  - Level of activity
  - Ability to care for needs independently or with assistance
  - Religious or spiritual beliefs and practices
- Legal history
- Mental status examination
- Strengths and deficits of the client
- Cultural beliefs and needs relevant to psychosocial care

Among the key aspects of this assessment are health status and interventions; mental status; psychiatric diagnoses (DSM-IV); somatic interventions for psychiatric symptoms; communication skills; support system availability and the client's willingness to accept support; community resource availability and the client's ability to gain access to these resources independently or with assistance; financial circumstances; ability to afford treatment and to purchase prescribed medication; availability of safe, affordable, habitable housing; access to and involvement in structured activity; ability to afford and prepare nutritious food; and possible legal entanglements.

Individual characteristics of clients will have an effect on these areas of concern. For example, a person for whom Vietnamese is a primary language will require the nurse to consider the implications of language and culture as the psychiatric nursing assessment is undertaken. The use of an interpreter and cultural consultant is essential when the nurse and the client are not from the same culture and may speak different languages. Refer to Chapter 5 for more on cultural diversity applied to psychiatric nursing.

Psychiatric Nursing Intervention Strategies

In the hospital setting, the focus of care is on stabilization, as defined by staff. In the community setting, treatment goals and interventions are *negotiated* rather than imposed on the client. Community psychiatric nurses must approach interventions with flexibility and resourcefulness to meet the broad range of needs of those who manage their symptoms of mental illness in the community. The complexity of navigating the mental health system and the social service funding systems is often overwhelming to clients. Interventions cannot be directed only toward discrete psychiatric symptoms but must also facilitate client access to, and continuation of support for, basic needs such as housing and nutrition (Murray et al. 1995).

An example of differences, in terms of treatment goals and nursing intervention strategies, between inpatient and community mental health settings is provided in Table 9–1. The table presents treatment approach, by setting, for clients who have established histories of mental illness and present with delusional thinking or hallucinatory experiences. Such clients are often fearful of care providers, resistant to taking medication, and reluctant to accept public assistance. They often have severely altered sleep patterns, racing thoughts, and poor concentration. Clients' behavior may be erratic or explosive when confronted, and they may have difficulty caring for their basic needs.

ROLES AND FUNCTIONS OF THE COMMUNITY PSYCHIATRIC NURSE

Psychiatric mental health nurses are educated at a variety of levels: associate (ADN), diploma (RN), baccalaureate (BSN), master's (MSN), advanced practice (APN), and doctoral (PhD). In addition to these levels of educational preparation, the specialty of psychiatric mental health nursing has access to a national certifying process through the American Nurses' Association's Credentialing Center. There are two levels of certification: the psychiatric mental health nurse (generalist) and the psychiatric mental health clinical specialist (advanced practice nurse). The clinical specialist certification is the only national certification for master's prepared advanced practice psychiatric mental health nurses. At this level, there is an option to subspecialize with a focus on children and adolescents or on adults (ANA 1994).

Combined education and expertise recognized by national certification provides a framework within which psychiatric nursing may determine the scope of practice. The American Nurses Association has published scope-of-practice statements for psychiatric mental health nursing and for psychiatric consultation and liaison nursing that further guide the differentiation among the levels of nursing practice (see Chapter 1).

Perhaps the most significant distinction among the multiple levels of preparation is the degree to which the nurse acts autonomously and provides consultation to

TABLE 9–1 CHARACTERISTICS, TREATMENT GOALS, AND INTERVENTIONS BY SETTING

SETTING	INPATIENT SETTING	COMMUNITY MENTAL HEALTH
Characteristics	▶ Locked unit possibly ▶ 24-hour supervision ▶ Access to multidisciplinary team supports ▶ Boundaries determined by staff ▶ Food and housekeeping and security services ▶ Milieu	▶ Locked apartment ▶ Boundaries determined by client ▶ Client may refuse to take medication ▶ Self-care, nutrition, and health care may be erratic ▶ Social isolation
Goal	▶ Stabilization of symptoms and return to community	▶ Maintenance of stability in community ▶ Client as an active member of treatment team ▶ Improved ability to function
Intervention Strategies	▶ Boundaries enforced by seclusion and restraint if necessary ▶ Develop short-term therapeutic relationship ▶ Within limits of setting, develop and implement a plan of care that attends to sociocultural context of individual ▶ Court-ordered medication ▶ Monitor and assist self care and nutrition ▶ Health assessment and intervention as needed ▶ Socialization activities provided and required as tolerated ▶ Conferences with family or significant others and discharge planning activities related to long-term treatment and housing	▶ Work with family or community resources such as police and landlord to gain access to apartment and client ▶ Negotiate access and boundaries with client ▶ Work with client and social support system to plan and implement care that is consistent with sociocultural belief system and context ▶ Negotiate consent for and adherence to taking medications as prescribed ▶ Establish, maintain, and use long-term therapeutic relationship ▶ Intervene using creative strategies ▶ Negotiate meaning of adequate self-care, nutrition, and health care with client and social support system (e.g., supply of fast-food meal vouchers versus home-cooked meals) ▶ Assist client in assessing for needed services from those available in community

other nurses, members of the treatment team, primary care practitioners, and providers outside the health care system. The nurse practice acts of individual states grant nurses authority to practice. As the national patchwork of practice acts is expanded, in keeping with the increased knowledge held within the profession of nursing, prescriptive authority and hospital privileges are becoming a delineation point between advanced practice and general practice psychiatric nursing (Carson 1993; Caverly 1996; Krauss 1993). Table 9–2 presents information regarding the roles of psychiatric nurses relevant to their education.

The scope of nursing practice, as related to educational preparation, is influenced by the increased emphasis on standardization of care and management by outcome. These factors have reduced the amount of expertise necessary to provide routine care (e.g., not long ago physicians were the practitioners who operated the equipment that measured blood pressure). As new technology enters everyday life, we find that medications previously available only by prescription are sold over the counter, and health care interventions are performed by lay people. Therefore, the descriptions provided in the following cases to differentiate the community psychiatric nursing roles in the treatment of clients with mental illness must be understood to have a certain fluidity and flexibility. The first case, that of Mr. Butler, describes the assessment and case management roles of the community psychiatric nurse and the psychiatric nurse practitioner as they work to meet the biopsychosocial needs of a person who is severely and persistently mentally ill.

Assessment and Intervention for Mr. Butler

- Mr. Butler has previously been diagnosed as suffering from schizophrenia. He has a history of both voluntary and involuntary psychiatric hospitalization. He does not trust mental health professionals and only reluctantly takes psychiatric medication. He lives in a subsidized apartment and receives intensive case management from staff at the local community mental health center. His family members are supportive in terms of financial help but are distant emotionally because of inability to predict the behavior they will encounter when they see him. His chief emotional tie was to an elderly cat, and the death of this pet has led to an increase in paranoid symptoms.
- Before his most recent hospitalization, Mr. Butler was distressed because his landlord threatened eviction if his apartment was not cleaned and fumigated. Mr. Butler was unwilling to permit the landlord to enter his

TABLE 9–2 COMMUNITY PSYCHIATRIC NURSING ROLES RELEVANT TO EDUCATIONAL PREPARATION

ROLE	DOCTORAL PREPARATION	MASTERS PREPARATION	BACCALAUREATE PREPARATION	ASSOCIATE DEGREE OR DIPLOMA PREPARATION
Practice	Nurse practitioner or clinical nurse specialist; manage consumer care and prescribe or recommend interventions.	Nurse practitioner or clinical nurse specialist; manage consumer care and prescribe or recommend interventions.	Direct nursing care for consumer and assist with medication management as prescribed.	Provide nursing care for consumer and assist with medication management as prescribed.
Consultation	Consultant to staff re assessment, plan of care, and pharmacologic or other interventions. Consult with family and consumer re treatment options. Consult with community to plan mental health services.	Consultant to staff re plan of care, to consumer and family re options for care; collaborate with community agencies re service coordination and planning processes.	Consult with staff re care planning, and work with nurse practitioner or MD to promote health and mental health care. Collaborate with staff from other agencies.	Consult with staff re care planning, and work with nurse practitioner or MD to promote health and mental health care. Collaborate with staff from other agencies.
Administration	Administrative or contract consultant roles within mental health agencies or mental health authority.	Administrative or contract consultant roles within mental health agencies or mental health authority.	Administrative roles within mental health agency or treatment team.	Leadership roles within mental health treatment team.
Research and education	Act as a research or teaching liaison with local university school of nursing. mentor nurse researchers and educators at clinical level.	Assume an educator or a research role within agency or mental health authority.	Participate in research at agency or mental health authority. Precept undergraduate nursing students.	Participate in research at agency or mental health authority. Precept undergraduate nursing students.

apartment, and when the issue was pressed by his case manager he refused further contact with the case manager. Subsequently, Mr. Butler stopped taking his medication, refused to leave his apartment, and ran out of food. The landlord complained that he was disturbing other tenants by constant yelling at all hours. Attempts to suggest hospitalization were met with increased agitation.

◗ The case manager followed steps to have Mr. Butler hospitalized involuntarily. Within 3 days, Mr. Butler had been restabilized on medication, interacted with staff and other clients in a socially comfortable manner, and was engaging in self-care activities. He was discharged back to the community 6 days after admission, with the plan that community mental health care would resume.

◗ Within weeks, the community psychiatric nurse noted that Mr. Butler had begun to miss appointments for medication management. He had never been a regular member of the daily clubhouse program and was still suspicious of his case manager because of the involuntary hospitalization. The nurse telephoned Mr. Butler, without response. At the next team meeting, the nurse arranged with the case manager to visit Mr. Butler at home. On the day of the visit, Mr. Butler presented as sedated, somewhat confused, and fearful. During the outreach to Mr. Butler's apartment, the nurse discovered that he had not been taking his medication as prescribed (a total of five: an antipsychotic, an anticonvulsant, a side effect medication, an antidiabetic medication, and an antihypertensive agent). All were to be taken at different times of the day. He had clearly missed multiple doses of each.

◗ The psychiatric mental health nurse sat with Mr. Butler and asked general questions about his well-being. During this discussion, she was able to ascertain his mental state and assess a recent history of change in health status. He agreed that she could check his blood pressure, which was elevated. The nurse sorted

Mr. Butler's medications and filled a reminder box with a 7-day supply divided into morning, afternoon, and evening doses. She and Mr. Butler contracted that he would take the medication in the box and she would keep the extra medication. The nurse also learned that Mr. Butler had not purchased food since discharge, and took him to the grocery store near his home. They selected food that required minimal preparation, and Mr. Butler agreed to eat at least once each day. He did have a large supply of coffee in the house, so they also problem-solved ways to reduce his daily consumption of 16 to 20 cups of coffee.

▸ On return to the community mental health center, the nurse stored the medication in a locked box for safety. She consulted with the case manager and the psychiatric nurse practitioner responsible for prescribing Mr. Butler's medication, informing both of Mr. Butler's elevated blood pressure and fragile mental state. The plan of care was revised so that the nurse assumed the responsibility for home visits and for ensuring that Mr. Butler was able to keep appointments with his primary care provider. The psychiatric nurse practitioner requested laboratory tests, including fasting blood glucose level, 12-hour anticonvulsant blood level, liver enzymes, electrolytes, and serum ammonia level. She also scheduled appointments to meet with Mr. Butler weekly until he stabilized.

Box 9–4 MULTIDISCIPLINARY TREATMENT TEAM (NONEXCLUSIVE LIST)

- Client
- Peer counselors
- Family members
- Employers
- Landlord
- Spiritual counselor
- Case manager
- Psychiatric nurse
- Psychiatric nurse practitioner
- Psychiatrist
- Psychiatric social worker
- Psychologist
- Occupational therapist
- Chiropractor
- Vocational rehabilitation therapist
- Nutritionist
- Primary care provider
- Recreation therapist
- Physical therapist

Member of Multidisciplinary Community Practice Team

The concept of using multidisciplinary treatment teams originated with the Mental Health Reform Act of 1963. The practice of psychiatric nursing was identified as one of the core mental health disciplines, along with psychiatry, social work, and psychology. This recognition permitted the allocation of resources to educate psychiatric nurses. It also acknowledged the particular contribution of psychiatric nursing. The team model provided a means of cross-fertilization among the disciplines. This led to enrichment and allowed for the development of a shared language among those providing mental health services (Chamberlain 1987; Peplau 1989).

In team meetings, each member is recognized for individual and discipline-specific expertise as the variety of professions represented on the multidisciplinary treatment team has grown. Generally the configuration of the team reflects the availability of fiscal and professional resources in the community. Box 9–4 presents a list of disciplines that may be represented on a multidisciplinary treatment team. Note that deference is still given to the authority of the psychiatrist as a director of the mental health team. This is in part related to the demands of regulatory and legal authorities, which historically have recognized only those practitioners with medical degrees (Talley and Brooke 1992; Safriet 1994). Increasingly, advanced practice nurses are assuming roles formerly considered the sole purview of medicine (Caverly 1996).

Recognition of the ability of nurses to have a voice in team treatment planning and to question the authority of other professionals was novel at the time it was implemented in community psychiatric practice; this level of professional performance was later modeled for the other nursing specialties. However, the multidisciplinary treatment team approach also led to some dilution of the nursing role embraced by psychiatric mental health nurses in the community. The autonomy of the role, the language of psychiatry and social services, and the respect available to the nurse in this setting created a professional dilemma. How could nurses in this actualized specialty of nursing (including entry educational levels) identify with nurses who functioned in institutional settings, followed physician orders, and received little recognition of their expertise?

In many cases, this conflict resulted in a schism between community psychiatric mental health nurses and their colleagues in other nursing specialties and settings. Community psychiatric mental health nurses in some parts of the United States sought job titles consonant with those of generic mental health practitioners in the community mental health system because of the perceived additional benefits. The improved lot of nursing in recent years has led to rethinking and revision of titling. In the current health and mental health care environment, identification as a nurse or (in particular) as an advanced practice nurse is usually considered preferable to other titling alternatives. Furthermore, the community psychiatric mental health nurse of today better integrates the multidisciplinary perspective with a strong nursing identity. The role incorporates case management, assessment and intervention, client advocacy, somatic therapies, community interaction, and systems intervention (Talley and Caverly 1994). As a team member, the community psychiatric mental health nurse, at all levels, is in a critical position to link the biopsychosocial components relevant to mental health care, and to do so in a manner that the client, significant others, and members of the treatment team can accept and understand.

Biopsychosocial Care Manager

The role of the community psychiatric mental health nurse includes the coordination of mental health, physical health, social service, educational service, and vocational realms of care for the mental health client. The reality of community mental health practice in the 1990s is that few clients present with uncomplicated symptoms of a single mental illness that can be either resolved or managed through brief psychotherapy and pharmacotherapy. The severity of illness with which individuals present, especially in the public sector, has increased and is correlated with increased substance abuse, poverty, and stress. In addition, there is well-documented evidence that the mentally ill not only experience greater risk for physical illness but also are less likely to receive timely and effective treatment (Farmer 1987; Talley 1988; Talley and Caverly 1994).

The 1980s brought increased emphasis on implementing case management, as a core mental health service and provider relationship, for the severely and persistently mentally ill in the community. In the private domain, case management, or "care management," has also found a niche. The intent is to charge case managers with designing individually tailored treatment services for clients, tracking needs for care, and facilitating connection with the range of services. Case management implies attention to and coordination of necessary services for the client, including "client identification and outreach, individual assessment, service planning, linking with services, monitoring of service delivery, and client advocacy" (Francis et al. 1995; Mellon 1994). Nursing and medicine are the only mental health disciplines possessing the knowledge, skill, ability, and legal authority to intervene in the full range of mental health care. This scope of practice, coupled with issues of personnel cost and availability, underscores the critical need for community psychiatric nurses to participate in coordination of care activities. Effective case management reduces unnecessary costly care by maintaining housing and providing creative alternatives to hospitalization (Bawden 1990; Francis et al. 1995; Mellon 1994).

Community tenure likewise increases when medications are taken as prescribed. Nurses are in a position to assist the client to manage medication, recognize side effects, and be aware of the interactions among drugs prescribed for physical illness and those for mental illness. Client education, and the efforts of prescribers to minimize both the number of medications and the frequency of daily dosing, increase the ability of clients to cooperate with treatment and to maintain stability (Omori et al. 1991; Meyer et al. 1991).

Psychiatric mental health nurses have not always valued their unique and important practice abilities. This is changing, and nursing is reclaiming direct care relationships with clients and embracing the advanced practice roles of the nurse practitioner in general and psychiatric specialties. This is a timely rediscovery, because health care reforms are likely to have a significant impact on the role of psychiatric nurses in the community (Huch 1995; Peplau 1989).

COMMUNITY RESOURCES

Community psychiatric mental health nurses originally practiced on site at a community mental health facility. As financial, health care, regulatory, cultural, and population changes have occurred, the location of practice has diversified. Nurses are providing primary mental health treatment at therapeutic day care centers, schools and school-based health centers, outpatient psychiatric hospital programs, and shelters. In addition to these more traditional environments for mental health care, psychiatric mental health nurses increasingly enter forensic settings as practitioners or consultants in drug and alcohol treatment centers, coroner's offices, and jails. Mobile mental health units have even been developed in some service areas. The characteristics of the client population, the geography, the community resources, and the personnel available are perhaps the greatest determinants of where community mental health nurses will be recruited to practice. These factors also influence expectations regarding the extent of preparation for community psychiatric mental health nursing practice (Osborne and Thomas 1991; Worley 1995).

Community Mental Health Centers

Community mental health centers (Box 9–5) were created in the 1960s and have since taken center stage for those who have no access to private care. The range of services available at such mental health centers varies, but generally there are emergency services, adult services, children's services, and elder services; there may also be a psychopharmacology clinic staffed by psychiatric nurses, psychiatric nurse practitioners, and psychiatrists.

Common components of mental health center services include groups such as life-skills psychoeducational classes, supportive day treatment groups, vocational rehabilitation groups, and clubhouse programs. Increasingly, dual diagnosis services for chemically dependent mentally ill clients are available at community mental health centers. Some organizations provide consultation services to nursing homes, manage adult residential facilities for the severely and persistently mentally ill, and provide emergency respite beds to prevent unnecessary hospitalization for clients experiencing crisis (Caverly 1991; Power 1991; Broskowski and Eaddy 1994).

- Nina is a psychiatric nurse who works in a medication clinic at a state-funded community mental health center. She is responsible for managing medications for a large caseload of relatively stable public-sector clients. In monthly half-hour appointments with clients, she assesses the client's response to the medication, looks for previously unrecognized side effects, and determines whether there is continued need for the medication. She also discusses general health care needs and psychosocial concerns such as marital stress or work-related problems. At times, difficulties with parenting or other family issues result in a client's referral to another provider at the clinic for specialized assessment.
- Most of the people Nina sees have known her for a long time and are open about their needs; some require careful probing about potential problem areas. It is essential that, when Nina refills a prescription, she feel confident it is a safe decision in the best interests of the client. She works using protocols established for the clinic. If she has concerns, Nina contacts the psychiatric nurse practitioner or the psychiatrist who is the primary prescriber for the client.

Goals of treatment might include the following:

- Assess response to prescribed medication and recognize side effects that will require intervention.
- Promote stable functioning in the community.
- Identify the need for additional services and assist the client to obtain them.

Homeless Shelters

Frequently, homeless shelters (Box 9–6) and community mental health centers affiliate to provide mental health

BOX 9–5 COMMUNITY MENTAL HEALTH CENTER

Tim is a 31-year-old man who was diagnosed as having bipolar disorder when he was a 19-year-old college student. In subsequent years he self-medicated with alcohol and failed to stabilize on lithium carbonate. Tim was hospitalized a number of times. At the age of 28, he became sober and engaged in regular psychopharmacologic management at the mental health center. He has now been employed full-time as a mechanic for over a year. He is married and expecting a first child in 4 months. His wife is also bipolar, and because of the pregnancy she has chosen to remain off her medication. Her mood disorder has remained remarkably stable, and she continues to be monitored closely. Even so, the situation has been very stressful for Tim. He has been having trouble sleeping and has noticed that his thoughts are racing at times. He is worried because he knows he is responsible for the welfare of his new family. He admits that he has been working as much overtime as he can to save money to buy baby supplies. The couple has no support from family because of the troubles they caused their parents while they were unstable and abusing substances.

The nurse recognizes that Tim appears more pressured than usual. He states that he has been taking his medication regularly, but that it seems not to be working as well as in the past. It is helpful for him to talk about the stress he is experiencing, and he does visibly calm during the interview; however, he is clearly in a hypomanic state.

Tim has been taking lithium carbonate, 1200 mg, at bedtime for the past year and a half. He has not changed his diet during this time and has not experienced side effects. Tim's most recent 12-hour lithium level was drawn 6 months ago, and at the time it was a relatively high 1.3 (range 0.5 to 1.5). The nurse determines that the dosage probably needs to be increased but would prefer to have a level drawn first. Since Tim took his medication at 10 PM last night and it is only 9 AM now, she sends him directly to the laboratory to have his blood drawn. She also increases the dose of lithium to 1500 mg at bedtime for the next week and reschedules to see Tim in 1 week. She plans to consult with his primary physician regarding her intervention.

Tim is comfortable with the plan and follows through with the intervention. Within a few days he notices that his thoughts are more collected and his sleep, while still disturbed, is much more restful. When he returns to the clinic the following week, he learns that his lithium level had dropped to 0.9. He appears more stable at the follow-up appointment. In spite of the improvement noted, the nurse schedules Tim to be seen every 2 weeks for the next month to ensure that he maintains his current stability.

1. Did the educational level of the nurse affect the nursing assessment or intervention with this client?
2. What additional considerations might be taken by the nurse in the future for this family?
3. What would you assess as the strengths of this family?

services to those who otherwise would not be noticed or receive treatment. In some cities, model programs provide funding for mental health services in shelter sites; other cities use community networking to patch together needed services for the disenfranchised. Shelters are of many different configurations, offering many targeted services to specific homeless populations.

The mental health needs at shelter sites vary with the clients who receive homeless care. Primary needs include mental health, substance abuse, and physical health assessment as well as triage to community services. In some instances, there is a need for care to be delivered on site because the client is reluctant to go to a mental health center. At times, the shelter staff transport disorganized or paranoid clients to appointments to ensure that they receive care (Caverly 1991; First et al. 1995; Mowbray et al. 1993).

▶ Erin is a psychiatric nurse who works 4 hours each day at the downtown emergency service center and 4 hours at the women's day shelter. She is employed by the city's homeless project but is part of a team of mental health professionals affiliated with the local community mental health center. Erin spends her day meeting with shelter residents who need help with public assistance paperwork or have questions about obtaining regular mental health care. She also has a group of clients whom she sees weekly to help manage the medications prescribed for them by staff at the mental health center. Sometimes people come to her because they have health problems and don't know where to go; they have no money and are not registered for medical coupons. She is able either to help with these needs or to arrange for appointments with providers who can help. Sometimes Erin actually drives residents to appointments to ensure their arrival on time. She is more likely to help change a bandage or check a wound than are the nurses at the mental health center. The residents appreciate her willingness to be flexible about her role. Erin practices good personal and professional boundaries but is comfortable with a broad definition of her practice.

Goals of treatment might include the following:

- Develop a trusting relationship with residents of the shelter in order to determine their needs for mental health care, physical health care, or social service intervention.
- Provide mental health and other health or social services on site to clients who need immediate intervention or who resist other services.
- Secure necessary services for clients who otherwise would not be likely to attain them.
- Assist residents to use their own resources as well as those offered to stabilize psychiatric symptoms.

BOX 9–6 HOMELESS SHELTER

Rose is a woman of unknown age. She is unkempt and communicates little with others. She uses the women's day shelter and sometimes sleeps at the main downtown shelter (when the weather is cold or wet). She is often seen talking to herself in a corner, and other residents give her a wide berth because she has a history of slapping people if they get too close. Most of the time she just stays to herself; when staff offer her food, she will always eat. She leaves without a word when the day shelter closes and returns regularly in the morning. Staff like her, but since they realize that she doesn't want to get too involved with them, they also give her a great deal of space.

The request for a psychiatric assessment came as a surprise, because the psychiatric nurse knew Rose would refuse to speak with her. The previous night, Rose was forced to leave the shelter because she became loud and unruly, screaming that the devil was eating her feet. She apologized for being profane, but no one heard her use profanity. She refused to be quiet. Once evicted, Rose remained in the street, walking back and forth and loudly complaining about her feet. Shelter staff considered calling the police or having her taken to the emergency department, but she left before the intervention could take place. Still, the behavior was not usual for Rose, and it was of concern.

The nurse found Rose the next morning sitting at her regular spot in the corner. Rose was still complaining under her breath about the devil eating her feet. The nurse decided that, rather than ask Rose about her mental state, she would ask to see her feet. Rose appeared nervous about this but consented, saying she was in great discomfort. With the wet shoes and socks removed, it became apparent that Rose's feet were darkly mottled and cold and had several open wounds where there was pressure from her shoes. The nurse offered Rose the opportunity to bathe her feet in warm water and found some clean socks. She asked Rose when her foot pain began, and Rose indicated it had been quite some time, but only recently the pain was so severe she was unable to stop thinking about her feet. The nurse contacted a health care clinic where free indigent care was available and arranged to take Rose to the clinic. In the course of this supportive work, Rose confided to the nurse that she had also been hearing voices more often lately and wondered if she should tell someone. The nurse suggested that they first take care of Rose's feet and then focus on the voices, and that there was probably something that would help quiet the voices. Rose looked grateful that someone understood.

1. Identify a positive approach this nurse took when assessing Rose's situation.
2. What lesson(s) did you learn from this case study that you might apply in your practice?

Mobile Mental Health Care Units

Mobile outreach units (Box 9–7) have sprung up in various areas throughout the United States to respond to those mentally ill clients who cannot effectively utilize traditional outpatient mental health services. Primm and Houck (1990) described Johns Hopkins Hospital Community Support Treatment and Rehabilitation (COSTAR), a mobile treatment unit serving inner-city Baltimore, Maryland. Treatment is pursued, "wooed," and supported in whatever setting clients find themselves or feel comfortable in: at home, in a public place, in a comfortable clinic, or in jail. Clients are sometimes assessed and treated in fast-food restaurants, receive fluphenazine decanoate (Prolixin Decanoate) injections in restaurant bathrooms, and are offered milkshakes and meals as rewards. If adherence to a prescribed medication schedule or dosing is a problem related to understanding rather than resistance, medications are packaged and labeled with the time and date to be taken. Creative problem solving and intervention planning is a hallmark of care provided by mobile mental health care teams.

In such a program, experienced nurses triage somatic complaints; monitor physical illnesses; provide psycho-education on topics such as substance abuse, nutrition, hygiene, sexual relations, and safer sex; and assist clients to manage symptoms of mental illnesses. Housing is ensured through active community case management coupled with a protective payee system to manage the client's funds. Intervention and psychoeducational efforts are directed toward both clients and those who make up their support systems. Recreation and social groups are valued as a means of developing social skills and a step toward pre-employment training. Other pre-employment activities include vocational rehabilitation and work training. In keeping with the philosophical base of such a program, case management staff are available by pager to clients and families or significant others (e.g., landlords, employers) 24 hours a day to permit emergency intervention or to avert a crisis.

- Jennifer provides emergency psychiatric evaluations and individual counseling as a member of a mobile treatment program. She and two primary health care providers travel in a van to rural areas of the state. In addition, there is a psychiatrist who travels with the team 1 week each month. The psychiatrist prescribes medications for the clients, who receive mental health care and case management from Jennifer throughout the month. She practices autonomously and provides consultation services to the family nurse practitioners with whom she works. Many of the individuals for whom she provides care are migrant workers. Jennifer speaks fluent Spanish and can effectively interview clients when interpreters are not available. Many of the people she sees are separated from their families and homesick. They are often living in austere circumstances, and depression is a common diagnosis. She is careful to evaluate for substance abuse disorders during all her assessments.
- Often Jennifer attempts to secure other social services for clients and their family members. Sometimes an intervention may be as simple as locating a source of infant formula for a mother who is unable to breast-feed. At other times, Jennifer must evaluate whether psychotic symptoms are due to a mood disorder, schizophrenia, or substance abuse. Jennifer has access to an on-line computer for literature and pharmacotherapy reference, and consults with the psychiatrist as necessary by telephone. She has standing orders that permit her to initiate pharmacological intervention in psychiatric emergencies.

Goals of treatment might include the following:

- Provide assessment and intervention for psychiatric and psychosocial disorders to a population that would

BOX 9–7 MOBILE CARE SETTING

A 37-year-old woman presents with a complaint of low energy, sadness, and poor concentration. She has a bruise on her face, and her arm is bandaged, but she refuses to have the wound evaluated. She is accompanied by her husband, who appears quite concerned. He is reluctant to leave her alone during the interview and she is adamant that he remain. He responds to questions directed to her and she defers to him. She shows signs of anxiety and hyperalertness when asked about her marriage and support system. A request that her husband leave the room creates a great deal of agitation, but he does leave. The woman is then asked direct questions about domestic violence.

Her only family is her husband, and she says he is a good man whom she will not speak against. She only wishes to feel better so that he won't be angry with her.

The nurse acknowledges the women's dilemma. She also confronts her regarding the need to be safe. The nurse provides education regarding domestic violence and the community resources available, should she wish to reach them. An appointment is scheduled for the following week when the mobile unit will again be in town. Before the woman's discharge, the nurse completes a risk assessment.

1. What are some of the ethical dilemmas presented in this case?
2. In situations such as these, what are some of the personal issues (self-assessment) you might want to look at when working with clients in similar situations? (See Chapter 15 for guidelines.)

otherwise have little or no access to mental health care.
- Provide differential diagnoses and recommend appropriate treatment to nonpsychiatric health care practitioners.
- Manage medications prescribed by another practitioner.

Forensic Settings

A small but growing number of nurses work with mentally ill offenders. Society has increased its efforts toward social control; consequently, we are seeing an increased use of correctional facilities to house the mentally ill. Deinstitutionalization has evidenced a "hydraulic effect" (i.e., as people are discharged from state mental hospitals, they enter the correctional institutions) (Reeder and Meldman 1991). Psychiatric mental health nurses are faced with a number of challenges, not least of which is the conflict arising around the provision of mental health care in an environment where the intent is punitive. Correction staff (from administrators to correction officers) often devalue or even resent the care the psychiatric nurse provides to the inmate. The inmate requesting mental health services is often viewed as enjoying an undeserved privilege or using manipulative behavior to seek drugs that will help make incarceration tolerable. The nurse is at the heart of this struggle, often needing to make difficult assessments both about inmates' needs and about the motivations behind the requests for service. The psychiatric nurse, to work successfully in a forensic setting (Box 9–8), must come with a background in crisis intervention and apply "a creative approach using a humanist, nonjudgmental philosophy" (Reeder and Meldman 1991).

The advocacy role of nursing is tested in this setting; there is a need to educate and collaborate with correction staff while integrating the agenda of care with that of incarceration. The necessity of a psychiatric nursing presence in correctional facilities cannot be overemphasized. As with any underserved and vulnerable population, there is a humanistic mandate to provide access to care, and in this circumstance there is an accompanying imperative need that care providers have a high level of expertise—including the ability to engage in a process to determine which problems require intervention.

Forensic psychiatric mental health nurses often find roles outside the confines of the correctional institution. Examples of such roles are seen in nurses who act as investigators to medical examiners or coroners, clinical forensic nurses who collect evidence from victims, nurses who evaluate clients as competency therapists, those who provide therapy to criminal defendants in pre-trial settings, and those who intervene after unexpected deaths to review evidence and care for survivors (Lynch 1993).

- Robert is a nurse who provides care to clients who have been incarcerated at the county jail. It is his responsibility to respond to referrals made by corrections and nursing staff for inmates who present with symptoms of psychiatric disorder, or who have reported on entry to the jail that they are currently taking a psychiatric medication. He is not a nurse practitioner, but jail protocols permit him to contact psychiatric providers for the inmate and accept orders for the continuation of medication. Robert also has access to standing orders that allow certain psychiatric medications to be dispensed as needed to inmates. Often the referrals he receives are for assessment of suicide risk in a newly incarcerated individual. He performs a standard risk assessment and a mental status examination, and also attempts to gather relevant psychosocial history if the inmate is cooperative.
- The challenges of Robert's work include distinguishing inmates who adopt psychiatric symptoms as a means of

BOX 9–8 FORENSIC SETTING

Julia has been arrested for possession with intent to sell narcotics. She has recently used heroin and is fearful of detoxing. Other prescribed medications include methadone maintenance and venlafaxine (Effexor), an antidepressant with a short half-life and withdrawal agitation. She informed the corrections officer that she would find a way to kill herself unless she could continue to receive the methadone and the Effexor. The nurse received a request to evaluate Julia the morning after she was incarcerated. At that time, she was irritable, impatient, sweating, and complaining of gastrointestinal distress. Her mood had become more labile than it had been at booking, and she was not amenable to being interviewed.

The nurse aborted the interview, ordered a toxicology screen, and contacted the practitioners who had been prescribing methadone and Effexor. It was established that Julia was truthful regarding her medication, and the nurse was then able to obtain medical orders for continued treatment during her incarceration. Julia was informed that she would receive her required medications and immediately contracted to remain safe from self-inflicted harm while incarcerated.

1. In what way would you have approached the same problem in a similar setting?
2. In another setting, would a different approach be more appropriate?
3. What personal issues might you want to be aware of (nurse's self-assessment) before assessing and intervening with (a) forensic clients or (b) clients with substance abuse problems in the community setting?

being removed to more private housing within the jail, recognizing drug-seeking behavior and substance withdrawal symptoms, and dealing with conflict between the agendas of care and punishment that separate him from the corrections staff with whom he works.

Goals of treatment might include the following:

- Assess the psychiatric status of inmates who present with psychiatric symptoms or are at risk for self-harm.
- Recommend appropriate placement within the facility to ensure the safety of inmates with psychiatric impairment and of those around them.
- Maintain medications and stable psychiatric status for inmates who have a psychiatric history.

Private Practice Settings

The advent of managed mental health care, and the expansion of legal scope for advanced practice psychiatric mental health nurses in many states, has encouraged a subgroup of nurses to enter the arena of private community practice (Box 9–9). The setting for this entrepreneurial practice varies, depending on the interest of the nurse, community need, and the characteristics of the community and client population. As third-party payers and other clients become familiar with the services offered by advanced practice psychiatric mental health nurses, there is a growing appreciation for the flexible, all-encompassing, biopsychosocial approach the advanced practice nurse brings to community mental health care. This is not to imply that all insurers recognize advanced practice; a number of reimbursement barriers continue to exist (Safriet 1994). The psychiatric mental health nurse serves a varied population of clients in a general practice utilizing a broad array of approaches from family and individual psychotherapy to pharmacotherapy. Subspecialization is increasingly common, and some nurses choose to work with a specific population such as survivors of trauma, children with learning disorders, persons suffering from chronic mental illness, or those with both physical and psychiatric illnesses. Advanced practice nurses in the field of psychiatric mental health have also begun to form and administer privately run multidisciplinary agencies (Caverly and Talley 1997; Caverly 1996).

◗ Carolyn is a psychiatric nurse practitioner with prescriptive authority. She has a full-time private practice serving persons who have mild to moderate mental illness, and who either are able to pay for services or are insured by the companies for which she is a preferred provider of psychiatric specialty care. She is thinking about discontinuing her relationship with the managed care organizations because she has concerns about the level of personal information they require her to provide regarding her clients. Her only reservation is that such a decision may result in the termination of long-standing relationships with clients because they would need to pay out-of-pocket for her services.

◗ Discomfort with this ethical dilemma has led Carolyn to to create a sliding fee scale and cultivate a clientele who prefer to pay independently for services. In addition to the clients who see her for therapy, she provides medication management for individuals who receive therapy from nonprescribing providers.

◗ Carolyn works primarily in her own office, but one afternoon each week she sees clients at a local AIDS residence facility. She has developed expertise in providing both pharmacological and psychotherapeutic intervention to persons with AIDS. She also occasionally visits a nursing home to provide mental health assessment of residents who are exhibiting psychiatric symptoms.

◗ Carolyn has a strong biopsychosocial background and conducts comprehensive assessments before she considers potential intervention strategies. She often orders laboratory or psychometric testing to ascertain the client's diagnosis and capacity to tolerate medication. She has a relationship established with two community laboratories and admitting privileges at the local psychiatric hospital. Since a large percentage of her practice consists of persons with both physical and mental health disorders, she has established a consulting relationship with a family nurse practitioner and with an internist. She usually obtains preliminary laboratory results before sending clients to one of these consultants for follow-up on a health-related concern. Among the routine laboratory tests she requests are those for thyroid-stimulating hormone, blood count, electrolytes, and liver enzymes.

Goals of treatment might include the following:

- Assessment for general psychiatric and mental health complaints.
- Psychotherapeutic or pharmacological intervention to stabilize or resolve psychiatric symptoms.
- Assistance to providers in planning and delivering care in a manner appropriate for the client.

Outpatient Substance Abuse Treatment Facilities

The incidence of mental illness among those who are also substance abusing is greater than 50% by most estimates. Identification of the dually diagnosed mentally ill chemical abuser (MICA) has led to the development of treatment services to accommodate these clients in both the mental health and substance abuse treatment settings (Box 9–10). However, because of different funding streams and treatment philosophies, there have often been significant gaps between the two systems. Psychiatric mental health nurses who have expertise in treatment of substance abuse have the ability to provide care that integrates the benefits of the two models and provides valuable consultation to the staff with whom they work.

BOX 9–9 NURSING HOME, PRIVATE PRACTICE NURSING CONSULT

Mr. Thomas is a 77-year-old man who has resided in a nursing care facility for 3 years after hip surgery and the death of his wife. He is pleasant and gregarious but has had repeated health problems. His current diagnoses include congestive heart failure, transient ischemic attacks, adult-onset diabetes, and severe osteoarthritis. He is receiving medications for each of these disorders but is seen only quarterly by the general practitioner at the nursing home. Within the past 2 months he has become increasingly confused and has been belligerent at times toward staff and residents. He becomes especially disturbed at night, but staff have noticed a change in his level of functioning throughout the day also. There is speculation that he is depressed because his grandson left for college 3 months ago. Until then, this grandson had visited Mr. Thomas every Sunday.

The psychiatric nurse practitioner was asked to meet with Mr. Thomas to assess his mental state and assess his presenting problems. Mr. Thomas appreciated the attention but became obstreperous when asked about the change in his behavior; however, he glowed when the topic of his grandson was broached. Review of the chart revealed the increased confusion, episodes of which were associated with loss of balance and visual disturbance. His blood glucose level was last checked 5 months previously when his medication was changed. Also, his arthritis medication has been changed and there has been no neurological evaluation in the past year. He has been complaining of physical discomfort more often since the medication change, and his sleep has been less consistent.

The nurse consultant's report recommended that Mr. Thomas receive a comprehensive physical assessment, including laboratory work-up and neurological examination. In the event of negative findings, the next step would be to try to engage Mr. Thomas in the available social activities at his resident community rather than immediately prescribing an antidepressant or antipsychotic medication. Mr. Thomas agreed to this plan.

1. In what way would you approach the same problem in a similar setting? Would your consult include recommendations for additional medication protocols?
2. Was the setting important to the decision-making process of the nurse?
3. What would be one concern for this client's future care? How could you address this concern?

▶ Kathryn is a psychiatric nurse who has also worked at an inpatient psychiatric facility and a chemical detoxification center. She currently works for an outpatient chemical dependency program, providing individual case management, counseling, and group therapy to clients who are both chemically dependent and mentally ill. She assists other counselors when they have questions about the medications their clients take, or about possible physical problems related to substance abuse. She does not have responsibility for medication dispensing or management; there are other nurses who work in a more traditional role dispensing methadone and naltrexone hydrochloride but have no counseling responsibilities. Kathryn sometimes works with probation officers or jail health personnel, and she has frequent contact with child protective services because she works with the mothers of small children. Occasionally she helps clients to find housing or to negotiate agreements with landlords to prevent eviction. Kathryn often finds herself in the position of enforcing the rules of the program, including termination of treatment when ongoing substance abuse is proved by drug testing.

Goals of treatment might include the following:

- Maintenance of sobriety.
- Stabilization of psychiatric symptoms and appropriate use of psychiatric resources.
- Stabilization of life style, including housing, family structure, and work or school.

Home Psychiatric Mental Health Care

Despite historical precedent, home health care (Box 9–11) is now considered an innovative treatment (Daudell-Strejc and Murphy 1995). Provision of community psychiatric nursing is closely linked to home health nursing, yet it has been rare for community psychiatric nurses to make home visits. Psychiatric nursing in the home has been viewed as a costly service and restricted to homebound, severely disabled clients. Clients who receive such care are usually elderly, physically impaired, or nonparticipators in traditional center-based community mental health care (Kimball and Williams-Burgess 1995). These individuals often have long-term severe mental problems as well as chronic physical problems (e.g., arthritis, diabetes). As community mental health agencies and bureaus become accountable for inpatient as well as outpatient costs of care, there is increased interest and willingness on the part of the organizations to provide this service as a means of reducing inpatient treatment days.

The mentally ill within the community are often vulnerable. They may lack family support, work skills, the ability to use public resources, and the cognitive or affective capacity to cope with daily living. Murphy and colleagues (1995) found that clients believed that community-based care meant increased personal freedom, self-selection of diet, greater mobility, more self-management, fewer prescribed medications, and less pressure to interact with people.

BOX 9–10 OUTPATIENT SUBSTANCE ABUSE SETTING

Roberta is a pregnant woman addicted to heroin who entered methadone treatment to decrease the risk to her unborn child. She is motivated to stay clean and sober. She is an adult survivor of incest and physical abuse; the pregnancy has brought these to the surface, causing significant depression. She currently has no housing and lives with her husband in single-room-occupancy hotels when they have money. He has a history of being physically abusive; Roberta is fearful he may harm her and the baby while she is pregnant, but she needs him to protect her on the streets and is ambivalent about leaving the relationship. She had an opportunity to stay at a women's shelter but chose not to leave her husband on the streets alone. She now regrets that decision.

The pregnancy is at month 7 and has been difficult. Roberta is fatigued and unable to sleep because of discomfort and inconsistent shelter. She has recurrent suicidal ideation but readily denies intention to hurt herself or her child. She has an earlier child, now 3 years old, who was taken by child protective services shortly after birth because of Roberta's heroin abuse during pregnancy. Her one focus now is on having a healthy baby and the opportunity to be a mother.

The nurse assessed Roberta's strengths and problem areas. Despite her motivation to be clean and sober, several circumstances threaten her ability to do so. Roberta exhibits symptoms of depression, but it is not clear whether these arise from psychiatric illness or situational factors. There is no concern that Roberta will volitionally harm herself or her baby, but her husband might. Priorities are identified as securing a stable place to live and arranging for consistent prenatal care. The nurse works with Roberta to develop a list of problems, identify means of approaching them, and look at available resources. Roberta is given the task of using a phone at the facility to call the organizations that may have services she needs.

Antidepressant medication is discussed, but, given the primacy of daily living needs, together they decide it is premature to consider medication before situational factors are addressed. Finally, the nurse confronts the issue of domestic violence. Roberta makes it clear that she has no intention of permitting her husband to hurt her while she is pregnant and that if he does she will immediately contact a women's shelter. She is given the shelter hotline number and encouraged to keep it where it will not be accessible to her husband. Plans are made for Roberta to enter the high-risk pregnancy program, to meet with her case manager twice a week, and to attend group twice weekly as she feels physically able.

1. What are some of the ethical issues the nurse might encounter in this situation? Which one would you grapple with first?
2. Are there cultural contradictions or ethical questions you might have (self-assessment) in order for you to plan and implement the best care for this client?
3. What other concerns would you have for this client?
4. What might you plan with Roberta in the future if she were to stay involved with the health care system?

A client's "resistance" to coming to a clinic for mental health care may be due to symptoms of psychiatric illness: the apathy or withdrawal of depression, the ambivalence or paranoid ideation associated with schizophrenia, or the anxiety related to agoraphobia. The downside of community-based care is the often difficult process of ensuring that those who need psychiatric services have access to them. Home mental health care improves the potential for many to receive treatment, but there will continue to be those who are reluctant to permit care providers into their home (Sullivan and Cohen 1990). A practice of having family members (or neighbors) of clients who are homebound or reclusive accompany professionals when they visit the client increases the probability that the professional will be granted access to the client's home (Peternelji-Taylor and Hartley 1993).

The environment in which a person chooses to live provides rich information about that person's culture, values, level of functioning, resources, and needs. Many aspects of assessment and intervention are facilitated through an outreach to the home. The realities with which an individual client must contend cannot be adequately appreciated when information is gleaned only through an interview at a mental health facility or an inpatient setting. The information obtained during a home visit can result in medication regimens being negotiated rather than merely ordered. Differential diagnoses are more easily made in the home because of the degree to which evidence of adaptive ability or dysfunction is present. For example, the depressed client's home may be organized but barren, while the organically impaired client's home may present random disorganization.

The concept of the professional as a guest in the home of the client requires nurses to rethink the manner in which the business of nursing is conducted. Bowers (1992) studied the community psychiatric nurse's interaction in a home visit and found it to be associated with a change in the dynamics of power and control. The client is firmly in charge and the nurses must use nonauthoritarian strategies, such as persuasion and negotiation, to intervene. Matters directed by the professional in the office (e.g., where to sit, whether there is music or television) must be worked out with clients when in their homes. The nurse must acknowledge that "because [clients are] on home ground, [they lay] down the rules, decide upon actions, and direct the visit" (Bowers 1992). Determining the areas in which it is appropriate to establish and exert oneself as the expert or to offer consultation and guidance is a skill nurses must develop.

Boundaries become important, albeit less clear, in the home setting, where there is inherently a greater degree of intimacy between nurse and client. It may be important for the psychiatric home health nurse to begin a visit by reinforcing or developing an informal relationship with the client. Efforts to accomplish this might include accepting refreshment offered by the client. This interaction can be a strain for the nurse who struggles to maintain distance and professional formality. However, there is great significance to the interaction that occurs during a home visit, and the therapeutic use of self in such a circumstance incorporates establishing connectedness, comfort, and emotional warmth through chatting about family issues or helping with small chores (e.g., mailing letters). The manner in which the nurse responds in a client's home is likely to be keenly observed and to have profound meaning to that individual or family, both positive and negative (Daudell-Strejc and Murphy 1995).

▸ Linda provides consultation to the city's Visiting Nurse Service (VNS). She is a psychiatric clinical specialist with a subspecialization in geropsychiatry. The local VNS predominantly serves an elderly, homebound, physically compromised population. This includes both rural and urban clients, as the county is quite large and diverse. She may be asked to assess whether an elderly man is capable of remaining in his home after having threatened the building manager with a golf club, to evaluate an elderly woman's complaint of abuse by a home living attendant, or to determine the ability of a confused elderly woman to continue to live independently in her own home.

▸ The variety of her work is what appeals to Linda. She is sometimes able to establish ongoing relationships with clients; at other times, she provides only consultation intended to help home health care nurses and their assistants to deliver appropriate care. She does not prescribe medication but does recommend pharmacological interventions to general practitioners. In most cases, there is no other psychiatric practitioner involved in the client's care; her assessments and recommendations are accepted by both nursing and medical providers.

Goals of treatment might include the following:

- Assess the diagnostic and functional status of the client.
- Determine the safety of the living situation.
- Ascertain the need for additional resources or redistribution of existing resources.
- Assess the need for, or response to, pharmacological intervention.
- Implement or recommend a psychosocial treatment plan.

BOX 9–11 HOME HEALTH CARE SETTING

Mrs. Avery is an 88-year-old woman who lives alone. She has recently had difficulty managing her diabetes, especially in taking her insulin appropriately. Her house is cluttered with stacks of old newspapers and there was a pan melted to the electric burner on the stove when the visiting nurse came for a regular visit. Apparently Mrs. Avery's limited olfactory sensation prevented her smelling the enamel burning on the pan, but she refuses to take it seriously, and won't agree to have someone stay at her home to assist her. Recently, she has called the police frequently to report crimes; when the police respond, they find no one in the vicinity and no evidence of damage. Mrs. Avery is hopeful the nurse consultant can help her rectify the problems with her neighbors by forcing them to move.

Mrs. Avery is alert and oriented. Her fund of knowledge is adequate and her thought processes are intact, although she is preoccupied with the perceived troubles her neighbors are causing. She shows no evidence of responding to internal stimuli, but she appears to have beliefs about her neighbors that are not reality based and becomes angry when these are challenged. Her insight and judgment are poor.

When her health status is discussed, Mrs. Avery proudly displays her new blood glucose monitoring device, but she doesn't know how to use it. Her insulin dosing has been erratic. A quick look in Mrs. Avery's refrigerator reveals a quart of milk, a bunch of celery, and a box of sweet rolls.

Mrs. Avery agrees to have the nurse meet with her neighbors to discuss her complaints. She also agrees to have the nurse arrange for more in-home assistance with blood glucose monitoring and diet management. Mrs. Avery remains socially isolated with the exception of her contact with police and home health nurses. She agrees to meet someone from the local senior center, so long as the first meeting occurs with the home health nurse present. The assessment and plan are provided to the home health agency and to the general practitioner who care for Mrs. Avery.

1. What are the ethical implications of the nurse's behavior?
2. How was the setting important in the decision-making process with Mrs. Avery?
3. Would the educational level of the nurse affect the nursing assessment or interventions?

ETHICAL ISSUES

As community psychiatric nurses assume greater autonomy and accountability for the care they deliver, ethical concerns become more of an issue. Ethical dilemmas are common in disciplines and specialties that care for the vulnerable and disenfranchised. Nurses who choose to become community psychiatric nurses have an obligation to develop a model for assessing the ethical implications of the clinical decisions required of them. In many cases, there is dissonance between what is best for the individual and what is in the best interest of the community or the general client milieu. State laws require reporting of some behaviors (e.g., child abuse), but often the information obtained from a client during psychiatric treatment is considered to be privileged. Psychiatric mental health nurses have an obligation to communicate clearly with clients about categories of information that fall beyond personal or professional understanding of privilege and that will not remain confidential. This standard is best communicated to the client before sensitive information is disclosed.

Each incident requiring ethical assessment is somewhat different, and the individual nurse brings personal insights to each situation. The role of the nurse is to act in the best interests of the client and of society, to the degree that this is possible. It is never acceptable for the nurse to seek self-gain from the relationship with a client, and there is most certainly an expectation of honesty in the relationship the nurse enters with the client. However, elements of justice, beneficence, and nonmaleficence are affected by the parameters of the nurse-client relationship and by the others who are a part of the equation. Ethical dilemmas arise in situations where there *is* no clear-cut ethical response. The nursing profession must find improved ways of supporting individual nurses as they struggle to find the best response to these difficult situations. Organized nursing has assisted in this process by addressing ethical dimensions in published practice standards and guidelines.

Ethical problems have been discussed in the literature, most often in relation to hospital settings. As psychiatric mental health nurses increasingly practice in independent home and community settings, important ethical concerns await identification and reflection. Three ethical problem areas experienced by community psychiatric nurses—moral uncertainty, dilemma, and moral distress—were studied by Forchuk in 1991. Ethical issues included "doing good, autonomy, maintaining client confidentiality, and avoiding deception." Community psychiatric mental health nurses indicated a belief in the client as decision maker, yet described an ownership for nursing actions (Forchuk 1991).

The issue of social control and the role assumed by community mental health professionals in maintaining social control is an important and constant ethical conflict for community psychiatric mental health nurses. The mentally ill are cared for in the community so long as they are able to maintain social standards of acceptable behavior. The community funds public-sector mental health care, and as such the community is the customer purchasing community mental health services. This is problematic for those who work in the public sector, because the desires of the community may not be consistent with the wishes of the individual client who is mentally ill. Like the public health model from which it has evolved, the health—or, in this case, the mental health and safety—of the community seems to supersede that of the individual. At the same time, community psychiatric mental health nurses are educated and socialized to care for individuals with mental illness. The power of the nurse in this dynamic process, and the often unacknowledged secondary agenda of community safety, cannot but affect the nature and experience of the relationship between the nurse and the client.

In the acute care setting the power differential inherent in psychiatric treatment is generally clear. In the community setting the nurse must consciously assess the effect of power and control on the long-term therapeutic relationship between nurse and client. Regulations have evolved to restrict the rights and privileges of those who suffer from mental illness. Each state has some version of an involuntary treatment act that permits professionals, sometimes community psychiatric nurses, to hospitalize and/or medicate persons against their will when sufficient grounds are evident. Key grounds for detention tend to be danger to self and to others (Whitley 1991). Refer to Chapter 4 for legal precedents. The following case presents a dilemma faced by the psychiatric nurse and shows one path that might be taken to resolve conflict. It is understood that, while the decision-making process may be explicit and consistent, the definition of **ethical dilemma** implies the lack of a clear right or wrong solution. Each nurse must weigh the issues and chart an action within an ethical frame of reference.

Ethical Conflict

- Sharon is a 34-year-old woman recently hospitalized after a suicide attempt. She has suffered from depression since the age of 14 and has experienced only rare, brief episodes of euthymic (normal) mood since that time. Sharon has been cooperative in taking antidepressant medications in spite of discomforts associated with side effects such as dry mouth, psychomotor stimulation, and blurred vision. Within the last year, she has been divorced, lost custody of her two young children, and become unemployed because she complained of workplace abuse.
- Sharon has recently been diagnosed with multiple sclerosis and has significant muscle weakness and pain attributed to this illness. The increased severity of Sharon's depressive symptoms, including fatigue and

suicidal intent, are thought to be directly related to her physical illness and the poor prognosis. Her general practitioner has become frustrated because Sharon is failing to follow through on treatment recommendations and physical therapy. He is also uncomfortable with her refusal to commit to a contract not to harm herself (refer to Chapter 24 for setting up a no-suicide contract). He has begun to disengage, and Sharon describes feeling hurt by this in spite of understanding the practitioner's reasons.

- As the primary mental health care provider for Sharon, the nurse feels an obligation to help Sharon clarify her own wishes for psychiatric treatment and to attempt to pursue mutually agreeable treatment goals. This has become more difficult since she expresses an almost constant suicidal intent. Sharon has promised that she will not overdose on the medications she receives from the mental health clinic because she doesn't want the nurse to feel responsible for her death. She is very clear, however, that she does intend to complete a successful suicide attempt at some undisclosed time.
- Sharon's thoughts are clear; she has made arrangements for her children to receive her belongings and has written them loving letters. She has also compiled albums that include their preschool report cards and pictures of the children and their mother together. In spite of her refusal to contract to be safe, she gives no indication that she is in immediate danger. She directly states that she appreciates the mental health care she is receiving and values her relationship with the nurse, but frankly does not wish to continue living. She asks that the nurse respect her decision.
- The fact that Sharon is so clearly considering her death, has a realistic understanding of her life circumstance, and has made what she believes to be an informed decision causes the nurse to feel uncomfortable, assuming that Sharon's decision is an indication of psychiatric impairment. The mental health center standard is that when clients refuse to contract to be safe from self-harm they must be hospitalized. If the individual declines a voluntary admission, the court-appointed mental health professionals are asked to detain the person.
- The nurse is aware that this is the treatment plan the agency expects her to pursue, and realizes that a history of depression, with past suicide attempts plus current suicidal ideation, is adequate grounds for a request that Sharon be detained. However, she chooses not to take this approach because she believes that such action will further distance Sharon from care. Also, Sharon says she would find involuntary treatment dehumanizing and that it would exacerbate her wish to die, and she indicates she would wait to be discharged and then complete her suicide plans. Given this knowledge, the nurse does not refer Sharon for an evaluation, and in fact does not explicitly discuss this decision with her manager. She believes that neither she nor her manager has the power to prevent Sharon from committing suicide, but that perhaps Sharon can be helped to consider alternatives and to create a series of reasons to delay taking action, thus allowing her to benefit from individual, group, and pharmacological interventions.
- Instead of seeking hospitalization for Sharon, the nurse increases the frequency of their appointments. She tries to reestablish a regular visitation schedule for Sharon and her children in order to strengthen Sharon's relationship with them, and to intervene with Sharon's ex-husband to ensure his cooperation (if not understanding). In conversations about the children or about parental suicide, the nurse comments about the wonderful qualities possessed by Sharon's children and the emotional trauma known to occur when a child's parent commits suicide. She offers to assist with transportation to physical therapy and health care appointments. While doing these things, she is careful to be honest in communicating her motives to Sharon. She expresses both concern and caring when she does this, and states that she personally values Sharon. At no time does the nurse promise not to seek involuntary psychiatric hospitalization; rather, she bases nursing actions, including commitment, on frequent assessment of imminent danger. She is also careful to evaluate for any indication that Sharon's desire to end her life is extended to the lives of her children.

ETHNIC AND CULTURAL CONSIDERATIONS

Culture is a concept that transcends mere ethnic diversity; its definition can include, but is not limited to, such elements as ethnicity, race, nationality, region, language, class, sexual orientation, and gender. Obviously, culture can be of tremendous significance when nurse and client are from different backgrounds; thus, psychiatric nurses are in great need of cultural awareness regarding their own biases and beliefs as they embark on community practice. It is a basic requirement that nurses become comfortable working with individuals, families, and communities who have diverse life experiences and understandings.

Community work frequently involves engagement with people who, because they are not acculturated, may have failed to secure services at a clinic or hospital. Migration and social change are considered the two primary stresses affecting the mental health of the world population (Lin 1986). Thus, it is not infrequent that immigrants suffer significant mental health disorders. Culturally sensitive and culturally competent assessment and intervention are necessary for effective mental health treatment, whether or not the practitioner is intimate with a given culture. The following case provides insight into ways culturally naive practitioners who have flexibility are able to seek out cultural brokers to assist in providing psychiatric care that is helpful to the client.

Cultural Context

▶ Sara is a community psychiatric nurse who works as a liaison practitioner with the local refugee clinic. She is experienced working with interpreters and is comfortable with clients from other cultures. Sara has requested an interpreter for her first appointment with an Eritrean client who is new to the clinic. She has no specific knowledge of Eritrea. The only available interpreter is Ethiopian. Unfortunately, Sara is not aware that there is significant struggle between the two African nations, and that animosity also exists between their nationals who are living in the United States. Worse, the Eritrean people generally distrust the Ethiopians.

▶ As the interview progresses, it becomes clear that the interpreter is unable to develop a relationship with the client. Either the client appears not to comprehend the questions or the answers are curt. Tension mounts in the room. Finally, the interpreter tells Sara that the situation is untenable. The interpreter is not interested in further victimizing the client by forcing him to reveal inadequacies to someone he perceives to be an enemy.

▶ Sara is grateful for the information, which helps her to understand why this interview was unproductive and the context for the client's presenting problems. She terminates the session, rescheduling at a time a non-Ethiopian interpreter will be available.

Goals of treatment might include the following:

- Utilize the interpreter as a cultural broker to learn about the Eritrean culture.
- Assess presenting psychiatric symptoms in the context of the client's culture.
- Plan intervention strategies that fit the client's cultural context.
- Utilize culturally relevent or available resources in implementing mental health care.

To be effective, the nurse must understand the client's culturally acceptable ways to resolve dysfunction. Kagawa-Singer and Chung (1994) suggest that therapists must do more than just "know the client's culture." The culture of the individual prescribes and defines not only what constitutes the healthy self but also the intra- and interpersonal ways in which the person achieves and maintains integrity and self-worth.

There are no cultural universals: each member of a culture has a personal interpretation of the cultural experience. Presumption of culturally appropriate care on the basis of stereotypes is never acceptable practice. Expression of disease varies with cultural identity and experience (Tabora and Flaskerud 1994). Psychiatric mental health nurses are accountable for understanding how the symptoms of an illness are expressed culturally and, conversely, what the meaning of a symptom is within the context of culture (Westermeyer 1985).

Interventions at a community level also need to be culturally competent; it is important that the intervention not be implemented using a template based on the dominant culture (Marin 1993). Sensitivity to clients includes consideration of their cultural values as well as an understanding of their culture's attitudes toward the identified needs and expected outcomes. Community interventions are most successful when approached from a collaborative, mutually respectful model.

Physiological and somatic differences between racial and ethnic groups are important considerations for those who prescribe or manage somatic therapies. Medications are prescribed in all cultures, but there are important differences in effective dosage levels and the potential for unwanted side effects (Lin 1986). In some instances, it is important to target physical rather than affective symptoms when recommending medications. For example, a woman may come to a clinic believing that the pain in her stomach and head is the problem; once domestic violence is ruled out, psychiatric and physical assessments suggest a diagnosis of posttraumatic stress disorder with depression and somatic symptoms. The pharmacotherapeutic intervention of choice is an antidepressant medication. However, if the woman must first accept depression as her primary problem, she may either decline treatment or agree to medication and not take it; it also becomes more likely that she will fail to return for future care. A more effective approach might be to offer medication that will help with the stomach pains and headache. The name of the drug, the side effects, and the benefits can be addressed in a routine fashion; the diagnosis of depression is downplayed. Treatment is then acceptable to the client, and both the physical symptoms and the psychiatric disorder improve.

THE CHANGING HEALTH CARE ENVIRONMENT

Community psychiatric nursing, like all the health care professions, will be affected by the changing health care environment. Health care spending has continued to grow, and some predict that it will reach 18% of the U. S. gross domestic product by the year 2000, and 32% by 2030. Health care purchasers (both private and public) press for revisions in health insurance that will compress costs associated with new and expensive technology, an aging population, and inefficient use and distribution of health care resources. Managed care as a way to distribute financial and health care resources favors outpatient services and a focus on prevention and wellness, rather than inpatient care (McLaughlin 1994). Policymakers demand greater proof of the effectiveness of a health care service before funding programs, yet are often isolated from the direct provision of mental health care, thus reinforcing fiscal aspects of mental health reforms to the possible detriment of the human aspects (Mechanic 1993, 1994).

Managed Care

The changing health care environment is a product of a number of forces: the globalization of our economy; the lack of state and local control in setting up many of the federally subsidized programs (e.g., Medicare and Medicaid), and the pressure on them to provide more care to the severely mentally ill; the efforts of the National Institute of Mental Health to direct its research focus toward biological understandings of mental illness; and a current mandate to focus once more on prevention. The National Alliance for the Mentally Ill emerged in the 1980s as a powerful voice for the mentally ill at state, local, and federal levels.

Within the health care delivery system, the array of health care provider disciplines has broadened. Health care management, through utilization reviews, put forth the concept that appropriate care is given in the appropriate setting by the appropriate provider. Geographical distribution of the health care workforce is changing the overall nature of the health care delivery system (McLaughlin 1994; Safriet 1994). Racial and ethnic minority groups are still underrepresented among health care providers; given the growing U. S. minority population, schools of nursing must grapple with the need to increase student and faculty diversity.

Previously, cost was driven by treatment decisions determined by the health care providers, who were paid directly by the insurance company or government program (e.g., Medicare, Medicaid) for the care or service provided to the client. The insurance company in turn approached the employers, who purchased the insurance for their employees.

The current health care environment embraces a managed care approach in which services are determined, provided, and monitored by a network of providers who are part of a health care company. Managed care companies define practice guidelines that frame the limits of services for which health care providers can receive reimbursement, and even dictate which medications will be provided for the client. Health care providers become just one part of the treatment triangle (client, provider, insurer), yet retain the responsibility for achieving good treatment outcomes in a cost-effective, timely manner. Hospital "downsizing" and emphasis on shorter hospital stays are contributing to projections that by the year 2000 there will be a surplus of physicians and hospital-based nurses in all specialties (except perhaps primary care) (Krauss 1993; McLaughlin 1994; Olson 1994).

Future Models

Future models of psychiatric mental health care suggest a separation between mental illness and mental health care. Mental illness will be addressed under the category of neurological disorders, along with Parkinson's disease, strokes, and schizophrenia. This new model encompasses a brain disease concept, with care being conceptualized and delivered on a neurological continuum that incorporates concepts of chronicity, persistence, and severity. Separating mental health and mental illness places diseases such as schizophrenia, bipolar disorder, and obsessive-compulsive disorder with other neurological diseases such as Parkinson's disease and multiple sclerosis. This model supports arguments for insurance parity for psychiatric disorders.

Mental health prevention and treatment will be designated social services; psychotherapy; stress management; preventive mental health care; and family, child, and adolescent behavioral and marital therapy delivered by persons working in social services. Psychiatric mental health nurses will be educated in either social services or neurological treatment. Psychiatric mental health service delivery will focus on the social networks necessary to support the level of function a client is capable of achieving.

Nurses at every level will have a larger role to play as this new model unfolds. There may be greater necessity for subspecialization in the area of brain disorders and somatic interventions or psychotherapy modalities. Nursing has enjoyed a long history of caring for the client in the home; with the shift to community-based care and home health care, the nurse is in an obvious position to play a crucial role (Mellon 1994). However, as nurses increase their presence in the field in general, and in home health care in particular, they need to become increasingly progressive, autonomous, and active in designing their role in the delivery of home health care (Bunn 1995; Worley 1995).

Interdisciplinary teams, as we know them today, may not exist in years to come because there will be no strict disciplines to define teams. All health care provider education may begin with a single core curriculum; the focus will be on outcome competencies rather than on degrees. Problem-based learning outlines a new approach to health care professional education that organizes curricula around problems, not disciplines; integrates theory and clinical learning; and emphasizes critical thinking skills as well as basic knowledge. Future professionals will skillfully adapt to change, reason critically, and treat holistically in an integrated approach to health care (Bruhn 1992).

To meet the challenge of the twenty-first century, Price and Capers (1995) suggest that for the associate degree nurse "educators must increase their focus on leadership development, include principles of home health nursing, increase content on gerontology, and introduce basic community health concepts." Bunn (1995) stated that "the emphasis on community-based mental health care will require not only a paradigm shift in the way educators and practicing nurses think but also result in a role transformation for nurses." Knowledge, skill, and increased role presence of all health professionals will be necessary as we embark on the twenty-first century.

SUMMARY

The community psychiatric mental health nurse has a history of home health nursing that dates back to the 1800s, when trained nurses visited homes in both urban and rural communities. A revolution in community mental health occurred after World War II and was in great part due to the combined effect of new psychotropic medications, a raised level of awareness and conscience about the conditions of institutions, and the normalization of mental health problems (as the armed services rejected or traumatized a great number of men). In response, mental health treatment began to shift to the community setting.

Community psychiatric mental health nurses have become service brokers for clients. In the community, clients direct their own lives, and thus treatment is a negotiated process. The nurse acts as a consultant to the client and the client's extended social support network.

The characteristics of treatment goals and intervention strategies within the community setting are consistent with hospital-based mental health nursing, except that a great deal more flexibility may be called for, as well as a constant demand for creative problem-solving skills. Nurses must demonstrate a number of personal attributes, such as an awareness of self as a therapeutic agent; flexible, creative problem-solving ability; calm presentation under stress; and the requisite knowledge and skills appropriate to the position. Community practice opportunities are varied, limited only by creativity, resources, the needs of the client population, the geography, and the community.

As mental health treatment becomes increasingly standardized, psychotropic medication is better understood to be an effective treatment. In the era of managed care, treatment has shifted to the community and into the homes of those afflicted with psychiatric mental health disorders.

It is predicted that psychiatric mental health nurses will become increasingly visible and viable as the emphasis in mental health treatment embraces the full biopsychosocial spectrum of disorders. The necessity for the psychiatric nursing profession to practice comfortably in neighborhood settings and community treatment agencies is becoming critical as health care resources become more limited. Entering the home of a client as a visitor/guest/clinician requires conscious preparation and ongoing reflection on the part of the community psychiatric mental health nurse. Treatment can be expected to incorporate innovative interventions, new psychotropic medications, and assertive outreach treatment modalities. Psychiatric mental health nursing beyond the confines of the hospital represents a tremendous challenge and an extraordinary opportunity for the discipline and specialty. The capacity to adapt and assume a flexible approach to the role plus a commitment to delivering appropriate and relevant care to clients will permit nurses without community expertise to assume and develop new psychiatric mental health nursing roles for the twenty-first century.

REFERENCES

American Nurses' Association (1994). *A statement on psychiatric– mental health clinical nursing practice and standards of psychiatric–mental health clinical nursing practice.* Washington, DC: American Nurses Publishing.

Bachrach, L. L. (1994). The chronic patient: The Carter Commission's contributions to mental health service planning. *Hospital and Community Psychiatry,* 45(6):527–528, 543.

Bawden, E. L. (1990). Reaching out to the chronically mentally ill homeless. *Journal of Psychosocial Nursing,* 28(3):9–13.

Bowers, L. (1992). Ethnomethodology II: A study of the community psychiatric nurse in the patient's home. *International Journal of Nursing Studies,* 29(1):69–79.

Broskowski, A., and Eaddy, M. (1994). Community mental health centers in a managed care environment. *Administration and Policy in Mental Health,* 21(4):335–351.

Bruhn, J. G. (1992). Problem-based learning: An approach toward reforming allied health education. *Journal of Allied Health,* 2(3):161–173.

Bunn, H. (1995). Preparing nurses for the challenge of the new focus on community mental health nursing. *Journal of Continuing Education in Nursing,* 26(2):55–59.

Callahan, D. (1994). Setting mental health priorities: Problems and possibilities. *Milbank Quarterly,* 72(3):451–470.

Carson, W. (1993). Prescriptive practice in the 1990's: A crazy quilt of overregulation. Unpublished manuscript. Washington, DC: Nurse Practice Counsel, American Nurses' Association.

Caverly, S. (1991). Coordinating psychosocial nursing care across treatment settings. *Journal of Psychosocial Nursing and Mental Health Services,* 29(8):26–29.

Caverly, S. (1996). The role of the psychiatric nurse practitioner. *Nursing Clinics of North America,* 31(3):449–463.

Caverly, S., and Talley, S. (1997). Roles and functions of psychiatric nurses in the community. In N. K. Worley (Ed.), *Mental health nursing in the community.* St. Louis: Mosby–Year Book.

Chamberlain, J. G. (1987). Update on psychiatric-mental health nursing education at the federal level. *Archives of Psychiatric Nursing,* 1(2):132–138.

Crosby, R. L. (1987). Community care of the chronically mentally ill. *Journal of Psychosocial Nursing,* 25(1):33–37.

Daudell-Strejc, D., and Murphy, C. (1995). Emerging clinical issues in home health psychiatric nursing. *Home Healthcare Nurse,* 13(2):17–21.

Farmer, S. (1987). Medical problems of chronic patients in a community support program. *Hospital and Community Psychiatry,* 38:745–749.

First, R. J., Wheeler, D. P., Belcher, J. R., and Johnson, D. (1995). Redefining the health care needs of persons who are homeless and mentally ill: Implications for diagnosis and treatment. *Journal of Applied Social Sciences,* 19(1):1–9.

Forchuk, C. (1991). Ethical problems encountered by mental health nurses. *Issues in Mental Health Nursing,* 12:375–383.

Francis, P., Merwin, E., and Fox, J. (1995). Relationship of clinical case management to hospitalization and service delivery for seriously mentally ill clients. *Issues in Mental Health Nursing,* 16:257–274.

Huch, M. H. (1995). Nursing and the next millennium. *Nursing Science Quarterly,* 8(1):38–44.

Kagawa-Singer, M., and Chung, R. C. (1994). A paradigm for culturally based care in ethnic minority populations. *Journal of Community Psychology,* 22:192–208.

Kimball, M. J., and Williams-Burgess, C. (1995). Failure to thrive: The silent epidemic of the elderly. *Archives of Psychiatric Nursing,* 9(2):99–105.

Krauss, J. B. (1993). Health care reform: Essential mental health services. American Nurses' Association. Washington, DC: American Nurses Publishing.

Lin, T. Y. (1986). Multiculturalism and Canadian psychiatry: Opportunities and challenges. *Canadian Journal of Psychiatry,* 31(7):681–690.

Lynch, V. A. (1993). Forensic nursing: diversity in education and practice. *Journal of Psychosocial Nursing and Mental Health Services,* 31(11):7–14.

Marcos, L. R. (1990). The politics of deinstitutionalization. In N. L. Cohen (Ed.), *Psychiatry takes to the streets: Outreach and crisis intervention for the mentally ill* (pp. 3–15). New York: Guilford Press.

Marin, G. (1993). Defining culturally appropriate community interventions: Hispanics as a case study. *Journal of Community Psychology,* 21:149–161.

McLaughlin, C. J. (1994). Health workforce issues and policy-making roles. In P. F. Larson, et al. (Eds.), *Health workforce issues for the 21st century* (pp. 1–22). Washington, DC: Association of Academic Health Centers.

Mechanic, D. (1993). Mental health services in the context of health insurance reform. *Milbank Quarterly*, 71(3):349–364.

Mechanic, D. (1994). Establishing mental health priorities. *Milbank Quarterly*, 71(3):501–514.

Mellon, S. K. (1994). Mental health clinical nurse specialist in home care for the 90s. *Issues in Mental Health Nursing*, 15:229–237.

Meyer, T. J., Van Kooten, D., Marsh, S., and Prochazka, A. V. (1991). Reduction of polypharmacy by feedback to clinicians. *Journal of General Internal Medicine*, 6(2):133–136.

Mowbray, C. T., Cohen, E., and Bybee, D. (1993). The challenge of outcome evaluation in homeless services: Engagement as an intermediate outcome measure. *Evaluation and Program Planning*, 16:337–346.

Murphy, L. N., Gass-Sternas, K., and Knight, K. (1995). Health of the chronically mentally ill who rejoin the community: A community assessment. *Issues in Mental Health Nursing*, 16:239–256.

Murray, R., et al. (1995). Components of an effective transitional residential program for homeless mentally ill clients. *Archives of Psychiatric Nursing*, 9(3):152–157.

Olson, D. P. (1994). The ethical considerations of managed care in mental health treatment. *Journal of Psychosocial Nursing and Mental Health Services*, 32(3):25–32.

Omori, D. M., Potyk, R. P., and Kroenke, K. (1991). The adverse effects of hospitalization on drug regimens. *Archives of Internal Medicine*, 151:1562–1564.

Osborne, O. H., and Thomas, M. D. (1991). On public sector psychosocial nursing: A conceptual framework. *Journal of Psychosocial Nursing and Mental Health Services*, 29(8):13–18.

Peplau, H. E. (1989). Future directions in psychiatric nursing from the perspective of history. *Journal of Psychosocial Nursing and Mental Health Services*, 27(2):18–28.

Peternelji-Taylor, C. A., and Hartley, V. L. (1993). Living with mental illness: Professional/family collaboration. *Journal of Psychosocial Nursing and Mental Health Services*, 31(3):23–28.

Power, J. (1991). Expanding the role of community mental health nurses. *Canadian Nurse*, 5:20–21.

Price, C. R., and Capers, E. S. (1995). Associate degree nursing education: Challenging premonitions with resourcefulness. *Nursing Forum*, 30(4):26–29.

Primm, A. B., and Houck, J. (1990). COSTAR: Flexibility in urban community mental health. In N. L. Cohen (Ed.), *Psychiatry takes to the streets: Outreach and crisis intervention for the mentally ill* (pp. 107–120). New York: Guilford Press.

Reeder, D., and Meldman, L. (1991). Conceptualizing psychosocial nursing in the jail setting. *Journal of Psychosocial Nursing and Mental Health Services*, 29(8):40–44.

Regier, D. A., et al. (1993). The de facto US mental and addictive disorders service system. *Archives of General Psychiatry*, 50:85–94.

Rochefort, D. A. (1993). *From poorhouses to homelessness: Policy analysis and mental health care.* Westport, CT: Auburn House.

Safriet, B. J. (1994). Impediments to progress in health care workforce policy: License and practice laws. *Inquiry*, 31:310–317.

Scales, C. J., Mitchell, J. L., and Smith, R. D. (1993). Survey report on forensic nursing. *Journal of Psychosocial Nursing*, 31(11):39–44.

Smith, C. M. (1995). Origins and future of community health nursing. In C. M. Smith and F. A. Maurer (Eds.), *Community health nursing: Theory and practice* (pp. 30–52). Philadelphia: W. B. Saunders.

Sullivan, A. M., and Cohen, N. L. (1990). The home visit and the chronically mentally ill. In N. L. Cohen (Ed.), *Psychiatry takes to the streets: Outreach and crisis intervention for the mentally ill* (pp. 42–60). New York: Guilford Press.

Tabora, B., and Flaskerud, J. H. (1994). Depression among Chinese Americans: A review of the literature. *Issues in Mental Health Nursing*, 15:569–584.

Talbott, J. A. (Ed.) (1981). *The chronic mentally ill.* New York: Human Sciences Press.

Talley, S. (1988). Basic health care needs of the mentally ill: Issues for psychiatric nursing. *Issues In Psychiatric Nursing*, 9:409–423.

Talley, S., and Brooke, P. S. (1992). Prescriptive authority for psychiatric clinical specialists: Framing the issues. *Archives of Psychiatric Nursing*, 6(2):71–82.

Talley, S., and Caverly, S. (1994). Advanced-practice psychiatric nursing and health care reform. *Hospital and Community Psychiatry*, 45(6):545–547.

Westermeyer, J. (1985). Psychiatric diagnosis across cultural boundaries. *American Journal of Psychiatry*, 142:798–805.

Whitley, M. P. (1991). Treatment dilemma: A political science perspective. *Journal of Psychosocial Nursing*, 29(8):35–39.

Worley, N. K. (1995). Community psychiatric nursing care. In G. W. Stuart and S. J. Sundeen (Eds.), *Principles and practice of psychiatric nursing* (5th ed.) (pp. 831–849). St. Louis: Mosby–Year Book.

SELF-STUDY AND CRITICAL THINKING

Matching questions

1. ________ Nurses who have a 2-year degree from an accredited school of nursing
2. ________ Nurses who have successfully completed 3 years at a school of nursing, with a traditional emphasis on clinical training
3. ________ Nurses who have a degree in nursing from a university setting after completing a 4-year program in nursing
4. ________ Nurses who have completed a 4-year, university-affiliated nursing degree program and have achieved national certification by the American Nurses Credentialing Center
5. ________ Nurses who have a master's degree in nursing from an accredited school and have achieved national certification by the American Nurses Credentialing Center
6. ________ Nurses who have a master's degree and a doctoral degree from the field of nursing or an allied field such as sociology, psychology, or public health

A. Associate Degree Nurse (ADN)
B. Diploma Nurse (RN)
C. Baccalaureate Degree Nurse (BDN)
D. Psychiatric Mental Health Clinical Specialist (RN, CS)
E. Doctoral Prepared Nurse (PhD)
F. Psychiatric Mental Health Nurse (RN, C)

Choose the correct answer.

7. The Community Mental Health Centers Act that President Kennedy signed into law in 1963
   A. Placed nurses at the forefront of the community mental health movement
   B. Reversed the trend toward home health care back to institutionalization
   C. Emphasized treatment within the community setting
   D. Helped initiate a returning mentally disabled servicemen act
8. The most significant influence allowing for treatment to move to the community setting was
   A. The discovery of psychotropic medication
   B. A new collaborative approach focusing on rehabilitation treatment by both staff and clients
   C. Television
   D. Identification of external causes of mental illness

9. Educated nurses who visited the homes of the sick in the 1800s paved the way for

   A. Community psychiatric mental health nurses
   B. Managed care
   C. Sectarian health care
   D. An interdisciplinary team approach

10. Community psychiatric nursing assessment does not include the following:

   A. Housing and financial stability
   B. Review of health history and mental status
   C. Reliance on the written report from the hospital rather than on the client's report
   D. Consideration of concerns expressed by the client's family

Write a short response.

11. If the client has authority to choose and in part direct mental health care, does the psychiatric mental health nurse have responsibility for treatment outcome? Justify your response.

12. Acceptable community psychiatric mental health nursing can be provided only by members of the same ethnic cultural background. Justify your response.

13. List four community settings in which the community psychiatric mental health nurse might work.

   A. client
   B. psychiatric Nurse Nutritionist
   C. spiritual councelor
   D. family members

14. List five members of an interdisciplinary team.

   A. primary care office
   B. Client worksite
   C. Youth Centers
   D. group homes
   E. private office

15. List important differences in possible nursing care interventions in the inpatient/hospital psychiatric unit versus community setting.

   A. suicidal precautions / continuous watch.
   B. use of restrants / if harm to others.
   C. ________________
   D. ________________
   E. ________________

16. Nurses must be aware of who their clients are. Which of the following might be the client of the community psychiatric mental health nurse?

    A. Mental health client
    B. The community
    C. Family member
    D. Landlord
    E. The legal system
    F. All of the above

17. Important attributes of the community psychiatric mental health nurse include

    A. ______
    B. ______
    C. ______
    D. ______
    E. ______

True or false

Place a T (true) or an F (false) in front of each statement.

18. ______ Community mental health nurses within the home setting find an important difference in "negotiating" treatment versus "ordering" treatment.

19. ______ Nurses in the home setting would turn off intrusive TV noise without asking permission from the client.

20. ______ Nurses would never go out of bounds of the traditional professional role in the home and perform an extra service such as hanging curtain rods for an elderly woman.

21. ______ Nurses would disregard the client's home environment in making an assessment of the client.

22. ______ Ethical dilemmas happen only in the inpatient hospital setting.

23. ______ Psychotropic medications are prescribed universally but have important dosage differences among culturally diverse populations.

24. ______ A psychiatric nurse working in the shelter setting must maintain boundaries and never assist a resident with health problems that are not specifically psychiatric in nature.

Critical thinking

25. In the chapter's case history of Mr. Butler (p. 225):

    A. What are the ethical aspects of the actions taken by the community psychiatric nurse?
    B. Why was the responsibility for home visits transferred to the community mental health nurse?
    C. Would it have been more logical to rehospitalize Mr. Butler?
    D. What other interventions might have been made?

26. Beth, age 11, has been living for a week in a house with other transients. Beth's aunt, a client of the community psychiatric nurse, just called to complain that Beth had stolen her jewelry and her medicine. The aunt, a client of the nurse, takes both

hypertensive and psychotropic medication. The aunt gave the following history of Beth and asked the nurse to intervene.

Beth is the second child of three in her family; her mother was using drugs at the time Beth was conceived and continues sporadically to use both drugs and alcohol. The children have been cared for by relatives over the years, but the aunt kicked Beth out of the house because of the theft. Beth's behavior has been increasingly out of control over the past few months, and she has been getting into difficulties with the law and with truant officers.

At the nurse's request, the aunt phoned the house to get Beth's permission for the nurse's visit. When the nurse arrived, she introduced herself and invited Beth to go with her to a fast-food restaurant. Beth agreed. The nurse told Beth about her relationship with Beth's aunt; she explained that the aunt had asked her to help Beth with her living situation, with school, and with anything else that Beth needed to help her feel better. Beth talked about her difficulty in finding a place to live and how hard it was to go to school. She was not sure where her mother was living. Beth and her aunt had gotten into a fight about Beth's not going to school, and Beth stole from her aunt because she felt angry and betrayed by her whole family. Beth was willing to let the nurse help her. Beth was too angry to stay with the aunt, so she chose to stay in a group home for adolescent girls until her mother could be found.

The nurse, with the help of the community agency, found her mother; the mother agreed to apply for housing, enter a drug and alcohol treatment program, and attend a parenting class so that she could have Beth live with her. The nurse then helped Beth enter a school close to her mother. She coordinated treatment with the school counselor to resolve school-related problems. Beth continued to see the community psychiatric nurse, who referred her for prescription of antidepressant medication (sertraline hydrochloride [Zoloft]) to help with her explosive anger, while she worked in therapy on issues of anger, abandonment, and neglect.

A. What was the ethical issue considered by the community psychiatric nurse when she asked the aunt to phone Beth and introduce the nurse? Should the nurse have taken the aunt with her to visit Beth?
B. Should Beth have been hospitalized? Why or why not?
C. Should Beth have been placed in a foster home and no effort made to rehabilitate her mother?
D. What are the implications if the nurse finds, or fails to find, Beth's siblings?

10

Communication Within Groups

CATHERINE M. LALA

OUTLINE

KEY TERMS AND CONCEPTS

The key terms and concepts listed here also appear in bold where they are defined or discussed in this chapter.

insight
feedback
resistance
acting out
behavioral group therapy
systematic desensitization
flooding
self-help groups
support groups
heterogeneous groups
homogeneous group

OBJECTIVES

After studying this chapter, the reader will be able to

1. Identify the basic concepts used in group therapy.
2. Describe the different roles group members may adopt within a group.
3. Discuss the approaches to group therapy for (a) time-limited groups, (b) therapeutic milieu groups, (c) behavioral group therapy, and (d) self-help groups.
4. Distinguish between the guidelines for establishing an inpatient versus an outpatient therapy group.
5. Contrast and compare the four phases of group development.
6. Act out one intervention for a group member who (a) monopolizes a group, (b), complains but rejects help, and (c) chronically helps others.
7. Apply, in a simulated group situation with classmates, useful interventions that a group leader could use when leading (a) a group for people with a serious and persistent mental illness, (b) a group for people with a mental disorder and a substance abuse problem (dual diagnosis), and (c) a group for people with eating disorders.

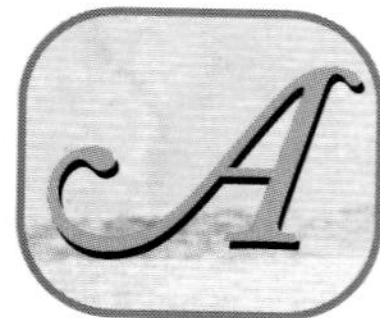

All humans, in order to live, strive for some personal connections in life. Infants are particularly sensitive to nonverbal behaviors, such as tenderness in touch. As growing children master language, they interpret verbal and nonverbal behaviors according to the frame of reference used in their family. Language defines thought. As individuals mature through experiences with significant role models and peers, they become members of school, social, or work groups; this membership gives them a sense of belonging to the larger society. Failure to experience positive group interactions leads to feelings of isolation and loneliness. Clients frequently use their experience in a group to help them find a way to resolve problems and to develop interpersonal skills—thereby increasing personal growth and fulfillment—and perhaps to redefine a satisfying emotional connection with others (L. Clarke, personal communication, 1993).

Nevertheless, many people are reluctant to join therapy groups and are initially fearful of being judged when they reveal personal information. Yalom (1983) stated that "clients often enter therapy with the disquieting feeling that their misery is unique or that they alone have certain frightening or unacceptable impulses or fantasies."

In the group, clients hear others share similar concerns, fantasies, and life experiences. The realization that they are not alone in their situation may offer considerable relief and a "welcome to the human race" experience. The name of this concept is *universality.* Universality is one of 10 curative factors of group therapy described by Yalom (1985) that can guide therapeutic interventions. Yalom's other curative factors of group therapy are

1. *Imparting of information.* Some groups, such as Alcoholics Anonymous (AA) and psychotherapy groups, help members learn about their symptoms and their interpersonal dynamics and about how working through problems in a trusting atmosphere leads to growth as an adult or individual.
2. *Instillation of hope.* Groups can instill hope in clients who are demoralized or pessimistic. Group members can gain hope from others with similar problems who have made positive changes in their lives through therapy.

3. *Altruism.* Learning that they can be useful to others leads members to value themselves more, prevents morbid self-absorption, and promotes self-growth.
4. *Corrective recapitulation of the primary family group.* Members are influenced in the group by their own histories. For example, the client initially perceives the behavior of other members as being like that of the client's siblings and the behavior of the group leader as being like that of the client's parents. When neither the members nor the leader responds as siblings or parents have in the past, the client begins to gain insight into his or her behavior (Naegle 1993). Through feedback and exploration, early conflicts can be resolved and growth can then take place.
5. *Development of socializing skills.* Group members can develop new socializing skills and can learn to correct maladaptive behavior through ongoing group interactions.
6. *Imitative behavior.* Imitative behavior is a powerful therapeutic tool through which a client identifies with the healthier aspects of the other group members or the leader and learns to imitate behaviors that the client wishes to develop (Wolfe 1993).
7. *Interpersonal learning.* Interpersonal learning in the group experience is gradually transferred to other situations in the person's life outside the group.
8. *Group cohesiveness.* Group cohesiveness relates to bonding or solidarity of the group members, the feelings of "we" instead of "I," and the fact that members are of value to each other. Cohesiveness is shown by regular group attendance and ability to communicate a full range of feelings (e.g., anger to joy) without the group's disintegrating.
9. *Catharsis.* Catharsis is the expression of feelings (intense negative as well as positive emotions) in a nonthreatening atmosphere.

Psychiatric nurses have many opportunities for observation and intervention. In primary psychiatric nursing, the nurse-client relationship is the cornerstone of all therapeutic nursing interactions. In a group setting, the nurse observes, interprets, and facilitates the client's relationships with others. The nurse-client relationship often affects a client's motivation and ability to feel safe in any kind of group. The nurse's experience in group therapy can motivate clients to continue in outpatient treatment.

The importance of nurses for detailing this effort and the expected outcomes cannot be underestimated. For many reasons, nursing staff members have not been sensitized to the importance of describing their practices in sufficient detail to allow others to replicate these practices (Van Servellen et al. 1992).

A protocol, or description, of the actual nursing care involved in a group includes

1. The clear, concise objectives of the group.
2. The method or means to evaluate the success of the group.
3. The organization of such features as

- Frequency of group meetings.
- Qualifications of group leaders.
- Descriptions of types of clients, their behaviors, and the diagnoses that are most suited to a type of group.

An example of a standard group protocol format is provided in Box 10–1.

After a group experience, when people are presented with qualitative outcome criteria such as a questionnaire based on curative factors of groups, they tend to respond in these ways:

I do not feel alone.
I need this.
Why don't they have more groups like this?
Extend the group to from 1 hour to 2.
I'm more able to open up.
After being in this group, I am more capable of reaching out to others.
This is my first time in a psychiatric hospital. I am in because of the encouragement of a friend. I told her, "I'm in a hole and I don't know how to get out." Now I tell people when I feel lonely and they come to visit. I know who I can count on.
If I want to change a behavior or something about myself, I'll try it in group first.

BOX 10–1 STANDARD GROUP PROTOCOL

- Title of the group
- Group activity staff (names and qualifications)
- Group format designer
- Group investigative team
- Consultants to the design and evaluation of this group activity
- Group leaders
- Purpose and goals of the group
- Conceptual/theoretical framework for the group
- Specific aims of the group
- Group format
- Specific group content and methods
- Client population (inclusion and evaluation criteria, including procedures for screening patients)
- Measurement of outcomes–description of measurement of outcomes (evaluation methods, tools, frequency of evaluations)
- Methods of documentation of group process and patient progress

Adapted from Van Servellen, G., et al. (1992). Methodological concerns in evaluating psychiatric nursing care modalities and a proposed standard of group protocol format for nurse-led groups. *Archives of Psychiatric Nursing,* VI(2): 117–124.

I used to feel I did not deserve caring messages. I used to make deflecting comments. I used to be self-effacing. Now, I can accept caring messages.

I used to consider friendship an inconvenience. Now, I reconsider this. I used to push people away. I feel more comfortable—maybe I can help someone else now.

Outcome criteria can also be used by an outside evaluator (e.g., another trained staff member) to help evaluate the effectiveness of the group. For example (Hamilton et al. 1993):

- Therapist gives feedback to group members about their behavior.
- Therapist facilitates interactions between group members.
- Therapist checks for understanding of what is being said.

ROLES NURSES PERFORM

The Nurse as Teacher

Nurses can teach groups of clients about managing chronic illness or specific rehabilitative or preventive health care. Examples of group teaching in a community setting are seminars on nutrition for senior citizens, stress management seminars, or exercise programs. Many wellness programs that are directed and coordinated by nurses provide an opportunity for increased nursing visibility in the community. Many facilities welcome new speakers and cultivate opportunities for new knowledge for their clients. With the increasing cost of health care, such programs can be seen as economical solutions to health care as well as opportunities to decrease social isolation.

Educational Preparation for Teaching a Group

Certification and credentialing programs exist for various kinds of groups. Teachers of groups would benefit from preparation of outlines and specification of goals and objectives. With the advent of managed care, groups need to be efficient since resources are finite. National health care trends indicate that the use of ambulatory, outpatient care is increasing. The nurse must couple knowledge of group process and content, which are described in this chapter, with an interest in helping others to learn. Supervision of the nurse is essential. Refer to Chapter 7.

Nurses need to be prepared to evaluate the outcomes of the groups. This may be easier to accomplish with education and psychoeducation groups than with therapy groups. A nurse can define key outcome quality indicators and can track those indicators over a period of time. For example, the key quality indicators for successful outcome (client education) in a medication education group could be any of the following: the client will (1) ask questions about medication, (2) maintain compliance while hospitalized, and (3) report side effects.

The group educator, who could be a nursing student with guidance or a basic-level or advanced-level nurse, can provide effective group education in a particular diagnosis, such as bipolar disorder. In a bipolar disorder group, a selected homogenous group on the inpatient unit could meet for up to two sessions per week. The support of the staff is obtained to promote group attendance. Box 10–2 is an example of an outline for leading a bipolar group.

The Nurse as Group Therapist

Nurses began to develop a role as leaders of group therapy in the 1960s. Peplau believed that nurses should work with other health professionals (e.g., psychiatric social workers, psychologists, psychiatrists) in the role of group psychotherapist.

Educational Preparation for Group Therapists

Individuals who conduct group psychotherapy need specific education and experience. The American Nurses' Association sets the standard for graduate study (masters degree or higher) for nurses, which includes the necessary theory, supervision, and clinical practice. On the bachelor and associate degree levels, nurses with an understanding of group therapy and process may be actively involved in leading therapeutic groups.

Training obtained through college courses, workshops, and ongoing clinical supervision is essential. Psychiatric clinical specialists can serve as role models and mentors for nurses who wish to learn about various types of groups. Group therapy always has a theoretical base; this base is one that the leader believes in, is educated in, and believes to be appropriate for the outcome criteria of the group.

Nurse group therapists need to have individual or peer-group supervision. In supervision, the nurse reviews the process of therapy with a more experienced therapist or with peers. Group work provides a rich learning environment. All psychotherapeutic work with clients—whether it is individual, couple, family, child, group, or any other type—requires interpersonal learning with a senior clinician who is trained in that particular therapy (Critchley and Maurin 1985). In *supervision*, a relationship exists between the supervisor and the supervisee that helps the supervisee become more therapeutic. The

BOX 10-2 BIPOLAR DISORDER SELF-MANAGEMENT GROUP

This group can be modified for both inpatient and outpatient settings. The purpose of a bipolar disorder group is:

1. To share information.
2. To teach self-management and coping with bipolar disorder.
3. To assist with improving interpersonal relationships (Pollack 1995).

MATERIALS

Flip chart/easel

RESOURCE MATERIALS

1. What is bipolar disorder? National Alliance for the Mentally Ill* (pamphlet)
2. Patient medication education sheets on: Lithium (Lithium Carbonate)
   Carbamazepine (Tegretol)
   Valproic Acid (Depakene)
   Pharmacopeia
3. Drug interactions—lithium and ibuprofen (Motrin)
4. Therapeutic drug levels—Laboratory information guide
5. Symptoms of bipolar disorder—National Depressive and Manic Depressive Association
6. Reading List, e.g.: Jamison, K.R. (1995). An unquiet mind. New York: A.A. Knopf.

Pollack (1995) provided the following format:

- Orientation to the group
- Introductions
- Review and discussion of group rules, such as "bring your feelings to the group," "group starts and ends on time," "be the chairperson of yourself"
- Presentation of the material on a chalkboard
- Group discussion
- Discussion about the session/evaluation by the patients and the therapist

GROUP TOPICS

- Understand bipolar disorder
- Relating to others
- Managing daily life
- Relating to one's self
- Managing other's reactions
- Knowing what to say in job interviews

Adapted from Pollack, L.E. (1995). Treatments of inpatients with bipolar disorders: a role for self-management groups. *Journal of Psychosocial Nursing,* 33:1.

*Alliance for the Mentally Ill of New York State, 260 Washington Avenue, Albany, New York 12210.

American Nurses' Association's *Standards of psychiatric–mental health nursing practice* (1994) states that

> The psychiatric mental health nurse engages in performance appraisal of own clinical practice and role performance with peers or supervisors on a regular basis, identifying strengths as well as areas for professional/practice development.

Clinical supervision should be ongoing throughout the nurse's experience as a group leader.

The Nurse as Co-Therapist

The use of a co-therapist can greatly benefit the beginning group therapist. For example, a co-therapist may be of help when anger escalates, when a client decides to leave the group, or when a client threatens to commit suicide. It is advantageous for the therapist and co-therapist to discuss their theoretical frameworks beforehand to establish if the frameworks are the same or at least compatible.

The co-therapists need to communicate about the group process and content as often as the group meets, both before and after each group session. Both therapists need to be aware of their reactions to each other. Feelings of competition or disagreement concerning interventions often emerge. At these times, supervision allows for clarification of the issues and helps the therapists work through them. Once the issues are in order, the therapists can focus once again on the group members and on the group process.

FEELING OF THERAPIST	POSSIBLE THERAPIST BEHAVIOR	IMPROVED THERAPIST BEHAVIOR
1. Feels left out, not understanding where the co-therapist is "leading" a client.	1. Begins to tell group members personal information.	1. Clarifies with the other therapist his or her confusion. Provides a model for other clients.
2. Has the same problem as a group member.	2. Asks the co-therapist in the group for a solution.	2. Works through the problem in his or her own supervision, joins therapy group on the outside.

BASIC GROUP CONCEPTS

Group therapy, by its very format, offers unique opportunities to experience and work through issues of intimacy and individuation. It is usually impossible for individuals to view themselves as existing alone and affecting no one after participating in group therapy for a significant period of time (Rutan and Waller 1979). Individuals are brought together in groups and are expected to work at their relationships with others in the group. The easy escape response of changing relationships is highly discouraged in favor of resolving conflicts in the group setting (Rutan and Waller 1993). Two tools that are commonly used in groups to bring about growth are insight and useful feedback.

Insight is categorized at four learning levels:

1. How one is seen by others
2. What one is doing in relation to others
3. Why one is doing what one is doing
4. Genetic insights

Useful **feedback** has the following characteristics:

- It is clear.
- It has a high degree of immediacy.
- It focuses on the sender of the message.
- It is affective (deals with emotions).
- It involves risky self-disclosure.
- It deals with the sender-receiver relationship.
- It is minimally evaluative (without judgments).

Clients come to therapy to make their futures better. They plan, think, and feel about what is store for them. Past, present, and future all have important places in treatment.

Common Group Phenomena

Groups are based on different models and theoretical orientations. However, they have the following in common (Morgan and Moreno 1973):

1. *Group acceptance.* Individuals feel that they are respected by, accepted by, and belong to the group.
2. *Reality testing.* Group members can monitor each person's reactions and behaviors, providing feedback in an open and nonthreatening manner.
3. *Universality.* Group members feel secure when they realize that they do not have unique problems and are not so different from other persons.
4. *Ventilation.* Group therapy provides an opportunity for ventilation of various emotions that would otherwise remain bottled up.
5. *Intellectualization.* Members gain insight into their problems by learning to examine or explore symptoms in themselves, as well as in other group members.
6. *Altruism.* Members give advice, support, and encouragement to one another.
7. *Transference.* The individual develops an emotional attachment to another person, such as the therapist or the members of the group.
8. *Interactions.* Group therapy provides group members with the opportunity to assert themselves to improve communication skills with others outside the group.

The therapist uses several techniques to "facilitate" communication:

1. *Communication.* Exploring what is vague, unclear, puzzling, contradictory, or incomplete.
2. *Confrontation.* Pointing out contradiction or incongruities, what is ignored, minimized, or even denied. Confrontation focuses on what is conscious in order to evoke preconscious material. It also increases social awareness and reality testing. The use of confrontation requires the client to be self-reflective.
3. *Interpretation.* Links conscious and preconscious material to assumed or hypothesized unconscious motivations in the here and now.

Roles of Group Members

The following are some roles that individuals adopt when they participate in a group. Each member may adopt more than one role:

- *Opinion giver:* States beliefs or values.
- *Opinion seeker:* Asks for clarification of beliefs or values.
- *Information giver:* Offers facts or personal experience.
- *Information seeker:* Asks for facts pertinent to what is being discussed.
- *Initiator:* Proposes new ideas on how the goal can be reached or how the problem can be viewed.
- *Elaborator:* Expands on another person's idea and takes the idea and works out what would happen if it were adopted.
- *Coordinator:* Brings together ideas and suggestions.
- *Orientor:* Keeps the group focused on goals or questions the direction taken by the group.

BOX 10–3 TERMS CENTRAL TO GROUP WORK

Group content—all that is said in the group
Group process—constant movement as members seek to reduce tensions that arise when people attempt to have their individual needs met while working to meet group goals; also includes all nonverbal behavior, such as yawning, facial expressions, and body posture
Confrontation—the process whereby problems or conflicts that have been covert are brought into the open
Covert content—the deeper, underlying meaning of messages or what is happening in the group
Dynamics—the ebb and flow of power and energy within a group
Feedback—letting group members know how they affect each other
Hidden agenda—individual, subgroup, or leader goals that are at cross purposes to the group's goals
Cohesiveness—the bond between members of a group, measured by the group's willingness to work toward common goals; members' sense of identification with the group
Conflict—open disagreement among members; may be positive, indicating involvement with the task, or negative, indicating frustration with an impossible task or intergroup conflict
Closed group—membership is restricted; no new members are added when others leave
Open group—a group in which new members are added as others leave
Subgroup—an individual or a small group that is isolated within a larger group and functions separately; members of a subgroup may have more loyalty, similar goals, or perceived similarities to one another than they do to the larger group

- *Evaluator or critic.* Examines possible group solutions against group standards and goals.
- *Clarifier.* Checks out what someone said by restating or questioning.
- *Recorder.* Acts as the group's memory (e.g., takes notes).
- *Summarizer.* Pulls together related ideas, restates suggestions, and offers decisions or conclusions.

Box 10–3 identifies terminology that is central to group work.

TYPES OF GROUPS AND GROUP THERAPIES

Many approaches to group therapy exist. Major types of groups and group therapies include

- Time-limited therapy groups.
- Reconstructive groups.
- Therapeutic milieu groups.
- Behavioral groups.
- Psychoeducational groups.
- Self-help groups.
- Spiritual groups.

Other groups not discussed in this chapter include problem-solving groups and children's groups.

Time-Limited Therapy Groups

In this age of managed care, time-limited group psychotherapy is conceptualized as its own modality and is no longer just a shorter version of traditional group therapy. Characteristics of short-term group therapy are as follows (Mackenzie 1993):

- There is an expectation that the time limit will increase the tempo of psychotherapeutic work and encourage rapid application to real-life circumstances.
- Careful assessment and selection are used to rule out clients who might be at risk for harm from an active approach.
- An explicit verbal agreement regarding circumscribed goals is openly negotiated between the client and the therapist.
- The therapist will intervene actively to develop and maintain a therapeutic climate and maintain a working focus on the identified goals.
- From an early point in therapy, there is an expectation that ideas will be actively applied to outside circumstances.
- The therapist will expect the client to assume responsibility for initiating therapy tasks and will encourage him or her to do so.
- There will be an encouragement to mobilize the use of outside resources that can reinforce positive changes.
- It is anticipated that the change process will continue after therapy terminates, and therefore that the full range of problematic issues need not be addressed within the therapy context.

The nurse therapist can assist in training nurses in the hospital or in a community mental health setting. To become successful group leaders of therapy groups, nurses need supervised training. A nurse is likely to succeed with therapy groups when he or she

1. Demonstrates the ability to enhance communication among group members (asks open-ended questions, directs members to each other, helps draw out the more silent members, protects vulnerable clients, and encourages problem solving).
2. Demonstrates therapeutic intervention or interventions to manage (a) the client who monopolizes the group, (b) the help-rejecting client, (c) the chronic-helper client.

3. Addresses the process of group when members are quiet for long periods.
4. Describes the underlying themes of groups to tie together common group experiences.
5. Tolerates aggression by directing angry feelings constructively.
6. Uses the curative factors of group therapy (Yalom) or another theoretical base.
7. Serves as a role model for (a) empathy and (b) interpersonal learning.
8. Communicates group content to other nursing staff.

Reconstructive Groups

The most common and widespread of the reconstructive groups is psychoanalytic group psychotherapy. The premise underlying psychoanalytic group therapy is that early interactions are believed to play a part in problems that people have as adults. According to psychoanalytic theory, a healthy balance must exist between the id, the ego, and the superego if an individual is to achieve satisfaction and competence in the areas of activity, work, play, and personal relationships.

Therapists use many concepts in psychoanalytic work. Important concepts include transference, countertransference, resistance, acting out, and insight. The concepts of transference and countertransference were introduced in Chapter 2. Resistance, acting out, and insight are discussed here.

Resistance is the unconscious use of thoughts, feelings, or behaviors that help clients avoid changing their view of reality. "A member of the group who does not accept the group in the first place . . . may simply walk out when things get unpleasant, not show up for sessions, or consistently come late to group" (Edelwich and Brodsky 1992).

Acting out occurs when unconscious wishes, needs, conflicts, and feelings are expressed in actions rather than words. For example, a woman who is married to a controlling husband may act out her unconscious anger toward her husband by entering into an extramarital affair.

Insight occurs when the client connects unconscious feelings, wishes, and conflicts to conscious behavior. An experience of emotional understanding can change both behaviors and underlying feelings.

The role of the therapist is to stimulate group interaction and group analysis of the interaction. The therapist does not do anything for the group members that they can do for themselves. The group leader helps make group members aware of defensive ways in which individual group members function and helps move clients toward emotional insight by mobilizing their defense mechanisms. In a psychoanalytic therapy group, members may be in individual therapy with the leader. Basic overall goals for psychoanalytic group therapy are shown in Table 10–1.

Therapeutic Milieu Groups

Therapeutic milieu groups aim to help increase clients' self-esteem, decrease social isolation, encourage appropriate social behaviors, and re-educate clients in basic living skills. These groups are often led by occupational or recreational therapists, although nurses frequently co-lead them. Examples of therapeutic milieu groups are recreational groups, physical activity groups, creative arts groups, self-care groups, and storytelling groups (Table 10–2).

Recreational Groups

Recreational groups focus on engaging in teamwork, learning how to spend leisure time, and increasing self-esteem by completing a project. Nostalgia groups encourage clients to talk about earlier years and about the good things in life. Exercise groups let clients experience physical and psychological release through physical exercise and games.

TABLE 10–1 PSYCHOANALYTICAL GROUP THERAPY

Target Population	Goals	Therapist's Activity	Frequency and Duration
People with ▶ Anxiety disorders ▶ Conversion disorders ▶ Dysthymia ▶ Behavioral problems (e.g., overeating, drinking, and smoking) ▶ Relationship problems ▶ Features of borderline personality disorder	*Overall goal:* Reconstruction of personality dynamics 1. Remove, modify, or retard existing symptoms 2. Mediate disturbed patterns of behavior 3. Promote positive personality growth and behavior	1. Challenges defenses 2. Interprets unconscious conflicts and dreams 3. Makes use of transference and countertransference phenomena	*Meets:* 1–3 times per week *For:* 1–3 or more years

From Wolberg, L. R. (1977). *The technique of psychotherapy* (3rd ed.). New York: Grune and Stratton.

TABLE 10–2 THERAPEUTIC MILIEU GROUPS

MILEIU GROUPS	TARGET POPULATION	GOALS	FREQUENCY AND DURATION
Activity groups (hospital) ▸ Recreational: current events, nostalgia, exercise, horticulture, pets, crafts ▸ Self-care: reality, cooking, grooming, discharge group, community meeting ▸ Creative arts: art, dance/movement, poetry, psychodrama, music, bibliotherapy ▸ Self-awareness: feelings (men's groups, women's group) ▸ Education: stress reduction, skills training, medication groups, assertiveness training, ways to increase self-esteem ▸ Physical activity	The psychiatric client in the hospital or in a day treatment program.	*Overall goal:* Increase in self-esteem: 1. Help clients manage time 2. Increase cooperation 3. Teach specific knowledge, skills, or both, related to patient's illness, treatment, or interpersonal communication (psychoeducational)	*Meets:* Once per week or more, often depending on the program

Physical Activity Groups

In many treatment programs for the mentally ill, exercise programs are typically prescribed by the recreational, occupational, or "activity" therapist. However, in any psychiatric treatment setting, a group of clients exists for which standard exercise tests and prescriptions are not effective and in some cases are actually contraindicated. In these cases, nurses are in the best position to offer guidance and prescriptions (Dexter 1992).

The nurse should discuss an exercise prescription with the client's psychiatrist and define with clients the kind of exercise they like best. Depending on the frequency, intensity, and duration of exercise, the following medical laboratory tests are recommended, along with a full history and physical examination by an internist for medical clearance.

A walking program helps provide an acceptable activity. Participants need a good pair of walking shoes, or, at minimum, a pair of sneakers. Walking is one of the most effective exercises for weight loss because it can be performed regularly, even by those who are deconditioned, overweight, or coping with special health concerns. In addition to its many health benefits, like lowered blood pressure, reduced risk of heart disease, and lowered blood cholesterol levels, walking has the lowest drop-out rate of any other fitness activity because it is safe, easy, and enjoyable.

Creative Arts Groups

The goal of creative arts therapy is for clients to get in touch with feelings and emotions through books, poems, music, and dance. Dance therapy, art therapy, and music therapy are helpful to clients who are demonstrating withdrawn behaviors and are not amenable to "talk" therapy. These groups with withdrawn clients are led by specially trained therapists.

Self-Care Groups

Examples of self-care groups include cooking groups, activities of daily living or grooming groups, medication groups, and client government groups. These types of groups educate clients and provide an opportunity for staff members to assess a client's ability to function in areas such as planning, budgeting, and other basic skills needed for living. Psychiatric nurses are the ideal professionals to teach in a medication education group for long-term self-management care. Sharing a concrete and objective "here-and-now" subject, such as medication information, in a group setting can also facilitate discussion of feelings of stigmatization, alienation, helplessness, and loss of self-control (Kuipers et al. 1988).

Storytelling Groups

Storytelling is an ancient art used to convey information, share feelings, and deliver certain life themes through the use of creativity and imagination (Wenckus 1994). The nurse educator can lead this group and encourages other group members to participate by encouraging them to ask the main character questions. The main character is a group member who volunteers.

Before each group, the therapist prepares an outline of questions for the main character. The following questions can be used:

- Where would you go if you were given a trip?
- Who would you meet?
- Would you buy gifts? What? For whom?
- Who would you write to?
- What would you do if money was no object?

Behavioral Groups

Behavioral group therapy can help members of a group eliminate certain undesirable behaviors. This type of group is led by a professional who is trained in behavioral therapy. The group is generally homogeneous (e.g., clients have the same phobias or the same compulsions). Behavioral therapy seeks to bring about change by altering the client's environment or the client's response to the environment.

The principles of behavioral therapy are guided by the tenets of behavioral theory. According to behavioral theorists, (1) the frequency of a specific behavior is influenced by a negative stimulus, a positive stimulus, or both; (2) events are associated when they occur together; and (3) through teaching and role modeling, new behaviors can be learned.

During behavioral group therapy, basic behavioral techniques, such as systematic desensitization and other anxiety-reducing regimens (e.g., flooding), are used (see Chapter 17).

Systematic desensitization involves having a client gradually approach the feared object or situation while the client is in a state of relaxation. **Flooding** is the process of saturating the client with the anxiety-producing experience without allowing the client to escape. This method causes the client to experience the anxiety, and usually within 5 to 20 minutes, the anxiety decreases.

During behavioral group therapy, clients discuss each person's problems, such as phobias, and how they interfere with the clients' quality of life. Each week, at the end of the session, the therapist gives clients individual homework assignments designed to help them overcome their undesirable behaviors. Clients are expected to complete their assignments and to report the results the following week. The homework begins with small, easy steps and progressively becomes more difficult.

An example of desensitization in a group in which all members have a fear of elevators would start with the leader talking group members through an imagined elevator ride. Next, the leader would walk the members to the elevator, and the next step would be the members' getting into the elevator. A subsequent step would be having the door close and immediately reopen, and then allowing clients to get out. Eventually, they would ride the elevator up one floor, then up several floors.

During these short, progressive steps, the group members would be encouraged to use stress-reduction techniques throughout the experience. Group support and encouragement are important aspects of behavioral group therapy (Table 10–3).

Psychoeducational Groups

Chapter 22 discusses psychoeducational groups for people with schizophrenia and people with severe and persistent mental illness.

Sexuality Groups

New York State has mandated acquired immunodeficiency syndrome (AIDS) education. AIDS has been identified as one of the most serious public health issues in the United States and throughout the world. Psychiatric diagnoses associated with AIDS include organic mental syndromes, adjustment disorder with depressed or anxious mood, panic disorder, major depression, psychoactive substance abuse, and sleep disorders.

Clients who, as a result of the manic phase of bipolar disorder or the abuse of substances, have used poor judgment in sexual liaisons are at high risk for AIDS and other sexually transmitted diseases. Topics for discussion include

TABLE 10–3 BEHAVIORAL GROUP THERAPY

Target Population	Goals	Therapist's Activity	Frequency and Duration
People with specific symptoms they want to modify, e.g. ▶ Phobias ▶ Sexual problems ▶ Passivity ▶ Smoking ▶ Overeating	*Overall goal:* Relief of a specific symptom or change in a specific behavior	1. Works to create new defenses 2. Uses an active and directive approach 3. Uses techniques of behavior modification	*Meets:* 1–3 times per week *For:* 6–12 sessions or more

- Acquired immunodeficiency syndrome.
- Modes of transmission and treatment of sexually transmitted diseases.
- Education on how to use a condom and other forms of "safer" sex.
- Sexuality and the use of psychotropic drugs.
- The effect of antidepressants on sexuality.

Know-Your-Body Groups

This type of group is ideal for medical and health-related topics and usually meets once a week. In a homogenous population, like a women's or men's group, the classes may focus on specific, gender-related health issues. A nurse is ideal for running these types of groups. Know-your-body groups are for people with serious and persistent mental illness who may have a limited knowledge of health care. Use of concrete terminology is needed to clarify fears and answer questions.

For example, an all-women know-your-body group might offer the following kinds of classes.

Breast self-examination	Demonstrate on plastic or foam breast model
Pap smear/mammogram	Obtain information on: ◗ How a pap smear is performed from gynecologist/nurse practitioner ◗ Mammography information from radiologist
Nutrition	Use the Food Guide Pyramid* ◗ Have members participate in cooking a lowfat, economical, balanced meal. Recreation therapy assistance would be helpful. This may improve social and interpersonal interaction and may assist in helping members delegate tasks and feel they are contributing, thereby increasing their self-esteem.
Osteoporosis	Preventive measures women can take.

*U.S. Department of Agriculture, Human Nutrition Information Services, August 1992, Leaflet No. 572.

The use of audiovisual materials is advocated for people who are predominantly visual in orientation. Giving clients a handout that visually or graphically reinforces what they have learned is helpful.

Physical Activity as a Group Experience

Recreation therapists often offer exercise programs for inpatients. However, nurses can offer exercise prescription and guidance in this area. Nurses who are certified by American Council on Exercise, Aerobic and Fitness Association of America (AFAA), or the American College of Sports Medicine are in an advantageous position. Both aerobic and nonaerobic exercises have been shown to reduce depression in people who are clinically diagnosed with depression. The nurse must remember that a client may have never exercised before. As with medications, the rule is "start low, go slow." Of course, the client must get medical clearance before beginning regular exercise.

When an exercise program is prescribed for psychiatric clients, the following factors need to be considered (Dexter 1992):

1. Health status
   - Excess or deficient body fat
   - Physical limitations or handicaps
   - Nutritional concerns (e.g., smoking, caffeine, alcohol)
   - Medication effects
2. Psychological issues
   - Specific symptoms (e.g., depression, mood swings)
   - Lack of motivation
   - Low self-esteem
   - Distorted self-image
   - Difficulty with structure, compliance, consistency
   - Difficulty with competition
   - Poor social skills
3. Sociocultural issues
   - Lack of successful past experience with exercise
   - Ideas about exercise related to such issues as family values, sex roles
4. Personal preference issues
   - Preference for solitary activities
   - Age, skills, interests

A walking group can be ideal for clients of any fitness level. Physicians often encourage recuperating clients to take a daily walk to strengthen their heart and back muscles and to increase their lung capacity. Walking stimulates blood circulation, reduces cholesterol and blood pressure levels, and helps prevent and control diabetes. It also reduces stress.

Information about proper walking technique can be found in commercial guidebooks, through a personal trainer, or through a community-based walking groups. High-risk clients (e.g., those who have anorexia nervosa) may need to achieve a specified weight gain before joining such a group. The goal of the group is to teach people to exercise without extremes.

Medication Groups

Medication groups are designed to teach clients about their medications, answer their questions, and prepare them for discharge. Clients are encouraged to know what medicines they are taking before they come to group. Resources provided by the leader might include pencils, an overhead projector, transparencies, and handouts. To promote medication compliance, one transparency (or handout) could ask

- What medicines are you taking now?
- What is the main action of these medications?
- What are the side effects of these medications?

The psychiatric mental health nurse informs clients about common side affects of their medications and describes treatment for these side effects. The United States Pharmacopeia (1993) presents client education sheets that list side effects in the following way:

- Common side effects that need not be reported to the doctor
- Side effects that need to be reported to the doctor
- Adverse effects

Clients are given a drug information sheet before they leave and are encouraged to review the material several times. Clients are encouraged to participate in treatment by being an informed consumer, and communication with the prescriber of the medication is stressed.

Box 10–4 gives an example of a medication group questionnaire that the group leader can use as a guide to understanding clients' teaching needs. Clients who have used particular medicines can be helpful to others who are weighing the risks and benefits of starting a medication. Box 10–5 gives a protocol for setting up a medication group.

For clients who have reading or cognitive difficulties, it is helpful to underscore the main advantages of each medication and possible side effects of their medication in one-on-one sessions.

BOX 10–4 MEDICATION GROUP QUESTIONNAIRE (Ciarmiello 1992)

1. a) The medications I am currently taking are:
   b) The dosages are:
2. I am fully aware of the actions of my medications.
3. My doctor and I have discussed why this (these) medication(s) are helpful and why I need them.
4. The times I take my medication(s) are:
5. The times I take my medication(s) when I am home are:
6. My doctor/nurse and I have discussed side effects.

Session 1

1. List three specific symptoms that may be reduced or eliminated by the use of medications.
2. Why is it important to take medication at the same time daily?

Self-Help Groups

Self-help groups are based on the premise that people who have experienced a particular problem are able to help others who have the same problem. Nurses may serve as resource people for their clients and need to be aware of the wide array of self-help groups available. Self-help groups are designed to serve people who have a common problem. One of their most important functions is to demonstrate to individuals that they are not alone in having a particular problem. Thus, these groups provide members with support, and their members help each other by telling their stories and providing alternative ways to view and to resolve problems.

A prototype for many self-help groups is the 12-step program developed by AA. The first step is admitting to having a problem (e.g., substance abuse, overeating, gambling). Integral to the program is the acknowledgment of a power higher than oneself. The first meeting is an open or general meeting at which several members tell their stories. As new members gain confidence and make a commitment to healing, they are encouraged to work through the 12 steps of the program with the help of a sponsor. The sponsor is an experienced member of AA who volunteers to be available for support whenever the sponsored individual needs special help (i.e., is tempted to drink alcohol).

The goal of AA is to maintain sobriety through group support, shared experiences, and faith in a power greater than oneself. AA and groups patterned after it (e.g., Narcotics Anonymous, Overeaters Anonymous) are led by group members. Often, one member makes a presentation, and other members share their experiences. To acknowledge one's experience verbally is to "take ownership" of a problem. In a study performed by Sheeren (1988), recovering alcoholic members of AA were asked to complete a questionnaire to assess the occurrence of relapse and its correlation to their level of involvement in the AA program. The findings showed that the greater the member involvement in AA, the lower the chance for relapse. The most significant areas of involvement were in reaching out to other members of AA for help and in making use of a sponsor (Sheeren 1988). Self-help groups such as these are spreading rapidly, and new ones are constantly being formed.

Not all self-help groups use the 12-step method, but all **support groups** are organized around one particular problem or crisis that has been experienced by all members of that group. A nurse may be included as a group member and may be asked to speak as a resource person, but unless the nurse has personally overcome the problem group that the members now have, the nurse would not be asked to lead the group.

Strategies used by group leaders include promotion of dialogue, self-disclosure, and encouragement among members (Kane et al. 1990). Concepts used in support groups include psychoeducation, self-disclosure, and mu-

BOX 10–5 EXAMPLE OF MEDICATION EDUCATION GROUP

GROUP
Medication Education Group

DESCRIPTIONS OF GROUP
A group for all clients, regardless of level of concentration, that prepares clients for self-management of medication on discharge.

CRITERIA FOR PATIENT SELECTION
Open to all clients, except those who are displaying the following behaviors: suicidal, homicidal, potential for assault.

MEDIA
Overhead transparencies, films, patient medication education sheets (Albany Medical Center).

PURPOSE
1. To educate clients on the primary function of their medications.
2. To provide information on side effects—that benefits can outweigh risks.
3. To describe a mechanism to negotiate relationships with health care workers.
4. To enhance a sense of control over treatment.

PROCEDURE
1. Orientation and introduction to the group
2. Brief description of major aspects of diagnoses.
3. Overview of antipsychotics and/or antidepressants.
4. Use of Albany Medical Center patient medication education sheets.
5. Use of the 1993 The United States Pharmocopeial Convention, Inc. patient education leaflets.
6. Specific open question period.

BEHAVIORAL OBJECTIVES
At the end of the 45-minute session, the patient will be able to
1. State one symptom they have that is treated by their medication.
2. Be able to ask at least one question about their medicine.
3. Identify one mechanism that helps with compliance with medicine.

CRITERIA FOR DISCHARGE
Not applicable

THEORETICAL JUSTIFICATION/FRAME OF REFERENCE
Recurrent episodes of acute mental illness may be related to defaulting behaviors (Davidhizar 1982). Although researchers have identified many methods to assist clients in following treatment regimens, none of the studies have shown a single intervention to be sufficient in maintaining long-term compliance (Haynes 1987). A comprehensive approach that uses a wide variety of interventions is most appropriate (Kuipers 1985).

Adapted from Davidhizar, R. E. (1982). Compliance by persons with schizophrenia: A research issue for the nurse. *Issues in Mental Health Nursing.* 4(3):233–255; Haynes, C. B., et al. (1987). A critical review of interventions to improve compliance with prescribed medications. *Patient Education and Counseling,* 10(2):156–166; Kuipers, J.C., et al. (1988). Designing a psychiatric medication education program. *Journal of Rehabilitation Research and Development,* 54(3):55–61; Collins-Colon, T. (1990). Do it yourself: Medication management for community based clients. *Journal of Psychosocial Nursing,* 28:6, 25–29.

tual support. These groups can also prevent physical, emotional, or social health problems; improve an individual's or a family's quality of life; and provide education necessary to further develop the member's potential.

◗ Bob and Jill, a married couple, are having difficulty conceiving a child. Their infertility is affecting their marriage, and they are depressed and angry. They begin to attend a RESOLVE group, in which everyone is having the same difficulty. Through the group process, they explore their options for having children or living child free. Bob and Jill realize they are not alone, and through the group they gain insights that help them deal with their anger and depression.

Examples of groups initiated by nurses include a support group for parents who have a child with a terminal illness or whose child has died and a support group for anorexics (Staples et al. 1990). Other self-help groups include Weight Watchers, Parents Without Partners, and National Alliance for the Mentally Ill. Some support groups have formed for those who are not in the mainstream population (e.g., Fat Women Unite, Coming Out). Characteristics of all these groups are peer support, group teaching, counseling, and use of shared experiences (Table 10–4).

Spiritual Groups

There is a growing awareness of the need to incorporate spiritual concerns and the spiritual process in healing, both mentally and physically. In recent years, the predominantly Judeo-Christian societies of the West have adopted some of the beliefs of Eastern religions, such as Hinduism, Buddhism, and Taoism. One example is the idea of karma (the law of cause and effect, sometimes loosely interpreted as "what goes around comes around"). There has also been increasing interest in, and respect for, the sometimes spiritually based healing practices of other cultures, including those indigenous to United States culture (e.g., Native American medicine).

A spiritual assessment tool (Burkhardt 1989) can be used in a group. Questions are grouped by categories. For example, the following questions relate to a person's ability to connect with others interpersonally. To assess inner strength:

- What brings you joy and peace in your life?
- What are your personal strengths?
- What life goals have you set for yourself?
- How aware were you of your body before you became sick?
- How has your illness influenced your faith?
- Does faith play a role in regaining your health?

To assess the degree of *interconnection* (e.g., positive self-concept, self-esteem, sense of self, ability to demonstrate love of self):

- How do you feel about yourself right now?
- What do you do to show love to yourself?
- Can you forgive yourself?

To assess a person's ability to *connect in life-giving ways* with family, friends, and social groups and to engage in the forgiveness of others:

- Who are the significant people in your life?
- Can you ask people for help when you need it?
- Do you belong to any groups?
- Can you share your feelings with others?
- What are some of the most loving things that others have done for you?
- What are the loving things that you do for other people?

TABLE 10–4 SELF-HELP GROUP THERAPY

TARGET POPULATION	GOALS	THERAPIST'S ACTIVITY	FREQUENCY AND DURATION
People who have experienced a common tragedy, crisis, illness or self-destructive behavior, e.g. **Support groups** ▸ Bereavement: for those who have experienced the loss of a loved one ▸ Rape: for those who have been raped ▸ Cancer: for those families and patients coping with the ramifications of cancer and its treatment ▸ RESOLVE: for couples experiencing infertility **Self-help groups** ▸ Alcoholics Anonymous (AA)—the prototype ▸ Gamblers Anonymous (GA) ▸ Overeaters Anonymous (OA) ▸ Narcotics Anonymous (NA) ▸ Co-Dependents Anonymous ▸ Adult Children of Alcoholics (ACOA)	*Overall goal:* Provision of support and encouragement of positive coping behaviors 1. Decrease feelings of isolation 2. Provide mutual support 3. Provide psychoeducation and health education 4. Reduce stress 5. Help people cease self-destructive behaviors or come to terms with an overwhelming event or situation	1. May or may not have a specific leader 2. Strengthens existing defenses 3. Is actively involved in the group process 4. Provides information to educate and give direction	*Meets:* Once or more per week *For:* Indefinite period of time, ongoing and open membership

ESTABLISHING A PSYCHOTHERAPY GROUP

This section discusses general guidelines for starting a psychotherapy group, as well as specifics for establishing inpatient and outpatient groups.

General Guidelines

The ideal number of clients in a psychotherapy group ranges from seven to ten. Having more than ten members is not recommended, because the group will subdivide, which is counterproductive. Too large a group can also create more opportunities for acting out, as opposed to working through issues.

Members should vary in age, gender, race, and psychodynamics. The presence of both male and female members helps members work through personal issues with persons of both genders. People have different personalities and coping styles, which helps members "try on" another member's way of dealing with an issue. Groups that have a mixture of personalities, coping styles, and psychodynamics are often referred to as **heterogeneous groups.**

Clients who should not be included in psychotherapy groups include those who are acutely psychotic, those with antisocial personality disorder, those experiencing drug or alcohol withdrawal, those who are actively using drugs or alcohol, and those who are violent. However, schizophrenic clients can greatly benefit from some modes of group therapy. Persons diagnosed with antisocial personality disorder should not be included in groups, because they are often disruptive to a psychotherapy group and are unable to relate in a way that is helpful to themselves or others (Lego 1996). Certain special groups may benefit people with antisocial traits. Other groups are effective for schizophrenics and people with addictions. Groups specific to these populations are discussed later in this chapter.

Group therapy may take place in an inpatient or an outpatient setting. Table 10–5 outlines the basic differences between inpatient and outpatient group therapy.

Inpatient Groups

One popular method of structuring an inpatient therapy group is by focusing on the here and now (Yalom 1985). The group therapist should

1. Provide instruction about the relevance of the here and now. Begin with a brief orientation for new clients: state that clients enter the hospital for different reasons and that everyone can benefit from examining how he or she relates to other people. Group members and the therapist or therapists provide feedback. Members have important and painful problems other than interpersonal ones, but given the brief duration of most inpatient hospitalizations, these problems may need to be addressed in individual therapy.
2. Provide spatial boundaries. No table is used. The group meets in the same place each time.
3. Start and end the session on time. Encourage clients and other therapists not to interfere with group time. Obtain administrative support.

TABLE 10–5 DIFFERENCES BETWEEN OUTPATIENT AND INPATIENT GROUP THERAPY

OUTPATIENT GROUPS	INPATIENT GROUPS
1. The group has a stable composition.	1. The group is rarely the same for more than one or two meetings.
2. Clients are carefully selected and prepared.	2. Clients are admitted to the group with little prior selection or preparation.
3. The group is homogenous regarding ego function, although conflicts and issues differ.	3. The group has a heterogenous level of ego functioning.
4. Motivated, self-referred clients make up the group; therapy is growth-orientated.	4. Clients are ambivalent, often there because they are in crisis and therapy is compulsory; therapy is relief oriented.
5. Treatment proceeds as long as required: 1–2 years, 50–100 meetings.	5. Treatment is limited to the hospital period: 1–3 weeks, with rapid patient turnover.
6. The boundary of the group is well maintained, with few external influences.	6. Continuous boundary interface with the milieu occurs.
7. Group cohesion develops normally, given sufficient time in treatment.	7. There is no time for cohesion to develop spontaneously; group development is aborted at an early stage.
8. Therapy is private.	8. Clients are open to observation and scrutiny by the milieu.
9. The leader allows the process to unfold; there is ample time to set group norms.	9. The group leader's structuring of the group is critical; passive analytical approaches lead to group disintegration.
10. No extragroup contact is encouraged.	10. Clients sleep, eat, and live together outside of the group; extragroup contact is endorsed.

Adapted from Leszcz, M. (1986). Inpatient groups. In A. J. Frances and R. E. Aoles (Eds.). *Psychiatric update* (Vol. 5). Washington, DC: American Psychiatric Press. Reprinted with permission. Copyright 1986 American Psychiatric Association.

4. Encourage clients to stay, but do not lock the door. If a client attempts to leave, ask him or her what is going on. Try to connect the behavior to a feeling. For example, a client who stated the day before that she isolates herself when she is feeling depressed would need encouragement to stay. If the client still leaves, follow up with the client after the group therapy session and find out more about the client's thoughts and feelings.
5. Be directive and decisive. For example, if a manic person monopolizes the group, suggest that the client stop talking and try listening to others.
6. If a client threatens to act out physically (e.g., by striking somebody), tell the client, "You may talk about your anger, but you cannot act on it in this group." Get help if the client becomes increasingly threatening, and escort the client from the room. Follow up after the group session, and do not allow the client to come back until the reason for the threatening behavior has been explored with the client's primary therapist.

An example of a basic protocol for an inpatient group could be

1. Orientation or preparation (3 to 5 minutes).
2. Agenda "go round": each member offers a personal agenda for the meeting (20 to 30 minutes).
3. Agenda "fitting": the therapist fits the agendas together by finding commonalties in the group.
4. Review.

In many inpatient settings, the group leader is often not the client's primary therapist. Information is obtained from the client, the primary therapist, and the chart. The nurse should keep in mind that the client's ease in communicating in the group setting is often based heavily on his or her feelings of comfort with the group leader.

Many clients have difficulty understanding that group therapy is indeed therapy, and they tend to feel that they need more one-on-one therapy. If the nurse therapist encounters this attitude, it is helpful for the nurse therapist to acknowledge that it is not unusual for the client to feel this way and that the client may be concerned about revealing information, experiencing rejection, or reliving a humiliating group experience. It is helpful to remind clients of the confidentiality of anything discussed in group therapy in order to build trust.

The nurse should encourage clients to discuss individual group issues with their therapists. If the client brings up any issues in group therapy that affect his or her safety, such as suicide, the nurse must discuss this with the client's therapist, the treatment team, or both. This situation is set up as part of the ground rules, and everyone knows this from the beginning.

It is often of little value for the client or the group for the nurse to mandate client attendance or for the client to use group therapy as a means of gaining a privilege, such as to obtain a day pass. Clients must take responsibility for their own needs. Better-functioning clients attend a group session regularly if it is run effectively and if the entire staff values group sessions and encourages clients. Yalom (1983) stated that

> patients who are . . . sincerely interested in doing something about their mental health gradually assimilate the ward values and soon have a difficult time justifying to themselves their failure to attend.

Yalom advocated mandatory attendance on inpatient units for heterogeneous team groups and homogeneous groups:

> The clinical facts of life are that if these groups were not mandatory, a significant proportion of patients would not attend. Patients who are withdrawn, frightened, depressed, hopeless, or drowsy because of medication would, if given a choice, opt to remain in their rooms, and an effective ward program would not be feasible.

A modification of group psychotherapy is therapy with the heterogeneous team group. A heterogeneous team group is one to which clients are assigned according to their order of admission instead of their suitability for a specific group. An advantage of this practice is that all clients are assigned to a group and are expected to attend group therapy. A disadvantage is that it is often difficult to lead sessions with such a group because of the wide range of psychopathological conditions of the group members. Often, members may be too ill during the first few days of hospitalization to receive any benefit from therapy.

A **homogeneous group** is one in which all members have the same diagnosis and similar levels of functioning. An example would be a group composed of people with schizophrenia. The advantages of the homogeneous group are that it provides more specific and appropriate therapy for persons who are disoriented and delusional and may be hallucinating and that it provides preparation for ongoing group work. One disadvantage of running both heterogeneous team groups and homogeneous groups on the same unit is that this practice can lead to further divisiveness on the inpatient unit.

Open inpatient psychotherapy groups do not usually pass through all stages of group development. An inpatient may be in group therapy for only two or three sessions. Although open therapy is of limited value for the client and the group, the client can still benefit from even a single session (Yalom 1985). Most clients have never been part of a group: with group therapy, clients have the opportunity to feel that they belong to something, often for the first time in their lives. With open psychotherapy groups, the inpatient group therapist must consider the life of the group to be only a single session (Yalom 1985). The therapist must be efficient, be active, and offer something useful for as many clients as possible during that session.

Outpatient Groups

Table 10–6 identifies specific nursing actions and rationales for organizing an outpatient psychotherapy group. Nurses often run outpatient psychotherapy groups in clinics, in community health units, and in private practice.

In outpatient psychoanalytic groups, prospective members are seen at least once individually before they are admitted to the group. The more times they are seen, the better. The rationale for this regimen is that a close tie develops between the client and the nurse; this tie helps the client remain in the group longer when the client becomes anxious. In contrast to pregroup preparation that occurs in an inpatient group, in an outpatient group, the client is often not prepared for what happens in group therapy or who will be there. Only a general statement is made (e.g., "The group is a place to discuss feelings, problems, or reactions") (Lego 1996). Setting general goals (e.g., wanting closer relationships, improving work life, relieving painful symptoms) is useful. It may be unrealistic to set goals that are too specific. Goal setting that is too specific is antithetical to the natural process of developing ongoing intimate relationships. Clients often have specific conscious goals that for a time are unobtainable because of unconscious factors. For instance, a woman may state that she wants to find a man and get married but may consistently choose to go out with men who are unsuitable (e.g., married men, men not interested in making a commitment).

Phases of Group Development

Groups, just like individuals, have an innate capacity for growth and development. Likewise, they have an ability to regress and to resist working effectively. Like individuals, groups have phases in which they move forward and

TABLE 10–6 OUTPATIENT PSYCHOTHERAPY GROUPS

NURSING ACTION	THEORETICAL RATIONALE
All prospective members are seen at least once individually before admission to the group.	All clients are initially screened for group. A tie often develops between the patient and the nurse. This tie can help the patient stay in the group, even as anxiety increases.
Clients are seen in group sessions and individual sessions as well.	Group psychotherapy produces anxiety, which spills over at times outside the group. This anxiety can motivate clients to explore their own reactions in individual sessions.
Before entering the group, the client is not prepared for what happens in the group session or who will be there. Only a general statement is made, such as, "The group is a place to discuss feelings, problems, or reactions."	If the client knows a great deal about the group in advance, spontaneous reactions are lost to exploration. These spontaneous reactions are "grist for the therapeutic mill."
Group members are not told about new members before the new members appear.	The spontaneous or irrational response of group members to the new member is useful for exploring (e.g., this may be reminiscent of the birth of a sibling).
Group members sit in chairs in a circle. No table is used, and no one sits on the floor.	All members should be visible to one another. This increases anxiety slightly, which leads to more irrational behavior and its subsequent observation. It also aids in the observation of nonverbal communication, which can then be explored.
The leader changes seats each session, causing other members to shift seats.	Members should not be able to find a comfortable "niche" in which they can hide.
Weekly sessions last 1 1/2 hours.	When groups meet only once a week, resistance builds between sessions, and it may take 45 minutes for work to begin. When groups meet daily, resistance is lower.
Sessions begin and end on time.	Clients pace their reactions according to this time frame. This pacing in itself is interesting to note (e.g., when a client reports in the last 5 minutes of the session that he has quit his job).
The same leader leads the group.	Group process is based on a balance of forces that takes the leader into account.
Observers, people who are not members of the group, do not sit in the group.	Changing leaders seriously changes this balance and makes interaction more superficial.
Open-ended groups are more effective than time-limited groups. The group continues indefinitely, with replacements made as members leave.	When members know only a certain number of sessions are left, they remain more controlled and superficial.

Adapted from Lego, S. (1984). Group therapy. In S. Lego (Ed.). *The American handbook of psychiatric nursing* (p. 208). Philadelphia: J.B. Lippincott.

TABLE 10–7 FOUR PHASES OF GROUP DEVELOPMENT

PHASE	DEFINITION	TASK ACTIVITY	INTERPERSONAL ACTIVITY
Forming	Group members concerned with their role, expectations, and what will happen in the group.	Members identify task and boundaries, e.g., issues of confidentiality, attendance	▸ Relationships are tested. ▸ Interpersonal boundaries are identified. ▸ Dependent relationship with leaders or other group members are formed.
Storming	Group members resistant to task and group influence.	Members respond emotionally to task, are often angry at leader or other members	▸ Intragroup conflict emerges.
Norming	Resistance to group overcome by members.	Members express intimate personal opinions and feelings around personal tasks.	▸ New roles are adopted. ▸ New standards evolve in group feelings. ▸ Cohesiveness develops.
Performing	Creative problem-solving occurs; solutions emerge.	Members direct group energy toward completion of tasks.	▸ Interpersonal structure of the group becomes tool to achieve its task. ▸ Roles become flexible and functional.

phases in which they fall back. Tuckman (1965) identified four phases that occur in small groups:

1. Forming
2. Storming
3. Norming
4. Performing

These are summarized in Table 10–7.

BEHAVIORS THAT POSE A CHALLENGE TO THE GROUP LEADER

Many defensive behaviors used by some clients interfere with their attaining satisfaction in their lives. At the same time, these behaviors can be disruptive to a group process and the development of group cohesion. Specific defensive and nonproductive behaviors or roles that some people carry out may become evident during the process of group psychotherapy. However, the therapist must carefully assess the group's readiness to have the therapist interpret such behavior for them. Clients are not always ready to hear insights, no matter how accurate these insights are. Premature interpretations can be ineffective and can impede therapy by misdirecting attention from the therapeutic work (Yalom 1983). The client who monopolizes the group, the client who complains but continues to reject help, the client who chronically helps others, and the disliked client often challenge a group leader.

The Person Who Monopolizes the Group

This person's compulsive speech is an attempt to deal with anxiety. As the client sees group tension grow, the client's level of anxiety rises and the client's tendency to speak increases even more. Therefore, no one else gets a chance to be heard, and other group members eventually lose interest and begin to withdraw.

▸ Holly is the most talkative member of the group until the nurse intervenes. Initially, Holly talks at length about her early experiences relating to the deaths of both her mother and her father and to having to live with her grandparents. The other members of the group become bored with the same old story, and they drift off. They have heard these stories many times, not only in group therapy but also during other activities.

Intervention

The leader asks group members why they have permitted the monopolizer to go on and on. This serves to validate the other members' feelings of anger. After the group members become angry, they may see how they, too, are responsible for allowing themselves to be victimized. Some members may be angry at the therapist for pointing out their passivity, but they may subsequently realize that they are responsible adults with the right to say what they feel. They may then discuss their fears of being assertive or of hurting the feelings of the monopolizer.

Placing responsibility on the group members also takes the therapist out of the authoritative position.

Group members may need help disclosing their own feelings and responses. The therapist encourages statements like "When you speak this way, I feel . . ." The therapist helps by saying that feelings are not right or wrong but simply exist. People feel less defensive with "I feel" statements than they do with "you are" statements. They help members feel like part of the group, not alienated from it.

The Person Who Complains But Continues to Reject Help

The client who complains but continues to reject help continually brings environmental or somatic problems to the group and often describes them in a manner that makes the problems seem insurmountable; in fact, the client appears to take pride in the insolubility of his or her problems. The client seems entirely self-centered. The group's attempts to help the person are continually rejected. The person who uses these tactics usually has highly conflicting feelings about his or her own dependency. Any notice from the therapist temporarily increases the client's self-esteem; on the other hand, the client has a pervasive mistrust toward all authority figures. Most clients who complain but continue to reject help have been subjected to severe deprivation early in their lives. For example, they may be orphans or may have been emotionally and physically abused.

▶ Michelle is always complaining about how horrible her relationship with her boyfriend is, and she manages to get the entire group worked up over this. Members tell her to leave him, not to spend all her time with him, and not to spend all her money on him, but each week she reports a new escapade or crisis. In every session, the group members become concerned and offer encouragement, advice, and solutions. Each time, the group becomes angry at her lack of change, and she is frustrated by her own inability to change. She asserts that the group is not helpful.

Intervention

The therapist agrees with the content of the client's pessimism and maintains a detached affect. If the client stays in the group long enough and the group develops a sense of cohesion, the therapist helps this individual recognize the pattern of his or her relationships. The therapist encourages the client to look at his or her "yes, but" behavior.

The Person Who Avoids Personal Issues by Helping Others

The client who chronically helps others is one who is overly helpful to others in an effort to defend against his or her own intense dependency needs. Because these dependency needs were never met during early childhood, clients are left with intense longings and unmet dependency needs as adults. These clients secretly wish that others would fulfill their wishes. They further have a need to have others treat them in a hostile way. Therefore, chronic helpers become consistently self-sacrificing in their dealings with others. Essentially, there is no way that anyone can fulfill their intense dependency needs. Their dependency is so great because they have subordinated all of their own needs to the needs of others. These people deny their own anger and needs and often tend to marry persons who cannot meet their dependency needs and who reject them through physical or emotional abuse or neglect (Light 1974).

▶ Sally always has a solution or a suggestion for everyone else's problem. She is adept at keeping the focus off herself and is always trying to "help" others in various ways. Psychodynamically, this practice allows her to avoid her own problems and to avoid making changes.

Intervention

The therapist helps clients experience their dysfunctional patterns of helpfulness and helps them experience their true feelings. The therapist could state how helpful this client has been to others in the group and then remark on the client's reluctance to ask for something personal from the group. The therapist could explore whether the client fears being rejected or feels that he or she does not have any right to seek help from the group. The client's behavior in the group is usually symbolic of the client's behavior outside the group.

The Disliked Person

Some people who are extremely self-centered, lack empathy or concern for other members of the group, are highly depressive, are angry, and refuse to take any personal responsibility can challenge the group leader and negatively affect the group process.

▶ Becky came to the support group on the inpatient psychiatric unit. She was very angry, stating "I don't know why I come to these groups anyway! They don't help." Becky was to be discharged the next day to a 28-day alcohol rehabilitation program. She had a previously scheduled dental appointment before the rehabilitation intake interview, and she was being strongly encouraged by her therapist to reschedule the appointment. The therapist feared she was at high risk for drinking again, since Becky stated that she constantly had the urge to drink. When Becky was confronted by a group member, who was an addictions therapist, about not being flexible and prioritizing her need for alcohol treatment, she exploded. "I thought this group was for support. This is outrageous!" Group members were obviously uncomfortable with her anger.

Clients who are severely narcissistic may have difficulty in group therapy for the following reasons:

- They have defense mechanisms that are resistant to treatment because they experience a wounding reaction to any comment perceived as criticism.
- They may be initially charming, then demanding.
- They may devalue the therapist and then feel elated.
- They may monopolize the group.

Intervention

The group therapist needs to listen to the content that is being avoided. Listening requires the participant-observer to stay therapeutically objective. Only then can the therapist be empathetic (Liebenberg 1990). In being empathetic, however, the therapist must be aware that a narcissistic client may fear excessive warmth because it stimulates possible erotic, homosexual, or castrating fears. Therapists need to empathize with the client.

DSM-IV CATEGORIES THAT MAY NOT BE SUITABLE FOR GROUP WORK

Group psychotherapy is appropriate for clients with many *Diagnostic and statistical manual of mental disorders*, 4th edition (DSM-IV) diagnoses. However, for people with the diagnosis of antisocial personality disorder or with strong paranoid traits, insight-oriented group psychotherapy is usually not appropriate. In addition, people with borderline personality disorders are not always appropriate therapeutic candidates, especially for the beginning group therapist.

The Antisocial Client

Some of the DSM-IV criteria that support a decision not to include clients with antisocial personality disorder in insight-oriented group psychotherapy include

- Failure to conform to social norms with respect to lawful behavior (e.g., stealing).
- Impulsiveness.
- Disregard for the truth, as indicated by repeated lying, use of aliases, or conning.
- Lack of remorse for actions.
- Tendency to use others for their own satisfaction.

People with antisocial personality disorders may benefit from a "tough love" group, in which constant, open confrontation of wrongdoing occurs. Such a group is oriented to the here and now and generally does not promote long-lasting change. The client usually does not gain insight but may conform to peer pressure. The client can benefit from a tough love group because it is action oriented and is a homogeneous group. Self-help groups such as AA, if appropriate, can be helpful. This beneficial effect may be due to the absence of a leader because the presence of a leader elicits feelings of resistance to authority. The antisocial client is self-serving and may consistently prevent the group from achieving any cohesion by the constant overt or covert "stirring up" of others. Chapter 19 provides a more elaborate discussion of antisocial personality disorder.

The Client with Paranoid Behaviors

People with strong paranoid traits consistently expect to be exploited or harmed by others and are reluctant to confide in others because they feel any information they share will be used against them. They therefore tend to avoid, or soon drop out of, group psychotherapy. Other personality traits that make it difficult for a paranoid person to benefit from group psychotherapy include the following:

- They are easily slighted and quick to react with anger or to counterattack.
- They read hidden, demeaning, or threatening meanings into benign remarks or events.
- They maintain grudges or are unforgiving of insults or slights.

▶ Kelly was one of eight people in the Clients' Rights Group. As the group leader discussed voluntary and involuntary status, Kelly began to raise her voice, asserting that her rights were violated. The group leader knew that Kelly's psychiatrist was asking the court to order her to be retained in the hospital because she was in an acute stage of her paranoia. The group leader asked Kelly to hold her comments until the discussion period at the end. Kelly became more irritable.

▶ The group leader realized she had been too authoritative in her first comment, and Kelly seemed to become more paranoid. She softened her voice tone and told Kelly that she would like to have her be a part of the group and that Kelly was understandably upset about the upcoming court day, yet the leader needed to get through the material. Kelly took this as a personal affront and yelled "Do you want me to be in group? Are you threatening to kick me out?" Other group members seemed anxious and impatient with Kelly's interruptions.

- In spite of attempts from the leader to tell Kelly she wanted her to stay, Kelly then focused on being picked on. She stated that she was more intelligent than the others and that they were just a bunch of naive followers. The group leader then asked her to leave, and Kelly left on her own.

When does one ask a client to leave group? Generally, persons who are paranoid and acutely psychotic may tolerate shorter, less provocative, less stimulating types of groups. It is helpful to process anxiety within the group and to follow up with the person who was asked to leave in order to help the person process possible feelings of rejection as soon after the group as possible. Chapter 19 provides a more complete discussion of paranoid personality disorder.

The Client with a Borderline Personality Disorder

Many people with the diagnosis of borderline personality disorder can gain insight in a psychotherapy group; however, because of their marked manipulativeness and self-destructive traits, they are not always appropriate group therapy candidates—especially for new group leaders. The rage of the person with borderline personality disorder may not be tolerated in a group setting. However, the use of a co-therapist could be helpful as long as the therapists acknowledge that they could be played against each other through this client's defense mechanism of splitting. Clients with borderline personality disorder feel safer when treatment is structured.

One problem encountered in group psychotherapy with a client who has borderline personality disorder is that the person with this disorder may become anxious as the group atmosphere becomes more cohesive, thereby increasing the potential for splitting the group. The benefit of group psychotherapy for this type of client is that the client may become less regressed in the group situation than in individual sessions because the group pressures the client to work things through instead of using avoidance and denial. For clients who are impulsive and action oriented (particularly those who are self-destructive), the action orientation of a group, as opposed to the one-to-one psychotherapy sessions, is often appealing (Leszcz 1989). Group members serve as a "mirror" and reflect back to the impulsive or self-destructive person how his or her actions affect the group.

The use of projective identification and exaggerated anger in a group setting by the client with borderline personality disorder is often a paradox and a defense. Clients with borderline personality disorder are discussed more fully in Chapter 19.

- A male client who stated that he wanted to learn to be close to others persisted in "tearing down" a female client who had asked the group for acknowledgment after she achieved a significant professional goal. After several group sessions, the man stated that he could not tolerate seeing this woman ask the group for recognition, which acknowledged her need for the group. He attacked her in the same fashion that he feared being attacked for his own neediness and his need of the group. He projected onto her his own contemptibility for his dependent, needful self and he adopted the position of ruthless persecutor, much as his parents had done with regard to his neediness. He elicited from the group intense hostility for his treatment, instead of the increased closeness he had said he wanted. Thus, he created the very atmosphere he dreaded (Leszcz 1989).
- The group therapist gently pointed out to the man that his criticizing actually served to distance him from others. The therapist then proceeded to ask him if someone significant in his past had criticized him excessively.
- At the same time, the group therapist acknowledged the risk that the woman took in asking for acknowledgment from the group. The group therapist neutralized the attack by indicating that the behaviors are reminiscent of not feeling acknowledged (by parents) or of actually being rejected. The man desired the recognition he had never received from his parents.

GROUP THERAPY FOR SPECIAL POPULATIONS

Three populations that some therapists have found amenable to alternative types of group therapy are those with serious and persistent mental illness, those with mental illness along with a concurrent substance abuse problem (dual diagnosis), and those with eating disorders.

The Seriously and Persistently Mentally Ill Client

A helpful form of therapy for persons with a severe long-term mental illness is therapy in a supportive group. In supportive group work, the goals are to help the clients better adapt to the environment by focusing on reality and to help them learn new behaviors to decrease isolation. The therapist needs to note early indications of the emergence of psychotic symptoms; such symptoms may indicate a need to change the client's treatment program. For example, nursing interventions aimed at decreasing anxiety may be implemented, or antipsychotic medication regimens may need to be changed.

When psychotic clients enter a group, the dynamics that develop can mobilize psychotic resistance, which then becomes the dominant group feature (Cohn 1988). Frosch (1983) stated that the major anxiety against which psychotic clients defend is *annihilation anxiety*—fear of dissolution of an already fragile self. At first, unacceptable aspects of the self are often projected onto the therapist in malignant forms. The therapist's task is to help the client perceive projected parts of his or her self as benign and useful rather than dangerous (Cohn 1988). To place a psychotic client in group therapy is to challenge the core around which defenses are constructed (i.e., the need to avoid new experiences). Several theoretical modalities that guide group interventions exist. Table 10–8 identifies some of the goals of supportive group work for schizophrenic clients. Chapter 22 also provides a discussion of this issue.

- One group member started to complain of how her "life stinks" and how "reality stinks" and left the group. The client had a history of persecutory delusions and had received news that she could not go home that day. Another group member became very anxious and said, "What is going on?" She rapidly got up and left the group. The remaining group members looked uneasy. One member started to hallucinate, as evidenced by her talking to herself.
- The group leader felt fearful as she realized that the group was literally decomposing before her eyes. Remembering that psychotic clients mirror fear that is manifested by the therapist and that they fear their aggressive impulses, she realized that she needed to think and keep one step ahead of the group. The fearful members had picked up some of the therapist's anxiety in addition to the aggression manifested by the client.
- The group leader told members that she would see each member who left the group and told people that it was okay for members to be upset. The members subsequently became less anxious and began to discuss their concerns about the effect their illnesses have on their lives and to focus on common areas of concern to work on.

The Client with a Dual Diagnosis (Mental Disorder with Co-Existing Substance Abuse)

Some inpatient psychiatric units recognize the importance of treating a person for both substance abuse and coexisting mental illness. The number of groups for clients diagnosed with both types of disorders (dual diagnosis) is increasing as a result of the recognition that substance abuse often exacerbates psychiatric symptoms and that the actual substance abuse is not detected unless an accurate assessment is performed.

The number of persons presenting with both a mental disorder and substance abuse has increased, particularly in urban and suburban areas (Office of Mental Health News 1991). A special program was started in 1988 at Buffalo (New York) General Hospital after it was noted that 40% of clients using the emergency services had dual diagnoses. Many of these clients were in crisis; had a history of resistance to treatment, denial of problems, and noncompliance with medication; were impulsive; and were concerned only with their immediate needs. This special program uses counselors who are available 24 hours a day and who have training in crisis intervention. The program continues to grow.

Edelwich and Brodsky (1992) advocated the use of group counseling, instead of group therapy, for drug and alcohol abusers. The rationale is that group counseling

- Is more action and task oriented.
- Emphasizes solving problems and making decisions rather than gaining insight. Group counseling has as its primary objectives behavioral change and skill acquisition.
- Is interactive, with an adherence to group process that is as rigorous as that of group psychotherapy (Edelwich and Brodsky 1992).

TABLE 10–8 SUPPORTIVE GROUP THERAPY FOR THE SEVERELY AND PERSISTENTLY MENTALLY ILL CLIENT

TARGET POPULATION	GOALS	THERAPIST'S ACTIVITY	FREQUENCY AND DURATION
▸ Schizophrenic clients ▸ Psychotic clients ▸ Seriously, persistently mentally ill clients ▸ Clients with cognitive impairment disorders	*Overall goal:* Better adaptation to environment 1. Decrease isolation 2. Increase involvement in group activities 3. Promote discussion relative to immediate life events and feelings in the group 4. Detect problems early 5. Focus on reality testing	1. Strengthens existing defenses 2. Is actively involved in the group process 3. May give advice and direction 4. Models appropriate behavior 5. Creates a safe environment	*Meets:* Once weekly *For:* 6 months or longer

It is recommended that the group leader have a background in group process, reality therapy, and rational-emotive therapy (see Chapter 2) (Ellis and Harper 1975). Glasser (1985) described four basic human needs and suggested questions the leader can use to assess each member in relation to these needs. Glasser's basic needs include those for (1) relationships and belonging; (2) self-esteem, power, and control; (3) fun and recreation; and (4) freedom and choices. Some examples of Glasser's (1985) questions are:

The need for relationships and belonging.

- Who are the important people in your life?
- How intimate are these relationships?
- Who can you talk to when you have a problem?

The need for self-esteem, power, and control.

- What do you want that you're not getting?
- What have you done in the past several days that improves your image of yourself?

The need for fun and recreation.

- When was the last time you had fun?
- How has your having fun in the past hurt other people?

The need for freedom and choices.

- What choices do you have in your life?
- What would you do if things did get better for you?

Some goals of groups that are composed of persons who have a mental disorder and substance abuse are to (Lala et al. 1992)

- Provide education about the processes of alcoholism, substance abuse, and addiction.
- Offer clients the opportunity to explore their issues with addiction.
- Identify issues related to relapse and discuss relapse prevention strategies.
- Encourage and motivate clients to use outpatient resources.

Many people are in the precarious position of using alcohol or other substances of abuse while balancing a job, managing their family life, or both. Often, the use of substances, including alcohol, is a symptom of underlying low self-esteem, depression, or unresolved grief and loss. The use of the substance may not be discovered until a crisis, such as a divorce or a car accident in which someone is hurt as a result of drunk driving, erupts. Because of the guilt and shame that are often associated with substance abuse by a person who was previously viewed as competent and judicious, a comprehensive treatment program is advocated, such as a 30-day alcohol or a substance rehabilitation treatment program. People need to be motivated to stay in these programs. These programs offer a multitreatment approach that uses individual, group, family, and spiritual therapies.

Gorski (1988) developed programs for relapse prevention—a cognitive system that addresses chemical addictions and dependencies as well as relapse prevention—by using cognitive, affective, behavioral, and situational techniques. Gorski advocated the involvement of spouses, older children, friends, and sponsors. See Chapter 25 for more on relapse prevention.

Table 10–9 gives an example of how a substance abuse education group may be structured and the kinds of issues that such a group addresses.

Empathy catalyzes the treatment process between the client and the nurse. A willingness to accept without judgment the client's subjectively processed views on reality is necessary for an understanding of the person's inner mental life (Kohut 1959).

TABLE 10–9 EXAMPLE OF A SCHEDULE FOR A SUBSTANCE ABUSE EDUCATION GROUP

TIME	TOPIC	OBJECTIVE
Week 1		
Monday	Addiction ◗ What it is ◗ What it is not	To identify parallels of addiction and mental illness
Friday	Introduction to recovery	To define recovery To identify parallels of addiction and mental illness in recovery
Week 2		
Monday	Introduction to relapse	To define relapse
Friday	Distortions in thinking and feeling	To identify thoughts and feelings that lead to reuse
Week 3		
Monday	The 12 steps	To identify a common framework to confront and aid in the recovery process
Friday	Physical aspects	To identify harmful effects of substances To identify dangers of medication and alcohol combinations To define cross-addiction
Week 4		
Monday	Preventing relapse	To define relapse prevention strategies To develop one fail-safe plan

Several questions would help in such a group. For example, if a client has insight into his or her destructive drinking pattern and is able to share this experience, the nurse can say, "Now that drinking is not working for you anymore, you are disillusioned, furious, and afraid. Let's talk about those feelings." Also, the nurse may say, "When you drink you feel you can do anything, be anything, and achieve anything, and that feels wonderful. No wonder you don't want to give it up." (Levin 1991).

Another experience for clients with dual diagnoses is shame and stigmatization. Many clients are taking medications that cause obvious side effects that draw attention, such as extrapyramidal symptoms, and further increase shame. For many clients, drinking is a misguided attempt to alleviate, or self-medicate, the symptoms of mental illness or the side effects of psychotropic medication. Nurses can help these clients experience rather than anesthetize their feelings of shame. "You felt so much shame when you realized that you were alcoholic and had a psychotic illness that you drank so you wouldn't feel your shame" (Levin 1991).

The Client with an Eating Disorder

Anorexia nervosa is an illness that is characterized by relentless pursuit of thinness in a misguided effort to control painful emotions (Casper 1985). The accompanying sense of well-being and control achieved through weight loss further reinforces this compelling need to lose even more weight. As a highly desirable characteristic, thinness then becomes integrated with the self-concept (see Chapter 26).

Group therapy can be a special way to assist clients with the transition from structured inpatient treatment to outpatient treatment that complements living in the community among peers and to lessen the sense of being "different." Since the rate of recidivism is highest within 2 weeks of discharge from the hospital, a group could provide a supportive context in which their needs can be met. Groups can decrease isolation, and weight and nutritional intake needs can be monitored and reinforced (Staples and Schwartz 1990).

The nurse must realize that the client with anorexia has a life-long illness, even after inpatient treatment. Anger in group can be manifested by a) lengthy periods of silence and b) verbal attacks on the leaders. Clients may have marked difficulty giving up their most valuable possession, their anorectic identity, and risk having nothing of personal value left. The nurse must work with recognizing the function of the "anorectic identity," that is, thinness as a defense against being nobody, and to patiently await a gradual redefinition of the self concept (Staples and Schwartz 1990).

A psychoeducation group may be the least intrusive approach for treating persons with eating disorders, in addition to a cognitive behavioral group, which has a higher rate of success than other group approaches (Wolfe 1995). The therapist neither expects nor solicits self-disclosure from clients. The goal is to effect change in cognitions, affects, and behaviors. Examples of topics for the group include

- Association between eating disorders and affective disorders.
- Physical complications.
- Cognitive, affective, and behavioral effects of starvation.
- Importance of normal eating patterns.
- Adverse effects of dieting, bingeing, or purging.
- Sociocultural pressures on women to be thin, to perform, and to please others.
- Coping strategies to deal with urges to binge.

SUMMARY

Nurses have many opportunities for professional, creative, and thoughtful work in groups. The beginning group therapist is encouraged to use modalities initially that concentrate on education (e.g., medication groups, know-your-body groups) on the inpatient psychiatric unit in order to become familiar with group dynamics, roles, and psychiatric diagnoses. Staff nurses in a hospital unit or in a community health center may run milieu groups, such as recreational, self-care, creative arts, storytelling, physical activity, and educational groups.

The advanced practitioners, such as clinical nurse specialists, are recommended to seek ongoing clinical supervision. Leading groups such as behavioral, cognitive, psychoanalytic, and family therapy requires specialized training and education. Beginning group therapists can benefit from observing such groups.

When working with groups, the nurse identifies the theoretical base that is the most comfortable for the nurse. To prepare clients adequately for therapy in an inpatient, psychotherapy group, the advanced-practice nurse needs to assess clients, provide a cognitive structure, and tell them what to expect. The focus is on the here and now and on relationships. The group psychotherapist is always active, analyzing both the group process and the content and continually striving to link the universal aspects of clients' common issues. The group becomes a microcosm of the inpatient unit, and the therapy group may be the first group with which a client feels a sense of belonging.

Outpatient groups that provide ongoing therapy, may be less structured, and tend to have the same members over an extended period of time, particularly those outpatient groups that are insight-oriented psychotherapy groups. Cognitive/behaviorally oriented groups are often more goal directed and clients may stay only until they meet their goal. The nurse therapist in an outpatient group may see the client for individual therapy as well. This therapist usually provides less structure and does less preparation than the inpatient therapist and generally has more time to see the group develop through the phases of uncertainty, overaggression, regression, and adaptation.

Significant learning challenges exist in group therapy with complex clients who have mental disorders; these can include people with borderline personality disorder, people with serious and persistent mental illness, people with both a mental disorder and substance abuse (dual diagnosis), and people with eating disorders. People with antisocial or strong paranoid traits do not respond well to therapy groups.

REFERENCES

American Nurses' Association (1994). *Standards of practice for psychiatric–mental health nursing practice.* Kansas City, MO: Author.

American Psychiatric Association (1994). *Diagnostic and statistical manual of mental disorders* (4th ed.). Washington, DC: Author.

Armstrong, S., and Rouslin, S. (1963). *Group psychotherapy in nursing practice.* New York: Macmillan Publishing Company.

Berne, E. (1966). *Principles of group treatment.* New York: Oxford University Press.

Burkhardt, M. (1989). Spirituality: An analysis of the concept. *Holistic Nursing Practice,* 3(3): 69.

Casper, R. (1985). Anorexia nervosa and bulimia. In W. Kelley (Ed.), *Practice of pediatrics.* Philadelphia: Harper & Row, 1985.

Ciarmiello, S. (1992). *Medication Group Questionnaire.* Unpublished material. Albany Medical Center, Albany, New York.

Clarke, L. (1993). Personal communication.

Cohn, B. (1988). Keeping the group alive: Dealing with resistance in a long term group of psychotic patients. *International Journal of Group Psychotherapy,* 38(3):319.

Critchley, D., and Maurin, J. (1985). *The clinical specialist in psychiatric mental health nursing* (pp 178–198). New York: John Wiley.

Dexter, N. (1992). *Physical exercise as a nursing intervention.* Unpublished paper. Stormant-Vail Regional Medical Center, Topeka, KS.

Edelwich, J., and Brodsky, A. (1992). *Group counseling for the resistant client.* New York: Lexington Press.

Ellis, A., and Harper, R. (1975). *A new guide to rational living.* North Hollywood: Wilshire.

Frosch, J. (1983). *The psychotic process.* New York: International Universities Press.

Glasser, W. (1965). *Reality Therapy.* New York: Harper & Row.

Glasser, W. (1985). *Control theory.* Scranton, PA: Harper Collins.

Gorski, T. (1988). *A guide for relapse prevention and the staying sober workbook: A serious solution for the problem of relapse.* Independence, MO: Independence Press.

Hamilton, J., et al. (1993). Quality assessment and improvement in group psychotherapy. *American Journal of Psychiatry 150*(2):316, 320.

Janssen, E. (1994). A self psychological approach to treating the mentally ill, chemical abusing, and addicted (MICAA) patient. *Archives of Psychiatric Nursing* 8(6):381–389.

Kanas, N. (1988). Therapy groups for schizophrenics: Patients on acute care units. *Hospital and Community Psychiatry,* 39(5):546.

Kane, C. F., DiMarino, E., and Jiminez, M. (1990). A comparison of short-term psychoeducational supports for relatives coping with chronic schizophrenia. *Archives of Psychiatric Nursing,* 4(6):343.

Kaplan, H. I., and Sadock, B. J. (1991). *Synopsis of psychiatry* (6th ed.). Baltimore: Williams & Wilkins.

Klein, R. (1993). Short-term group psychotherapy. In H. I. Kaplan and B. J. Saddock (Eds.), *Comprehensive group psychotherapy* (pp. 256–270). Baltimore: Williams & Wilkins.

Kohut, H. (1959). Introspection, empathy and psychoanalysis: An examination between mode of theory and observation. *Journal of the American Psychiatric Association,* 14:459–483.

Kuipers, J., et al. (1988). Designing a psychiatric medication education program. *Journal of Rehabilitation Research and Development,* 54(3):55.

Lacquer, H. P. (1972). Mechanisms of change in multiple family therapy. In C. J. Sager and H. S. Kaplan (Eds), *Progress in group and family therapy.* New York: Brunner/Mazel.

Lala, C., Shannon, S., and Williams, G. (1992). *Drug/alcohol education group outline.* Unpublished material. Albany Medical Center.

Lego, S. (ed.) (1996). *Psychiatric nursing—A comprehensive reference* (2nd ed.). Philadelphia: Lippincott-Raven.

Lego, S. (1984). *The American handbook of psychiatric nursing.* Philadelphia: J. B. Lippincott.

Leszcz, M. (1986). Inpatient groups. In A. J. Frances and R. E. Aoles (Eds.), *Psychiatry update* (p. 729). Washington, DC: American Psychiatric Press.

Leszcz, M. (1989). Group psychotherapy of the characterologically difficult patient. *International Journal of Group Psychotherapy,* 39(3):311.

Levin, J. (1991). When the patient abuses alcohol. In H. Jackson (Ed.), *Using self-psychology in psychotherapy* (pp. 203–221). Northvale, NJ: Jason Aronson.

Liebenberg, B. (1990). The unwanted and unwanting patient. In B. E. Roth, W. N. Stone and H. O. Kibel (Eds.). The difficult patient in group. Group psychotherapy with borderline and narcissistic disorders (pp. 311–322). Madison, CT: International Universities Press.

Light, N. (1974). The chronic helper in group therapy. *Perspectives in Psychiatric Care,* 12:129–139.

Mackenzie, K.R. (1993). Time-limited group theory and technique. In A. Alonso and H. Swiller (eds.), *Group therapy in clinical practice* (pp. 423–444). Washington, DC: American Psychiatric Press.

Morgan, A. J., and Moreno, J. W. (1973). *The practice of mental health nursing: A community approach.* Philadelphia: J. B. Lippincott.

Naegle, M. (Ed.). (1993). *Substance abuse education in nursing* (Vol. III, press publication no. 15-2464). New York: National League for Nursing.

Office of Mental Health News, New York State, Summer, 1991.

Peplau, H.E. (1991). *Interpersonal relations in nursing—A conceptual frame of reference for psychodynamic nursing.* New York: Springer Publishing.

Plimley, C., et al. (1991). Dual diagnosis: Mentally ill chemical abusers need professionals working together (pp 7, 13). Office of Mental Health News.

Pollack, L. (1995). Treatment of inpatients with bipolar disorder: A role for self-management groups. *Journal of Psychosocial Nursing,* 33:1, 11–16.

Rutan, J. S., and Waller, S. (1993). *Psychodynamic group psychotherapy* (2nd ed.). New York: Guilford Press.

Rutan, J. S., and Alonso, A. (1979). Group therapy. In A. Lazare (Ed.), *Outpatient psychiatry: Diagnosis and treatment.* Baltimore, MD: Williams & Wilkins.

Satir, V. (1984). *Conjoint family therapy.* Palo Alto: Science Behavior Books.

Sheeren, M. (1988). The relationship between relapse and involvement in Alcoholics Anonymous. *Journal of Studies on Alcohol,* 29:104.

Staples, N., and Schwartz, M. (1990). Anorexia nervosa support group: Providing transitional support. *Journal of Psychosocial Nursing,* 28(2):6.

Tuckman, B. (1965). Developmental sequence in small groups. *Psychological Bulletin,* 63.

United States Pharmacopoeia (1993). Patient Education Leaflets—Introductory version. United States Pharmacopeial Convention.

Van Servellen, G., et al. (1992). Methodological concerns in evaluating psychiatric nursing care modalities and a proposed standard group protocol format for nurse-led groups. *Archives of Psychiatric Nursing,* 6(2):117–124.

Wenckus, E. (1994). Storytelling: Using an ancient art to work with groups. *Journal of Psychsocial Nursing,* 32:7, 30–32.

Wolberg, L. R. (1977) *The technique of psychotherapy* (3rd ed.). New York: Grune & Stratton.

Wolfe, B.E. (1995). Eating disorders: Symptoms and syndromes. Psychiatric nursing conference sponsored by Contemporary Forums, Boston, May 12, 1995.

Wolfe, M. (1993). Group modalities in the care of clients with drug and alcohol problems. In M. A. Naegle (Ed.). *Substance abuse education in nursing* (Vol. III, pp. 6–7). New York: National League for Nursing Press.

Yalom, I. (1983). *Inpatient group psychotherapy.* New York: Basic Books.

Yalom, I. (1985). *The theory and practice of group psychotherapy.* New York: Basic Books.

Further Reading

Beeber A. (1991). Psychotherapy with schizophrenics in team groups. A system model. *American Journal of Psychotherapy,* 45:78.

Captain, C. (1989). Family recovery from alcoholism: Mediating family factors. *Nursing Clinics of North America,* 24:55.

Collins-Colon, T. (1990). Do it yourself: Medication management for community based clients. *Journal of Psychosocial Nursing,* 28:6.

Delgado, M. (1983). Hispanics and psychotherapy groups. *International Journal of Group Psychotherapy,* 33(4):503.

Flaskerud, J. (1989). Psychiatric nurses' needs for AIDS information. *Perspectives in Psychiatric Care,* 25(3,4):3.

Janssen, E. (1994). A Self-Psychological Approach to treating the mentally ill, chemical abusing, and addicted (MICAA) patient. *Archives of Psychiatric Nursing* 8(6):381–389.

Kanas, N. (1988). Therapy groups for schizophrenics: Patients on acute care units. *Hospital and Community Psychiatry,* 39(5):546.

Kapur, R., et al. (1986). Group psychotherapy in an acute inpatient setting. *Psychiatry,* 49(4):337–349.

Kuipers, J., et al. (1988). Designing a psychiatric medication education program. *Journal of Rehabilitation,* 54(3):55.

Minkoff, K. M. D. (1990) *Parallels between alcoholism addiction and major mental illness: Active use and stages of recovery.* Woburn, MA: Choate Symnes Health Services.

Piccinino, S. (1990). The nursing care challenge: Borderline patients. *Journal of Psychosocial Nursing,* 28(4):22.

Van Sevellen, G., et al. (1991). Nursing-led group modalities in a psychiatric inpatient setting: A program evaluation. *Archives of Psychiatric Nursing,* 5(3):128.

SELF-STUDY AND CRITICAL THINKING

Match each group term with the correct definition.

1. ________ Ebb and flow of power or energy.
2. ________ Group in which new members are added as others leave.
3. ________ Process by which a problem that has been hidden is brought into the open.
4. ________ Deeper, underlying meaning of messages of what is happening in the group.
5. ________ All that is said in a group.
6. ________ The nonverbal actions that vary, depending on the level of anxiety in meeting individual goals while working to meet group goals.
7. ________ Two or more individuals in a group that join together. They may have more loyalty to each other than they do to the larger group.
8. ________ Membership is restricted and often time limited.

A. Group content
B. Group process
C. Subgrouping
D. Covert content (communication)
E. Confrontation
F. Open group
G. Closed group
H. Dynamics

Match each group role with the correct definition.

9. ________ Asks for clarification of beliefs and values
10. ________ Checks out what someone said by questioning and restating
11. ________ Keeps the group focused on goals and questions directions
12. ________ Asks for facts pertinent to what is being discussed
13. ________ Examines possible group solutions against group standards
14. ________ States beliefs and values

A. Information seeker
B. Evaluator
C. Orientor
D. Clarifier
E. Opinion seeker
F. Opinion giver

True or false

If false, correct the statement.

15. ________ For treatment of an alcoholic to be successful, it is helpful for the alcoholic's family to receive some kind of family therapy.
16. ________ For the family of an alcoholic, family-centered nursing services can be just as effective as family therapy.
17. ________ A client should not be included in an inpatient group if he or she can attend only two sessions.
18. ________ Confidentiality is essential in all aspects of inpatient group therapy, even if a client reveals suicidal thoughts.

19. __________ Group members are encouraged to stay, even when they want to leave, once the group session has started.

20. __________ The group therapist encourages a client to talk about his or her feelings if the client threatens to do something violent.

Multiple choice

Select the correct answer.

21. The primary goal of the inpatient group therapist is
    A. To focus on the here and now
    B. To examine interpersonal relationships within the group
    C. To be proactive and create a structure for the group
    D. All of the above

22. Countertransference is
    A. The client's feelings or reactions toward the therapist
    B. The therapist's feelings or reactions toward the client
    C. The underlying meaning in group interaction
    D. The content of an interaction

23. Self-help groups
    A. Can use a nurse as a leader or group member only if he or she has had a similar problem and has resolved it
    B. Often meet without a designated leader
    C. Provide mutual support
    D. All of the above

24. Self-help groups, such as Alcoholics Anonymous, Co-Dependents Anonymous, and the National Alliance for the Mentally Ill, can
    A. Prevent physical, emotional, or social health problems
    B. Improve an individual's or a family's quality of life
    C. Provide education to develop an individual's potential
    D. All of the above

Critical thinking

25. Construct a formula for a medication teaching group that would cover information useful for your client or clients.
26. If possible, co-lead this group with a staff member or a fellow student with instructor guidelines.
27. Role play with classmates (one acting as group leader) a group experience in intervening with a client who (a) monopolizes, (b) complains but rejects help, and (c) chronically helps others.
28. Identify which milieu groups are offered in your clinical setting and ask to either co-lead or participate in at least two, with your instructor's guidance.

11

Communication Within Families

JEANNEMARIE G. BAKER

OUTLINE

KEY TERMS AND CONCEPTS

The key terms and concepts listed here also appear in bold where they are defined or discussed in this chapter.

double bind theory
strategic model of family therapy
structural model of family therapy
family systems theory

family triangles
nuclear family
flexibility
boundaries
clear boundaries
diffused or enmeshed boundaries
rigid or disengaged boundaries
multigenerational issues
sociocultural context
genogram
psychoeducational family therapy

OBJECTIVES

After studying this chapter, the reader will be able to

1. Contrast and compare several diverse forms of family.
2. Discuss the characteristics of a healthy family and give a clinical example.
3. Differentiate between functional and dysfunctional family patterns of behavior as they relate to the five family functions.
4. Describe the dynamics of stability versus change within the family life cycle.
5. Identify five family theorists and their contributions to the family therapy movement.
6. Analyze the meaning and value of the family's sociocultural context when assessing and planning intervention strategies.
7. Construct a genogram by use of a three-generation approach.
8. Formulate seven outcome criteria that a counselor and family might develop together.
9. Identify some strategies for family intervention.
10. Distinguish between the nursing intervention strategies of a basic level nurse and a certified nurse specialist regarding counseling/psychotherapy and psychobiological issues.

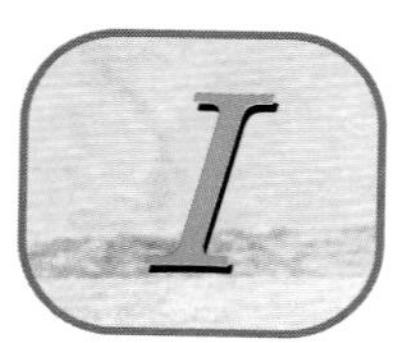

In the late 1940s and early 1950s, with the psychoanalytic movement firmly established as a mode of treatment for mental and emotional disturbances, new approaches began to exert an influence. It was at this time that the development of the interpersonal field of behavior began to take shape. In addition, more attention was being focused on sociocultural factors as they influenced human behavior. Also, small-group psychology, communications theory, and general systems theory became critical areas of exploration. Other societal changes, emerging especially in the late 1950s and 1960s, included a greater emphasis on consumerism, the women's movement, individual rights, and antiracism.

THE DEVELOPMENT OF THE FAMILY SYSTEMS PERSPECTIVE

In clinical settings, therapists were beginning to notice the effects of the social milieu on their clients. The therapeutic community was established as a treatment modality at this time, and group therapy and psychodrama were developed. All of these changes were rooted in observations of the client and viewing treatment in terms of social systems. An *interactive* (interpersonal) rather than an *indwelling* (intrapsychic) model of mental illness was becoming more widely accepted. These influences paved the way for an interest in the family system as it related to psychiatric disorders.

One of the original shapers of family theory and therapy was Haley (1980), who was associated with the Mental Research Institute in Palo Alto, California, where the double bind theory was developed. The **double bind theory** describes a situation in which two conflicting messages are given simultaneously on two levels, verbal and nonverbal. Since the messages conflict, people find themselves in a double bind, in which no acceptable response exists. For example, a recently divorced and lonely mother says to her teenaged daughter, "Go on out, have fun with your friends. I'll be just fine." However, the nonverbal message is that the mother will be left alone and lonely. The nonverbal message is made clear by the mother's dejected face, slumped posture, and sad tone of voice. The daughter is now in a no-win situation. If she goes out with her friends, she will feel guilty for leaving her mother alone. If she stays home with her mother, she will miss out on the friendships and activities that are important for teenage development.

Virginia Satir (1972, 1983), a leading theorist of the same era, moved the focus from the patient's symptom to the patient's position and relationships within the family.

The Milan Group, especially Palazolli, Cecchin, and Prata, established the use of paradox (i.e., "Don't Change") as a way to work with families. Probably more than anyone, Minuchin (1974), a structural therapist, established the legitimacy of family therapy within psychiatry. Bowen (1985) was a leading proponent of the family systems model; he underplayed problem resolution, focusing instead on the long-term differentiation process of individual family members. Table 11–1 provides an overview of various family theorists and their approaches.

The terms *strategic* and *structural* are used to identify a framework from which specific therapists operate. A **strategic model of family therapy** assumes that by changing any single element in the family system, change can be brought about in the entire system. Briefly, the aim of strategic therapy is to change the patterns, the rules, and the meaning of family interactions. For example, in the Gomez family, whom you will read about shortly, a pattern of communicating, partly cultural, exists that excludes any discussion with the children. All decisions, whether or not they involve the children, are made without consulting the children. Consequently, the children in this family often feel powerless, and the 12-year-old has begun to engage in destructive behavior at school, which has precipitated a visit to a family therapist. A family therapist using the strategic model might work with the family to change their rigid pattern of communicating, allowing the children to be present when important decisions are being made. The children could comment and offer suggestions on how issues could be resolved. This could result in a resolution of the 12-year-old's negative behavior by giving him a sense of control over aspects of his life and a more positive outlet for being heard and recognized. This intervention would result in a systemic change in the way the Gomez family communicates.

The **structural model of family therapy** is based on a normative concept of a healthy family, emphasizing the boundaries between family subsystems and the establishment and maintenance of a clear hierarchy based on parental competence. A therapist using the structural model with the Gomez family, rather than focusing on changing a specific pattern, would highlight the importance of boundaries between the parental and sibling subsystems (children). At the same time, the therapist would emphasize the importance of flexibility in the family system that would allow for the changes inherent to normal growth and development.

The aims of **family systems theory** are to decrease emotional reactivity and to encourage differentiation among individual family members (i.e., increase each member's "sense of self"). In family therapy, no one model exists; all the shapers of family theory have made substantial contributions to the field of family therapy. In addition, all techniques are not applicable to all problems, and the experienced clinician must be discerning. However, many concepts are widely used in working with

TABLE 11–1 FAMILY THEORISTS

THEORIST	FRAMEWORK	INTERVENTION STRATEGY
Minuchin	**Structural model** of organizational patterns, boundaries, and subsystems; scapegoating	Restructure dysfunctional triangles; clarify boundaries; structure role-appropriate subsytems
Satir	**Structural model** of family relationships. Focuses on intergenerational picture, sees self-esteem as a critical factor; an individual's symptoms express family pain.	Use of nurturing, identify communication patterns
Haley	**Strategic model;** family is organized hierarchically with inequality of power; life cycle perspective, double binds	Plan therapeutic moves rather than respond to what is happening.
Bowen	**Family systems model:** focuses on long-term differentiation and process, less emphasis on problem resolution; emphasizes the family of origin's relationship patterns.	Objective is to change one's perspectives and current relationships with key family members, promote separation and individuation of members, encouraage rational rather than irrational thoughts and behaviors.
Milan Group (Palazolli, Cecchin, Prata)	**Strategic model:** focuses on use of paradox, challenges family about present situation, relationships, and problem.	Use circular questioning; formulate systematic hypotheses; maintain neutrality; prescribe rituals.
Carter	**Multicontextual model:** family life cycle stage; multigenerational issues; sociocultural context.	View family in a sociocultural context of gender, race, ethnicity, class, religion, and sexual orientation, as well as in a context of their particular life cycle stage and multigenerational issues.

families. The concepts of the identified patient, the family triangle, and the nuclear family emotional system are discussed here. Table 11–2 identifies other concepts relevant to family work.

The Identified Patient

The "identified patient," or *index person,* is the individual in the family whom everyone regards as "the problem." This problem family member generally bears most of the family system's anxiety. When a family comes for treatment, the presenting problem must be addressed before the underlying systematic problem is dealt with. The family member who is the identified patient is not always the one who initially seeks help from inpatient or outpatient services.

Nurses generally tend to be more aware of the biophysical aspects of an individual than of the interpersonal aspects. Understandably, nurses also tend to subscribe to the medical model of cause-and-effect thinking. However, when a client is assessed in the context of family, the nurse clinician must think in a less linear way (cause and effect) and more in terms of a circular causality. In circular causality, the presenting problem is viewed from many different perspectives. For example, the nurse considers a particular family's stressors and strengths in light of the family's current life cycle stage, its sociocultural context and multigenerational issues, and the family's impact on the presenting problem. Thus, there is more than one perspective to be considered when looking at the identified patient from a family system's perspective. The focus is on the family system's anxiety.

▶ Eight-year-old Tommy, who is hyperactive and disruptive at school and at home, is brought to the community mental health clinic to be evaluated for attention-deficit hyperactivity disorder. The nurse clinician performs an assessment and finds that a great deal of turmoil exists within the family. The family is composed of a heterosexual couple (married and the parents of the three children) and a grandmother. Tommy's father has just lost his job, and his grandmother was recently diagnosed with bladder cancer. Tommy's mother is

TABLE 11–2 CENTRAL CONCEPTS OF FAMILY

Homeostasis	Tendency of a system to maintain a dynamic equilibrium around some central tendency and to undertake operations designed to restore that equilibrium when it is threatened in some way.
Boundaries	Clear boundaries are those that maintain distinctions between individuals within the family and between the family and the outside world. Clear boundaries allow for balanced flow of energy between members. Roles of children and parent or parents are clearly defined. Diffuse or rigid boundaries are more often seen in families with problematic functioning. Enmeshed versus disengaged, and degree of flexibility and individuation: enmeshed boundaries are the result of the fusion or blending together of individuals so that the distinct person fails to emerge.
Triangulation	When two-person relationships tend to be stressful and unstable, the tendency is to draw in a third person to stabilize the system by forming a coalition in which the two join the third.
Complementary	Members of the system fit together as a functional whole, in which there is an interdependent fit or balance, e.g., responsibility and irresponsibility.
Scapegoating	A form of displacement whereby a family member (usually the least powerful) is blamed for another's or other family members' distress. The purpose is to keep the focus off the painful issues and the problems of the blamers. In a family, the blamers are often the parents, and the scapegoat a child.
Double bind	A positive command (often verbal) followed by a negative command (often nonverbal), leaving the recipient confused, trapped, and immobilized since there is no way to act.
Hierarchy	The function of power and its structures in families, differentiating parental and sibling roles and generational boundaries.
Family life cycle	The family's developmental process over time; refers to the family's past course, its present tasks, and its future course.
Differentiation	Developing a strong identity and sense of self while at the same time maintaining an emotional connectedness with one's family or origin.
Sociocultural context	The framework for viewing the family in terms of the influence of gender, race, ethnicity, religion, economic class, and sexual orientation.
Multigenerational, emotional transition process	The continuation and persistence from generation to generation of certain emotional interactive family patterns, e.g., reenactment of fairly predictable and almost ritual-like patterns; repetition of themes or toxic issues; and repetition of reciprocal patterns, e.g., overfunctioner and underfunctioner.

planning to file for separation because of constant, unresolved arguments with her husband. The nurse clinician who views this family from a position of circular causality would not focus solely on Tommy but would view Tommy's symptoms as a function of many difficult losses and transitions that are stressing the entire family's coping mechanisms.

▶ The nurse identifies the multiple stressors in this family, believing that Tommy's symptoms of hyperactivity and acting out are related to the severe stresses in the family system. Once the issues within the family are addressed and plans are made to deal with these issues, perhaps Tommy's symptoms will subside. She refers the couple to a family therapist. In the meantime, she encourages the couple to focus more on their own issues and less on Tommy's behavior. An appointment is made to go to the clinic in 1 month, where Tommy will be reevaluated.

Family Triangles

Bowen (1985) described a relationship process in families that can be seen as a system of interlocking triangles. In relationships between two people, the major tension lies in the struggle between closeness and independence. When the tension in a close twosome builds, a third person (child, friend, parent) is brought in to help lower the tension. The **family triangle** then becomes the basic building block of interpersonal relationships. All triangles contain a close side, a distant side, and a side in which conflict or tension exists between two people (Andrus 1996). The intensity of the triangling process varies among families and within the same family over time; this is because triangles are related to lack of emotional stability. *Differentiation* refers to the ability of the individual to establish a unique identity and still remain emotionally connected to the family of origin. The lower the level of differentiation in a family, the higher the tension, and the more important the role of triangling is to the lowering of tension and the preservation of emotional stability. As the family becomes stressed, for whatever reasons, the anxiety in the system gets triggered, and the triangles become more active.

The Arturo family described in the following vignette has a low level of differentiation. Their enmeshment is such that if one member of the family becomes anxious over an upcoming job interview, all the family members experience anxiety. In order to bind that anxiety, individuals begin to interact with other family members in whatever their preferred patterns of operation are. Some of these maneuvers may include arguing, becoming helpless, refusing to speak to certain family members, and being unable to be alone.

▶ When Grampa Arturo experienced a mild heart attack that required hospitalization, the entire family was thrown into a state of anxiety and chaos, which rendered them helpless and unable to make clear decisions. Grampa's daughter Helena was predicting his impending death. Her husband Emilio, although concerned about his wife's father, felt Helena was being unreasonable. Both Helena and Emilio engaged in angry arguments over Helena's "unreasonableness" and Emilio's "stubbornness." Their two adult children were brought into the argument (triangled in) and were expected to take sides, as usual.

▶ The family's stress over the possible loss of Grampa Arturo was bound by means of activation of the familiar triangles, which are set in motion whenever this family faces the possibility of change. (Emilio and Helena rehash each other's personality flaws, and their children are drawn into the argument.) This family's intense anxiety about the highly charged issue of the possible loss of Grampa Arturo is not their focus; rather, they fall back on the family system's established patterns of interaction.

▶ The first task of the nurse in this situation is to calm down the system by setting guidelines for family communication. For example, each individual is given the opportunity to express his or her concerns, thoughts, and feelings regarding the crisis situation. Therefore, every member's concerns and issues get heard and acknowledged by the other family members. The nurse can then work with the family and explore with them ways to deal with the crisis, taking a more constructive and effective approach.

When working with families, nurse clinicians need to avoid becoming triangled into the family's system. The nurse's personal work on his or her own differentiation process is an important way to maintain emotional stability in the face of a chaotic family situation, where the nurse's own issues may be playing out. Holding the family members accountable for themselves—making clear that the responsibility for change is theirs and not that of the nurse clinician—is a way of remaining clear of their triangles. For example, the nurse clinician could become triangled in to the Arturo family system in any number of ways: perhaps the nurse recently experienced the loss of a grandparent; or maybe the nurse belongs to an enmeshed family system, in which the children are regularly drawn into spousal arguments; or perhaps stubbornness is an unresolved issue for the nurse. Any of these possibilities could allow the nurse to become triangled into a family system, making good therapeutic intervention difficult, if not impossible. The likelihood is great that nurse clinicians will become triangled into others' (e.g., the Arturo family's) family systems to engage in their own family battles. Nurse clinicians need to make regular concerted efforts to self-reflect (self-assessment) and to understand their own personal family issues through therapy or supervision. *Regular supervision is always recommended when nurse clinicians work with individuals, couples, or families.* Supervision can be conducted with peer professionals, in groups, or privately with a more experienced clinician. One indication that a nurse clinician is being triangled in is that his or her level of anxiety is greater than the situation warrants.

The Nuclear Family Emotional System

The term **nuclear family** refers to a parent or parents and the children under the parents' care. Bowen (1985) developed the concept of a *nuclear family emotional system*, which is defined as the flow of emotional processes within the nuclear family. In this concept, symptoms are viewed as belonging to the nuclear family emotional system rather than to any one individual. Within the system, a distinction is made between conventional medical (psychiatric) diagnosis and family diagnosis; rather than viewing a symptom as reflecting a "disease" that is confined to a "client," Bowen identified an emotional process that transcends the boundaries of a client and encompasses the family relationship system. The earlier example of 8-year-old Tommy, who was believed by his family and others to have attention-deficit hyperactivity disorder, is one in which Tommy's symptoms could be viewed as reflecting the family's conflicts and changes.

Many different models, theories, and therapies have been developed to enable people to be considered within a family context. Some therapists are committed to just one theory and interpret family activity exclusively through its concepts. Other therapists are eclectic in their approach, combining concepts from different theories in their treatment of families. The nurse can draw from many theories as he or she develops a general understanding of the concepts related to families.

THE FAMILY

The family is the primary system to which a person belongs, and in most cases, it is the most powerful system to which a person may ever belong. Birth, puberty, marriage, and death are all considered to be family experiences. The family can be the source of love or hate, pride or shame, security or insecurity. Although individual family members have roles and functions, the overriding value in families lies in the relationships between family members. It is these family relationships that provide the primary context of human development. "Family" comprises the entire emotional system of at least three, and frequently four, generations. In their discussion of the changing family life cycle, Carter and McGoldrick (1989) emphasized the intergenerational connectedness of the family as being one of our greatest human resources.

Most people no longer live in families that conform to the prevailing cultural ideal of the 1950s. The definition of family has become more complicated over the past 2 decades, and the traditional family with a breadwinner, a housewife, and children now represents only a small minority of families. Today, many configurations of family exist. In some families, there is a single parent; in some families, both parents are gay or lesbian; in other families, the grandparents are the main caregivers; in other families, no one is related, but the members have come to live together for mutual support; and in still other families, the members are blended through divorce and marriage.

Characteristics of a Healthy Family

Two primary characteristics are essential to healthy family functioning: flexibility and boundaries.

Flexibility is critical. A flexible family is able to recognize the need for change as members move through the family life cycle. Flexibility is the key factor for negotiating normal transitions within the family life cycle as well as those within the individual life cycle. Inherent in this process of being flexible is the ability to come up with available options to cope with a situation that requires change and restructuring. The more rigid and inflexible a family, the fewer the available options for change. Also, the flexible family tends to function more openly as a system, allowing for differences and for challenging ideas without family members feeling threatened or fearful about losing control or losing their identity. In flexible families, individuals are free to express their thoughts and emotions. The family that is flexible adapts to changes, thereby maintaining continuity and promoting the psychosocial growth of its individual members.

Boundaries are the means by which a family differentiates among its members. **Boundaries** are rules that define who participates in a particular family function, how they participate, and the role that they play. Boundaries function to protect differences in the system. Boundaries also separate the family from the outside world and give it a unique identity. The development of interpersonal skills depends on the siblings' freedom to grow and evolve without interference by the parent or parents. For example, fighting among siblings can enable development of negotiating skills. Generally, healthy families are ones in which the boundaries are well defined without being too rigid.

Family Functions

Healthy families provide individuals with the tools that guide how they will function in intimate relationships, in the workplace, within their culture, and in society generally. These tools are acquired through the activities that are associated with family life. These activities can be divided into five functions: (1) management, (2) boundary, (3) communication, (4) emotional-supportive, and (5) socialization (Roberts 1983). Although family counselors may use various assessment strategies, these five areas are always included. Table 11–3 presents an assessment tool

TABLE 11–3 FAMILY FUNCTION CHECKLIST

Client Family ______________ Date of Assessment ______________

Family Functions	Observed Behavior	Assessed Need Level (I–IV)	Suggested Nursing Responses
I. *Management function* A. Use of power for all family members			
B. Rule making clear, accepted			
C. Fiscal support adequate			
D. Successful negotiations with extrafamilial systems			
E. Future planning present			
II. *Boundary function* A. Clear individual boundaries			
B. Clear generational boundaries			
C. Clear family boundaries			
III. *Communication function* A. Straight messages			
B. No manipulation			
C. Expression of positive and negative feelings safely			
IV. *Emotional-supportive function* A. Mutual positive regard			
B. Deals with conflict			
C. Uses resources for all family members			
D. Allows growth for all family members			
V. *Socialization function* A. Children growing and developing in a healthy pattern			
B. Mutual negotiation of roles by age and ability			
C. Parents feeling good about parenting			
D. Spouses happy with each other's role behavior			

Roberts, F. B. (1983). An interaction model for family assessment. In I. W. Clements and F. B. Roberts (Eds.), *Family health: a theoretical approach to nursing care* (p. 202). New York: John Wiley.

that the family counselor can use to evaluate Roberts' five functions. The following sections explain these functions more fully.

Management Function

Every day in every family, decisions are made regarding issues of power, rule making, and provision of financial support. Other management issues include future planning and goods allocation (who gets what within the family). In healthy families, it is usually the adults in the family who agree as to how these functions are to be performed. In families with a single parent, these management functions may sometimes become overwhelming, and single parents can benefit from discussions with other adults. In more chaotic families, an inappropriate member, such as a teenager or a grandparent, may be the one who makes these decisions. Although children learn decision-making skills as they mature and increasingly make decisions and choices about their own lives, they should not have to take on this responsibility for the family of origin.

Boundary Function

Boundaries functions maintain a distinction between individuals in the family. Boundaries may be clear, diffuse, rigid, or inconsistent. **Clear boundaries** are well understood by all members of the family; they help to define the roles of members within the families and allow for differences between members. To a great extent, a person's emotional, social, and physical functioning are related to his or her level of role differentiation within the family and the amount of anxiety within the family system (Cooley 1995).

Diffused, or **enmeshed, boundaries** refer to a blending together of the roles, thoughts, and feelings of the individuals so that clear distinctions between family members fail to emerge. The members of a family that operates with diffused, rigid, or inconsistent boundaries are more prone to psychological or psychosomatic symptoms. A common phenomenon within families with diffuse boundaries is that individuals expect other members of the family to know what they are thinking ("Why did you take that? You know I wanted it.") and to believe they know what other family members are thinking ("I know exactly why you did that").

Rigid, or **disengaged, boundaries** are those in which the rules and roles are adhered to no matter what; thus, rigid boundaries prevent family members from trying out new roles or, in some cases, from taking on more mature functions as time goes on. In families in which rigid boundaries predominate, isolation may be marked. The family is often cut off from the community and outside influences, and even from each other.

▸ Lucy Manero is a single parent with two preschool-aged children. The family is living on public assistance. Lucy is a teenage mother who is working toward a general equivalency degree and who also works "under the table" part time as a seamstress. Her mother, Maria, watches the children for Lucy, and discipline is a hot issue between Lucy and Maria.

If the boundary functioning of this family were clear, Lucy and Maria would have worked out an arrangement in which Maria would be in charge of disciplining the children when Lucy is away and when both Lucy and Maria are present, Lucy would make the decisions without interference from Maria. The children would be made aware of these arrangements and would clearly understand who is in charge and when. They would know that Lucy and Maria have different operating styles, to which they would learn to adjust. If the boundary functioning of this family were blurred, Lucy and Maria would likely be interfering with each other's mode of discipline, which undoubtedly would lead to tension between them as their anxiety levels increase, and angry outbursts around many issues would eventually ensue. The children, in turn, would become confused as to where their loyalties lie and would probably engage in manipulative behaviors because of the unclear boundaries. If the boundary functioning of this family were rigid, Lucy and Maria would likely have great difficulty agreeing on issues of discipline if their perceptions of rules and roles differed. The children would probably be triangled into a double bind position between a warring mother and daughter in which no correct response exists. All family members would likely become stuck in this established, rigid pattern with no available alternatives.

Communication Function

Communication patterns are extremely important in family life. Healthy communication patterns include clear and comprehensible messages (e.g., "I would like to go now," or "I don't like it when you interrupt what I'm saying"). Healthy communication within the family encourages members to ask for what they want and to express their feelings appropriately. Feelings of affection and conflict are both openly expressed. Family members are able to ask for what they want and get the attention they need without resorting to manipulation to get their needs met. When communication among family members is not clear, it cannot be used as a means to solve problems or to resolve conflict; therefore, the cardinal rule for effective and functional communication in families is "Be clear and direct in saying what you want and need."

As simple as this may seem, it is one of the hardest skills to activate in a family system. To be direct, individuals must first have a sense that the self is respected and loved; this sense entitles them to take a stand and to set boundaries with others. The consequences for being clear and direct may be unpleasant in a family system in which boundaries are enmeshed and confusion is the norm. To attempt to change a family pattern is to pit oneself against the status quo. Saying what one wants and needs is especially difficult when one believes that family members should already know—especially if the family member is a spouse, a parent, or a close sibling. In fact, most family members cannot read each other's minds, although emotionally undifferentiated members may think that this is possible. The following is a spousal situation that shows how easily communication can be misunderstood when clear and direct messages are not sent.

▸ Mary would like to spend more time with her husband John on the weekends; however, John always seems to be busy with projects around the house or talking with friends on the telephone. Mary feels that he does not notice her, or maybe is not interested in her, so she spends a lot of time working out or playing tennis. John figures that Mary is doing what she wants to do, and that it makes her happy, so he contents himself by finding things to do alone. The net result is that Mary and John spend little time together.

▸ Mary finally confronts John clearly and directly about his "disinterest" in her, saying what she wants and needs, which is her desire to spend more time together on the weekends. John replies that he had no idea she felt that way. He had thought she enjoyed the way things were. Actually, he, too, would like to have more time together. What a learning experience for them both!

Box 11–1 identifies some unhealthy communication patterns.

Emotional-Supportive Function

All families encounter conflicts, and no family is 100% "functional." However, in a healthy family, feelings of affection are generally uppermost, and anger and conflict do not dominate the family's pattern of interaction. Healthy families are concerned with each other's needs, and most of the family members' emotional and physical needs are met most of the time. When people's emotional needs are met, they feel support from those around them and are free to grow and explore new roles and facets of their personalities. A family that is dominated by conflict and anger alienates its members, leaving them isolated and fearful. This is not an atmosphere in which personality growth can take place, so this family would not be considered functional.

BOX 11–1 EXAMPLES OF DYSFUNCTIONAL COMMUNICATION

Manipulating
Instead of asking directly for what one wants, family members manipulate others into getting what they want. For example, a child starts a fight with a sibling in order to get attention. Another example is a family member's making requests with strings attached, so that the other person has a difficult time refusing the request, "If you do this for me then I won't tell Daddy that you are getting poor grades in school."

Distracting
In order to avoid functional problem solving and resolve conflicts within the family, family members introduce irrelevant details into problematic issues.

Generalizing
When dealing with problematic family issues, members use global statements, like "always" and "never," instead of dealing with specific problems and areas of conflict. Family members may say "Harry is always angry" instead of "Harry, what is upsetting you?"

Blaming
Family members blame others for failures, errors, or negative consequences of an action in order to keep the focus off of themselves. This is a response to fear of being blamed by others.

Placating
Family members "pretend" to be inadequate but well meaning in order to keep peace in the family at any price. "Don't yell at the children, dear, I put the shoes on the stairs."

Socialization Function

It is within families that each member learns socialization skills. People learn how to interact, negotiate, and plan; they adopt coping skills. This is most evident in the socialization of children. Children learn how to function effectively within their family, and then they apply those skills in society. Parents are socialized into their family role by the demands of each child throughout the developmental stages of their children. The role of the parents changes again when the children mature and leave home, and the partners may renegotiate the pattern of their lives together. As time goes on, the parents may need their adult children's help if they become less able to care for their needs. Each phase brings new demands and requires new approaches to deal with changes as people become socialized into new roles. Families have difficulty negotiating role change, and changes often increase the stress within families for a time. In response to the family's developmental life cycle, healthy families use flexibility to adapt to new roles.

The Family Life Cycle

The life cycle of the individual takes place within the family life cycle, which is the primary context of human development. The family is a system that moves through time, and family stress is often the greatest at transition points from one stage to another of the family developmental process. Symptoms are most likely to appear when an interruption or a dislocation occurs in the unfolding family life cycle; this interruption or dislocation could be a serious illness, death, or divorce. At these times, therapeutic efforts often need to be directed toward helping family members reorganize so that they can then proceed developmentally. Unlike all other organizations, families incorporate new members only by birth, adoption, or marriage, and members can leave only by death. If no way can be found to function within the system, the pressures of family membership with no available exit can, in the extreme, lead to mental illness or suicide. The development of symptoms should be viewed not only as a response to an interruption or a dislocation in the family life cycle but also as a solution to a stressful situation. This model takes a traditional family approach and would need to be modified for less traditional family consultations.

Six main stages exist in the changing family life cycle: (1) launching the single young adult, (2) joining families through couple formation, (3) becoming parents—families with young children,, (4) families with adolescents, (5) launching children and moving on, and (6) families in later life. Table 11–4 elaborates the stages in the life cycle of the family.

Launching the Single Young Adult

Three required changes need to take place in this stage. The primary task for the young adult during this stage is

TABLE 11–4 THE STAGES OF THE FAMILY LIFE CYCLE

Family Life Cycle Stage	Emotional Process of Transition: Key Principles	Second-Order Changes in Family Status Required to Proceed Developmentally
1. Leaving home: Single young adults	Accepting emotional and financial responsiblity for self	a. Differentiation of self in relation to family of origin b. Development of intimate peer relationships c. Establishment of self regarding work and financial independence
2. The joining of families through marriage: The new couple	Commitment to a new system	a. Formation of marital system b. Realignment of relationships with extended families and friends to include spouse
3. Families with young children	Accepting new members into the system	a. Adjusting marital system to make space for child(ren) b. Joining in childrearing, financial, and household tasks c. Realignment of relationships with extended family to include parenting and grandparenting roles
4. Families with adolescents	Increasing flexibility of family boundaries to include children's independence and grandparent's frailties	a. Shifting of parent-child relationships to permit adolescent to move in and out of system b. Refocus on midlife marital and career issues c. Beginning shift toward joint caring for older generation
5. Launching children and moving on	Accepting a multitude of exits from and entries into the family system	a. Renegotiation of marital system as dyad b. Development of adult-to-adult relationships c. Realignment of relationships to include in-laws and grandchildren d. Dealing with disabilities and death of parents (grandparents)
6. Families in later life	Accepting the shifting of generational roles	a. Maintaining own and/or couple functioning and interests in face of physiological decline; exploration of new familial and social role options b. Support for a more central role of middle generation c. Making room in the system for the wisdom and experience of the elderly, supporting the older generation without overfunctioning for them d. Dealing with the loss of spouse, siblings, and other peers in preparation for own death. Life review and integration.

From Carter, E., and McGoldrick, M. (1989). *The changing family life cycle: A framework for family therapy* (2nd ed., p. 15). Boston: Allyson and Bacon.

to come to terms with his or her family of origin, which profoundly influences how all succeeding stages of the family life cycle will be carried out. Recall that *differentiation* refers to the ability of the individual to establish a unique identity and yet still remain emotionally connected to one's family of origin. The second change entails the development of intimate peer relationships. The third change requires that the young adult establish himself or herself regarding work and financial independence.

Joining Families: The Couple

This stage requires commitment to a new system. Two changes in family status are required. The first is the formation of a couple or marital system, which may entail setting limits with intrusive in-laws, disentangling from an enmeshed family of origin, and struggling for balance regarding intimacy. The second required change involves realigning relationships with extended families and friends to include both spouses.

Becoming Parents: Families with Young Children

Three changes in family status are required at this stage: an adjustment of the marital system to make space for children; a joining in child rearing, financial and household tasks; and a realignment of the relationships with the extended family to include the new roles of parenting and grandparenting. This shift requires that the adults now move up a generation and become caretakers to the younger generation. A common problem that occurs during this stage, and that can continue into successive stages, is the setting up of a triangle among the two parents and the child, in which one parent is overinvolved with the child and the other plays a more peripheral role. In this situation, the child eventually becomes the means by which the parents communicate with each other about issues they cannot deal with directly. In other words, spousal conflicts may be brought into the parental arena, where they clearly do not belong.

◗ Six-year-old Lisa is having trouble making friends. Her mother, Susan, has been feeling anxious and helpless as she tries to find ways to engage Lisa with other youngsters. Susan develops an overprotectiveness with Lisa that further inhibits Lisa from venturing out to make friends. Susan feels that her husband Bill is uncaring and disinterested because he thinks that she should be more relaxed about Lisa's social life, letting things develop naturally. Bill's job requires that he travel most of the week, so he is not involved with Susan's daily experiences and struggles with Lisa.

◗ In the spousal arena, Susan and Bill have been avoiding intimacy for almost a year. Susan is angry with Bill for spending so much time with his parents, which further casts him in a peripheral role in their nuclear family, and Bill is angry with Susan, sensing her rejection of him.

◗ Both parents are feeling isolated and alienated and are consequently angry at each other. Neither Bill nor Susan addresses this issue directly. Instead, they play out their anger in the parental arena as they battle over how to handle Lisa's social isolation.

Figure 11–1 diagrams this family triangle.

Families with Adolescents

Three basic changes in family status are required in this stage. Perhaps the most dramatic is the gradual shifting of parent-child relationships to permit the adolescent to move in and out of the system. The flexibility of family boundaries needs to increase; these boundaries must now become permeable. Parents can no longer maintain complete authority at this stage, and this adjustment may be difficult. Adolescents open the family to a whole array of new values as they bring friends and new ideas into the family. Families who are threatened by this are often stuck in an earlier view of their children. Creating more flexible boundaries that will allow adolescents to be dependent at times, and to experiment with increasing degrees of independence at other times, can put special strains on all family members.

The second change in family status at this stage requires a refocusing on midlife couplehood and career issues. One or both spouses may be experiencing a midlife crisis that is characterized by the exploration of personal, career, and marital dissatisfactions. An intense renegotiation of the marriage often occurs at this time. The third required change at this stage involves beginning a shift toward jointly caring for the older generation.

Launching Children and Moving On

This stage in the changing family life cycle requires an overall acceptance of a multitude of exits from, and en-

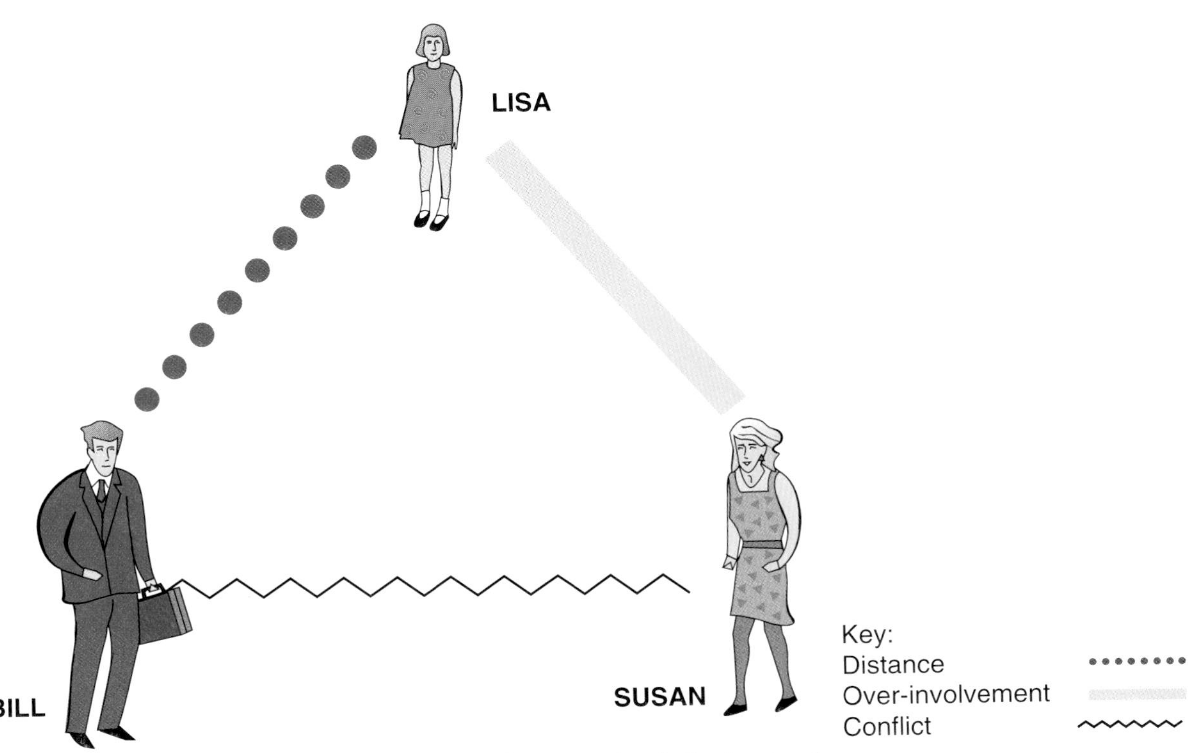

Figure 11–1 Example of a family triangle.

tries into, the family system. These include the launching of grown children, the entry of their spouses and children, and the leavetakings as grandparents grow ill and die. Four changes in family status are required at this stage: (1) the renegotiation of the marital system as a dyad, (2) the development of adult-to-adult relationships between grown children and their parents, (3) the realignment of relationships to include in-laws and grandchildren, and (4) the need to deal with the disabilities and death of parents and grandparents. This last is considered to be the newest, longest, and most problematic of all the phases in the family life cycle. Because of the low birthrate and long life span of most adults, parents launch their children almost 20 years before retirement and must then find other life activities.

In some situations, solidification of the marriage or couplehood has not taken place by this time, and reinvestment in the relationship is not possible. In these families, in order to preserve the family unit by maintaining a balance in the system, the family may mobilize itself to keep the last child at home. This may also happen in a single-parent family situation when the parent does not have close relationships and interests outside the family. At other times, the partners may choose to go their separate ways after child rearing is concluded.

The Family in Later Life

Four changes in family status occur at this stage. One is maintaining self or couple functioning and interests in the face of physiological decline. This may be a time of exploration of new familial and social role options. A second change is that of allowing the middle generation to assume a more central role. The third change is that of making room in the system for the wisdom and experience of the elderly by supporting the older generation without taking over for them. The fourth required change in family status involves dealing with the loss of spouse, siblings, and other peers and preparing for one's own death, which often includes a review of life to achieve an integration of meaning.

With an understanding of the normative issues and inherent problems of the changing family life cycle, the nurse clinician has a basis for approaching a patient's presenting problem and assessing the available resources of the patient's family. For example, the family in which the grandmother is critically ill with terminal cancer may be in the life cycle stage of a family with adolescents. The nurse may wonder if the issue of control is not a predominant one for this family as parents grapple with the loss of authority over their teenagers, a possible midlife crisis of their own, and the impending loss of an important family elder. The nurse clinician then needs to evaluate the degree of flexibility within the family, as this directly affects the availability of alternatives in managing such disruptions in the family life cycle.

If the family is a closed system, in which the nuclear family is their primary source of support, the extended family is either not available or not involved, and community supports are not accessed, then other family members could become symptomatic in some way. Often, it is the teenagers who demonstrate symptoms, such as getting involved with drugs or getting into trouble at school; these problems often serve as a mechanism to diffuse the stress and anxiety in the family system as the family tries to maintain a homeostatic balance. At other times, it may be a parent who uses alcohol or drugs to self-medicate and temporarily feel relief of overwhelming feelings in a difficult situation. Since people are living longer and losses are often greater as people outlive friends and family members, a family at this stage benefits from a keen assessment and the availability of appropriate resource information and support.

ASSESSMENT STRATEGIES IN FAMILY THERAPY

Various techniques developed by family therapists are used by practitioners to generate useful family data. Essential information regarding sociocultural issues, past medical and mental illness, family interactions and communication styles, and areas of stress within the family need to be obtained before planning and intervention can take place.

Carter and McGoldrick (1989) developed a model for marital and family assessment that includes three important areas of consideration:

1. Stage of the family life cycle
2. Multigenerational issues
3. Sociocultural context

Much of the information regarding these important areas of assessment can be obtained through the construction of a multigenerational genogram, which is discussed later in the chapter.

Multigenerational Issues

The influence of family is not restricted to the members of a household. Family comprises the entire emotional system of at least three, and frequently four, generations; this means that they have **multigenerational issues.** Through this intergenerational system, various patterns (e.g., geographical distance, suicide, divorce, addiction, affairs, grief, triangles, and loss) are passed down through the generations. The messages and legacies of the multigenerational family relate in some way to the client's presenting problem. For example, in a family with adolescents in which the grandmother is terminally ill with cancer, if a pattern of addiction is already established in the family, the impending loss of an important family figure may exacerbate an incipient addiction in one of the family members. An astute nurse may express concern to the family regarding this possibility, perhaps preventing the development of a serious problem. This family may also have a preferred pattern of dealing with grief by using denial and by not allowing the outward expression of painful feelings. If this is the case, the nurse guides the family into learning about other, more acceptable and healthier, ways of dealing with grief, because unexpressed feelings of grief may lead to further symptomatic behaviors in other family members.

Sociocultural Context

The family must be viewed not as an isolated unit but in a **sociocultural context,** in which the issues of gender, race, ethnicity, class, sexual orientation, and religion are equally considered. Each of these contextual issues affects the family's specific values, norms, traditions, roles, and rules. For example, in the family with adolescents, the way the family relates to the terminally ill family member may be decidedly different in a first-generation Italian-American Catholic family than in an Asian family or than in an African American Baptist family. Therefore, the nurse clinician needs to ask the question, How does this family's cultural and religious beliefs affect the patient's presenting problem and what impact does it have on the family's available options?

In regard to gender, for example, the position of women in United States society needs to be understood in terms of job opportunity, earning power, and status, which for most women are secondary to those of men. Gender and culture must be viewed together since the relative status of males and females differs according to culture. In particular, people from Asian and Latin cultures living in the United States have difficulty understanding American gender roles. In the context of race and ethnicity, it is extremely important that nurses be aware of and understand the mores, practices, and beliefs of the many different cultures that currently make up America's fabric (refer back to Chapter 5). This sensitivity prepares the nurse clinician to make effective interventions for families in times of crisis or psychiatric emergency. Since our American society does not outwardly make class distinctions (as do the British, for example), viewing the family in the context of class may not come easily and indeed may be downright uncomfortable; in fact, class is often considered by most therapists to be the "last taboo." Yet, although it is unspoken, most Americans do have a definite sense of the class to which they belong. It is most often defined in terms of money, education, and taste, and only with gentle questioning do these defining issues come to the fore.

Sexual orientation is another part of the context that often gets overlooked. When gathering family information, the nurse must ask questions regarding sexual orientation (e.g., in terms of long-term relationships). Finally, the context of religion figures prominently in a large percentage of the population, and within this context are many issues regarding why a person becomes ill and how that person should be treated. When the family is viewed in a sociocultural context, religion is an important issue for consideration.

Constructing a Genogram

The **genogram** is an efficient format that provides a clinical summary of information and relationships across at least three generations. It is an invaluable family assessment tool that incorporates the three important areas of consideration in the evaluation of a family: (1) the stage of the family life cycle, (2) the multigenerational issues, (3) and the sociocultural context. The genogram provides a graphic display of complex patterns, as well as a source of hypotheses that indicate how the presenting problem connects to the family context and the evolution of the family over time (McGoldrick and Gerson 1985). Patterns of illness, shifts in relationships, and changes in structure are easily noted by use of the genogram. The physical, social, and emotional functioning of family members is interdependent; therefore, change in one part of the family system results in changes in other parts. This concept of *homeostasis* is a pivotal one in family systems thinking. The family system constantly pushes toward stability (i.e., maintaining the status quo) in the continuing face of change. This move toward stability is compelling, and for families with a rigid style of operating, maintaining stability can become very problematic because of inflexibility and limited alternatives for adjusting to the inevitable changes that are part of every family life cycle. The genogram reflects the family system's adaptation to its total context at a given moment.

Bowen (1985) provided much of the conceptual framework for the analysis of genogram patterns. He proposed that the family is organized according to generation, age, sex, roles, functions, and interests, and that where each individual fits into the family structure influences the family functioning, the relational patterns, and the type of family formed in the next generation. He further contended that sex and birth order shape sibling relationships and characteristics. Also, some issues tend to be played out from generation to generation through persisting interactive emotional patterns. A major concept is that of triangling, which was discussed earlier. Recall that triangling occurs when a two-person relationship tends to be unstable, and under stress, the tendency of those in the relationship is to draw in a third person to stabilize the system by forming a coalition by which the two join in relation to the third.

In creating a genogram, the nurse clinician is able to map the family structure and record family information. This information should include demographics such as location, occupation, and educational level. Functional information regarding medical, emotional, and behavioral status is also recorded. Finally, critical events must be noted (e.g., important transitions, moves, job changes, separations, illnesses, and deaths). Figure 11–2 provides an example of a genogram derived from the data from the following vignette of the Schneider family.

▶ Hank and Catherine Schneider are both college educated, and each suffers from intermittent depression. Hank is an only child whose father died of a heart attack at age 55, Hank's present age. Hank's mother committed suicide at age 35. This is a toxic subject in Hank's family of origin. In Catherine's family of origin, she is the eldest, born after three miscarriages. Much pressure and expectation were placed on Catherine. Catherine's brother Mike was born 4 years after Catherine. Their mother died during Mike's birth. Mike never finished high school, has a serious alcohol addiction, and has had three marriages that ended in

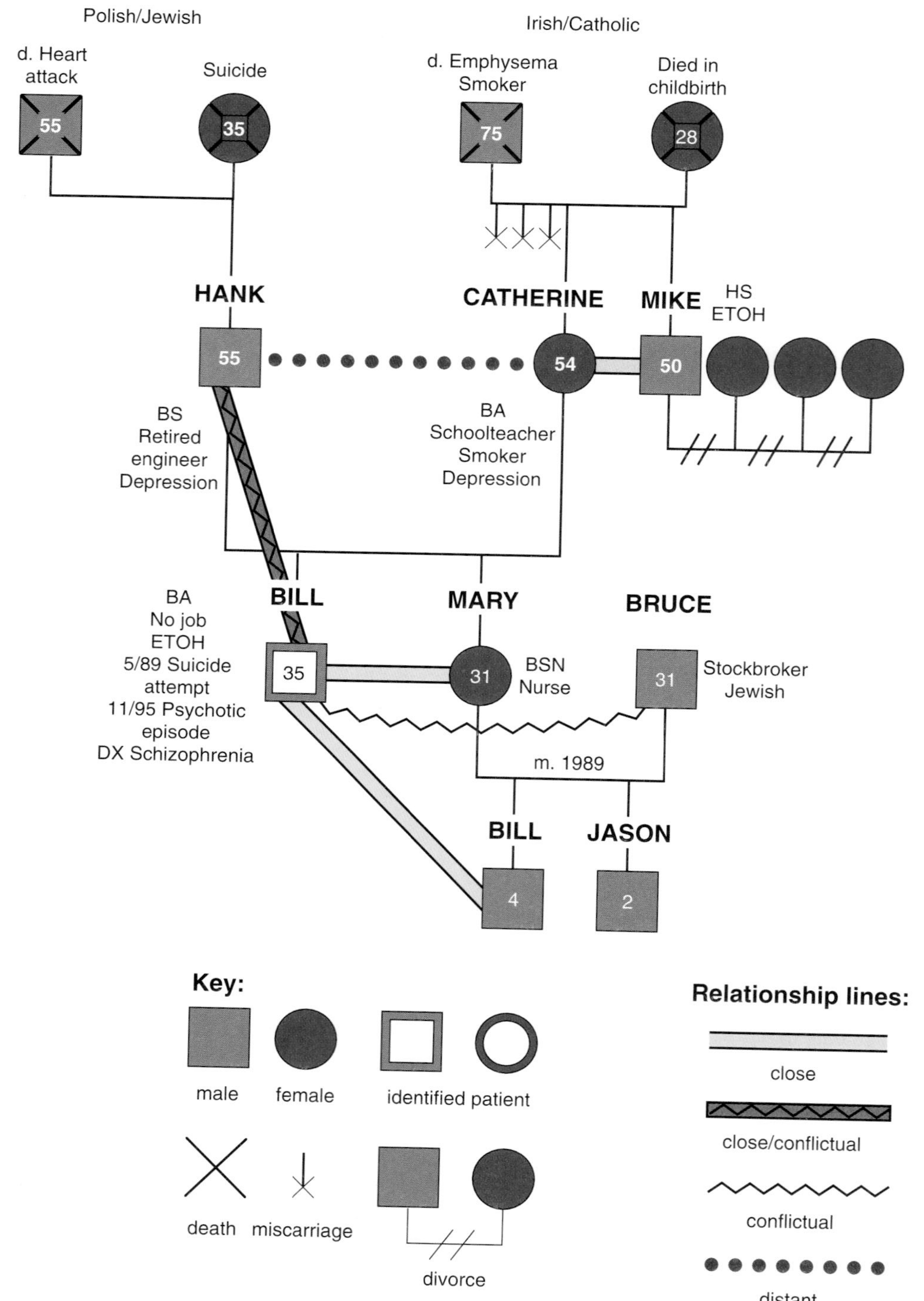

Figure 11–2 Genogram of the Schneider family.

divorce. One can speculate about the level of guilt Mike may feel regarding the loss of his mother.

- Hank and Catherine have two children, Bill and Mary. Bill, the identified patient, is 35 years old, has a college degree, and has not been able to hold down a job. He also has an addiction to alcohol. In 1989, Bill made a suicide attempt. In November 1995, Bill experienced a psychotic episode for which he was hospitalized and was diagnosed as having schizophrenia. His younger sister, Mary, has a college degree and works as a nurse. She married Bruce in 1989, the year that Bill attempted suicide. Mary and Bruce have two young children, aged 4 and 2 years.

Other Assessment Strategies

Other tools are available to help the practitioner assess how the family functions as a unit and identify individual member's perceptions of how the family communicates; deals with emotional issues, such as anger, conflict, and affection; works together as a unit to plan and solve problems; makes the important decisions for the family; and functions generally. A focused interview, one in which the nurse can ask these questions directly, or an assessment device can be used to obtain this information.

Table 11–5 presents the McMaster Family Assessment Device, which is a 60-item self-report designed to assess the family functions just mentioned. This assessment tool can give the nurse an idea of the range of issues that are helpful when the nurse is identifying areas that need change so that the family can function in a healthier and more satisfying way for all of its members. It should be used only by practitioners trained in family assessment and intervention strategies. Students might use this assessment device after discussing with their instructor the suitability of this tool for use with their particular client.

DIAGNOSES

Families have many needs at different times in their development. Family life often involves new members, deaths, mental and physical illness, economic reverberations, developmental crisis, and unanticipated changes or decline. Severe dysfunctional patterns (e.g., marked relational conflict, sexual misconduct, abuse, violence, and suicide) exist within many families that cause physical or mental anguish to the members.

Numerous nursing diagnoses are useful in working with families. Box 11–2 identifies some useful family nursing diagnoses. DSM-IV (APA 1994) has also identified areas that can be used to target medical or psychiatric attention. These areas come under the heading "other conditions that may be a focus of clinical attention." These DSM-IV categories are listed below:

DSM-IV AREA	COMMENTS
Relational Problems	Relational problems related to a mental disorder or a generic medical condition, sibling relational problem or problems
Problems related to abuse or neglect	Includes physical and sexual abuse and neglect of a child, and physical or sexual abuse of an adult
Bereavement	Bereavement may cause considerable impairment and complications
Identity problems	
Religious or spiritual problems	
Age-related decline	
Acculturation problems	

PLANNING

Outcome Criteria

In developing a plan of care (Clements 1983), the practitioner first:

- Defines with the family their goals and decides whether the goals are realistic and obtainable.
- Realizes that it is improvement (e.g., improving communication among members, reducing family stress, helping members achieve appropriate roles), rather than perfection, that the family members are striving for.
- Praises each family member as each new gain is made.
- Reviews past accomplishments when a family member is frustrated after having a setback.

BOX 11–2 POSSIBLE NURSING DIAGNOSES FOR FAMILY INTERVENTIONS

Altered parenting
Sexual dysfunctioning
Altered family processes
Altered family processes: alcohol
Caregiver role strain
Risk for caregiver role strain
Parental role conflict
Spiritual distress (distress of the human spirit)
Impaired adjustment
Ineffective denial
Ineffective family coping: disabling/comprised
Ineffective management of therapeutic regimen: families
Knowledge deficit
Impaired verbal communication
Defensive coping

TABLE 11–5 McMASTER FAMILY ASSESSMENT DEVICE

Instructions: Following are a number of statements about families. Please read each statement carefully, and decide how well it describes your own family. You should answer according to how you see your family. For each statement there are four (4) possible responses:

Strongly Agree (SA)	Check SA if you feel that the statement describes your family very accurately.
Agree (A)	Check A if you feel that the statement describes your family for the most part.
Disagree (D)	Check D if you feel that the statement does not describe your family for the most part.
Strongly Disagree (SD)	Check SD if your feel that the statement does not describe your family at all.

Try not to spend too much time thinking about each statement, but respond as quickly and honestly as you can. If you have trouble with one, answer with your first reaction. Please be sure to answer every statement and mark all your answers in the space provided next to each statement.

STATEMENTS	SA	A	D	SD
1. Planning family activities is difficult because we misunderstand each other.	____	____	____	____
2. We resolve most everyday problems around the house.	____	____	____	____
3. When someone is upset the others know why.	____	____	____	____
4. When you ask someone to do something, you have to check that they did it.	____	____	____	____
5. If someone is in trouble, the others become too involved.	____	____	____	____
6. In times of crisis we can turn to each other for support.	____	____	____	____
7. We don't know what to do when an emergency comes up.	____	____	____	____
8. We sometimes run out of things that we need.	____	____	____	____
9. We are reluctant to show our affection to each other.	____	____	____	____
10. We make sure members meet their family responsibilities.	____	____	____	____
11. We cannot talk to each other about the sadness we feel.	____	____	____	____
12. We usually act on our decisions regarding problems.	____	____	____	____
13. You only get the interest of others when something is important to them.	____	____	____	____
14. You can't tell how a person is feeling from what they are saying.	____	____	____	____
15. Family tasks don't get spread around enough.	____	____	____	____
16. Individuals are accepted for what they are.	____	____	____	____
17. You can easily get away with breaking the rules.	____	____	____	____
18. People come right out and say things instead of hinting at them.	____	____	____	____
19. Some of us just don't respond emotionally.	____	____	____	____
20. We know what to do in an emergency.	____	____	____	____
21. We avoid discussing our fears and concerns.	____	____	____	____
22. It is difficult to talk to each other about tender feelings.	____	____	____	____
23. We have trouble meeting our bills.	____	____	____	____
24. After our family tries to solve a problem, we usually discuss whether it worked or not.	____	____	____	____
25. We are too self-centered.	____	____	____	____
26. We can express our feelings to each other.	____	____	____	____
27. We have no clear expectations about toilet habits.	____	____	____	____
28. We do not show our love for each other.	____	____	____	____
29. We talk to people directly rather than through go-betweens.	____	____	____	____
30. Each of us has particular duties and responsibilities.	____	____	____	____
31. There are lots of bad feelings in the family.	____	____	____	____
32. We have rules about hitting people.	____	____	____	____

TABLE 11–5 McMASTER FAMILY ASSESSMENT DEVICE *(Continued)*

STATEMENTS	SA	A	D	SD
33. We get involved with each other only when something interests us.	___	___	___	___
34. There's little time to explore personal interests.	___	___	___	___
35. We often don't say what we mean.	___	___	___	___
36. We feel accepted for what we are.	___	___	___	___
37. We show interest in each other when we can get something out of it personally.	___	___	___	___
38. We resolve most emotional upsets that come up.	___	___	___	___
39. Tenderness takes second place to other things in our family.	___	___	___	___
40. We discuss who is to do household jobs.	___	___	___	___
41. Making decisions is a problem for our family.	___	___	___	___
42. Our family shows interest in each other only when they can get something out of it.	___	___	___	___
43. We are frank with each other.	___	___	___	___
44. We don't hold to any rules or standards.	___	___	___	___
45. If people are asked to do something, they need reminding.	___	___	___	___
46. We are able to make decisions about how to solve problems.	___	___	___	___
47. If the rules are broken, we don't know what to expect.	___	___	___	___
48. Anything goes in our family.	___	___	___	___
49. We express tenderness	___	___	___	___
50. We confront problems involving feelings.	___	___	___	___
51. We don't get along well together.	___	___	___	___
52. We don't talk to each other when we are angry.	___	___	___	___
53. We are generally dissatisfied with the family duties assigned to us.	___	___	___	___
54. Even though we mean well, we intrude too much into each other's lives.	___	___	___	___
55. There are rules about dangerous situations.	___	___	___	___
56. We confide in each other.	___	___	___	___
57. We cry openly.	___	___	___	___
58. We don't have reasonable transport.	___	___	___	___
59. When we don't like what someone has done, we tell them.	___	___	___	___
60. We try to think of different ways to solve problems.	___	___	___	___

From Schutle, N. S., and Malouff, J. M. (1995). *Sourcebook of adult assessment strategies.* New York: Plenum Press. Brown University/Butler Hospital Family Research Program, © 1982.

- Ensures that goals and interventions are congruent with the family's culture, life style, and values.

Although different theories are held and a wide variety of methods are used by different therapists, the goals of family therapy are basically the same. These goals (Steinglass 1995) are to

- Reduce dysfunctional behavior of individual family members.
- Resolve or reduce intrafamily relationship conflicts and conflicts between the family and its extended family.
- Mobilize family resources and encourage adaptive family problem-solving behaviors.
- Improve family communication skills.
- Heighten awareness and sensitivity to other family members' emotional needs and help family members meet the needs of their members.
- Strengthen the family's ability to cope with major life stressors and traumatic events, including chronic physical or psychiatric illness.
- Improve integration of the family system into the societal system, e.g., school, medical facilities, workplace, and especially the extended family.

Other goals families might have when working with a nurse in psychoeducational interventions or in community or self-help groups, as well as through professional counseling, might include

- Learning to accept the illness of a family member.
- Learning to deal effectively with an ill member's symptoms, such as hallucinations, delusions, poor hygiene, physical limitations, paranoia, and aggression.
- Understanding what the medications can and cannot do and when the family should seek medical advice.
- Assistance in locating community resources.
- Reducing family anxiety and restoring or gaining a sense of control and balance in family life.

Nurse's Feelings and Self-Assessment

Nurses must be well trained when working with families in a counseling situation because the potential for multiple transferences and triangulations is high. Therefore, a nurse educated at the advanced practice level or a certified clinical specialist with special training in family work is usually best qualified to conduct family therapy. However, all nurses interact with families, whether in hospital acute care settings or in community-based settings. Most nurses come from a family, and since no family is perfect, all nurses are subject to forming triangles when anxious, to becoming defensive when personal family anxieties are aroused, or to experiencing role blurring or loosening of self-boundaries when sensitive personal issues and conflicts are triggered.

Often, when working with families, the nurse is most helpful when he or she is able to draw back and recognize when a personal issue is increasing anxiety levels. When the nurse believes that he or she is getting drawn into the family dynamics rather than maintaining an objective stance, discussing these issues with a professional peer or supervisor is extremely important in order to maintain effectiveness. The nurse should identify a time when he or she reacted intensely (positively or negatively) to either a client or a client's situation. How was this issue dealt with later in conference? Common issues with which health care workers may intensely identify are alcohol or drug use, family abuse, codependency issues, rescue fantasies, and lifestyles. These and many other issues that evoke strong feelings need to be addressed before the nurse is able to see the client and the client's situation and needs clearly. Self-assessment is a crucial component of effective nursing care not only in psychiatric nursing but also in other nursing specialties.

INTERVENTIONS

Family Interventions

Family therapy is viewed by professionals as appropriate for most situations, with the possible exception of family violence or abuse. Many therapists are hesitant to treat such families because the therapist is unable to ensure that the material that arises from couples therapy and family therapy will not lead to more violence when the family returns home (Steinglass 1995).

However, in most other situations, family therapy is useful, especially when it is combined with psychopharmacology in the treatment of families who have a member with a mental illness, such as bipolar disorder, depression, and schizophrenia. However, not all families can afford the money or the time for traditional family therapy. Therefore, many families greatly benefit from psychoeducational family therapy and from self-help groups. The first part of this section introduces the student to (1) traditional family therapy intervention strategies, (2) psychoeducational groups, and (3) self-help groups that may benefit families and family members.

Traditional Family Therapy

Family therapists use a wide variety of theoretical philosophies and techniques to bring about change in dysfunctional patterns of behavior and interaction. Some therapists may focus on the here and now, while others may rely more heavily on the family's history and reports of what happened between sessions. Most family therapists use an eclectic approach, drawing on a variety of techniques that are designed to fit the particular personality and strengths of the family (Steinglass 1995).

Multiple-family group therapy is often used with families who have a hospitalized family member in an inpatient setting. These groups can help family members identify and gain insight into their own problems as they are reflected in the problems of other families. Several families meet in one group with one or more therapists, usually once a week until their ill family member is discharged; these groups often continue for a specific period of time after the client is discharged.

Psychoeducational Family Therapy

Psychoeducational groups have proved immensely effective, especially as a family treatment modality combined with other modalities (e.g., psychopharmacology). One of the most successful areas of psychoeducational family training is schizophrenia. Some studies have shown that psychoeducational family therapy reduces the long-term need for rehospitalization by as much as 50 to 80% (Steinglass 1995). Chapter 22 provides more detail on the content and process of psychoeducational groups for people with schizophrenia and their families.

The primary goal of **psychoeducational family therapy** is the sharing of mental health care information. Family education groups help family members better understand their member's illness, prodromal symptoms (symptoms that may appear before a full relapse), medications needed to help reduce the symptoms, and more. The modes of psychoeducational family meetings or multiple family meetings allow feelings to be shared and strategies for dealing with these feelings to be developed. Painful issues of anger or loss, feelings of stigmatization or sadness, and feelings of helplessness can be shared and put in a perspective that the family and individual members can deal with more satisfactorily. Psychoeducational family groups are extremely useful for people with all kinds of mental as well as medical disorders.

Self-Help Groups

Self-help groups can be divided into two types. One type is for groups of people who have a personal problem or social deprivation. The second is for families with a member who has a specific problem or condition. Self-help groups acknowledge the needs of family members. Some groups may focus on families with healthy members, while others offer assistance to families whose members may be experiencing a health disorder or crisis. Most health professionals are aware that for any developmental event, life crisis, or health disorder, a comparable mutual-aid group exists. These health professionals are in the best position to help their clients and their families find additional support and information. For many people, self-help groups can be healing. Table 11–6 provides a partial list of self-help groups.

Nursing Interventions

The roles of the psychiatric mental health nurse (RN, C) and the clinical specialist (RN, CS) vary in the ways in which the nurse clinician works with families in both the hospital and the community settings. Differences exist in counseling and psychobiological interventions. The basic-level nurse clinician may provide counseling by use of a problem-solving approach for a problem that represents an immediate family difficulty related to health or well-being. The advanced practice nurse, a certified clinical specialist who has postgraduate training in family therapy, may conduct private family therapy sessions. As to psychobiological interventions, the advanced practice certified specialists may have prescriptive authority (in accordance with their state practice act and their qualifications).

The roles of the entry-level nurse and the staff nurse, although different in scope from the of the psychiatric mental health nurse and the clinical specialist, are equally important, especially in promoting and monitoring a family's mental health. Developing and practicing good listening skills and regarding family members in a positive, nonjudgmental way are critically important skills for all levels of nurses.

An important function of entry-level and staff nurses is to assess cues from various family members that indicate the degree and the amount of stress the family system is experiencing. These critical observations need to be readily reported so that appropriate interventions may be made in a timely manner. Some indicators of stress in a family system are (1) an inability by the family or a family member to process and act on certain recommended treatment directives, (2) various somatic complaints among family members, (3) a high degree of anxiety, (4) depression, (5) problems in school, and (6) drug use.

Promoting and monitoring a family's mental health can occur in virtually any setting and often requires making the most of an opportune moment. It does not have to be a formal meeting. Sometimes, an informal conversation (therapeutic encounter) can have the greatest effect. A few general guidelines help the nurse clinician be nonjudgmental in the information presented, as well as in tone of voice and questions asked. For example, the question "Don't you think you should at least try to comply with your medical regimen?" would probably cause the patient to tune the nurse out, while the question "Tell me what this medical regimen of yours is like" could open the door to understanding and problem solving in a collaborative rather than a hierarchical way. The nonblaming manner promotes open and flexible communication among all professionals and family members in the caregiving system. If other family members are involved in the conversation, be it on the hospital unit or in a family therapy session, the nurse should get each member's view of how the individual member's medical regimen affects the way the family functions and what the individual members see as a possible solution to the problem.

A second guideline for the nurse clinician is to impart information that is clear and understandable to all family members and to allow them to choose and decide what to do with the information. This is both a respectful and an empowering way to work with families, which indicates to them that they are the ones who are accountable and responsible for however they choose to use the information.

Third, it is imperative that the perspective of each family member is elicited and heard. Often, some family members hear another member's view for the first time in this democratic forum, and many times, they are surprised ("I didn't know you felt that way"). The more family input there is, the more options usually exist for alternative ways of managing problematic situations. This approach defines the family as the central psychosocial unit of care. The following vignette provides an example of maintaining neutrality and of hearing from all members.

▶ Ms. Conway, the head nurse on the adolescent psychiatric unit, was concerned about all the negative comments the staff members were making regarding the fact that none of Chip's family had been in to visit him for over a week. In fact, she was concerned that Chip was picking up the staff's feelings as well. After many attempts, Ms. Conway finally reached Chip's mother by telephone and began to assess the situation. She

TABLE 11–6 EXAMPLES OF SELF-HELP GROUPS FOR INDIVIDUALS AND FAMILIES

NAME OF GROUP	TARGET POPULATION
Al-Anon	Families of alcoholics
Alcoholics Anonymous (AA)	
Alzheimer's Disease and Related Disorders Foundation	Caregivers of a family member with Alzheimer's disease
Arthritis Foundation	
Child Abuse Prevention—Kid's Peace	
Committee to Combat Huntington's Disease	
Compassionate Friends	Parents of children who have died
Depression After Delivery	Women with postpartum depression
Des-Action	People who are unaware that they have been exposed to diethystilbesterol
Epilepsy Foundation	
Hodgkin's Disease and Lymphoma Organization	
Hypoglycemia Lay Group	
International Association of Laryngectomies	
Make Today Count	Clients and family members of people with life-threatening illness
Mended Hearts	Clients and families of people who have had heart surgery
Myasthenia Gravis Foundation	
Naim Conference	Catholic widows and widowers
Narcotics Anonymous	
National Alliance for the Mentally Ill (NAMI)	
National Amputation Foundation	
National Depressive and Manic Association—National Victim's Center	
National Multiple Sclerosis Society	
National Organization for Victim's Assistance	
National Organization of Mothers of Twins Clubs	
National Paraplegia Foundation	
National Society for Autistic Children	
Neurotics Anonymous (Serendipity)	Clients and family members of people with emotional problems
Parents Anonymous	Parents who abuse their children
Parents, Families, Friends of Lesbians and Gays (PFLAG)	
Parents of Large Families	
Parents of Prematures	
Parents Without Partners	Single parents
People with AIDS Coalition	
The Phoenix Society	Burn victims and their families
Post-Partum Education for Parents	Support and discussion group for new parents
Pills Anonymous	Individuals addicted to sedatives, tranquilizers, and other mood-changing substances
Reach for Recovery	
Recovery Inc.—The Association of Nervous and Former Mental Patients	
Suicide Prevention Hotline	
Survivors	Relatives and friends of suicide victims
United Cerebral Palsy Association	
United Ostomy Association	

discovered that Chip's mom is divorced and is working double shifts to meet the family's expenses. There is a 2-year-old at home and a set of twins in the fourth grade.

◗ Chip's mom was planning to visit on the weekend, but the babysitter called to say she was sick. Once Ms. Conway was able to see the situation from another perspective, that this was a family with young children that was struggling to make ends meet, she called a staff meeting to address the situation.

Further interventions in this situation would be to process (problem solve) with Chip and his mother what is realistic for each of them regarding visiting. Perhaps an extended family member or a friend can visit when the mother cannot. Longer-range planning for supervision for Chip when he is discharged should also be discussed as family supports are identified and assessed.

Unfortunately, the negative comments about family members by staff occur all too often. This can present a difficult situation for the student, who is entering the "culture" of the unit as an outsider and who realizes the negative effects that this behavior has on family members. An intervention is in order; however, it would be appropriate for the student to first seek supervision from the instructor, so that the most effective approach can be planned out beforehand. One useful technique is for the student to ask questions of the head nurse and staff in such a way that alternative ways to view the family in a broader perspective are embedded in the questions. An example of this might be "Has anyone had a chance to contact Chip's mom to see if there are any problems?" or "I wonder what it's like for Chip's mom to have her son in a psychiatric unit?"

Case Management

Although the nursing profession has always interacted with families to some degree in the process of meeting a client's needs, our current knowledge of family systems dictates that the family be the primary focus when the management of the individual client is planned. The family's culture, ethnicity, socioeconomic status, and stage of family life cycle, as well as its unique patterns and beliefs about illness, all affect an individual's progress and response to case management. The family is the most powerful group to which an individual may ever belong, and it is vital that the nurse not discount or ignore the importance of the family's influence on its members when planning care.

To a great extent, case management entails teaching, giving appropriate referrals and offering emotional support.

◗ David Gardiner, age 21, is leaving the hospital after having experienced his first psychotic episode while taking his final exams before graduation from college. David is being discharged back to his family, which consists of his mother and father; his maternal grandfather, who has been recently bedridden; and a younger brother Todd, who is 17 years of age. David's diagnosis is paranoid schizophrenia. The nurse takes a psychoeducational approach with the family.

◗ Issues and needs are addressed by the nurse during family meetings while David is still hospitalized, and later in follow-up family therapy after discharge. Initial interventions involve imparting information about David's mental illness through reading materials and discussion. The nurse also gives the family information and telephone numbers of psychosocial support groups and affiliation with a local chapter of the National Alliance for the Mentally Ill (NAMI).

◗ The nurse maintains ongoing assessment of the family's strengths and weaknesses, including family supports as well as community support. She identifies some of the areas that may need to be addressed during the next few meetings.

◗ Some of these issues include reorganizing family roles to accommodate a family member with a newly diagnosed, severe and persistent mental illness; managing their bedridden grandfather; attending to Todd's probable fears that he, too, may have this illness; dealing with potential parental guilt feelings from a genetic point of view; planning how to mobilize should David experience another psychotic episode; managing medication and stressing the importance of compliance; dealing with concerns about David's future and formulating realistic expectations; coping with feelings of loss for what was, and what was hoped for; and, finally, maintaining the integrity and functioning of the spousal subsystem.

◗ The nurse discusses these and other issues with the family and identifies where and how these issues can best be addressed. For example, the visiting nurse was called in to evaluate the grandfather's situation and need for support in the home, and a multiple family psychoeducation group was formed to continue the family's understanding of David's illness, to learn ways to cope with common problems that may arise, and to provide a place for the family to share their feelings of loss and grief.

Psychobiological Issues

The nurse is often the first to explain to the family the purpose for a prescribed medication as well as the desired effects and possible side effects and adverse reactions. The following situation took place at the time of discharge.

◗ Susan Harris, a 45-year-old account executive and mother of three teenagers, had been referred by her physician to the mental health center for acute depression. The psychiatrist there had prescribed an antidepressant. Routinely, new clients are seen by the nurse clinician for a review of medications as a part of the health teaching. Unfortunately, the nurse clinician was engaged with another client in crisis at the time and missed meeting with Susan and her husband.

- One week later, Susan made an appointment with the clinical specialist for symptoms of insomnia and lack of sexual desire, which was a concern for both Susan and her husband. She feared that she was getting worse and "going crazy." During the appointment, the nurse clinician reviewed the side effects and adverse reactions of antidepressants with Mrs. Harris. She informed Mrs. Harris that the medication she was taking might take 3 weeks or longer to take effect. She also explained that common side effects of the group of medications she was taking (selective serotonin reuptake inhibitors) were sleeplessness and lowered sexual drive. They discussed ways to combat these side effects (see Chapter 20). The nurse urged Susan to continue taking the medication; however, if the side effects were to continue, the medication could be changed. Susan was due to visit the clinic 2 weeks later for follow-up. The nurse urged Susan to discuss the side effects of the medication with her husband and encouraged him to come with her to the clinic at her next appointment.

Certainly, the more information the family has at its disposal, the less anxiety will distort their observations and decision making after discharge. Because of untoward circumstances in this case, the nurse clinician on the unit did not review Susan's medication with her before she was discharged. The clinical specialist needs to closely monitor Susan to determine whether her symptoms represent an exacerbation of her depression or a reaction to the antidepressant medication. If Susan is having a reaction to the medication, the nurse may consult with a physician and try another medication.

FAMILIES IN CRISIS

Chronic Illness

The diagnosis of a chronic illness generally produces some form of crisis or disorganization in the family, and it is therefore useful to examine the stressful events that are already confronting the family, the meaning the family ascribes to the illness, and the family's resources for managing these current stressors, as well as those that will arise during the course of the illness and its treatment (Rolland 1994).

Every family experiences life cycle stressors associated with the transitions in the development of the family as a whole and in the development of each member. A chronic illness adds new stressors to those already present. For example, the financial burden of medical and/or psychiatric treatment exists. When the client is an adult and is the primary income earner, the family may lose income. Another potential stressor is the management of the client at home. For example, when the client is a child, the illness may require the parent or parents to take time away from work or from the care of the client's siblings in order to accompany the child to clinic appointments.

It is very important that the nurse clinician define the stressor or stressors as the family sees them within their cultural, socioeconomic, and experiential perspective. The particular meanings that family members ascribe to a chronic illness vary according to the family's view of the world, the family's beliefs about health or illness, and the family members' previous experience with illness. The nurse needs to ask him- or herself the following questions:

- Does the family view the world as relatively safe, predictable, and subject to some degree of control?
- Does the family believe that the illness is the result of the individual's poor health habits or personal weakness?
- Is sickness associated with dependence, incompetence, or helplessness?
- How effectively has the family coped with previous illness?

Financial, social, personal, and mental resources for coping need to be assessed (Carter and McGoldrick, 1989). Without health insurance or a health maintenance policy that pays for the cost of treating an illness, a family may be forced to deplete savings, accumulate large debts, or even move to less expensive housing, with the attendant disruption of neighborhood and school relationships; in general, this situation requires lowering of the family's standard of living. A related financial resource is the flexibility of the adult family members' work schedules. Some family members may lose income, or even their jobs, if they take time away from work when the client needs additional care at home or in the hospital.

If the patient is a child and neither parent can take time from work, someone else must be available to take the child to the doctor and administer medications. In addition, someone must be available to act as a surrogate parent to the child's healthy siblings so that their lives can continue as normally as possible. A family's social network may include grandparents, uncles and aunts, neighbors, friends, co-workers, members of the family's church or synagogue, and parents of the healthy siblings' friends. If the chronically ill client is an adult, social resources may include a member of the extended family or a friend who is willing to assume some of the client's roles within the family. Alternative sources of support are an important area to assess.

Personal resources include self-esteem, the family member's individual sense of physical and emotional well-being, intelligence, education, and the belief that every individual can influence events.

Mental resources include flexibility and management of affect. The many demands of a chronic illness in a family member may necessitate changes in family roles, routines, and boundaries. These demands for change are additional stressors to which the family must adapt, and the lack of family flexibility may engender even more stressors.

Regarding the management of affect, when a chronic illness is diagnosed, family members experience a variety of feelings about the illness, the client, the family, and their own health. Some of the feelings experienced include sadness, irritation, resentment, anger, anxiety, depression, worry about the client, fear of death (the serious illness of a sibling threatens a child's own bodily integrity and creates fears and uncertainties about one's own health and mortality), jealously, guilt, and inadequacy. Family members must go through a process of mourning in which the loss of the client and the family as it once was and might have been is mourned. To cope effectively, family members need to find ways of managing these feelings where the tendency is to either rely on previous family rules or to develop new rules that either permit or alter the expression of these feelings. When a family does not permit an expression of affect from its members, other avenues may be pursued, such as exercise, involvement in projects of some sort, or withdrawal into solitude. Aggressiveness and self-destructive behaviors engaged in outside of the family are other potential means of expressing the family's prohibited affect. Acting out behaviors can include school problems, increased domestic violence, incest, substance abuse, depression, and psychosomatic disorders.

Illness is a disruption in the family life cycle. With this disruption comes anxiety about the ill member's well-being, the burden of constant caretaking, and loss of family income. These are common illness-related experiences that strain the family's coping abilities. A triangle can emerge around the management of the illness, especially if care responsibilities are assumed more and more exclusively by one family member and are relinquished by others. The family's preoccupation with illness can shape or delay critical life cycle tasks. For example, a parent who is ill may require that the eldest daughter who is now in college to return home to deal with caretaking responsibilities or to ease the family's financial burdens, effectively putting her own life cycle task on hold. Finally, decisions about whom members can marry, when they can leave home, and whether they should have children can be powerfully influenced by the presence of an illness. Box 11–3 offers some guidelines for working with families who have an ill family member.

BOX 11–3 GUIDELINES FOR WORKING WITH FAMILIES WITH AN ILL FAMILY MEMBER

1. Clarify and normalize the impact of the illness on the family.
2. Empower the family to believe in its own capacities for problem solving and illness management.
3. Change the problem-generating narrative about the client, the family, and the disease. Reframe behavior (look at it from a broader perspective) in your own mind in order to be more effective and helpful.
4. Help the family to identify emotional and concrete resources both inside and outside the family.
5. Encourage the family to become connected to community support systems in order to relieve isolation.
6. Impart clear medical information.
7. Help client and family to map the pre-illness and post-illness structure in order to help the family to return as much as possible to their pre-illness state of functioning.
8. Help client and family plan for the future while the ill person can participate.

Adapted from Walker, G. (1991). *In the midst of winter.* New York: W. W. Norton.

Family Loss

The family who is facing a loss of some sort is a family in crisis. The loss may be related to divorce, relocation, loss of a job, illness, entering school, dropping out of school, marriage, homosexual declaration, or death. All changes in life, those that are desired as well as those that are not, involve loss. This process of change and loss requires that the family give up or alter certain roles and relationships, expectations, and dreams and make way for new ones. This progress helps put the loss in perspective so that the family can move on with their lives.

The process of mourning is essential for the family to move on. If this process is not recognized and does not take place, the family is likely to revert to a previous stage of functioning or get stuck in the same stage where healthy growth and development becomes stymied.

One Family in Crisis

- The Langer's nuclear family includes their daughter Joan, age 25, who with her husband Kevin is expecting a first child in 1 month; their son Bill, age 21, who is a senior in college; Mrs. Langer, age 48, who is a substitute teacher; Mr. Langer, age 52, who recently retired because of company downsizing; and grandmother Goldman, age 83, Mrs. Langer's mother, who is recovering from a broken hip. The Langers are Jewish and attend a reformed synagogue.
- Bill Langer was completing his final year of college when he began to hear disturbing voices telling him of his "special powers." He left school to join an ashram, where his symptoms escalated. The voices led Bill to stab himself in the abdomen, and he was rushed to the

CASE STUDY: Ortega Family

The Ortega family has just arrived on the locked unit of a large city psychiatric hospital. Maria Ortega is an 18-year-old female college student and the eldest of four siblings. She is admitted through the emergency department after having slashed her wrists and losing a lot of blood. Her parents and extended family members are talking loudly, crying hysterically, and pacing about the waiting area. Having finished the usual admitting procedures, the nurse clinician now turns her attention to the family members.

ASSESSMENT

The tendency for some families in a time of crisis is to overreact and be unable to focus on the problem at hand. This may happen in families in which the boundaries are blurred and unclear, and individuation of family members is not well defined. The primary initial goal was to calm down the family system. Chairs were provided for everyone, and the nurse clinician proceeded to talk in a soft, slow, emphatic manner, answering any questions that the family had. Once the nurse clinician joins with the family in this way, she then began to construct a genogram as she asked the family for information. During this process, the nurse clinician discovered that the youngest child in the Ortega family, Tony, age 4, has an autistic disorder. Maria was Tony's primary caretaker before she left for college. The family was stressed both financially and emotionally because of the "loss" of Maria before the present emergency.

NURSING DIAGNOSIS

Maria's suicide attempt seems to be related to her depression and feelings of hopelessness. These feelings appear to originate from what is taking place in the family system. The nursing diagnosis was: **altered role performance related to loss of financial and caregiving support.**

PLANNING

Although Maria would most likely be in the hospital for a few days, family therapy sessions were to begin on the unit, and follow-up sessions would take place at the community mental health center after discharge. **Outcome criteria** included helping the family stabilize and meet their needs, allowing Maria to leave home and become an independent young adult. **Short-term goals** centered around helping the family identify alternative ways to deal with Tony's care and the management of Maria's tuition.

INTERVENTION

Once Maria is discharged, the family decides to continue with family therapy sessions in a community mental health clinic, where they meet weekly with a certified specialist. Here, the work that was begun during hospitalization is continued, where the family, which is no longer in a crisis situation, is able to work toward making changes that will prevent a similar situation from occurring. If the clinical specialist is licensed for prescriptive privileges, she would take over the management of Maria's antidepressant medication prescribed by the hospital psychiatrist. Otherwise, she would report her observations and progress to the medicating psychiatrist when necessary.

The family is eventually able to work together and find ways to expand their financial resources. With information they obtain from the nurse, they are able to contact two community resources that increase their understanding of how to work with Tony as well as ways to divide up the responsibility for Tony's care so the family does not seem so overwhelmed.

EVALUATION

Shortly after discharge, Maria stops taking the antidepressant. She states the the problem is no longer overwhelming and that once her anxiety and feelings of helplessness subsided, so did her suicidal thoughts.

hospital. During his convalescence, Bill jumped from a fourth-story window, which resulted in injuries leading to paraplegia. The Langer family was devastated. Bill was a bright and promising young musician for whom his family held great expectations.

When meeting with this family, the nurse clinician's assessment included information regarding the family's life cycle stage, multigenerational issues, sociocultural context of the family, and family stressors and strengths.

The life cycle stage of this family is that of launching children and moving on. Bill's launching was unsuccessful. His present condition is preventing him from moving on. It also prevents the other family members from doing the same, as they focus on the crisis situation and immediate and long-term changes and adjustments that are required. Renegotiating the marital system as a dyad will be put on hold, and the development of adult-to-adult relationships between parent and child will be thwarted because of Bill's situation of once again being dependent on his parents. Grandmother's caretaking may be disrupted, owing to this more pressing priority. Susan, who is establishing her own nuclear family, may be pulled back into the system of her family of origin to assist in the adjustment around the crisis. The entire family system has become unbalanced by the crisis. Alternative patterns of operating must be negotiated by the family members so that a new balance can be struck to deal with these sudden changes in their lives. The function of the nurse clinician is to help the family to recognize the extent of the disruption in their family life cycle and to discover alternatives for dealing with the disruption.

The nurse clinician discerned two significant multigenerational issues that were critical to helping this family make changes. One was that a pattern of suicide existed in this family on both sides. Bill's paternal uncle and his maternal grandfather committed suicide. Second, a pervasive family belief that "women are the strong ones and the men are the weak ones" existed. This theme could have limited the possible alternatives for action in this family, perhaps overburdening the women and underestimating the potential of the men.

The sociocultural context of the Langer family aided the nurse in her assessment of potential strengths and weaknesses. The Langers were religious Jews. Families with strong religious ties often find that their religion a tremendous source of strength in times of crisis. This family was involved and connected to the greater community and its resources, which also broadened their options. They were financially solvent, which provided a certain security. In addition, the Langers were outspoken and proactive when it came to solving problems; they asked many questions and sought out experts. When these kind of strengths are present, families can access a variety of options that will help them find alternatives for making difficult adjustments.

The process of rebalancing the family system after such a disruption will take time. However, timely interventions by the nurse clinician can make a tremendous difference in providing the family with direction and with the belief that they are indeed capable of adapting to these untoward changes in the family's life cycle.

The brief case study on page 298 describes a family systems intervention during an acute crisis in the hospital setting.

SUMMARY

The aim of family systems theory is to decrease emotional reactivity among family members and to encourage differentiation among individual family members.

The primary characteristics that are essential to healthy family functioning are flexibility and clear boundaries.

The six main stages in the changing family life cycle are (1) launching of the single young adult, (2) joining of families through couple formation, (3) becoming parents—families with young children, (4) families with adolescents, (5) launching children and moving on, and (6) the family in later life.

The genogram is an efficient clinical summary and format for information and relationships across at least three generations.

The family's culture, ethnicity, socioeconomic status, and life cycle stage, as well as its unique patterns and beliefs about illness, all affect the individual patient's progress and response to case management.

The impact of the family and the family's effect on the health and progress of the ill family member is invaluable. It is imperative that the nurse clinician assess the identified patient in the context of the family. Using a multicontextual framework, the nurse clinician observes the stage of the family life cycle, the multigenerational issues, and the family's sociocultural status. The nurse clinician must continually be sensitive to the many different perspectives of individual family members in terms of how they view the problem and what their ideas are regarding negotiating within the family system to accommodate to the changes required.

REFERENCES

American Psychiatric Association (1994). *Diagnostic and statistical manual of mental disorders* (4th ed.). Washington, DC: American Psychiatric Association.

Andrus, K. (1996). Family therapy. In V. B. Carson and E. N. Arnold (Eds.), *Mental health nursing: The nurse-patient journey*. Philadelphia: W. B. Saunders.

Bowen, M. (1985). *Family therapy in clinical practice*. New Jersey: Jason Aronson.

Carter, B., and McGoldrick, M. (Eds.) (1989). *The changing family life cycle: A framework for family therapy* (2nd ed.). Boston: Allyn & Bacon.

Clements, I. (1983). Stress adaptation. In I. W. Clements and F. B. Roberts (Eds.), *Family health: A theoretical approach to nursing care* (pp. 133–144). New York: John Wiley.

Cooley, M. (1995). A family perspective in community health nursing. In C. M. Smith and F. A. Mauer (Eds.), *Community nursing: Theory and practice* (pp. 205–220). Philadelphia: W. B. Saunders.
Haley, J. (1980). *Leaving home.* New York: McGraw-Hill.
McGoldrick, M., and Gerson, R. (1985). *Genograms in family assessment.* New York: W. W. Norton.
Minuchin, S. (1974). *Families and family therapy.* Cambridge, MA: Harvard University Press.
Roberts, F. B. (1983). An interaction model for family assessment. In I. W. Clements and F. B. Roberts (Eds.), *Family health: A theoretical approach to nursing care* (pp. 189–204). New York: John Wiley.
Rolland, J. (1994). *Families, illness, and disability: An integrative treatment approach.* New York: Basic Books.
Satir, V. (1972). *Peoplemaking.* Palo Alto, CA: Science and Behavior Books.
Satir, V. (1983). *Conjoint family therapy.* Palo Alto: Science and Behavior Books.
Steinglass, P. L. (1995). Family therapy. In H. I. Kaplan and B.J. Sadock (Eds.), *Comprehensive textbook of psychiatry* VI (Vol. 1, pp. 1838–1846). Baltimore: Williams & Wilkins.

Further Reading

Brown, F. H. (Ed.) (1991). *Reweaving the family tapestry: A multigenerational approach to families.* New York: W.W. Norton.
Coalition of Psychiatric Nursing Organizations (1994). *A statement on psychiatric-mental health clinical nursing practice.* Washington, D.C.: American Nurses Publishing.
Kerr, M.E., and Bowen, M. (1988). *Family evaluation.* New York: W.W. Norton.
Luepnitz, D.A. (1988). *The family interpreted.* New York: Basic Books.
McGoldrick, M., Pearce, J.K., and Giordano, J. (Eds.) (1982). *Ethnicity and family therapy.* New York: Guilford Press.
Pittman, F.S. (1987). *Treating families in transition and crisis.* New York: W.W. Norton
Rosen, E.J. (1990). *Families facing death: Family dynamics of terminal illness.* New York: Lexington Books.
Simon, F.B., Stierlin, H., and Wynne, L.C. (1985). *The language of family therapy: A systematic vocabulary and source book.* New York: Family Process Press.

SELF-STUDY AND CRITICAL THINKING

Definitions

1. Define the following terms as they apply to the family systems theory:
   A. Triangles
   B. Boundaries
   C. Sociocultural context
   D. Homeostasis

Critical thinking

2. Use a family from your clinical experience. Evaluate this family's functional/dysfunction status using the five family functions described in the text, e.g., management, boundary, communication, emotional-supportive, and socialization functions.
3. Using the same family from above, create a genogram that identifies their stage in the family life cycle and describe the sociocultural context of this family.
4. Create your own personal genogram, including at least three generations. Be sure to include
   A. Location, occupation and educational level
   B. Critical events, such as births, marriages, moves, job changes, separations, divorce, illnesses, death
   C. Relationship patterns, such as cut-offs, distancing, over-involvement, and conflict
5. Make time to be together with your family (however that is defined by you) and review the McMaster Family Assessment Guide to see how you all view your family dynamics.
6. Identify two stressful topics or areas within your family. Using reframing, try to see these stressful events in a more positive and healthy light that can allow you alternative ways of experiencing or behaving in these situations.
7. A family has just found out that their young son is going to die. The parents have been fighting and blaming each other for ignoring the child's ongoing symptoms of leg pain, which was eventually diagnosed as advanced cancer. There are two other siblings in the family. How would you as the primary nurse apply family concepts to help this family? What would be an outcome criterion? What would be two of the short-term goals?

12

Communication with Angry and Aggressive Clients

CARROL ALVAREZ

OUTLINE

KEY TERMS AND CONCEPTS

The key terms and concepts listed here also appear in bold where they are defined or discussed in this chapter.

anger
aggression
ineffective individual coping, overwhelmed
ineffective individual coping, maladaptive pattern
posttrauma response
validation therapy

OBJECTIVES

After studying this chapter, the reader will be able to

1. Compare and contrast three theories that explore the nature of aggression.
2. Demonstrate with a classmate two verbal interventions for potential aggression for each of eight specific client populations.
3. Write out a medication protocol that includes the major classifications of medications used for potentially aggressive clients.
4. Describe four criteria for the use of seclusion or restraint rather than verbal intervention.

5. Act out with classmates a simulated situation in which the sample restraint protocol is used. (Omit step 5 in the protocol if you are without instructor supervision.)
6. Discuss and elaborate on three principles that you would consider when planning interventions for clients whose culture is different from your own; do this with classmates who represent at least three different cultural backgrounds, sharing examples from each culture.
7. Role play with classmates by using understandable but unhelpful responses to anger and aggression in clients; discuss how these responses can affect nursing interventions.
8. Describe three steps to prevent long-term effects resulting from client anger and aggression toward nurses. Discuss what health team members do in such cases with members in your psychiatric clinical facility.

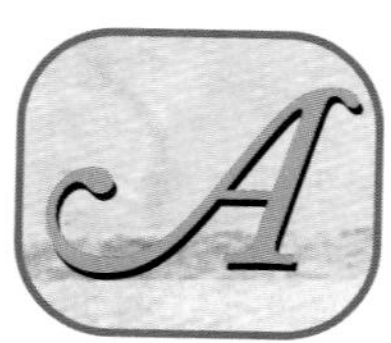

Anger and **aggression** are difficult targets for nursing intervention, particularly if their focus is the nurse, because they imply threat and thereby readily elicit emotional and personal responses. Nurses are inevitably asked to deal with anger and aggression because they are universal emotions. Anger is included in all descriptions of primary emotions and is one of six that can generally be identified across cultures via facial expression (Ekman 1972). In addition, while anger and aggression are more obvious in some people than others, both are responses to perceptions of threat or loss of control; the need for health care and the environments in which health care is typically provided readily precipitate feelings of personal peril and lack of control.

Anger and aggression are the last two stages of a response that begins with feelings of vulnerability and then uneasiness. Clients often communicate their anxiety before escalating to anger. Nursing interventions for anger and aggression begin at these early stages, with accurate assessment of clients' behaviors, appropriate intervention, and care to reassess that the intervention was effective. Impulsive clients may move quickly through these early stages, such that a display of anger is their first sign of distress. Quick and accurate intervention nevertheless prevents aggression, which in most instances is the physical attempt to take control.

THEORY

Another Look at Old Theory

Early theories of aggression developed from preexisting theories of drive (Freud 1933) and instinct (Lorenz 1966). Both the drive and the instinct theories led to a view that anger was an innate driving force that was essential to survival under some circumstances (e.g., hunting and warfare) and that repressing it would be unhealthy. This view led to therapies in which clients were encouraged to express their anger. Expression (i.e., "getting it all out"), not a search for solutions and resolution, became the treatment goal (Rappaport 1967).

Research has since shown that simple expression of anger is not beneficial to clients. Rather, expression of anger can lead to increased anger and to negative physiological changes. For example, subjects in one study described feeling increased anger and showed increased physiological correlates of anger when they described an event using loud and fast speech, as compared with descriptions of the same event that were soft and slow; these changes were true even when the event being described was neutral in content (Siegman et al. 1990; Siegman 1993). Similar affective and physiological correlates were seen when subjects articulated angry thoughts while discussing provocative events (Davison et al. 1991).

The physiological changes associated with anger expression are significant because they reflect a cardiac reactivity in men that has been shown to be associated with coronary heart disease. In other research, the opposite approach to anger—repression—has been associated with essential hypertension and cardiac reactivity in women (Gentry 1985; Julius et al. 1985; Manuck et al. 1985; Anderson and Lawler 1995). These negative cardiovascular effects have been shown not to occur when provocative events are handled assertively or when participants respond reflectively, constraining anger while trying to solve the underlying problem (Harburg et al. 1991; Anderson and Lawler 1995). Total repression of anger, however, has been linked with immunological problems and some forms of cancer (Esterling et al. 1990; Jensen 1987; Temoshok 1987).

Finally, family therapists have suggested that the venting of anger in ongoing relationships solves nothing and may serve to maintain dysfunctional interaction patterns. The possibility of developing more constructive interactional strategies is then diminished (Burman et al. 1993).

Clearly, the simple expression of anger is not useful. However, other anger management techniques that can be taught have been shown to be beneficial. These techniques are derived from two theoretical bases.

Behavioral Theory

Early behaviorists held that emotions, including anger, were learned responses to environmental stimuli (Skinner 1953). Social learning theorists adapted this theory through research that showed that children learn aggression by imitating others and that people repeat behavior that is rewarded (Bandura 1973). Thus, children who watch television violence learn violent ways of resolving problems. Not only is television violence portrayed as an option for resolving conflict, but 73% of violent acts are also shown without negative consequences (National Television Violence Study Council 1996). When parents are not present or are too preoccupied to teach their children alternative ways of dealing with problems, the range of skills learned by the children for managing frustration remains limited. Similarly, children who grow up in angry families learn to respond to frustration with anger and violence. Anger and aggression in the family and on television have two intrinsic rewards: (1) frequently, they accomplish the purpose of keeping the angry person in control while those around the person are intimidated; (2) they also provide for the relief of pent-up distress. Children and young adults with mental problems may be unable to process anger management skills taught by parents and schools.

Bandura's research suggested that emotional arousal would have an increased probability of expression as aggression when the context predisposed to aggression; this has implications for milieu therapy in particular. Staff attitudes have been shown to set the context within which emotional arousal occurs. For example, a rigid intolerance of affect and an authoritarian style by nurses have been associated with assault (Soloff 1983; Cooper and Mendonca 1989; Durivage 1989). Alternatively, a client may receive increased status and approval from other clients because of intimidation and threats that remain unaddressed by staff. The milieu is thus predisposed the rewarding of arousal when it is discharged via anger or aggression.

Cognitive Theory

Novaco's research (1976, 1985) described how cognitions drive anger. Individuals appraise events as threatening, and this cognition leads to the emotional and physiological arousal necessary to take action. Although threat is usually understood as an alert to physical danger, Beck (1976) noted that perceived assault on areas of personal domain, such as values, moral code, and protective rules, can also lead to anger. For example, anger and aggression are generated around moral issues, such as whether women have a right to abortion. People with frequent anger are often those who are vigilant for signs of threat (e.g., gang members who scan their environment for signs of disrespect). Such signs are cognitively interpreted as threats to status.

Similarly, clinic clients who have been kept waiting for long periods of time without explanation may interpret this as neglect and a lack of respect. Anger may escalate when the initial appraisal is followed by cognitions such as "They have no right to treat me this way. I am a person too." These additional cognitions become the drivers of the escalation, until successful interventions are used or until those who are angry take action. As Novaco (1985) noted, cognition and mood interact and can become mutually reinforcing; the later cognitions increase the anger, which validates the cognitions. The resulting action may take the form of assault. In some individuals, the period of escalation can be rapid.

Novaco stated that "there is no direct relationship between external events and anger. The arousal of anger is a cognitively mediated process" (1985, p. 210). An event may generate fear, hurt, humiliation, or powerlessness in some individuals (however, subsequent cognitions may then generate anger as a response to "being made to feel this way"), while generating anger in others. An event is more likely to lead to anger and then to aggression if the event is perceived as threatening (Beck 1976). This function is thus adaptive and ideally leads to self-preservation in circumstances of genuine danger (e.g., war). This adaptive function is likely the reason that anger is a primary and universal emotion. However, problems result when the same escalation process of cognition-emotion-action, or cognition-emotion-cognition–more emotion–action, occurs in social settings where physical danger is not present.

Nurses, of course, are not immune to anger. A client who is shouting angrily may reasonably be appraised as a potential threat. This appraisal may lead to anger on the nurse's part, as well as an impulse for self-protection. One study found that the nurse's response to anger from a client varied according to the interpretation given to the client's anger and to the nurse's self-appraised ability to manage the situation. Only when self-efficacy was perceived as adequate did the nurse move to help the client. When self-efficacy was not seen as adequate, nurses showed a decreased ability to process the client's message and a decreased ability to problem-solve (Smith and Hart 1994).

Biological Theory

Physiological correlates of anger include increased pulse, respiration, and finger temperature; blood pressure, both systolic and diastolic, may also increase. These changes can be seen when actors are asked to move facial muscles that lead to expressions commonly recognized as anger (Ekman et al. 1983; Levenson, Ekman, and Frieson 1990). As noted earlier, such changes also occur when a neutral topic is described with a loud and rapid speech pattern and when a situation is cognitively appraised as threatening. These widely variant ways of stimulating a sense of anger have led one author to hypothesize that none of the elements of anger—physiological correlates, cognitive appraisals, speech rate and volume, facial expression, or emotion—are secondary consequences of the experience; each represents an integral dimension of anger (Siegman et al. 1990).

All dimensions may therefore be centrally mediated. This suggestion is supported by the fact that many neurological conditions are associated with anger and aggression. For example, certain brain tumors, Alzheimer's disease, temporal lobe epilepsy, and traumatic injury to certain parts of the brain result in changes to personality that include increased violence. Twenty-five percent of people with brain injury have severe behavior disorders, including aggression, that disrupt their lives (Jacobs 1987). In fact, a series of studies have shown a relationship between impulsive aggression and low levels of the neurotransmitter serotonin (Brown et al. 1989). Serotonin is not localized to any one area of the brain and has been implicated in major depression as well as certain behaviors in people with personality disorders. The specific sites of these various serotonin effects in the brain, and the determinants of which response occurs when levels are low, are the subjects of continued study.

✓ One site known to be associated with aggression is the limbic system, which mediates primitive emotion and behaviors that are necessary for survival. The limbic system contains several structures that appear to have a role in the production of aggression. For example, in animal studies, stimulation of the amygdala produces rage responses, while lesions in the same structure produce docility. The temporal lobe of the brain shares some structures with the limbic system. Here, in the temporal lobe, memory is thought to be integrated; memory of previous insult is important in the cognitive appraisal of threat in the face of new stimuli. This lobe is also the source of complex partial seizures, which include aggressive behavior. The role of serotonin levels within these structures is not clear. The results of studies suggest that serotonin affects the impulsivity of action in response to anger (Virkkunen et al. 1994).

Finally, research findings indicate that violence is a function of both childhood environment and genetics. One review of adoption studies concluded that genetic factors explain more of the difference in antisocial behaviors than environmental factors. In general, when an adopted child had either an alcoholic or an antisocial biological parent, the presence of a poor adoptive environment resulted in a greater increase in antisocial behavior, including violence, than would be expected from the simple sum of the two effects (Cadoret 1982; Cadoret et al. 1985). In another study, adoptees with criminality in both their biological and their adoptive parents were 14 times more likely to be criminal than those without this parental history (Cloninger et al. 1982). Such studies have looked at three factors that are typically associated with aggression and violence: alcoholism, criminality, and antisocial personality disorder. Results of this research have been similar and consistent (Dahl 1994; DiLalla and Gottesman 1991).

ASSESSMENT

Accurate and early assessment can identify client anxiety before it escalates to anger and aggression. Such assess-

BOX 12–1 CUES TO POTENTIAL AGGRESSION

Verbal
Morose silence
Short responses
Illogical responses
Easily frustrated
Loud, demanding, threatening tone
Demeaning remarks
Negative response to rules or requests
Clipped or pressured speech
Direct warning or threat
Nonverbal, facial expression
Tense jaws
Clenched teeth
Lip biting
Lip quivering
Frowning
Vigilance
Intense focus
Staring
Dilated pupils
Flushed or blanched face
Pulsing carotid
Nonverbal, breathing
Rapid
Shallow
Irregular
Nonverbal, body language and posture
Shift from relaxed to tense
Hand twisting
Fist clenching and unclenching
Fist clenching
Pacing
Stony withdrawal
Confrontive, straight-on stance
Aggressive leaning forward
Tension-release gestures, e.g., pounding or kicking
Affect and attitude
Anxiety
Mistrust
Suspiciousness
Fear
Sarcasm
Overt hostility

ment also leads directly to the appropriate nursing diagnosis and intervention. Client expressions of anxiety or anger generally look similar. Both may involve increased rate and volume of speech, increased demands, irritability, frowning, redness of face, pacing, and twisting of hands or clenching and unclenching of fists. A complete list of such cues is provided in Box 12–1. Simple observation of these signs, however, does not provide the information necessary to drive the appropriate intervention. Taking an accurate history of the client's background and usual coping skills, as well as gathering the client's perception of the issue (if possible), are required.

Clients' perceptions, such as the belief that they are being made to wait unnecessarily in a clinic waiting room, often provide a useful point of intervention. In this example, the nurse may apologize for the wait (thereby validating the client's distress), explain the reason, and offer to provide updates at regular and predictable intervals. In other situations, the client's perception may be vague, constantly changing, or otherwise of less use. For example, a client recently admitted to an inpatient medical unit may have multiple complaints, all of which are communicated in a loud and angry voice. Additional client history can let the nurse know if this client has generally useful coping skills that either are not readily available or have failed in the crisis of the acute illness, or it can let the nurse know if the client has a limited range of coping at baseline. For example, if a history reveals that the client generally responds to stress by jogging or working out, the nurse might empathize with this additional loss brought about by the hospitalization, might work with the client to devise another strategy for the length of the admission, or might work with the physical therapy department to create a program of modified physical activity that would not harm the client. If the client's usual coping skills are poor, different types of interventions must be designed.

NURSING DIAGNOSIS

Two nursing diagnoses are important when potential aggression is identified. The first is **ineffective individual coping.** Because this diagnosis alone does not lead logically to a plan for intervention, in this text, it is broken down into three subcategories based on cause: (1) **ineffective individual coping, *overwhelmed;*** (2) **ineffective individual coping, *maladaptive pattern;*** and (3) **ineffective individual coping, *psychotic.*** These three types of ineffective coping represent three major ways in which clients become overwhelmed, anxious, and angry. Clients may have coping skills that are adequate for day-to-day events in their lives but are overwhelmed by the stresses of illness or hospitalization. Other clients may have a pattern of maladaptive coping, which consists of a set of coping strategies that have been developed to meet unusual or extraordinary situations (e.g., abusive families). Finally, some clients may have coping styles that reflect psychotic thought processes.

Ideally, intervention occurs at the point of ineffective individual coping. Nurses work with clients to support or teach ways of coping that will decrease anxiety and distress. However, clients may escalate quickly or may mask early signs of distress; nurses may be distracted and may miss those early signs, even when they are visible. Other clients may be acutely intoxicated and not amenable to early nursing interventions. In these situations, the problem with anger may not be resolved before the potential for violence exists. When this diagnosis is used, de-escalation of anger is the primary nursing intervention. Seclusion or restraint may be necessary to ensure the safety of clients and staff.

PLANNING

Planning Outcome Criteria

Having clearly defined outcome criteria (goals) when interventions are planned for angry and aggressive clients is important for identifying the behaviors that staff would encourage and identify if their interventions have been successful. Different outcome criteria have been outlined for meeting anger and aggression in different settings under different conditions in the intervention section in this chapter. Therefore, specific outcome criteria are included in the intervention section to correlate with a variety of settings and nursing diagnoses.

Nurse's Feelings and Self-Assessment

The nurse's ability to intervene safely in situations of anger and potential violence depends on his or her awareness of self. Without this awareness, nursing interventions are marked by impulsive or emotion-based responses, which are generally nontherapeutic and may be harmful. Self-awareness includes knowledge of personal responses to anger and aggression, of norms brought from the nurses' own families, and of norms brought from the larger society. In addition, staff must be aware of personal dynamics that may trigger emotions and reactions that are not therapeutic with specific clients. Finally, nurses must assess situational factors (e.g., fatigue) that may decrease normal competence in the management of complex client problems. Self-assessment introduces objectivity and awareness into nurse-client interactions, which are prerequisites for planned, theory-based interventions.

Nurses' responses to angry or threatening clients can escalate along a continuum similar to that of clients. Depending on their level of comfort, nurses may respond with professional concern, sympathy, anxiety, fear, or anger of their own. However, the more a nursing intervention is prompted by emotion, the less likely it is to be therapeutic. For example, a nurse who interprets client anger as a threat and becomes frightened may respond with flight or with inappropriate aggression before assessing the situation and the self's competence to deal with it.

Nurses' responses may also reflect norms from their families of origin. In some families, anger is responded to with attempts at peacemaking; in others, anger is responded to aggressively, with attempts to maintain domination. Some families ignore anger, leaving its antecedents and consequences unaddressed, while others respond to it with strict rules of allowed and forbidden behaviors. These responses are usually learned early (Bandura 1973) and are often unexamined; many people remain unaware that alternative responses exist that are both possible and permissible. Even those who, in adulthood, have altered their approach to the presence of anger may find old patterns resurfacing when their stress is increased. These unexamined responses by nurses can strongly influence their limit-setting styles as well as their impulsive reactions when they feel threatened. Similarly, nurses' responses may reflect those of the society or culture in which they were reared.

Nurses also have personal issues that they bring to potential conflict. Certain types of clients may lead to feelings of dislike, irritability, or fear in the nurse. If these feelings remain unexamined, they influence interactions with clients who have these characteristics; anger and aggression may be precipitated or escalated. Similarly, certain types of interactions or settings may trigger intense personal feelings in the nurse. If these precipitants to discomfort are known in advance, the nurse is less surprised when they occur and can also develop a self-management strategy for their occurrence.

Finally, situational events can effect nursing interventions. Staff may be dealing with such issues as sleep deprivation, fatigue, conflict with co-workers, and burnout. Acknowledging these issues allows the nurse to re-examine the response to a client or to negotiate a reassignment of clients for a time. At the least, the nurse can better assess how he or she may be contributing to the conflict, with an intent to change those attitudes and behaviors.

Self-assessment ideally promotes calm, theory-based responses to client anger and potential aggression. These responses are further supported by the following techniques:

- Deep breathing
- Relaxation of muscles that are not in use
- Empathetic interpretation of the client's distress
- Review of intervention strategies

In settings in which staff can reasonably expect episodes of client anger and aggression, staff must have regular teaching and practice of verbal and nonverbal interventions. This fosters increased confidence in the nurse's own abilities and those of co-workers.

Care of Staff

Nurses who are the focus of anger and aggression and nurses who work in environments in which potential anger is a theme are at risk for **posttrauma response** (PTR). PTR is a set of normal reactions to the experience of an overwhelming, unusual, and threatening event. These reactions have a biologic basis and are marked by such signs as

- Intrusive memory of the event.
- Sleep disturbance.
- Feelings of responsibility for the event.
- Embarrassment.
- Heightened startle response.
- Increased vigilance.
- Increased anxiety.
- A sense of isolation.

Nurses can continue to experience such signs for as long as 6 weeks after the event. Occasionally, such signs may be present 6 months or even 1 year after the event (Ryan and Poster 1989).

Nurses may experience PTR after events that do not include anger and aggression. Such events include criticism from a peer or a needle stick. However, because anger is so linked to threat, nurses are more at risk when they face angry clients and family members.

Assessment of threat is individual. One staff member may feel comfortable in a situation that is the source of distress to another. Interpretation of threat is in part a function of previous life experience, job experience, and sense of competency. PTR can be increased when other staff members minimize the distress that a nurse has experienced because they did not respond to the situation in the same way.

Support and intervention help prevent PTR symptoms from becoming chronic, resulting in posttraumatic stress disorder. This support can take several forms. A meeting of all staff should take place immediately after a show of force, in which a client has been secluded or restrained against his or her will. A review of the process takes place at this time. In addition, people are allowed to describe their feelings about the events leading up to, during, and after the show of force. Checking of perceptions occurs, as does emotional support for anyone experiencing distress.

A similar meeting, often called a *critical incident debriefing*, can be held after any event of anger or aggression that is experienced by a staff group. In this type of debriefing, review of the events occurs only for the purpose of gathering information from individuals who were involved and getting a common picture of what occurred. Administrative reviews, for the purpose of identifying system or process problems, and decisions about where blame might be assigned, must occur at another time. Participants are invited to share their responses to the described event. Teaching is provided regarding normal PTR and the anticipated recovery time.

Critical incident debriefing allows for mutual support among staff and decreases feelings of isolation. Discussion of events allows participants to sort, clarify, and provide meaning to elements that may have seemed chaotic or unclear at the time of their occurrence. PTR teaching normalizes and validates what nurses are experiencing. One nurse on a psychiatric unit was still experiencing sleep disturbance and a sense of uneasiness at work 2 weeks after a verbal assault by a client. Because she believed such signs would be gone after 3 days, the nurse was questioning her emotional health; information about PTR was useful to her and was a source of relief.

Such debriefing need not occur in groups. Individual nurses may seek out critical incident debriefing for themselves. In settings in which formal critical incident debriefing is not available, nurses may receive the same benefit from talking with a nurse manager, peers, or an advanced practice psychiatric mental health nurse. Others may choose to discuss these events with friends or family. Dealing with such events as they occur prevents the development of chronic symptoms and decreases the chance of cumulative stress (commonly called *burnout*).

Cultural Issues

Research on anger, aggression, culture, and ethnicity is limited and often contradictory; it frequently focuses specifically on criminal populations, with findings that may not be generalizable to noncriminal members of the same ethnic groups (Lyon et al. 1992; Valdez et al. 1995). Research on domestic violence that has included ethnicity as one of the variables suggested that ethnicity is not a predictor of either more or less violence among couples and families (Gin et al. 1991; Kua and Ko 1991; White and Koss 1991).

One group, African American men, is known to be overly represented in the criminal justice system, but the reasons for this are controversial and are probably a function of several factors, including socioeconomic issues, community breakdown, short-term and long-term effects of racism, and hopelessness. One author suggested that as African Americans experience repeated harm and loss due to racism, they begin to have a cognitive appraisal style of threat or challenge that leads to either passive or active negative emotions; these lead in turn to increased physical, psychological, and social illnesses (Outlaw 1993).

Other authors have suggested that American society itself is more violent than other societies because it was founded in rebellion, expanded at the expense of Native Americans and African slaves, responded with violence to each new wave of immigration, and experienced similar unrest at times of economic downturn (Blue and Griffith 1995). A better understanding of the histories of other societies would allow for a more balanced comparison, however.

One study reported not how ethnicity correlated with violence on inpatient psychiatric units but how it correlated with the accuracy of staff prediction of client violence. Nonwhite clients and male clients were the groups in which violence was overpredicted most often (McNiel and Binder 1995). This outcome suggests that in the absence of clear markers for clients who are at risk for violence (other than a history of violence), racial and gender biases may occur.

Despite the lack of compelling research evidence on culture, ethnicity, and violence, we know that intercultural differences and beliefs can lead to friction and conflict if they are not acknowledged and addressed. For example, new immigrants often come with an unfamiliarity with diseases that are regularly diagnosed in this country; they also may have a different understanding of what causes those diseases. Clients may distrust the health care system, either because of its briskness and unfamiliarity or because of earlier negative experiences. For example, the parents who bring a child into a clinic for treatment of an injury may be puzzled when, as part of the assessment, the clinician does a physical examination and then begins to ask questions about the child's nutritional status and eating habits. If this discrepancy between client intention and clinician response is not explained, the parent may be reluctant to bring the child back to the clinic at another time.

A common practice among some Southeast Asian groups is "coining." For example, parents of Vietnamese children have been reported for child abuse when health care workers saw the bruises left by coining, which is the rubbing of the skin with a coin to make the symptoms of viral infections vanish. In this example, parental use of folk medicine in an attempt to care for the child led to temporary removal of the child from the home and to long-lasting distrust of the health care system. In the earlier example, the parents may simply move to a different health care provider. In the example of coining, the parents became reluctant to use any services of the mainstream culture.

In psychiatry, these kinds of differences can lead to similarly profound errors. For example, some Asian cultures believe in, and talk to, spirits. If a client from one of these cultures is brought into the emergency department (ED) for evaluation of an apparent depressive episode with psychotic features after the death of a loved one, the clinician must either be culturally competent for that client's system of values or have access to consultation from someone who is. The risk is unnecessary hospitalization and medication, in addition to increased distress and distrust by the client.

Various cultural and racial groups have varying perspectives on the origins of disease, the origins of behaviors, the appropriateness of certain behaviors at specific times, and the origins and appropriateness of emotions that might be considered mental health problems in this country. In addition, diversity exists within ethnic and cultural groups. For example, the health beliefs of urban immigrant members of some Asian cultures are different than those of rural members of the same culture. Diagnosis and treatment of mental illnesses in these groups cannot be accurately accomplished without an awareness of these differences and without culturally competent resources. When treatment is attempted without this kind of assistance, the results include errors that lead to distrust, alienation, friction, conflict, anger, and aggression.

INTERVENTION

Inpatient Medical and Surgical Settings

Ineffective Individual Coping, Overwhelmed

Clients with acute illnesses that require hospitalization are particularly vulnerable to anxiety. The inpatient setting predisposes to both a loss of control and a lack of privacy; these feelings occur against the background of serious illness that may have an uncertain outcome. Clients with westernized concepts of medicine, including client autonomy as a key component of treatment, may worry that they are not being given pertinent information by the treatment team. Families from certain Asian and Latin cultures may believe that they must be vigilant to prevent the treatment team from giving negative information to the client or to prevent the team from requesting that the client make a treatment decision in isolation from the family.

In addition, potential friction exists at the boundary at which the requirements of the institution meet the personality of the client; for example, many inpatient settings are now nonsmoking environments. In addition, one client's usual sleep-wake cycle may include remaining awake until after midnight and arising at midmorning. Another client may rely on a partner or caregiver for activities that the nursing staff see as pertinent for resumption of independent function.

Clients also experience a peculiar type of sensory deprivation, in which they may be bombarded with sensory information that is difficult to interpret while they experience diminished stimulus heterogeneity, social isolation, and diminished kinesthetic input. These phenomena represent three of four criteria for sensory deprivation, which impairs clients' ability to cope and increases their irritability (Suedfeld 1969; Oster 1976).

For some clients, anger occurring under these circumstances may represent failure of usual healthy coping strategies. However, for others, the anger may represent clients' normal means of coping. These latter clients often have marginal adaptive skills before hospitalization. Their skills have frequently been learned in settings such as dysfunctional families and the streets. If these clients have a history of chemical dependence, their ability to learn healthy coping strategies has been further impeded.

A careful assessment, with history and information from family, determines whether client anger is a usual or an unusual way of managing stress. Interventions for clients whose usual coping strategies are healthy involve finding ways to re-establish or substitute similar means of dealing with the hospitalization. This problem solving occurs in collaboration with the client, in which the nurse acknowledges the client's distress, validates it as understandable under the circumstances, and indicates a willingness to search for solutions. Validation includes making an apology to the client when appropriate, such as when a promised intervention (e.g., changing a dressing by a certain time) has not been delivered.

This collaboration cannot occur unless nurses recognize their own self-protective responses to angry clients, including the wish to avoid contact with them, impatience, and frustration. Unrecognized, these understandable but unhelpful responses on the part of nurses can result in negative cycles of staff-client conflict in which the client feels increasingly misunderstood and ignored, and therefore increasingly hostile, while staff wish to further avoid or to punish. These negative interactive cycles interfere with the provision of empathic care; they ultimately lead to burnout in nurses.

Finally, clients who have become angry may be unable to moderate this emotion enough to problem-solve with their nurses; others may be unable to communicate the source of their anger. Often, the nurse, knowing the client and the context of the anger, can make an accurate guess at what feeling is behind the anger. Naming this feeling can lead to a dissipation of the anger, can help the client to feel understood, and can lead to a calmer discussion of the distress. Some of the feelings that can precipitate anger are listed in Box 12–2.

BOX 12–2 FEELINGS THAT MAY UNDERLIE ANGER

Discounted
Embarrassed
Frightened
Found out
Guilty
Humiliated
Hurt
Ignored
Inadequate
Insecure
Not heard
Out of control of the situation
Rejected
Threatened
Tired
Vulnerable

◗ A 41-year-old woman with a long history of peripheral vascular disease and of surgeries for vascular grafts and repair of graft occlusions is admitted to the hospital with severe pain in her left foot. Tests reveal that vessels to the foot are occluded. Additional surgery is ruled out, and medication is prescribed. Unfortunately, the medication is ineffective, and the foot begins to necrose. Physicians then discuss amputation with the client. The client refuses the surgery, demands a series of unproved alternative therapies, and is extremely angry with all members of the hospital staff. The treatment team becomes increasingly impatient to schedule further surgery before the necrosis worsens and the client begins to experience systemic signs of infection. This impatience aggravates the client's feelings of being out of control and erodes her belief that she is a competent partner in her treatment.

◗ This conflict ends via nursing intervention. The nurse is aware that before her disability from progressive vascular disease, the client was employed for many years as a buyer at a local department store. The nurse knows, too, that the client's family lives some distance from the hospital and is unable to visit regularly. Finally, the nurse understands that when the client was admitted, she had expected medical intervention once more to save her leg. Nursing intervention is twofold. First, the client's anger and unwillingness to discuss her condition end when the nurse names her feelings of fear and being out of control. Once the client's anger is reduced, the nurse is able to help her negotiate more time for the final decision; this allows the client to complete her anticipatory grieving (including stages of denial, anger, and bargaining). In this interval, the client's wish to explore alternative therapies is addressed via second and third medical opinions; she is also able to consult further with her family.

Outcome criteria, along with interventions and rationales, for clients whose normal, healthy coping resources are overwhelmed are presented in Table 12–1.

Ineffective Individual Coping, Maladaptive Pattern

Clients whose coping skills were marginal before hospitalization need a different set of interventions than those described earlier. Clients who usually cope well can either use their standard coping strategies once the barriers have been removed or generate useful alternatives. Clients with maladaptive coping are poorly equipped to use alternatives when their initial attempts to cope are unsuccessful or are found to be inappropriate. Such clients frequently manifest anger and aggression. For some, anger and intimidation are primary strategies used to obtain short-term goals. For others, the anger occurs when limited or primitive attempts at coping are unsuccessful and alternatives are unknown. For these clients, anger is a particular risk in inpatient settings.

In addition to the stressor of acute illness, these clients are often worried that they will be judged negatively or treated unfairly by hospital professionals. Also, clients with chemical dependence are anxious about being cut off from their substance of choice; they likewise have well-founded concerns that any physical pain may be inadequately addressed. Chemically dependent clients, in particular, may become engaged in conflicts with staff when the clients seem to disregard treatment advice or engage in behaviors that are incompatible with recovery. For these clients, recovery is often a secondary goal; this situation can frustrate those staff for whom it is a primary goal. Finally, many clients with maladaptive coping also have personality styles that externalize blame. That is,

TABLE 12–1 INTERVENTION GUIDELINES
Ineffective Individual Coping: OVERWHELMED

Short-Term Outcomes

1. The client will describe his or her concerns to the nurse before becoming angry.
2. The client will describe and use one method for decreasing his or her stress level while in the hospital.

Intervention	Rationale
1. With the client, assess his or her usual means of coping. Adapt or build on these for use in the hospital. Refer to physical therapy or recreation therapy as appropriate.	1. Allows for support of usually functional coping strategies and those with which the patient is most proficient.
2. With the client, assess those aspects of the hospitalization that cause the most concern. Design a plan that addresses these concerns.	2. Intervenes into those environmental factors that have contributed to overwhelming the patient's usual coping methods.
3. Assess for sensory deprivation. Provide for increased heterogeneity of stimuli, to the extent possible.	3. Allows for intervention into a common but silent stressor of hospitalized patients.
4. Respond to client anxiety or anger with active listening and validation of client distress. Apologize if appropriate.	4. Allows the patient to feel heard and understood; builds trust.
5. Name likely feeling underlying patient anger.	5. Names the real issue; often dissipates anger.

they see the source of their discomfort and anxiety as being outside themselves; relief must therefore also come from an outside source (e.g., the nurse).

As noted previously, an adequate nursing history allows for early identification of clients who need special care plans. This recognition also decreases the potential for staff frustration by altering expectations of clients' coping abilities.

Initial client anxiety can be addressed with a respectful approach that establishes a sense of mutual collaboration. Respect can be maintained if nurses operate from the following assumptions (Linehan 1993a):

- Clients are doing the best they can.
- Clients want to improve.
- Client behaviors make sense within their world view.

In addition, baseline anxiety can be moderated by the provision of comfort items before they are requested (e.g., coffee, deck of cards); this can build rapport and acts symbolically to reassure. Anxiety can also be minimized by reducing ambiguity. This strategy includes clear and concrete communication. Providing clarity about what the nurse can and cannot do is most usefully ended with an offer of something within the nurse's power to provide (i.e., leaving the client with a "yes").

Interventions for anxiety might also include the use of distractions, such as magazines, action comics, and video games. Generally, distractions that are colorful and do not require sustained attention work best, although this varies according to the client's interests and abilities. Finally, clients with a high level of baseline anxiety and limited coping skills are helped when their interactions with the treatment team are predictable; this might include speaking with the physician at a specific time each day or having the client see a single spokesperson from the treatment team each day.

Because these clients have limited coping skills, nursing interventions include teaching alternative behaviors and strategies. For clients who externalize blame, such teaching may best be preceded by a gentle challenge. The challenge serves to engage the client's interest in teaching that might otherwise be seen as irrelevant (Doren 1996).

▶ A 21-year-old man who was in an automobile accident is bedridden with a pelvic fracture. During his first day of admission, he yells at each nurse who walks by his room, using expletives in his demands that the nurse enter the room. The nurse who is assigned to the client for the evening stops in his doorway after he yells at her and asks in mild disbelief "Is this working for you? Do nurses really come in here when you yell at them that way?" The client responds sullenly, justifying his behavior by complaining about his care. However, the nurse's challenge has caught his attention, and she goes on to suggest (i.e., teach) alternative strategies for contacting her and other nurses. The strategies are immediately put into use by the client.

▶ This intervention is also important in that the nurse has taught a couple of strategies, providing the client with choices and thus with more control.

Anger may be communicated via long-term verbal abuse. If attempts to teach alternatives have not been successful, three interventions can be used. The first is to leave the room as soon as the abuse begins; the client can be informed that the nurse will return in a specific amount of time (e.g., 20 minutes), when the situation is calmer. A matter-of-fact, neutral manner is important because fear, indignation, and arguing are gratifying to many verbally abusive clients. Alternatively, if the nurse is in the midst of a procedure and cannot leave immediately, the nurse can break off conversation and eye contact, completing the procedure quickly and matter-of-factly before leaving the room.

Withdrawal of attention to the abuse is successful only if a second intervention is also used. This step requires attending positively to nonabusive communication by the client. Interventions can include discussing non–illness-related topics, responding to requests, and providing emotional support.

Finally, clients who are regularly verbally abusive may respond best to the predictability of routine, such as scheduled contacts with the nurse (e.g., every 30 minutes or every 60 minutes). Use of such contacts provides nursing attention that is not contingent on the client's behavior and therefore does not reinforce the abuse. This intervention works only to the extent that the nurse maintains the scheduled contacts as agreed on. In addition, other staff members must be informed of the care plan so that they do not inadvertently sabotage it by responding to incidental requests by the client. Of course, the client's illness or injury may sometimes require nursing visits for assessment or intervention outside the scheduled contact times. These visits can be carried out in a calm, brief, matter-of-fact manner. This care plan is best negotiated with the client and can be seen as supportive in that it attempts to address client anxiety about getting needs met (anxiety that is reflected in the verbal abuse and also manifested by frequent angry demands) through the predictability of the nurse's contacts.

Again, appropriate interventions can be difficult when the nurse is feeling threatened. Remaining matter of fact with clients who habitually use anger and intimidation can be difficult because these people are often skillful at making personal and pointed statements. It is important for the nurse to remember that clients do not know their nurses personally and thus have no basis on which they can make accurate judgments. Nurses can also vent their own responses elsewhere, with other staff or family members or via critical incident debriefing.

Short-term outcome criteria, along with interventions and rationales, for clients with maladaptive coping are presented in Table 12–2.

TABLE 12–2 INTERVENTION GUIDELINES
Ineffective Individual Coping: MALADAPTIVE PATTERN

Short-Term Outcomes

1. The client will participate in recommended treatment.
2. The client will describe his or her concerns without losing control.
3. The client will make requests to his or her assigned nurse.
4. The client will talk about topics that are not conflict-related.

Intervention	Rationale
1. Use matter-of-fact, neutral approach.	1. Does not reinforce or gratify the client's maladaptive behaviors; does not add the nurse's affect to the issue.
2. Avoid control battles. If the client is noncompliant with treatment, perform chart teaching of rationale for treatment. Chart client's refusal.	2. Control battles with clients are perceived as a challenge and generally lead to escalation of the conflict.
3. If the client is noncompliant with treatment, suggest collaboration on a daily routine, to include a) Tasks that client is to perform independently, or b) Routine times for treatment. Once developed, post this in the client's room.	3. Daily routine provides predictability for the client; collaboration increases the likelihood of the client's following through.
4. If the client is verbally abusive, let him or her know you will be back when the situation is calmer—at least 20 minutes. Return when time is up. Make contact with the client at other, calmer times (consider implementing number 7, below). Provide social reinforcement at these times (e.g., coffee, conversation about non–conflict related topics, support, validation of distress).	4. Removes all attention and reinforcement of verbal abuse; provides reinforcement for appropriate behaviors; allows for building of alternative coping skills.
5. Calmly point out when the client's behavior is not achieving his or her stated goal; then teach alternate, more acceptable methods of attaining that goal.	5. Catches the client's attention with a gentle challenge, then offers an opportunity for learning alternate skills.
6. Ask the client's family, or recreation therapy department, to provide distractions.	6. Provides an external, nonpharmacological intervention to increase the client's comfort and decrease distress.
7. Schedule contacts with the client so that nurse-client contacts are routine, predictable, not contingent on the client's behavior.	7. Allows client contacts to be made in a manner that is not contingent on the client's behavior; addresses client concerns about being neglected; builds trust.
8. Provide pain medications as ordered. Avoid prn scheduling if possible. Refer complaints about pain medication to the physician (i.e., stay out of the middle).	8. Conflicts about pain medications lead to control battles and to increased client focus (even perseverance) on both the pain and the medication.
9. Communicate care plan to all staff, for consistency.	9. Inconsistency in carrying out the plan of care can lead to intermittent reinforcement of the client's maladaptive behaviors, thereby increasing their frequency.

prn, as needed.

Ineffective Individual Coping, Psychotic

In clients with a history of psychiatric illnesses that include psychosis, their psychotic symptoms are often exacerbated by hospitalization for physical problems. This increase is a function of increased anxiety as well as altered environment. Psychotic symptoms, such as auditory hallucinations and delusions, are disturbances of perception, and unfamiliar environments, such as hospital units, increase the stress for clients who have difficulty interpreting external cues. In addition, such clients are known to be largely unable to interpret the emotions or the intent of others via commonly recognized cues in facial expression (Feinberg et al. 1986). Hospital staff are therefore another source of potential threat.

Anger or aggression may be a client response to an increase in psychotic symptoms. Because an increase in these symptoms may not be immediately apparent to nurses, ongoing assessment of apparent client comfort, client agitation, and level of client preoccupation with internal stimuli is important.

Antipsychotic medications are the intervention of choice with these clients. Antianxiety agents are also useful for managing periods of increased anxiety or agitation in clients with these illnesses (Wolkowitz and Pickar 1991). Clients with severe and persistent psychotic illnesses may also have symptoms, called *negative symptoms*, of withdrawal, flatness of affect, latency of response, and restricted speech. These symptoms are less amenable to treatment with medication than are the more obvious positive symptoms (e.g., hallucinations, delusions, thought disorder) but are less likely to result in aggression. Chapter 22 provides more information on positive and negative symptoms.

Psychotic symptoms may also be seen in clients without histories of psychiatric illness but who, as a result of their illness or injury, have a metabolic disturbance (e.g., electrolyte imbalance), sleep deprivation, impaired neurological functioning, or medication side effects. These clients do not have a psychiatric illness; rather, they are delirious. Their hallucinations tend to be visual, olfactory, or tactile rather than auditory. Delusions are rare. Delirium is discussed in the section on cognitive deficits in Chapter 23.

Short-term outcome criteria, along with nursing interventions and rationales, for clients with psychotic disturbances due to psychiatric illnesses are presented in Table 12–3.

Inpatient Psychiatric Settings

Inpatient psychiatric settings have historically been seen as particularly prone to violence. Early psychiatric hospitals were built away from urban centers to protect people from the unpredictability of the clients. However, not all psychiatric clients are potentially violent, and aggression appears to be correlated less with certain illnesses than with certain client characteristics. For example, the best single predictor of violence is a history of violence in a particular client (Davis 1991; Davis and Boster 1988). A second significant risk factor is impulsivity (Rossi et al. 1986; Berkowitz 1982, 1983).

TABLE 12–3 INTERVENTION GUIDELINES
Ineffective Individual Coping: PSYCHOTIC

Short-Term Outcomes

1. The client will check out delusions and hallucinations with staff, rather than acting on them.
2. The client will recognize the need to manage psychotic symptoms.
3. The client will refrain from behaviors that are intrusive or frightening to other clients.

Intervention	Rationale
1. Assess client's distress from delusions and hallucinations at each contact.	1. Allows for ongoing assessment, early intervention.
2. Decrease sensory stimulation: ▸ Put client in private room, or bed farthest from doorway. ▸ Limit number of visitors present at one time. ▸ Do not put the client in the TV room. ▸ Turn on the television for specific programs only (i.e., not on continuously). ▸ Do not place client in chair at the nurse's station.	2. Decreases the possibility of client's being overwhelmed by environmental stimuli; decreases number of stimuli available for perceptual distortion.
3. Provide as much structure and predictability to the client's day as possible. Post a schedule in the client's room; include mealtimes, bath time, awake time, bed time.	3. Decreases number of decisions that must be made by the client; decreases possibility of client's being overwhelmed by uncertainty; increases client's sense of security.
4. Teach client management techniques for auditory hallucinations (find out what techniques client finds helpful): ▸ Asking for prn medication ▸ Using radio with earphones ▸ Humming	4. Provides client with skills that may interrupt anxiety provoking symptoms.
5. When client is tangential, gently refocus as necessary.	5. Provides external structure to help client communicate his or her thoughts and concerns.
6. Provide frequent, short, reality-oriented contacts; give clear and simple directions or explanations.	6. Provides reminders of what is real; does so in a manner that does not add excessive external stimuli.
7. Use prn medications as ordered for increased distress or agitation.	7. Provides for use of appropriate pharmacotherapy.
8. Provide nonconfrontive reality orientation when client is talking about hallucinations and delusions (e.g., "Gee, I don't hear anything.")	8. Provides reminder of what is real, but does so in a manner that is not challenging or invalidating.
9. Empathize with client's underlying fear and anxiety (e.g., "It must be frightening to think those things are happening.")	9. Validates client's affective response to symptoms; allows client to feel understood; builds trust.

prn, as needed.

The context of anger and aggression has also been reported as a factor. In one study, clients identified conflict with staff as the most common reason for violence (Sheridan et al. 1990). In another study, impulsive behavior by psychotic clients was not a function of symptoms such as hallucinations and delusions but was a result of interactions with staff that involved setting of limits or imposition of rules (Gallop et al. 1992).

Given these factors, research on the relationship of client anger to nursing styles of limit setting is pertinent. In one study, six interpersonal styles were studied: (1) belittlement, (2) platitudes, (3) solutions provided without options, (4) solutions provided with options, (5) affective involvement without options, and (6) affective involvement with options. A belittling style of limit setting might be simply telling an angry client that she or he is (i.e., the behavior is) *inappropriate*. Providing solutions without options might be telling a client to take a time-out away from others. Affective involvement with options might consist of acknowledging the client's anger, followed by asking whether the client would be helped by a time-out or whether talking the issue out with a staff member would be more useful.

This study found that nursing styles of setting limits were powerful moderators of situational anger, regardless of the client's diagnosis or impulsivity. For all clients, belittlement was more likely to precipitate anger than were other styles. Affective involvement with options was the strategy that was least likely to generate anger. For non-impulsive clients, three styles were effective without causing anger: (1) solutions with options, (2) affective involvement without options, and (3) affective involvement with options. For clients with high levels of impulsivity, however, only the third style kept anger at a low level. Interestingly, with these clients, empathy alone (i.e., affective involvement without options) was not sufficient (Lancee et al. 1995).

If staff can identify clients who have a potential for violence, early intervention becomes possible. Nurses can work with the clients to recognize their early signs of anger and can teach them strategies to manage the anger and to prevent aggression. Because anger has a strong cognitive component, cognitive interventions are helpful. Cognitive techniques can be taught in groups (Gerlock 1994) or individually (Reeder 1991). Both state and trait anger have been decreased via the use of cognitive therapy groups. While anger is often an attempt to regain or maintain control, it generally works only for the short term. Cognitive therapy can provide an alternative means of control that works for the long term as well.

◗ A 19-year-old man has a 2-year history of quadriplegia. This client also has a history of drug abuse that began in grade school, an inability to set or work toward long-term goals, and a primary coping style of anger and intimidation. The client is admitted to an inpatient psychiatric unit because of increasing suicidal ideation. He clearly communicates to staff that his preferred means of coping with anger is to "cuss people out" and run into them with his wheelchair. However, in the hospital, the consequence of wheelchair assaults is that the client is secluded in his room, which he finds intolerable. The client requests that someone work with him on anger management, so that he can have the increased control afforded by the ability to develop alternatives.

◗ Via cognitive therapy, this client is taught to identify the thoughts and beliefs he uses to drive his anger. These typically relate to feeling unheard by the staff; secondarily, he often believes that staff purposely act to increase their control at his expense. The client is taught to look at each situation to find proof either for and against his beliefs (e.g., in neutral observations of a particular staff member, did this person act like a "control freak"?). He then learns to substitute more reality-based interpretations of events and interactions. Finally, the client is taught to generate options for action in the situation; he then lists the pros and cons of those options. These are interventions developed by Beck (Beck 1976; Beck et al. 1979) and Beck and Freeman (1990). Because cognitive therapy is a specialized therapy learned in part through supervised clinical practice, cognitive interventions would be enhanced by the consultation of an advanced practice nurse with expertise in this modality.

◗ Because this client is intelligent and motivated to gain increased personal control, he learns these techniques quickly. In addition, once it becomes clear that issues of feeling unheard and out of control underlay most episodes of anger, the client is able to target those issues for problem solving. He rapidly develops effective and appropriate ways to make himself heard and understood. He also becomes adept at communicating when he feels out of control and at finding ingenious ways of negotiating control on issues that are particularly important to him. The client's suicidal impulses, which occur when he is frustrated, also diminish.

Finally, because interpersonal friction has been identified as a primary source of anger and aggression on psychiatric units, teaching at-risk clients ways to address potentially conflictual interactions is helpful. For example, Linehan (1993b) developed a teaching module on interpersonal effectiveness that has been shown to decrease self-harm behaviors in clients with borderline personality disorder, when it is used as a part of her 8-month outpatient program. The effectiveness of this module when used alone and with other populations has not been studied. It is developed for use with a highly impulsive diagnostic group. Clients are taught to recognize behaviors that complicate difficult interactions (e.g., shouting, threatening). Handouts that accompany the module provide structured ways to think about these interactions.

Homework sheet number 1, in particular, teaches clients facing a potentially provoking interaction to identify their goal for the interaction, their goal for the state of the relationship at the end of the interaction, and their goal for the way they will feel about themselves. Then, teaching that not all goals can be met in all interactions, the handout asks clients to prioritize those three goals (Linehan 1993b, p. 129).

Short-term outcome criteria along with nursing interventions and rationales for potentially angry clients on psychiatric units are presented in Table 12–4.

Inpatient Psychiatric Milieu

The inclusion of the milieu as part of inpatient treatment occurred after World War II as a result of the work by Jones (1953). Jones focused on the social organization of psychiatric units, including such factors as authority structure, staff and client roles, and communication and decision-making patterns. He used these components to develop a community that increased client roles in their treatment and in the culture of the unit. Jones believed that unit culture could be used to promote client learning; problems that occurred on the unit would be used as learning situations that could be applied to normal environments.

Twenty years later, Moos (1974a, 1974b) developed the Ward Atmosphere Scale to rate unit cultures and to assess the effects of those atmospheres on clients. This rating scale was developed when inpatient units had lengths of stay that were months or years long. Currently, lengths of stay are much shorter. Nevertheless, unit milieu continues to be an important component of client treatment, particularly as it relates to anger and aggression.

As noted previously, the milieu of the inpatient psychiatric unit provides the context within which arousal occurs. Rigid intolerance and authoritarian styles on psychiatric units have been correlated with increased violence (Cooper and Mendonca 1989; Durivage 1989). This is consistent with the trend noted in a more recent study, in which the unit with the lowest score on autonomy, as measured by the Ward Atmosphere Scale, had the greatest number of assaults; the unit with the fewest assaults had the highest scores on autonomy (Lanza et al. 1994).

Units with little structure or with a structure that is unpredictable have also been correlated with increased violence. One study reported that peaceful units were

TABLE 12–4 INTERVENTION GUIDELINES
Potential for Violence: INPATIENT PSYCHIATRIC SETTINGS

Short-Term Outcomes

1. The client will not harm or threaten others while hospitalized.
2. By discharge, the client will state one method of managing violent impulses.
3. The client will follow unit rules.

Intervention	Rationale
1. Evaluate client for low-stimulation protocol and private room. Obtain information about client's history of violence.	1. Decreases overstimulation as source of anxiety, anger, and aggression; history provides the best information about cues to client aggression.
2. Orient client to unit rules and safety goals. Reassure client of his or her safety. Set expectation of appropriate behavior and be consistent in following up these expectations. Contract with client for appropriate behavior.	2. Provides client with information about the unit's requirements and provides clear behavioral expectation; contract allows for collaborative approach to potential violence and increases likelihood of client adherence.
3. Set limits on inappropriate expression of anger and hostility when they occur. Teach alternatives.	3. Limits prevent escalation; teaching allows for development of appropriate skills.
4. Recognize behaviors that indicate that client is escalating and intervene to de-escalate the situation. Teach client early recognition of these behaviors.	4. Provides early intervention and interrupts escalation; teaches client how to do the same.
5. Assess need for medication and effectiveness of medication for agitation or increased psychotic symptoms.	5. Provides for use of appropriate pharmacotherapy.
6. Assess client at each contact.	6. Provides for early intervention.
7. In the case of threats to specific people in the community, follow hospital protocol for warning.	7. Addresses the professional duty to warn.
8. Seclude or restrain for safety as necessary. Advance client to room seclusion schedule as he or she demonstrates behavioral control.	8. Provides for safety of client and staff when all other interventions have been unsuccessful.
9. Assess for referral to anger management program at discharge.	9. Facilitates client's pursuit of therapy on this issue after discharge.

characterized by staff availability and frequent staff-client interaction. Unit structure was treatment oriented and predictable; group therapy meetings and other components of the ward environment occurred at regularly scheduled times. Interventions for potential violence were supportive, nonpunitive, and encouraged the client to regain control.

In contrast, units that were violent despite having client populations that were similar to those on the peaceful units were characterized by a chaotic staff organization and a haphazard use of routines and schedules. Therapeutic interactions were minimal. No early recognition of increasing client tension occurred, and intervention for aggression tended to be punitive. Staff did not debrief regarding these interventions and were thus unable to identify antecedents to the aggression or ways to improve on the interventions themselves (Katz and Kirkland 1990).

Other elements of milieu that have been correlated with increased client aggression have been unit policies that allow clients to vent anger toward staff and a low staff-to-client ratio (Lanza 1988; Lanza et al. 1994). The latter issue is typically outside the direct control of staff nurses; it may require creativity in staffing patterns, scheduling of unit activities, types of therapeutic interventions (e.g., an increase in therapy and therapeutic education groups), and client assignments. Nurses must also take the responsibility for documenting the effects of low staff-to-client ratios.

Similarly, Watson (1992) discussed the disruption that may be caused to the milieu when the strictures of third-party reimbursement lead to organizational changes and program changes that are not consistent with the values of staff. For example, clients may be discharged earlier in their treatment, while they are still in transition out of their psychiatric crises. These changes can interrupt nursing goals for clients, decrease the group cohesiveness that is so useful in milieu therapy, and increase the effort required to maintain a specific unit culture.

In this context, the community meeting, which is an intrinsic part of milieu therapy, may best undergo both a change in focus and an increase in importance. Traditionally, this meeting has included time for clients to make community decisions and to give feedback to others about their progress in treatment. Shorter stays may change the focus to one of orientation of clients to the unit culture and to the problem-solving of issues common to the unit community. In shorter-stay groups, new patients are oriented to the unit and its rules, and all patients are expected to participate in solving immediate, here-and-now problems occurring on the unit (e.g., conflict about television watching and scheduling during Monday night football). These are short-term goals that hopefully result in increased skill acquisition by patients. As patients learn how to address the television scheduling conflict, they learn how to address other kinds of conflicts as well (over time). The latter task allows staff to facilitate problem solving in a manner that teaches skills and enhances the effective use of these skills; in this way, clients are assisted in skill building and in becoming better members of all their communities.

In summary, therapeutic elements of the inpatient milieu include accessibility of staff (including a reasonable staff-to-client ratio), frequent staff-client interactions that are supportive and therapeutic, and predictable unit structure. Treatment focus includes problem solving, and clients are encouraged to maintain control of their anger. Regular community meetings may be part of the unit structure and serve to communicate the unit culture. Client autonomy is nurtured, as are client successes in communication and socialization. Although one study faulted psychiatrists' leadership when these elements were lacking on units, all are clearly within the scope of nursing practice and can thus reasonably be seen as the responsibility of the nurse.

Of course, these elements must all be present in the context of a safe environment. An inpatient unit must be free of weapons and objects that can be readily used in aggression.

Emergency Department Settings

Emergency departments are, almost by definition, fear-producing environments. Clients come to the ED because they believe themselves to be in physiological danger, from either illness or injury. Once in the ED, clients relinquish their well-being to professionals, who are often rushed. Communications may be hurried or incomplete. In addition, a subgroup of ED clients are likely to have psychiatric problems or chemical dependence. In one study of ED trauma clients, 88% of those with penetrating trauma and 50% of those with blunt trauma were found to have preexisting psychiatric or behavioral problems (Whetsell et al. 1988). These contextual factors predispose to anxiety that, if unaddressed, can lead to anger and aggression.

Again, early assessment and intervention are important for prevention. Signs of increasing anxiety and anger include fidgeting, increasing volume of voice, change in tone of voice, continued questioning, frequent demands, criticism, and pacing. Most of these cues can be seen as attempts to gain control of the situation or to avoid abandonment by keeping the nurse close by (Nield-Anderson and Doubrava 1993). The goals of intervention are (1) reduction of anxiety via the reduction of ambiguity, (2) establishment of a sense of mutual collaboration based on trust and honesty, and (3) increase in the client's or relative's sense of personal control.

Several interventions are particularly pertinent in the ED and have been well described in the literature (Kinkle 1993; Nield-Anderson and Doubrava 1993). Clients and family members who are always addressed by name feel less anonymous. Lengthy waits are more tolerable if they are predicted, explained, and interrupted by periodic updates. For particularly anxious or irritable clients and families, these updates may be most effective if they are provided in a predictable and agreed-on fashion (e.g., every 20 minutes). Offering coffee or other beverages during the wait (if not contraindicated for the client) or informing family members where these might be obtained lets people know that their comfort and concerns are considered important. Also, the earlier a client is allowed to tell his or her story, the more likely it is the client will feel heard and attended to.

Certain clients may come into the ED already angry. These are likely to be clients who have been involved in a fight or have been injured while committing a crime. These clients are admitted in a heightened state of excitability, and the usual ED environment intensifies that. Interventions include decreasing sensory stimulation (to the extent possible) while addressing client needs and concerns, speaking calmly and matter-of-factly, and keeping voice tone neutral. Such clients may be challenging and personal in their remarks; again, it is important that the nurse not respond defensively or with irritation or impatience. For some clients, an angry or frightened response is gratifying. For others, such responses simply serve to increase their feelings of being out of control and thereby further their escalation.

Client: (shouting) I want my methadone now, you white bitch!

Nurse: (although startled by the client's outburst, taking a deep breath, keeping voice low and calm) I need to check the physician's order, Mr Roy. If he has written the order, I'll get your methadone within the next 15 minutes. If he hasn't, I'll let him know that you are waiting, and I'll be back in 10 minutes to let you know what's going on.

As noted earlier, maintaining a calm professional tone in the face of insults or escalating anger can be difficult. The nurse may require a time-out or may wish to negotiate with another nurse for a change in client assignment. Personal insults are most usefully seen as signs of the client's emotional state or as clues to the client's ability and style of coping.

Finally, any ED client may be acting under the influence of drugs or alcohol. These clients may have three problems: (1) potential emotional lability, (2) inability to receive verbal and written information accurately, and (3) inability to perceive the extent of their illness or injury accurately. If the nurse is caring for an intoxicated man who knows of his illness or injury but is yelling or cursing, the nurse may take his or her hands off the client, step back, and wait. This can be followed by an indirect statement of limit setting (e.g., "I can't work while you are yelling"). Direct limit setting often leads to increased aggression, particularly if the client interprets the limit setting as judgment or criticism. The nurse can also try an appeal to the client's egocentrism (e.g., "I thought you would *want* me to be working on your leg. You said you were worried about it"). Verbal communication must be brief and concrete. If the client is unaware of the illness or injury or is so out of control that approach is risky, and if intervention cannot wait, restraints are likely to be the only option.

Short-term outcome criteria, along with nursing interventions and rationales, for potentially angry clients in the ED are presented in Table 12–5.

Outpatient Settings

Outpatient settings, because they are less acute than inpatient settings, are generally less associated with anger and assault. Because of this, staff may be surprised and annoyed when a client does become angry. Clients at risk for becoming angry are those who are anxious, those who must endure unusually long waits, and clients with poor social and coping skills.

Interventions include

1. Showing concern.
2. Allowing the client to express feelings and describe problems.
3. Acknowledging the client's distress.
4. Actively listening and collaborating, including
   - Asking questions to clarify.
   - Restating the problem.
   - Restating the feelings or naming the underlying feelings.
   - Taking notes, if necessary, to keep the details clear (this will also give the message that the problem is being taken seriously).
5. Collaborating with the client on how to resolve the problem.

Angry clients may become tangential; staying focused on the main problem is important. So, too, is admitting and apologizing for any mistakes.

Occasionally, clients make inappropriate requests, such as asking that a disability or insurance form be competed inaccurately. The possibility of this experience is increased now that nurses are serving in advanced practice roles, operating independently in clinics and private practice. Nursing interventions include

- Explaining the difference between subjective and objective findings.
- Speaking in concrete terms: explaining what is being seen in the examination and must therefore be reported.
- Letting the client know that just as the nurse would not lie to the client, the nurse will not lie on the form.
- Validating the fact that the client has personal reasons for making the request, although the nurse cannot accede to them.

Cognitive Deficits

A client group that is particularly at risk for acting aggressively is that with cognitive deficits. Such deficits may

TABLE 12–5 INTERVENTION GUIDELINES
Potential for Violence: EMERGENCY DEPARTMENT

Short-Term Outcomes

1. The client and family will report the status of their wait in the emergency department.
2. The client and family will have comfort attended to while waiting.
3. The client and family will describe their concerns or distress without losing control.
4. The client who is admitted in an already aroused state will become calmer via environmental intervention.
5. The client who is admitted in an intoxicated state will allow staff to provide emergency care without conflict

Intervention	Rationale
1. Provide periodic updates to clients and families while they are waiting.	1. Decreases anxiety by keeping client and family informed of their status; builds trust.
2. Offer coffee to family members or let them know where they can find it if the wait is long. Offer comfort items (e.g., blanket) to client.	2. Decreases anxiety by letting client and family know that their needs are being considered.
3. Provide client and family an opportunity to tell their story at the earliest point possible. Assess for increasing distress at each nursing contact. Validate client and family concerns as understandable under the circumstances.	3. Allows client and family to feel that they have been heard and that their concerns are known; frequent assessment allows for early intervention; validation allows client and family to feel understood.
4. Speak calmly and matter-of-factly; keep voice tone neutral. Decrease sensory stimulation to the extent possible. Provide predictable contacts to the extent possible.	4. Sets a tone of calmness and control; does not add the nurse's affect to the environmental stimuli; decreases overstimulation as a source of distress; builds trust.
5. If client is yelling and illness or injury is not life threatening, remove your hands from client and step back until he or she has quieted.	5. Provides opportunity for client to regain control without the added stress and stimulation of personal contact and invaded personal space.
6. Make an indirect statement of limit setting (e.g., "I can't work while you are yelling.").	6. Sets limit in nonchallenging manner.
7. Appeal to client's egocentrism (e.g., "I thought you would want me to be working on your leg—you said you were worried about it.").	7. Speaks to client's self-interest.
8. Keep verbal communication brief and concrete.	8. Keeps environmental stimulation at a minimum; provides information in forms that client can most easily manage and understand.
9. Use restraints as necessary for client and staff safety.	9. Provides for safety of client and staff when all other interventions have been unsuccessful.

result from delirium, brain injury, or illnesses associated with aging (e.g., Alzheimer's disease, multi-infarct dementia). Delirium is a side effect of certain metabolic dysfunctions, such as electrolyte imbalance; it is time limited, ending when the underlying disorder is treated. Delirium is marked by clouded consciousness; decreased ability to shift, focus, and sustain attention to environmental stimuli; and disorientation. Hallmark symptoms include a short onset and waxing and waning of symptoms (American Psychiatric Association 1994).

Alzheimer's disease and multi-infarct dementia are progressive diseases of brain deterioration. The onset is slow and these diseases are ultimately fatal. Brain injury may be traumatic, or the result of illnesses such as carcinoma. Although symptoms and prognoses of such injuries are highly variable, depending on the cause and the affected area, they often have the following elements in common with delirium and illnesses such Alzheimer's disease: decreased impulse control, emotional lability, and decreased ability to interpret information from the environment. Clients who are unable to understand their environment can become anxious, frightened, angry, and assaultive. Their situation is analogous to that of an individual who remembers falling asleep at home but awakens in the morning in a train station in another country, surrounded by strangers and noise, with no recollection of coming there.

Traditional approaches to disorientation and to the agitation that it can cause have relied heavily on reality orientation and medication. Reality orientation consists of providing the correct information to the client about place, date, and current life circumstances. For many clients, this is comforting because it reminds them of pertinent information and helps them feel grounded. For others, reality orientation does not work and may cause further escalation. A client who does not understand the environment may also not be able to recognize or trust the caregiver. If the client is feeling frightened and threatened, information from a seeming stranger is suspect and becomes part of the confusion. Some disoriented clients believe that they are young and feel the need to return to important tasks that are specific to those earlier years. For example, an elderly woman may insist that she has babies at home that she needs to care for. This client is likely to become more agitated if the nurse tries to tell her that her babies have grown up and that there is no home to return to. A woman who believes that she is 23 years old and has babies at home would not be calmed by being told that she is 78 and has no babies. It is often more helpful in such a case to try and reflect back to clients their feelings and show understanding and concern for their plight. For example:

Nurse: Mrs. Green, you miss your children, and this can be a lonely place.

Sedating medication may calm agitation, but it also acts to further cloud a client's sensorium, making disorientation worse. A negative spiral of disorientation, agitation, medication, clouded consciousness, and further disorientation that leads to additional agitation and more medication may result. The outcome of such a spiral is generally oversedation—and possibly a hastened death from diseases related to inactivity.

Alternative interventions exist. Orientation aides, such as a calendar and a clock, can provide easy reference and increased autonomy; they must be prominent and must be easily read by clients with diminished eyesight. Because such clients have difficulty interpreting environmental stimuli, another set of interventions involves making the environment as simple, predictable, and comfortable as possible. Simplicity includes decreasing sensory stimuli. In the hospital, this might include placing the client's bed away from doorways that enter onto the hall and choosing not to turn on the television. Predictability can be provided by making each day's activity schedule as much like that of the previous day as possible; the days' schedule can be prominently posted in the client's room. Comfort might include familiar photographs, familiar objects from home, and a rocking chair; the latter can provide a rhythmic source of self-soothing.

If a client becomes agitated, a calm and unhurried approach is important to avoid further increasing the client's fear. A client who is uncertain of the surroundings feels further threatened by the rush toward him or her of one or more strangers who also appear agitated (i.e., staff). The steps for making contact with an agitated, disoriented client (catastrophic reaction) are listed in Box 12–3.

Episodes of agitation have been decreased in number and in intensity for clients with age-related dementias and in clients with head injuries as the result of identification of the antecedents and consequences of such episodes (Teri and Logsdon 1990; Uomoto and Brockway 1992). Once antecedents are understood, interventions are often obvious.

BOX 12–3 COGNITIVE DEFICITS

The Catastrophic Reaction: Making Contact

Cognitive deficits result in
- A decreased ability to interpret sensory stimuli.
- A decreased ability to tolerate sensory stimuli.

Striking out represents fear or the feeling that the environment is out of control

A second agitated person (e.g., staff) leads to increased agitation.

Therefore

1. Face the client from within 2 feet, remaining as calm and unhurried as possible.
2. Say the client's name.
3. Gain eye contact.
4. Smile.
5. Repeat 2) through 4) several times if necessary, to gain and maintain contact.
6. Use gentle touch, keep voice soft (the person often matches this tone and lowers his or her voice also).
7. Ask the client if he or she needs the bathroom.
8. Help the client regain a sense of control—ask what he or she needs.
9. Validate the client's feelings: "You look upset. This can be a confusing place."
10. Use short, simple sentences; complex explanations just represent more noise.
11. Decrease sensory stimulation.
12. Use rhythmic sources of self-stimulation, e.g., humming, a rocking chair.

Adapted from Rader, J., Doan, J., Schwab, M. (1985). How to decrease wandering, a form of agenda behavior. *Geriatric Nursing,* 6(4):196–199.

▸ An 81-year-old woman with Alzheimer's disease always becomes agitated during her morning care; this comes to be a time dreaded among her caregivers. Careful observation of the antecedents to episodes of agitation reveals a natural course to the morning problems. The client is initially calm when care begins. However, one staff person gives morning care to the client and her roommate at the same time, moving between the two. Observation of the process reveals that the client becomes distracted by cues being given to her roommate and often startles when the caregiver returns to her. As this process continues over several minutes, the client becomes increasingly distressed and then agitated. When her care is provided by one person who remains with her throughout the process, the client's morning agitation ends.

Consequences of agitation may also be a factor if they serve to reinforce the behaviors. For example, an elderly man who loves ice cream and who becomes calm when it is given to him becomes agitated more often when ice cream is routinely used to stop his angry behaviors. Previously high-functioning clients who have suffered a cerebral insult can be taught to monitor for individual signs of impending anger and to implement predesigned responses (e.g., taking a time-out).

Finally, clients who misperceive their setting or life situation may be calmed by **validation therapy** (Feil 1992). This intervention begins where clients are and grounds them where they feel most secure. Rather than attempting to re-orient the client, the nurse asks him or her to further describe the setting or situation that the client has reported as a problem (e.g., the need to return home). During the conversation, the nurse can comment on what appears to be underlying the client's distress, thus validating it. For example, the elderly woman who believes that she needs to return home to care for her children is asked to tell the nurse more about her children. The nurse may note that the client misses her children and that the current setting gets lonely at times. As nurses show interest in aspects of the client's life, they establish themselves as safe, understanding persons. In turn, the client often becomes calmer and more open to redirection. As they reminisce in this fashion, clients often bring themselves into the present: "Of course, they're all grown and doing well on their own now." Refer to Chapter 23 for more on interventions for people with cognitive impairments.

Box 12–4 provides a framework for a validation therapy.

BOX 12–4 COGNITIVE DEFICITS: VALIDATION THERAPY

This therapy lets you begin emotionally where the client is.

This therapy "grounds" the client where he or she feels most secure.

Reality orientation is the first intervention. Resistance to this may represent an increased feeling by the client that the environment makes no sense.

Therefore

1. Make the connection as described in Box 12–3.
2. Repeat some part of what the client has said: "You need to go home to fix dinner for your children?"
3. Reflect what seems to be the underlying feeling (usually related to a lack of connectedness or security): "You miss your children. And this can be a lonely place."
4. Continue to talk with the client about the topic (e.g., the children); this establishes you as a safe, understanding person.
5. As the client becomes calmer and more secure, redirect him or her (e.g., back to the client room).
6. Provide a parting reinforcer (e.g., food, rocking chair), an esteem-enhancing comment, or a reassuring comment.
7. Provide orienting information again only if the person requests it.

Adapted from Rader, J., Doan, J., Schwab, M. (1985). How to decrease wandering, a form of agenda behavior. *Geriatric Nursing,* 6(4):196–199.

Psychobiological Interventions

Medication for anger and aggression best targets the underlying cause of the anger. For example, antipsychotic medication is used for clients whose hallucinations, delusions, or thought disorder drive their anger. Similarly, manic clients who are irritable and show poor impulse control are helped by treatment with mood-stabilizing medications, such as lithium. In both these examples, benzodiazepines may be used until the primary medication has reached a therapeutic blood level or has had sufficient time to take effect.

In the absence of psychotic symptoms, antipsychotic medications are not the best choice for the treatment of aggression. This use relies solely on the sedative effects of the drug and it places clients at risk for side effects, including the permanent and disfiguring tardive dyskinesia.

Benzodiazepine use for aggression is always short term. With long-term use, clients develop tolerance to its sedative effects, are at increased risk for side effects, and may develop psychological dependence on the drug. In a small number of clients, benzodiazepines have led to paradoxical rage responses, indicating that careful observation is necessary when these drugs are used for calming agitated, aggressive clients.

Unfortunately, the psychological mechanisms contributing to anger are not always clear. In many cases, nurses rely on empirical research about the effects of medication on anger in various client populations. For example, fluoxetine was found to decrease anger in clients with borderline personality disorder, independent of changes in their depression (Salzman et al. 1995). This effect is likely a function of the role serotonin has been found to play in impulsive aggression. Fluoxetine has also been found to decrease sudden attacks of anger in a subgroup of depressed clients for whom such anger was an added symptom (Fava et al. 1993).

Impulsive anger related to brain injury, either from trauma or illnesses such as stroke, has been found to respond to beta blockers (e.g., propranolol). In many of the clinical trials reported with these clients, beta blockers were successful after multiple failed attempts with antipsychotics, benzodiazepines, anticonvulsants, and lithium. Improvement was marked or moderate in as many as 75% of clients in some reports (Williams et al. 1982; Greendyke et al. 1984). An 8-week trial may be necessary with beta blockers. In addition, these drugs can increase blood levels of certain antipsychotic medications, leading to increased side effects or toxicity. Other common side effects are bradycardia, hypotension, and occasional depression.

Haloperidol (Haldol)	• Should be limited to psychosis-induced violence. • Not to be used for aggression alone for more than 6 weeks.
Lorazepam (Ativan)	Initially 1 to 2 mg orally or intramuscularly every hour until calm. Taper at 10% a day from highest dose to avoid withdrawal symptoms unless the drug is used less than a week. Not to be used for aggression alone for more than 6 weeks.
Trazodone (Desyrel)	Acutely lowers aggression and agitation in demented or mentally retarded clients without impairing cognition. Doses up to 500 mg have been used.

All psychoactive drugs must be used with caution, and with elderly clients, drugs are usually given in doses lower than what would normally be considered therapeutic. Elderly clients are often sensitive to psychiatric medications; they have side effects and toxic effects more quickly than younger clients. Treatment effects can regularly be seen at lower-than-usual doses. For these clients, pharmacotherapy is best begun slowly and dosages raised gradually.

Similarly, clients of differing ethnic groups and of differing national origin respond differently from each other in both the treatment effects and the side effects of medications, including psychiatric medications. These differences are in part a function of differing drug effects at the cellular level and are thought to result from both genetic and environmental factors (e.g., diet). Pharmacotherapy is again best begun slowly, with dosages raised gradually; several drug trials may be required before the most useful regimen is found. As with all clients, concern must be taken for client reports of effects and side effects; translators and experts in the client's culture may be necessary for these reports to be obtained most accurately (Lin et al. 1995).

Maxmen and Ward (1995) stated that it is important to identify whether the presenting behavior is acute aggression or chronic aggression.

Acute aggression can be medically managed best by either (Maxmen and Ward 1995).

Chronic aggression is a more common problem, and aggression may diminish only after a therapeutic dose level of the appropriate medication exists for about 4 to 8 weeks. Clients should be informed about this time lag. Drugs used to treat clients with chronic aggression include propranolol, anticonvulsants (carbamazepine, valproic acid), lithium, and buspirone. Caution is taken when chronic aggression is treated with antipsychotics (risk of tardive dyskinesia, hypotension, oversedation), and benzodiazepines, which rarely halt chronic violence and may trigger paradoxical rage reaction (Maxmen and Ward 1995).

A summary of medications used in the treatment of persistent aggression is given in Table 12–6.

TABLE 12–6 PSYCHOTROPIC TREATMENT OF CHRONIC AGGRESSION

GENERIC GROUP	INDICATIONS	COMMENTS
Beta blockers, e.g., propranolol	Recurrent or chronic aggression in organically based violence, e.g. ▸ Alzheimer's disease ▸ Stroke ▸ Huntington's disease Psychosis in which aggression is unrelated to psychotic thought	Often used in high doses (120–240 mg/day). Consistent and effective results may take 4–8 weeks.
Anticonvulsants	Bipolar disorder Borderline personality disorder Conduct disorder Episodic dyscontrol Posttraumatic stress disorder (PTSD) Central nervous system disorder	Carbamazepine—monitor bone marrow suppression and blood abnormalities Valproic acid—monitor liver function and platelets.
Lithium	Mania-associated violence Uncontrolled rage triggered by nothing or minor stimuli, e.g., borderline personality disorder, PTSD	Effective for violence in prisoners and mentally retarded. Does not affect aggressive behavior until therapeutic blood levels are reached
Buspirone (BuSpar)	Cognitively impaired populations and possibly prison populations	Nonsedating and nonaddicting. Effectiveness takes 4–10 weeks to decrease aggression.
Nadolol	Diminishes assaultiveness in chronic paranoid schizophrenia	Few reports.
Trazodone	Aggression and agitation in demented and mentally retarded (does not impair cognition).	Do not use in males who cannot report priapism. Monitor for orthostatic hypotension.

Adapted from Maxmen, J. S., and Ward, N. G. (1995). *Psychotropic drugs fast facts* (2nd ed., pp. 233–236). New York: W. W. Norton. Copyright © 1995 by Nicholas J. Ward and the Estate of Jerrold S. Maxmen. Copyright © 1991 by Jerrold S. Maxmen. Reprinted by permission of W. W. Norton & Company, Inc.

Risk for Violence: Use of Restraints

At times, the best early assessment and intervention, whether behavioral or medicinal, is unsuccessful in calming an aggressive client. If that client presents risk to himself or others, seclusion or restraint is necessary. Use of seclusion or restraint in these circumstances demonstrates the value of human life by preventing clients from harming themselves or others.

Seclusion is the involuntary confinement of a client alone in a room, which the client is prevented from leaving, for a specific period of time. The goal of seclusion is never punitive. Rather, as noted earlier, *the goal is safety of the client and others.* Certain clients are able to control their aggression without restraint as long as they are alone or are in an environment of very low stimulation. Other clients may be coming out of a period of time in restraints and may need a period of time in seclusion in order to make a successful transition back onto the unit or into the normal living environment. As a part of this transition, clients may be placed on a schedule that alternates periods of seclusion with increasing time in the ward community (e.g., 45 minutes in seclusion, alternating with 15 minutes out, followed by 30 minutes in seclusion and 30 minutes out).

Seclusion or physical restraint is not used unless alternative interventions have been considered, including verbal intervention, behavioral care plan, medication, decrease in sensory stimulation, removal of a particular problematic stimulus, presence of a significant other, frequent observation, and use of a sitter. Seclusion or restraint are used in circumstances where the client

- Presents a clear and present danger to self.
- Presents a clear and present danger to others.
- Has been legally detained for involuntary treatment and is thought to be an escape risk.
- Requests to be secluded or restrained.

The mechanism for placing an aggressive client in restraints requires having an adequate number of staff available, all of whom have been trained in restraint procedures. Staff who work in areas where potentially aggressive clients are regularly treated, such as EDs and sychiatric units, are required to have regular training and practice in restraint procedures. Such training and practice increase staff proficiency in the use of restraints and decrease the possibilities of injury to staff or clients.

Clients may not be held in seclusion or restraint without a physician's order. Once in restraint, clients must be directly observed at frequent, regular intervals for level of awareness, level of activity, safety within the restraints, hydration, toileting, nutrition, and comfort. The frequency of observation is mandated by licensing and accreditation agencies. Refer to Chapter 4 for more on the legalities of seclusion and restraints and Chapter 21 for more on the procedure.

A sample restraint protocol is given in Table 12–7.

EVALUATION

Evaluation of the care plan is essential with clients who are potentially angry and aggressive. A well-considered plan has specific outcome criteria goals (e.g., see Tables 12–1 through 12–5). Evaluation provides information about whether the interventions have met these goals; if they have not, the plan must be adjusted. The plan is also individualized. For example, an initial care plan may include assessment of the environmental stimuli that precede a client's agitation. Once these have been identified, the plan provides interventions that are specific to those stimuli. However, the plan can work only if staff evaluate the effectiveness of this approach by noting whether the agitation has decreased or disappeared. Evaluation may reveal that the client's agitation has decreased except for specific situations. The plan can then be adjusted to include these situations.

Evaluation allows staff to recognize the aspects of the plan that work and provides information about the aspects that do not. With this information, the plan can be continually improved, such that the ultimate goal—safety for clients and staff—is met.

SUMMARY

Anger and aggression are difficult targets for nursing intervention. Since these two emotions are universal, nurses benefit from an understanding of how the angry and aggressive client should be handled. An understanding of client cues to escalating aggression, appropriate goals for intervention for individuals in a variety of situations, and helpful nursing interventions is important for nurses in any setting.

Numerous theories exist that help explain why anger for some gets out of control; the theories can help us understand what triggers and escalates aggression in various individuals. As opposed to older beliefs, it has been found that "getting it all out" is not, after all, a useful way to diminish anger. On the contrary, it has been found that the expression of anger can lead to increased anger and to negative physiological changes. There are, however, two theories of anger and aggression that have led to useful management techniques that are beneficial for clients who escalate out of control. These two theories are the (1) behavioral theory and (2) cognitive theory of anger and aggression. A third theory of anger and aggression is biological theory, which helps explain why some people

TABLE 12–7 SAMPLE RESTRAINT PROTOCOL

ACTION	INFORMATION
1. Use verbal interventions whenever possible to help prevent aggressive or destructive client behavior. Verbally try to persuade the client not to follow through with the violent act: a. Provide reassurance. b. Offer an alternative. c. Identify the danger and consequence of the intended action. d. Establish the limits.	
2. If verbal interventions are unsuccessful, call for a show of force.	A show of force often results in the client's reconsidering his or her action. A minimum of eight people is gathered, and a leader is designated.
3. The designated leader will a. Assign staff to clear all clients and visitors from the area. b. Assign staff to obtain restraints.	
c. Maintain communication with the client throughout the procedure or designate someone else to do this.	Only the person designated to talk with the client during the procedure should do so.
d. Decide when to restrain the client.	The client may choose to walk to a seclusion room.
e. Make limb assignments; include at least one staff member at the client's head, at each arm, and at each leg.	
4. Approach client as a group. The person assigned to talk with client states the purpose of the action and talks the client through the procedure. a. Reassure the client. b. Give the client the opportunity to regain control.	A coordinated approach promotes safety, decreases confusion, and decreases client and staff anxiety.
5. Physically immobilize the client when the leader gives the order.	Use a predetermined command, e.g., "Hands on."
a. Hold the legs at the ankle and above the knee, and hold the arms at the wrist and above the elbow.	
b. Lift the client by the assigned limb and carry to the bed or stretcher when directed by the leader.	Direct pressure over kneecap or elbow may cause injury.
c. Place the client in a supine position.	
d. Avoid applying pressure on the client's neck or mouth.	If the client spits, a towel may be loosely placed over his or her mouth.
e. Assess the client's airway and the ability to breathe.	Do not obstruct or compromise airway.
6. Apply restraints in the following order: waist, both wrists, both ankles.	Place restraints so that they are secure but do not abrade the skin or decrease circulation.
7. Search the client for dangerous objects.	
8. Process (review with others) the restraint procedure on its completion.	The leader is responsible for calling a post-restraint debriefing.
9. Complete an incident report, including the client behavior that resulted in the use of restraint and the other interventions that were attempted first.	
10. Obtain a physician's order for restraint within 1 hour of the use of restraint.	
11. Ensure client comfort: a. Check restraints every 15 minutes and document on the patient restraint flowsheet. b. Institute comfort measures, e.g., offering fluids and providing for elimination at regular intervals. Document on the flowsheet. c. Evaluate the client's need for medication.	Frequent position changes, massages of skin, and range of motion exercises prevent prolonged pressure against blood vessels or peripheral nerves.
12. Protect the client from others while he or she is in the highly vulnerable restrained state.	
13. Use verbal interventions with the client to help diminish the time in restraints. a. Provide a short period for the client to become calm. b. Explore with the client the events that caused him or her to lose control. c. Problem-solve and explore alternatives.	
14. Gradually remove physical restraints in order to test the client's control. Document the client's response.	Remove one limb at a time, at regular intervals. Remove waist and wrist restraint together; remove these last.

are more prone to anger and aggressive behavior than others in terms of genetic inheritance and some medical conditions (temporal lobe epilepsy, traumatic head injury, Alzheimer's disease).

It is helpful for health care workers to know what cues should be looked for and what should be assessed when a client's anger is escalating (verbal cues, nonverbal cues that include facial expression, breathing, body language, and posture). A client's past aggressive behavior is also an important indicator to future aggressive episodes.

Working with angry and aggressive clients is a challenge for all nurses, and a careful understanding and recognition of one's personal responses to angry or threatening clients can be crucial. We all possess personal dynamics that may trigger emotions and reactions that are not always therapeutic with specific clients. Unexamined responses to angry clients, even though they reflect those of society or the nurse's personal culture, may strongly influence unhelpful or even provocative responses to threatening clients. Certain types of clients may evoke feelings of dislike, irritability, or fear in the nurse. If these feelings remain unexamined, they can influence interactions that may precipitate or even escalate aggressive or angry behavior.

After a threatening event, a critical-incident debriefing meeting to review the process and allow people to describe their feelings can help prevent PTR in staff and help gather information to help minimize similar future events.

Many approaches are effective in helping clients de-escalate and maintain control. For clients with ineffective individual coping, different interventions exist for clients who are overwhelmed, have maladaptive patterns of coping, and are psychotic. In addition, there are different settings in which staff approach and milieu management are extremely important in helping to de-escalate client anger. These interventions may be different in the inpatient psychiatric setting than they would be for the ED or even for outpatient settings.

For clients with cognitive deficits, a whole different set of interventions can be extremely useful in allaying a client's anxiety and minimizing aggressive behavior. At times, specific medications may be useful, and at other times, usually as a last resort when other interventions have been tried and failed, restraints may be needed to protect the safety of the client as well as other clients and the staff. Each unit has a clear protocol for the safe administration of restraints and for the humane management of care during the time the client is restrained, as well as clear guidelines for understanding the client's legal rights.

REFERENCES

American Psychiatric Association (1994). *Diagnostic and statistical manual of mental disorders* (4th ed.). Washington, DC: American Psychiatric Association.

Anderson, S., and Lawler, K. (1995). The anger recall interview and cardiovascular reactivity in women: An examination of context and experience. *Journal of Psychosomatic Research*, 39(3):335–343.

Bandura, A. (1973). *Aggression: A social learning analysis*. New York: Prentice Hall.

Beck, A. (1976). *Cognitive therapy and the emotional disorders*. New York: International Universities Press.

Beck, A., et al. (1979). *Cognitive therapy of depression*. New York: Guilford Press.

Beck, A., and Freeman, A. (1990). *Cognitive therapy of personality disorders*. New York: Guilford Press.

Berkowitz, L. (1982). Aversive conditions as stimuli to aggression. In L. Berkowitz (Ed.), *Advances in experimental psychology*. San Diego: Academic Press.

Berkowitz, L. (1983). In R. G. Green and E. I. Donnerstein (Eds.), *Aggression: Theoretical and empirical views* (Vol. 1). New York: Academic Press.

Blue, H., and Griffith, E. (1995). Sociocultural and therapeutic perspectives on violence. *Psychiatric Clinics of North America*, 18(3):571–587.

Brown, C., et al. (1989). Blood platelet uptake of serotonin in episodic aggression. *Psychiatry Research*, 27(1):5–12.

Burman, B., Margolin, G., and John, R. (1993). America's angriest home videos: Behavioral contingencies observed in home reenactments of marital conflict. *Journal of Consulting and Clinical Psychology*, 61(1):28–39.

Cadoret, R. (1982). Genotype-environmental interaction in antisocial behavior. *Psychological Medicine*, 12:235–239.

Cadoret, R., et al. (1985). Alcoholism and antisocial personality disorder: Interrelationships, genetic and environmental factors. *Archive of General Psychiatry*, 42:161–167.

Cloninger, C., et al. (1982). Predisposition to petty criminality in Swedish adoptees: II. Cross-fostering analysis of gene-environment interaction. *Archives of General Psychiatry*, 39:1242–1249.

Cooper, A., and Mendonca, J. (1989). A prospective study of patients' assaults on nursing staff in a psychogeriatric unit. *Canadian Journal of Psychiatry*, 34(5):399–404.

Dahl, A. (1994). Heredity in personality disorders: An overview. *Clinical Genetics*, 46:138–143.

Davis, D., and Boster, L. (1988). Multifaceted therapeutic interventions with the violent psychiatric inpatient. *Hospital and Community Psychiatry*, 39(8):867–869.

Davis, S. (1991). Violence by psychiatric inpatients: A review. *Hospital and Community Psychiatry*, 42:585–590.

Davison, G., et al. (1991). Relaxation, reduction in angry articulated thoughts, and improvements in borderline hypertension and heart rate. *Journal of Behavioral Medicine*, 14(5):453–468.

DiLalla, L., and Gottesman, I. (1991). Biologic and genetic contributors to violence: Widom's untold tale. *Psychological Bulletin*, 109(1):125–129.

Doren, D. (1996). *Understanding and treating the psychopath*. Northvale, NJ: J. Aronson.

Durivage, D. (1989). Assaultive behavior: Before it happens. *Canadian Journal of Psychiatry*, 34(5):393–397.

Ekman, P. (1972). *Darwin and facial expression: A century of research in review*. New York: Academic Press.

Ekman, P., Levenson, R., and Friesen, W. (1983). Autonomic nervous system activity distinguishes among emotions. *Science*, 221(4616):1208–1210.

Esterling, B., et al. (1990). Emotional repression, stress disclosure responses, and Epstein-Barr viral capsid antigen titers. *Psychosomatic Medicine*, 52(4):397–410.

Fava, M., et al. (1993). Anger attacks in unipolar depression: I. Clinical correlates and response to fluoxetine treatment. *American Journal of Psychiatry*, 150(8):1158–1163.

Feil, N. (1992). *Validation: The Feil method*. Cleveland: Edward Feil Productions.

Feinberg, T., et al. (1986). Facial discrimination and emotional recognition in schizophrenia and affective disorders. *Archives of General Psychiatry*, 43(3):276–279.

Freud, S. (1933). *New introductory lectures on psychoanalysis*. New York: Morton.

Gallop, R., McCay, E., and Esplen, M. (1992). The conceptualization of impulsivity for psychiatric nursing practice. *Archives of Psychiatric Nursing*, 6(6):366–373.

Gentry, W. (1985). Relationship of anger-coping styles and blood pressure among black Americans. In M. A. Chesney and R. H. Roseman (Eds.), *Anger and hostility in cardiovascular and behavioral disorders* (pp. 139–147). Washington, DC: Hemisphere Publishing.

Gerlock, A. (1994). Veterans' responses to anger management intervention. *Issues in Mental Health Nursing*, 15(4):393–408.

Gin, N., et al. (1991). Prevalence of domestic violence among patients in three ambulatory care internal medicine clinics. *Journal of General Internal Medicine*, 6(4):317–322.

Greendyke, R., Schuster, D., and Wooten, J. (1984). Propanolol in the treatment of assaultive patients with organic brain disease. *Journal of Clinical Psychopharmacology*, 4:282–285.

Harburg, E., et al. (1991). Anger-coping styles and blood pressure in black and white males: Buffalo, New York. *Psychosomatic Medicine*, 53(2):153–164.

Jacobs, H. (1987). The Los Angeles head injury survey: Project rationale and design implications. *Journal of Head Trauma Rehabilitation*, 2(3):37–50.

Jensen, M. (1987). Psychobiological factors predicting the course of breast cancer. *Journal of Personality*, 55(3):317–342.

Jones, M. (1953). *The therapeutic community*. New York: Basic Books.

Julius, S., Schneider, R., and Egan, B. (1985). Suppressed anger in hypertension: Facts and problems. In M. A. Chesney and R. H. Rosenman (Eds.), *Anger and hostility in cardiovascular and behavioral disorders* (pp. 127–135). Washington, DC: Hemisphere Publishing.

Katz, P., and Kirkland, F. (1990). Violence and social structure on mental hospital wards. *Psychiatry*, 53:262–277.

Kinkle, S. (1993). Violence in the ED: How to stop it before it starts. *American Journal of Nursing*, 93(7):22–24.
Kua, E., and Ko, S. (1991). Family violence and Asian drinkers. *Forensic Science International*, 50(1):43–46.
Lancee, W., et al. (1995). The relationship between nurses' limit-setting styles and anger in psychiatric inpatients. *Psychiatric Services*, 46(6):609–613.
Lanza, M. (1988). Factors relevant to patient assault. *Issues in Mental Health Nursing*, 9:239–258.
Lanza, M., et al. (1994). Environmental characteristics related to patient assaults. *Issues in Mental Health Nursing*, 15:319–335.
Levenson, R., Ekman, P., and Friesen, W. (1990). Voluntary facial action generates emotion-specific autonomic nervous system activity. *Psychophysiology*, 27(4):363–384.
Lin, K., Anderson, D., and Poland, R. (1995). Ethnicity and psychopharmacology: Bridging the gap. *Psychiatric Clinics of North America*, 18(3):635–648.
Linehan, M. (1993a). *Cognitive-behavioral treatment of borderline personality disorder.* New York: Guilford Press.
Linehan, M. (1993b). *Skills training manual for treating borderline personality disorder.* New York: Guilford Press.
Lorenz, K. (1966). *On aggression.* New York: Bantam Books.
Lyon, J., Henggeler, S., and Hall, J. (1992). The family relations, peer relations, and criminal activities of Caucasian and Hispanic-American gang members. *Journal of Abnormal Child Psychology*, 20(5):439–449.
Manuck, S., et al. (1985). Behavioral factors in hypertension: Cardiovascular responsivity, anger, and social competence. In M. A. Chesney and R. H. Rosenman (Eds.), *Anger and hostility in cardiovascular and behavioral disorders* (pp. 149–172). Washington, DC: Hemisphere Publishing.
Maxmen, J. S., and Ward, N. G. (1995). *Psychotropic drugs fast facts* (2nd ed.). New York: W. W. Norton.
McNeil, D., and Binder, R. (1995). Correlates of accuracy in the assessment of psychiatric inpatients' risk of violence. *American Journal of Psychiatry*, 152(6):901–906.
Moos, R. (1974a). *Evaluating treatment environments.* New York: John Wiley.
Moos, R. (1974b). *Ward Atmosphere Scale manual.* Palo Alto, CA: Consulting Psychologists.
National Television Violence Study Council (1996). National violence study: Council statement. Studio City, CA: MediaScope.
Nield-Anderson, L. and Doubrava, J. (1993). Defusing verbal abuse: A program for emergency department triage nurses. *Journal of Emergency Nursing*, 19(5):441–445.
Novaco R. (1976). The functions and regulations of the arousal of anger. *American Journal of Psychiatry*, 133(10):1124–1127.
Novaco, R. (1985). Anger and its therapeutic regulation. In M. A. Chesney and R. H. Rosenman (Eds.), *Anger and hostility in cardiovascular and behavioral disorders* (pp. 203–222). New York: McGraw-Hill.
Oster, C. (1976). Sensory deprivation in geriatric patients. *Journal of the American Geriatrics Society*, 24(10):461–463.
Outlaw, F. (1993). Stress and coping: The influence of race on the cognitive appraisal processing of African-Americans. *Issues in Mental Health Nursing*, 14:399–409.
Rappaport, D. (1967). *The collected papers of David Rappaport.* New York: Basic Books.
Reeder, D. (1991). Cognitive therapy of anger management: theoretical and practical considerations. *Archives of Psychiatric Nursing*, 5(3):147–150.
Rossi, A., et al. (1986). Characteristics of psychiatric patients who engage in assaultive or other fear-inducing behaviors. *Journal of Nervous and Mental Disease*, 174(3):154–160.
Ryan, J., and Poster, E. (1989). The assaulted nurse: Short-term and long-term responses. *Archives of Psychiatric Nursing*, 3(6):323–331.
Salzman, C., et al. (1995). Effect of fluoxetine on anger in symptomatic volunteers with borderline personality disorder. *Journal of Clinical Psychopharmacology*, 15(1):23–29.
Sheridan, M., et al. (1990). Precipitants of violence in a psychiatric inpatient setting. *Hospital and Community Psychiatry*, 41(7):776–780.
Siegman, A. (1993). Cardiovascular consequences of expressing, experiencing, and repressing anger. *Journal of Behavioral Medicine*, 16(6):539–569.
Siegman, A., Anderson, R., and Berger, T. (1990). The angry voice: Its effects on the experience of anger and cardiovascular reactivity. *Psychosomatic Medicine*, 52(6):631–643.
Skinner, B. (1953). *Science and human behavior.* New York: Macmillan.
Smith, M., and Hart, G. (1994). Nurses' responses to patient anger: From disconnecting to connecting. *Journal of Advanced Nursing*, 20(4):643–651.
Soloff, P. (1983). Seclusion and restraint. In J. Lion and W. Reid (Eds.), *Assaults within psychiatric facilities* (pp. 241–264). New York: Grune & Stratton.
Suedfeld, P. (1969). Introduction and historical background. In J. P. Zubeck (Ed.), *Sensory deprivation: 15 years of research* (p. 4). New York: Appleton-Century-Crofts.
Temoshok, L. (1987). Psychoimmunology and AIDS. *Clinical Immunology Newsletter*, 9:113–116.
Teri, L., and Logsdon, R. (1990). Assessment and management of behavioral disturbances in Alzheimer's disease. *Comprehensive Therapy*, 16(5):36–42.
Uomoto, J., and Brockway, J. (1992). Anger management training for brain injured patients and their family members. *Archives of Physical Medicine and Rehabilitation*, 73(7):674–679.
Valdez, A., et al. (1995). Illegal drug use, alcohol and aggressive crime among Mexican-American and white male arrestees in San Antonio. *Journal of Psychoactive Drugs*, 27(2):135–143.
Virkkunen, M., et al. (1994). CSF biochemistries, glucose metabolism, and diurnal activity rhythms in alcoholic, violent offenders, fire setters, and healthy volunteers. *Archives of General Psychiatry*, 51(20):20–27.
Watson, J. (1992). Maintenance of therapeutic community principles in an age of biopharmacology and economic restraints. *Archives of Psychiatric Nursing*, 6(3):183–188.
Whetsell, L., Patterson, C., and Young, D. (1989). Pre-injury psychopathology in trauma patients. *Journal of Trauma*, 2(8):1158–1161.
White, J., and Koss, M. (1991). Courtship violence: Incidence in a national sample of higher education students. *Violence and Victims*, 6(4):247–256.
Williams, D., et al. (1982). The effect of propranolol on uncontrolled rage outbursts in children and adolescents with organic brain dysfunction. *Journal of the American Academy of Child Psychiatry*, 21:129–135.
Wolkowitz, O., and Pickar, D. (1991). Benzodiazepines in the treatment of schizophrenia: A review and reappraisal. *American Journal of Psychiatry*, 148(6):714–126.

SELF-STUDY AND CRITICAL THINKING

Write a short response.

1. Describe the importance of predictability with clients who are potentially angry. Give one clinical example of the use of predictability.
2. Withdrawal of attention to verbally abusive behaviors works only if the strategy is accompanied by what additional intervention?
3. Modulation of sensory stimulation can be an important nursing intervention for potential anger. Describe one instance in which sensory stimulation should be increased. Describe one instance in which sensory stimulation should be decreased.
4. What are the four criteria for the use of seclusion or restraint rather than verbal interventions?
5. What assumptions does Linehan suggest in order for clinicians to maintain an empathetic approach to clients with maladaptive coping patterns?
6. List and briefly describe three key concepts that explain anger and aggression.
7. What potential problems are presented by the presence of drugs or alcohol in a client in the emergency department?

True or false

Write in T—if true or F—if false. If false, explain why and correct statement.

8. The following limit-setting statements would be likely to work with an irritable, impulsive psychiatric client:

_________ Loud music can be disturbing to other clients.
_________ I know that music sounds better when it's played at top volume, but you can't play it that loudly on the unit.
_________ You like it better loud, don't you? It's too loud for the dayroom. Would you like the earphones, or would listening to it in your room be better?
_________ Either use the earphones or go to your room to listen to your music.

9. Which of the following statements about expressing one's anger are true?

_________ Expressing anger when it occurs is always useful because it prevents long-term health effects caused by holding anger in.
_________ Briefly withholding anger while searching for a solution to the provocation leads to the fewest cardiac complications.There are no physiologic consequences to making an angry facial expression in order to emphasize a point in an argument.
_________ Interventions to client anger can be made at a cognitive, behavioral, or physiologic level.
_________ A client with a severe personality disorder and a long history of chemical dependence cannot learn anger management skills.
_________ Teaching a client to pound on his or her pillow when angry is one strategy for decreasing potential client aggression.
_________ A client who raises his or her voice will likely continue to escalate in anger unless convinced to speak more softly.

Multiple choice

10. Which of the following clients present special considerations when medications are being used to treat impulsive aggression?

A. Young adults
B. Middle-aged women
C. The elderly
D. Anyone who is not from the dominant ethnic group
E. Those with a psychotic illness

11. Which of the following statements about ethnicity and aggression are true?

A. Research has not supported a link between ethnicity and aggression.
B. African American men are overrepresented in the criminal justice system.
C. Ethnicity is one factor leading to overprediction of violence on inpatient psychiatric units.
D. Manifestations of the basic psychiatric illnesses such as schizophrenia are straightforward, independent of patients' ethnicity or culture.
E. In general, each culture's views of illness and health care are homogeneous within the culture.

Critical thinking

12. A 79-year-old woman is admitted to the medical unit of a hospital with increasing shortness of breath and irregular pulse. The client, despite her difficulties and obvious anxiety, is gracious with the nurses and shows a delightful sense of humor;

she is fully oriented. An admitting examination is performed, and medications are prescribed. During her first night on the unit, the client is found wandering in the hall, agitated and believing she is in danger. When approached by the nurse, the client hits at her. What would the first nursing intervention be?

What additional interventions might be used?

What nursing assessments would be important once the client has become calm?

What medications would ideally be used for the client's agitation? Based on what considerations?

13. A 24-year-old man is admitted to an inpatient unit because of command hallucinations telling him to kill himself. The client has a 5-year history of schizophrenia. Staff notes that the client is irritable and has a history of assault. What interventions should be built into the care plan?
14. A psychiatric nurse is threatened over the period of 2 days by a client whose aggression has led to his remaining in restraint during that time and requiring frequent checks for comfort and safety as well as basic nursing care. The nurse has had a nightmare in which the client is chasing him and also has had intrusive images of the client standing behind him. When discussing these signs, the nurse wonders if he is foreseeing his future. What interventions should be made?

Part II

Foundations in Practice

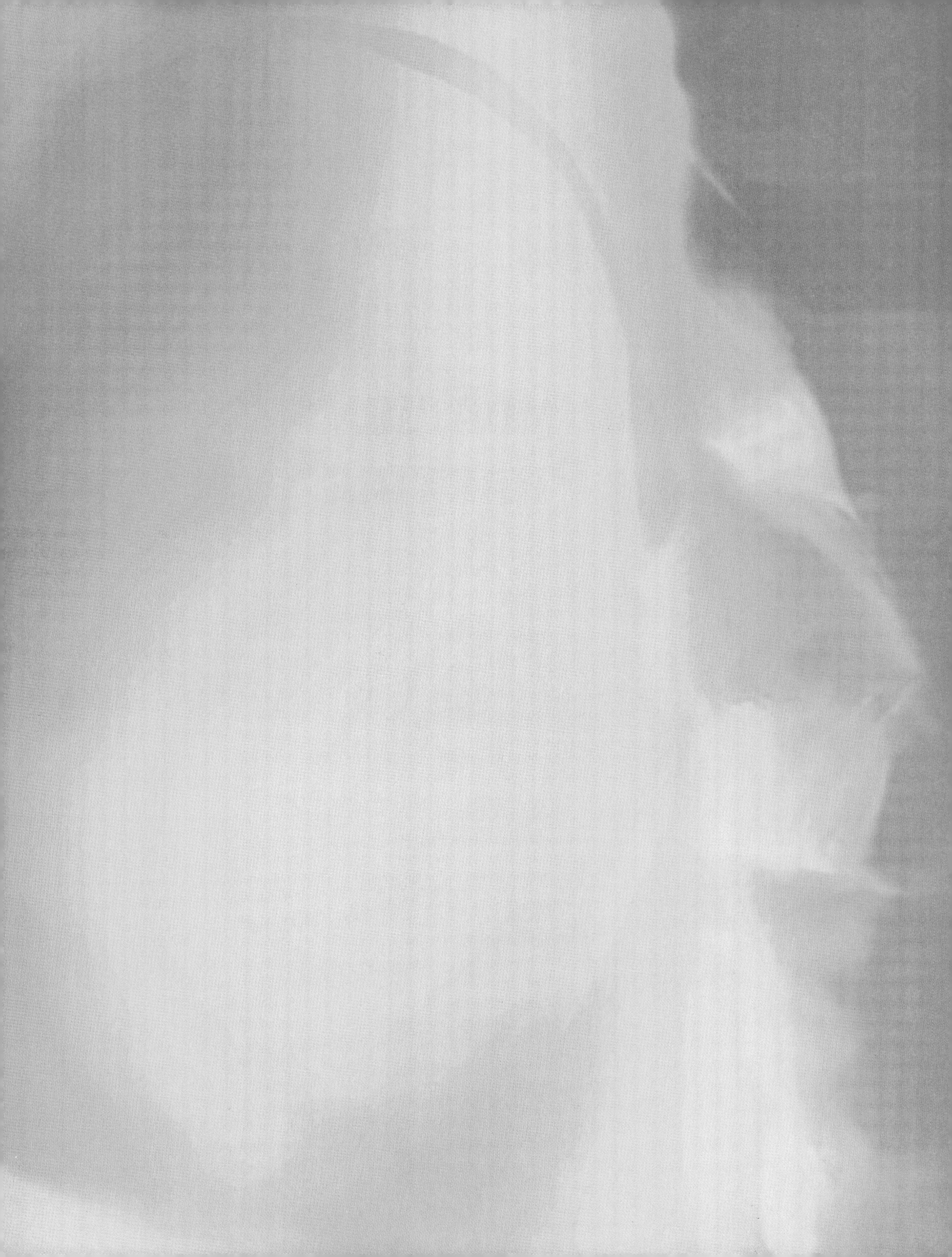

UNIT THREE

Stress and People in Crises

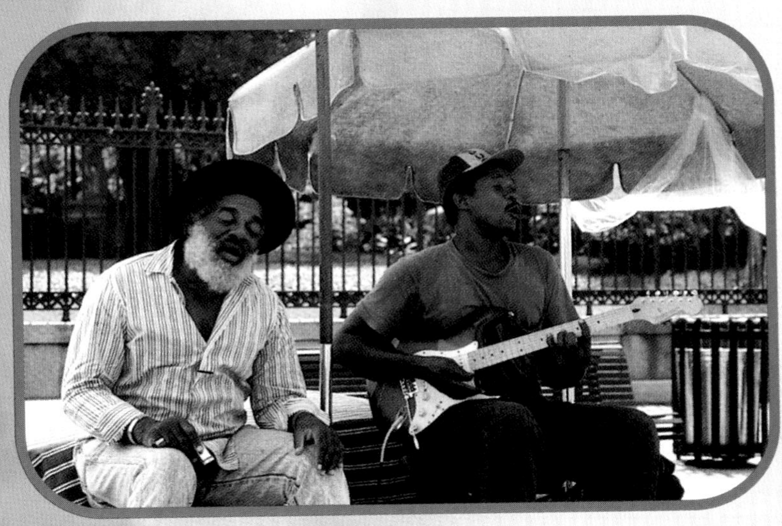

. . . drag your thoughts away from your troubles—by the ears, by the heels, or any other way, so you can manage it; it's the healthiest thing a body can do.

MARK TWAIN, *THE AMERICAN CLAIMANT*

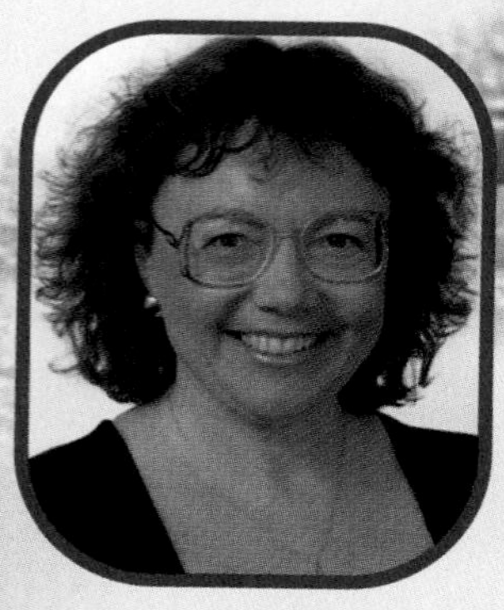

A Nurse Speaks

Maureen H. McCracken

I am a holistic psychiatric mental health clinical nurse specialist certified by the American Nurses' Association in Adult, Adolescent, and Child Mental Health Nursing in Herndon, Virginia. I am also a Healing Touch Practitioner and Instructor certified by the American Holistic Nurses Association. In my private practice, I provide psychotherapy and Healing Touch (HT) (an eclectic course of energy work developed by Janet Mentgen, RN) and a few other complementary health modalities. HT, my focus for this article, is a modern version of the ancient art of laying on of hands. HT is heart-centered work using the practitioner's hands and intention to bring balance and harmony into the human energy system. Used in combination with psychotherapy, it can accelerate emotional, mental, and spiritual healing. HT may work where words fail. In work with couples, it can at times bring a deeper understanding than discussion. At other times I find it may break through an impasse when preverbal memories need to be released.

When do I do HT with my psychotherapy clients? What is it like?

Clients may benefit from HT when they are anxious; when they are in a manic or depressed phase; when they are grieving or going through a major life transition such as birth, death, divorce, or even graduation. They may also benefit when in troubled relationships. HT is also preventive. Frequently I will offer HT when physical conditions are present and the client would benefit from alleviation of pain or infection. HT induces the relaxation response, reduces anxiety, reduces the perception of pain (in some cases, eliminating it entirely), and may accelerate wound healing physically, mentally, emotionally, and spiritually. It is believed to work on the autonomic nervous system, particularly the parasympathetic and neuroendocrine systems.

Therapeutic Touch (TT) was brought into the nursing field 20 years ago by Dolores Krieger, PhD. TT is now taught in 70 countries and in more than 80 universities. If the client has not been watching the recent television and radio presentations regarding alternative medicine, Therapeutic and Healing Touch, she may feel reassured to know that TT has been used in nursing for over 20 years and is one of the most widely researched topics in the nursing community.

In psychotherapy, the word "touch" can be a risky one to use owing to transference, ethical/professional issues, and sexual abuse issues. Fortunately, HT or TT can be used entirely off the body (2 to 12 inches off the body) and is being used in hospitals and outpatient settings for a variety of purposes, particularly for reducing anxiety and pain. Unlike other psychotherapists, nurses are specifically licensed to touch, and HT is an effective, noninvasive, natural, nonpharmaceutical, and economical technique.

The first time I ever used HT was with a nurse who was coming to see me for depression. One day she came after dental surgery with a jaw so swollen she couldn't speak. I offered HT after inquiring whether she had heard of TT. She had heard of it and was very interested in it. I spent 10 to 15 minutes "unruffling" (gentle, rhythmical vertical hand movements) the field outside her jaw, which totally eliminated the pain, and she was able to talk for the rest of the session.

I have used HT in a family session. A mother of a hyperactive, oppositional child came to me with depression, irritability, and screaming attacks. She brought the child with her and was not sure if she could continue to provide care for this child because of her high blood glucose and high blood pressure. She feared that she would have a stroke or go into diabetic coma. I worked with her for about 45 minutes using HT techniques. During the treatment, the child played quietly with a dollhouse. After the session, the mother felt calm. She reported to me at the next visit that her blood glucose and pressure had lowered by 10 to 20 points.

A young man came to see me who had been diagnosed with an obsessive-compulsive disorder—rituals and obsessions that interfered with his job and marital relationship. Although I was using cognitive techniques with him, HT seemed to him to provide the most benefit. He ended therapy after four sessions in control of his symptoms.

One young woman suffered from chronic headaches and depression. Her history included severe sexual and emotional abuse. At one time, she had gone to her doctors every day for headaches. Amitrex had failed, and sometimes the only thing that worked was intravenous Demerol. With HT treatment, she was able to reduce her doctor's visits to once a week.

HT came into my life with the grace of an oncoming storm when my life needed healing. I signed up for one weekend of training and went on as if on a trajectory to complete the training through the instructor level. It has brought joy and healing into my life. Additionally, I have met a host of like-minded sisters and brothers across the country. It has stilled panic attacks and freed others from pain. It has brought healing into my clients' relationships and my own. I took to it like a duck to water and plan to keep on paddling.

13

Reducing Stress and Anxiety

ELIZABETH M. VARCAROLIS

OUTLINE

KEY TERMS AND CONCEPTS

The key terms and concepts listed here also appear in bold where they are defined or discussed in this chapter.

- stress
- distress
- eustress
- physical stressors
- psychological stressors
- anxiety
- fear
- normal anxiety
- acute (state) anxiety
- chronic (trait) anxiety
- empathy
- primary anxiety
- secondary anxiety
- mild anxiety

moderate anxiety
severe anxiety
panic level of anxiety
Benson's relaxation techniques
meditation
guided imagery
therapeutic touch (TT)
cognitive restructuring-reframing
assertiveness training
progressive muscle relaxation (PMR)
biofeedback

OBJECTIVES

After studying this chapter, the reader will be able to

1. Recognize the short- and long-term physiological consequences of stress.
2. Analyze the ways in which culture can affect a person's perception and reaction to stress and give examples.
3. Differentiate among five categories of coping and give at least two examples of each.
4. Explain how it is helpful for nurses to be able to name an emotion someone is experiencing when stressed, using the emotion anger as an example.
5. Teach a classmate or client two simple techniques to help lower stress and anxiety.
6. Discuss what is meant by normal anxiety.
7. Differentiate between the meanings of the following concepts: (a) anxiety and fear, (b) primary and secondary anxiety, (c) acute and chronic anxiety.
8. State three defining characteristics for a person in each of the following levels of anxiety: (a) mild, (b) moderate, (c) severe, (d) panic.
9. Formulate basic outcome criteria (goals) for a person in each of the above levels of anxiety.
10. Demonstrate at least four nursing interventions and give rationales for a person in each of the following levels of anxiety: (a) mild to moderate, (b) severe to panic.

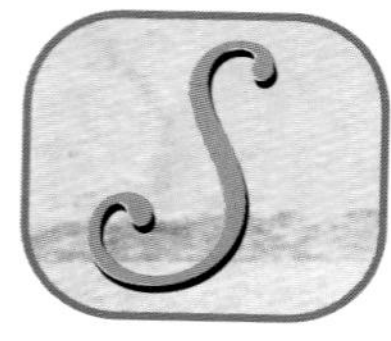

Stress is a universal experience and a component in all our lives, yet it is defined differently by different scholars. Selye (1993) defines **stress** as "the nonspecific (that is, common) result of any demand upon the body." Other definitions of stress describe the "occasions of sympathetic nervous system arousal, as well as the noxious nature of the stress stimulus and the attempts to remove it" (Mandler 1993). Stress may be chronic (e.g., poverty), transitory (e.g., noise), or highly individual (e.g., a bad relationship with a significant other) (Katlin et al. 1993).

STRESS

Hans Selye in 1956 popularized a physiological version of stress as *general adaptation syndrome (GAS)*. It is now believed that GAS occurs in two stages: (1) an initial adaptive response (fight or flight) and (2) the eventual maladaptive consequences of prolonged stress (Table 13–1) (Rossi 1993). Stress produces a wide array of psychological and physiological responses. Table 13–2 identifies some of the objective findings, behavioral manifestations, and subjective states experienced over time as a reaction to stress. The body reacts physiologically in the same manner, whether the stress is real or perceived and whether it is of a physical, psychological, or social nature.

Figure 13–1 shows the short-term (initial adaptive response) and long-term (eventual maladaptive consequences) *physiological* effects of stress on the hypothalamus (brain)-pituitary (endocrine) and the sympatho-adrenomedullary systems. A variety of chronic physical disorders (e.g., hypertension, diabetes) and numerous physical diseases have been linked to long-term, sustained stress.

In 1974 Selye distinguished between the *psychological* reactions of *distress* and *eustress*. According to Selye, **distress** is destructive to health. Selye's distress concept included three types: harm/loss, threat, and challenge. **Eustress** is demonstrated by a person's confidence in the ability to master given demands or tasks with success. Eustress is not harmful to a person's health and may even enhance a sense of well-being (Selye 1974). "Psychological stress focuses on the negative emotions, though the positive emotions of eustress often serve as breathers, . . . sustainers and restorers that replenish damaged resources" (Lazarus et al. 1980).

Selye's psychological reactions can be further described as follows:

- *Distress:* negative, draining energy (anxiety, depression, confusion, helplessness, hopelessness, fatigue)

TABLE 13–1 REACTIONS TO STRESS OVER TIME

Initial Adaptive Response			Prolonged Stress Response		
Seconds	**Minutes**	**Hours**	**Days**	**Weeks**	**Years/Decades**
▶ Cannon's fight-or-flight response	▶ **Complex adaptive response:** Mind-body messengers: e.g., epinephrine, cortisol		▶ **Prolonged stress response:** Mind-body messengers		
				↑Addictions	
	↑Energy mobilization and use		↑Fatigue	↑Myopathy	↑Steroid diabetes
	↑Cognition and performance		↕Sleep	↑Depression	↓Memory and learning
	↑Cardiovascular tone		↑Stress hypertension		
	↑Cardiopulmonary tone		↑Respiratory problems		
	↑Stress analgesia		↑Opportunistic infections		
	↓Immune system		↑Psychogenic ulcers		
	↓Digestion		↓Libido	Impotence, anovulation	
	↓Sexuality				
	↓Growth				

Adapted from Rossi, E. L. (1993). *The psychobiology of mind-body healing.* New York: W. W. Norton; and Sapolsky, R. M. (1990). Stress in the wild. *Scientific American,* 262:116–123.

▶ *Eustress:* positive, motivating energy (happiness, hopefulness, peacefulness, purposeful movement)

Stressors

It is important to keep in mind that a variety of dissimilar situations (e.g., emotional arousal, fatigue, fear, loss, humiliation, loss of blood, and even great and unexpected success) are all capable of producing stress and triggering the stress response (Selye 1993). There are no factors that can be singled out as the cause of stress reaction; however, as we have seen, stressors can be divided into two categories, physical and psychological.

Physical stressors include environmental conditions such as cold, trauma, and excessive cold or heat, as well as physical conditions such as infection, hemorrhage, hunger, and pain. **Psychological stressors** include divorce, loss of a job, unmanageable debt, death of a loved one, and retirement, as well as changes we might consider to be positive, such as marriage or unexpected success. One of the most widely adopted methods for identifying and evaluating personal psychological stressors is the Holmes and Rahe social readjustment rating scale. Holmes and Rahe (1967) published this life-change scale as a means of monitoring the level of stressful life events over a given period (1 year). This scale has been used extensively to evaluate people's situations and their susceptibility to physical and mental illness (see Box 14–1 in Chapter 14 for the life-event scale). Subsequent to Holmes and Rahe's contribution, a variety of scales have been devised to measure stressful life events that are conceptualized in different ways. These scales also show stressful life events to be related to a wide variety of physical and mental disorders (Brown and Harris 1989; Dohrenwend and Dohrenwend 1974, 1983; Lazarus and DeLongis 1983).

Researchers have looked at the degree to which various life events upset a specific individual. They found that it is the *perception* of a recent life event that determines the person's emotional and psychological reactions

TABLE 13–2 FIGHT-OR-FLIGHT

Fight-or-Flight Response
Objective Findings
1. Increased heart rate 2. Increased blood pressure 3. Increased oxygen consumption 4. Peripheral vasoconstriction 5. Sweat gland stimulation (hands, feet, axillae) 6. Pupil dilation 7. No endorphin release 8. Minimal or absent slow alpha waves on EEG, no theta waves 9. Increased blood lactate levels (associated with high anxiety) 10. Increased blood glucose, free fatty acid, and cholesterol level
Behavioral Manifestations
Frequent urination, restlessness, sleeplessness, hostility, motor incoordination, repetitive questioning, disorganized loud speech, scattered thoughts.
Subjective Stress
Tension; fear; frustration; difficulty concentrating; "pressured," shaky, or jittery feeling; confusion; desire to flee; butterflies in stomach; nausea; irritability; depression; pounding heart

EEG, electroencephalogram.
Data from Benson, H. (1985); and Varcarolis (1996).

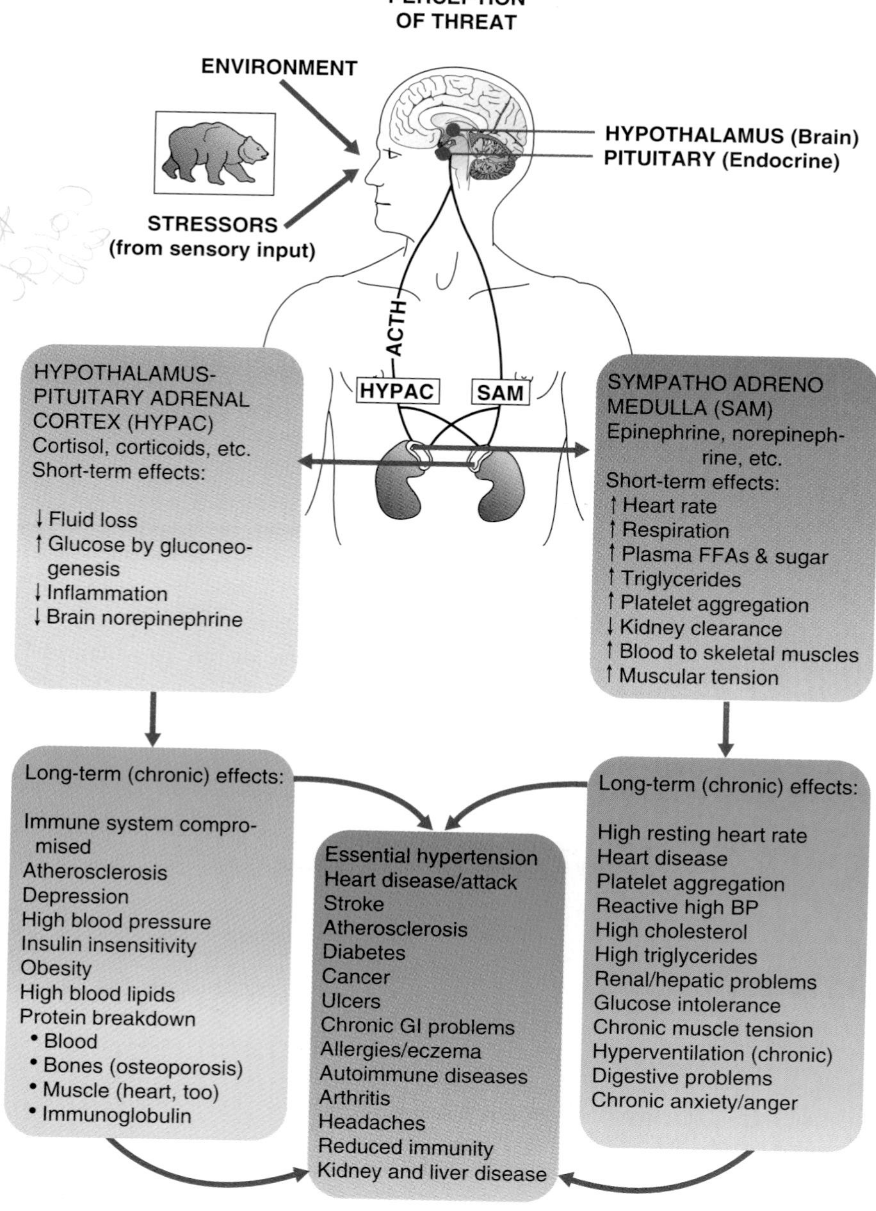

Figure 13–1 The stress response. BP, blood pressure; FFAs, free fatty acids. (From Brigham, D.D. (1994). *Imagery for getting well: Clinical applications of behavioral medicine.* New York: W.W. Norton.)

to it (Rahe 1995). A man in his forties who has a new baby, has just purchased a home, and is laid off with 6 months' severance pay may feel the stress of the event (lost job) more intensely than a man who is 62 years of age, financially secure, and asked to take an early retirement.

The Holmes and Masuda (1972) updated life event and social readjustment scale is a helpful tool for evaluating clients in crisis and looking at events that affect a client's life during a time of either physical or emotional stress. Often we focus only on the presenting symptoms. The use of this tool can help the nurse assess more accurately a person's stress threshold and potential for future illness. If you want to check yourself on this stress scale, refer to Box 14–1.

Stress and Coping

Mediating Factors

Behavioral responses to stress and anxiety are affected by such factors as age, sex, culture, life experiences, and life style. These are all elements that may work to lessen or increase the degree of emotional or physical influence and the sequelae to stress. Social support, however, is one mediating factor that has been heavily researched and has significant implications for nurses and other health care professionals. The fact that strong social support from significant others can enhance mental and physical health and act as a significant buffer against distress has been well documented in the literature. Studies have found strong correlations between lower mortality rates and intact support systems (Fawzy 1995).

The proliferation of self-help groups attests to the need people have for social supports, and the explosive growth of a great variety of support groups reflects the effectiveness of such groups for many people. Many of the support groups currently available are for people going through similar stressful life events, such as the prototype Alcoholics Anonymous (AA), Gamblers Anonymous (GA), Reach for Recovery (for cancer patients), Parents Without Partners (PA), to note but a few. See Appendix E for a list of self-help groups and telephone numbers. Table 11–7 in Chapter 11 also identifies a large variety of self-help groups. It is important, however, to differentiate between social support relationships of high quality and those of low quality. Low-quality support relationships may, and often do, negatively affect a person's coping effectiveness in a crisis. High-quality relationships have been linked with less loneliness, more supportive behavior, and greater life satisfaction (Hobfall and Vaux 1993). High-quality emotional support is a critical factor in enhancing a person's sense of control and rebuilding feelings of self-esteem and competency. Supportive relationships of high quality have the following characteristics: (1) they are relatively free from conflict and negative interactions; and (2) they are close, confiding, and reciprocal (Hobfall and Vaux 1993).

Cultural Considerations

Each culture emphasizes certain problems of living more than others, and interprets problems differently from other cultures. For example, there are differences across cultures in what is considered dangerous, how to manage violations of the social code, and what reactions are permissible in given experiences. These sociocultural variations influence how a stressful event is appraised as well as how the emotion produced by such an event is regulated (Lazarus 1993). So how, and to what extent, people interpret an event as stressful is greatly influenced by specific cultural variables.

Culture also plays a role in how people experience stressors in their life, and how that experience dictates the kind of interventions that will be useful. For example, the idea that stress leads to an emotional state that may result in somatic discomfort is not necessarily shared by the rest of the world. The Western European and North American cultures do subscribe to a psychophysiological view of stress and somatic distress. However, the overwhelming majority of Asian, African, and Central American peoples "not only express subjective distress in somatic terms, but actually experience this distress somatically, such that psychological interpretations of suffering may not be much use cross-culturally" (Gonzalez et al. 1995). The authors go on to say that psychotherapeutic principles can and do apply cross-culturally, but an astute therapist must be mindful of cultural differences. The following vignette illustrates this point:

◗ A 62-year-old Puerto Rican woman was referred for evaluation of incapacitating abdominal pain for the previous 9 months, since a medical diagnostic evaluation of this pain was negative. The pain had begun approximately 1 month after her substance-abusing son had been jailed for killing his lover, whom the patient loved "like a daughter." The patient expected that the psychiatrist would prescribe medication that would take her pain away, and she was initially distressed to learn that she was expected to talk about her life. While not ruling out the use of medication, the therapist explained to her that her pain might be related to the wrenching emotional ordeal of the past year. The therapist made it a point to validate her pain and took great care not to imply that the pain was "merely" the expression of unacknowledged emotion. In particular, he told her that he understood her pain to be very real and that he did not expect her pain to be gone overnight. This approach allowed the patient to engage in a course of brief psychotherapy during which her conflicted feelings about her substance-abusing offspring were examined, though these feelings were never specifically identified as the cause of her pain. Eventually the patient felt strong enough to make drastic changes in her role as enabler of her children, at which point she reported that her pain was much improved. (Gonzalez et al., 1995, p. 60.)

Stress and Defense Mechanisms

A number of defense mechanisms were introduced in Chapter 2. Recall that stress leads to increased anxiety, which then triggers some form of relief behavior. Defense mechanisms, or coping styles, are automatic psychological processes that protect the individual against anxiety and from the awareness of internal or external dangers or stressors (APA 1994, p. 751). Defense mechanisms are relief behaviors used by everyone. They serve to lower anxiety, maintain ego function, and protect one's sense of self.

High levels of anxiety can disturb problem solving and learning as well as perception and functioning. Unconscious defensive maneuvers are mobilized so that an individual can continue to meet personal and social goals in acceptable ways. All defense mechanisms are mobilized by the ego, with the exception of regression. In regression, the ego itself (personality) is relegated to a less mature, although more comfortable, mode of operation. Most defense mechanisms are mobilized on an unconscious level. A notable exception is suppression, which uses the conscious mind.

Adaptive use of defense mechanisms helps people lower anxiety to achieve goals in acceptable ways. Maladaptive use of defense mechanisms may lead to distortions in reality and self-deception that can interfere with individual growth and interpersonal satisfaction. Determination of the effective use of defense mechanisms is based on frequency, intensity, and duration of use.

Sigmond Freud and his daughter Anna Freud outlined most of the defense mechanisms that we acknowledge today. The following summarizes five of their most important properties (Vaillant 1994):

1. Defenses are a major means of managing conflict and affect.
2. Defenses are relatively unconscious.
3. Defenses are discrete from one another.
4. Although often the hallmarks of major psychiatric syndromes, defenses are reversible.
5. Defenses are adaptive as well as pathological.

Over the years, researchers have hypothesized that defense mechanisms could be organized into a hierarchy of relative psychopathology. Devised by Vaillant (1994), Table 13–3 arranges specific defense mechanisms into four general classes of psychopathology. The ones identified as immature defenses are often associated with the personality disorders.

Definitions of many common defense mechanisms follow. They are presented in the order of Vaillant's hierarchy. Actually, all defense mechanisms except sublimation and altruism can be used in both healthy and not-so-healthy ways. (Sublimation and altruism are always healthy coping mechanisms.) Most people use a variety of defense mechanisms, and not always on the same level. Again, the adaptive or maladaptive use of defense mechanisms is determined for the most part by their frequency, intensity, and duration of use.

TABLE 13–3 DEFENSES ORGANIZED INTO HIERARCHY OF PSYCHOPATHOLOGY

CATEGORY	DEFENSE
Mature defenses	Suppression Altruism Humor Sublimation
Neurotic (intermediate) defenses	Intellectualization, isolation Repression Reaction formation Displacement, somatization Undoing, rationalization
Immature defenses	Passive aggression Acting out Dissociation Projection
Psychotic defenses	Denial (of external reality) Distortion (of external reality)

Adapted from Vaillant, G. (1994). Ego mechanisms of defense and personality psychopathology. *Journal of Abnormal Psychology*, 103 (1): 44–50.

MATURE DEFENSES

Altruism. Emotional conflicts and stressors are dealt with by meeting the needs of others. As opposed to being self-sacrificing, with altruism the person receives gratification either vicariously or from the response of others (APA 1994). Six months after losing her husband in a car accident, Jeanette began to spend one day a week doing grief counseling with families who had lost a loved one. She found that she was very effective in helping others in their grief, and obtained a great deal of satisfaction and pleasure from helping others work through their pain.

Sublimation. Sublimation is an unconscious process of substituting constructive and socially acceptable activity for strong impulses that are not acceptable in their original form. Often, these impulses are sexual or aggressive in nature. A man with strong hostile feelings may choose to become a butcher, or he may be involved with rough contact sports. A person who is unable to experience sexual activity may channel this energy into something creative, like painting or gardening.

Humor. The individual deals with emotional conflicts or stressors by emphasizing the amusing or ironic aspects of the conflict or stressor (APA 1994). A man goes to an interview that means a great deal to him. He is being interviewed by the top executives of the company. He has recently had foot surgery and, in entering the interview room, he stumbles and loses his balance. There is a stunned silence, and then the man states calmly, "I was hoping I could put my best foot forward." With everyone laughing, the interview continues in a relaxed manner.

Suppression. Suppression is the conscious denial of a disturbing situation or feeling. A student who has been studying for the state board examinations says "I can't worry about paying my rent until after my exam tomorrow."

NEUROTIC (INTERMEDIATE) DEFENSES

Repression. Repression is the exclusion of unpleasant or unwanted experiences, emotions, or ideas from conscious awareness. "Forgetting" the name of a former husband and "forgetting" an appointment to discuss poor grades are examples. Repression is considered the cornerstone of the defense mechanisms, and it is the first line of psychological defense against anxiety.

Displacement. Transfer of emotions associated with a particular person, object, or situation to another person, object, or situation that is nonthreatening is called displacement. The frequently used example—boss yells at man, man yells at wife, wife yells at child, child kicks the cat—demonstrates a successive use of displaced hostility. The use of displacement is common but not always adaptive. Spousal, child, and elder abuse are often cases of displaced hostility.

Reaction-Formation. In reaction-formation (also termed *overcompensation*), unacceptable feelings or behaviors are kept out of awareness by developing the opposite behavior or emotion. For example, a person who harbors hostility toward children becomes a Scout leader.

Somatization. Transforming anxiety on an unconscious level to a physical symptom that has no organic cause is a form of somatizing. Often the symptom functions to obtain attention or as an excuse. For example, a professor develops laryngitis on the day he is scheduled to defend a research proposal to a group of peers. A woman who doesn't want to go out with her boss's brother calls to say "her back went out" and she can't make the date (and, in fact, her back is sore).

Undoing. Undoing makes up for an act or communication (e.g., giving a gift to "undo" an argument). A common behavioral example of undoing is compulsive handwashing. This can be viewed as cleansing oneself of an act or thought perceived as unacceptable.

Rationalization. Rationalization consists of justifying illogical or unreasonable ideas, actions, or feelings by developing acceptable explanations that satisfy the teller as well as the listener. Common examples are "If I had Lynn's brains, I'd get good grades too" or "Everybody cheats, so why shouldn't I?" Rationalization is a form of self-deception.

IMMATURE DEFENSES (PERSONALITY DISORDERS)

Passive Aggression. A passive aggressive individual deals with emotional conflict or stressors by indirectly and unassertively expressing aggression toward others. On the surface, there is an appearance of compliance that masks covert resistance, resentment, and/or hostility (APA 1994). With passive aggression, resistance is expressed through procrastination, inefficiency, and stubbornness, especially in response to assigned tasks or demands for independent action (Gunderson and Phillips 1995). Sam promises his boss that he is working on the presentation for important clients, even though he constantly "forgets" to bring in samples of the presentation. The day of the presentation, Sam calls in sick with the "flu."

Acting Out Behaviors. An individual deals with emotional conflicts or stressors by actions rather than reflections or feelings (APA 1994). For example, a person may lash out in anger verbally or physically to distract the self from threatening thoughts or feelings (e.g., powerlessness). The verbal or physical expression of anger can make a person feel temporarily less helpless or vulnerable (i.e., more powerful and more in control). By lashing out at others, an individual can transfer the focus from personal doubts and insecurities to some other person or object. This is an example of a destructive coping style. When Harry was turned down a third time for a promotion, he went to his office and tore apart every client file in his file cabinet. His initial feeling of worthlessness and lowered self-esteem related to the situation was interpreted by Harry to mean "I am no good." This thinking resulted in Harry's quickly transforming these painful feelings into actions of anger and destruction. Temporarily, Harry felt more powerful and less vulnerable.

Dissociation. A disruption in the usually integrated functions of consciousness, memory, identity, or perception of the environment is known as dissociation. A young mother who watched her son get run over by a car was taken to a neighbor's house while the police dealt with the accident. Later she told the policeman "I really don't remember what happened. The last thing I remember was going out the door to check on Johnny." At that moment, to protect herself from an unbearable situation, she split off the threatening event from awareness until she could begin to deal with her feelings of devastation.

Devaluation. Emotional conflicts or stressors are dealt with by attributing negative qualities to self or others (APA 1994). When devaluing another, the individual then appears good by contrast. A woman who is very jealous of a co-worker says "Oh yes, she won the award. Those awards don't mean anything anyway, and I wonder what she had to do to be chosen." In this way she minimizes the other's accomplishments and keeps her own fragile self-esteem intact.

Idealization. Emotional conflicts or stressors are dealt with by attributing exaggerated positive qualities to others (APA 1994). Idealization is an important aspect of the development of the self. Children who grow up with parents they can respect and idealize develop healthy standards of conduct and morality (Merikangas and Kupfer 1995).

When people idealize and overvalue a person in a new relationship, they are sure to be disappointed when the object of the idealization turns out to be human. This leads to a great deal of disappointment and painful lowering of self-esteem. Such individuals may then end up devaluing and rejecting the object of their affection to protect their own self-esteem. This pattern can be repeated over and over on a job, within friendships, and within marriages. Mary met the most "wonderful and perfect" man. No one could tell Mary that Jim was nice but had some quirks, like everyone else. Mary wouldn't listen. When Jim failed to live up to Mary's expectations of giving her constant attention, adoration, and gifts, Mary was devastated. Shortly thereafter, she was saying that Jim was, like all men, a brute, and that she wanted no more to do with such an insensitive person.

Splitting. Splitting is the inability to integrate the positive and negative qualities of oneself or others into a cohesive image. Aspects of the self and of others tend to alternate between opposite poles: e.g., good, loving, worthy, nurturing; or bad, hateful, destructive, rejecting, worthless (APA 1994). This is prevalent in personality disorders, especially the borderline ones. Alice viewed her therapist as the most wonderful, loving, and insightful therapist she had ever had. When her therapist refused to write her a prescription for Valium, Alice shouted at her that she was the "stupidest, most uncaring and thickheaded person" and she demanded another therapist "right away."

Projection. A person unconsciously rejects emotionally unacceptable personal features and attributes them to other people, objects, or situations through projection. This is the hallmark of "blaming" or "scapegoating," which is the root of prejudice. People who always feel that others are out to deceive or cheat them may be projecting onto others those characteristics in themselves that they find distasteful and cannot consciously accept.

Projection of anxiety can often be seen in systems (family, hospital, school, business). In a family in which there are problems, the child is often "scapegoated," and the pain and anxiety within the family are projected onto the child: "the problem is Tommy." In a larger system in which anxiety and conflict are present, the weakest members are scapegoated: "the problem is the nurses' aides, the students, the new salesman" (Miller and Winstead-Fry 1982). When pain and anxiety exist within a system, projection can be an automatic relief behavior. Once the cause of the anxiety is identified, changes in relief behavior can ensue, and the system can become more functional and productive.

PSYCHOTIC (SEVERE) DEFENSES

Denial. Denial involves escaping unpleasant realities by ignoring their existence. For example, a man might believe physical limitations to be a negative reflection on one's "manhood." Thus, he may deny chest pains, even though heart attacks run in his family, because of a threat to his self-image as a man. A woman whose health has deteriorated because of alcohol abuse denies she has a problem with alcohol by saying she can stop drinking whenever she wants.

The term *psychotic denial* is used when there is gross impairment in reality testing. A schizophrenic man who says he wants to stay out of the hospital tells the nurse it is his medication, not the cocaine, that makes him frankly psychotic and aggressive. Refer to Table 13–4 for more defense mechanisms.

A Stress and Coping Model

There are a number of coping models in the literature. Rahe (1993) developed a model that is useful in conceptualizing the various stages of the stress response. This presentation is limited for clarity's sake.

STEP 1: STRESS RESPONSE AND PATTERNS. Step 1 is the assessing of recent life events (refer again to Box 14–1 for the Holmes and Masuda life event scale). The life events are filtered through people's perception of the life events they are experiencing. For example, a young unmarried woman who is struggling with a new job would likely perceive an unplanned pregnancy as a more stressful event than would a married woman who was financially comfortable and had been planning a family.

STEPS 2 AND 3: PSYCHOLOGICAL DEFENSES AND PSYCHOPHYSIOLOGICAL RESPONSES. When people experience a number of stressful life events at the same time, they employ a variety of defense mechanisms, including denial, projection, displacement, and repression, as previously discussed. We all experience stress every day and use a variety of defense mechanisms to lower our anxiety and stress levels. However, when defense mechanisms do not lower our anxiety and stress levels, a number of psychophysiological responses may come into play. These psychophysiological defenses are divided into responses that are (1) in our own awareness, such as headache or muscle tension; and (2) out of our awareness, such as increased blood pressure or an increase in lipids. Other responses may be psychological in nature, such as depression (Rahe 1995).

Most people, when faced with stressful life events of a mild to moderate nature, use a variety of psychological defenses briefly and go on to other successful coping strategies as outlined in Step 4. A person is at an elevated risk for near-future illness, however, if he or she is under overwhelming stress, experiencing multiple stressors, or using inadequate coping skills, or if there are other exacerbating circumstances (Rahe 1995).

STEP 4: RESPONSE REDUCTION. People use a variety of ways to cope with life stressors, and a number of factors can act as mediators for stress in our lives, such as life satisfaction (work, family, hobbies, humor) and social supports. Rahe (1995) identifies four categories of coping that people use as stress buffers:

1. Health-sustaining habits (e.g., medical compliance, proper diet, relaxation, pacing one's energy)
2. Life satisfactions (e.g., work, family, humor, spiritual solace, arts, nature)
3. Social supports
4. Response to stress

Response to Stress. Lazarus and Folkman (1984) categorized responses to stress and thereby created a useful model for evaluating coping styles. They formulated three positive and three negative stress response styles. *Positive* coping styles include

1. Problem solving (figuring out how to deal with the situation).
2. Utilizing social support (calling in others who are caring and may be helpful in dealing with the situation).
3. Looking for the "silver lining" (reframing the situation to see the positive as well as the negative sides and how to use the situation for one's advantage).

Negative coping styles of Lazarus and Folkman (1984) include

1. Avoidance (choosing not to deal with the situation, letting negative feelings and situations fester and continue to become chronic).

TABLE 13–4 DEFENSE MECHANISMS

MILD USE	EXTREME EXAMPLE
Repression	
Man forgets wife's birthday after a marital fight.	Woman is unable to enjoy sex after having pushed out of awareness a traumatic sexual incident from childhood.
Sublimation	
Woman who is angry with her boss writes a short story about a heroic woman. By definition, use of sublimation is always constructive.	None
Regression	
4-year-old with a new baby brother starts sucking his thumb and wanting a bottle.	Man who loses a promotion starts complaining to others, hands in sloppy work, misses appointments, and comes in late for meetings.
Displacement	
Patient criticizes a nurse after his family fails to visit.	Child who is unable to acknowledge fear of his father becomes fearful of animals.
Projection	
Man who is unconsciously attracted to other women teases his wife about flirting.	Woman who has repressed an attraction toward other women refuses to socialize. She fears another woman will make homosexual advances toward her.
Compensation	
Short man becomes assertively verbal and excels in business.	Individual drinks when self-esteem is low to diffuse discomfort temporarily.
Reaction-Formation	
Recovering alcoholic constantly preaches about the evils of drink.	Mother who has an unconscious hostility toward her daughter is overprotective and hovers over her to protect her from harm, interfering with her normal growth and development.
Denial	
Man reacts to news of the death of a loved one: "No, I don't believe you. The doctor said he was fine."	Woman whose husband died 3 years ago still keeps his clothes in the closet and talks about him in the present tense.
Conversion	
Student is unable to take a final examination because of terrible headache.	Man becomes blind after seeing his wife flirt with other men.
Undoing	
After flirting with her male secretary, a woman brings her husband tickets to a show.	Man with rigid and moralistic beliefs and repressed sexuality is driven to wash his hands when around attractive women to gain composure.
Rationalization	
"I didn't get the raise because the boss doesn't like me."	Father who thinks his son was fathered by another man excuses his malicious treatment of the boy by saying "He is lazy and disobedient," when that is not the case.
Identification	
5-year-old girl dresses in her mother's shoes and dress and meets daddy at the door.	Young boy thinks a pimp in the neighborhood with money and drugs is someone to look up to.

Table continued on following page

TABLE 13–4 DEFENSE MECHANISMS *(Continued)*

MILD USE	EXTREME EXAMPLE
Introjection	
After his wife's death, husband has transient complaints of chest pains and difficulty breathing—the symptoms his wife had before she died.	Young child whose parents were overcritical and belittling grows up thinking that she is not any good. She has taken on her parent's evaluation of her as part of her self-image.
Suppression	
Business man who is preparing to make an important speech that day is told by his wife that morning that she wants a divorce. Although visibly upset, he puts the incident aside until after his speech, when he can give the matter his total concentration.	A woman who feels a lump in her breast shortly before leaving for a 3-week vacation puts the information in the back of her mind until after returning from her vacation.

2. Self-blame (blaming the self keeps the focus on minimizing one's self-esteem and prevents positive action toward resolution or working through the feelings related to the event).
3. Wishful thinking (a form of denial that involves thinking that things will resolve by themselves and that "everything will be fine").

STEP 5: ILLNESS BEHAVIORS AND ILLNESS MEASURES. When psychological defenses are ineffective and attempts at coping are unsuccessful, a person is at high risk for near-future illness (Rahe 1995). The illness behaviors, such as a headache or stomachache, often lead to recognition of the symptoms of hypertension or ulcers. A positive response to the recognition of illness behaviors is that of seeking medical treatment and the adoption of compliance behaviors to seek symptom relief.

Stress and Emotions

Lazarus (1993, p. 23) states that "if we know that a person is experiencing psychological stress, we have useful information, but it is far more useful to know that a person feels angry, anxious, guilty, sad, relieved, loving, etc." According to Lazarus, each of these emotions tells us something different about the situations the person is facing. It helps us understand more about people's

1. Subjective appraisal of the situation (how they view what is happening).
2. Goal commitment and beliefs (what they want to happen and believe about the situation).
3. Coping ability (how a troubled person-environment situation is being coped with).

For example, when people are experiencing anger, they may be experiencing a personal slight; guilt shows that a person feels blameworthy for a moral transgression; pride indicates that the person's self-esteem or ego identity has been enhanced. Information obtained by expanding the concept of stress to include emotions can be far more revealing about a person's condition and the clinical implications (Lazarus 1993).

If the clinician observes that a person experiences one emotion frequently, such as anger, we have learned one of two things: either the person is often placed in situations that provoke the emotion; or the personality factors, such as goals or beliefs, make that person vulnerable to that particular recurrent emotion (Lazarus 1993).

Lazarus views the identifying of emotions as being congruent with the current cognitive therapy of depression. Cognitive therapy makes an effort to change a person's dysfunctional beliefs that lead to chronic or recurrent emotional distress, such as that of depression.

Lazarus (1991) and others (e.g., Frijda 1986) postulate that for most emotions there are *core relational themes* and what are termed *action tendencies.* A core relational theme is the evaluation of what is happening in terms of one's well-being. For example, when a person is experiencing anger, the core relational theme is that of being slighted or demeaned. The core relational theme for anxiety is that of facing an uncertain or existential threat. The core relational theme for guilt is that of having transgressed a moral imperative. Action tendencies refer to the psychological mobilization to cope with a threat.

Table 13–5 displays some common emotions, their core relational themes, and their action tendencies. Knowing the emotion that a person is feeling can be helpful in looking at the person's interpretation of what is happening and clarifying what the person believes to be an appropriate action to relieve his or her stress. This gives the counselor important information and directions for further assessment and appropriate planning with the client that can reduce the client's stress in healthy and self-enhancing ways. For example, if the client is experiencing anger, the goal might be to help restore self-esteem. If a client is feeling anxious or fearful, the goal would be to help restore a feeling of safety.

TABLE 13–5 CORE RELATIONSHIP THEMES OF SOME "NEGATIVE" EMOTIONS

EMOTION	CORE RELATIONSHIP THEMES	ACTION TENDENCIES
Anger	A demeaning offense against me and mine, leads to wounded self-esteem, decreased sense of worth, decreased social esteem.	Attack those who hurt you/yours, verbally or physically—or desire to attack. Vengeance to restore one's injured self-esteem.
Fright	Immediate, concrete, and overwhelming threat.	Flight or escape
Guilt	Self-blame, having transgressed a moral imperative.	Internalize guilt: Make amends, atone for what one has done
	We should have done otherwise.	Externalize guilt: Blame the victim
Shame	Failure to live up to an ego ideal, leads to a sense of failure.	Hide evidence of one's failure—withdraw from social supports to hide "failure."
Anxiety	Facing an uncertain, unnamed threat—existential threat.	When one does not know what will happen and what to do about it, often a psychological paralysis sets in

Adapted from Lazarus, R. S. (1993). Why we should think of stress as a subset of emotion. In L. Goldberger and S. Breznitz (Eds.), *Handbook of stress: Theoretical and clinical aspects* (2nd ed.) (pp. 21–39). New York: Free Press. Adapted with the permission of The Free Press, a division of Simon & Schuster. Copyright © 1982, 1993 by The Free Press.

Implications for Stress Management

Siegman's (1993) experiments with angry, anxious, and sad voices indicated that people have control over their negative emotions when they learn to modify their vocal tone. For example, when people are anxious or angry, they can lessen these emotions both psychologically and physically by speaking slowly and softly. When people are angry or anxious, they experience an increase in blood pressure, heart rate, cortisol, and epinephrine. They also raise their voice, accelerate their speech, and interrupt others. The heightened levels of blood pressure, heart rate, and catecholamines only further intensify their angry voice as well as their feeling of anger or anxiety. An angry voice will further intensify and escalate the nature of the person's emotions, so that eventually the anger turns into rage and anxiety into panic. By learning to speak more slowly and softly, people can lower their feelings of stress as well as their cardiac arousal (Siegman 1993). Therefore, nurses and their clients can learn to lessen their feelings of anger and other stress-related emotions when they purposely reduce their speech rate and the loudness of their voice. Conversely, when people are feeling sad or depressed, speaking in a loud, forceful voice can significantly attenuate these emotions as well as their physical manifestations. Siegman (1993) quoted findings demonstrating that people have the ability to modify their negative emotions, as well as their physiological manifestations of stress, by control of expressive vocal behavior. These findings have important implications for stress management and the avoidance of stress-related illnesses.

ANXIETY

Stress is a state produced by a change in the environment that is perceived as challenging, threatening, or damaging to a person's well-being. Stress can lead to a variety of psychological responses, the most common of which is probably anxiety.

Anxiety is a universal human experience that is a stranger to no one. It is the most basic of emotions. A basic principle in psychiatric nursing is that "all behavior is purposeful, meaningful, and can be understood" (Burd 1968). Dysfunctional behavior is often a defense against anxiety. When behavior is recognized as dysfunctional, interventions to reduce anxiety can be initiated by the nurse. As anxiety decreases, dysfunctional behavior will frequently decrease, and vice versa.

Anxiety is experienced on four levels: mild, moderate, severe, and panic anxiety. It can be broken down into three categories—normal, acute, and chronic—and it can be operationally defined.

Hildegard Peplau, one of the first nurse theorists, identifies anxiety as one of the most important concepts in psychiatric nursing. Nurses can use the concept of anxiety to explain many clinical observations. Peplau (1968) conceptualized an anxiety model useful to the practice of nursing. Conceptualizing anxiety using Peplau's model has led to principles that serve as guides in nursing intervention. This conceptual basis of anxiety can be used by nurses as a framework to guide therapeutic approaches to clients in any setting.

Anxiety can be defined as a feeling of apprehension, uneasiness, uncertainty, or dread resulting from a real or a perceived threat whose actual source is unknown or unrecognized.

Fear is a reaction to a specific danger, whereas anxiety is a vague sense of dread relating to an unspecified danger. The body reacts in similar ways physiologically, however, to both anxiety and fear.

An important distinction between anxiety and fear is that anxiety attacks us at a deeper level than fear. Anxiety invades the central core of the personality. It erodes the individual feelings of self-esteem and personal worth that contribute to a sense of being fully human.

Normal anxiety is a healthy life force that is necessary for survival. It provides the energy needed to carry out the tasks involved in living and striving toward goals. Anxiety motivates people to make and survive change. It prompts constructive behaviors, such as studying for an examination, being on time for job interviews, preparing for a presentation, and working toward a promotion.

Acute (state) anxiety is precipitated by an imminent loss or change that threatens an individual's sense of security. It may be seen in performers before a concert. For example, Barbra Streisand admits to experiencing acute anxiety before live concerts. Patients preparing for surgery often experience acute anxiety. The death of a loved one can stimulate acute anxiety when there is great disruption in one's life. In general, crisis involves the experience of acute anxiety. Acute anxiety is also referred to as *state anxiety*.

Chronic (trait) anxiety is anxiety that the person has lived with for a time. Ego psychologists suggest that in a nurturing environment the developing personality incorporates the parents' positive attributes, thus allowing the child to tolerate anxiety. When conditions for personality growth are less than adequate, positive values may not be incorporated, and the child may become anxiety-ridden, a state that often covers up overwhelming, angry, and hostile impulses (Sullivan 1953). A child may demonstrate chronic anxiety by a permanent attitude of apprehension or by overreaction to all unexpected environmental stimuli. In adults, chronic anxiety may take the form of chronic fatigue, insomnia, discomfort in daily activities, and discomfort in personal relationships. Poor concentration may interfere with effective work functioning. When the subjective feelings of anxiety become too overwhelming, anxiety is unconsciously placed out of awareness (repressed) and is expressed in behavioral characteristics or symptoms. *Trait anxiety* is another name for chronic anxiety.

An understanding of the types, levels, and defensive patterns used in response to anxiety is basic to psychiatric nursing care. This understanding is essential for assessing and planning interventions to lower a client's level of anxiety, as well as one's own, effectively. With practice, one becomes more skilled both at identifying levels of anxiety and the defenses used to alleviate it, and at evaluating the possible stressors contributing to increases in a person's level of anxiety.

Theories of Anxiety

Anxiety is a response to a stressful situation. As stated, stress can be defined as a perceived threat to an expectation, thereby triggering anxiety. The result is some form of relief. Therefore:

STRESS → ↑ ANXIETY → RELIEF BEHAVIOR
(defense mechanisms / coping behaviors)

Stress can be psychological, social, spiritual, or physical. Anxiety can be an appropriate or inappropriate response and can result in healthy relief behaviors or psychiatric symptoms. Thus, anxiety may be experienced as (1) a *symptom* involving a subjective feeling of apprehension or nervousness, (2) a *syndrome* involving both psychic and somatic symptoms, or (3) *primary disease*, such as generalized anxiety disorder or phobic disorder. As a symptom or syndrome, anxiety may be "normal" in certain circumstances. It may be "abnormal" when its severity is inappropriate or when it occurs in inappropriate circumstances.

There is no one etiological theory of anxiety that explains all the clinical and biological data. Various theories have made contributions to possible etiological factors in the development of anxiety. Three major theories are (1) psychodynamic, (2) behavioral, and (3) biological.

Psychodynamic Theory

As reviewed in Chapter 2, Freud proposed that anxiety is the result of *unconscious* psychic conflicts. When these *intrapsychic* conflicts, or forbidden impulses (sexual or aggressive), threaten to become conscious, anxiety is experienced. Anxiety then becomes a *signal* to the ego to take defensive action to repress anxiety. When the use of defense mechanisms is successful, anxiety is lowered and a sense of security returns. However, if the conflict is intense and the anxiety level high, the defense mechanisms may be experienced as symptoms, such as phobias, regression, or ritualistic behaviors.

Harry Stack Sullivan (1953) believed that anxiety results from *interpersonal conflicts* rather than from an intrapsychic process. He stated that anxiety is linked to the anxiety experienced in infancy and early childhood. The infant's first experiences with emotional discomfort and acute anxiety become the prototype for future emotional distress. For example, a child reared by hostile and rejecting parents may later react with painful anxiety when treated in a cold or critical manner by another individual. Past experiences leave people vulnerable to anxiety in the present, and specific events or interpersonal exchanges can trigger underlying anxiety. Two principles basic to nursing practice are based on Sullivan's theory of anxiety.

First, anxiety can be communicated interpersonally. It is communicated from one person to another via empathy (Sullivan 1953). **Empathy** is the ability to feel for and with another and to understand the other's experience. An example of anxiety transferred from person to person via empathy is what may occur in mass crisis situations. In such situations, people in high levels of anxiety need to be attended to first to avoid the spread of anxiety, which could lead to group panic and confusion.

Second, anxiety is an energy (Peplau 1968). We cannot see anxiety in others; instead, behavior expresses the anxiety that a person feels. No one wants to experience uncomfortable levels of anxiety. Relief behaviors are those that discharge the energy of anxiety. Familiar behaviors, such as movement, talking, and meditation, are examples of relief behaviors used to lessen the experience of anxiety. There are considered healthy relief behaviors; there are also unhealthy ones (e.g., drugs, alcohol, unprotected sex, undue risk taking).

Rollo May (1983) stated "Anxiety is the apprehension cued off by a threat to some value that the individual holds essential to his existence as a personality." These threats consist of those to biological integrity, such as food or shelter, and those to psychological well-being, such as loss of respect or freedom. A person experiencing an unconscious conflict may become anxious, although the reason for the anxiety may not be known. People modify their relationships with others constantly to keep anxiety as low as possible, thereby maintaining a feeling of emotional security. Anxiety caused by psychological factors (intrapsychic or interpersonal conflict) is referred to as **primary anxiety.**

Behavioral Theory

The success of behavioral therapy techniques in the treatment of phobias and obsessive-compulsive behaviors supports the theory that anxiety is a result of a learned, or conditioned, response. According to behavioral theory, anxiety results from a system of responses to a particular stimulus. Over time, an individual develops a learned, or conditioned, response to certain stimuli. This assumption has given rise to the concept that anxiety can be learned and unlearned as a result of experience. Some behavioral therapists have regarded Freud's *signal* theory as identical to that of the learned conditioned response. Chapter 17 discusses behavioral interventions used effectively in the treatment of certain anxiety disorders, such as phobias.

Biological Theory

There is an increasing body of knowledge supporting the hypothesis that manifestations of anxiety may be due to physiological abnormalities. Diagnostic decisions need to be made when one is confronted with anxiety symptoms in order to determine whether the anxiety is (1) secondary to a medical disorder; (2) secondary to a pervasive psychiatric disorder, such as depression; or (3) a primary anxiety disorder, such as a phobia.

In up to 40% or more of cases, anxiety may be a warning of an underlying physiological process. That is, the anxiety is caused by a physical disease or abnormality, *not* by an emotional conflict. Anxiety secondary to a physical condition is termed **secondary anxiety.** For example, people with certain neurological disorders (multiple sclerosis, brain tumor), endocrine disorders (thyroid, pituitary, diabetes), circulatory disorders (anemia, coronary insufficiency), drug intoxication or withdrawal, and other disorders may experience anxiety due to physiological processes (Popkin 1995).

Several promising studies have focused on the neuroanatomy and biochemistry of normal and pathological anxiety states. (Chapter 17 identifies specific studies relevant to anxiety disorders.) Although these preliminary investigations do not show conclusive cause-and-effect relationships at present, it is a rich field for future research (Kaplan and Sadock 1995).

Assessment of Anxiety

Assessing the presence of problematic levels of anxiety may or may not be easy. For example, a person in acute anxiety may demonstrate obvious signs and symptoms of distress and may be experiencing the anxiety subjectively: "I feel so upset." Alternatively, a person might not be aware of experiencing anxiety; instead, the anxiety might be repressed from conscious awareness but expressed in some other form of relief behavior. For example, a woman who is unaware of experiencing anxiety related to feelings of inadequacy might be displacing her anxiety as anger toward her family. A man who is unaware of experiencing anxiety related to low self-esteem might compensate by drinking or taking drugs to feel better temporarily. Established patterns of dealing with anxiety may be observed by noting specific relief behaviors a person uses.

Levels of Anxiety

Levels of anxiety range from mild to moderate to severe to panic. Peplau's (1968) classic delineation of these four levels of anxiety is based on Sullivan's work. Assessment of a client's level of anxiety is basic to therapeutic intervention in any setting—psychiatric, hospital, or community. Determination of specific levels of anxiety can be used as guidelines for intervention (Table 13–6). Anxiety is experienced on a continuum from mild to moderate to severe to panic, and overlapping can and does occur. Use Table 13–6 as a guide for making observations.

Mild Anxiety

Mild anxiety occurs in the normal experience of everyday living. The person's ability to perceive reality is brought into sharp focus. A person sees, hears, and grasps more information, and problem solving becomes more effective. A person may display such physical symptoms as slight discomfort, restlessness, irritability, or mild tension-relieving behaviors (e.g., nail-biting, foot or finger tapping, fidgeting).

TABLE 13–6 ANXIETY LEVELS

MILD	MODERATE	SEVERE	PANIC
		Perceptual Field	
Perceptual field can be heightened	Perceptual field narrows. Person grasps less of what is going on.	Perceptual field greatly reduced.	Unable to focus on the environment.
Is alert and can see, hear, and grasp what is happening in the environment.	Can attend to more *if pointed out by another* (selective inattention).	Focus is on details or one specific detail. Attention is scattered.	Experiences the utmost state of terror and emotional paralysis. Feels he "ceases to exist."
Can identify things that are disturbing and are producing anxiety.		Completely absorbed with self.	In panic, hallucinations or delusions may take the place of reality.
		May not be able to attend to events in the environment *even when pointed out by others.*	
		In severe and panic levels of anxiety, the environment is blocked out. It is as if these events are not occurring.	
		Ability to Learn	
Able to effectively work toward a goal and examine alternatives.	Able to solve problems but not at optimal ability.	Unable to see connections between events or details.	May be mute or have extreme psychomotor agitation leading to exhaustion.
	Benefits from guidance of others.	Distorted perceptions.	Disorganized or irrational reasoning.
Mild and moderate levels of anxiety can alert the person that something is wrong and can stimulate appropriate action.		**Severe and panic levels prevent problem solving and finding effective solutions. Unproductive relief behaviors are called into play, thus perpetuating a vicious cycle.**	
		Physical or Other Characteristics	
Slight discomfort Attention-seeking behaviors Restlessness Irritability or impatience Mild tension-relieving behavior: foot or finger rapping, lip chewing, fidgeting	Voice tremors Change in voice pitch Difficulty concentrating Shakiness Repetitive questioning Somatic complaints, e.g., urinary frequency and urgency, headache, backache, insomnia Increased respiration rate Increased pulse rate Increased muscle tension More extreme tension-relieving behavior: pacing, banging hands on table	Feelings of dread Ineffective functioning Confusion Purposeless activity Sense of impending doom More intense somatic complaints, e.g., dizziness, nausea, headache, sleeplessness Hyperventilation Tachycardia Withdrawal Loud and rapid speech Threats and demands	Experience of terror Immobility or severe hyperactivity or flight Dilated pupils Unintelligible communication or inability to speak Severe shakiness Sleeplessness Severe withdrawal Hallucinations or delusions likely Out of touch with reality

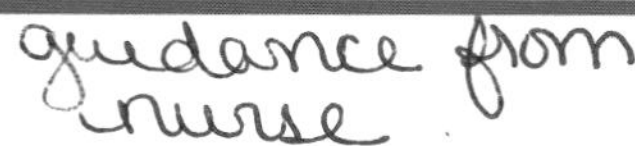

Moderate Anxiety

As anxiety escalates, the perceptual field narrows, and some details are excluded from observation. The person in **moderate anxiety** sees, hears, and grasps less information than someone not in that state. Individuals may experience *selective inattention*, in which only certain things in the environment are seen or heard unless they are brought to the person's attention. Although the ability to think clearly is hampered, learning and problem solving can still take place, though not at an optimal level. At the moderate level of anxiety, the person's ability to problem-solve is greatly enhanced by the supportive presence of another. Physical symptoms include tension, pounding heart, increased pulse and respiration rate, perspiration, and mild somatic symptoms (gastric discomfort, headache, urinary urgency). Voice tremors and shaking may be noticed. Mild or moderate anxiety levels can be constructive, because anxiety can be viewed as a signal that something in the person's life needs attention.

Severe Anxiety

The perceptual field of a person experiencing severe anxiety is greatly reduced. A person in **severe anxiety** may focus on one particular detail or many scattered details. The person may have difficulty noticing what is going on in the environment, even when it is pointed out by another. Learning and problem solving are not possible at this level, and the person may be dazed and confused. Behavior is "automatic" and aimed at reducing or relieving anxiety. The person may complain of increased severity of somatic symptoms (headache, nausea, dizziness, insomnia), trembling, and pounding heart. The person may also experience hyperventilation and a sense of impending doom or dread.

Panic Level of Anxiety

Feelings of panic are very painful. The **panic level of anxiety** is the most extreme form and results in markedly disturbed behavior. The person is not able to process what is going on in the environment and may lose touch with reality. The behavior that results may be manifested by confusion, shouting, screaming, or withdrawal. Hallucinations, or false sensory perceptions, such as seeing people or objects that are not there, may be experienced by people in panic levels of anxiety. Physical behavior may be erratic, uncoordinated, and impulsive. Automatic behaviors are used to reduce and relieve anxiety, although such efforts may be ineffective. Acute panic may lead to exhaustion. Review Table 13–6 to identify the levels of anxiety in relation to (1) perceptual field, (2) ability to learn, and (3) physical and other defining characteristics.

HOLISTIC APPROACHES FOR REDUCING STRESS AND ANXIETY

The Nurse's Response

Nurses not only work constantly with people in high-stress situations but also spend their working hours in environments reflecting high levels of anxiety. Anxiety can be experienced by clients, clients' families, and health care workers. Mild to moderate anxiety reactions are commonly seen in clients on the medical and surgical units, as well as in the obstetrical, gynecological, and pediatric settings. Severe to panic levels of anxiety can be seen in emergency departments and intensive care units. Severe and panic levels of anxiety are frequently observed in the psychiatric setting.

Working with people in high levels of anxiety can be uncomfortable and intimidating at times for all staff members, but especially for students new to the psychiatric setting. Because anxiety is communicated from person to person through the process of empathy, strong emotions will be experienced by nurses working with clients in any hospital or community setting.

At times, nurses may find that before they are ready to interact with a client, personal feelings need to be sorted out so that therapeutic communication between nurse and client can be at its most effective. Identifying levels of anxiety in the client and in oneself, and dealing with strong and sometimes confusing countertransferential feelings triggered by certain client behaviors, can all be greatly facilitated by working closely with the instructor. Ideally, staff members should have supervision available to increase the effectiveness of care and prevent burnout.

Counseling Techniques

Perhaps one of the most helpful and meaningful experiences for a person in uncomfortable levels of stress and anxiety is a calm and caring human presence. The calmness of another helps deflect some of the anxious person's anxiety. The feeling that someone cares helps lessen the feelings of isolation and aloneness and offers a connection to stability.

Specific communication techniques are based on assessment of the client's specific needs; many of the techniques suggested for people in mild to moderate levels of anxiety are also appropriate for people in other levels, and vice versa. As mentioned earlier, one self-intervention when faced with stress in the form of anger or anxiety is to speak slowly and softly. This can help reduce both psychological and physical reactions to stress. This is also an effective tool to teach clients.

Mild to Moderate Levels of Anxiety

A person in mild to moderate levels of anxiety is still able to problem-solve; however, the ability to concentrate decreases as anxiety increases. The nurse can help the client focus and solve problems with the use of specific communication techniques, such as employing open-ended questions, giving broad openings, and exploring and seeking clarification. These techniques can be useful to a client experiencing mild to moderate anxiety. Closing off topics of communication and bringing up irrelevant topics can increase a person's anxiety and are tactics that usually make the *nurse* feel better, not the client.

Reducing the anxiety level and preventing escalation of anxiety to more distressing levels can be aided by a calm presence, recognition of the anxious person's distress, and willingness to listen. Evaluation of effective past coping mechanisms is useful. Often the nurse can help the client to consider alternatives to problem situations and offer activities that may temporarily relieve feelings of inner tension.

Table 13–7 offers concrete examples of appropriate nursing interventions and rationales for patients in mild to moderate levels of anxiety. Refer to the first case study at the end of the chapter; it demonstrates a nurse's use of counseling techniques with a young woman in moderate levels of anxiety.

Severe To Panic Levels of Anxiety

A person in severe to panic levels of anxiety is unable to solve problems and may have a poor grasp of what is happening in the environment. Unproductive relief behaviors may take over and the person may not be in control of his or her actions. Extreme regression or running about aimlessly may be behavioral manifestations of the person's intense pain. The nurse is concerned with the client's safety and, at times, the safety of others. Physical needs (e.g., fluids and rest) have to be met to prevent exhaustion. Anxiety reduction measures may take the form of removing the person to a quiet environment where there is minimal stimulation, and providing gross motor activities to drain off some of the tension. The use of medications may have to be considered, but both medications and restraints should be used only after other more personal and less restrictive interventions have failed to decrease anxiety to safer levels. Although communication may be scattered and disjointed, themes can often be heard, and the nurse can address these themes. The feeling that one is understood can decrease the sense of isolation and also reduce anxiety.

Because the person in severe to panic levels of anxiety is unable to solve problems, communication techniques suggested for the person in mild to moderate levels of anxiety are not always effective. Because clients in severe to panic anxiety levels are out of control, they need to know that they are safe from their own impulses. *Firm, short, and simple statements are useful.* Reinforcing commonalities in the environment and pointing out reality when there are distortions can also be useful interventions for the severely anxious person. Table 13–8 suggests basic nursing interventions for the client in severe to panic levels of anxiety. Refer to the second case study at the end of the chapter for a demonstration of appropriate counseling techniques for an elderly man in severe anxiety.

TABLE 13–7 MILD TO MODERATE LEVELS OF ANXIETY

INTERVENTION	RATIONALE
Nursing Diagnosis: Moderate anxiety related to situational event or intrapsychic conflict, as evidenced by increase in vital signs, moderate discomfort, narrowing or perceptual field, and selective inattention	
1. Help the client identify anxiety. "Are you comfortable right now?"	1. Validate observations with the client, name the anxiety, and start to work with the client to lower anxiety.
2. Anticipate anxiety-provoking situations.	2. Escalation of anxiety to a more disorganizing level is prevented.
3. Use nonverbal language to demonstrate interest, e.g., lean forward, maintain eye contact, nod your head.	3. Verbal and nonverbal messages should be consistent. The presence of an interested person provides a stabilizing focus.
4. Encourage client to talk about his or her feelings and concerns.	4. When concerns are stated out loud, problems can be discussed and feelings of isolation decreased.
5. Avoid closing off avenues of communication that are important for the client. Focus on the client's concerns.	5. When staff anxiety increases, "changing the topic" or "offering advice" is common but leaves the person isolated.
6. Ask questions to clarify what is being said. "I'm not sure what you mean. Give me an example."	6. Increased anxiety results in scattering of thoughts. Clarifying helps the client identify thoughts and feelings.
7. Help the client identify thoughts or feelings before the onset of anxiety. "What were you thinking right before you started to feel anxious?"	7. Helps the client identify thoughts and feelings, facilitates problem solving.
8. Encourage problem solving with the client.	8. Encouraging clients to explore alternatives increases sense of control and decreases anxiety.
9. Assist in developing alternative solutions to a problem through role play or modeling behaviors.	9. Encourage the client to try out alternative behaviors and solutions.
10. Explore behaviors that have worked to relieve anxiety in the past.	10. Encourage the mobilization of successful coping mechanisms and strengths.
11. Provide outlets for working off excess energy (e.g., walking, pingpong, dancing, exercises).	11. Physical activity can provide relief of built-up tension, increase muscle tone, and increase endorphins.

TABLE 13–8 SEVERE TO PANIC LEVELS OF ANXIETY

INTERVENTION	RATIONALE
Nursing Diagnosis: Severe to panic levels of anxiety related to severe threat, as evidenced by verbal or physical acting out, extreme immobility, sense of impending doom, inability to differentiate reality (possible hallucinations or delusions), and inability to problem solve	
1. Maintain a calm manner.	1. Anxiety is communicated interpersonally. The quiet calm of the nurse can serve to calm the client. The presence of anxiety can escalate anxiety in the client.
2. Always remain with the person in acute severe to panic levels of anxiety.	2. Alone with immense anxiety, a person feels abandoned. A caring face may be the only contact with reality when confusion becomes overwhelming.
3. Minimize environmental stimuli. Move to a quieter setting and stay with the client.	3. Further escalation of anxiety to self and to others in the setting is prevented.
4. Use clear and simple statements and repetition.	4. A person has difficulty concentrating and processing information with severe to panic levels of anxiety.
5. Use a low-pitched voice, speak slowly.	5. A high-pitched voice can convey anxiety. Low pitch can decrease anxiety.
6. Reinforce reality if distortions occur, e.g., seeing objects that are not there or hearing voices when no one is present.	6. Anxiety can be reduced by focusing on and validating what is going on in the environment.
7. Listen for themes in communication.	7. In severe to panic levels of anxiety, verbal communication themes may be the only indication of the client's thoughts or feelings.
8. Attend to physical and safety needs when necessary, e.g., warmth, fluids, elimination, pain relief, need for family contact.	8. High levels of anxiety may obscure the client's awareness of physical needs.
9. Because safety is an overall goal, physical limits may need to be set. Speak in a firm, authoritative voice: "You may not hit anyone here. If you can't control yourself, we will help you."	9. A person who is out of control is often terrorized. Staff must offer the client and others protection from destructive and self-destructive impulses.
10. Provide opportunities for exercise, e.g., pacing with nurse, punching bag, ping-pong.	10. Physical activity helps channel and dissipate tension and may temporarily lower anxiety.
11. When a person is constantly moving or pacing, offer high caloric fluids.	11. Prevent dehydration and exhaustion.
12. Assess the person's need for medication or seclusion after other interventions have been tried and have not been successful.	12. Prevent exhaustion and physical harm to self and others.

Stress and Anxiety Reduction Techniques

Nurses are learning a great variety of stress and anxiety reduction techniques and teaching clients alternative ways of handling anxiety and stress. Some of the benefits of stress reduction have been compiled by Varcarolis (1996):

1. Alter the course of certain medical conditions such as high blood pressure, arrhythmias, arthritis, cancer, and peptic ulcers.
2. Decrease the need for medications such as insulin, analgesics, and antihypertensives.
3. Diminish or eliminate the need for unhealthy and destructive behaviors such as smoking, addictions to drugs, insomnia, and overeating.
4. Increase cognitive functions such as learning, concentration, and study habits.
5. Facilitate the Lamaze method of childbirth.
6. Enhance the effectiveness of therapeutic touch (TT).
7. Break up static patterns of thinking and allow fresh and creative ways of perceiving life events.
8. Increase the sense of well-being through endorphin release.

Nurses use the relaxation techniques mentioned below in all areas of nursing practice, as well as in dealing with their own home or workplace stressful environments. For example, a study of preoperative cardiac catherization patients showed that relaxation techniques could reduce the amount of preoperative medication (diazepam [Valium]) needed (Warner et al. 1992). Relaxation techniques are used successfully by nurses in critical care areas to help patients cope with their symptoms and treatment (Heath

1992). Relaxation techniques and progressive muscle relaxation (PMR) are taught to elderly clients to help treat areas of anxiety, altered comfort, or sleep pattern disturbances (Weinberger 1991).

Some stress reduction techniques used by nurses in their practice include relaxation techniques, meditation, imaging and visualization, TT, cognitive-restructuring and reframing, PMR, and biofeedback. These techniques, with the exception of biofeedback, can be taught to clients in any setting with the consent of the client's physician. Be aware that some of these techniques may have contraindications.

Benson's Relaxation Techniques

Herbert Benson (1985) outlined specific techniques that enable most people to elicit what he referred to as the *relaxation response*. Essentially, **Benson's relaxation techniques** teach the client how to switch from the sympathetic mode (fight-or-flight response) of the autonomic nervous system to a state of relaxation (the parasympathetic mode). Follow the steps in Box 13–1 to practice the relaxation response.

Many students find that by using these techniques on a regular basis, they are able to reduce examination anxiety and increase concentration and retention. Although many of these stressors cannot be removed, the level of stress can be reduced. Personal perception of an experience can be altered and new coping skills learned through stress reduction techniques. Feelings of anxiety and stress can be decreased by a student's choosing to become actively involved in stress reduction techniques (Davidhizer 1991). Students are encouraged to teach friends and family members these techniques. Practicing with others can enhance results.

Benson's relaxation techniques have been used successfully in conjunction with meditation and visual imagery to treat numerous disorders, such as diabetes, high blood pressure, migraines, cancer, and peptic ulcers.

Any client who is to be taught relaxation techniques should obtain the knowledge and consent of his or her physician. Snyder (1984) cautions against the use of relaxation techniques with certain clients. For example:

1. Depressed persons may experience further withdrawal.
2. Hallucinating and delusional patients may lose contact with reality altogether.
3. The toxic effects of some medications may be enhanced.
4. Some patients in pain may have a heightened experience of pain corresponding to the increase in body awareness.

Other techniques to induce relaxation have been developed. Some have an internal focus (e.g., meditation, guided imagery, TT). Some techniques are based on teaching a person effective coping abilities, such as cognitive restructuring and assertive communication skills. Others (e.g., PMR, biofeedback) have an external focus.

BOX 13–1 BENSON'S RELAXATION TECHNIQUE

The nurse instructs the client as follows:

1. Choose any word or brief phrase that reflects your belief system, such as "love," "unity in faith and love," "joy," "shalom," "one God," "peace."
2. Sit in a comfortable position.
3. Close your eyes.
4. Deeply relax all your muscles, beginning at your feet and progressing up to your face. Keep them relaxed.
5. Breath through your nose. Become aware of your breathing. As you breathe out, say your word or phrase silently to yourself. For example, breath IN . . . . OUT, "phrase," IN . . . . OUT, "phrase," etc. Breathe easily and naturally.
6. Continue for 10 or 20 minutes. You may open your eyes and check the time, but do not use an alarm. When you finish, sit quietly for several minutes, at first with your eyes closed and then with your eyes open. Do not stand up for a few minutes.
7. Do not worry about whether you are successful in achieving a deep level of relaxation. Maintain a passive attitude and permit relaxation to occur at its own pace. When distracting thoughts occur, try to ignore them by not dwelling on them, and return to repeating your word or phrase. With practice, the response should come with little effort. Practice the technique once or twice daily, but not within 2 hours after any meal, since the digestive process seems to interfere with the elicitation of the relaxation response.

From Benson, H. (1985). *The relaxation response* (2nd ed.). New York: William Morrow.

INTERNAL FOCUS

Meditation. Meditation follows the basic guidelines described for the relaxation response. It is a discipline for training the mind to develop greater calm and then using that calm to bring penetrative insight into one's experience. Meditation can be used to help people reach their deep inner resources for healing, calm the mind, and operate more efficiently in the world. It can help people develop strategies to cope with stress, make sensible adaptive choices under pressure, and feel more engaged in life (Kabat-Zinn 1993). Meditation elicits a relaxation response by creating a hypometabolic state of quieting the sympathetic nervous system. Some people meditate using a visual object or a sound to help them focus. Others may find it useful to concentrate on their breathing while meditating. There are many meditation techniques, some with a spiritual base, such as Siddha meditation. Meditation is easy to practice anywhere.

Guided Imagery. Used in conjunction with the relaxation response, **guided imagery** is a process whereby a person is led to envision images that are both calming and health enhancing. The content of the imagery exercises is shaped by the person helping with the imagery process. If a person has dysfunctional images, he or she can be helped to generate more effective and functional coping images to replace the depressogenic or anxiety-producing ones. For example, athletes have discovered that the use of positive coping and successful images can lead to an increase in performance (Freeman and Reinecke 1993).

Imagery tapes are commonly found in many kinds of stores (e.g., music, book); however, people can make their own tapes, using soothing music in the background. A common imagery technique used for deep relaxation is to lead the individual into a positive sensory experience. For example, a person will pick a favorite spot, one that is beautiful and quiet and that gives the person joy (e.g., a beach). It can be a real or imaginary place. The person is then asked to *see* in his mind the soft blue of the sky, *feel* the warm sand under his back, *smell* the fresh salty ocean breeze, and *feel* it brush his face and hair while *hearing* the soothing sounds of the waves in the background. Refer to Box 17–3 in Chapter 17 for a guided imagery script.

Imagery techniques are an effective tool used for many medical conditions. They are an effective means of relieving pain for many people. Pain is reduced by producing muscle relaxation, focusing the person away from the pain; for some, imagery techniques are healing exercises in that they not only relieve the pain, but in some cases diminish the source of the pain (Matassarin-Jacobs 1993). Guided imagery is used with cancer patients to help them reduce their chronic high levels of cortisol, epinephrine, and catecholamines (which prevent the immune system from functioning effectively) and produce beta-endorphins (which increase pain thresholds and enhance lymphocyte proliferation) (Brigham 1994). Guided imagery is used for all sorts of healing. Often tapes are made specifically for clients and their specific situation. However, there are many healing tapes available to clients and to health care workers.

Therapeutic Touch (TT). Krieger (1979) developed a nursing model for using **therapeutic touch (TT)** from the ancient practice of "laying on of hands," although the practitioner does not actually touch the patient. TT is based on the assumptions of Eastern medicine that illness or pain are merely blockages in the body's energy field. Through intentional "manipulation," these energy field blocks can be removed (Brigham 1994). A nurse who is specially trained in this therapeutic stress reduction technique goes into a meditative state in order to enter the energy field of the client, and to passively visualize the free flow of energy from the client with the intent to support or promote healing. The practitioner follows three steps during the process of TT: centering, scanning, and rebalancing. (Refer to Box 13–2 for a centering technique used by some practitioners.) The practitioner's focus is to create a state of harmony and balance that promotes self-healing in the client (Beare and Myers 1994).

Clients receiving TT have been found to require less pain medication, describe greater pain reduction, and report longer periods of pain relief. Research has demonstrated that TT can promote wound healing, and some practitioners have reported accelerated bone healings also (Mackey 1995). Preliminary studies suggest that TT may significantly reduce anxiety, improve affect, and bolster the immune system by diminishing the immunosuppressive effects of stress (Mackey 1995). TT is currently part of 80 nursing curricula in the United States and abroad and is being taught to hospital nursing staff around the world (Mackey 1995).*

Cognitive Restructuring-Reframing. Cognitive restructuring-reframing has been found to be posi-

BOX 13–2 HOW TO CENTER YOURSELF

Centering, the most fundamental aspect of therapeutic touch, is for some the most difficult to master. If you have never experienced a meditative state, it may take time and practice to develop the skill. Following are guidelines for "centering".

1. Sit comfortably and close your eyes or focus on one spot on the floor.
2. Take a deep breath in through your nose, filling your lungs. Hold it for a second or two, feeling the stillness.
3. Exhale completely, while quietly telling yourself to relax.
4. Allow all tension, anxiety, and extraneous thoughts to leave your mind and body. As you exhale, imagine a tall oak tree standing in the sunlight, firmly rooted to the earth, taking energy in from the sun.
5. Take another deep breath. Exhale deeply, as you picture tension flowing out of your body through your feet and into the ground.
6. As you concentrate on your breathing, you will start to become focused.
7. Take another breath and exhale, reaching deep within yourself to the center of your being. As you allow yourself to become centered and focused, you will experience inner peace and wholeness.

With practice and experience, you will be able to center yourself within one or two deep breaths.

From Mackey, R. B. (1995). Discover the healing power of therapeutic touch. *American Journal of Nursing,* 95(4): 27–32. Used with permission of Lippincott-Raven Publishers, Philadelphia, PA.

*For more information on Therapeutic Touch workshops near you, contact Nurse Healers Professional Associates, Inc., PO Box 444, Allison Park, PA 15101-0444. Voice Mail (412) 355-8476.

tively correlated with greater positive affect and higher self-esteem (Fawzy 1995). Cognitive restructuring includes the restructuring of irrational beliefs, replacing the worried self-statement ("I can't pass this course, I can't pass this course") with more positive self-statements ("If I choose to study, I will increase my chances of success"). Cognitive restructuring and cognitive reframing are techniques commonly used in cognitive therapies, e.g. Albert Ellis' Cognitive Behavioral Approach (REBT).

Reframing is a healthy stress-reduction tool and a technique used by some counselors for a variety of purposes. When used to reduce stress, imagery may be used along with cognitive reframing. The goal of reframing is to change a participant's perceptions of stress through cognitive restructuring. The desired result is to restructure a disturbing event or experience to one that is less disturbing and in which the client can have a sense of control. When the perception of the disturbing event is changed, there is less stimulation to the sympathetic nervous system, which in turn reduces the secretion of cortisol and catecholamines, which destroy the balance of the immune system (Brigham 1994).

Cognitive distortions often include overgeneralizations ("He always," "I'll never") and "should" statements ("I should have done better," "He shouldn't have said that"). The following are some examples of cognitive restructuring-reframing anxiety-producing thoughts (Ellis and Harper 1975):

Irrational belief: I'll never be happy until I am loved by someone I really care about.

Positive statements: a. If I do not get love from one person, I can still get it from others and find happiness that way.
b. If someone I deeply care for rejects me, that will seem unfortunate, but I will hardly die.
c. If the only person I truly care for does not return my love, I could devote more time and energy to winning someone else's love and probably find someone better for me.
d. If no one I care for ever cares for me, I can still find enjoyment in friendships, in work, in books, and in other things.

Irrational belief: He should treat me better, after all I do for him.

Positive statement: I would like him to do certain things to show that he cares. If he chooses to continue to do things that hurt me after he understands what those things are, I am free to make choices about leaving or staying in this hurtful relationship.

Often, cognitive restructuring is done along with progressive relaxation.

Assertiveness Training. Assertiveness is a learned behavior that includes standing up for one's rights without violating the rights of others. **Assertiveness training** has proved to be a successful way of decreasing stress, anxiety, and conflict resulting from stressful interpersonal relationships, although some may experience the initial training and practice as somewhat stressful (Beare and Myers 1994). It has been demonstrated that when people openly and honestly express their needs, feelings, and desires, while respecting the feelings and rights of others, stress and anxiety are considerably lowered.

The concept of assertiveness is different from that of aggressiveness or passivity. When people are aggressive, as we learned earlier in the chapter, their behavior escalates; their voice becomes loud; they interrupt others; and physiologically their heart rate, blood pressure, and levels of certain stress-related hormones are raised. This in turn can escalate stress and anxiety in others, so that it becomes impossible to effectively problem solve or come together in a respectful understanding toward a solution. In extreme situations, escalating anger can lead to physical violence. When people suppress their feelings or are passive, they suffer high levels of anxiety, discomfort, or depression and develop physical problems (Brigham 1994).

Brigham identifies four situations and formulas for assertive communications:

Formula 1 (Simple Assertion)

a. It is simply an open, honest, direct statement of a request, an opinion, a question, a feeling, or a need.

EXAMPLES:

"No, I don't think that is the best plan of action."
"Right now, I need some help with this."
"Yes, I do like the way she handled that situation."

Formula 2 (Empathetic Assertion)

a. Show understanding and recognition of the other person's feelings, yet
b. Assertively state what one needs.

EXAMPLES:

"(a) I know you are concerned that I will be hurt by this decision, (b) but I need to make this decision myself."

Formula 3 (Feeling Assertive)

a. Nonaccusingly describe the situation or behavior in question.
b. State one's feelings (not opinions), and
c. Ask for a change.

EXAMPLES:

"(a) When I am criticized in front of others, (b) I feel embarrassed and hurt, (c) I'd prefer that if you need to tell me something, you do it in private."

Formula 4 (Confrontational Assertion)

a. Ask for private time to talk.
b. Point out the facts in a nonaccusing manner.
c. Check areas in which you may not understand the situation.
d. Ask for the changes you need.

EXAMPLES:

"(a) I need to talk to you privately. (b) It seems to me that our communication is not what it has been in the past. I notice that you watch TV while I am telling you things that are important to me. (c) It seems to me that we just aren't as close. Am I off base? (d) I'd like to find out what the problem is so we can get our relationship back on track."

EXTERNAL FOCUS

Progressive Muscular Relaxation (PMR). Progressive muscular relaxation (PMR) is a technique that can help patients achieve deep relaxation. The premise behind PMR is that deep relaxation can occur when muscle contraction is almost completely eliminated. Jacobson (1974), who first developed PMR, devised a program of instruction wherein systematic tensing and releasing of various muscles, and learning to discriminate between sensations of tension and relaxation, occur. The technique can be learned and practiced in hospitals as well as in the community for patients with a variety of conditions (Table 13–9).

Many training sessions are usually needed for mastery of PMR. For best results the student should receive live instruction and proceed only with the approval of a physician.

Biofeedback. In recent years, behavioral researchers have been exploring the clinical use of biofeedback as a means of improving somatic functioning. Biofeedback is the American culture's counterpart to Zen, yoga, and transcendental meditation. Americans seem to be impressed with science, technology, and electronic equipment, and biofeedback procedures and instruments correspond to these interests.

A visit to the commercial exhibit area of any psychological or psychiatric convention will reveal a plentiful display of complex biofeedback apparatus, touted as an efficient, even miraculous, means of helping people control one or another bodily-mental state. Basically, by using sensitive instrumentation, **biofeedback** gives a person prompt and exact information, otherwise unavailable, on muscle activity, brain waves, skin temperature, heart rate, blood pressure, and other bodily functions. This particular internal physiological process is detected and amplified by a sensitive recording device. It is assumed that a person can achieve greater voluntary control over phenomena once considered to be exclusively involuntary, if he or she knows instantaneously, through an auditory or visual signal, whether a somatic activity is increasing or decreasing. Because anxiety has generally been viewed as a state involving the autonomic (involuntary) nervous system, and because psychophysiological disorders afflict organs innervated by this system, it is obvious why researchers and clinicians became intrigued with biofeedback. Indeed, biofeedback was for a time virtually synonymous with behavioral medicine.

In a series of studies at Harvard Medical School, Shapiro and associates (1970) and Schwartz (1973) demonstrated that human volunteers could achieve sig-

TABLE 13–9 MUSCLE GROUPS AND SUGGESTIONS FOR PROGRESSIVE RELAXATION

1. Right/left hand and forearm: Begin with your dominant side. Make a very tight fist.
2. Right/left upper arm: Press your elbow down into the arm rest. While pressing down, try to move your upper arm toward your ribcage.
3. Right/left hand and forearm: Same as 1.
4. Right/left upper arm: Same as 2.
5. Forehead: Raise your eyebrows as high as you can. If this does not cause tension, make a deep frown.
6. Middle face: Wrinkle your nose and shut your eyelids tightly together.
7. Jaws: Clench your teeth and pull back the corners of your mouth. At the same time, press your tongue against the roof of your mouth.
8. Neck: Pull your chin toward your chest with the muscles in the front of your neck while simultaneously pulling your head back with the muscles in the rear of your neck.
9. Shoulders and upper back: Pull your shoulders back as though you were trying to touch your shoulder blades together. An alternative movement is to shrug your shoulders. Raise your shoulders as though you were trying to touch your ears with the tops of your shoulders.
10. Stomach: Pull the muscles of your stomach inward while at the same time pressing them downward. This makes your stomach hard, as you would if you were preparing to be hit in the stomach.
11. Right/left thigh: Try to bend your knee forward with the muscles of the back of your thigh while at the same time bending in the opposite direction with the muscles on the top of your thigh.
12. Right/left calf: Bend your foot toward your shin as though you were trying to touch your shin with your toes. (This is the opposite movement from pointing your toes.)
13. Right/left thigh: Same as 11.
14. Right/left calf: Same as 12.

Adapted from Jacobson, E. (1974). *Progressive relaxation* (3rd ed.). Chicago: University of Chicago Press.

nificant short-term changes in blood pressure and heart rate. They found that some subjects could even be trained to increase their heart rate while decreasing blood pressure. Achievement of this fine-grained control lent impetus to biofeedback work with human beings and awakened hope that certain clinical disorders might be alleviated in this way.

What is not yet clear, however, is whether, through biofeedback, clinically significant results can be achieved. In the move from analog to the more challenging world of the clinic, at least three vital questions must be asked. First, can persons whose systems are *malfunctioning* achieve the same biofeedback control over bodily events that normal subjects can acquire? Second, if actual patients can achieve some degree of control, will it be enough to make a significant difference in their condition? Third, can the control achieved by patients hooked up to and receiving immediate feedback from a remarkable apparatus be carried over to real-life situations in which they will have no special devices to inform them of the state of the bodily functions that they have learned to control?

Research in patients suffering from essential hypertension has been somewhat encouraging, but results have not been certain enough to establish biofeedback as a standard treatment for the condition (Shapiro and Surwit 1979). Moreover, some (Blanchard et al. 1976) believe that relaxation training, which is often given along with biofeedback, does more to reduce blood pressure than the biofeedback itself, a conclusion drawn in reviews by Emmelkamp (1986), O'Leary and Wilson (1975), and Reed and colleagues (1986). A study by Canino and associates (1994) found a significant reduction in both systolic and diastolic values both after treatment and at 6 months' follow-up, using a combination of biofeedback, PMR, and anxiety management training.

Biofeedback has been used in an attempt to control migraine, an extremely debilitating headache suffered by 10% of the general population. Although there are two competing schools regarding the best way to use biofeedback in treating migraine headaches, there have been positive results in reducing their severity. Tension headaches, believed to be caused by excessive and persistent tension in the frontalis muscles of the forehead and in the muscles of the neck, have also been handled within this framework, the standard treatment entailing feedback of tension in the frontalis muscles. For example, Holroyd and colleagues (1984) found that *believing* that one was reducing frontalis tension via biofeedback was associated with reduction in tension headaches, whether or not such reductions were actually being achieved. Enhanced feelings of self-efficacy and internal control appear to have inherent stress-reducing properties. It is possible that biofeedback strengthens the sense of control, thereby reducing general anxiety levels and ultimately reducing tension headaches.

Attempts have also been made, with mixed success, to alleviate other medical problems by means of biofeedback. Increasing finger temperature, which dilates the blood vessels in the hand, has been found somewhat useful in helping people with Raynaud's disease, in which blood flow to the extremities is reduced by spasms of small peripheral arteries (Surwit 1982). Biofeedback has also been used to increase and enhance muscular control in such neuromuscular disorders as cerebral palsy and post-stroke paralysis (Basmajian 1977). If a neuromuscular dysfunction is caused by the faintness of muscle movement in damaged tissues, amplifying these proprioceptive signals by biofeedback might make the patient aware of them and possibly allow control (Runck 1980). For example, a study by Brucker and Bulaeva (1996) found biofeedback useful for increasing voluntary electromyographic responses in clients with long-term spinal cord injury. Moreover, with the increasing recognition of the role of stress in a variety of medical illnesses, including diseases affected by immune dysfunction, biofeedback has emerged as one of the strategies used in stress management. Although it is uncertain whether it is necessary to use complex instrumentation required for proper biofeedback of minute levels of muscle tension or certain patterns of electroencephalographic activity, it has been confirmed that teaching people to relax deeply and to apply these skills to real-life stressors can be helpful in lowering stress levels.*

Stress and Anxiety Reduction Activities

Music

Music and emotion may share certain essential characteristics, allowing music to resonate with that of emotional experience. Music is common to all people and cultures. Certain impressions and emotions are often communicated more successfully through music than through the spoken word. In fact, simultaneous singing and rhythmic movement facilitate the initiation and fluency of speech (Borchgrevink 1993).

In medicine, music is used as an alternative channel of communication in aphasia and developmental disorders, as well as in psychotherapy. Gerdner and Swanson (1993), in a sample of elderly clients, found that music can be used successfully as an alternative approach to management of confusion and agitation. By altering affective, cognitive, and sensory processes, music therapists as part of multidisciplinary hospice teams use music to promote the quality of life for terminally ill clients and their family members (Mandel 1993). The need to cope with disease, psychosocial integration, and promotion of positive resources for self-healing are all regarded as indications for music therapy (Escher et al. 1993).

*The author would like to thank Dr. Julius Trubowitz for his contribution of the biofeedback section of this chapter.

Pets

Peaceful contact with beloved pets can bring joy, laughter, and stress reduction, a fact known to all pet owners. Pets make us feel happy. They provide an outlet for the expression of warm and affectionate feelings toward a safe and trusting being. The use of pets in nursing homes has long been known to bring out withdrawn individuals and aid socialization. Pets soothe us, so it is not surprising that spending time with them can help reduce high blood pressure in some individuals. A study by Friedmann and Thomas (1995) supported previous findings that pet ownership and social supports are significant predictors of survival among clients with coronary artery disease. For many, being around pets greatly improves their quality of life.

Exercise

Regular exercise is a great stress buster for many people. High levels of epinephrine can be drained off physically instead of being internalized onto visceral targets (stomach, intestines) or affecting somatic functions (gastric secretion, vasoconstriction). Exercise helps reduce muscle tension and may also increase endorphin release. It has long been known that, for some depressed people, a brisk walk or other form of enjoyable exercise can help increase endorphin production and thus improve mood. There is a great deal of data that indicates a positive correlation between physical exercise and lowered levels of acute measures of anxiety (Brown 1990). In clinical work with clients who have performance anxiety, about 33% said that exercise was the single most useful maneuver during their encounter with anxiety-arousing situations (Stoyva and Carlson 1993).

Tai chi, a slow-moving and nonvigorous form of exercise, can aid in the attainment of deep psychological and physical relaxation. It is one of the best known of China's martial arts. When practiced seriously, tai chi affects a large part of a person's thought and behavior, and with increasing skill the experience becomes one of meditation in action.

Breathing Exercises

Within the past several years, there has been increasing evidence that respiratory retraining, usually in the form of learning abdominal (diaphragmatic) breathing, has some definite merits in the modification of stress and anxiety reactions (Stoyva and Carlson 1993). One breathing exercise that has proved helpful for many clients with anxiety disorders is in two parts, as follows:

First, shift to relaxed, abdominal breathing. Breathe in by the mouth, hold for 3 seconds, and breathe out slowly through the nose.

Second, with every breath, turn attention to the muscular sensations that accompany the expansion of the belly.

The second part helps clients interrupt trains of thought, thereby quieting mental noise. With increasing skill, this becomes a tool for dampening the cognitive processes likely to set off stress and anxiety reactions. In clinical work with people who have performance anxiety, 50% reported breathing exercises to be useful during the feared situation (Stoyva and Carlson 1993).

CASE STUDY 1: USE OF COUNSELING IN MODERATE LEVELS OF ANXIETY

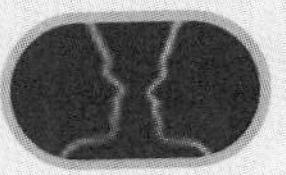

In the following case study, the first name of the client is used, while the surname is used for the nurse. This is to help avoid confusion. In the clinical setting, we would clarify how the client prefers to be addressed, by either first name or surname. Personal choice is often influenced by age, culture, previous experience, sex, or other personal considerations.

Donna James, a 24-year-old recently married woman, was brought to the hospital for vaginal bleeding during her fourteenth week of pregnancy. The medical team was unable to save the baby. Donna learned about the loss of her baby early that morning.

That evening, after dinner trays had been served, Jane Johnson, the evening nurse, went in to check Donna's vital signs. She found the dinner tray untouched and Donna crying. Ms. Johnson introduced herself and said "You're crying. May I help?" Donna started talking rapidly in a high-pitched voice, asking Ms. Johnson several times when she could go home. She said "I didn't know I'd be so upset." Donna's pulse rate was 112 and her respiration rate 26. She stated that she was not hungry and had a terrible headache. Ms. Johnson checked her for signs of shock and bleeding, but the physical assessment findings were normal.

ASSESSMENT

From her data, Ms. Johnson assessed Donna's anxiety level as moderate: she had repeatedly asked the same question in a high-pitched voice, she had an increase in pulse and respiration rates, she was crying, and she complained of lack of appetite and

Continued on following page

CASE STUDY 1: USE OF COUNSELING IN MODERATE LEVELS OF ANXIETY *(Continued)*

a headache. Further assessment and intervention could increase Donna's comfort and prevent her anxiety from escalating. Ms. Johnson said "I understand that this is a very difficult time for you." She told Donna that when she was finished taking her other client's vital signs, in about a quarter of an hour, she would be back to spend 15 minutes with her.

OBJECTIVE DATA

1. Increase in pulse and respiration rates (pulse, 112; respiration, 26)
2. Change in voice pitch
3. Crying—relief behavior
4. Repetitive questioning

SUBJECTIVE DATA

1. "I didn't know I'd be so upset."
2. "I have a terrible headache."
3. "I'm not hungry."

NURSING DIAGNOSIS

From her data, Ms. Johnson devised the following nursing diagnosis:

Anxiety (moderate), possibly related to Donna's feelings about the termination of her pregnancy (situational crisis), as evidenced by crying and somatic complaints.

However, more data would be needed.

PLANNING

Because general goals focus on decreasing anxiety, preventing further escalation of anxiety, and facilitating effective problem solving for a person in a moderate level of anxiety, Ms. Johnson proposed the following short-term outcomes.

1. Client's anxiety level will be mild by 11 PM, with the aid of nursing interventions.

Ms. Johnson planned to spend time with Donna to gather more data. Donna needed to discuss her feelings and concerns further and to mobilize some of her usual coping patterns.

INTERVENTION

When Ms. Johnson returned, she pulled the curtain around the bed. She leaned forward and sat where eye contact was possible. Ms. Johnson told Donna she had 15 minutes to spend with her. At first, Donna's talk shifted from topic to topic, and it was difficult for Ms. Johnson to identify Donna's feelings.

DIALOGUE	THERAPEUTIC TOOL/COMMENT
Nurse: I came back because you appeared upset. Were you? **Donna:** Yes . . . the baby . . . we wanted the baby, but my husband says we can have more . . . he's quite right, I guess. My mother-in-law blames the whole thing on me . . . says I'm too irresponsible and that we can't afford a family right now. I did want the baby . . . my husband is so worried about all the bills. He just got a job last month, you know. He couldn't come to see me because he is working overtime. My mother-in-law phones, but I could tell she wanted to get off the phone.	Initially, the nurse provides privacy and decreases the environmental stimuli.

Ms. Johnson demonstrates concern for Donna by

a. Making the observation that she understands that Donna may be feeling anxious.
b. Coming back at the time she had indicated.

CASE STUDY 1: USE OF COUNSELING IN MODERATE LEVELS OF ANXIETY *(Continued)*

c. Letting Donna talk about how she is feeling. She did not assume what Donna was feeling or why. She neither cut Donna off nor offered advice.
d. Letting Donna talk, listening for themes.

At first, Ms. Johnson sat with Donna, nodding and listening carefully to what was being said and listening for themes. Ms. Johnson waited until she had more data, then began to redirect and comment on what was being said.

DIALOGUE		THERAPEUTIC TOOL/COMMENT
Nurse:	It sounds as if there is a lot going on, but no one seems available for you now.	The nurse listens to the content of what Donna is saying and tries to focus on the themes. Crying can be a healthy release of tension. It is an excellent time to identify feelings because at that time feelings are close to the surface.
Donna:	My husband is a good man, he's very concerned with the bills. We were just starting to save some money *(begins to cry)*.	
Nurse:	Tell me what you're feeling right now.	
Donna:	Lonely . . . I feel so alone.	
Nurse:	What usually helps you when you're feeling lonely?	The nurse assesses past coping mechanisms that have been helpful.
Donna:	My husband . . . talking to my husband. He's my best friend.	
Nurse:	Since he's not here now, perhaps it will help if we talk.	The nurse offers her assistance.

Ms. Johnson and Donna continued to talk. Donna talked about the lack of support she felt from her mother-in-law and her feelings of being left alone by her husband because of his new job. They talked together about the possibility of Donna's finding a part-time job that would help the financial situation. Donna would have an opportunity to be part of a social network other than her immediate family if she worked. Ms. Johnson wondered if the actual loss of the baby was only a part of what was bothering Donna, who explained that once the bleeding had started, they had prepared themselves for the loss.

After 15 minutes, Ms. Johnson said that their time was up, but that she would come back before the end of the shift at 11 PM and spend 10 more minutes with her. Ms. Johnson asked Donna about her headache. Donna said that she felt much better and that her headache was gone. She appeared more relaxed and her vital signs had returned to baseline. Her voice was softer and more natural, and she was no longer easily distracted. Donna said she felt she was now able to get some rest.

When Ms. Johnson went back at 11 PM, Donna was asleep. When Ms. Johnson reported off duty, she asked the day shift to evaluate the need for further referrals before discharge.

EVALUATION

The goal was that Donna's anxiety level would be reduced to mild by 11 PM with the aid of nursing intervention. This was an appropriate and realistic short-term goal (outcome) set within a realistic time frame and, most important, it was measurable.

Ms. Johnson noted that one of Donna's somatic complaints (headache) was gone, her vital signs were back to baseline, her speech was no longer rapid and forced, her thoughts were more coherent, and she was now asleep. Ms. Johnson determined that the stated short-term goal was met.

CASE STUDY 2: COUNSELING TECHNIQUES FOR A PERSON IN SEVERE LEVELS OF ANXIETY

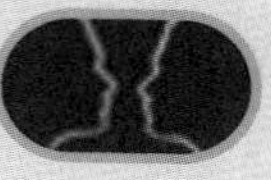

Tom Michaels, a 63-year-old man, came into the emergency department (ED) with his wife Anne, who had taken an overdose of sleeping pills and antidepressant medications. Ten years before, Anne's mother had died, and since that time Anne had suffered several episodes of severe depression with suicidal attempts. She had needed hospitalization during these episodes. Anne Michaels had been released 2 weeks previously after treatment for depression and threatened suicide.

Tom had long established a routine of giving his wife her antidepressant medications in the morning and her sleeping medication at night and keeping the bottles hidden when he was not at home. Today, he had forgotten to hide the medications before he went to work. His wife had taken the remaining pills from both bottles with large quantities of alcohol. When Tom returned home for lunch, Anne was comatose.

In the ED, Anne suffered a cardiac arrest and was taken to the intensive care unit (ICU).

Tom appeared very jittery. He moved about the room aimlessly. He dropped his hat, a medication card, and his keys. His hands were trembling, and he looked around the room, bewildered. He appeared unable to focus on any one thing. He said over and over, in a loud, high-pitched voice, "Why didn't I hide the bottles?" He was wringing his hands and began stamping his feet, saying "It's all my fault. Everything is falling apart."

Other people in the waiting room appeared distracted and alarmed by his behavior. Tom appeared to be oblivious to his surroundings.

ASSESSMENT

Russell Brown, the psychiatric nurse clinician working in the ED, came into the waiting room and assessed Tom's behavior as indicative of a severe anxiety level. After talking with Tom briefly, Mr. Brown believed nursing intervention was indicated.

Mr. Brown based his conclusion on the following assessment of the client.

OBJECTIVE DATA

1. Unable to focus on anything
2. Purposeless activity (walking around aimlessly)
3. Oblivious to his surroundings
4. Confused and bewildered
5. Unproductive relief behavior (stomping, wringing hands, dropping things)

SUBJECTIVE DATA

1. "Everything is falling apart."
2. "Why didn't I hide the bottles?"
3. "It's all my fault."

NURSING DIAGNOSIS

Mr. Brown formulated the following nursing diagnosis:

Anxiety (severe) related to the client's perception of responsibility for his wife's coma and possible death, as evidenced by inability to focus, confusion, and the feeling that "everything is falling apart."

PLANNING

Mr. Brown thought that if he could lower Tom's anxiety to a moderate level, he could work with Tom to get a clear picture of his situation and place the events in a more realistic perspective. He also thought that Tom needed to talk to someone and share some of his pain and confusion in order to sort out his feelings. Mr. Brown identified two short-term goals (outcomes):

1. Client's anxiety will decrease to moderate levels by 4 PM.
2. Client will talk about his feelings and plans by 4 PM.

INTERVENTION

Mr. Brown took Tom to a quiet room in the back of the ED. He introduced himself to Tom and said he noticed that Tom was upset. He said "I will stay with you." At first, Tom found it difficult to sit down and continued pacing around the room. Mr. Brown sat quietly and calmly, listening to Tom' self-recriminations. He listened carefully to what Tom was saying and what he was not saying, to identify themes.

After a while, Tom became calmer and was able to sit next to Mr. Brown. Mr. Brown offered him orange juice, which he accepted and held tightly.

Mr. Brown spoke calmly, using simple, clear statements. He used communication tools that were helpful to Tom in sorting out his feelings and naming them.

CASE STUDY 2: COUNSELING TECHNIQUES FOR A PERSON IN SEVERE LEVELS OF ANXIETY *(Continued)*

DIALOGUE	THERAPEUTIC TOOL/COMMENT
Tom: Yes . . . yes . . . I forgot to hide the bottles. She usually tells me when she feels bad. Why didn't she tell me?	
Nurse: You think that if she had told you she wanted to kill herself you would have hidden the pills?	The nurse asks for clarification on Tom's thinking.
Tom: Yes, if I had only known, this wouldn't have happened.	
Nurse: It sound as if you believe you should have known what your wife was thinking without her telling you.	Here the nurse clarifies Tom's expectations that he should be able to read his wife's mind.
Tom: Well . . . yes . . . when you put it that way . . . I just don't know what I'll do if she dies.	

When Mr. Brown thought that Tom had discussed his feelings of guilt sufficiently, he asked Tom to clarify his thinking about his wife's behavior. Tom was able to place his feelings of guilt in a more realistic perspective. Next, Mr. Brown brought up another issue—the question of whether Tom's wife would live or die.

DIALOGUE	THERAPEUTIC TOOL/COMMENT
Nurse: You stated that if your wife dies, you don't know what you will do.	Reflecting.
Tom: Oh God *(he begins to cry)*, I can't live without her . . . she's all I have in the world.	
Silence.	
Nurse: She means a great deal to you.	The nurse reflects Tom's feelings back to him.
Tom: Everything. Since her mother died, we are each other's only family.	
Nurse: What would it mean to you if your wife died?	The nurse asks Tom to evaluate his feelings about his wife.
Tom: I couldn't live by myself, alone. I couldn't stand it. *(Starts to cry again.)*	
Nurse: It sounds as if being alone is very frightening to you.	The nurse restates in clear tones Tom's experience.
Tom: Yes . . . I don't know how I'd manage by myself.	
Nurse: A change like that could take time adjusting to.	The nurse validates that if Tom's wife died it would be very painful. At the same time, he implies hope that Tom could work through the death, in time.
Tom: Yes . . . it would be very hard.	

Again, Mr. Brown gave Tom a chance to sort out his feelings and fears. Mr. Brown helped him focus on the reality that his wife might die and encouraged him to express fears related to her possible death. After a while, Mr. Brown offered to go up to the ICU with Tom to see how his wife was doing. On arrival at the ICU, Anne, although still comatose, was stabilized and breathing on her own.

Continued on following page

CASE STUDY 2: COUNSELING TECHNIQUES FOR A PERSON IN SEVERE LEVELS OF ANXIETY *(Continued)*

After arrival at the ICU, Tom started to worry about whether he had locked the door at home. Mr. Brown encouraged him to call neighbors and ask them to check the door. At this time, Tom was able to focus on everyday things. Mr. Brown made arrangements to see Tom the next day when he came in to visit his wife.

The next day, Mrs. Michaels regained consciousness, and she was discharged 1 week later. At the time of discharge, Tom and Anne Michaels were considering family therapy with the psychiatric nurse clinician once a week in the outpatient department.

EVALUATION

The first goal was to lower anxiety from severe to moderate within a given time. Mr. Brown could see that Tom had become more visibly calm: his trembling, wringing of hands, and stomping of feet had ceased, and he was able to focus on his thoughts and feelings with the aid of Mr. Brown.

The second short-term goal set for Tom was that he would talk about his feelings and plans within a given time. Tom was able to identify and discuss with the nurse feelings of guilt and fear of being left alone in the world if his wife should die. Both these feelings were overwhelming him. He was also able to make tentative plans with Mr. Brown for the future.

SUMMARY

Stress is a universal experience. Selye popularized the now-famous general adaptation syndrome (GAS). Stress elicits an initial adaptive response (defense mechanisms or relief actions of some sort), and most of the time these suffice to lower people's stress levels so that they can continue with their lives. However, stress can lead to chronic psychological and physiological responses (eventual maladaptive consequences) when not mitigated at an earlier stage. There are basically two categories of stressors: physical (heat, hunger, cold, noise, trauma) and psychological (death of a loved one, loss of job, school, humiliation).

Age, sex, culture, life experience, and life style are all important in identifying the degree of stress a person is experiencing. However, perhaps the most important factor to assess is a person's support system. Studies have shown that social and intimate supports of high quality can go a long way to minimize the long-term effects of stress.

Cultural differences exist in the ways people perceive an event as stressful and in the appropriate behaviors to deal with a stressful event. There are a variety of stress coping models; the one chosen in this chapter was that of Rahe.

Information about a person's emotional experience and needs can be gained by assessing the feelings the person is experiencing under stress. Some of the emotional needs (core relational themes) and action needs (action tendency) have been outlined by Lazarus. The way in which voice tone can influence the emotions of both the person who is experiencing the emotion and those around that person has been briefly discussed, citing the findings from Siegman's research.

Stress can be psychological, social, or biological. Anxiety can be rational or irrational, and the relief behavior can be adaptive or take the form of symptoms or syndromes.

Physiologically, the body reacts to anxiety and fear by the arousal of the sympathetic nervous system. Specific symptoms include rapid heartbeat, increased blood pressure, increased pulse rate, diaphoresis, peripheral vasoconstriction, restlessness, repetitive questioning, feelings of frustration, and difficulty concentrating.

The nurse learns to assess the level of anxiety a person is experiencing. For example, anxiety is assessed as mild to moderate or severe to panic. Different levels may indicate the need for different goals and nursing interventions.

Anxiety is not a constant state; it can be conceptualized on a continuum. Anxiety follows specific principles, which can be used as guides for planning effective nursing care. Specific nursing interventions are useful to people in moderate levels of anxiety; other nursing interventions are useful to those experiencing severe to panic levels of anxiety. The ability to evaluate personal levels of and reactions to anxiety is a process that can be learned. The ability to assess personal anxiety, as well as the anxiety of others, enables nurses to increase their effectiveness in interpersonal exchanges with clients, peers, and others. Application of the conceptual model of anxiety during implementation of the nursing process has been illustrated in two case studies.

Nurses are being trained in a great variety of holistic, noninvasive approaches to relieve people's stress. It is well accepted through replicated studies that the reduction of chronic stress is beneficial in many ways. For example, lowering the effects of chronic stress can alter the course of many physical conditions; decrease the need for some medications; diminish or eliminate the need for unhealthy and destructive behaviors such as smoking, insomnia, and drug addictions; and increase a person's cognitive functioning. An array of stress reduction techniques are available to the nurse clinician.

REFERENCES

American Psychiatric Association (1994). *Diagnostic and statistical manual of mental disorders* (4th ed.). Washington, DC: American Psychiatric Association.

Basmajian, J. V. (1977). Learned control of single motor units. In G. E. Schwartz and J. Beath (Eds.), *Biofeedback: Theory and research*. New York: Academic Press.

Beare, P. G., and Myers, J. L. (1994). *Principles and practice of adult health nursing* (2nd ed.). St. Louis: C. V. Mosby.

Benson, H. (1985). *The relaxation response* (2nd ed.). New York: William Morrow.

Blanchard, E. B., et al. (1976). Evaluation of biofeedback in the treatment of borderline essential hypertension. *Journal of Applied Behavior Analysis*, 12:99–109.

Borchgrevink, H. M. (1993). Music, brain, and medicine. *Tidsskrift for den Norske Laegeforening*, 133(30):3743.

Brigham, D. D. (1994). *Imagery for getting well: Clinical applications of behavioral medicine*. New York: W. W. Norton.

Brown, G. W., and Harris, T. (1989). *Social virgins of depression: A study of psychiatric disorders in women*. New York: Free Press.

Brucker, B. S., and Bulaeva, N. V. (1996). Biofeedback effect on electromyography responses in patients with spinal cord injury. *Archives of Physical Medical Rehabilitation*, 77(2):133.

Burd, S. F. (1968). Effects of nursing intervention in anxiety of patients. In S. F. Burd and M. A. Marshall (Eds.), *Some clinical approaches to psychiatric nursing*. New York: Macmillan.

Canino, E., et al. (1994). A behavioral treatment program as a therapy in control of primary hypertension. *Acta Cientifica Venezolana*, 45(1):30.

Davidhizer, R. (1991). How to stay sane as a student of nursing. *Imprint*, 38(4):96.

Dohrenwend, B. S., and Dohrenwend, B. P. (1974). *Stressful life events: Their nature and effects*. New York: John Wiley.

Dohrenwend, B.S., and Dohrenwend, B.P. (1983). Life stress and illness: Formulation of the issues. In B.S. Dohrenwend and B.P. Dohrenwend (Eds.), *Stressful life events and their contexts*. New Brunswick, N.J.: Rutgers University Press.

Ellis, A., and Harper, R. A. (1975). *A new guide to rational living*. North Hollywood, CA: Wilshire.

Emmelkamp, P. M. G. (1986). Behavior therapy with adults. In S. L. Garfield and E. Bergin (Eds.), *Handbook of psychotherapy and behavior change* (3rd ed.). New York: John Wiley.

Escher, J., et al. (1993). Music therapy and internal medicine. *Schweizerische Rundschau für Medizin Praxis*, 82(36):957.

Fawzy, F. I. (1995). Behavior and immunity. In H. I. Kaplan and B. J. Sadock (Eds.), *Comprehensive textbook of psychiatry/VI* (Vol. 2, pp. 1559–1570). Baltimore: Williams & Wilkins.

Freeman, A., and Reinecke, M. A. (1993). *Cognitive therapy of suicidal behavior: A manual for treatment*. New York: Springer.

Friedmann, E., and Thomas, S. A. (1995). Pet ownership, social support, and one-year survival after acute myocardial infarction in the Cardiac Arrhythmia Suppression Trial. *American Journal of Cardiology*, 76(17):1213.

Frijda, N. H. (1986). *The emotions*. Cambridge, MA: University Press.

Gerdner, L. A., and Swanson, E. A. (1993). Effects of individualized music on confused and agitated elderly patients. *Archives of Psychiatric Nursing*, 7(5):284.

Gonzalez, C. A., Griffith, E. E. H., and Ruiz, P. (1995). Cross-cultural issues in psychiatric treatment. In G. O. Gabbard (Ed.), *Treatment of psychiatric disorders* (2nd ed.) (Vol. 1, pp. 55–74). Washington, DC: American Psychiatric Press.

Gunderson, J. G., and Phillips, K. A. (1995). Personality disorders. In H. I. Kaplan and B. J. Sadock (Eds.), *Comprehensive textbook of psychiatry/VI* (Vol. 2, pp. 1425–1462). Baltimore: Williams & Wilkins.

Heath, A. H. (1992). Imagery: Helping ICU patients control pain and anxiety. *Dimensions of Critical Care Nursing*, 11(1)57.

Hobfall, S. E., and Vaux, A. (1993). Social support: Social resources and social context. In L. Goldberger and S. Breznitz (Eds.), *Handbook of stress: Theoretical and clinical aspects* (2nd ed.) (pp. 685–705). New York: Free Press.

Holmes, T. H., and Masuda, M. (1972). Life events and social readjustment scale. *Psychosomatic Medicine* in Psychology Today, April p 71.

Holmes, T. H., and Rahe, R. H. (1967). The social readjustment rating scale. *Journal of Psychosomatic Research*, 11:213.

Holroyd, K., et al. (1984). Change mechanisms in EMG biofeedback training: Cognitive changes underlying improvements in tension headache. *Journal of Consulting and Clinical Psychology*, 52:1039.

Jacobson, E. (1974). *Progressive relaxation* (3rd ed.). Chicago: University of Chicago Press.

Kabat-Zinn, J. (1993). Meditation. In B. Moyers (Ed.), *Healing and the mind* (pp. 115–144). New York: Doubleday.

Kaplan H. I., and Sadock, B. J. (1995). *Synopsis of psychiatry* (6th ed.). Baltimore: Williams & Wilkins.

Katlin, E. S., Derit, S., and Wine, S. K. F. (1993). In L. Goldberger and S. Breznitz (Eds.), *Handbook of stress: Theoretical and clinical aspects* (2nd ed.) (pp. 142–157). New York: Free Press.

Krieger, D. (1979). *The therapeutic touch*. New Jersey: Prentice Hall.

Lazarus, R. S. (1991). *Emotion and adaptation*. New York: Oxford University Press.

Lazarus, R. S. (1993). Why we should think of stress as a subset of emotion. In L. Goldberger and S. Breznitz (Eds.), *Handbook of stress: Theoretical and clinical aspects* (2nd ed.) (pp. 21–39). New York: Free Press.

Lazarus, R. S., and DeLongis, A. (1983). Psychological stress and coping in aging. *American Psychologist*, 38:245.

Lazarus, R. S., and Folkman, S. (1984). *Stress, appraisal, and coping*. New York: Springer.

Lazarus, R. S., Kanner, A. D., and Folkman, S. (1980). A cognitive-phenomenological analysis. In R. Pluchik and H. Kellerman (Eds.), *Theories of emotion. Vol. 1: Emotion: theory, research and experience*. New York: Academic Press.

Mackey, R. B. (1995). Discover the healing power of therapeutic touch. *American Journal of Nursing*, 95(4):27.

Mandel, S. E. (1993). The role of the music therapist on the hospice/palliative care team. *Journal of Palliative Care* 9(4):37.

Mandler, G. (1993). Thought, memory and learning: Effects of emotional stress. In L. Goldberger and S. Breznitz (Eds.), *Handbook of stress: Theoretical and clinical aspects* (2nd ed.) (pp. 40–55). New York: Free Press.

Matassarin-Jacobs, E. (1993). Pain assessment and intervention. In J. M. Black and E. Matassarin-Jacobs (Eds.), *Luckmann and Sorensen's medical-surgical nursing: a psychopharmologic approach* (4th ed.) (pp. 311–358). Philadelphia: W. B. Saunders.

May, R. (1983). Anxiety and stress. In H. Selye (Ed.), *Selye's guide to stress research* (Vol. 2). New York: Scientific and Academic Editions.

Merikangas, K. R., and Kupfer, D. J. (1995). Mood disorders: Genetic aspects. In H. I. Kaplan and B. J. Sadock (Eds.), *Comprehensive textbook of psychiatry/VI* (Vol. 1, pp. 1102–1115). Baltimore: Williams & Wilkins.

Miller S., and Winstead-Fry, P. (1982). Family systems theory in nursing practice. Reston, VA: Reston Publishing Company.

O'Leary, K. D., and Wilson, G. G. (1975). *Behavior therapy: Application and outcome*. Englewood Cliffs, NJ: Prentice Hall.

Papkin, M. K. (1995). Consultation-liaison psychiatry. In H. I. Kaplan and B. J. Sadock (Eds.), *Comprehensive textbook of psychiatry/VI* (6th ed.) (pp. 1592-1606). Baltimore, MD: Williams & Wilkins.

Peplau, H. E. (1968). A working definition of anxiety. In S. F. Burd and M. A. Marshall (Eds.), *Some clinical approaches to psychiatric nursing*. New York: Macmillan.

Rahe, R. H. (1995). Stress and psychiatry. In H. I. Kaplan and B. J. Sadock (Eds.), *Comprehensive textbook of psychiatry/VI* (Vol. 2, pp. 1545–1559). Baltimore: Williams & Wilkins.

Rahe, R. H. (1993). Acute versus chronic post-traumatic stress disorder. *Integrative Physiological and Behavioral Science*, 28(1):45.

Reed, S. D., Katkin, E. S., and Goldband, S. (1986). Biofeedback and behavioral medicine. In F. H. Kanfer and A. P. Goldstein (Eds.), *Helping people change: A textbook of methods* (3rd ed.). Elmsford, NY: Pergamon.

Rossi, E. L. (1993). *The psychobiology of mind-body healing: New concepts of therapeutic hypnosis* (2nd ed.). New York: W. W. Norton.

Runck, B. (1980). *Biofeedback—Issues in treatment assessment*. Rockville, MD: National Institute of Mental Health.

Sapolsky, R. M. (1990). Stress in the wild. *Scientific American*, 262:116.

Schwartz, G. E. (1973). Biofeedback as therapy: Some theoretical and practical issues. *American Psychologist*, 28:666.

Selye, H. (1974). *Stress without distress*. Philadelphia: J. B. Lippincott.

Selye, H. (1993). History of the stress concept. In L. Goldberger and S. Breznitz (Eds.), *Handbook of stress: Theoretical and clinical aspects* (2nd ed.) (pp. 7–17). New York: Free Press.

Shapiro, D. and Surwit, R. S. (1979). Biofeedback. In O. E. Pomerleau and J. P. Brady (Eds.), *Behavioral medicine: Theory and practice*. Baltimore: Williams & Wilkins.

Shapiro, D., Tursky, B., and Schwartz, G. E. (1970). Control of blood pressure in man by operant conditioning. *Circulation Research*, 26:127.

Siegman, A. W. (1993). Paraverbal correlates of stress: Implications for stress identification and management. In L. Goldberger and S. Breznitz (Eds.), *Handbook of stress: Theoretical and clinical aspects* (2nd ed.) (pp. 274–299). New York: Free Press.

Snyder, S. H. (1984). Progressive relaxation as a nursing intervention: An analysis. *Advances in Nursing Science*, 6:47.

Stoyva, J. M., and Carlson, J. G. (1993). A coping/rest model of relaxation and stress management. In L. Goldberger and S. Breznitz (Eds.), *Handbook of stress: Theoretical and clinical aspects* (2nd ed.) (pp. 724–756). New York: Free Press.

Sullivan, H. S. (1953). *The interpersonal theory of psychiatry*. New York: W. W. Norton.

Surwit, R. S. (1982). Behavioral treatment of Raynaud's syndrome in peripheral vascular disease. *Journal of Consulting and Clinical Psychology*, 50:922.

Vaillant, G. E. (1994). Ego mechanisms of defense and personality psychopathology. *Journal of Abnormal Psychology*, 103(1):44.

Varcarolis, E. M. (1996) Relaxation. In S. Lego (Ed.), *Psychiatric Nursing: A comprehensive reference* (pp. 143–153). Philadelphia: JB Lippincott.

Warner, C. D., et al. (1992). The effectiveness of teaching relaxation techniques to patients undergoing elective cardiac catheterization. *Journal of Cardiovascular Nursing*, 6(2):66.

Weinberger, R. (1991). Teaching the elderly stress reduction. *Journal of Gerontologic Nursing*, 17(10):23.

SELF-STUDY AND CRITICAL THINKING

True or false

If false, change the statement to make it true.

1. ________ The concepts that anxiety (1) is energy and (2) can be communicated interpersonally come from *psychodynamic theory.*
2. ________ Secondary anxiety originating from physiological abnormalities or processes is consistent with *behavioral/learning theory.*
3. ________ Anxiety is a learned response, and learned responses to anxiety can be unlearned. This is a basic premise of *biological theory.*

Matching questions

4. ________ A feeling of dread resulting from a threat whose source is unknown.
5. ________ Anxiety precipitated by an imminent loss or change.
6. ________ Anxiety that a person has lived with for a long time and that possibly results from inadequate nurturing.
7. ________ Anxiety that is triggered by a physiological process.
8. ________ The ability to feel for and with another and understand the other's experience.

A. Fear
B. Primary anxiety
C. Chronic anxiety
D. Empathy
E. Normal anxiety
F. Anxiety
G. Secondary anxiety
H. Acute anxiety

Identify levels of anxiety.

9. Rosa is extremely agitated. She is pacing up and down, complaining of nausea and headache, and is unable to concentrate on anything but her lost cat. She is in the ________________ level of anxiety.
10. Neil is having difficulty taking in what is going on around him since he heard his promotion was denied. His heart is pounding and his hands are diaphoretic. He finds a friend, who helps him look at his situation and figure out his alternatives. He is in the ________________ level of anxiety.
11. Gary tells his neighbors that he has been chosen by God to bring peace to the world and that God speaks to him all the time. He is too disorganized to work at a steady job but sometimes helps neighboring farmers harvest their crops. He is in the ________________ level of anxiety.
12. Denise is told she has been chosen to compete in the final rounds of the championship spelling bee in her state. She starts planning her strategy by making up study time schedules and lists of words to go over, and she becomes very intent on her goal of doing her best. She is in the ________________ level of anxiety.

13. A man who is to have open heart surgery in the morning starts to complain of palpitations and nausea and has difficulty articulating, and his speech jumps from one topic to the next. He can hardly take in what is going on around him unless it is pointed out to him. He is in the ____________ level of anxiety. State three interventions that would be useful to this client and give the rationale for each intervention.

    A. ____________ R. ____________
    B. ____________ R. ____________
    C. ____________ R. ____________

14. A woman comes into the emergency room after having been beaten by a mugger. She is incoherent, says she feels like she is going to die, and vacillates between periods of withdrawal and crying and screaming. She is in the ____________ level of anxiety. State at least three interventions a nurse could use with a person in this level of anxiety and give the rationale for each intervention.

    A. ____________ R. ____________
    B. ____________ R. ____________
    C. ____________ R. ____________

Critical thinking

15. Assess your level of stress using the life-events scale found in Box 14–1 and evaluate your potential for illness in the coming year. Identify stress reduction techniques, described toward the end of the chapter, that you think would be useful for you to learn.
16. Teach a classmate the breathing technique identified in this chapter. Have the classmate teach you how to center yourself (Box 13–2).
17. Assess a classmate's coping styles in terms of ego defense mechanisms and social support systems. Have the same classmate assess yours. Discuss the relevance of both of your findings.
18. Using Figure 13–1, explain to a classmate the short-term effects of stress on the sympatho-adreno-medulla system, and if the stress is not relieved, identify the term effects. Have the classmate summarize what you have just told him or her.
19. Have a classmate explain to you, using Figure 13–1, the short-term effects of stress on the hypothalamus-pituitary-adrenal cortex, and if the stress becomes chronic, the eventual long-term effects. Summarize to your classmate your understanding of what was just presented.
20. Discuss with your classmate one patient you have cared for in the hospital who had one of the stress-related diseases identified in Figure 13–1, and see if you can identify some stressors in that person's life, and possible ways that that person could lower his or her chronic stress levels.

14

Crisis and Crisis Intervention

Elizabeth M. Varcarolis

OUTLINE

KEY TERMS AND CONCEPTS

The key terms and concepts listed here also appear in bold where they are defined or discussed in this chapter.

crisis
crisis intervention
maturational crisis
situational crisis
adventitious crisis
phases of crisis
primary care
secondary care
tertiary care

OBJECTIVES

After studying this chapter, the reader will be able to

1. Differentiate among the three types of crises discussed in this chapter and give an example of each from your own experience.
2. Diagram Caplan's four phases of crises.
3. Delineate at least six aspects of crisis that have relevance for nurses involved in crisis intervention.
4. Develop a handout including areas to assess during crisis, with at least two sample questions for each area.
5. Evaluate your stress points using the Holmes and Masuda life events scale.
6. Describe three qualities the nurse can develop that can greatly enhance effective crisis intervention.
7. Discuss the common problems health care professionals may have when starting crisis intervention, and discuss at least two interventions for each problem.
8. Compare and contrast the differences among primary, secondary, and tertiary intervention, including appropriate intervention strategies.
9. Analyze four situations that can precipitate a crisis in an individual with severe and persistent mental health problems.
10. Explain to a classmate four potential crisis situations, common in the hospital setting, that a client may face. Give concrete examples of how they can be minimized

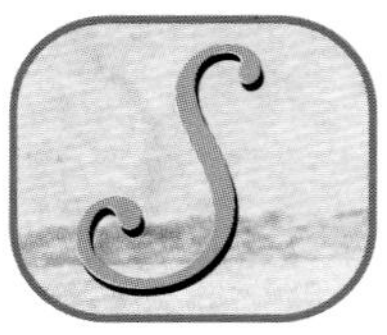

tress by itself does not constitute a crisis, but often a stressful event or the perception of such an event may precipitate a crisis. A **crisis** is an acute, time-limited phenomenon experienced as an overwhelming emotional reaction to a stressful situational, developmental, or societal event, or to the perception of that event. One person may perceive a stressful event as disastrous, whereas another person may view the same event as a challenge. For example, one woman upon finding that she is pregnant may experience anxiety and depression, whereas another woman will feel joy and excitement.

Life events, such as marriage, job promotion, the death of a spouse, or loss of a job, can be viewed as potential crises and may lead to psychological or physical illness (Holmes and Masuda 1972). Anxiety usually characterizes the reaction to crisis, but other emotions (e.g., depression, anger, fear) may also be involved.

A crisis itself is not a pathological state, and being in crisis is not pathological. It is a struggle for equilibrium and adjustment when problems are perceived as insolvable. A crisis presents both a danger to personality organization and a potential opportunity for personality growth. The outcome depends on how the individual perceives and deals with the crisis and what outside supports are available at the time the crisis occurs.

As anxiety escalates in response to a stressful event, relief behaviors are elicited. When a person's usual defense mechanisms are not able to lower or maintain anxiety, personality disorganization and interferences with daily living may follow. When the ability to cope with stress is hampered, anxiety may rise to severe or panic levels and may therefore interfere with problem solving. A person experiencing a psychiatric emergency of this sort needs immediate help in the form of **crisis intervention.** Basic steps in the development of a crisis are shown in Figure 14–1. Crisis intervention (1) is short-term, (2) focuses on solving the immediate problem, (3) aims to reestablish former coping patterns and problem-solving ability, and (4) is usually limited to a 4- to 6-week period after which resolution will be attained.

Nurses, perhaps more than any other group, deal with people who are experiencing disruption in their lives. People often undergo increased amounts of stress and anxiety in the medical/surgical, pediatric, obstetrical, and emergency department settings, as well as in the formal psychiatric setting. An understanding of what constitutes a crisis and a basic knowledge of crisis intervention enable the nurse to cope effectively with potential and actual crisis situations. The ability to recognize a crisis and intervene in a timely manner can influence the quality and course of another person's life.

THEORY

Crisis theory was developed in the early 1940s by Erich Lindemann, who conducted a classic study of the grief reactions of close relatives of victims in the Coconut Grove nightclub fire. This study formed the foundation of crisis theory and clinical intervention. Lindemann observed that "acute grief was the normal reaction to a distressing situation" (Ewing 1978). Lindemann showed that preventive intervention in crisis situations could eliminate or decrease serious personality disorganization and devastating psychological consequences from the sustained effects of severe anxiety.

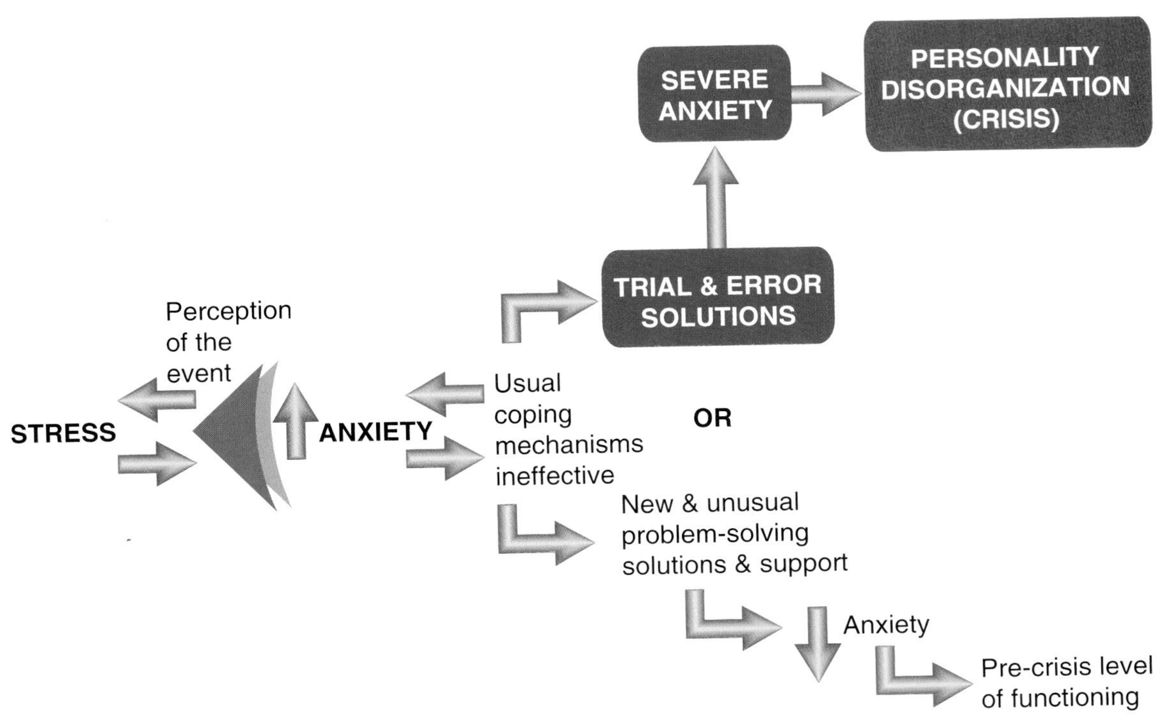

Figure 14–1 Phases in the process of crisis.

In the early 1960s, Gerald Caplan (1964) defined crisis theory and outlined crisis intervention. Since that time, our understanding of crisis and effective intervention has been refined and enhanced by numerous clinicians and theorists.

In 1961, a report from the Joint Commission on Mental Illness and Mental Health spoke about the need for community mental health centers throughout the country. This report stimulated the establishment of crisis services, which are now an important part of mental health programs in hospitals and communities.

The following ways of looking at crisis are derived from established crisis theory and constitute a sound knowledge base for the application of the nursing process to a crisis. An understanding of these three areas of crisis theory enables application of the nursing process: (1) types of crisis, (2) phases of crisis, and (3) aspects of crisis that have relevance for nurses.

Types of Crisis

Three basic types of crisis situations have been identified: (1) maturational, (2) situational, and (3) adventitious.

Maturational Crisis

A process of maturation occurs throughout the life cycle. Erikson identified eight stages of growth and development in which specific maturational tasks must be mastered. Each of these stages constitutes a crisis in personal growth and development (see Chapter 2.)

Each developmental stage can be referred to as a **maturational crisis.** When a person arrives at a new stage, formerly used coping styles are no longer appropriate, and new coping mechanisms have yet to be developed. For a time, the person is without effective defenses. This often leads to increased anxiety, which may be seen in variations in the person's normal behavior. Temporary disequilibrium may affect interpersonal relationships, body image, and social and work roles (Hoff 1995). Successful resolution of these tasks leads to development of basic human qualities. Erikson believed that the way these crises are resolved at one stage affects the ability to pass through subsequent stages, because each crisis provides the starting point for moving to the next stage. If a person lacks support systems and adequate role models, successful resolution may be difficult or may not occur. Unresolved problems in the past and inadequate coping mechanisms can adversely affect what is learned in each developmental stage. When a person is experiencing severe difficulty during a maturational crisis, professional intervention may be indicated.

Alcohol and drug addiction are examples of how progression through the maturational stages can be interrupted. This phenomenon is too often seen among teenagers today. When the addictive behavior is controlled (by the late teens), the young person's growth and development will resume at the point at which it was interrupted. A young person whose addiction is arrested at 19 years of age could have the social and problem-solving skills of a 14-year-old. Often these teenagers do not receive treatment, and their adult coping skills are diminished or absent.

Situational Crisis

A **situational crisis** arises from an external rather than an internal source. Examples of external situations that could precipitate a crisis include loss of a job, the death of a loved one, abortion, a change of job, a change in financial status, "coming out" as to homosexual orientation, divorce, the addition of new family members, pregnancy, and severe physical illness.

These situations were first referred to as "life events" by Holmes and Masuda (1972). Each event is assigned stress points that, when totaled, may predict the risk for illness. A high point count can act as a predictor of physical or psychological illness. Holmes and Masuda's Life Events and Social Readjustment Scale (Box 14–1) can be a useful tool for evaluating potential crisis situations and for planning primary intervention.

Some authors refer to these events as critical life problems because these problems are encountered by most people during the course of their lives. Whether these events precipitate a crisis depends on such factors as the degree of support available from caring friends and family members, a person's general emotional status, and a person's ability to understand and cope with the meaning of the stressful event.

As in all crises or potential crisis situations, the stressful event involves a loss or change that threatens a person's self-concept and self-esteem. To varying degrees, successful resolution of a crisis depends on resolution of the grief associated with the loss.

BOX 14–1 LIFE EVENTS AND SOCIAL READJUSTMENT SCALE

DIRECTIONS

Using yourself or a client as the subject, place a check mark on the line to the left of each event that has occurred in the subject's life during the past year. If the event has occurred more than once, place a check mark for each occurrence, then add up the accumulated points.

	Event	POINTS
____	1. Death of a spouse	100
____	2. Divorce	73
____	3. Marital separation	65
____	4. Jail term	63
____	5. Death of a close family member	63
____	6. Personal injury or loss	53
____	7. Marriage	50
____	8. Firing from work	47
____	9. Marital reconciliation	45
____	10. Retirement	45
____	11. Change in health of family member	44
____	12. Pregnancy	40
____	13. Sexual difficulties	39
____	14. New family member	39
____	15. Business readjustment	39
____	16. Change in financial state	38
____	17. Death of a close friend	37
____	18. Change to a different line of work	36
____	19. Change in number of arguments with spouse	35
____	20. Mortgage over $100,000	31
____	21. Foreclosure of mortgage or loan	30
____	22. Change in responsibilities at work	29
____	23. Son or daughter leaving home	29

	Event	POINTS
____	24. Trouble with in-laws	29
____	25. Outstanding personal achievement	28
____	26. Spouse beginning or stopping work	26
____	27. Beginning or ending school	26
____	28. Change in living conditions	25
____	29. Revision of personal habits	24
____	30. Trouble with boss	23
____	31. Change in work hours or conditions	20
____	32. Change in residence	20
____	33. Change in schools	20
____	34. Change in recreation	19
____	35. Change in religion or spiritual activities	19
____	36. Change in social activities	18
____	37. Mortgage or loan less than $100,000	17
____	38. Change in sleeping habits	16
____	39. Change in number of family get-togethers	15
____	40. Change in eating habits	15
____	41. Vacation	13
____	42. Christmas or High Holidays	12
____	43. Minor violations of the law	11
	Subject's total	____

FIND THE SUBJECT'S LIFE CRISIS LEVEL AMONG THE FOLLOWING:

150–199	Mild risk
200–299	Moderate risk
300 or more	Major risk

Adapted from Holmes, T. H., and Masuda, M. (1972). Psychosomatic syndrome. *Psychology Today*, April:72.

Adventitious Crisis

An **adventitious crisis,** or crisis of disaster, is not a part of everyday life; it is unplanned and accidental. Adventitious crises may result from (1) a natural disaster (e.g., flood, fire, earthquake), (2) a national disaster (e.g., war, riot, internment in concentration camps), or (3) a crime of violence (e.g., rape, murder, spousal or child abuse).

Recent literature identifies numerous studies related to the psychological sequelae suffered by people after bombings, hurricanes, earthquakes, and the witnessing of traumatic deaths of others. Common phenomena experienced were posttraumatic stress disorder and depression. The need for psychological first aid (crisis intervention) and debriefing after any crisis situation cannot be overstressed for all age groups (children, adolescents, adults, and the elderly) (Leach 1995; Garrison et al. 1995; Karanci and Rustemli 1995; Goenjiian et al. 1995; Urano et al. 1995).

A person may be experiencing two types of crisis situation simultaneously. For example, a 51-year-old woman may be going through a midlife crisis when her husband dies suddenly of cancer, or a 14-year-old girl may be forced to move away from her friends because of a parent's job transfer to another state.

Phases of Crisis

Caplan (1964) identified four distinct **phases of crisis:**

1. A person confronted by a conflict or problem that threatens the self-concept responds with increased feelings of anxiety. The increase in anxiety stimulates the use of problem-solving techniques and defense mechanisms in an effort to solve the problem and lower anxiety.
2. If the usual defensive response fails, and if the threat persists, anxiety continues to rise and produce feelings of extreme discomfort. Individual functioning becomes disorganized. Trial-and-error attempts at solving the problem and restoring a normal balance begin.
3. If the trial-and-error attempts fail, anxiety can escalate to severe and panic levels, and the person mobilizes automatic relief behaviors, such as withdrawal and flight. Some form of resolution (e.g., compromising needs or redefining the situation to make an acceptable solution) may be made in this stage.
4. If the problem is not solved, anxiety can overwhelm the person and lead to serious personality disorganization. This maladaptive response can take the form of confusion, immobilization with fear, violence against others, or suicidal behavior, as well as yelling or running about aimlessly (Robinson 1973; Hoff 1989).

Refer again to Figure 14–1 for a diagram of the phases of crisis.

Aspects of Crisis That Have Relevance For Nurses

Here are the specific aspects of crisis theory that are basic to crisis intervention:

1. A crisis is self-limiting and is usually resolved within 4 to 6 weeks (Aguilera 1994; Croushore et al. 1981).
2. The resolution of a crisis results in one of three different functional levels. The person will emerge at a higher level of functioning, the same level of functioning, or a lower level of functioning.
3. The goal of crisis intervention is to maintain the precrisis level of functioning (Aguilera 1994).
4. The form of resolution of the crisis depends on the actions of the subject and the intervention of others (Ewing 1978).
5. During a crisis, people are often more open to outside intervention than they are at times of stable functioning (Ewing 1978). With intervention, the person can learn different adaptive means of problem solving to correct inadequate solutions.
6. The person in a crisis situation is assumed to be mentally healthy and to have functioned well in the past but is presently in a state of disequilibrium.
7. Crisis intervention deals with the person's present problem and resolution of the immediate crisis only (Aguilera 1994). Dealing with material not directly related to the crisis can take place at a later time. Crisis intervention deals with the "here and now."
8. The nurse must be willing to take an active, even directive, role in intervention, in direct contrast to what occurs in conventional therapeutic intervention techniques, which stress a more passive and nondirective role (Hoff 1995).
9. Early intervention probably increases the chances for a better prognosis.
10. The client is encouraged to set realistic goals and plan an intervention with the nurse that is focused on the current situation.

Hoff (1995) stated that the probability of positive crisis outcomes is enhanced by the following basic steps of crisis management, which closely follow the nursing process:

1. Psychosocial assessment of the individual's or family's crisis, including evaluation of victimization, trauma, and the risk of suicide or assault on others
2. Development of a plan with the person or family in crisis
3. Implementation of the plan, drawing on personal, social, and material resources
4. Follow-up and evaluation of the crisis management process and outcomes

ASSESSMENT

A person's equilibrium may be adversely affected by one or more of the following: (1) an unrealistic perception of the precipitating event, (2) inadequate situational supports, or (3) inadequate coping mechanisms (Aguilera 1994). It is crucial to assess these factors when a crisis situation is evaluated, because data gained from the assessment are used as guides for both the nurse and the client to set realistic and meaningful goals, as well as to plan possible solutions to the problem situation.

After determining whether there is a need for external controls because of suicidal or homicidal ideation or gestures, the nurse assesses three main areas: the client's perception of the precipitating event, the client's situational supports, and the client's personal coping skills.

Assessing the Client's Perception of the Precipitating Event

The nurse's initial task is to assess the individual or family and the problem. The more clearly the problem can be defined, the better is the chance that an effective solution will be found.

Sample Questions To Ask

A number of authors (Croushore et al. 1981; King 1971) suggest sample questions:

- Has anything particularly upsetting happened to you within the past few days or weeks?
- What was happening in your life before you started to feel this way?
- What leads you to seek help now?
- Describe how you are feeling right now.
- How does this problem affect your life?
- How do you see this problem affecting your future?

▶ Laura, a 15-year-old girl, is brought to the emergency room after slashing her wrists. She was found by her mother, who returned home early from a date. Her mother called the police, and they rushed Laura to the hospital. After Laura is seen by the medical personnel, she is interviewed by the psychiatric nurse working in the emergency department. The nurse speaks calmly. She introduces herself and tells Laura she would like to spend some time with her. The nurse states "It looks as if things are pretty overwhelming. Is that how you're feeling?" The nurse makes the observation that things must be very bad if Laura wants to kill herself. Laura sits slumped in a chair with her hands in her lap and her head hanging down. There are tears in her eyes.

Example: Assessing Laura's Perception of the Precipitating Event

Nurse: Laura, tell me what has happened.

Laura: I can't. . . I can't go home . . . no one cares . . . no one believes me . . . I can't go through it again.

Nurse: Tell me what you can't go through again, Laura. (Laura starts to cry, shaking with sobs. The nurse sits quietly for a while, offers Laura some tissues, then speaks.)

Nurse: Laura, tell me what is so terrible. Let's look at it together.

▶ After a while, Laura starts telling the nurse that when she was 9 years old her mother had a boyfriend. When her mother was out of the house, the boyfriend would touch her. Eventually, he forced her to have sex with him. He threatened Laura that if she told anyone he would kill her. When she was 11 years old, the boyfriend moved to another state. Two weeks ago, Laura's mother said the old boyfriend was coming back to live with them. Laura, terrified, told her mother what had happened years ago, but her mother called her a liar. Her mother said that if it came to a choice between Laura and the boyfriend, the mother would take the boyfriend.

Assessing Situational Supports

The client's support systems are assessed to determine the resources available to the person. Does the stressful event involve important people in the support system? Is the client isolated from others or are there family and friends who can provide the vital support? Family and friends may be called upon to aid the individual by offering material or emotional supports: for example, lending money, offering services, or being available to give affection and understanding. If these resources are not available, the counselor/nurse acts as a temporary support system while relationships with individuals or groups in the community are established.

Sample Questions To Ask

Aguilera (1994) suggests some questions:

- With whom do you live?
- To whom do you talk when you feel overwhelmed?
- Whom can you trust?
- Who is available to help you?
- Where do you go to worship (or talk to God), to school, or to other community-based activities?
- During difficult times in the past, who did you want most to help you?
- Who is the most helpful?

Example: Assessing Laura's Situational Supports

Nurse: Laura, who can you go to? Do you have any other family?

Laura: No. My dad left when I was 6. We stay pretty much alone. My mom doesn't allow my brother and me to play with other kids.

Nurse: Do you have anyone you can talk to?

Laura: No, I really don't have any friends. All the other kids think I'm stuck-up. I don't fit in too well, I guess. My mom would never let me go out, anyway. There are always things to do at home.

Nurse: What about your place of worship, or your teachers at school?

Laura: The teachers are nice, but I can't tell them things like this. Besides, they wouldn't believe me either.

Assessing Personal Coping Skills

In crisis situations, it is important to evaluate the person's level of anxiety. Common coping mechanisms may be overeating, drinking, smoking, withdrawing, seeking out someone to talk to, yelling, fighting, or engaging in other physical activity (Croushore et al. 1981). The potential for suicide or homicide must be assessed. If the client is suicidal, homicidal, or unable to take care of personal needs, hospitalization should be considered (Aguilera 1994).

Sample Questions to Ask

- What do you usually do to feel better?
- Did you try it this time? If so, what was different?
- Have you thought of killing yourself or someone else?
- What helped you through difficult times in the past?
- What do you think might happen now?

Example: Assessing Laura's Personal Coping Style

The nurse learns that Laura does very well in school, especially in math. Laura explains that when she studies, she can forget her problems and get lost in other worlds. Getting good grades also has another reward: it is the only time her mother says anything nice about her. Her mother boasts to her boyfriends about how bright her daughter is.

Nurse: What do you think would help your situation?

Laura: I don't want to die . . . I just don't know where to turn.

The nurse tells Laura that she wants to work with her to find a solution, and that she is concerned for Laura's safety and well-being.

NURSING DIAGNOSIS

A person in crisis may exhibit various behaviors that indicate a number of human problems. For example, when a person is in crisis, the nursing diagnosis of ineffective individual coping is often evident. Because anxiety levels may escalate to moderate or severe levels, the ability to solve problems is usually impaired, if it is present at all. **Ineffective individual coping** may be evidenced by inability to meet basic needs, inability to meet role expectations, alteration in social participation, use of inappropriate defense mechanisms, or impairment of usual patterns of communication. Possible etiologies or "related to's" for ineffective individual coping could include situational crises, inadequate support systems, maturational crises, multiple life changes, inadequate coping methods, unrealistic perceptions, and unmet expectations (Doenges and Moorehouse 1988).

Altered thought processes may be evidenced by altered attention span; distractibility; or disorientation to time, place, person, circumstance, and events. Altered thought processes in a crisis situation could be "related to" psychological conflicts or impaired judgment.

Because change in one member of a family almost always affects all the members, altered family process is a probable diagnosis. **Altered family process** can be "related to" a situational or developmental crisis of one or more members. Altered family process may be evidenced by subjective data regarding feelings of confusion or objective data identified by the nurse. For example, the family may no longer be able to help each other or the member in crisis to meet physical or emotional needs. The family may have difficulty adapting or responding to the changes or traumatic experience of the member in crisis. The family's ability to make decisions or accomplish developmental tasks may be impaired. Communications may become confused, and inability to express feelings may be evident.

Anxiety (moderate/severe/panic) is always present, and the nurse works with the client to lower the anxiety to a level at which the client is able to start problem solving and making effective plans for dealing with the crisis situation. Anxiety can be "related to" many etiologies, such as situational or maturational crises, threat to self-concept, threat to or change in health status (role functioning or socioeconomic status), and physiological factors (hyperthyroidism or use of some medications).

The assessment of Laura's (1) perception of the precipitating event, (2) situational supports, and (3) personal coping skills gives the nurse enough data to formulate two diagnoses and to work with Laura in setting goals and planning interventions.

Example: Nursing Diagnosis for Laura

The nurse formulates the following nursing diagnoses:

- ***Anxiety (moderate/severe):*** related to rape-trauma syndrome, as evidenced by ineffectual problem solving and feelings of impending doom.

- ***Ineffective family coping:*** compromised, related to Laura's perception of inadequate understanding by her mother and fear of renewed sexual assault.

PLANNING

Planning involves both (1) planning for short-term goals and long-term outcomes and (2) nurse's feelings and self-assessment.

Planning Outcome Criteria

Planning realistic goals is done together with the client or family. Goals are made to fit within the person's cultural and personal values. Without the client's involvement, the goals may be irrelevant or unacceptable solutions to that person's crisis. For example, a nurse new to crisis intervention who suggests that a woman leave her husband because he beats her may be surprised to find that the woman has different goals. Thus, goals are always made with the client, and they have to be congruent with clients' needs, values, and (in some instances) cultural expectations. The nurse evaluates goals for safety and works on contingency plans when necessary. The basic task in all potential crisis situations is to resolve the presenting problem and to support the person who is in crisis in an attempt to regain a pre-crisis level of functioning. Defining realistic goals gives the client a sense of control, which can decrease the impact of the crisis. Then, the nurse and client plan together acceptable means of meeting the goals.

The client—not the nurse—solves the problem. Important assumptions when working with a person in crisis (Hoff 1995) are that

- The person is in charge of his or her own life.
- The person is able to make decisions.
- The crisis counseling relationship is one between partners.

The nurse helps the client refocus to gain new perspectives on the situation. The nurse supports the client during the process of finding constructive ways to solve or cope with the problem. The client is involved in setting both the long-term outcomes and the short-term goals, as well as in planning intervention.

Nurse's Feelings and Self-Assessment

All types of people may be involved in helping individuals in crisis. For example, people from various professional backgrounds are trained in crisis intervention—police, teachers, welfare workers, clergy, social workers, and psychologists, as well as nurses. Crisis intervention is often practiced unwittingly by people without formal training, such as bartenders, concerned bystanders, friends, and neighbors. People can play a crucial role in the successful resolution of a crisis by responding spontaneously with concern and caring.

Beginning practitioners in crisis intervention often face common problems that must be worked through before they become comfortable and competent in the role of a crisis counselor. Four of the more common problems are the counselor's

1. Needing to be needed.
2. Setting unrealistic goals for clients.
3. Having difficulty dealing with the issue of suicide.
4. Having difficulty terminating.

Refer to Table 14–1 for examples and results of these problems, appropriate interventions, and desired outcomes. It is crucial in beginning crisis intervention that supervision be made available as an integral part of the training process. The supervisor should be an experienced professional; this could be a peer, a teacher, or a supervisor.

Personal Qualities That Enhance Nursing Effectiveness

Nurses need to monitor personal feelings and thoughts constantly when dealing with a person in crisis. It is important to recognize one's own level of anxiety to prevent closing off the expression of painful feelings by the client. Because a client's situation or anxiety level may trigger uncomfortable levels of anxiety in the nurse at times, the nurse tends to repress such feelings to maintain personal comfort. When the nurse is not aware of personal feelings and reactions, she or he may unconsciously prevent the expression of the painful feelings in the client that are precipitating the nurse's own discomfort. Thus, closing off feelings in the client can render the nurse ineffective. However, specific personal attributes in the nurse can contribute favorably to the outcome of an individual in crisis (Donlon and Rockwell 1982).

CARING. The caring nurse has profound respect for the human condition and believes that people in crisis should have the opportunity to ease their pain and to alter their situation. A cold and technical approach will bring little success with a person in crisis.

LISTENING. This specifically refers to

1. Hearing what the client says and does not say in the conversation.
2. Listening carefully to nonverbal expressions as well as verbal ones.
3. Monitoring what goes on in the interaction between the client and the nurse.
4. Identifying one's own feelings during the interaction with the client.

Listening is facilitated by looking at the person who speaks. Feedback can be given by clarifying what the per-

TABLE 14–1 COMMON PROBLEMS FACED BY BEGINNING PRACTITIONERS

EXAMPLES	RESULTS	INTERVENTIONS	OUTCOME
Problem 1. ***Counselor needing to feel needed.*** **Feels total responsibility to "care for" or "cure" client's problems.**			
Nurse • Allows excessive phone calls between sessions • Gives direct advice without sufficient knowledge of client's situation • Attempts to influence life style of client on a judgmental basis	Client becomes more dependent on nurse and relies less on own abilities Nurses reacts to client's not getting "cured" or taking advice by projecting feelings of frustration and anger onto client	Nurse • Evaluates with an experienced professional nurse's needs versus client's needs • Discourages dependency by client • Encourages goal setting and problem solving by client • Takes control only if suicide or homicide is a possibility	Client is free to grow and problem-solve own life crises Nurse's skills and effectiveness grow as comfort with role and own goals are clarified
Problem 2. ***Counselor setting unrealistic goals for clients.*** **Goals become nurse's goals and not mutually determined goals for the client.**			
Nurse • Expects physically abused woman to leave battering partner • Expects man who abuses alcohol to stop drinking when loss of family or job is imminent	Nurse feels anxious and responsible when expectations are not met; anxiety resulting from feelings of inadequacy are projected onto client in the form of frustration and anger	Nurse • Examines with an experienced professional realistic expectations of self and client • Reevaluates client's level of functioning and works with client on his level • Encourages setting of goals by client	Nurse's ability to assess and problem-solve increases as anger and frustration decrease Client feels less alienated, and a working relationship can ensue
Problem 3. ***Counselor having difficulty dealing with suicidal client.***			
Nurse selectively inattends by • Denying possible clues • Neglecting to follow up on verbal suicide clues • Changing topic to less threatening subject when self-destructive themes come up	Client is robbed of opportunity to share feelings and find alternatives to intolerable situation Client remains suicidal Nurse's crisis intervention ceases to be effective	Nurse • Assesses her own feelings and anxieties with help of an experienced professional • Evaluates all clues or slight suspicions and acts on them, e.g., "Are you thinking of killing yourself?" If yes, nurse assesses a. Suicide potential b. Need for hospitalization	Client experiences relief in sharing feelings and evaluating alternatives Suicide potential can be minimized Nurse becomes more adept at picking up clues and minimizing suicide potential
Problem 4. ***Counselor having difficulty terminating*** **after crisis has resolved.**			
Nurse tempted to work on other problems in client's life in order to prolong contact with client	Nurse steps into territory of traditional therapy without proper training or experience.	Nurse • Works with an experienced professional to a. Explore own feelings regarding separations and termination b. Reinforce crisis model; crisis intervention is a preventive tool, not psychotherapy	Nurse becomes better able to help client with his feelings when nurse's own feelings are recognized Client is free to go back to his life situation or request appropriate referral to work on other issues of importance to him

Data from Finkleman, A. W. (1977). The nurse therapist: Outpatient crisis intervention with the chronic psychiatric patient. *Journal of Psychosocial Nursing and Mental Health Services*, 8:27, 1977; and Wallace, M. A., and Morley, W. E. (1970). Teaching crisis intervention. *American Journal of Nursing*, 7:1484.

son is saying. This is done by repeating a short summary to the client, who agrees with or corrects the nurse's impression. Refrain from judging or moralizing, but try to understand the other person's experience. The importance of having someone listen during a difficult time cannot be overstressed; it helps a person in discouraging levels of anxiety to feel connected.

CREATIVITY AND FLEXIBILITY. A helping person must be able to look at another person's crisis situation from various angles and to work with the client to find possible solutions. Each individual is unique, and one's perception of a situation is filtered through cultural, family, and personal traditions and beliefs. The possible alternatives must be compatible with these traditions and beliefs. What is helpful for one person is often not appropriate for another. There are no simple solutions for people in crisis. The nurse must be able to view the situation from the client's perspective (have empathy) and work with the client to identify alternatives that will be effective in lowering anxiety and facilitating normal functioning.

Example: Planning the Intervention With Laura

A social worker is called. Laura, the nurse, and the social worker meet together. All agree that Laura should not be in the home if the boyfriend returns. The nurse then meets with Laura and her mother; however, Laura's mother continues to berate Laura for lying. She states that she does not care what Laura says, she has her own life to live. She says if Laura doesn't like it, she can move out. The nurse and Laura set three goals together:

1. A safe environment will be found for Laura before the boyfriend comes to live with the mother.
2. At least two support systems will be made available to Laura within 24 hours.
3. Continued evaluation and support will be available until the immediate crisis is over (6 to 8 weeks).

After talking with the nurse and the social worker, Laura seems open to the possibility of going to a foster home. She also agrees to talk to a counselor at her school. The nurse sets up an appointment when she, Laura, and the counselor can meet. The nurse will continue to see Laura twice a week.

INTERVENTION

Crisis intervention has two basic thrusts. First, external controls may be applied for protection of the person in crisis if the person is suicidal or homicidal. Second, anxiety reduction techniques are used, so that inner resources can be put into effect.

During the initial interview, the person in crisis first needs to gain a feeling of safety. Solutions to the crisis may be offered, so that the client is aware of other options. Feelings of support and hope will temporarily diminish anxiety. The nurse needs to play an active role by indicating that help is available. Help is conveyed by the competent use of crisis skills and genuine interest and support. It is not conveyed by the use of false reassurances and platitudes, such as "everything will be all right."

Crisis intervention requires a creative and flexible approach through the use of traditional and nontraditional therapeutic roles. The nurse may act as educator, adviser, and model.

Counseling Strategies

There are three levels of nursing care in crisis intervention: primary, secondary, and tertiary. Psychotherapeutic nursing interventions in crisis are directed toward these three levels of care.

PRIMARY CARE. Primary care promotes mental health and reduces mental illness in order to decrease the incidence of crisis. On this level the nurse can

1. Work with an individual to recognize potential problems by evaluating the stressful life events the person is experiencing.
2. Teach an individual specific coping skills such as decision-making, problem-solving, assertiveness skills, meditation, and relaxation skills, to handle stressful events.
3. Assist an individual to evaluate the timing or reduction of life changes in order to decrease the negative effects of stress as much as possible. This may involve working with a client to plan environmental changes, make important interpersonal decisions, and rethink changes in occupational roles.

SECONDARY CARE. Secondary care establishes intervention during an acute crisis to prevent prolonged anxiety from diminishing personal effectiveness and personality organization. The nurse works with the client to assess the client's problem, support systems, and coping styles. Desired goals are explored and interventions planned. Secondary care lessens the time a person is mentally disabled during a crisis. Secondary level care occurs in hospital units, emergency rooms, clinics, or mental health centers, usually during daytime hours.

TERTIARY CARE. Tertiary care provides support for those who have experienced and are now recovering from a disabling mental state. Social and community facilities that offer tertiary intervention include rehabilitation centers, sheltered workshops, day hospitals, and outpatient clinics. Primary goals are aimed at facilitating optimal levels of functioning and preventing further emotional disruptions. People with severe and persistent mental problems are often extremely susceptible to crisis, and community facilities provide the structured environment that can help prevent problem situations.

Example: Performing Secondary Crisis Intervention With Laura

- The nurse meets with Laura twice weekly during the next 4 weeks. Laura is motivated to work with the social worker and the nurse to find another place to live. The nurse suggests several times that Laura start to see a counselor in the outpatient clinic after the crisis is over, where she could talk about some of her pain. Laura is not interested, however, and says she will talk to the school counselor if she needs to talk.
- Three weeks after the attempted suicide, foster placement is found for Laura. The couple seems very interested in Laura, and Laura appears happy about the attention she is receiving.

CRISIS INTERVENTION FOR THE SEVERELY AND PERSISTENTLY MENTALLY ILL

Clients with a severe long-term mental illness also experience crises. The incidence of crisis may be increased in this population because of the nature of severe and persistent mental illness. Crisis theory and intervention can be adapted successfully with clients who have long-term mental illness. Five characteristics of people with a severe and persistent mental illness have been identified (Finkelman 1977):

1. Inadequate problem-solving ability
2. Inadequate communication skills
3. Low self-esteem
4. Poor success with endeavors such as work, school, family, and social relationships
5. Inpatient or outpatient treatment for at least 2 years

Although the client's illness is in the chronic state, there are healthy and unhealthy aspects of the client's personality. It is important to stress the healthy aspects, rather than the pathological aspects, during assessment of this client. Some of the major differences between the person who has long-term and severe difficulties in living and the mentally healthy person are outlined in Table 14–2.

Potential Crises in the Severely and Persistently Mentally Ill

People usually have a number of coping responses they use when stressed in their everyday world. Any kind of change in our routines or lives constitutes some degree of stress. For the person with limited abilities, even slight change might increase the potential for a full-blown crisis. Four common potential crisis situations for the severely and persistently mentally ill client have been identified (Finkelman 1977):

1. Change in treatment approaches, such as change in routine of treatment, therapist's absence due to vacation or illness, or change in appointment time.
2. Problems or changes at work, at school, or with the family, and anniversaries of significant or traumatic events in the person's life.
3. Lack of money, inadequate transportation, and problems meeting basic needs.
4. Sexual relationships for people unsure about their own sexual identity are always a source of anxiety. These feelings can be compounded in severely and persistently ill clients if there are other complications (e.g., pregnancy, impotence).

Adapting the Crisis Model

Traditionally, crisis intervention refers to disequilibrium in the functioning of otherwise mentally healthy persons. The goal is to prevent temporary difficulty in functioning from progressing to severe personality disorganization. Intervention and support can help people find the way

TABLE 14-2 MENTALLY HEALTHY VERSUS A SEVERELY AND PERSISTENTLY MENTALLY ILL PERSON IN CRISIS

MENTALLY HEALTHY PERSON	SEVERELY AND PERSISTENTLY MENTALLY ILL PERSON
1. Has realistic perception of potential crisis event.	1. Because of chronically high anxiety state, potential crisis event is usually distorted by minimizing or maximizing the event.
2. Has healthy ego boundaries, good problem-solving abilities.	2. Inadequate ego functioning assumes inadequate problem-solving abilities; nurse becomes more active in assisting person with this task.
3. Usually has adequate situational supports.	3. Person often has no family or friends and may be living an isolated existence.
4. Usually has adequate coping mechanisms. Defense mechanisms can be used as support to lower anxiety.	4. Because ego functioning in chronic patients is poor, coping mechanisms are usually inadequate or poorly utilized.

Data from Finkleman, A. W. (1977). The nurse therapist: Outpatient crisis intervention with the chronic psychiatric patient. *Journal of Psychosocial Nursing and Mental Health Services*, 8:27.

back to their previous level of functioning. People with severe and long-term mental health problems, however, are readily susceptible to crisis. The nurse must be able to adapt the crisis model to this group. These adaptations include focusing on the client's strengths, modifying and setting realistic goals with the client, taking a more active role in the problem-solving process, and using direct interventions, such as making arrangements the person would ordinarily be able to make.

EVALUATION

Goals are compared with the outcomes for the effectiveness of the crisis intervention. This is usually done 4 to 8 weeks after the initial interview, although it can be done in a shorter time frame. If the intervention has been successful, the person's level of anxiety and ability to function should be at pre-crisis levels. Often, a person chooses to follow up additional areas of concern, and referral to other agencies for more long-term work is made. Crisis intervention often serves to prepare a person for further treatment.

Example: Evaluating Laura's Crisis

- After 6 weeks, Laura and the nurse decide that the crisis is over. Laura remains aloof and distant. The nurse evaluates Laura as being in a moderate amount of emotional pain. Laura feels she is doing well, however, and feels more secure and accepted. The nurse's assessment indicated that Laura had other serious issues (e.g., the issue of her earlier sexual assaults), and the nurse strongly suggests to Laura that she could benefit from further counseling. The decision, however, is up to Laura. Laura says she is satisfied with the way things are, and again states that if she has any problems she will see her school counselor.
- *Postscript.* Two years later, Laura is continuing to do well in school and is planning to go to a local community college for computer programming. Laura gets along well with her foster parents, and plans are being made for adoption. Laura remains aloof. She has no close friends and continues to throw her energy into her studies. For the present, she is getting pleasure from her academic accomplishments, and she has security and warm attention in her new home environment. If at a later date she decides there are other things for her to work out, she knows the resources that are available in her community.

CASE STUDY: WORKING WITH A PERSON IN CRISIS

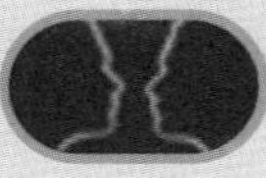

Ms. Greg, the psychiatric nurse consultant, was called to the neurological unit. She was told that Mr. Raymond, a 43-year-old man with Guillain-Barré syndrome, was presenting a serious nursing problem, and the staff requested a consult.

The head nurse said that Mr. Raymond was hostile and sexually abusive to the nursing staff. His abusive language, demeaning attitude, and angry outbursts were having an adverse effect on the unit as a whole. The other nurses stated that they felt ineffective and angry and that they had tried to be patient and understanding; however, nothing seemed to get through to him. The situation had affected the morale of the staff and, the nurses believed, the quality of their care.

Mr. Raymond, a Native American, was employed as a taxicab driver. Six months before his admission to the hospital, he had given up drinking after years of episodic alcohol abuse. He was engaged to a woman who visited him every day.

He needed a great deal of assistance with every aspect of his activities of daily living. His muscle weakness had progressed to the point that he was essentially paralyzed. At the time the consult was made, he could breathe on his own, but he had to be turned and positioned every 2 hours. He was fed through a gastrostomy tube.

ASSESSMENT

Ms. Greg gathered data from Mr. Raymond and the nursing staff and spoke with Mr. Raymond's fiancée.

MR. RAYMOND'S PERCEPTION OF THE PRECIPITATING EVENT

During the initial interview, Mr. Raymond spoke to Ms. Greg angrily, using profanity and making lewd sexual suggestions. He also expressed anger about needing a nurse to "scratch my head and help me blow my nose." He still could not figure out how his illness suddenly developed. He said the doctors told him that it was too early to know for sure if he would recover completely, but that the prognosis was good.

MR. RAYMOND'S SUPPORT SYSTEM

Ms. Greg spoke with Mr. Raymond's fiancée. Mr. Raymond's relationships with his fiancée and with his Native American

CASE STUDY: WORKING WITH A PERSON IN CRISIS *(Continued)*

culture group were strong. With minimal ties outside their reservation, neither Mr. Raymond nor his fiancée had much knowledge of outside supportive agencies.

MR. RAYMOND'S PERSONAL COPING SKILLS

Mr. Raymond came from a strongly male-dominated subculture in which the man was expected to be a strong leader. His ability to be an independent person with the power to affect the direction of his life was central to his perception of being acceptable as a man.

Mr. Raymond felt powerless, out of control, and enraged. He was handling his anxiety by displacing these feelings onto the environment, namely, the staff and his fiancée. This redirection of anger temporarily lowered his anxiety and distracted him from painful feelings. When he intimidated others through sexual profanity and hostility, he felt temporarily in control and experienced an illusion of power. He used displacement to relieve his painful levels of anxiety when he felt threatened.

Mr. Raymond's use of displacement was not adaptive, because the issues causing his distress were not being resolved. His anxiety continued to escalate. The effect his behavior was having on others caused them to move away from him. This withdrawal further increased his sense of isolation and helplessness.

NURSING DIAGNOSIS

On the basis of her assessment, Ms. Greg identified three main problem areas and formulated the following nursing diagnoses:

Ineffective individual coping related to inadequate coping methods, as evidenced by inappropriate use of defense mechanism (displacement)

- Anger directed toward staff and fiancée
- Profanity and crude sexual remarks aimed at staff
- Frustration and withdrawal on the part of the staff
- Continued escalation of anxiety

Powerlessness related to cultural differences and lack of control over his health care environment, as evidenced by frustration over inability to perform previously uncomplicated tasks

- Angry over nurses' having to "scratch my head and blow my nose"
- Minimal awareness of available supports in larger community

Ineffective staff coping related to exhaustion of staff supportive capacity toward client, as evidenced by staff withdrawal and limited personal communication with client

- Staff felt ineffective.
- Morale of staff was poor.
- Nurses believed that the quality of their care was adversely affected.

PLANNING

PLANNING OUTCOME CRITERIA

Ms. Greg spoke to Mr. Raymond and told him she would like to spend time with him for 15 minutes every morning and talk about his concerns. She suggested that there might be alternative ways he could handle his feelings, and community resources could be explored. Mr. Raymond gruffly agreed, saying "You can visit me, if it will make you feel better." They made arrangements to meet at 7:30 AM for 15 minutes each morning.

Continued on following page

CASE STUDY: WORKING WITH A PERSON IN CRISIS *(Continued)*

For each nursing diagnosis the following short-term goals were set:

NURSING DIAGNOSIS	SHORT-TERM GOAL
1. **Ineffective individual coping** related to inadequate coping methods, as evidenced by inappropriate use of defense mechanisms (displacement)	1. Mr. Raymond will be able to name and discuss at least two feelings about his illness and lack of mobility (by the end of the week).
2. **Powerlessness related** to lack of control over health care environment, as evidenced by frustration over inability to perform previous tasks	2. Mr. Raymond will be able to name two community organizations that could offer him information and support (by the end of 2 weeks).
3. **Ineffective staff coping** related to exhaustion of staff supportive capacity toward client, as evidenced by staff withdrawal and limited personal communication	3. Staff and nurse consultant will discuss reactions and alternative nursing responses to Mr. Raymond's behavior (twice within the next 7 days).

Ms. Greg created a nursing care plan (Nursing Care Plan 14–1) and shared it with the staff.

INTERVENTION

The following morning, Ms. Greg went into Mr. Raymond's room at 7:30 AM and sat by his bedside. At first, Mr. Raymond's comments were hostile.

DIALOGUE	THERAPEUTIC TOOL/COMMENT
Nurse: Mr. Raymond, I'm here as we discussed. I'll be spending 15 minutes with you every morning. We could use this time to talk about some of your concerns.	Nurse offers herself as a resource, gives information, and clarifies her role and client expectations. Night was the most difficult time for Mr. Raymond. In the early morning he would be the most vulnerable and open for therapeutic intervention and support.
Mr. R: Listen, sweetheart, my only concern is how to get a little sexual relief, get it?	
Nurse: Being hospitalized and partially paralyzed can be overwhelming for anyone. Perhaps you wish you could find some relief from your situation.	Nurse focuses on the process "need for relief" and not the sexual content. Encourages discussion of feelings. Sexual issues are often challenging to new nurses, and discussing your feelings and appropriate interventions with an experienced professional is important for your own growth and to the quality of the care you give.
Mr. R: What do you know, Ms. Know-it-all? I can't even scratch my nose without getting one of those fools to do it for me . . . and half the time those bitches aren't even around.	

CASE STUDY: WORKING WITH A PERSON IN CRISIS *(Continued)*

Nurse:	It must be difficult to have to ask people to do everything for you.	Nurse restates what the client says in terms of his feelings. Continues to refocus away from the environment back to the client.
Mr. R:	Yeah . . . the other night a fly got into the room and kept landing on my face. I had to shout for 5 minutes before one of those bitches came in, just to take the fly out of the room.	
Nurse:	Having to rely on others for everything can be a terrifying experience for anyone. It sounds extremely frustrating for you.	Nurse acknowledges that frustration and anger would be a normal and healthy response for anyone in this situation. Encourages the client to talk about these feelings instead of acting them out.
Mr. R:	Yeah . . . it's a bitch . . . like a living hell.	

Ms. Greg continued to spend time with Mr. Raymond in the mornings. He was gradually able to talk more about his feelings of anger and frustration and was less apt to act with hostility toward the staff. As he began to feel more in control, he became less defensive about others caring for him.

After 2 weeks, Ms. Greg cut her visits down to twice a week. Mr. Raymond was beginning to get gross motor movements back but was not walking yet. He still displaced much of his frustration and lack of control on the environment, but he was better able to acknowledge the reality of his situation. He could identify what he was feeling and talk about those feelings briefly.

DIALOGUE		THERAPEUTIC TOOL/COMMENT
Nurse:	What's happening? Your face looks tense this morning, Mr. Raymond.	Nurse observes the client's clenched fists, rigid posture, and tense facial expression.
Mr. R:	I had to wait 10 minutes for a bedpan last night.	
Nurse:	And you're angry about that.	Nurse verbalizes the implied.
Mr. R:	Well, there were only two nurses on duty for 30 people, and the aide was on her break . . . You can't expect them to be everywhere . . . but still . . .	
Nurse:	It may be hard to accept that people can't be there all the time for you.	Nurse validates the difficulty of accepting situations one does not like when one is powerless to make changes.
Mr. R:	Well . . . that's the way it is in this place.	

Continued on following page

CASE STUDY: WORKING WITH A PERSON IN CRISIS *(Continued)*

NURSES' FEELINGS AND SELF-ASSESSMENT

Ms. Greg met with the staff twice. The staff discussed their feelings of helplessness and lack of control stemming from their feelings of rejection by Mr. Raymond. They talked of their anger about Mr. Raymond's demeaning behavior, and their frustration about the situation. Ms. Greg pointed out to the staff that Mr. Raymond's feelings of helplessness, lack of control, and anger at his situation were the same feelings the staff was experiencing. Displacement of the helplessness and frustration by intimidating the staff gave Mr. Raymond a brief feeling of control. It also distracted him from his own feelings of helplessness.

The nurses became more understanding of the motivation for the behavior Mr. Raymond employed to cope with moderate to severe levels of anxiety. The staff began to focus more on the client and less on personal reactions, and decided together on two approaches they could try as a group. First, they would not take Mr. Raymond's behavior personally. Second, Mr. Raymond's feelings that were displaced would be refocused back to him.

EVALUATION

After 6 weeks, Mr. Raymond was able to get around with assistance, and his ability to perform his activities of daily living was increasing. Although Mr. Raymond was still angry and still felt overwhelmed at times, he was able to identify more of his feelings. He did not need to act them out so often. He was able to talk to his fiancée about his feelings, and he lashed out at her less. He was looking forward to going home, and his boss was holding his old job.

Mr. Raymond contacted the Guillain-Barré Society, who made arrangements for a meeting with him. He was still thinking about Alcoholics Anonymous but believed he could handle this problem himself.

The staff felt more comfortable and competent in their relationships with Mr. Raymond. The goals had been met. Mr. Raymond and Ms. Greg both believed that the crisis was over, and the visits were terminated. Mr. Raymond was given the number of the crisis unit and encouraged to call if he had questions or felt the need to talk.

NURSING CARE PLAN 14–1 A PERSON IN CRISIS: MR. RAYMOND

NURSING DIAGNOSIS

Ineffective individual coping: related to inadequate coping methods, as evidenced by inappropriate use of defense mechanisms (displacement).

Supporting Data

- Anger directed at staff and fiancée
- Profanity and crude sexual remarks aimed at staff
- Isolation related to staff withdrawal
- Continued escalation of anxiety

Outcome Criteria: By discharge, Mr. Raymond will state he feels more comfortable discussing difficult feelings.

SHORT-TERM GOAL	INTERVENTION	RATIONALE	EVALUATION
1. Mr. Raymond will be able to name and discuss at least two feelings about his illness and lack of mobility (by the end of the week).	1a. Nurse will meet with client for 15 minutes at 7:30 AM each day for a week.	1a. Night was usually the most frightening for client; in early morning, feelings were closer to surface.	GOAL MET Within 7 days, Mr. Raymond was able to speak to nurse more openly about feelings of anger and frustration.
	1b. When client lashes out with verbal abuse, nurse will remain calm.	1b. Client perceives that nurse is in control of her feelings. This can be reassuring to client and can increase client's sense of security.	
	1c. Nurse will consistently redirect and refocus anger from environment back to client, e.g., "It must be difficult to be in this situation."	1c. Refocusing feelings offers client opportunity to cope effectively with his anxiety and decreases need to act out toward staff and fiancée.	
	1d. Nurse will come on time each day and stay for allotted time.	1d. Consistency sets stage for trust and reinforces that client's anger will not drive nurse away.	

NURSING DIAGNOSIS

Powerlessness: related to health care environment, as evidenced by frustration over inability to perform previous tasks.

Supporting data

- Angry over nurses having to "scratch my head and help me blow my nose"
- Minimal awareness of available supports in larger community

Outcome Criteria: By discharge, Mr. Raymond will have contacted at least one outside community support.

Continued on following page

NURSING CARE PLAN 14–1 A PERSON IN CRISIS: MR. RAYMOND *(Continued)*

SHORT-TERM GOAL	INTERVENTION	RATIONALE	EVALUATION
1. By end of 2 weeks, Mr. Raymond will be able to name at least two community organizations that can offer information and support.	1a. Nurse will spend time with client and his fiancée. Role of specific agencies and how they may be of use will be discussed.	1a. Both client and fiancée will have opportunity to ask questions with nurse present.	GOAL MET By end of 10 days, Mr. Raymond and his fiancee could name two community resources they were interested in.
	1b. Nurse will introduce one agency at a time.	1b. Gradual introduction allows time for information to sink in and minimizes feeling of being pressured or overwhelmed.	At end of 6 weeks, Mr. Raymond had contacted the Guillain-Barré Society.
	1c. Nurse will follow up but not push or persuade client to contact any of the agencies.	1c. Client is able to make own decisions once he has appropriate information	

NURSING DIAGNOSIS

Ineffective staff coping: related to feelings of helplessness, as evidenced by staff withdrawal and limited personal communication.

Supporting Data

- Staff state they feel inadequate.
- Morale of staff is poor.
- Nurses state that the quality of their care is adversely affected.

Outcome Criteria: By the end of 3 weeks, staff will state that interactions with Mr. Raymond are comfortable and effective.

NURSING CARE PLAN 14–1 A PERSON IN CRISIS: MR. RAYMOND *(Continued)*

SHORT TERM GOAL	INTERVENTION	RATIONALE	EVALUATION
1. Staff and nurse will meet for 15 minutes twice by end of week to discuss reactions and alternative nursing responses to Mr. Raymond's behavior.	1a. Specific time for staff meeting is set aside and participation encouraged.	1a. Action gives message that meeting is serious and input from entire staff is needed to plan effective intervention.	GOAL MET By end of 7 days, staff had met twice to discuss feelings and reactions toward Mr. Raymond.
	1b. Staff is encouraged to identify commonalities in their feelings and how these feelings are affecting their level of care.	1b. Sharing can minimize feelings of isolation and guilt over angry feelings. Examining reactions to client behaviors and possible client motivation for behavior can facilitate staff problem solving.	Staff planned to redirect feelings back to client.
	1c. Nurse will support group planning of effective nursing actions.	1c. When anxiety is lowered, staff is able to discuss as a unit the aspects of client's behavior they view as a problem. Interventions can then be carried out with consistency and mutual support.	Staff planned to make an effort to remember that Mr. Raymond's remarks were a defensive reaction. By end of 6 weeks, staff stated they felt more comfortable and competent in their care of Mr. Raymond.

SUMMARY

A crisis is not a pathological state but a struggle for emotional balance. It can offer the opportunity for emotional growth, or it can lead to possible personality disorganization. Early intervention during a time of crisis greatly increases the possibility of a successful outcome. There are three types of crisis: maturational, situational, and adventitious, as well as specific phases in its development. Crisis and crisis intervention are based on certain assumptions:

1. A crisis is usually resolved within 4 to 6 weeks.
2. Crisis intervention therapy is short term, from 1 to 6 weeks, and focuses on the present problem only.
3. Resolution of a crisis takes three forms: a person emerges at a higher level, at pre-crisis level, or at a lower level of functioning.
4. Social support and intervention can maximize successful resolution.
5. Crisis therapists take an active and directive approach with the client in crisis.
6. The client takes an active role in setting goals and planning possible solutions.

Traditionally, crisis intervention is aimed at the mentally healthy person who is functioning well but is temporarily overwhelmed and unable to function. However, people who have long-term and persistent mental problems are also susceptible to crisis, and the crisis model can be adapted for their needs also.

The steps in crisis intervention are consistent with the nursing process (assessment, nursing diagnosis, planning, intervention, and evaluation). Each has specific goals and tasks.

Specific qualities in the nurse that can facilitate effective intervention are a caring attitude, flexibility in planning care, an ability to listen, and an active approach.

Nurses' ability to be aware of their own feelings and thoughts is crucial in working with a person in crisis. The availability of peer supports and supervision to discuss the questions that normally arise is essential for the beginning crisis counselor. Learning crisis intervention is a process, and there are certain problems all health care professionals must deal with to improve their skills.

The basic goals of crisis intervention are to reduce the individual's anxiety level and to support the effort to return to a normal level of functioning.

REFERENCES

Aguilera, D. C. (1994). *Crisis intervention: Theory and methodology* (7th ed.). St. Louis: C. V. Mosby.
Caplan, G. (1964). *Symptoms of preventive psychiatry*. New York: Basic Books.
Croushore, T., et al. (1981). *Using crisis intervention wisely*. Philadelphia: Nursing 81 Books, Intermed Communications.
Doenges, M., and Moorehouse, M. (1988). *Nurses' pocket guide: Nursing diagnoses with interventions* (2nd ed.). Philadelphia: F. A. Davis.
Donlon, P. T., and Rockwell, D. A. (1982). *Psychiatric disorders, diagnosis and treatment*. Bowie, MD: Robert J. Brady.
Ewing, C. P. (1978). *Crisis intervention as psychotherapy*. New York: Oxford University Press.
Finkelman, A. W. (1977). *The nurse therapist: Outpatient crisis intervention with the chronic patient*. Journal of Psychosocial Nursing and Mental Health Services, 8:27.
Garrison, C. Z., et al. (1995). *Posttraumatic stress disorder in adolescents after Hurricane Andrew*. Journal of American Academy of Child and Adolescent Psychiatry, 34(9):1193.
Goenjiian, A. K., et al. (1995). Psychiatric comorbidity in children after the 1988 earthquake in Armenia. *Journal of American Academy of Child and Adolescent Psychiatry*, 34(9):1174.
Hoff, L. A. (1989). *People in crisis: Understanding and helping* (3rd ed.). Menlo Park, CA: Addison-Wesley.
Hoff, L. A. (1995). *People in crisis: Understanding and helping* (4th ed.). San Francisco: Jossey-Bass.
Holmes, T. H., and Masuda, M. (1972). Psychosomatic syndrome. *Psychology Today*, April:72.
Karanci, A. N., and Rustemli, A. (1995). Psychological consequences of the 1992 Erzincan (Turkey) earthquake. *Disasters*, 19(1):8.
King, J. M. (1971). The initial interview: Basis for assessment in crisis intervention. *Perspectives in Psychiatric Care*, 6:247.
Leach, J. (1995). Psychological first aid: A practical aide-memoire. *Aviation-Space and Environmental Medicine*, 66(7):668.
Robinson, L. (1973). Psychiatric emergencies. *Nursing* 73(7):43.
Urano, R. J., et al. (1995). Longitudinal assessment of posttraumatic stress disorder and depression after exposure to traumatic death. *Journal of Nervous and Mental Disorders*, 183(1):36.
Wallace, M. A., and Morley, W. E. (1970) Teaching crisis intervention. *American Journal of Nursing*, 7:1484.

SELF-STUDY AND CRITICAL THINKING

Matching questions

Match the situation with the type of actual or potential crisis.

1. ________ New baby is brought into household
2. ________ Person is raped
3. ________ Adult celebrates 50th birthday
4. ________ House burns down
5. ________ Child or spouse is battered
6. ________ Girl becomes a teenager

A. Maturational
B. Situational
C. Adventitious

Match the appropriate intervention to the appropriate level of intervention.

7. ________ Teach problem solving
8. ________ Attend rehabilitation center
9. ________ Assess precipitating events
10. ________ Teach assertiveness training

A. Primary
B. Secondary
C. Tertiary

True or false

Place a T or an F next to each statement. Correct the false statements.

11. ________ A crisis situation can last up to 4 months before it is resolved.
12. ________ The goal of crisis therapy is to have the person obtain a higher level of functioning.
13. ________ Crisis therapy deals with the person in the present situation and with the person's immediate presenting problems.
14. ________ A person in crisis has always had problems and does not cope well in his or her usual life situations.

15. __________ A crisis situation can offer the opportunity for personality growth, or the potential for personality deterioration.

16. __________ Intervention rarely has any effect on the resolution of a crisis.

17. __________ The nurse counselor must take a firm and direct approach with a person in crisis.

18. __________ It is necessary for the nurse counselor to do all the planning and make all the decisions for the person in crisis because the person is often too disorganized.

Completion

Complete the statements by filling in the appropriate information.

19. Three personal qualities that can enhance a nurse's effectiveness in a crisis are

A. ____________________
B. ____________________
C. ____________________

20. Three ways you can demonstrate concern and show that you are listening are

A. ____________________
B. ____________________
C. ____________________

21. Identify two self-interventions a nurse can use if problems arise when crisis counseling is started.

Problem	**Intervention**
A. Needing to feel needed	1. __________
	2. __________
B. Setting unrealistic goals	1. __________
	2. __________

Complete the statements by filling in the appropriate information.

22. Four experiences that could potentiate a crisis in a person with a chronic mental problem are

A. ____________________
B. ____________________
C. ____________________
D. ____________________

23. Four common crisis situations that a nurse may encounter in a general hospital are

A. ____________________
B. ____________________
C. ____________________
D. ____________________

Critical thinking

Write a short paragraph in response to the following:

24. After you determine whether a person is homicidal or suicidal or both, identify the three important areas in the assessment. Give examples of two questions in each area that need to be answered before planning can take place.
25. Clara, 22, a senior in nursing school, tells her nursing instructor that her mother (aged 45) has just lost her job. Clara's mother has been drinking heavily for years and tells Clara she can't cope anymore; she wants to leave and "find herself." Clara has a 12-year-old sister, Joy, and her mother tells Clara that it is time for Clara to start taking some responsibility and earning a living. Clara's father was killed 8 years ago in a hit-and-run accident by a drunken driver.

    A. How many different types of crises are going on with this family? Discuss the crises in light of each individual in this family.
    B. If this family came for crisis counseling, what areas would you assess and what kinds of questions would you ask in order to assess each member's individual needs and the needs of the family as a unit (perception of event, coping styles, social supports)?
    C. Formulate some tentative goals you might set in conjunction with the family.
    D. Identify and name appropriate referral agencies in your area that would be useful if this family were willing to expand their resources and stabilize.
    E. How would you set up follow-up visits for this family? Would you see them together, alone, or in a combination during the crisis period (4 to 6 weeks)? How would you decide whether follow-up counseling was indicated?

15

Families in Crisis: FAMILY VIOLENCE

KATHLEEN SMITH-DIJULIO

OUTLINE

KEY TERMS AND CONCEPTS

The key terms and concepts listed here also appear in bold where they are defined or discussed in this chapter.

family violence
perpetrator
vulnerable person
crisis situation
physical violence
battering
endangerment
sexual violence

emotional violence
neglect
economic maltreatment
health care record
primary prevention
secondary prevention
tertiary prevention
shelters/safe houses

OBJECTIVES

After studying this chapter, the reader will be able to

1. Discuss the epidemiological theory of violence in terms of stresses on the perpetrator, vulnerable person, and environment that could escalate anxiety to the point at which violence becomes the relief behavior.
2. Contrast and compare three characteristics of perpetrators with three characteristics of a vulnerable person.
3. Name three indicators of (a) physical violence, (b) sexual violence, (c) neglect, and (d) emotional violence.
4. Make up a story of economic maltreatment using personal observations and the text.
5. Describe four areas to assess when interviewing a person who has experienced family violence.
6. Formulate four nursing diagnoses for the survivor of violence, and list supporting data from the assessment.
7. Formulate three nursing diagnoses for the perpetrator, and list supporting data from the assessment.
8. Formulate two short-term outcomes (goals) for both the survivor of abuse and the perpetrator.
9. Discuss three interventions that would be appropriate in dealing with both the victim and the perpetrator.
10. Write out a safety plan, including the essential elements, for an abused spouse.
11. Compare and contrast primary, secondary, and tertiary levels of intervention, giving two examples of intervention for each level.
12. Identify two common emotional responses you might experience when faced with a person subjected to family violence.
13. Describe at least three possible referrals for a violent family (child, adult, elder) and write down the telephone numbers of the corresponding agencies in your community.
14. Name and discuss three psychotherapeutic modalities that are useful for violent families.

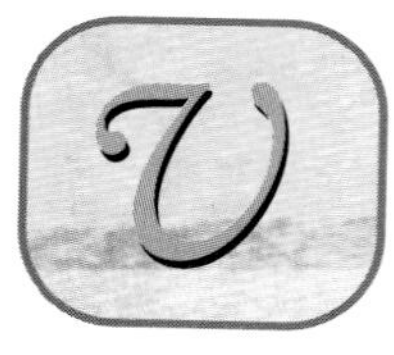

Violence is a complex, multifaceted phenomenon that is not only tolerated but also socially sanctioned throughout American society. It is the root of many of our social ills. Violence is considered America's number one public health issue. A violent family is one in which at least one family member is using physical or sexual force against another, resulting in physically or emotionally destructive injury, or both (Campbell and Campbell 1993). Family violence occurs in a variety of forms with alarming frequency, affecting family members of all ages. An act of family violence occurs in the United States every 15 seconds—more frequently than any other crime (Chez 1994). The secondary effects of violence, such as anxiety, depression, and suicide, are health care issues that can last a lifetime. Family violence is common in childhood histories of juvenile delinquents, runaways, violent criminals, prostitutes, and those who in turn are violent toward others (Irons 1993; Warren et al. 1994). Exposure to violence can adversely affect children's development in many areas, including their ability to function in school, emotional stability, orientation toward the future, and future sexual enjoyment. Abused adolescents report more psychopathological changes, poorer coping and social skills, a higher incidence of dissociated identity disorder, and poorer impulse control than do other adolescents. A legacy of violence can leave a lifetime of emotional scars if intervention and support are not available. Box 15–1 identifies some of the sequelae of family violence.

It has been estimated that half of all Americans have experienced violence in their families. Battering is the single largest cause of injury to women in the United States. Two to 4 million women are beaten by their partners each year. Of these, 2000 to 4000 will die as a result of their injuries (AAFP 1994). Violence toward infants is one of the leading causes of postneonatal mortality (Ludwig and Kornberg 1992). It has been estimated that between 1 and 2 million older Americans annually, or more than one in ten elderly persons living with a family member, are maltreated (Lachs and Fulmer 1993). Distinct service delivery systems and social policies have developed to address these problems, yet one type of violence is a fairly strong predictor of another, especially for

BOX 15–1 LONG-TERM EFFECTS OF FAMILY VIOLENCE

People involved in family violence are found to have higher levels of

- Depression
- Suicidal feelings
- Self-contempt
- Inability to trust
- Inability to develop intimate relationships in later life

Victims of severe violence are also at higher risk for experiencing recurring symptoms of posttraumatic stress disorder related to the unresolved trauma:

- Flashbacks
- Dissociation—out-of-body experiences
- Poor self-esteem
- Compulsive or impulsive behaviors (e.g., substance abuse, spending money, gambling, and promiscuity)
- Multiple somatic complaints

Children who witness violence in their homes

- After the age of 5 or 6 years show an indication of identifying with the aggressor and losing respect for the victim
- Are at greater risk for developing behavioral and emotional problems throughout their lives

Some mental and behavioral disorders are associated with violence in childhood:

- Depressive disorders
- Posttraumatic stress disorder
- Somatic complaints
- Low self-esteem
- Phobias (agoraphobia, social and specific phobias)
- Antisocial behaviors
- Child or spouse abuse

Adolescents are more likely to have behavioral symptoms such as

- Failing grades
- Difficulty forming relationships
- Increased incidence of theft, police arrest, and violent behaviors
- Seductive or promiscuous behaviors
- Running away from home

spousal and child abuse (McKay 1994). This connection calls for more coordinated efforts of prevention and intervention.

Violence within family, trust, or dependency relationships represents a serious misuse of power. Violence can also occur in gay and lesbian relationships. Domestic violence is the third largest health problem for gay men, following substance abuse and AIDS. Violence between siblings is one of the most common and unrecognized forms of domestic violence. Another alarming and often unreported form of domestic violence is that of children toward parents. Although often not reported or even discussed, violence toward men by women also occurs and also goes unrecognized as a problem.

Violence within families is seldom recognized by outsiders, including nurses. The United States Objectives for the Year 2000 call for the extension of "protocols for routinely identifying, testing, and properly referring victims" seen in emergency departments and primary care settings (Public Health Service 1989). The American Nurses' Association has published *Position statement on physical violence against women*, which supports the Healthy People 2000 Objectives and calls for increased education about violence against women for all health professionals (Bullock et al. 1989). The Joint Commission on Accreditation of Healthcare Organizations (JCAHO) requires staff education in domestic violence and maltreatment of elders as well as standards of care to guide clinical practice.

The nurse is often the first point of contact for people experiencing family violence and thus is in an ideal position to contribute to prevention, detection, and effective intervention. Because of their numbers, the variety of their practice locations, and the nature of their practice, nurses are in close contact with a large segment of the population who are at risk for violent episodes (Ross and Hoff 1994). The Nursing Network on Violence Against Women encourages the development of a nursing practice that focuses on health issues relating to the effects of violence on women's lives. Altering the pattern of violence against women can also affect child abuse, because the main predictor of violence toward children is violence toward their mothers.

Ultimately, the general tolerance of violence in the United States must be addressed if long-lasting changes are to be made. It took until 1967 for all states to enact laws against child abuse, and only since 1978 have battered women been able to expect protection in most communities. All states have systems for investigating elder mistreatment; 47 have mandatory reporting laws. Awareness and public concern continue to grow. However, laws and awareness are not enough to decrease the incidence of family violence in the United States. We also need police support and enforcement and a judicial system that enforces the consequences. As long as families live in crisis and social changes are not forthcoming, the conditions exist for violence to occur.

One fourth of all children living in this country do not have adequate food. Parents raising children in poverty (a large proportion of whom are single women) are not likely to have the skills or resources to teach their children to function effectively as adults. Family stress is often constant. For example, some parents of children living in poverty cannot financially support their families because of long-term unemployment. Other parents cannot be permanent family members without jeopardizing their families' public assistance payments, and therefore cannot maintain their role as responsible adults.

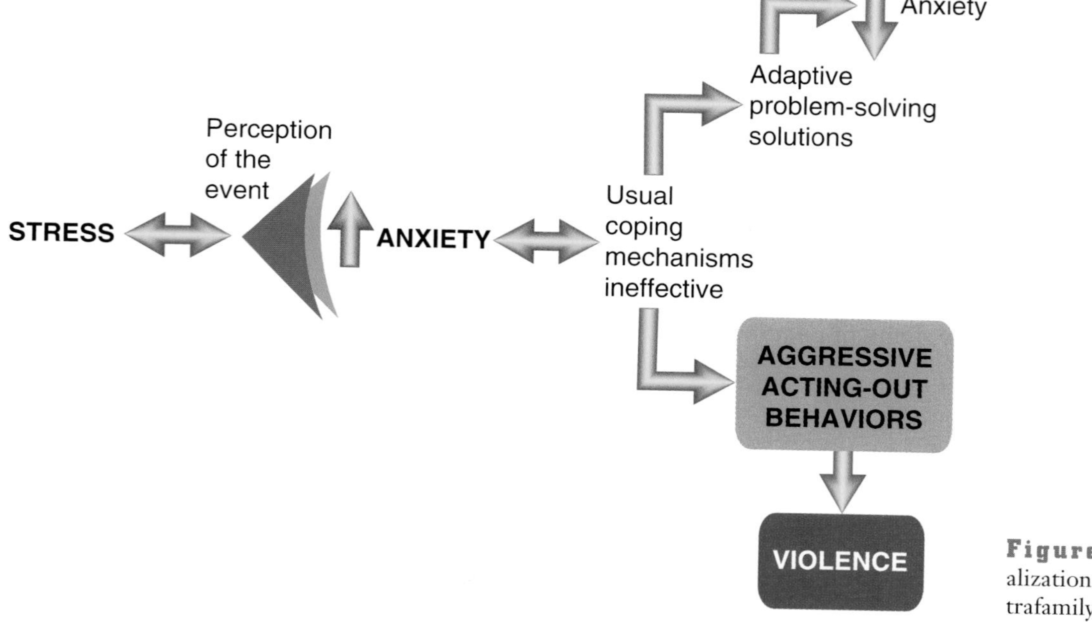

Figure 15–1 Conceptualization of the process of intrafamily abuse.

Smaller family units, often working mothers in one-parent households, and a higher life expectancy have changed the character of the family structure and thus the support for older adults. It is frequently the "young-old" children (those in their fifties and sixties) who take care of their "old-old" parents (those in their seventies and older). In addition, this sandwich generation is still coping with the demands of their own growing offspring. Family violence as a maladaptive crisis response to stress and anxiety is conceptualized in Figure 15–1. Social factors that reinforce violence include the wide acceptance of the hitting of children (corporal punishment); the celebration of increasingly violent movies, video games, and comic books; the violent themes in rap music; and the increase in the total volume of pornography (which is strongly associated with physical abuse of women) (Cramer and McFarlane 1994).

THEORY

Family violence refers to physical injury or mental anguish inflicted by one family member upon another or the deprivation of essential services by a caregiver. To be more effective in working with victims, the nurse needs an understanding of conditions for violence and types of maltreatment.

Conditions for Violence

Abuse occurs across all segments of American society and is reinforced by the society and the culture. The actual occurrence of violence requires (1) a perpetrator; (2) someone who by age or situation is vulnerable, i.e., children, women, the elderly, and the mentally ill or physically challenged person; and (3) a crisis situation.

The Perpetrator

The propensity for violence is rooted in childhood and manifested by a general lack of self-regard, dissatisfaction with life, and inability to assume adult roles. Witnessing family violence, experiencing family violence, and poor parenting are contributing factors.

Deficiencies in patterns of family functioning in households experiencing violence are a result of many factors. There is usually a lack of role modeling as well as a lack of knowledge about the characteristics of healthy relationships. There is uncertainty about what it is realistic to expect of self, spouse, an older adult, or children. **Perpetrators,** those who initiate violence, often consider their own needs to be more important than anyone else's, and look toward others to meet their needs.

These same families, already highly stressed, often have even greater demands placed on them by geographical moves, job changes or losses, an ill child or other family member, or an elder adult who moves in and needs care. Violent families are often socially isolated from support systems. This isolation may be a result of mobility patterns, characteristics that alienate others, and social stresses that cut families off from potential and actual supports.

In addition to these general characteristics, specific characteristics of violent parents and those who maltreat elders are listed in Boxes 15–2 and 15–3.

Family abuse has many scenarios. In cases of women assaulting their partners, many are attempting to protect themselves from violence initiated by their spouse

BOX 15–2 CHARACTERISTICS OF VIOLENT PARENTS

- A history of violence, neglect, or emotional deprivation as a child
- Family authoritarianism: raise children as they were raised by their own parents
- Low self-esteem, feelings of worthlessness, depression
- Poor coping skills
- Social isolation (may be suspicious of others): few or no friends, little or no involvement in social or community activities
- Involved in a crisis situation: unemployment, divorce, financial difficulties
- Rigid, unrealistic expectations of child's behavior
- Frequent use of harsh punishment
- History of severe mental illness, such as schizophrenia
- Violent temper outbursts
- Looking to child for satisfaction of needs for love, support, and reassurance (often unmet because of parenting deficits in family of origin)
- Projection of blame onto the child for their "troubles" (e.g., stepparent may project hostility toward new mate onto a child)
- Lack of effective parenting skills
- Inability to seek help from others
- Perception of the child as bad or evil
- History of drug or alcohol abuse
- Feeling of little or no control over life
- Low tolerance for frustration
- Poor impulse control

Data from Warner, C. G. (Ed.). (1981). *Conflict intervention in social and domestic violence.* Bowie, MD: Robert J. Brady.

BOX 15–3 CHARACTERISTICS OF ELDER ABUSERS

PHYSICAL AND PSYCHOLOGICAL VIOLENCE

The perpetrator may have

- A history of mental illness
- A recent decline in mental status
- Recent medical problems
- A financial dependence on the victim
- Shared living arrangements with the victim
- A history of alcohol or drug abuse
- Pathological family dynamics

NEGLECT

The perpetrator may

- Abuse alcohol or drugs
- Not live with the victim
- Not have a decline in mental status
- Not have recent medical problems
- Not experience the victim as a source of stress

FINANCIAL MALTREATMENT

The perpetrator may

- Abuse alcohol or drugs
- Be a distant relative
- Be financially dependent on the victim
- Be greedy

Data from Wolf, R. S., and Pillemer, K. A. (1989). *Helping elderly victims: The reality of elder abuse.* New York: Columbia University Press; and Wolf, R. S. (1990). Elder abuse: Scope, characteristics, and treatment. *Nurse Practitioner Forum,* 1(2):102.

(Gelles and Straus 1988). Other less common cases may involve a frail elderly man married to a much younger woman. Men may fear ridicule if they expose the problem of violence (Sadock 1995). There are also teenagers who are violent toward their parents. Since the most common occurrence of spousal abuse is the pattern of a man inflicting violence upon his female partner, for simplicity that will be the model used here; however, the principles discussed apply to any member of a household who is violent toward another member (e.g., siblings, same sex partners, extended family members). Violence toward children and older adults will be considered separately.

▸ A 53-year-old man came to the ambulatory care clinic looking very fatigued and complaining of pain in his left shoulder "since last night." Holding his left arm close to his side, he averted his eyes from those of the receptionist, nurse, and doctor. When asked if anything had occurred that might have caused the pain, he answered "I fell." Asked why he had not sought care last night, he stated "I . . . I . . . thought it would go away overnight."

▸ Upon further examination and x-ray, it was determined that the patient had sustained a fractured clavicle. Additional direct, supportive questioning elicited the information that the patient had been injured when pushed down the stairs by his 17-year-old stepson.

Violent men are found in all segments of society. They believe in male supremacy, being in charge, and being dominant. "Acting out" physically makes them feel more in control, more masculine, and more powerful. Parent-child interactions, peer-group experiences, observations of the partner dyad, and the influence of the media (television, comics, video games, movies) all support the same message: males can expect to be in a position of power in relationships and may use physical aggression to maintain that position (Birns et al. 1994). Extreme pathological jealousy is characteristic of an abusive male. Many refuse to allow their partners to work outside the home; others demand that their partners work in the same place as they so that they can monitor activities and friendships. Many accompany their partners to and from all activities and forbid them to have personal friends or to participate in recreational activities outside the home. When this is not possible, the man may restrict mobility by monitoring the odometer and keeping clock watches. Even with such restrictions, these men accuse their partners of infidelity. Many perpetrators maintain their possessiveness by controlling the family finances to the extent that there is barely enough money for daily living. These men may appear to outsiders as ordinary doctors, machinists, lawyers, salesmen, executives, and plumbers—or even police officers, judges, and politicians. Men who commit domestic violence may be found among a larger pool of men with poor problem-solving skills; in addition, they seem to have borderline or antisocial personality traits and histories of abuse as children (Else et al. 1993). However, they may exert their control in subtle ways not evident at first to outsiders.

Individuals are more likely to engage in family violence when intoxicated. Alcohol and other drugs may play a disinhibitory role in disregarding social rules that prohibit violence against children, women, and the elderly, whom perpetrators view as weak and inferior. Unfortunately, the consumption of alcohol and drugs is often used as a rationalization by the victim to excuse the behavior ("He was drunk and he didn't know what he was doing"). In fact, when drug and alcohol use are reduced or eliminated, family violence still occurs.

Both male and female perpetrators perceive themselves as having poor social skills. They describe their relationships with their spouses as being the closest they have ever known, which is typical in enmeshed and codependent relationships. They lack supportive relationships outside the marriage. When not being violent, perpetrators have been described as remorseful, childlike, and yearning to be nurtured.

The Vulnerable Person

The **vulnerable person** is the one in the family unit on whom violence is perpetrated. In some situations, violence does not occur until after the legal marriage of couples who have lived together or dated for a long time. Perhaps this reflects the notion of women as property legally bound to the husband by the marriage ceremony.

Pregnancy often serves to increase violence even further according to Sadock (1995). An estimated 15% to 25% of women experience violence during pregnancy. One reason may be that the husband resents the added responsibility that a baby requires, or he may resent the relationship that the baby will have with his mate. Violence also escalates when the wife makes a move toward independence, such as visiting friends "without permission," getting a job, or going back to school. Women are at greatest risk for violence when they attempt to leave the relationship.

Children are most likely to be abused if they are under 3 years of age; are perceived as being "different" because of temperamental traits, congenital abnormalities, or chronic disease (Devlin and Reynolds 1994); remind the parents of someone they do not like (perhaps an ex-spouse); are different from the parents' fantasy of what the child "should" be like; or are a product of an unwanted pregnancy. Interference with emotional bonding between parents and child (e.g., with a premature birth or prolonged illness requiring hospitalization) has also been found to increase the risk of possible future abuse. Adolescents are abused at least as frequently as children, yet are often overlooked; in some situations they may be blamed for their maltreatment because society views the teenage years as rocky.

Elder adults may become vulnerable because of being in poor mental or physical health or being disruptive (e.g., a person with Alzheimer's disease) (Vida 1994). The dependency needs of elderly persons are usually what put them at risk for abuse. The typical victim is female, over 75 years of age, white, living with a relative, and having a physical and/or mental impairment (All 1994). Another scenario is the elder male cared for by a daughter whom he abused as a child, and who now is abusive toward him. Dealing with the problems of the elderly can be stressful for adult caregivers at the best of times, but in families in which violence was a coping strategy, the potential for abuse is great.

The Crisis Situation

Anyone may be at risk for abuse in a **crisis situation,** one that puts stress on a family with a violent member. Stressful life events tax coping skills, leaving the perpetrator incapable of dealing with what is going on. A person with good impulse control who can solve problems and has a healthy support system is less likely to resort to violence. Social isolation due to frequent moves or an inability to make friends contributes to ineffective coping during crisis situations. Refer to Chapter 14 for more on crisis and crisis intervention.

The Cycle of Violence

The intensity of violence alternates with periods of safety, hope, and trust. This pattern has been described as a process of escalation/de-escalation.

The *tension-building stage* is characterized by minor incidents such as pushing, shoving, and verbal abuse. During this time the woman does not say that the abuse is unacceptable, for fear more severe abuse will follow. The abuser then rationalizes that his abusive behavior is acceptable.

As the tension escalates, both spouses may try to reduce it. The batterer may try to reduce the tension with the use of alcohol or drugs. The vulnerable person may try to reduce the tension by minimizing the importance of the incidents ("I should have had the house neater . . . dinner ready.") A woman may also try to reduce the tension by somatizing, thus perpetuating the "poor-me" image.

During the *acute battering stage*, the perpetrator releases the built-up tension by brutal and uncontrollable beatings. He is unable to control the degree of destructiveness inflicted on the victim. Severe injuries can and do result. The perpetrator may have amnesia and may not remember what happened during the battering. The victim usually depersonalizes the incident and is able to remember the beatings in detail. After the beatings, both are in shock.

The *honeymoon stage* may be characterized by kindness and loving behaviors. The perpetrator, at least initially, feels remorseful and apologetic and may bring presents, make promises, and tell the victim how much she is loved and needed. The victim usually believes the promises, feels needed and loved, and drops any legal proceedings or plans to leave that may have been initiated during the acute battering stage. Unfortunately, without intervention the cycle will repeat itself. The honeymoon stage will fade away as tension starts to build.

When *escalation/de-escalation* occurs, conditions of anger and fear escalate until an incident of violence occurs, after which there is a diffusion of tension and a brief feeling of safety. Over time, the periods of calmness and safety are briefer and the periods of anger and fear are more intense. There are periods of stability, but the violence increases over time.

Without treatment, violence never diminishes and almost always escalates in frequency and intensity. With each repeat of the pattern, the self-esteem of those experiencing the violence becomes more and more eroded. The victim either believes the violence was deserved or accepts the blame for it. This can lead to feelings of depression, hopelessness, immobilization, and self-deprecation.

Types of Maltreatment

Five specific types of maltreatment have been identified: (1) physical violence, (2) sexual violence, (3) emotional violence, (4) neglect, and (5) economic maltreatment.

Physical Violence

Physical violence includes both battering and physical endangerment. Physical **battering** refers to physical assaults, such as hitting, kicking, biting, throwing, and burning. Physical **endangerment** is reckless behavior toward a vulnerable person that could lead to serious physical injury (e.g., leaving an immobilized elderly person alone for long periods or allowing a child to play in an environment where toxic chemicals are within reach).

Sexual Violence

Sexual violence toward children covers any sexual approach or sexual act, whether explicit or implicit. This form of violence, usually perpetrated by a father or stepfather against his daughter (incest), is now reported in such numbers that it may well be the most common form of violence toward children. It has been reported to occur with similar frequency across all cultures (Finkelhor 1994). Box 15–4 lists forms of sexual abuse of children. Childhood sexual abuse destroys an individual's positive self-concept and can interfere with the learning of self-care skills. (Sexual abuse of adults is usually referred to as sexual assault, or rape, and is discussed in Chapter 16.)

Emotional Violence

Emotional violence kills the spirit and the ability to succeed later in life, to feel deeply, and to make emotional contact with others. It can take the form of

- Terrorizing an individual through verbal threats.
- Demeaning an individual's worth.
- Blatant or subtle hostility and hatred directed toward an individual.
- Persistently ignoring an individual and her or his needs.
- Consistently belittling and criticizing an individual.
- Withholding warmth and affection from an individual.
- Threatening an individual with abandonment or institutionalization (nursing home, psychiatric hospital).

BOX 15–4 FORMS OF SEXUAL ABUSE OF CHILDREN

Touching, fondling, and physically exploring child's genitalia
Masturbation by male perpetrator against child's perineum, buttocks, abdomen, or thighs
Manual masturbation of perpetrator by child
All combinations of oral-genital contact between child of either sex and adult of either sex
Actual or attempted anal intercourse with child of either sex
Actual or attempted vaginal intercourse (without force)
Forceful attempt at vaginal intercourse, with local or general trauma
Exhibitionism
Voyeurism
Exploitation of children in preparation of sexually suggestive or pornographic materials

Data from Ghent, W. R., DaSylva, N. P., and Farren, M. E. (1985). Family violence: Guidelines for recognition and management. *Canadian Medical Association Journal,* 132(5): 545.

Neglect

Neglect can be physical, developmental, or educational. *Physical neglect* is failure to provide the medical, dental, or psychiatric care needed to prevent or treat physical or emotional illnesses. *Developmental neglect* is failure to provide emotional nurturing and the physical and cognitive stimulation needed to ensure freedom from developmental deficits. The physical consequences of neglect are typically overshadowed by the associated disruption in the child's critical areas of development (e.g., trust, attachment, self-control, moral and social judgments). *Educational neglect* occurs when a child's caretakers deprive the child of the education available in accordance with the state's education laws.

Children and adolescents are most often the victims of neglect, as manifested by such things as abandonment, inattention to health care, inadequate supervision (including permitting or condoning maladaptive behavior such as substance abuse), deprivation of necessities, educational neglect, and emotional neglect. Neglect of the elderly is also a disturbing phenomenon. Caregivers may withhold proper medical care, allow their elderly family member to live in unsafe conditions, and let him or her go without sufficient food or clothing.

Economic Maltreatment

Economic maltreatment refers to using another's resources, without permission, for one's personal gain. This can occur, for example, when family members deplete an elderly person's resources without the person's knowledge, as well as when a controlling husband squanders his wife's income or refuses to allow her access to money because he wants to maintain her dependence on him. Other examples include the theft of Social Security or pension checks, the use of threats to enforce the signing or changing of wills or other legal documents, and coercion in any financial matter (Lachs and Pillemer 1995).

ASSESSMENT

Persons experiencing violence present in every health care setting, including outpatient clinics, community health centers, emergency departments, general hospitals, physicians' offices, and nursing homes. Complaints may be vague and can include insomnia, abdominal pain, hyperventilation, headache, or menstrual problems (Parker 1995). Sensitivity is required on the part of the nurse, who might suspect family violence. Awareness of the nurse's feelings and attention to the process and setting of the interview are important to facilitate accurate assessment of physical and behavioral indicators of family violence.

The Process and Setting of the Interview

Important and relevant information about the family situation can be gathered by routine assessment conducted with tact, understanding, and a calm, relaxed attitude. Important interviewing guidelines are listed in Box 15–5. A person who feels judged or accused of wrongdoing is most likely to become defensive, and any attempts at changing coping strategies in the family are thwarted. In this vein, it is better to ask about ways of solving disagreements or methods of disciplining children rather than use the words *abuse* or *violence*, which appear judgmental and thus are threatening to the family.

When interviewing, sit near the abused client and spend some time establishing a rapport before focusing on the details of the violent experience. Reassure the client that he or she did nothing wrong. The interview should be nonthreatening and supportive, never suggestive of a trial or inquisition. The person who experienced the violence should be allowed to tell the story and not be interrupted. Establishing trust is crucial if the client is to feel comfortable enough to self-disclose. Verbal approaches may include the following:

- Tell me about what happened to you.
- Who takes care of you? (for children and dependent elders)

BOX 15–5 INTERVIEW GUIDELINES

DO'S

- Conduct the interview in private
- Be direct, honest, and professional
- Use language the client understands
- Ask the client to clarify words not understood
- Be understanding
- Be attentive
- Inform the client if you must make a referral to Child/Adult Protective Services, and explain the process
- Assess safety and help reduce danger (at discharge)

DONT'S

- Do *not* try to "prove" abuse by accusations or demands
- Do *not* display horror, anger, shock, or disapproval of the perpetrator or situation
- Do *not* place blame or make judgments
- Do *not* allow the client to feel "at fault" or "in trouble"
- Do *not* probe or press for answers the client is not willing to give
- Do *not* conduct the interview with a group of interviewers
- Do *not* force a child to remove clothing

- What happens when you do something wrong? (for children) *or* How do you and your partner/caregiver resolve disagreements? (for women and the elderly)
- What do you do for fun?
- Who helps you with your child(ren), parent?
- What time do you have for yourself?

An interview built on concern and carried out in an atmosphere that is nonjudgmental is most effective. Such statements as "It must be difficult to care for three small children when there is little food in the house" or "Being responsible for two elderly parents without the help of family or friends must be hard on you" are useful for eliciting important data that help the nurse plan more effective alternatives and coping strategies. When the perpetrator is informed that a referral to child or adult protective services has been made, for example, it should be emphasized that the referral is not punishment but an attempt to safeguard the victim and obtain help for the family.

Questions that are open-ended and require a descriptive response can be less threatening and elicit more relevant information than questions that are direct or can be answered "yes" or "no." Here are some examples for approaching parents:

- What arrangements do you make when you have to leave your child alone?
- How do you discipline your child?
- When your infant cries for a long time, how do you get him or her to stop?
- What about your child's behavior bothers you the most?

Openness and directness about the situation can strengthen the relationship with those experiencing violence. The Nursing Research Consortium on Violence and Abuse has developed a five-question assessment tool (Box 15–6) that has been used extensively to assist in the routine identification of domestic violence. It can be used in clinical settings without requesting permission. The following vignette illustrates the key points for assessing a woman in crisis at the initial interview, as well as suggested follow-up.

BOX 15–6 ABUSE ASSESSMENT SCREEN

1. Have you ever been emotionally or physically abused by your partner or someone important to you? Yes ________ No ________
   If yes, by whom? ________________
   Number of times ________________
2. Within the past year, have you been hit, slapped, kicked, or otherwise physically hurt by someone?
   Yes ________ No ________
   If yes, by whom? ________________
   Number of times ________________
3. Since you have been pregnant, have you been hit, slapped, kicked, or otherwise physically hurt by someone?
   Yes ________ No ________
   If yes, by whom? ________________
   Number of times ________________
4. Within the past year, has anyone forced you to have sexual activities?
   Yes ________ No ________
   If yes, by whom? ________________
   Number of times ________________
5. Are you afraid of your partner or anyone listed above?
   Yes ________ No ________

The Abuse Assessment Screen was developed by the Nursing Research Consortium on Violence and Abuse, 1989. Its reproduction and use is encouraged.

- Darnell Peters is a 42-year-old married woman in a relationship she describes as "bad for a long time. We don't communicate." She is brought to the emergency department by ambulance with lacerations to her face and swollen eyes, lips, and nose. She tells the nurse that her husband had been in bed asleep for hours before she joined him. On getting into bed, she attempted to redistribute the blankets. Suddenly, he leaped from the bed, started punching her in the face, and began to throw her against the wall. She called out to her 11-year-old son to call the police. The police arrived, called an ambulance, and took Mr. Peters to jail.
- The nurse takes Mrs. Peters to an individual examination room (to emphasize confidentiality) to assess the whole problem. Mrs. Peters states that their relationship is always stormy. "He is always putting me down and yelling at me." He started hitting her 5 years ago when she became pregnant with her second and last child. The beatings have increased in intensity over the past year, and this emergency department visit is the fifth this year. Tonight is the first time she has ever called the police.
- Mrs. Peters has visibly lost control. Periods of crying alternate with periods of silence. She appears apathetic and depressed. The nurse remains calm and objective. After Mrs. Peters has finished talking, the nurse explores alternatives designed to help her reduce the danger when she is discharged. "I'm concerned that you will be hurt again if you go home. What options do you have?" Acknowledging the escalating intensity of the violence, Mrs. Peters is able to make arrangements with a shelter to take her and her two children in until after she has secured a restraining order.
- The nurse charts the abuse referrals. Careful and complete records help ensure that Mrs. Peters will receive proper follow-up care, and will assist Mrs. Peters

when and if she pursues legal action (see the later section, "Maintaining Accurate Records").

When determining the need for further help, it is also useful to assess (a) violence indicators, (b) levels of anxiety and coping responses, (c) family coping patterns, (d) support systems, (e) suicide potential, (f) homicide potential, and (g) drug and alcohol use.

Assessing Types of Maltreatment

ASSESSING PHYSICAL VIOLENCE. A series of minor complaints, such as headaches, "back trouble," dizziness, and "accidents," especially falls, may be covert indications of violence. Overt signs of battering include bruises, scars, burns, and other wounds in various stages of healing, particularly around the head, face, chest, arms, abdomen, back, buttocks, and genitalia (Devlin and Reynolds 1994). Signs of violence may not be clearly manifested (Box 15–7). Injuries seen in emergency departments, clinics, and offices that should arouse the nurse's suspicion are listed in Box 15–8. A physician's office or clinic may be one of the few places a person experiencing violence is allowed to go. Sickness is viewed as a legitimate excuse for seeking professional help. **If the explanation does not match the injury seen, or if the client minimizes the seriousness of the injury, violence may be suspected.** The key to identification is a high index of suspicion.

Nonspecific bruising in older children is common. Any bruises on an infant under 6 months of age should be considered suspicious. A specific type of abuse to which young children are susceptible is *shaking*. They are more vulnerable because of their relatively large head size and weight; weak neck muscles; thin, friable central nervous system vasculature; and soft, less myelinated brain tissue. The baby who has been shaken may often present with respiratory problems. If the pulmonary examination is not normal, the possibility of rigorous shaking must be considered. Full bulging fontanelles and a head circumference greater than the 90th percentile are also suggestive. Shaking can cause intracranial hemorrhage leading to cerebral edema and death (Butler 1995).

Ask clients directly, but in a nonthreatening manner, whether the injury has been caused by someone close to them. Observe the nonverbal response, such as hesitation or lack of eye contact, as well as the verbal response. Then ask specific questions, such as "When was the last time it happened?" "How often does it happen?" "In what ways are you hurt?"

BOX 15–8 PRESENTING PROBLEMS OF VICTIMS OF FAMILY VIOLENCE

IN THE EMERGENCY DEPARTMENT

- Bleeding injuries, especially to head and face
- Internal injuries, concussions, perforated eardrums, abdominal injuries, severe bruising, eye injuries, strangulation marks on neck
- Back injuries
- Broken or fractured jaws, arms, pelvis, ribs, clavicle, legs
- Burns from cigarettes, appliances, scalding liquids, acids
- Psychological trauma, anxiety, attacks of hyperventilation, heart, palpitations, severe crying spells, suicidal tendencies
- Miscarriages

AMBULATORY CARE SETTINGS

- Perforated eardrums, twisted or stiff neck and shoulder muscles, headache
- Depression, stress-related conditions (e.g., insomnia, violent nightmares, anxiety, extreme fatigue, eczema, loss of hair)
- Talk of having "problems" with husband or son, describing him as very jealous, impulsive, or an alcohol or drug abuser
- Repeated visits with new complaint
- Bruises of various ages and specific shapes (fingers, belt)

IN BOTH SETTINGS

- Observe for signs of stress due to family violence: emotional, behavioral, school, or sleep problems and increased aggressive behavior
- Injuries to a pregnant woman
- Recurrent visits for injuries attributed to being "accident prone"

BOX 15–7 PHYSICAL SYMPTOMS INDICATING POSSIBLE FAMILY VIOLENCE

CHIEF COMPLAINTS WITHOUT PHYSICAL CAUSE

- Headache
- Abdominal pain
- Insomnia
- Choking sensation
- Chest pain
- Back pain
- Dizziness
- "Accidents"

PRESENTING PROBLEMS (SIGNS OF HIGH ANXIETY AND CHRONIC STRESS)

- Agitation
- Hyperventilation
- Panic attack
- Gastrointestinal disturbances
- Hypertension
- Physical injuries

Data from Swanson, R. W. (1984). Battered wife syndrome. *Canadian Medical Association Journal,* 130(6):709.

Along with recognition of the indicators of physical violence, nurses note the alleged method of injury. Inconsistent explanations serve as a warning that further investigation is necessary. Vague explanations, such as "She fell from a chair (a lap, down the stairs)," "He was running away," or "The hot water was turned on by mistake," should alert the nurse to possible violence.

ASSESSING SEXUAL VIOLENCE. Sexual violence toward children and dependent elders has been receiving more attention and concern. It is estimated that one in four females and one in ten males will be sexually abused as children. Increasing age of the child is a risk factor, with a dramatic increase occurring around 10 years of age (Finkelhor 1993).

▶ Ms. Randall, 83, is admitted from an adult foster home for evaluation of deterioration in her mental status. She is confused and disoriented to time and place and is unable to give a coherent history. Blood and urine are collected for diagnostic evaluation. The laboratory report notes semen in the urine. Adult Protective Services is called to begin an investigation into the adult family home.

ASSESSING EMOTIONAL VIOLENCE. Whenever physical or sexual violence is occurring, emotional violence also occurs. It may also exist alone. When there is emotional violence, low self-esteem, anguish, and isolation are instilled in place of love and acceptance. Intimidation or threats may be used to keep those experiencing emotional maltreatment from revealing their plight, causing victims to react to the nurse with passivity, withdrawal, or discounting the impact of their experience. Emotional violence is less obvious and more difficult to assess than physical violence.

ASSESSING NEGLECT. Neglect may stem from both benign and hostile causes. When a person does not meet another's needs because of a lack of resources, the neglect is benign and can usually be reversed with education and support. Neglect may also stem from hostility, however, signaling a serious disturbance in the caregiving relationship. In such a case, education is not sufficient, and more rigorous interventions are needed to safeguard the child or older adult from permanent physical and emotional harm. Neglected children and elders often appear undernourished, dirty, and poorly clothed. Neglect is also manifested by inadequate medical care, such as lack of immunizations or untreated medical conditions.

ASSESSING ECONOMIC MALTREATMENT. At times, money may serve as a motive for keeping the older adult at home, even if institutionalization is recommended. If the elderly are no longer able to care for their funds, the family may use some for their own personal purposes, thus restricting the older adult or not allowing him or her to meet basic needs. When the elder is compelled to use all personal resources in return for care, maltreatment is occurring.

Assessing the Level of Anxiety and Coping Responses

Nonverbal responses to history taking can be indicative of the victim's anxiety level. The identification of anxiety levels is described in Chapter 13. Hesitation, lack of eye contact, and vague statements, such as "It's been rough lately," indicate that the situation is difficult to talk about.

Agitation and anxiety bordering on panic are often present in women experiencing violence. They may be apprehensive of imminent doom, with good reason, as their husbands threaten violence, death, or mutilation. Because they live in terror, battered women remain vigilant, unable to relax or sleep. When they do sleep, they may have nightmares of danger and violence. Signs of the effect of living with chronic stress and severe levels of anxiety may be present (e.g., hypertension, irritability, gastrointestinal disturbances).

▶ A woman coming to the walk-in clinic with bilateral corneal abrasions raised the index of suspicion of an astute nurse who noted the vague responses to history questions and the client's unrelenting checking of the clock followed by urgently stating "I've got to get home." Upon further questioning, the woman revealed that she was often quite fatigued because of caring for her five children under 7 years of age. Yet her husband, who worked until 2 AM, expected her to be awake when he came home from work and have a warm meal ready in the oven. "He hits me if I'm asleep." She had taped her eyes open so that even if she were lying down when he came home she would look awake. "I didn't even think about taking my contacts out."

The coping mechanisms many battered women employ to live in violent and terrifying situations often prevent the dissolution of the marriage. These coping mechanisms present in the form of beliefs or myths (Table 15–1). Because of feelings of confusion, shame, despair, and powerlessness, victims may withdraw from interaction with others.

Having elderly victims relate the events of an average day can supply essential information about how they are coping, and clarify for the interviewer their experience of isolation. As a result of isolation, their self-esteem plummets further, and any sense of control over their lives is lost.

People experiencing violence frequently become quite defensive of their loved ones, even if they are abusive. It is crucial that the nurse allow them to maintain any defensive rationalizations that they have developed to protect their family members, even if the violent behavior is obvious. Abuse victims are not likely to accept care if they feel that the nurse is critical either of them or of their loved ones. However, although nurses must not appear critical, they do have both a legal and ethical obligation to report what they observe or assess—always in the case

TABLE 15-1 MYTH VERSUS FACT: FAMILY VIOLENCE

MYTH	FACT
1. The victim's behavior often causes violence.	1. The victim's behavior is ***not*** the cause of violence. Violence is the abuser's pattern of behavior, and the victim cannot learn how to control it.
2. Men have the right to keep their wives/children in line.	2. No person has the right to beat or hurt another person.
3. Spouse abuse is a minor problem.	3. There is a *real* danger that a woman may be killed by a violent partner.
4. Battered women are masochistic and like to be beaten. (The abuse cannot be that bad or they would leave.)	4. Women do not like, ask, or deserve to be abused. Economic considerations are usually the only reason they stay.
5. Family violence is most prevalent in those from poor working-class backgrounds who are usually poorly educated.	5. Violence occurs in families from all socioeconomic, religious, cultural, and educational backgrounds.
6. The family is sacred and should be allowed to take care of its own problems.	6. Intervention in family violence is justified because it always escalates in frequency and intensity, can end in death, and is passed on to future generations.
7. Abused women tacitly accept the abuse by trying to conceal it, by not reporting it, or by failing to seek help.	7. When attempting to disclose their situation, many women are met with disbelief. This discourages them from persevering.
8. Myths abused women believe: "I can't live without him." "If I hadn't done . . ., it wouldn't have happened." "He will change." "I stay for the sake of the children." "His jealousy and possessiveness proves he really loves me."	8. These myths are coping mechanisms women use to allay panic in a situation of random and brutal violence. They give the illusion of control and rationality.
9. Alcohol and stress are the major causes of physical and verbal abuse.	9. This myth offers an explanation of and tolerance for battering. There are no excuses and it is not acceptable behavior. Abuse is a learned behavior, not an uncontrollable reaction. People are abusive because they have acquired the belief that violence and aggression are acceptable and effective responses to real or imagined threats.
10. Violence occurs only between heterosexual partners.	10. Gay and lesbian partners experience violence for reasons similar to those in heterosexual partners.
11. Pregnancy protects a woman from battering.	11. Battering frequently begins or escalates during pregnancy.

of child abuse, and in most states for elder abuse (Campbell 1994). Legislation is currently being considered for spousal abuse.

Assessing Family Coping Patterns

When assessing family violence, the nurse should show a willingness to listen and avoid any judgmental tone. Questioning about memories of early family relationships can provide additional information about attitudes in the home and the way they might influence coping.

Attitudes about children, women, and the elderly, and the roles and duties of each, should be considered further. The nurse notes whether the perpetrator views these roles in a negative light. In our society, responsibility for care of children and the elderly usually falls on the woman. If there are disputes, she is generally expected to mediate between the needs of her spouse and those of the child or older person. This burden may be difficult to bear physically and emotionally, and may set her up for violence. The problem is compounded if the partner refuses to share in the responsibility, while still feeling accountable. Living with children and older adults in the same household can cause frustration, stress, and anger. Unless there are appropriate outlets for stress, violence can occur.

Assessing Support Systems

The person experiencing violence is usually in a dependent position, relying on the perpetrator (spouse, parent, other family member, or caregiver) for basic needs. Such situations foster isolation from others. Contacts to the outside are often controlled by the perpetrator, thus reducing connections to other family members or friends. Those victimized by violence may feel unworthy and believe that no one else could possibly want to have anything to do with them, a reflection of their low self-esteem. Alternatively, they might isolate themselves from others in a strategic effort to protect themselves from any actual or potentially unsupportive response. Feelings of shame and disgrace also prevent victims from talking to others, including social agency supports or the criminal justice system. Children's options are especially limited, as are those of the physically and mentally challenged. Assessing for support should focus on intrapersonal, interpersonal, and community resources (e.g., the school system for school-age victims).

Assessing Suicide Potential

A person experiencing violence may feel so trapped in a detrimental relationship, yet so desperate to get out, that suicide may seem the only answer. The threat of suicide may also be used by an emotionally violent person in an attempt to manipulate the partner or spouse into caving in to demands ("Don't leave me or I'll kill myself" or "I took all my pills . . . I said I would the next time you were late").

A suicide attempt may be the presenting symptom in the emergency department. It has been estimated that at least 10% of abused women attempt suicide (Walker 1980). With sensitive questioning conducted in a caring manner, the nurse can elicit the history of violence. Often the overdose is with a combination of alcohol and other central nervous system depressants, tranquilizers, or sleeping medications that have been prescribed in previous visits to physicians' offices, clinics, or emergency departments.

When the crisis of the immediate suicide attempt has been resolved, careful questioning to determine lethality is in order. (See Chapter 24 for suicide assessment.) For example, if the client still feels that life is not worth living, has a suicide plan, and has the means to carry it out, admission to an inpatient psychiatric unit must be considered. On the other hand, if the client is talking about future plans and hanging in there "for the sake of the children," outpatient referrals are appropriate. Each situation needs to be dealt with individually.

Assessing Homicide Potential

Inquire whether the client feels safe to go home, and if so, whether a safety plan is in place for when the violence recurs. Certain factors place a vulnerable person at greater risk for homicide from continuing and escalating violence:

- The presence of a gun in the home
- Alcohol and drug abuse
- The perpetrator also being violent in other situations (harmed pets, beat a spouse when she was pregnant, forced sex upon her)
- The perpetrator being extremely jealous and obsessive about his relationship with the victim and trying to control all her daily activities (Campbell 1995).

Persons victimized by violence should be asked if they have ever felt like killing the perpetrator, and if so whether they have the current desire and means to carry it out. If the answer is "yes," intervention is required.

Assessing Drug and Alcohol Use

A person experiencing violence may self-medicate with alcohol or other drugs as a way of escaping a dreadful situation. The drugs are usually central nervous system depressants (e.g., benzodiazepines) prescribed by physicians in response to the battered person's presentation with vague complaints, which are often stress related (e.g., insomnia, gastrointestinal upsets, feeling jittery, difficulty concentrating).

The level of intoxication can be determined by history, physical examination, and blood alcohol level. If the battered woman is intoxicated on presentation, allow her to sober up before instituting referral. Referral information will not be understood or assimilated if she is intoxicated. She should not be discharged with her husband.

Assess for a chronic alcohol or drug problem (refer to Chapter 25) and provide appropriate treatment referrals. Choices of treatment can include both inpatient and outpatient options.

Maintaining Accurate Records

Because of the possibility of legal action, it is essential that the **health care record** contain an accurate and detailed description of the victim's medical history, the psychosocial history of the family, and observations of the family interactions during the interviews. Especially important in documenting findings from initial assessment are (1) verbatim statements of who caused the injury and when it occurred; (2) a body map to indicate size, color, shape, areas, and types of injuries, with explanations; and (3) physical evidence, when possible, of sexual abuse. Procedures for evidence collection must be carefully followed or legal action can be thwarted. If the battered client consents, take photos. If the beating has just occurred, ask the client to return in a day or two for more photos; bruises may be more evident at that time. The client must be assured of the confidentiality of the record and of its power should legal action be initiated. Even if intervention does not occur at this time, the record is begun; the next provider will not have to stumble across the problem and will be in a better position to offer support.

NURSING DIAGNOSIS

Nursing diagnoses are focused on the underlying causes and symptoms of family violence. There are usually a number of areas of concern and problems resulting from the violence as well as the safety issue. Violence is a situational crisis with attendant threats to physical, emotional, and psychological health and, ultimately, life. **Risk for injury to self or other, Anxiety,** and **Fear** are nursing diagnoses that apply. **Coping, ineffective family: disabling, Powerlessness,** and **Caregiver role strain** are others. Feelings of helplessness, hopelessness, and powerlessness contribute to the diagnosis of **Body image disturbances** and **Self-esteem disturbances.** The crisis of family violence precipitates **Altered family process** or **Altered parenting** as the family system becomes less able to meet the emotional, physical, or security needs of its members.

Pain related to physical injury or trauma would most certainly take high priority and need immediate attention.

PLANNING

The identification of desired outcomes and designing of nursing interventions that facilitate achieving those outcomes should be developed as much as possible in collaboration with the survivor and primary support person. These outcomes should be continually reassessed and revised as new information about the survivor's needs emerges. A comprehensive plan can also be the coordinating framework for the work of an interdisciplinary team.

Planning Outcome Criteria

With each nursing diagnosis, long- and short-term outcomes (goals) are identified. They are directed toward the client and the perpetrator in specific circumstances. Diagnoses with possible outcomes for child, female, and elderly survivors are listed.

Altered family process related to feelings of rage and helplessness associated with the illness of one parent and difficulty with finances.

LONG-TERM OUTCOMES

- By (date), parents will state that group meetings with other parents who have battered are useful.
- Parents and child will share in two planned pleasurable activities twice a day when child returns home.

SHORT-TERM GOALS

- Within 24 hours, parents will be able to name and call three agencies that can help financially during the crisis.
- By end of first interview, parents will be able to name two places they can contact to discuss feelings of rage and helplessness.
- Within 2 weeks, parents will be able to name three alternative actions to take when feelings of helplessness and rage start to surface.

Altered family process related to inadequate marital relationship (applies only if the perpetrator acknowledges a problem for which he wants help and demonstrates steps toward change verified by the spouse).

LONG-TERM OUTCOMES

- Perpetrator will state that he realizes he must change in order to stay with his family.
- Perpetrator will join and attend a group for spouses who batter.
- Within 3 months, couple will state that they want to join a couples therapy group.
- Couple will be able to name three possible effects that family violence may have on their children.
- Within 6 months, couple will state that violence has ceased altogether.

SHORT-TERM GOALS

- Client will state that she is interested in knowing about family treatment modalities.
- Client will state that she no longer chooses to live in a situation with violence.
- Client will name three places she can call to receive counseling for herself or her family.

Altered Family Process related to demands of caring for a dependent elder.

LONG-TERM GOALS (OUTCOMES)

- Family members will state that they will meet with the nurse on a weekly basis for counseling starting (date).
- Abuser will meet with other family members and discuss feelings on care of elderly by (date).
- Family members will meet together and discuss alternatives for care of elderly by (date).
- Client and family will meet together and discuss resources and supports they feel are important to them by (date).
- Family members will demonstrate, instead of violence, two appropriate methods of dealing with frustration.

SHORT-TERM GOALS

- Family members will meet together and discuss alternative ways of dealing with elderly client by (date).
- Family members will name two strategies for avoiding physical or emotional violence toward client by (date).
- Family members will name two support services to whom they can turn for help by (date).
- One other family member or support person will spend time with elder and relieve abuser of caregiving duties by (date).

Risk for injury, self or others relates to mate's poor impulse control.

LONG-TERM OUTCOMES

- Within 3 weeks, client will state that she believes she does not deserve to be beaten.

- Within 3 weeks, client will state that she has joined a women's support group or is having family counseling.
- Client will state that her living conditions are now safe from spouse abuse *or*
- Within 2 months, client will state that she has found safe housing for herself and children.

SHORT-TERM GOALS

- After initial interview, client will name four community resources she can contact (hotlines, shelters, support groups, neighbor, crisis center, spiritual adviser who does not support violence).
- After initial interview, client will describe a safety plan to be used in future violent situations.
- Client will state her right to live in a safe environment.
- Client will state the dangers to her and her children in her home situation.
- Client will state that she knows how to obtain a restraining order.

Risk for injury related to violent parent.

LONG-TERM OUTCOME

- Child will know what plans are made for his or her protection and will state them to nurse after decision is made by health care team.

SHORT-TERM GOALS

- Child will be safe until adequate home and family assessment is made by (date).
- Child will be treated by physician and receive medical care for injuries within 1 hour.
- Child will participate with therapist (nurse, social worker, counselor) for purpose of therapy and emotional support (art, play, group, or other) within 24 hours.

Caretaker role strain related to being a dependent elder

LONG-TERM OUTCOMES

- Client will state that caregiver has provided adequate food, clothing, housing, and medical care by (date).
- Client will be free of physical signs of abuse by (date).

SHORT-TERM GOALS

- Client will state that he or she feels safer and more comfortable by (date) *or*
- Client will ask to be removed from violent situation by (date).
- Client will name one person who can be called for help by (date).

Nurse's Feelings and Self-Assessment

In all areas of psychiatric nursing and counseling, the nurse should be aware of personal emotions and thoughts. Strong negative feelings can cloud one's judgment and interfere with assessment and intervention, no matter how well the nurse tries to cover or deny feelings. Perhaps more than in any other situation, intense and overwhelming feelings may be aroused by working with those experiencing violence. The nurse may also have come from a violent environment and thus identify too closely with the victim; old personal issues around the abuse may surface, further clouding judgment. Common reactions include (1) intense protective feelings and sympathy for those affected and (2) anger and outrage toward the perpetrator.

Intense feelings of sympathy and protectiveness triggered by the pain and vulnerability of the person who is victimized may lead to "rescue fantasies" in the nurse. When this happens, the nurse projects personal emotional needs onto the victim, and the tendency is to be the "savior." When the rescue contract is not fulfilled, the victim is left more isolated than ever.

Outrage and anger toward perpetrators may lead to ignoring their needs. In the case of violence against children, parental support and involvement in a treatment plan may be the best options for stopping the violence. In the case of elder maltreatment, many caregivers are well intentioned but lack the economic, social, educational, or psychological resources to provide the care required.

One attitude worth challenging is that family conflict resolution is a private, family matter. Nurses are probably in people's homes more than any other professionals. If nursing care of families does not include assessing for and intervening with violence, it is unlikely that violence will be identified as a problem (Campbell and Campbell 1993).

Interdisciplinary team conferences can be especially helpful in clarifying reactions and neutralizing intense emotions. Information from physicians, psychologists, nurses, and social workers can assist in refocusing efforts to work constructively with a family in crisis. Sharing perceptions and feelings with other professionals can help reduce feelings of isolation and discomfort for nurses.

The more thought the nurse gives to the issue of family violence before encountering someone experiencing it, the more effective will be the subsequent interaction. Acknowledging accepted myths is the first step in at least putting them aside in working with a person experiencing violence, and it eventually allows the counteracting of these myths with facts. Myths have served to perpetuate acceptance of violence (Chez 1994). Look again at Table 15–1 for some myths regarding spouse abuse and facts that counter them.

Awareness of personal feelings in response to those experiencing violence stimulates examination of personal views toward violence and the status of children, women, and elders. This is most effectively done through professional or peer supervision. An understanding of the dynamics of violence is crucial to effective nursing intervention. It is advisable for nurses working with people involved in family violence to review their cases with other professionals in peer supervision or with a clinical supervisor. Violence can evoke strong and frequently irrational feelings. Nurses need to sort out their own strong feelings through professional or peer supervision before they can work effectively with their clients.

Nurses are members of society and have been socialized to live within the social norms that contribute to the treatment of children, women, and the elderly as second-class citizens. Some nurses may still believe that it is acceptable for parents to hit children and for men to physically beat women. American society is violent, and some nurses may have come to accept violence as a way of life. Nurses react in large measure as a result of the way they have been socialized. Some nurses have grown up in violent households; some may currently live in violent homes. Awareness of individual feelings and reactions facilitates caregiving in that the nurse can consciously and deliberately respond to the victim rather than get sidetracked into having to deal with personal reactions in the work setting. Common responses of health care professionals to violence are listed in Box 15–9. These feelings need to be recognized when they arise and dealt with in supervision for therapeutic intervention to be maximized. All the feelings listed seem "natural" or "normal" as a response to caring for someone who has experienced violence. The student or practitioner new to this setting needs to be aware that these feelings may overpower the nurse's ability to be therapeutic, and supervision with a more experienced professional is vital during these times.

INTERVENTION

Nurses are reluctant to intervene with violent families both because of beliefs about the privacy of families and because of discomfort and fear. However, the moral foundations of the nurse's role as caregiver place nurses in an ideal position to empower and assist families for whom violence is a major concern (Henderson and Ericksen 1994). In addition, nurses have a legal responsibility and are mandated to report suspected or actual cases of child abuse. At present, most states have mandatory reporting laws for elder abuse. Some are beginning to mandate reporting of violence against women. When child or elder abuse is suspected, a report is made to the protective agency designated by each state. The appropriate agency may be the state or county child welfare agency, law enforcement agency, juvenile court, or county health department. Each state has specific guidelines for reporting, including whether the report can be oral or written, or both, and specifying the time that can elapse after suspicion of abuse or neglect (immediately, 24 hours, or 48 hours). Every battered woman is a crime victim, and assault with a weapon is reportable in most states. Also, approximately 40 states have marital rape statutes (Sheridan 1993).

An example follows of a case to report.

- Two nurses who work in a family practice clinic are suspicious of child abuse. A 12-year-old girl has recurrent urinary tract infections. She is always accompanied to clinic visits by her father, who even goes into the bathroom with her when she is producing urine samples. He answers all questions for her even when they are directed toward her. He has recently refused the next diagnostic test for attempting to ascertain the reason for the recurrent infections.
- After pressure by the nurses, the physician agrees to ask the girl some questions in private. The nurses think the physician has discounted the problem, asked

BOX 15–9 COMMON RESPONSES OF HEALTH CARE PROFESSIONALS TO VIOLENCE

FEELING	SOURCE
Anger	Anger may be felt toward the person responsible for the violence, toward those who allowed it to happen, and toward society for condoning its occurrence through attitudes, traditions, and laws.
Embarrassment	The victim is a symbol of something close to home: the stress and strain of family life unleashed as uncontrollable anger.
Confusion	Our cherished view of the family as a haven of safety and privacy is challenged.
Fear	A small percentage of perpetrators are dangerous to others.
Anguish	The nurse may have experienced family violence.
Helplessness	The nurse may want to do more, to eliminate the problem, to cure the victim.
Discouragement	Discouragement may result if no long-term solution is achieved.
"Blame the victim" mentality	Lay people as well as health care workers can get caught up in "blaming the victim" for not having the house neat, food on time, clothes neat. There is never an excuse for violence, and no one has the right to hurt another person. "Blaming the victim" can occur when health care professionals feel overwhelmed. Supervision is a must for therapeutic intervention.

superficial questions, and dismissed their concerns. They attempt to get the girl alone for a discussion, but to no avail. After consultation with clinical resources, they decide to report their concerns to Children's Protective Services. They inform the father, who becomes outraged at their accusations and threatens to change doctors. The nurses try to reassure him about the nature of the referral, to no avail. Subsequent investigation confirms the likelihood of sexual abuse, and the child is placed in temporary foster care with follow-up counseling. The father refuses treatment and 4 months later leaves the family.

This case illustrates that a reasonable basis for suspecting maltreatment, not proof, is all that is required to report. Nurses must attempt to maintain both an appropriate level of suspicion and a neutral, objective attitude. One can be too concerned and jump to conclusions (which is what the physician in this case thought the nurses were doing) or not concerned enough and rationalize an incomplete examination to avoid confrontation (which is what the nurses thought the physician was doing). Given these opposing stances, the case was reported, as required by law and ethical standards, and Children's Protective Services was given the opportunity to sort it out.

Immunity from criminal or civil liability is provided when reporting is mandated. On the other hand, a nurse can be held civilly and criminally liable if a case of suspected abuse is not reported (Lewin 1994). There may be a risk to the ongoing health care relationship, but the nurse must hold the client's safety and health (mental, physical, and emotional) as most important. Nonetheless, it is vitally important not to jump immediately to intervention when abuse is mentioned. Nurses have been known to skip the assessment and planning phases of the nursing process because of the feelings this problem engenders.

Competency may be a consideration in a situation of elder mistreatment. Unless incompetency has been established legally, elders have the right to self-determination. Some institutions and health care agencies have developed guidelines for dealing with actual or suspected situations of mistreatment. These protocols list possible behaviors or conditions of the elderly and the most appropriate intervention. The establishment of such protocols is highly recommended because it gives support to the nurse's actions.

Quality nursing care for those experiencing violence must be culturally sensitive (Sue and Sue 1990). The nurse must be aware of the cultural issues that may affect response to violence and to intervention. For example, Cambodian women control their responses to stress and violence through nonconfrontation and withdrawal, which are designed to restore equilibrium (Frye and D'Avanzo 1994). Culture is important because it is central to how people organize their experience. Even the most acculturated people have a tendency to revert to their cultural past in organizing coping strategies after a stressful event (Campbell et al. 1993). If there is a language barrier, the nurse should speak slowly and clearly in English, without using jargon, and allow time for the response. If no English is spoken, a trained medical interpreter should be provided. A family member should *not* be used, to ensure confidentiality and to protect the person from future retaliation.

Primary prevention consists of measures taken to prevent the occurrence of family violence. Identifying people at high risk, providing health teaching, and coordinating supportive services to prevent crises are examples of primary prevention. Specific strategies include (1) reducing stress, (2) reducing the influence of risk factors, (3) increasing social support, (4) increasing coping skills, and (5) increasing self-esteem (Andrews 1994).

Nurses can engage in educational programs that heighten public and professional awareness of violence. One example is group-based instruction for children on personal safety, which is a common approach for prevention of child sexual abuse. This prevention program is most effective for children 7 to 12 years of age and also contributes to secondary prevention (see below), as it gives children an opportunity to disclose past or present abuse (Daro 1994). School nurses or community health nurses can play a major role in these programs. The rate of spontaneous recovery after a child's disclosure of sexual abuse is high when a supporting adult is present. Age, developmental level, intrapersonal resources, and the circumstances of the abuse affect the extent of the consequences (Briere and Elliott 1994; Larson et al. 1994). Nurses can assist families facing this crisis by counseling them regarding the strengths in the family and how to make use of them in this time of crisis. Ongoing support during the acute adjustment period should be given to those who are more at risk for long-term negative effects (Beutler et al. 1994)

Community health nurses are also in a position to assess family functioning in the home during visits for such matters as assisting children with chronic health problems. In addition, the community health nurse and clinic nurse maintain contact with the family over time, which allows for assessment of changes. They are also in an excellent position to connect parents to appropriate resources in the community that can meet their needs.

Secondary prevention involves early intervention in abusive situations to minimize their disabling or long-term effects. Nurses can establish screening programs for individuals at risk, participate in the medical treatment of injuries resulting from violent episodes, and coordinate community services to provide continuity of care (Ross and Hoff 1994). Stress and depression can be reduced with supportive psychotherapy, support groups, and pharmacotherapy. Social dysfunction or lack of information can be addressed by counseling and education. Caregiver burden can be reduced by assistance in caregiving, nursing, or housekeeping or (in cases in which caregiving needs exceed even optimized caregiver capacity) placement of the patient in a more appropriate setting (Vida 1994). Secondary prevention is most often carried out in an outpatient setting. The following vignette illustrates a successful secondary prevention effort.

- Billy, age 4, is brought into the physician's office by 15-year-old Mary, the children's babysitter, with second-degree burns on his right hand. Mary frequently babysits for Billy and his younger brother Jimmy, age 2, and older brother Tom, age 6. Mary appears apprehensive and says she is very concerned. Mary tells the nurse that the children have told her in the past that Billy's mother has threatened them with burning if they do not behave. Billy told her that his mother once held his hands on a cold stove and told him that if he was bad, she would burn him. Mary is shocked that Billy's mother would do such a thing, but at the same time she mentions she feels guilty for "telling on Ms. J."
- Mary also states that the older brother told Mary what had happened but was afraid that if his mother found out, she would burn him also. Mary says she is aware that the mother hits the children, but she did not believe that anyone would burn her own child.
- The nurse reports what happened to the physician, and the mother is called and asked to come to the office.
- Billy appears frightened and in pain. The nurse asks Mary to come with Billy while she examines him.

Nurse: Tell me about your hand, Billy. *Billy looks down and starts to cry.*
Nurse: It's OK if you don't want to talk about it, Billy.
Billy: *Not looking at the nurse, he says softly,* My mommy burned my hand on the stove.
Nurse: Tell me what happened before that happened.
Billy: Mommy was mad because I didn't put my toys away.
Nurse: What does your mommy usually do when she gets mad?
Billy: She yells mostly; sometimes she hits us. Mommy is going to be so mad at Tommy for telling.
Nurse: Tell me about the hitting.
Billy: Mommy hits us a lot since Daddy left us. *Billy starts to cry to himself.*

- On examination, the nurse notices a ringed pattern of burns across Billy's right palm like the burner of an electric stove. There are blisters on the fingers. Billy appears well-nourished and properly dressed. He is at his approximate developmental age except for some language delay.
- Because of the physical evidence and history, there is strong suspicion of child abuse. Children's Protective Services is notified, and the family situation is evaluated for possible placement of Billy in protective custody. The initial evaluation concludes that there is no indication of serious potential harm to the child and that Billy should return home.
- The mother, who was initially defensive, starts to cry and states, "I can't cope with being alone and I don't know where to turn." The intervention that the nurse facilitates centers around caring for Billy's immediate health needs; finding supports for the mother to help her cope with crises; providing a counseling referral for the mother to learn alternative ways of expressing anger and frustration; informing the mother of parents' groups; providing referrals to play groups or day care for the children to help increase their feelings of self-esteem and security; and providing a break, and perhaps some instruction in parenting, for the mother.

Tertiary prevention involves nurses facilitating the healing and rehabilitative process by counseling individuals and families; providing support for groups of survivors; and assisting survivors of violence to achieve their optimal level of safety, health, and well-being (Ross and Hoff 1994). Tertiary interventions often occur in mental health settings.

Counseling (Basic Level)

Counseling interventions include crisis intervention and the promotion of growth. It is useful to emphasize that people have a right to live without fear of violence or physical harm, and without fear of assault. The role of the nurse is to support the victim, counsel about safety, and facilitate access to other resources as appropriate. By listening, giving support, discussing options, and describing other ways of living, the nurse initiates an awareness of other possibilities.

All women experiencing violence should be counseled about developing a safety plan, a plan for a fast escape when violence recurs. They should be asked to identify the signs of escalation of violence and to pick a particular sign that will tell them in the future that "now is the time to leave." If children are present, they can all agree on a code word that, when spoken by their mother, means "it is time to go." If she plans ahead, she may be able to leave before the violence occurs. She should plan where she is going and how she will get there. The nurse should suggest that she have a bag already packed for herself and her children with a few articles of clothing, essential toiletry items, money for cab fare and phone calls, identification cards, insurance information, and a list of referral sources with their telephone numbers (Box 15–10). (In many, but by no means all, communities, there is a 24-hour telephone number provided by the Domestic Abuse Warning Network, or help can be reached through a national hotline. People who answer the phone have information on the services available for battered women.) The packed bag should be kept in a place where the perpetrator will not find it. Often, the perpetrator will terrorize

BOX 15–10 EXAMPLE OF A SAFETY PLAN

Suggest that the victim

- Hide money
- Hide extra set of house and car keys
- Establish code with family and friends
- Ask neighbor to call police if violence begins
- Remove weapons
- Have available:
  social security numbers (his, yours, children)
  rent and utility receipts
  birth certificates (yours and children)
  driver's license (yours and children)
  bank account numbers
  insurance policies
  marriage license
  valuable jewelry
  important phone numbers
- Hide bag with extra clothing (and whatever children will need) perhaps at a neighbor's

the mother by going through her belongings (purse, dresser). If such information is found, he might beat her. One suggestion is to put the phone number on the back of his photo in her wallet.

If the mother chooses to leave, **shelters** or **safe houses** are available in many communities (although, sadly, only at half the rate of animal shelters—a reflection on our social values). They are open 24 hours a day and can be reached through hotline information, hospital emergency rooms, YWCAs, or the local office of the National Organization for Women (NOW). The address of the house is usually kept secret to protect the women from attack by their mates. Besides protection, many of these safe shelters provide important education and consciousness-raising functions. The woman should be given the number of the nearest available shelter, even if she decides for the present to stay with her partner. Referral phone numbers may be kept for years before the decision to call is made. Having the number all that time contributes to thinking about options.

Case Management

Community mental health centers are becoming increasingly involved in the delivery of services to victims and perpetrators of domestic violence (Jordan and Walker 1994). Nurses working in these settings have the opportunity to be case managers to coordinate community, medical, criminal justice, and social systems in order to provide comprehensive services for violent families. Strategies must encompass needs for housing, child care, economic stability, physical and emotional safety, counseling, legal protection, career development or job training, education, ongoing support groups, and health care (Loring and Smith 1994). The myriad of agencies and people that those seeking help have to reach can be daunting and confusing. A nurse functioning in a case manager role can assist the client in choosing the best options for her and coordinating the interventions of several agencies. Suggestions for interventions for common assessment domains and community resources are listed in Table 15–2.

Milieu Therapy

Interventions are geared toward stabilizing the home situation and maintaining a violence-free environment. The interventions offered should leave options for growth, increase in self-esteem, and a higher quality of life for all family members. Providing and maintaining a therapeutic environment in the home ideally involves three levels of help for violent families:

1. Provide the family with economic support, job opportunities, and social services, such as family service agencies.
2. Arrange social support in the form of a public health nurse, lay home visitor, day care teacher, school teacher, social worker, respite worker, or any other potential contact person who has a good relationship with the family.
3. Encourage and provide family therapy.

Day care centers for small children or elders can help relieve the caregiver, although many people cannot afford the cost. Homemakers, brought into the home to help with direct household assistance, can reduce feelings of being overwhelmed.

Amundson (1989) describes an intensive home-based crisis interaction and family education program developed by clinical nurse specialists in mental health nursing. The program accepts only families referred by Children's Protective Services in which at least one child is in imminent danger of being placed in foster, group, or institutional care. The goal is to prevent out-of-home placement of children by means of intensive, in-home intervention that teaches families new problem-solving skills for avoiding future crises.

Self-Care Activities (Basic Level)

The primary goal of intervention is empowerment (Chez 1994). Supporting the client to act on her own behalf can decrease feelings of helplessness and hopelessness. Giving referral numbers and providing an opportunity for her to call from your office, or inquiring at the next visit whether she was successful in reaching the appropriate agency, demonstrates confidence in her ability to take care of herself.

Specific referrals regarding emergency money and legal counseling should be made available to each woman. Legal assistance can take the form of an order for protection, an injunction, a civil suit, or criminal charges. Vocational counseling is another referral that may be appropriate. Social workers can provide detailed referral options.

Battered women should be given referrals to parenting resources that enable them to explore alternative approaches to discipline (i.e., no hitting, slapping, or other expressions of violence). It is distressing to see women in shelters use these methods with their children. Such behavior perpetuates the idea that violence solves problems, and passes the problem of violence on to the next generation.

Health Teaching (Basic Level)

Health teaching is one of the most important aspects of primary prevention. The first line of intervention is prevention, through teaching people additional ways of coping. In families at risk for violence, health teaching includes meeting with both the client and the family and discussing associated risk factors. The client, caregiver, and family need to learn to recognize behaviors and situations that might trigger violence.

Normal developmental and physiological changes should be explained to enable family members to gain a more positive view of the victim and the crisis situation. Gaining a more complete understanding can help family

TABLE 15–2 VICTIMS OF VIOLENCE—NURSING NEEDS ASSESSMENT AND INTERVENTION

	Assessment	Intervention	
Domain	**Nursing Assessment**	**Nursing Education/ Intervention**	**Community Agencies**
Physiological	Brief head-to-toe assessment	Appropriate medical follow-up	Community clinics Medical staff referrals
	Nutritional habits	Healthy dietary practices Basic food groups Food availability	WIC (Women, Infants, and Children) services Community food shelves
	Sleep patterns	Impact of sleep deprivation	Counseling, crisis nursery
	Chemical dependency/use	Encourage access to counseling/ support groups	Referrals to AA, counselors, community agencies supporting rehabilitation
	Sexual assault	Assess for immediate physical needs	Sexual assault advocates
Psychological/ sociocultural	Self-esteem	Affirm: You don't deserve it/You didn't cause it	Battered women's resources
	Coping skills/needs	Need to take care of self Relaxation techniques Pursue things she enjoys	Community women's courses, groups, public library
	Support system (family, friends)	Emphasize need to access Provide opportunity to call Help identify support services	Support groups Stress management classes Crisis nursery Battered women's groups and shelters
	Depression	Offer support Validate: It is part of the abuse cycle Evaluate severity: candidate for posttraumatic stress disorder?	Counseling, psychotherapy Resources at place of employment
Educational	Understanding/perception of abuse	Definitions/characteristics: What constitutes abuse, escalating characteristics	Battered women's resources
	Literacy		Community education
	Language/hearing barriers		Interpreter services, hearing society
Financial	Is there need for money? (transportation, food, medical care, basic needs)		Social services Battered women's resources Counseling, employment, clothing community resources Medical assistance/AFDC

TABLE 15–2 VICTIMS OF VIOLENCE—NURSING NEEDS ASSESSMENT AND INTERVENTION *(Continued)*

	ASSESSMENT	INTERVENTION	
Domain	**Nursing Assessment**	**Nursing Education/ Intervention**	**Community Agencies**
Legal	Desire for legal action	Facilitate contact of law enforcement Advise of resources available	Battered women's advocates Law enforcement
	Legal questions		Judicare or local attorney resources Legal clinics Battered women's resources
Safety	Fear level	Safety plan: ▶ Self-defense ▶ Emergency numbers ▶ Self-protection during abuse: curl into ball, hold head, scream loudly ▶ Have children or neighbors call 911	Community self-defense classes Women's shelter and advocates
	Safety level: ▶ Does she feel safe? ▶ Has there been a recent increase in violence? ▶ Has she been choked? ▶ Is there a weapon in the house? ▶ Has he used/threatened to use a weapon? ▶ Has he threatened to harm the children? ▶ Has he threatened to kill her?	Counsel regarding long-range plans: ▶ Discuss potential for escalation and increased risk ▶ Discuss awareness of options, considering risk Escape plan: ▶ Where will she go? ▶ How will she get there? ▶ What does she need to leave? ▶ Hide an "escape kit" that is easily accessible: ▶ papers, money, documents ▶ phone numbers, including number of women's shelter ▶ clothing, glasses, medications ▶ keys	Child protection Women's shelter and advocates
	Safety of children	Presence of child abuse	Child protection

*Battered women's advocates and shelter staff members are excellent resources for any of the above needs.
AFDC, Aid to Families with Dependent Children.
Developed by Marlene Jezierski, R. N. From Jezierski, M. (1994). Abuse of women by male partners: Basic knowledge for emergency nurses. *Journal of Emergency Nursing*, 20(5):361.

members broaden their insight and thus increase their compassion. They may then begin to anticipate new stress situations and be able to prepare for them before a crisis occurs.

Educating family members to analyze their respective roles and develop suggestions for realignment or redistribution of responsibilities is important for effecting change in a violent situation. The process includes assessing the need for role changes in all family members, identifying role conflicts, clarifying expectations, and strengthening the ability of family members to perform their individual roles. Refer to Chapter 11 for family interventions.

Nurses who work on a maternity unit are often in a position to spot potential violence in new families and initiate appropriate interventions, including education about effective parenting as well as coping techniques. Information about these interventions should be shared with the client's ambulatory care nurse for appropriate monitoring and follow-up. Parents who are candidates for special attention include

1. New parents whose behavior toward the infant is rejecting, hostile, or indifferent.
2. Teenage parents, most of whom are children themselves and who require special help and guidance in handling the baby and discussing their expectations of the baby and their support systems.
3. Retarded parents, for whom careful, explicit, and repeated instructions on caring for the child and recognizing the infant's needs are indicated.
4. Parents who grew up watching their mother being beaten. This is the biggest risk factor for perpetuation of family violence.

Nurses can also recognize the vulnerable child. When it is known that specific children are at risk, referrals to community resources are in order. These may include emergency child care facilities, emergency telephone numbers, numbers of 24-hour crisis centers or hotlines, and respite programs in which volunteers take the child for an occasional weekend so that parents can get some relief. Public health nurses can make home visits; such visits allow assessment of potential violence in the crucial first few months of life. This early period is when the style of parent-child interactions is set for later life. Important factors for the public health nurse to assess are noted in Box 15–11. Such observations made by nurses in clinic and public health settings are fundamental in case finding and evaluation.

Psychotherapy (Advanced Level)

Psychotherapy is carried out by a nurse who is educated at the master's level in psychiatric nursing and certified or eligible for certification. Therapy is most effective after crisis intervention, when the situation is less chaotic and tumultuous. A variety of therapeutic modalities are available for violent families. The principles used when working with them are the ones used with other client groups: empowerment, therapeutic communication, validation, support, and respect for client autonomy (Henderson and Ericksen 1994).

Individual Therapy

The goals of individual therapy for a survivor center on helping the person recognize feelings about experiencing violence, about the self, and about options. It affords a survivor the process of internal change and rebuilding. Expected outcomes include an increase in self-esteem and affirmation that no one deserves to experience violence. The fourth edition of the *Diagnostic and statistical manual of mental disorders* (DSM-IV) includes a section on problems related to abuse or neglect under the category "Conditions That May Be a Focus of Clinical Attention."

People who experienced violence as a child or who have left a violent relationship may choose individual therapy to work out symptoms of depression, anxiety, somatization, or posttraumatic stress disorder (Hall et al. 1993; Seng and Peterson 1995; Walling et al. 1994). Many of the psychological symptoms shown by battered women can be understood as complex survival strategies and responses to violence. This constellation of symptoms has been referred to as the "battered woman syndrome" (the posttraumatic stress disorder category in DSM-IV) (Jackson 1994). Disclosure of violence has been found to worsen psychiatric symptoms in an adult psychiatric population because of hostile and rejecting responses from significant others in the survivor's social network, including the therapist (McNulty and Wardle 1994; Weaver et al. 1994).

Box 15–11 FACTORS TO ASSESS DURING A HOME VISIT

FOR CHILD

Responsiveness to infant's crying
Responsiveness to infant's signals related to feeding
Caregiver's facial expressions in response to infant
Holding of child
Playfulness of caregiver with infant
Type of physical contact during feeding
Temperament of infant: average, quiet, or active
Parent's attitudes signaling possible warnings:

- Complaints of inadequacy as a parent
- Complaints of inadequacy of child
- Fear of "doing something wrong"
- Attribution of badness to newborn
- History of a destructive childhood
- Misdirected anger
- Continued evidence of isolation, apathy, anger, frustration, projection
- Adult conflict

Environmental conditions:

- Sleeping arrangements
- Child management
- Home management
- Use of supports (formal and informal)

Need for immediate services for situational (economics, child care), emotional, or educational information:

- Sharing information about hotlines, babysitters, homemakers, parent groups
- Sharing information about child development
- Child care and home management

FOR ELDER

Environmental conditions:

- House in poor repair
- Inadequate heat, lighting, furniture, cooking utensils
- Presence of garbage or vermin
- Old food in kitchen
- Lack of assistive devices
- Locks on refrigerator
- Blocked stairways
- Victim lying in urine, feces, or food
- Unpleasant odors

Medication:

- Medication not being taken as prescribed

Data from Galbraith 1986; Elder abuse 1991.

Individual therapy is often indicated for the perpetrator also, particularly when an individual psychopathological process is identified. Many perpetrators meet the DSM-IV criteria for intermittent explosive disorder, which involves repeated episodes of assault or destruction of property out of proportion to precipitating stressors that cannot be accounted for by another mental disorder, the physiological effects of a substance, or a general medical condition. Differential diagnoses for intermittent explosive disorder include antisocial personality disorder, borderline personality disorder, a psychotic disorder, or a manic episode (Murphy 1994). Therapy for the perpetrator is most effective when it is court mandated, because then the perpetrator is more likely to stay the course of treatment.

Family Therapy

Because family violence is a symptom of a family in crisis, each part of the family system needs attention. Also, because change in one member of the family system effects change in the whole system, support and understanding are needed by all members. Family interventions may maximize positive interactions among family members. Family therapy should take place *only* if the violence is recent and if *both* partners agree to be involved. The perpetrator should have taken steps to control violent behavior that are verified by the survivor.

Expected outcomes are that the perpetrator will recognize inner states of anger and learn alternative ways of dealing with anger. Intermediate goals are that members of the family will openly communicate and learn to listen to each other.

Group Therapy

Therapy groups provide assurances that one is not alone and that positive change is possible. Because many survivors have been isolated over time, they have been deprived of validation and positive feedback from others. Working in a group can help diminish feelings of isolation, strengthen feelings of self-esteem and self-worth, and increase the potential for realistic problem solving in a supportive atmosphere.

Self-help groups serve a vital function for many people. Hotlines provide emergency resources and information on how to contact self-help groups within the community, such as Parents Anonymous.

The real problem in a violent relationship is the perpetrator. Nurses engaged in therapy with perpetrators have a **duty to warn** potential victims if they conclude that the perpetrator is a danger (Campbell 1994). Refer to Chapter 4 for legal guidelines. In groups for perpetrators, the men are taught to recognize signs of escalating anger and learn ways of channeling their anger nonviolently. Men who have never discussed problems with anyone before are encouraged to discuss their thoughts and feelings. Sharing with others who have similar problems can help minimize feelings of isolation and allow mutual problem solving for handling overwhelming feelings of pain, low self-esteem, and rage. These feelings often stem from some kind of loss. Untended mourning and grief (usually from childhood deprivations and victimization) get translated into anger, rage, and violence. Group therapy can help create a community of healing and restoration.

EVALUATION

Failures in interventions with abusive families are often due not to our lack or theirs but to deficits in the social, economic, and political systems in which we live. Being valued and protected as a child or elder and valued as a woman is not merely a privilege but a right. Nurses can direct their interventions to the social environment and can question, among other things, the acceptance of corporal punishment as a technique for guiding behavior in children, the unequal burden of caregiving responsibilities placed on women, the low priority given to education and preparation for parenthood, and the belief that one has little social value if one is elderly.

Evaluation of brief interventions can be based on whether the survivor acknowledges the violence, is willing to accept intervention, and/or is removed from the violent situation. With more long-term intervention, evaluation should be made by all members of the health care team on an ongoing basis. Because violence is a symptom of a family in distress, diagnosis, interventions, and evaluation should ideally be carried out by a multidisciplinary team that includes a physician, a nurse, a social worker, an attorney, and perhaps a psychiatrist.

Evaluation of established outcomes (goals) can lead to the formulation of new goals when old ones are reached, or to changes in intervention if desired outcomes have not been met. The goals of changing family interactions and reducing the incidence of violence in the family are a primary focus of evaluation. Outcomes are being met when changes are noted in decreased evidence of violence, in healthier coping patterns used by the victim or the family, or in the support systems available. When these changes are positive, the nurse may continue to work with the family as a resource person or facilitator. When such changes are not noted or are negative, the nurse works with the family to reevaluate the agreed-upon outcomes and the interventions originally set for their attainment.

The following is a case study of family violence.

CASE STUDY: WORKING WITH A FAMILY EXPERIENCING VIOLENCE

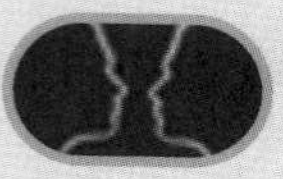

Mrs. Rob, an 84-year-old woman recently widowed, moved to her son's apartment 3 months ago. She had been living alone in her third-floor walk-up in the city. Because of her declining health, crime in the neighborhood, and three flights of stairs to climb, and with her son John's encouragement, she went to live with him. He and his wife, Judy, who have been married for almost 20 years, have five children 6 to 18 years of age, all living in a rather cramped three-bedroom apartment.

Mrs. Rob was being cared for by the visiting nurse, who monitored her blood pressure and adjusted her medication. Over a series of visits, the nurse, Ms. Green, noticed that Mrs. Rob was looking unkempt, pale, and withdrawn. While taking her blood pressure, the nurse observed bruises on Mrs. Rob's arms and neck. When questioned about the bruises, Mrs. Rob appeared anxious and nervous. She said that she had slipped in the bathroom. Mrs. Rob became increasingly apprehensive and stiffened up in her chair when her daughter-in-law, Judy, came into the room asking when the next visit was. The nurse noticed that Judy avoided eye contact with Mrs. Rob.

When the injuries were brought to Judy's attention, she responded by becoming angry and agitated, blaming Mrs. Rob for causing so many problems. She would not explain the reason for the change in Mrs. Rob's behavior or the origin of the bruises to the nurse. She merely commented, "I have had to give up my job since my mother-in-law came here. It's been difficult and crowded ever since she moved in. The kids are complaining. We are having trouble making ends meet since I gave up my job. And my husband is no help at all."

ASSESSMENT

Ms. Green suspected that Mrs. Rob was experiencing mistreatment and spoke of the case with her team at the visiting nurse center. The nurse identified objective and subjective data that supported suspected elder mistreatment.

OBJECTIVE DATA

1. Physical symptoms of violence (i.e., bruises, unkempt appearance, withdrawn attitude)
2. Stressful, crowded living conditions
3. No eye contact between Mrs. Rob and her daughter-in-law
4. Economic hardships leading to stress
5. No support for the daughter-in-law from rest of family for care of Mrs. Rob
6. Mrs. Rob unable to make decisions

SUBJECTIVE DATA

1. Mrs. Rob states she "slipped in the bathroom," but physical findings do not support explanation.
2. Daughter-in-law states, "It's been difficult and crowded ever since she moved in."
3. Mrs. Rob exhibits withdrawn and apprehensive behavior.

NURSING DIAGNOSIS

On the basis of the data, the nurse formulated the following nursing diagnoses:

1. **Risk for injury** related to increase in family stress, as evidenced by signs of violence.
   - Mrs. Rob states she slipped in the bathroom, but physical findings do not support that explanation
   - Physical symptoms of violence present (bruises, unkempt appearance, withdrawn attitude)
   - Stressful, crowded living conditions
2. **Ineffective individual coping** related to helplessness, as evidenced by inability to meet role expectations.
   - Mrs. Rob appears unkempt, anxious, depressed
   - Mrs. Rob exhibits withdrawn and apprehensive behavior
   - Mrs. Rob is unable to make decisions
3. **Risk for violence** related to increased stressors within a short period, as evidenced by probable elder abuse and feelings of helplessness verbalized by primary caregiver.
   - Judy states, "It's been difficult and crowded ever since she moved in"
   - No eye contact between Judy and Mrs. Rob
   - Signs and symptoms of physical abuse on elder
   - "My husband is no help at all"

CASE STUDY: WORKING WITH A FAMILY EXPERIENCING VIOLENCE *(Continued)*

4. **Caregiver role strain** related to extreme feelings of being overwhelmed and of helplessness.
   - Family not helping with care of mother-in-law; burden of care on Judy
   - Economic hardships leading to stress when Judy gave up job to care for Mrs. Rob

PLANNING

The nurse discusses several possible goals with members of her team, giving attention to the priority of goals and to whether they are realistic in this situation.

NURSE'S FEELINGS AND SELF-ASSESSMENT

Ms. Green has been in a number of situations with violent families, but this was the first time she encountered elder maltreatment. She discussed her reactions with the other team members. She was especially angry at Judy, although she was able to understand the daughter-in-law's frustration. The team concurred with Ms. Green that there seemed to be potential for positive change with this family. If abuse did not abate, more drastic measures would need to be taken and legal services contacted.

INTERVENTION

Violence toward elders is a signal of a family in crisis. Ms. Green knew she had to address the needs of the whole family to effect change within the family system. She focused on Mrs. Rob's physical safety first, then on Mrs. Rob's strengths to work within the family system. It was evident that Judy was overwhelmed with multiple stressors, and interventions for her and the rest of the family were vital for effective change.

Ms. Green continued to meet with the family on a weekly basis. Interventions were mapped out, with input from the family. Although it was difficult at first to get the husband involved, he became more active when his feelings of helplessness and guilt began to fade. Ms. Green encouraged the children to participate, and many useful suggestions came from their observations and ideas.

This family seemed motivated to change their circumstances because all members were feeling overwhelmed and helpless. Although suggestions regarding outside services were initially met with some resistance, other services were contacted. Judy stated that she found weekly counseling a great help. The Friendly Visitors Service allowed Judy some time to herself each week. Refer to Nursing Care Plan 15–1 for specific interventions for this family.

EVALUATION

Eight weeks after the nurse's initial visit, Mrs. Rob appeared well groomed, friendly, and more spontaneous in her conversation. She commented, "Things are better with my daughter-in-law." No bruises or other signs of physical violence were noticeable. She was considerably more outgoing and even took the initiative to contact an old friend. She had talked openly with her son and daughter-in-law about stress in the family. Mrs. Rob said that she went out for a walk when her daughter-in-law, Judy, appeared tense, and returned to find the tension had lessened. Neither Mrs. Rob nor her family had initiated plans for alternative housing.

As a further result of the nurse's intervention, Judy was more in control of her emotions. Although she did on occasion yell at her mother-in-law, she felt this was no longer the same uncontrolled, explosive anger. Verbalizing her feelings to her husband helped alleviate her frustrations. Judy was seeing a counselor at the community center and was planning to look for a part-time job to "get out of the house."

The family members gradually began to communicate with one another. Mrs. Rob's other son and his family were contacted for assistance. Although this son had not yet offered to share some of the responsibility for taking care of his mother, he did agree to give some financial support. The family continued to meet with the nurse.

NURSING CARE PLAN 15–1 A FAMILY INVOLVED WITH VIOLENCE

NURSING DIAGNOSIS

Risk for injury: related to increase in family stress, as evidenced by signs of abuse

Supporting Data

- States that she slipped in the bathroom
- Physical symptoms of abuse (bruises, unkempt appearance, withdrawn attitude)
- Stressful, crowded living conditions

Outcome Criteria: Client will be well nourished and free from signs of physical abuse by (date).

SHORT-TERM GOAL	INTERVENTION	RATIONALE	EVALUATION
1. Client will state the abuse is decreased by (date).	1a. Assess severity of signs and symptoms of abuse and potential for further injury on weekly visits. 1b. Discuss with client factors leading to abuse and concern for physical safety.	1a. Determines need for further intervention. 1b. Validates situation is serious and increases client's knowledge base.	*GOAL MET* Client says she is no longer abused in family situation
2. In 1 week client will name two persons she can call in case of further abuse.	2. Discuss with client support services such as hotlines and crisis units to call in case of emergency situation.	2. Maximizes client's safety through use of support systems.	

NURSING DIAGNOSIS

Ineffective individual coping: related to helplessness, as evidenced by inability to meet role expectations

Supporting Data

- Appears unkempt, anxious, depressed
- Exhibits withdrawn and apprehensive behavior
- Unable to make decisions
- Remaining in battering situation
- Denial of seriousness of abusive situation

Outcome Criteria: Client will have definite plans for alternatives to present living situation within 1 month.

SHORT-TERM GOAL	INTERVENTION	RATIONALE	EVALUATION
1. Client will identify three of her personal strengths by (date).	1a. Approach client in positive, nonjudgmental manner. 1b. Assist client to develop effective coping skills. 1c. Assist client to identify personal assests.	1a. Encourages disclosure and development of relationship. 1b. Redirects self-assessment to positive skills. 1c. Can help increase self-esteem.	*GOAL MET* Client has identified personal strengths and made two behavioral changes. She has not made any definite plans for a change in living situation. She says she is feeling a little better about living with son's family.

NURSING CARE PLAN 15–1 A FAMILY INVOLVED WITH VIOLENCE (Continued)

SHORT-TERM GOAL	INTERVENTION	RATIONALE	EVALUATION
2. Client will make one decision about the future by (date).	2a. Encourage client to examine situation and alternatives. 2b. Reinforce client's use of problem-solving skills.	2a. When in a dependent situation, individuals may have difficulty making decisions. 2b. Encourages client to function at optimal level.	
3. Client will state two behavioral changes to be carried out by (date).	3a. Explore with client ways to make changes. 3b. Assist client in making decisions for action for future.	3a. Directs assessment to positive areas. 3b. Can help improve self-esteem.	

NURSING DIAGNOSIS

Risk for violence: by abuser related to increased stressors within a short time as evidenced by aggressive behaviors

Supporting Data

- States "It's been difficult and crowded ever since she moved in"
- No eye contact with Mrs. Rob
- Signs and symptoms of physical abuse on mother-in-law

Outcome Criteria: By (date) abuser will state that she has control over her feelings and is not abusing Mrs. Rob.

SHORT-TERM GOAL	INTERVENTION	RATIONALE	EVALUATION
1. Abuser will name three conditions that contribute to her loss of control with Mrs. Rob by (date).	1. Nurse will meet with abuser and encourage problem-solving approach.	1. Develops abuser's problem-solving abilities and explores alternatives.	*GOAL MET* Abuser has not abused Mrs. Rob. Daughter-in-law states "I feel better about dealing with stressful situations."
2. Abuser will have used three new coping behaviors with Mrs. Rob by (date).	2a. Encourage abuser to verbalize feelings about Mrs. Rob and understand which conditions lead to stress so that they can be avoided. 2b. Encourage development of alternative behaviors. 2c. Reinforce positive approaches suggested by abuser.	2a. Positive approach to deal with stress. 2b. Acceptable manner of dealing with stress. 2c. Increases abilities to deal with stress.	
3. Abuser will seek counseling by (date).	3. Encourage abuser's use of counseling, reinforcing benfits and needs gained from such a regular intervention.	3. Increases coping abilities.	
4. Abuser will name three support services she can call on, and will have used one by (date).	4a. Explore with abuser available support services. Encourage use. 4b. Initiate referrals for support services.	4a. Increases knowledge of resources. 4b. Provides needed support.	

Continued on following page

NURSING CARE PLAN 15–1 A FAMILY INVOLVED WITH VIOLENCE *(Continued)*

NURSING DIAGNOSIS

Caretaker role strain: related to extreme feelings of being overwhelmed and helpless

Supporting Data

- Family not helping with care of mother-in-law; it is being left to daughter-in-law, who states "My husband is not being any help at all"
- Economic hardships leading to stress when wife gave up job to care for elder

Outcome Criteria: Client and family members will meet together and discuss mutual expectations and actions they wish to share by (date).

SHORT-TERM GOAL	INTERVENTION	RATIONALE	EVALUATION
1. Family members will meet for counseling with nurse on a regular basis by (date).	1a. Nurse will meet with family members and encourage problem solving of present situation. 1b. Nurse will suggest that family members meet together on regular basis for problem solving and support.	1a. Family members have opportunity to verbalize their feelings about present situation, offering different perspectives. 1b. Family will solve problems together.	*GOAL MET* Family members are meeting regularly.

Outcome Criteria: Family members will share the responsibilities of caring for Mrs. Rob by (date).

SHORT-TERM GOAL	INTERVENTION	RATIONALE	EVALUATION
1. Family will identify supports and resources they feel are important to them by (date).	1a. Nurse will assist family in identifying support services available, then select appropriate services. 1b. Nurse will contact suggested services for family when requested.	1a. Support services can provide assistance to the family. 1b. Nurse can provide needed support and expertise.	*GOAL PARTIALLY MET* No other outside family member is providing the half-day respite for Mrs. Rob's immediate family. The family has identified support services and contacted one agency.
2. One other family member will spend half a day per week with Mrs. Rob by (date).	2. Family will meet together and discuss responsibility for care of Mrs. Rob and make suggestions for more support by family members. Nurse will act as facilitator in discussion, if necessary.	2. Family will problem-solve and explore avenues for needed assistance.	

SUMMARY

Family violence occurs across all age groups and can be predicted with some accuracy by examining the characteristics of perpetrators, vulnerable people, and situations in which violence is likely. Maltreatment can be physical, sexual, emotional, economic, or caused by neglect. Violence in families follows predictable stages; unless interventions are applied, violence will grow in frequency and intensity. Assessment includes identifying indicators of mistreatment, levels of anxiety, coping mechanisms, support systems, and suicide and homicide potential as well as alcohol and drug abuse.

Suspicion or actual evidence of violence must be carefully documented and then reported to the appropriate authorities. Strong and irrational responses by health care professionals are common in working with abuse victims. Knowing about these reactions and how to reduce intense feelings increases the nurse's therapeutic effectiveness.

Intervention occurs at primary, secondary, and tertiary levels. Primary intervention aims at preventing abuse and the use of violence as a coping strategy. Early recognition and secondary intervention in cases in which abuse has already occurred but is not an ingrained habit can greatly reduce the subsequent incidence of abuse. Tertiary intervention involves nurses facilitating the healing and rehabilitative process through counseling; group work; and assisting survivors of violence to achieve their optimal level of safety, health, and well-being. Evaluation and follow-up interventions are vital to the promotion of family growth and individual safety.

REFERENCES

All, A. C. (1994). A literature review: Assessment and intervention in elder abuse. *Journal of Gerontological Nursing*, 20(7):25.

American Academy of Family Physicians (1994). Commission on Special Issues and Clinical Interests. *Domestic violence: A family affair.* AAFP White Paper. Boston: American Academy of Family Physicians.

Amundson, M. F.(1989). Family crisis care: A home-based intervention program for child abuse. *Issues in Mental Health Nursing*, 10(3/4):285.

Andrews, A. B. (1994). Developing community systems for the primary prevention of family violence. *Family Community Health*, 16(4):1.

Beutler, L. E., Williams, R. E., and Zetzer, H. A. (1994). Efficacy of treatment for victims of child sexual abuse. *The Future of Children*, 4(2):156.

Birns, B., Cascardi, M., and Meyer, S.-L. (1994). Sex-role socialization: Developmental influences on wife abuse. *American Journal of Orthopsychiatry*, 64(1):50.

Briere, J. N., and Elliott, D. M. (1994). Immediate and long-term impacts of child sexual abuse. *The Future of Children*, 4(2):54.

Bullock, L. F. C., et al. (1989). Breaking the cycle of abuse: How nurses can intervene. *Journal of Psychosocial Nursing*, 27(8):11.

Butler, G. L. (1995). Shaken baby syndrome. *Journal of Psychosocial Nursing*, 33(9):47.

Campbell, D., and Campbell, J. (1993). Nursing care of families using violence. In J. C. Campbell and J. Humphreys (Eds.), *Nursing care of survivors of family violence* (2nd ed.) (p. 290). St. Louis: C. V. Mosby.

Campbell, J. C. (1994). Domestic homicide: Risk assessment and professional duty to warn. *Maryland Medical Journal*, 43(10):885.

Campbell, J. C. (1995). Prediction of homicide of and by battered women. In J. C. Campbell (Ed.), *Assessing dangerousness.* Thousand Oaks, CA: Sage.

Campbell, J. C., McKenna, L. S., Torres, S., et al. (1993). Nursing care of abused women. In J. C. Campbell and J. Humphreys (Eds.), *Nursing care of survivors of family violence* (2nd ed.) (p. 250). St. Louis: C. V. Mosby.

Chez, N. (1994). Helping the victim of domestic violence. *American Journal of Nursing*, 94(7):33.

Cramer, E., and McFarlane, J. (1994). Pornography and abuse of women. *Public Health Nursing*, 11(4):268.

Daro, D. A. (1994). Prevention of child sexual abuse. *The Future of Children*, 4(2):198.

Devlin, B. K., and Reynolds, E. (1994). Child abuse: How to recognize it, how to intervene. *American Journal of Nursing*, 94(3):26.

Elder abuse (1991). Risk factors help identify victims, burned out caregivers. *Geriatrics*, 46(10):23.

Else, L., et al. (1993). Personality characteristics of men who physically abuse women. *Hospital and Community Psychiatry*, 44(10):54.

Finkelhor, D. (1993). Epidemiological factors in the clinical identification of child sexual abuse. *Child Abuse and Neglect*, 17:67.

Finkelhor, D. (1994). The international epidemiology of child sexual abuse. *Child Abuse and Neglect*, 18(5):409.

Frye, B. A., and D'Avanzo, C. D. (1994). Cultural themes in family stress and violence among Cambodian refugee women in the inner city. *Advances in Nursing Science*, 16(3):64.

Galbraith, M. (Ed.) (1986). *Elder abuse: Perspectives on an emerging crisis* (Vol. III). Kansas City, KS: Mid-America Congress on Aging.

Gelles, R., and Straus, M. (1988). *Intimate violence.* New York: Simon & Schuster.

Hall, L. A., et al.(1993). Childhood physical and sexual abuse: Their relationship with depressive symptoms in adulthood. *IMAGE: Journal of Nursing Scholarship*, 25(4):317.

Henderson, A. D., and Ericksen, J. R. (1994). Enhancing nurses' effectiveness with abused women. *Journal of Psychosocial Nursing*, 32(6):11.

Irons, T. G. (1993). Documenting sexual abuse of a child. *Emergency Medicine*, (5):57.

Jackson, J. K. (1994). Understanding survival responses of battered women. *Maryland Medical Journal*, 43(10):871.

Jordan, C. E., and Walker, R. (1994). Guidelines for handling domestic violence cases in community mental health centers. *Hospital Community Psychiatry*, 45(2):147.

Lachs, M. S., and Fulmer, T. (1993). Geriatric emergency care, recognizing elder abuse and neglect. *Clinics in Geriatric Medicine*, 9:665.

Lachs, M. S., and Pillemer, K. (1995). Abuse and neglect of elderly persons. *New England Journal of Medicine*, 332(7):437.

Larson, C. S., et al.(1994). Sexual abuse of children: Recommendations and analysis. *The Future of Children*, 4(2):4.

Lewin, L. (1994). Child abuse: Ethical and legal concerns for the nurse. *Journal of Psychosocial Nursing*, 32(12):15.

Loring, M. T., and Smith, R. W. (1994). Health care barriers and interventions for battered women. *Public Health Reports*, 109(3):328.

Ludwig, S., and Kornberg, A. E. (Eds.) (1992). *Child abuse: A medical reference.* New York: Churchill Livingstone.

McKay, M. M. (1994). The link between domestic violence and child abuse: Assessment and treatment considerations. *Child Welfare*, 73(1):29.

McNulty, C., and Wardle, J. (1994). Adult disclosure of sexual abuse: A primary cause of psychological distress. *Child Abuse and Neglect*, 18(7):549.

Murphy, C. M. (1994). Treating perpetrators of adult domestic violence. *Maryland Medical Journal*, 43(10):877.

Parker, V. F. (1995). Battered. *RN*, 58(1):26.

Public Health Service (1989). *Goals for Year 2000. Promoting health/preventing disease: Year 2000 objectives for the nation, draft for review and comment, September 1989.* Washington, DC: U.S. Department of Health and Human Services.

Ross, M. M., and Hoff, L. A. (1994). Teaching nurses about abuse. *Canadian Nurse*, 90(6):33.

Sadock, V. (1995). Physical and sexual abuse of adults. In H. I. Kaplan and B. J. Sadock (Eds.), *Comprehensive textbook of psychiatry IV* (Vol. 2) (pp. 1729–1737). Baltimore: Williams & Wilkins.

Seng, J. S., and Peterson, B. A. (1995). Incorporating routine screening for history of childhood sexual abuse into well-woman and maternity care. *Journal of Nurse-Midwifery*, 40(1):26.

Sheridan, D. J. (1993). The role of the battered woman specialist. *Journal of Psychosocial Nursing*, 31(11):31.

Sue D. W., and Sue D. (1990). *Counseling the culturally different: Theory and practice* (2nd ed.). New York: John Wiley.

Vida, S. (1994). An update on elder abuse and neglect. *Canadian Journal of Psychiatry*, 39(8)(Suppl. 1):S34.

Walker, L. (1980). *The battered woman.* New York: Harper & Row.

Walling, M. K., et al. (1994). Abuse history and chronic pain in women. II. A multivariate analysis of abuse and psychological morbidity. *Obstetrics and Gynecology*, 84(2):200.

Warren, J. K., Fary, F., and Moorhead, J. (1994). Self-reported experiences of physical and sexual abuse among runaway youths. *Perspectives in Psychiatric Care*, 30(1):23.

Weaver, P. L., et al. (1994). Adult survivors of childhood sexual abuse: Survivor's disclosure and nurse therapist's response. *Journal of Psychosocial Nursing*, 32(12):19.

*Wolfe, D. A., and Korsch, B. (1994). Witnessing domestic violence during childhood and adolescence: Implication for pediatric practice. *Pediatrics*, 94(4):594.

Further Reading

Aravams, S. C., et al. (1993). Diagnostic and treatment guidelines on elder abuse and neglect. *Archives of Family Medicine*, 2:371.

Becker, J. V. (1994). Offenders: Characteristics and treatment. *The Future of Children*, 4(2):176.
Burgess, A. W., Hartman, C. R., and Kelley, S. J. (1990). Assessing child abuse: The TRIADS checklist. *Journal of Psychosocial Nursing*, 28(4):6.
Chiocca, E. M. (1995). Shaken baby syndrome: A nursing perspective. *Pediatric Nursing*, 21(1):33.
Dubowitz, H., and King, H. (1995). Family violence: A child-centered, family-focused approach. *Pediatric Clinics of North America*, 42(1):153.
Dunning, S. (1994). Elder abuse is our fight, too. *RN*, 57(8):76.
Fulmer, T. (1991). Elder mistreatment: Progress in community detection and intervention. *Family Community Health*, 14(2):26.
Gage, R. B. (1991). Examining the dynamics of spouse abuse: An alternative view. *Nurse Practitioner*, 16(4):11.
Gazmararian, J. A. (1995). The relationship between pregnancy intendedness and physical violence in mothers of newborns. *Obstetrics and Gynecology*, 85(6):1031.
Gelles, R. J., and Straus, M. A. (1988). *Intimate violence*. New York: Simon & Schuster.
Glaister, J. A. (1994). Clara's story: Post-traumatic response and therapeutic art. *Perspectives in Psychiatric Care*, 30(1):17.
Guidry, H. M. (1995). Childhood sexual abuse: Role of the family physician. *American Family Physician*, 51(2):407.
Holtzworth-Munroe, A., and Stuart, G. L. (1994). Typologies of male batterers: Three subtypes and the differences among them. *Psychological Bulletin*, 116(3):476.
Holz, K. A. (1994). A practical approach to clients who are survivors of childhood sexual abuse. *Journal of Nurse-Midwifery*, 39(1):13.
Hyman, A., Schillinger, D., and Lo, B. (1995). Laws mandating reporting of domestic violence. *Journal of the American Medical Association*, 273(22):1781.
Jecker, N. S. (1993). Privacy beliefs and the violent family. *Journal of the American Medical Association*, 269(6):776.
Kantor, G. K., and Straus, M. A. (1990). The "drunken bum" theory of wife beating. In M. A. Straus and R. J. Gelles (Eds.), *Physical violence in American families* (p. 203). New Brunswick, NJ: Transaction Press.
Kennedy, L. (1994). Women in crisis. *Canadian Nurse*, 90(6):26.
Lobel, K. (Ed.) (1986). *Naming the violence: Speaking about lesbian battering*. Seattle: Seal Press.
Mareth, T. R. (1994). Psychiatric investigation of allegations of child sexual abuse. *Military Medicine*, 159:487.
McFarlane, J., and Parker, B. (1994). An assessment and intervention protocol. *MCN: American Journal of Maternal Child Nursing*, 19:321.
Monaco, J. E., and Brooks, W. G. (1994). The critical care aspects of child abuse. *Pediatric Clinics of North America*, 41(6):1259.
Noel, N. L., and Yam, M. (1992). Domestic violence: The pregnant battered woman. Nursing Clinics of North America, 27(4):871.
Novello, A. C., and Soto-Torres, L. E. (1992). Women and hidden epidemics: HIV/AIDS and domestic violence. *The Female Patient*, 17:17.
Parker, B., and McFarlane, J. (1991). Identifying and helping battered pregnant women. *MCN: American Journal of Maternal Child Nursing*, 16:161.
Parker, B., et al. (1993). Physical and emotional abuse in pregnancy: A comparison of adult and teenage women. *Nursing Research*, 42(3):173.
Pence, D. M., and Wilson, C. A. (1994). Reporting and investigating child sexual abuse. *The Future of Children*, 4(2):70.
Sampselle, C. M., et al. (1992). Prevalence of abuse among pregnant women choosing certified nurse-midwife or physician providers. *Journal of Nurse-Midwifery*, 37(4):269.
Scott, C. J., and Matricciani, R. M. (1994). Joint Commission on Accreditation of Healthcare Organizations standards to improve care for victims of abuse. *Maryland Medical Journal*, 43(10):891.
Smilkstein, G., Aspy, C. B., and Quiggins, P. A. (1994). Conjugal conflict and violence: A review and theoretical paradigm. *Clinical Research and Methods*, 26(2):111.
Spaccarelli, S. (1994). Stress, appraisal, and coping in child sexual abuse: A theoretical and empirical review. *Psychology Bulletin*, 116(2):340.
Tilden, V. P., et al.(1994). Factors that influence clinicians' assessment and management of family violence. *American Journal of Public Health*, 84(4):628.
Weiler, K., and Buckwalter, K. C. (1992). Geriatric mental health: Abuse among rural mentally ill. *Journal of Psychosocial Nursing*, 30(9):32.
Wissow, L. S. (1990). *Child advocacy for the clinician: An approach to child abuse and neglect*. Baltimore: Williams & Wilkins.

SELF-STUDY AND CRITICAL THINKING

Completion

1. How would you respond to a colleague who stated, "I don't think it's any of our business what people do in the privacy of their own homes"?

____
____
____
____

2. Congratulations! You successfully convinced your colleagues to routinely assess for family violence. Now they want to know how to do it. What would you tell them?

____
____
____
____

3. Your HMO's routine health screening form for adolescents, adults, and elders has just been changed to include questions about family violence. How would you respond to patients who indicate on this form that family violence occurs in their home?

____
____
____
____

Multiple choice

Choose the answer that most accurately completes the statement.

4. Which factor can signal conditions for family abuse?

   A. A family illness
   B. A parent who has been drinking
   C. A child who is highly gifted in an "average to below-average" household
   D. A parent who comes from another country
   E. All of the above

5. Which of the following are common characteristics of abusing parents?

   A. Unrealistic expectations of child's behavior
   B. Lack of effective parenting skills
   C. Male gender
   D. Poor coping skills
   E. Alcoholic
   F. All of the above

Matching

Match the example on the left with the type of abuse listed in the right column.

6. ________ "You no good slut. I wish you were never born."

7. ________ Joe says children don't know how to behave unless you give them good healthy spankings.

8. ________ Tom says life is the best teacher. His children don't need schools.

9. ________ As Sally ate her lunch at the park, she noticed a man near her with his penis sticking out of his pants.

10. ________ Henrietta refused to get her child counseling even though it had been recommended by her child's teacher, the principal, and concerned friends.

11. ________ The playground equipment in George's backyard was in a dangerous state of disrepair, yet eight of his children and neighborhood children continued to play on it. "They'll survive" was his attitude.

12. ________ When Joannie misbehaved, she would get locked in her closet for hours at a time.

13. ________ Martha never played with her baby and rarely touched him, feeling that he could do just fine for himself.

A. Physical battering
B. Physical endangerment
C. Sexual violence
D. Physical neglect
E. Developmental neglect
F. Educational neglect
G. Emotional violence

Multiple choice

Choose the most appropriate answer.

14. For assessing whether a child's safety or security needs are being met, which remark would be appropriate to ask parents?
    A. What do you do when you get angry with your child?
    B. Did you graduate from high school?
    C. How did this happen?
    D. Describe your marriage.
15. Circle all of the following myths a woman may believe that keep her locked into an abusive relationship:
    A. She stays "for the sake of the children."
    B. "He will change."
    C. She deserves the beatings once in a while.
    D. No one has the right to harm or beat another.
16. Questioning the acceptance of violence in America and modeling nonviolent problem-solving strategies are examples of what level of intervention?
    A. Primary
    B. Secondary
    C. Tertiary

Write brief responses in answer to the following:

17. List two possible nursing diagnoses for a victim of spouse abuse and one goal for each.
    1. Nursing Diagnosis:
       Goal:
    2. Nursing Diagnosis:
       Goal:
18. List three common responses a nurse might experience when working with a woman in a violent relationship that would warrant peer supervision or clinical supervision.
    1.
    2.
    3.
19. Identify three areas to assess for when evaluating the effectiveness of intervention in family violence.
    1.
    2.
    3.

Critical thinking

20. Write out a safety plan that could be adopted with other clients.
21. Identify at least four referrals in your community for a battered person.
22. Identify two referrals in your community for a violent person, partner, or parent.

16

Rape

KATHLEEN SMITH-DIJULIO

OUTLINE

KEY TERMS AND CONCEPTS

The key terms and concepts listed here also appear in bold where they are defined or discussed in this chapter.

spousal/marital rape
acquaintance/date rape
rape-trauma syndrome
acute phase
long-term reorganization phase
expressed style of coping
controlled style of coping
compound reaction
silent reaction
blaming-the-victim phenomenon

OBJECTIVES

After studying this chapter, the reader will be able to

1. Define sexual assault (rape) and differentiate between its subtypes.
2. Discuss the reasons that rapes go unreported.
3. Distinguish between the acute and long-term phases of the rape-trauma syndrome and identify some common reactions during each phase.
4. Identify and give examples of five areas to assess when working with a person who has been sexually assaulted.
5. Formulate two long-term and two short-term outcomes for the nursing diagnosis *rape-trauma syndrome*.
6. Analyze your thoughts and feelings regarding the myths about rape and its impact on survivors.
7. Teach a peer five counseling techniques that are useful when working with a person who has been sexually assaulted.
8. Describe the role of the sexual assault nurse examiner to a colleague.
9. Discuss the responsibilities of the nurse when a rape survivor is discharged from the emergency department, citing specific referrals from your community.
10. Develop a handout delineating the nurse's role when staffing a rape-crisis hotline.
11. Discuss the long-term psychological effects of sexual assault that might lead to a survivor's seeking psychotherapy.
12. Identify three outcome criteria that would signify successful interventions for a person who has suffered a sexual assault.

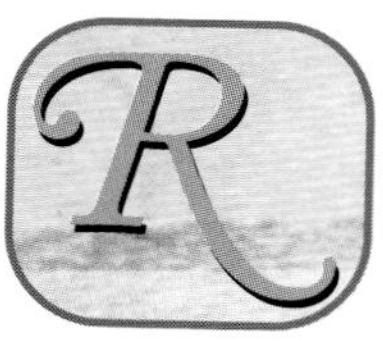

Rape is an act of violence, and sex is the weapon used by the perpetrator. Rape engulfs its victims in fear, causing severe panic reactions. After being traumatized, the person raped often carries an additional burden of shame, guilt, fear, anger, distrust, and embarrassment.

Rape, also referred to as *sexual assault*, is nonconsensual vaginal, anal, or oral penetration, obtained by force, by threat of bodily harm, or when a person is incapable of giving consent (Koss 1993). It is usually men who rape, and most of those raped are women. When men are raped, the rape is generally perpetrated by a heterosexual male.

A male who is raped is more likely to have physical trauma and to have been victimized by several assailants than is a female. Reported homosexual rape occurs primarily in closed institutions, such as prisons and maximum-security hospitals. Estimates are that 0.5% to 3% of inmates (homosexual or heterosexual) are sexually assaulted (Sadock 1995). The psychodynamics are the same as those of heterosexual rape, and males experience the same devastation and sequelae as do females. Since women are more frequently assaulted sexually, this chapter uses the female pronoun throughout; however, the principles discussed apply to anyone who is raped.

THEORY

Sexual assault is one of the fastest-growing violent crimes in the United States. There were 105,000 *reported* rapes in the United States in 1993 (U.S. Department of Justice 1994). Because rape is notoriously underreported, it is estimated that a woman is raped in the United States every 5 minutes (U.S. Department of Justice 1994).

Stranger rape is what most people envisage when they think of sexual assault, yet this is the least common type. Notable subtypes that occur much more frequently are spousal/marital rape and acquaintance/date rape (Davis et al. 1993; Hampton 1995). In recent years the courts have recognized **spousal** (or **marital**) **rape,** in which the perpetrator (nearly always the male) is married to the person raped. With **acquaintance** (or **date**) **rape,** the perpetrator is known to, and presumably trusted by, the person raped. The incidence of rape peaks among females 16 to 19 years of age. The incidence of date rape is estimated to be as high as 20% (Hampton 1995). Nonetheless, many thousands of women over 50 years of age are raped every year (Tyra 1993). The psychological and emotional sequelae of rape seem to vary depending on the level of intimacy of the perpetrator. Sexual distress is more common among women who have been sexually assaulted by intimates; fear and anxiety are more common in those assaulted by strangers; depression occurs in both groups (Ullman and Siegel 1993).

Some estimates are that only 25% of rapes are reported; others put the proportion as low as 10%. One major reason for the underreporting of rape is that the victim, as well as the rapist, goes on trial. Rape is the only crime in which the victim is required to prove innocence. Women have historically been held responsible for the occurrence of rape. Common beliefs persist that if the woman had not, for example, been so careless, been drinking, dressed so provocatively, or stayed out so late, she would not have been raped. Additionally, women have usually been required to show evidence of resisting rape.

The fact that a woman is more likely to be raped by someone she knows than by a stranger also inhibits reporting. Because it involves the violation of trust, rape by an acquaintance or marital partner has a dire psychological impact. In addition, victims may be threatened with another attack or with death if they report the rape.

Another reason that rapes go unreported lies in the social taboos against talking about sexuality—especially forced and violent sexual crimes. Men who are raped are even less likely to report it than women, owing to the general lack of acceptance by society of sex between two men. Thus, those raped are victimized not only by the crime itself but also by society's reactions. Personal anguish and grief also keep the raped person from seeking emergency medical care and reporting the crime. Finally, reporting of rape may be delayed (or may not occur at all) because of impaired cognitive processing, altered states of consciousness, or cognitive dissonance (Burgess et al. 1995).

Feminists have done a great deal to raise the consciousness of individuals and of American society as a whole to the fact that women are people, not property, and should be accorded the same rights and privileges as men. This change is evidenced in laws such as those that allow a wife to bring rape charges against her husband. Formerly it was believed that a man was entitled to sex in a relationship, no matter how he obtained it. Nurses have a role to play in facilitating a re-examination of issues that precipitate and support violent acts (Duchscher 1994).

Most people who are raped suffer severe and long-lasting emotional trauma. Five features of the assault experience contribute to psychological trauma:

1. The assault is sudden and arbitrary.
2. The assault is perceived as life-threatening.
3. The main purpose of an assault is to violate a person's physical integrity and render him or her helpless.
4. The assault forces participation in the crime.
5. The assault overwhelms normal coping strategies.

Long-term psychological effects of sexual assault may include the development of depression, suicide, anxiety, and fear; difficulties with daily functioning; low self-esteem; sexual dysfunction; and somatic complaints in many survivors. Incest victims may experience a negative self-image, depression, eating disorders, personality disorders, self-destructive behavior, and substance abuse (Boutcher and Gallop 1996). Timely intervention can greatly help to minimize the devastating sequelae of rape.

Boutcher and Gallop (1996) cite studies indicating that a history of sexual abuse in psychiatric clients is associated with a characteristic pattern of symptoms that may include depression, anxiety disorders, chemical dependency, suicide attempts, self-mutilation, compulsive sexual behavior, and psychotic-like symptoms.

The **rape-trauma syndrome** is a variant of posttraumatic stress disorder and consists of (1) an acute phase and (2) the long-term reorganization process that occurs after an actual or attempted sexual assault. Each phase has separate symptoms.

Acute Phase of Rape-Trauma Syndrome

The **acute phase** of the rape-trauma syndrome occurs immediately after the assault and may last for a couple of weeks. This is the stage seen by emergency department personnel. Nurses are the clinicians most involved in dealing with these initial reactions. During this phase, there is a great deal of disorganization in the person's life style, and somatic symptoms are common (Kimerling and Calhoun 1994). This disorganization can be described in terms of impact reactions, somatic reactions, and emotional reactions (Table 16–1).

The most common initial reaction is shock, numbness, and disbelief. Outwardly, the person may appear self-contained and calm and may make remarks such as "It doesn't seem real" or "I don't believe this really happened to me." Sometimes, cognitive functions may be impaired, and the traumatized person may appear extremely confused and have difficulty with concentrating and decision making. Alternatively, the person may become hysterical or restless, or may cry or even smile. These reactions to crisis are typical and reflect cognitive, affective, and behavioral disruptions.

People who have experienced an emotionally overwhelming event may need to deny its impact. Denial of the horror and impact of the event in this case is an adaptive and protective reaction that gives the person time to prepare for the reality of the event. Examples of such denial may be found in such statements as "I don't want to talk about it" or "I just want to forget what happened." Behaviors that minimize the magnitude of the event include reluctance to seek medical attention and failure to follow up with legal counsel.

Long-Term Reorganization Phase of Rape-Trauma Syndrome

The **long-term reorganization phase** of rape-trauma syndrome occurs 2 or more weeks after the rape. Nurses who initially care for the survivors can help them anticipate and prepare for the reactions they are likely to experience (Burgess 1995; Burgess and Holstrom 1974). These include the following:

1. Intrusive thoughts of the rape break into the survivor's conscious mind during the day and during sleep. These thoughts commonly include anger and violence toward the assailant, flashbacks (re-experiencing the traumatic event), dreams with violent content, and insomnia.
2. Increased motor activity follows, such as moving, taking trips, changing telephone numbers, and making frequent visits to old friends. This activity stems from the fear that the assailant will return. Anxiety, mood

TABLE 16–1 ACUTE PHASE OF RAPE-TRAUMA SYNDROME

Impact Reaction	Somatic Reaction	Emotional Reaction
Expressed Style	Evidenced within first several weeks after a rape	▸ Fear of physical violence and death
Overt behaviors	**Physical Trauma**	▸ Denial
▸ Crying, sobbing	▸ Bruises (breasts, throat, or back)	▸ Anxiety
▸ Smiling, laughing, joking	▸ Soreness	▸ Shock
▸ Restlessness, agitation, hysteria	**Skeletal Muscle Tension**	▸ Humiliation
▸ Volatility, anger	▸ Headaches	▸ Fatigue
▸ Confusion, incoherence, disorientation	▸ Sleep disturbances	▸ Embarrassment
▸ Tenseness	▸ Grimaces, twitches	▸ Desire for revenge
Controlled Style	**Gastrointestinal**	▸ Self-blame
Covert reactions	▸ Stomach pains	▸ Lowered self-esteem
▸ Confusion, incoherence, disorientation	▸ Nausea	▸ Shame
▸ Masked facies	▸ Poor appetite	▸ Guilt
▸ Calm, subdued appearance	▸ Diarrhea	▸ Anger
▸ Shocked, numb, confused, disbelieving appearance	**Genitourinary**	
▸ Distractibility, difficulty making decisions	▸ Vaginal itching	
	▸ Vaginal discharge	
	▸ Pain or discomfort	

Data from Burgess 1995; Burgess and Holstrom 1974.

swings, crying spells, and depression are likely to be observed.

3. Fears and phobias develop as a defensive reaction to the rape. Typical phobias include
   - Fear of the indoors (if the rape occurred indoors).
   - Fear of the outdoors (if the rape occurred outdoors).
   - Fear of being alone (common for most women after an assault).
   - Fear of crowds—"Any person in the crowd might be a rapist."
   - Fear of sexual encounters and activities. Many women experience acute disruption of their sex life with partners. Rape is especially disruptive for those with no previous sexual experience.

As mentioned, the consequences of sexual assault may be severe, debilitating, and long term. Intervention and support for the survivor can help prevent some of the sequelae mentioned: anxiety, depression, suicide, difficulties with daily functioning and interpersonal relationships, sexual dysfunction, and somatic complaints.

ASSESSMENT

Once the rape survivor is at the emergency department, the attention received depends on the protocol of the particular hospital. Ledray and Arndt (1994) suggest the following interventions:

- Treatment and documentation of injuries
- Treatment and evaluation of sexually transmitted diseases (STDs)
- Pregnancy risk evaluation and prevention
- Crisis intervention and arrangements for follow-up counseling
- Collection of medicolegal evidence while maintaining the proper chain of evidence

The nurse talks with the survivor, the family or friends who accompany the survivor, and the police, to gather as much data as possible for assessing the crisis. The nurse then assesses the survivor's (1) level of anxiety, (2) coping mechanisms used, (3) available support systems, (4) signs and symptoms of emotional trauma, and (5) signs and symptoms of physical trauma. Information obtained from the assessment is then analyzed and nursing diagnoses are formulated. An independent nursing role of Sexual Assault Nurse Examiner or Forensic Nurse Specialist successfully accomplishes all of these activities.

The Sexual Assault Nurse Examiner/Clinician completes the full evidentiary examination, evaluates the survivor's risk of pregnancy, and offers preventive care; treats prophylactically for STDs; provides crisis intervention; and ensures that injuries are treated by appropriate medical personnel (Ledray 1993). With a consistent as well as experienced corps of nurses conducting most of the rape examinations, the quality of the forensic evidence increases dramatically, which enables the judicial system to prosecute rapists more effectively (Thomas and Zachritz 1993).

Assessing the Level of Anxiety

Assessing, understanding, and evaluating reactions and feelings after rape are essential nursing skills. Because of the personal threat to safety and security, the survivor can be assumed to be experiencing acute anxiety. If nurses are sensitive to this fact, they will take their time. Support, reassurance, and appropriate therapeutic techniques can help diminish anxiety.

Depending on the individual's intra- and interpersonal resources, the anxiety level may range from moderate to panic. (These levels are discussed in Chapter 13.) It is important to take cues from the client. *Do not initiate touching*, as this may further increase the survivor's anxiety level. If the survivor reaches out and makes the first contact, then touch is acceptable. Touch might take the form of a hand on the arm or hand, or holding the client when she cries.

The presence of a supportive, helpful person can assist in diminishing anxiety caused by the rape. If a third party is present, the survivor's permission should be obtained before a history is taken in front of someone else. The third party should be there only for support, not to answer questions. If the third party interferes with the history-taking process or seems to make the survivor uncomfortable, he or she should be asked to wait in another area.

Assessing Coping Mechanisms Used

Everyone has ways of dealing with stressful situations. The same coping skills that have helped the survivor through other difficult problems will be used in adjusting to the rape. In addition, new ways of getting through difficult times may be developed, for both the short- and long-term adjustment.

Behavioral responses include crying; withdrawing; smoking; wanting to talk about the event; acting hysterical, confused, disoriented, or incoherent; and even laughing or joking. These behaviors are examples of an **expressed style of coping** (Table 16–1).

Cognitive coping mechanisms are the thoughts people have that help them deal with high anxiety levels. If thoughts are verbalized, the nurse will know what the survivor is thinking. If not, the nurse can ask questions such as "What do you think might help now?" or "What can I do to help you in this difficult situation?"

Assessing Support Systems Available

The availability, size, and utility of a survivor's social support system need to be assessed. The nurse should ask whether there are family or friends with whom the survivor feels safe and in whom she can confide. However, family, neighbors, and friends (generally the people considered valuable supports) are the people most often involved in perpetrating the unwanted sexual experiences. Pay careful attention to verbal and nonverbal cues the survivor may be communicating regarding persons in her social network. For example, someone the survivor knows may suggest that he or she has a spare room where the survivor can spend the night so as not to be alone, yet the survivor seems hesitant. Be certain that the source of the hesitancy is privately explored before railroading the survivor into doing something that might be detrimental. The hesitancy could be due to increased anxiety and decreased ability to make decisions, or it could be due to fear of finding herself in another sexual assault situation.

◗ Ms. Ruiz, age 18, is brought to the emergency department by a concerned neighbor. She was found wandering aimlessly outside her house, sobbing, and muttering "He had no right to do that to me." Because of Ms. Ruiz's distraught appearance and her statement, the triage nurse suspects sexual assault and brings the victim to the office of the psychiatric nurse, Ms. Wong. Ms. Wong introduces herself, explains her role, and states that she is there to help. Ms. Wong then asks Ms. Ruiz what happened. After careful, sensitive, nonthreatening questioning, Ms. Ruiz divulges that she had been out with her boyfriend, who raped her and then dropped her off at her house. Because no one else was at home and she was so upset and afraid, she did not go inside, and the neighbor, Ms. Green, had seen her outside.

◗ After the entire history and examination are completed, plans for discharge are discussed. Ms. Ruiz states that no one will be home until Sunday night, 2 days away, and that she does not feel comfortable calling any friends because she does not want them to know what has happened. The neighbor, Ms. Green, had told the nurse earlier that Ms. Ruiz could stay with her family.

Nurse: Earlier, your neighbor, Ms. Green, told me that you are welcome to spend the weekend with her family.

Ms. Ruiz: *(Loudly, sharply, with eyes wide)* Oh, no, I couldn't do that.

Nurse: You don't seem to like that idea.

Ms. Ruiz: Oh, I just wouldn't want to bother them.

Nurse: Ms. Green seems quite concerned about your welfare.

Ms. Ruiz: Oh, yes, she's very nice. *(Pause)*

Nurse: But not someone you would want to spend the weekend with?

Ms. Ruiz: Her children are too noisy. I've got homework to do.

Nurse: You might not get the quiet you need to study. *(Pause)* Yet you also do not want to be alone?

Ms. Ruiz: *(Wringing a tissue in her hands, head hanging, soft voice)* I can't go in that house anymore.

Nurse: Something about being in that house disturbs you?

Ms. Ruiz: Mr. Green *(deep sigh, pause)* used to . . . uh . . . take advantage of me when I used to babysit his children.

Nurse: Take advantage?

Ms. Ruiz: Yes . . . *(sobbing)* he used to force me to have sex with him. He said he'd blame it on me if I told anyone.

Nurse: What a frightening experience that must have been for you.

Ms. Ruiz: Yes.

Nurse: I can see why you would not want to spend the night there. Let's continue to explore other options.

▶ A suitable place to stay is finally arranged. Ms. Ruiz is given counseling referrals that will help her deal with the process of reorganization from the current rape experience as well as to begin to explore her feelings about past sexual abuse she has suffered at the hands of her neighbor.

Assessing Signs and Symptoms of Emotional Trauma

Nurses work most frequently with sexual assault survivors in the emergency department soon after the rape has occurred. The triage nurse makes the initial assessment. Rape is a psychological emergency and should receive immediate attention (University of Louisville 1995). A special waiting area, separate from the general lobby, should be provided. This kind of focused supportive attention helps the rape survivor begin to feel safe and at ease. Some emergency departments provide Sexual Assault Nurse Examiners/Clinicians who are specially trained to meet the myriad needs of the sexual assault survivor (Ledray and Arndt 1994).

The extent of the psychological and emotional trauma sustained may not be readily apparent from behavior, especially if the person uses the **controlled style of coping** during the acute phase of the rape trauma (Table 16–1) (Burgess 1995). Ill-informed staff may wonder whether the person was actually raped. That skepticism may be communicated, serving to increase the survivor's anxiety and lower her self-esteem. It is important to remember that despite the person's apparent response, *psychological and emotional trauma is always experienced during and after an assault.* Nurses are never in the position of judging the validity of a rape.

A nursing history should be conducted and properly recorded. When obtaining a history, the nurse needs to determine only the details of the assault that will be helpful in addressing the immediate physical and psychological needs of the victim.

The nurse should allow the survivor to talk at a comfortable pace. Pose questions in nonjudgmental, descriptive terms. Refrain from asking "why" questions. Relating the events of the rape will most likely be traumatic and embarrassing. The nurse should assess the type as well as the time, place, and circumstances of the assault. What occurred? For example, was there

- Fondling?
- Oral penetration or attempted penetration?
- Vaginal penetration or attempted penetration?
- Rectal penetration or attempted penetration?
- Ejaculation? Where? On or in the body?

If suicidal thoughts are expressed, the nurse should assess what precautions are needed by asking direct questions such as "Are you thinking of harming yourself?" and "Have you ever tried to kill yourself before this attack occurred?" If the answer is "yes," the nurse must make a thorough suicide assessment (plan, means to carry it out) as described in Chapter 24.

Assessing Signs and Symptoms of Physical Trauma

Most medicolegal evidence that must be collected is designed to document trauma. Practitioners must provide psychological support while collecting and preserving potentially crucial legal evidence such as hair, skin, and semen samples. Determination of the presence of sperm or semen may help to identify the assailant. The most characteristic physical signs of sexual assault are injuries to the face, head, neck, and extremities. Any noted injuries should be carefully documented, preferably on a body map. Vaginal and perineal injury and other trauma are usually absent, and there may be no evidence of sperm on physical examination.

The nurse takes a brief gynecological history, including date of last menstrual period, the likelihood of current pregnancy, and any history of venereal disease. If the victim has never undergone a pelvic examination, the steps will need to be explained. The nurse plays a crucial role in giving support and minimizing the trauma of the examination.

Although the medical examination helps to determine whether any injury occurred and is used to collect evidence for identification and prosecution of the rapist, the survivor may feel that it is another violation of her body. Recognizing this, the nurse can explain the examination procedure in a way that will be reassuring and supportive. Allowing the survivor to participate in all decisions affecting care helps her regain a sense of control over her life.

The survivor has the right to refuse either a legal or a medical examination. ***Consent forms must be signed for***

photographs, pelvic examination, and whatever other procedures might be needed to collect evidence and provide treatment. The correct preservation of body fluids and swabs is essential, especially because new techniques, such as DNA (genetic) fingerprinting, may identify the rapist. A water-moistened speculum is used to preserve all evidence. A shower and fresh clothing should be available to the survivor immediately after the examination, if possible.

It is becoming a common practice (because it is cost effective and because many survivors are lost to follow-up after the emergency department visit) to eliminate baseline STD data collection and treat prophylactically for syphilis, chlamydiosis, and gonorrhea, according to guidelines from the CDC (Ledray and Arndt 1994).

Human immunodeficiency virus (HIV) exposure is an ever-growing concern of sexual assault survivors. The risk of exposure varies with the type of assault and the rate of infection in the area. In high-risk areas, such as New York, California, New Jersey, and Florida, and for high-risk anal assaults, testing is especially important (Ledray and Arndt 1994). When the risk of transmission is low, routine HIV testing is not required. However, the concern should always be addressed and the rape survivor given the information needed to evaluate the likely risk. With this information a person and sexual partner(s) can make educated choices about HIV testing and safer-sex practices until testing can be done in 6 months (Ledray and Arndt 1994).

About 3% to 5% of women who are raped become pregnant as a result. Prophylaxis with ethinyl estradiol and norgestrel (Ovral) can be offered, but if the survivor is likely to seek aftercare, she may want to wait to initiate intervention until results of a pregnancy test are obtained or until her next period is due. If Ovral is the choice, an antiemetic should be given to prevent regurgitation (Ledray and Arndt 1994).

All data must be carefully documented, including verbatim statements by the survivor, detailed observations of emotional and physical status, and all results from the physical examination. All laboratory tests performed should be noted and findings recorded as soon as they are available.

NURSING DIAGNOSIS

Rape-trauma syndrome is the nursing diagnosis that applies to the physical and psychological effects resulting from an episode of sexual assault. It includes an acute phase of disorganization of the survivor's life style and a long-term phase of reorganization. The diagnosis has application regardless of the setting in which the survivor is encountered. This syndrome comprises the following subcomponents, presented along with their defining characteristics.

RAPE-TRAUMA SYNDROME: COMPOUND REACTION. Compound reaction can occur in survivors with previous or current physical, emotional, or social difficulties and who are suffering rape-trauma syndrome. Symptoms of **compound reaction** include

- All symptoms listed under rape-trauma syndrome (Table 16–1).
- Reliance on alcohol or other drugs.
- Reactivated symptoms of previous conditions, such as physical or psychiatric illness.

RAPE-TRAUMA SYNDROME: SILENT REACTION. Silent reaction is a complex stress reaction to rape, in which an individual is unable to describe or discuss the rape. Symptoms include

- Abrupt changes in relationships with men.
- Nightmares.
- Increasing anxiety during the interview, such as blocking of associations, long periods of silence, minor stuttering, or physical distress.
- Marked changes in sexual behavior.
- Sudden onset of phobic reactions.
- No verbalization of the occurrence of rape.

PLANNING

Planning care for a person who has survived a sexual assault includes (1) identifying realistic outcomes and (2) the nurse's feelings and self-assessment.

Planning Outcome Criteria

Client-centered outcomes (goals) for alleviating the survivor's discomfort and distress originate from the nursing diagnosis. The goals are both short and long term. Short-term goals are those that the nurse and the survivor can achieve while working together to relieve the symptoms exhibited during the acute phase of the rape-trauma syndrome. Long-term outcomes (goals) are those that will allow the survivor to begin to reorganize her life after the immediate crisis.

Examples of short-term goals could be as follows:

Rape-trauma syndrome: acute phase. The survivor will

- Begin to express reactions and feelings about the assault before leaving the emergency room.
- Have a short-term plan for handling immediate situational needs.
- List common physical, social, and emotional reactions that often follow a sexual assault before she leaves the emergency department.
- Speak to a community-based rape-victim advocate in the emergency department.
- State the results of the physical examination completed in the emergency department.

TABLE 16–2 MYTH VERSUS FACT: RAPE

Myth	Fact
1. Many women really want to be raped.	1. No women ask to be raped—no matter how they are dressed, what their behavior is, or where they are at any given time. Studies show that violence toward women in the media leads to attitudes that foster tolerance of rape.
2. Most rapists are oversexed.	2. Sex is used as an instrument of violence in rape. Rape is an act of aggression, anger, or power.
3. Most women are raped by strangers.	3. 57% of rape victims are raped by someone they know and who is a part of their extended family.
4. No healthy adult female who resists vigorously can be raped by an unarmed man.	4. Most men can overpower most women because of differences in body build. Also, the victim may panic, making her actions less effective than usual.
5. Most charges of rape are unfounded.	5. There is no evidence to show that there are more false reports for rape than for other crimes. Most rape victims do not even report the rape.
6. Rapes usually occur in dark alleys.	6. Over 50% of all rapes occur in the home.
7. Rape is usually an impulsive act.	7. Most rapes are planned; over 50% involve a weapon.
8. Nice girls don't get raped.	8. Any woman is a potential rape victim. Victims range in age from 6 months to 90 years.
9. There was not enough time for a rape to occur.	9. There is no minimal time limit that characterizes rape. It can happen very quickly.
10. Do not fight or try to get away because you will just get hurt.	10. There are no verifiable data to substantiate the theory that a victim will be injured if she tries to get away.
11. Only females are raped.	11. There is a growing number of male rape victims—not necessarily just men in prisons or in the homosexual community.
12. Rape is a sexual act.	12. Rape is a violent expression of aggression, anger, and need for power.

Data from Costin 1985; Helen 1984; Sadock 1995.

- State that she will keep a follow-up appointment with the nurse, rape-victim advocate, or social worker on (date).

Examples of long-term goals could be as follows:

Rape-trauma syndrome: long-term reorganization phase. The survivor will

- Discuss the need for follow-up crisis counseling and other support by (date).
- State that the acuteness of the memory of the rape subsides over time and is less vivid and less frightening within 3 to 5 months.
- State that the physical symptoms (e.g., sleep disturbances, poor appetite, and physical trauma) have subsided within 3 to 5 months.

Nurse's Feelings and Self-Assessment

As members of society, nurses have been exposed to the various myths and judgments that exist about rape. Nurses' attitudes influence the physical and psychological care administered to rape survivors. Knowing the myths and facts surrounding rape can increase nurses' awareness of their personal beliefs and feelings regarding rape. Nurses who examine their personal feelings and reactions before encountering a rape survivor are better prepared to give empathetic and effective care. This process is the same as that described for caring for survivors of other types of violence (see Chapter 15).

Belief in myths about rape is perpetuated by society's tendency to deny and minimize the perceived injury and to blame survivors for what happened to them. Unfortunately, nurses are not immune from the **blaming-the-victim phenomenon.** Acceptance of myths coincides with beliefs that women's social roles and rights should be more restricted than those of men. The extent to which some of these beliefs might still be held by individuals of different cultural groups depends on their level of acculturation to the predominant American culture. Nurses' attitudes and beliefs are factors that can influence the care of sexual assault victims. Table 16–2 compares rape myths and facts.

INTERVENTION

The circumstance of rape can be the most devastating experience in a person's life and constitutes an acute adventitious crisis. It is a total violation of the person's body and will. Typical crisis reactions reflect cognitive, affective, and behavioral disruptions. For survivors to return to their previous level of functioning, it is necessary for them to fully mourn their losses, experience anger, and work through their terrifying fears.

Counseling (Basic Level)

The rape survivor may be too traumatized, ashamed, or afraid to come to the hospital. For this reason, most communities provide telephone hotlines on a 24-hour basis.

Cultural definitions of what constitutes rape may also affect the decision to seek treatment (Lefley et al. 1993). Hispanic females, enculturated in the spirit of *marianismo* (the ennoblement of female chastity), may be particularly traumatized by rape because of a greater tendency to view themselves as both culpable and tainted by sexual assault. Ongoing energy is invested in trying to block the traumatic event through avoidance and obsessive-compulsive mechanisms (Lefley et al. 1993). This, of course, is maladaptive and may contribute to posttraumatic stress disorder.

The likelihood of African American women seeking help may depend on their assessment of whether rape treatment is regarded positively in their communities. Support groups provided by community mental health centers or churches may be more acceptable than individual psychotherapy (Lefley et al. 1993; Matthews 1994). For some survivors, the role of a parish nurse may be the survivor's greatest resource.

Counseling in the Emergency Department or Crisis Center (Basic Level)

Nurses' attitudes about sexual assault can have an important therapeutic impact. The most effective approach is to provide nonjudgmental care as well as maximal emotional support. This means that displays of shock, horror, disgust, surprise, or disbelief are not appropriate. Crisis management is the practice of primary prevention of psychiatric disorders. Confidentiality is, of course, crucial. Sexual assault cases are not to be discussed, except with the medical personnel involved, without the victim's consent. Records must be carefully guarded against any unauthorized access.

The most helpful things the nurse can do are to listen and let the victim talk. When the nurse listens carefully and empathically, the survivor's distress can be heard. A woman who feels understood is no longer alone; she then feels more in control of her situation.

It is especially important to help the survivor and her significant others separate issues of vulnerability from blame (Ledray and Arndt 1994). Although the person may have made choices that made her more vulnerable, she is not to blame for the rape, no matter what she did. She may, however, decide to avoid some of those choices in the future (e.g., walking alone late at night or excessive use of alcohol). Focusing on one's behavior (which is controllable) allows the survivor to believe that similar experiences can be avoided in the future.

- Mary has come to see that it was not her fault that she was raped. However, she is now adamant about not walking from the bus stop alone late at night, and from now on will take a cab, get a lift from a friend, or take a safer alternative route when going home.

Using reflective communication techniques (see Chapter 7) to respond to the expressed psychological themes is helpful. Examples of helpful and unhelpful responses follow.

A woman states, "I am so mad at myself. I should have never gone out tonight."

- Helpful response — You believe if you had made a different decision earlier this evening, this wouldn't have happened.
- Unhelpful response — Your actions had nothing to do with what happened.

If the survivor consents, involve her support system (e.g., family or friends), and discuss with them the nature and trauma of sexual assault and possible delayed reactions that may occur.

One survivor expressed it this way:

- "It takes a few days to hit you. It was bad. It was really rough for my husband. I needed to be reassured. I needed to be told that there was nothing I could do to prevent it. Understanding helps."

Social support effectively moderates somatic symptoms and subjective health ratings. The survivor who is able to confide comfortably in one or two friends or family members, especially immediately after the assault, is likely to experience fewer somatic manifestations of stress (Kimerling and Calhoun 1994). Family and friends may need support and reassurance as much as the survivor does. This is especially true for those from traditional cultures (Lefley et al. 1993). The long-standing cultural myth that women are the property of men still prevents some people from empathizing with the woman's severe psychic injury and from being supportive. She is, instead, often thought of as "devalued." Table 16–3 summarizes the main counseling techniques used by an educated nurse working with a rape survivor. Follow-up care is strongly encouraged.

Self-Care Activities (Basic Level)

When preparing the survivor to go home, give all referral information and follow-up instructions in writing, detailing likely physical concerns and emotional reactions, le-

TABLE 16–3 NURSING INTERVENTIONS AND RATIONALES: VICTIMS OF RAPE

INTERVENTION	RATIONALE
1. Do not leave the person alone.	1. Prevents increase in isolation, escalation of anxiety.
2. Maintain a nonjudgmental attitude.	2. Decreases emotional burden.
3. Provide nonjudgmental care.	3. Lessens feelings of shame and embarrassment.
4. Maximize emotional support ▶ Stay with the victim ▶ Show concern for the victim's needs	4. Prevents further disorganization ▶ Shows concern for the victim's needs ▶ Validates the worth of the person
5. Ensure confidentiality.	5. Encourages sharing the event and protects a person's self-concept and sense of control.
6. Encourage the person to talk through empathetic listening.	6. Helps the person sort out thoughts and feelings. Lowers anxiety by reducing feelings of isolation.
7. Allow negative expression of affect and behavioral self-blame.	7. Reinforces the victim's value as a human being.
8. Encourage problem solving when anxiety lowers to moderate levels.	8. Increases the person's sense of control.
9. Engage the support system (e.g., family and friends) when appropriate.	9. Provides warmth and feelings of safety when shock wears off and the acute disorganization phase begins. The focus should remain on returning the victim to psychological well-being.
10. Emphasize that the person did the right thing to save his or her life.	10. Helps reduce guilt and maintain self-esteem.
11. Arrange for support follow-up.	11. Acknowledges that healing takes time.

Data from Burgess and Holstrom 1973; Braen 1989; Sadock 1995.

gal matters, victim compensation, and ways that family and friends can help. Legal referrals (i.e., names of attorneys who specialize in rape cases and options for low-cost legal assistance) can also be given.

Case Management (Basic Level)

Caring for the survivor is not completed in a single visit. Her emotional state and other psychological needs should be reassessed by phone or personal contact within 24 to 48 hours after discharge from the hospital. Repeat referrals should be made for needed resources or support services at this time. Effective crisis intervention and continuity of care require outreach activities and services beyond the emergency medical setting.

Survivors may seek help from medical professionals rather than from mental health professionals because medical treatment is more socially sanctioned and they are likely to be experiencing the physical sequelae of stress (Kimerling and Calhoun 1994; Beebe et al. 1994; Golding 1994). Being aware of this, the office nurse can make a more focused assessment of stress-related symptoms and/or depression and ascertain the need for mental health referral. Reporting symptoms and seeking medical treatment are adaptive coping behaviors and can be reinforced as such.

Follow-up visits should occur at least 2, 4, and 6 weeks after the initial evaluation. At each visit, the survivor should be assessed for psychological progress, venereal disease, and pregnancy.

Counseling on the Crisis Hotline (Basic Level)

Nearly all communities provide 24-hour crisis telephone services. Some provide 24-hour hotlines for rape victims (e.g., Rape Relief in Seattle). The hotline may be used for information and referral, or as a prelude to a personal contact for future telephone counseling.

The phone counselor talks briefly with the person to determine where she is, what has happened, and what kind of help she needs. The counselor provides empathic listening and the survivor is further encouraged to go to the hospital. She is advised not to wash, change clothes, douche, brush teeth, or eat or drink anything, all of which might destroy evidence. The survivor is urged to call the police. The police can take the survivor to the emergency department or the police and rape advocate can meet the survivor at the emergency department. Over the phone, the counselor can also encourage the survivor to make necessary decisions about communications with family and friends and can give information about what to expect from the hospital and the police. However, all of this communication is better done in person, if possible. The main focus of the telephone contact is on the immediate steps the survivor may take. The counselor provides the necessary information for the victim to make decisions. Unfortunately, survivors frequently wish to remain anonymous, and some do not want any immediate or follow-up counseling. However, they may change their minds in the future, and having made contact and received referrals gives them the option of following up at another time if they choose.

Psychotherapy (Advanced Level)

Survivor

Most rape survivors are eventually able to resume their previous lives after supportive services and crisis counseling. However, many carry with them a constant emotional trauma: flashbacks, nightmares, fear, phobias, and other symptoms associated with posttraumatic stress reaction (see Chapter 17). Some people who survive rape may be susceptible to a psychotic episode or an emotional disturbance so severe that hospitalization is required. Others whose emotional life may be so overburdened with multiple internal and external pressures may require individual psychotherapy.

Depression and suicide ideation are frequent sequelae of rape (Kimerling and Calhoun 1994). Depression is more common in those who do not disclose the assault to significant others because of concerns about being stigmatized, having children living at home, or having a pending civil lawsuit (Mackey et al. 1992). Any exposure to stimuli related to the traumatic event may activate a reliving of the traumatic state.

Rape survivors are likely to benefit from group therapy or support groups (Koss 1993). These modalities may be particularly beneficial for survivors from cultures that are group oriented rather than individualistic, and for women who derive much of their self-definition from cultural norms (Lefley et al. 1993). Group therapy can make the difference between a person coming out of the crisis at a lower level of functioning or gradually adapting to the experience with an increase in coping skills (Welch 1995).

Rapist

Research (Sadock 1995) has categorized rapists into the following separate groups:

CATEGORIES OF RAPIST	MOTIVATION OF RAPISTS
Sexual sadists	Aroused by the pain of their victim
Exploitative predators	Using victims as objects for their gratification in an impulsive way
Inadequate men	Obsessed with sexual fantasies and believing that no woman has the right to refuse a sexual encounter
Men who displace their anger	Anger and frustration against other persons or situations are used to relieve pent-up aggression or fear, a way to regain a feeling of power

It has been reported that convicted rapists are part of a subculture of violence. In the United States, about 71% of arrested rapists have criminal histories, including records of assault, robbery, and homicide. Statistics show that most men who commit rapes are between 25 and 44 years of age; 51% are white and tend to rape white victims; 47% are black and tend to rape black victims; and the other 2% come from other races (Sadock 1995).

Psychotherapy is essential for rapists for behavior change to occur. Unfortunately, most do not acknowledge the need for behavior change, and therapy programs and techniques are in their infancy. To date, there is no single method or program of treatment that has been found to be totally effective. Research is needed to evaluate those few programs that have been developed.

EVALUATION

Completion of the process of reorganization after a rape crisis can be evaluated by assessing sleeping and eating patterns, the presence or absence of phobias, motor behavior, relationships, self-esteem, and the presence or absence of somatic reactions (DiVasto 1985). The survivors are recovered if they are

1. Sleeping well, with very few instances of episodic nightmares or broken sleep.
2. Eating as was their pattern before the rape.
3. Calm and relaxed or only mildly suspicious, fearful, or restless.
4. Getting support from family and friends. Some strain might still be present in relationships, but it should be minimal.
5. Generally positive about themselves. On occasion, doubts about self-worth may occur.
6. Free from somatic reactions. If mild symptoms persist and minor discomfort is reported, the survivor should be able to talk about it and feel in control of the symptoms.

In general, the closer the survivor's life style is to the pattern that was present before the rape, the more complete the recovery has been.

CASE STUDY 16–1: WORKING WITH A PERSON WHO HAS BEEN RAPED

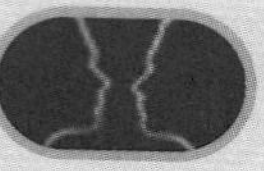

Latisha Smith, a 36-year-old single mother of two, went out one evening with some friends. Her children were at a slumber party and she "needed to get away and have a little rest and relaxation." She and her friends had gone bowling. Later in the evening, Latisha was tired and ready to go home. A man who had joined the group offered to take her home. She had seen the man at the bowling alley before but did not know much about him. Not in the habit of going home alone with men she did not know, she hesitated. A friend whom she trusted encouraged her to go with James because he was a nice man.

James drove Latisha home. He then asked if he could come into her house to use the bathroom before driving the long distance to his house. She reluctantly agreed and sat on the living room couch. After using the bathroom, James sat next to Latisha and began to kiss her and fondle her breasts. As she protested, James became more forceful in his advances. Latisha was confused and frightened. She managed to get away from him briefly, but he began grabbing, squeezing, and biting her. He told her gruffly, "If you don't do what I say, I'll break your neck." She screamed, but he proceeded to rape her. James became nervous that the noise would alert the neighbors and raced out of the house. A neighbor did in fact arrive just after James fled. The neighbor called the police and then brought Latisha to the local hospital emergency department for a physical examination, crisis intervention, and support.

In the emergency department, Latisha was visibly shaken. She kept saying, over and over, "I shouldn't have let him take me home. I should have fought harder, I shouldn't have let him do this."

The nurse took Latisha to a quiet cubicle. She didn't want Latisha to stay alone and asked the neighbor to stay with her. The nurse then notified the doctor and the rape-victim advocate. When the nurse came back, she told Latisha that she would like to talk to her before the doctor came. Latisha looked at her neighbor and then down. The nurse asked the neighbor to wait outside for a while and said she would call her later.

Latisha: It was horrible. I feel so dirty.
Nurse: You have had a traumatic experience. Do you want to talk about it?
Latisha: I feel so ashamed, I should have never let that man take me home.
Nurse: You think that if you hadn't gone home with a stranger this wouldn't have happened?
Latisha: Yes . . . I shouldn't have let him do it to me anyway, I shouldn't have let him rape me.
Nurse: You mentioned that he said he would break your neck if you didn't do as he said.
Latisha: Yes, he said that . . . he was going to kill me, it was awful.
Nurse: It seems you did the right thing in order to stay alive.

As the nurse continued to talk with Latisha, her anxiety level seemed to lessen. The nurse talked to Latisha about the kinds of experiences rape victims often have after the rape, and explained that the reactions she might have 2 or 3 weeks from now are normal in these circumstances. The nurse continued to collect the necessary information. She said that the doctor would want to examine Latisha, and explained the procedure to her. She then asked Latisha to sign a consent. While preparing Latisha for examination, the nurse noticed bite marks and bruises on both breasts. She also noted Latisha's lower lip, which was cut and bleeding. After the examination, Latisha was given clean clothes and a place to shower.

ASSESSMENT

The nurse organized her data into subjective and objective components.

OBJECTIVE DATA

1. Crying and sobbing
2. Bruises and bite marks on each breast
3. Lip cut and bleeding
4. Rape reported to the police

SUBJECTIVE DATA

1. "He was going to kill me."
2. "It was horrible. I feel so dirty."
3. "I shouldn't have let him rape me."

NURSING DIAGNOSIS

The nurse formulated the following diagnosis:

1. Rape-trauma syndrome
   - "I shouldn't have let him rape me."
   - "He was going to kill me."
   - Crying and sobbing
   - Bruises and bite marks on both breasts
   - Rape reported to the police
   - "It was horrible. I feel so dirty."

CASE STUDY 16–1: WORKING WITH A PERSON WHO HAS BEEN RAPED (Continued)

PLANNING

OUTCOME CRITERIA

The nurse devised a plan of care for Latisha, based on the nursing diagnosis and the nurse's training as a crisis counselor.

NURSING DIAGNOSIS	LONG-TERM OUTCOME	SHORT-TERM GOALS
1. *Rape-trauma syndrome*	1. Within 5 months Latisha will state that she thinks less about the rape, is sleeping better, feels safer, and is functioning at her previous level.	1a. Latisha will begin to express emotional reactions and feelings before she leaves the emergency department. 1b. Latisha will be able to list possible socioemotional reactions following sexual assault. 1c. Latisha will have written referrals for legal, medical, and crisis counseling before she leaves the emergency department. 1d. Latisha will have a follow-up appointment with the gynecology clinic and the rape advocate-counselor for weekly meetings before she leaves the emergency department. 1e. Latisha's anxiety level will go from severe to moderate before she leaves the emergency department.

NURSE'S FEELINGS AND SELF-ASSESSMENT

The nurse had worked with rape survivors before and had helped develop the hospital protocol. It took a while for her to be able to remain neutral as well as responsive, because her own anger at rapists had initially interfered. She also remembers a time when a woman came in stating that she was raped but was so calm, smiling, and polite that the nurse initially did not believe her story. She had not, at that point, examined her own feelings or dealt with the popular societal myths regarding rape. It was only later, when she had talked to more experienced health care personnel, that she learned that crisis reactions can seem bizarre, confusing, and contradictory.

The nurse learned that staying with the survivor, encouraging her to express her reactions and feelings, and listening were effective methods of reducing feelings of anxiety. Once the nurse learned through supervision and peer discussion to let go of her personal anger at the attacker and her ambivalence toward the survivor, her care and effectiveness improved greatly. All of this growth took time and support from more experienced nurses and other members of the health care team.

Continued on following page

CASE STUDY 16–1: WORKING WITH A PERSON WHO HAS BEEN RAPED (Continued)

INTERVENTION

Latisha stated that she felt more comfortable after taking a shower and talking to the nurse. She seemed less confused and better able to concentrate, and she began to discuss what she would tell her children. Specific interventions are found in Nursing Care Plan 16–1.

It was decided that Latisha's neighbor would stay with her overnight. Latisha had an appointment the following week with the nurse counselor and with a women's health nurse practitioner in the outpatient clinic. She was also given written information about legal counseling, crisis groups, and other community follow-up services for rape survivors.

The nurse documented Latisha's physical and emotional status, including verbatim responses, as well as the results of the physical examination and tests. The nurse called Latisha the next morning and encouraged her to call back if she had any further questions.

EVALUATION

Latisha kept her counseling appointment with the nurse counselor at the community mental health center as well as her appointment with the women's health nurse practitioner. She continued with the counseling for several months. For a time, she experienced acute anxiety attacks when she went out at night, and she had new locks put on all her windows and doors. After 3 months, she expressed interest in a group that was forming in the next town for women who had been raped; however, she said that she didn't know if she could go because it started at 6 PM. The counselor told her that arrangements could be made for a volunteer to take her there and back until she felt safer going out at night.

After 4 months, Latisha stated that she did feel safer and had been out at night twice in the past week. She was not comfortable yet, but said she was making progress. She told the counselor that she was not ready to date. The group had been a great help to her. She continued to call the nurse counselor about once every 2 weeks to report on her progress.

Latisha said she was functioning well as a mother and in her job. After 5 months, the flashbacks ceased and she started sleeping throughout the night without nightmares.

NURSING CARE PLAN 16–1 A SURVIVOR OF SEXUAL ASSAULT

NURSING DIAGNOSIS

Rape-Trauma Syndrome

Supporting Data

- "I shouldn't have let him rape me."
- "He was going to kill me."
- Sobbing and crying
- Bruises and bites on both breasts
- Rape reported to police
- "It was horrible, I feel so dirty."

Outcome Criteria: Within 5 months, survivor will state that she thinks less about the rape, is sleeping better, feels safer, and is functioning at her previous level.

SHORT-TERM GOALS	INTERVENTION	RATIONALE	EVALUATION
1. Survivor will begin to express emotional reactions and feelings before she leaves the emergency room.	1a. Nurse remains neutral and nonjudgmental and assures survivor of confidentiality.	1a. Lessens feelings of shame and guilt and encourages sharing of painful feelings	1. *GOAL MET* Survivor discussed feelings of shame, self-blame, and fear. Continues counseling with rape-victim advocate.

NURSING CARE PLAN 16–1 A SURVIVOR OF SEXUAL ASSAULT *(Continued)*

SHORT-TERM GOALS	INTERVENTION	RATIONALE	EVALUATION
	1b. Nurse does not leave survivor alone.	1b. Deters feelings of isolation and escalation of anxiety	
	1c. Nurse allows negative expressions and behavioral self-blame—uses reflective techniques.	1c. Fosters feelings of control	
	1d. Nurse assures survivor she did the right thing to save her life.	1d. Decreases burden of guilt and shame	
	1e. When anxiety level is down to moderate, nurse encourages problem solving.	1e. Increases survivor's feeling of control in her own life (when in severe and panic levels, a person cannot problem-solve)	
2. Survivor will be able to list possible socioemotional reactions following sexual assault.	2. Nurse tells survivor of common reactions experienced by people in long-term reorganization phase, e.g., phobias, flashbacks, insomnia, increased motor activity.	2. Helps survivor anticipate reactions and understand them as part of recovery process	2. *GOAL MET* Survivor was able to state five possible future reactions.
3. Survivor will state that she will keep a follow-up appointment with the gynecology clinic and rape advocate or counselor before she leaves the emergency room.	3a. Nurse explains emergency room procedure to survivor.	3a. Lowers anticipatory anxiety	3. *GOAL MET* Survivor kept appointments with gynecology clinic and rape advocate.
	3b. Nurse explains physical examination.	3b. Allows for questions and concerns; victim may be too traumatized and may refuse	
	3c. Nurse has survivor sign consent form.	3c. Follows legal protocol	
	3d. Nurse (or female rape-victim advocate) stays with survivor during examination.	3d. Often decreases isolation and anxiety	
	3e. Nurse explains role of rape-victim advocate.	3e. Awareness of supports and why they are needed	
	3f. Nurse gives results of gynecological and physical examination to survivor.	3f. Enables survivor to participate in decision and to understand need for follow-up care	
	3g. Nurse documents all physical and emotional data (with verbatim remarks) and lists laboratory tests.	3g. Needed for both medical and legal follow-up	

Continued on following page

NURSING CARE PLAN 16–1 A SURVIVOR OF SEXUAL ASSAULT *(Continued)*

SHORT-TERM GOALS	INTERVENTION	RATIONALE	EVALUATION
4. Survivor's anxiety level will lessen from severe to moderate before she leaves the emergency room or counseling center.	4a. Nurse gives written referrals for legal, medical, and crisis counseling. 4b. Nurse informs survivor he or she will call her tomorrow AM. 4c. Nurse makes plans so that survivor is not alone for a few days.	4a. Minimizes increase in anxiety level 4b. Validates concern for her feelings and safety 4c. Helps decrease anxiety and increase feelings of safety	4. *GOAL MET* Survivor was able to start making future plans and stated that she felt less anxious. Survivor called nurse to "check in." Nurse plans to have conferences with survivor.

SUMMARY

In recent years, rape survivors have begun to receive the attention they deserve from the health care system, along with the empathy and support they need. A rape survivor experiences a wide range of feelings, which may or may not be exhibited. Feelings of fear, degradation, anger and rage, helplessness, and nervousness are common. Long-term sequelae, such as sleep disturbances, disturbed relationships, flashbacks, depression, and somatic complaints, are also common.

The circumstances of the initial medical evaluation may be frightening and stressful. Police interrogation, repeated questioning by health professionals, and the physical examination itself all have the potential to add to the trauma of the sexual assault. As one survivor stated, "The last thing I wanted was a pelvic exam. I had been violated already." Nurses, in their role of case managers, can serve to minimize repetition of questions and support the survivor as she goes through the entire ordeal. After resolution of the immediate crisis, survivors require long-term health care that can include counseling to minimize the long-term effects of the rape and to assist in an early return to a normal living pattern.

Although community resources may vary considerably, most metropolitan areas now have special programs to assist rape survivors. Such assistance usually includes advice on the management of the acute crisis, as well as guidelines for the collection of evidence and preparation for trial should legal action follow.

REFERENCES

Beebe, D. K., et al. (1994). Prevalence of sexual assault among women patients seen in family practice clinics. *Family Practice Research Journal*, 14(3):223.

Boutcher, F., and Gallop, R. (1996). Psychiatric nurses' attitudes toward sexuality, sexual assault and rape, and incest. *Archives of General Psychiatric Nursing*, X(3):184.

Braen, G. R. (1989). The adult female survivor of sexual assault. *Hospital Medicine*, 25(12):43.

Burgess, A. W. (1995). Rape trauma syndrome: A nursing diagnosis. *Occupational Health Nursing*, 33(8):405.

Burgess, A. W., Fehder, W. P., and Hartman, C. R. (1995). Delayed reporting of the rape victim. *Journal of Psychosocial Nursing*, 33(9):21.

Burgess, A. W., and Holstrom, L. L. (1973). The rape victim in the ER. *American Journal of Nursing*, 73(10):1740.

Burgess, A. W., and Holstrom, L. L. (1974). Rape trauma syndrome. *American Journal of Psychiatry*, 131:981.

Costin, F. (1985). Beliefs about rape and women's social roles. *Archives of Sexual Behavior*, 14(4):319.

Davis, T. C., Peck, G. Q., and Storment, J. M. (1993). Acquaintance rape and the high school student. *Journal of Adolescent Health*, 14:220.

DiVasto, P. (1985). Measuring the aftermath of rape. *Journal of Psychosocial Nursing*, 23(2):33.

Duchscher, J. E. B. (1994). Acting on violence against women. *Canadian Nurse*, 90(6):21.

Golding, J. M. (1994). Sexual assault history and physical health in randomly selected Los Angeles women. *Health Psychology*, 13(2):130.

Hampton, H. L. (1995). Care of the woman who has been raped. *New England Journal of Medicine*, 332(4):234.

Helen, M. (1984). Rape: Some facts, myths and responses. *Australian Nurses Journal*, 13(8):42.

Kimerling, R., and Calhoun, K. S. (1994). Somatic symptoms, social support, and treatment seeking among sexual assault victims. *Journal of Consulting and Clinical Psychology*, 62(2):333.

Koss, M. P. (1993). Rape. *American Psychologist*, 48(10):1062.

Ledray, L. E. (1993). Sexual assault nurse clinician: An emerging area of nursing expertise. *AWHONNS Clinical Issues in Perinatal and Women's Health Nursing*, 4(2):180.

Ledray, L. E., and Arndt, S. (1994). Examining the sexual assault victim: A new model for nursing care. *Journal of Psychosocial Nursing*, 32(2):7.

Lefley, H. P., et al.(1993). Cultural beliefs about rape and victims' response in three ethnic groups. *American Journal of Orthopsychiatry*, 63(4):623.

Mackey, T., et al. (1992). Factors associated with long-term depressive symptoms of sexual assault victims. *Archives of Psychiatric Nursing*, 6(1):10.

Matthews, N. A. (1994). *Confronting rape*. New York: Routledge.

Sadock, V. (1995). Physical and sexual abuse of adults. In H. I. Kaplan and B. J. Sadock (Eds.), *Comprehensive textbook of psychiatry IV* (Vol. 2, pp. 1729–1737). Baltimore: Williams & Wilkins.

Thomas, M., and Zachritz, H. (1993). Tulsa sexual assault nurse examiners (SANE) program. *Journal of Oklahoma State Medical Association*, 86(6):284.

Tyra, P. A. (1993). Older women: Victims of rape. *Journal of Gerontological Nursing*, 19(5):7.

Ullman, S. E., and Siegel, J. M. (1993). Victim-offender relationship and sexual assault. *Violence and Victims*, 8(2):121.

University of Louisville (1995). The victim of rape: Conducting a medico-legal examination. A Continuing Education monograph.

U.S. Department of Justice (1994). *Uniform Crime Reports 1993*. Washington, DC: U.S. Government Printing Office.

Welch, M. (1995). Clients' experiences of depression during recovery from traumatic injury. *Clinical Nurse Specialist*, 9(2):92.

Further Reading

Andrews, J. (1992). Sexual assault aftercare instructions. *Journal of Emergency Nursing*, 18(2):152.

Antognoli-Toland, P. (1985). Comprehensive program for examination of sexual assault victims by nurses: A hospital-based project in Texas. *Journal of Emergency Nursing*, 11(3):132.

Dubin, W. K., and Weiss, K. J. (1991). *Handbook of psychiatric emergencies*. Springhouse, PA: Springhouse.

Ellis, G. M. (1994). Acquaintance rape. *Perspectives in Psychiatric Care*, 30(1):11.

Gallese, L. E., and Treuting, E. G. (1981). Help for rape victims through group therapy. *Journal of Psychosocial Nursing*, 19:20.

Hanson, K. A., and Gidycz, C. A. (1993). Evaluation of a sexual assault prevention program. *Journal of Consulting and Clinical Psychology*, 61(6):1046.

Hendricks-Matthews, M. K. (1993). Survivors of abuse: Health care issues. *Primary Care*, 20(2):391.

Jezierski, M. (1992). Sexual assault nurse examiner: A role with lifetime impact. *Journal of Emergency Nursing*, 18(2):177.

Kaplan, H. I., and Sadock, B. J. (Eds.), *Comprehensive textbook of psychiatry IV.* Baltimore: Williams & Wilkins.

Lederle, D. J., DiGirolamo, J., and Poskins, P. (1985). Rape crisis services. *Illinois Medical Journal*, 167(4):305.

Ledray, L. E. (1990). Counseling rape victims: The nursing challenge. *Perspectives in Psychiatric Care*, 26(2):21.

MacFarlane, E., and Hawley, P. (1993). Sexual assault: Coping with crisis. *Canadian Nurse*, 89(6):21.

Mayer, R. A., and Boggio, N. T. (1992). The adolescent rape victim. *Emergency Medicine*, 24(3):98.

Mims, F. H., and Chang, A. S. (1984). Unwanted sexual experiences of young women. *Journal of Psychosocial Nursing*, 22(6):7.

Rose, D. S. (1986). "Worse than death": Psychodynamics of rape victims and need for psychotherapy. *American Journal of Psychiatry*, 143:817.

Ruckman, L. M. (1992). Rape: How to begin the healing. *American Journal of Nursing*, 92(9):48.

Sampselle, C. M. (1991). The role of nursing in preventing violence against women. *Journal of Obstetric, Gynecologic, and Neonatal Nursing*, 20(6):481.

Schwartz, I. L. (1991). Sexual violence against women: Prevalence, consequences, societal factors, and prevention. *American Journal of Preventive Medicine*, 7(6):363.

Smith, S. B. (1995). Restraints: Retraumatization for rape victims? *Journal of Psychosocial Nursing*, 33(7):23.

Struckman-Johnson, C., and Struckman-Johnson, M. (1994). Men pressured and forced into sexual experience. *Archives of Sexual Behavior*, 23(1):93.

Thompson, V. L. S., and West, S. D. (1992). Brief report. Attitudes of African American adults toward treatment in cases of rape. *Community Mental Health Journal*, 28(6):531.

Tintinalli, J. E. (1985). Clinical findings and legal resolution in sexual assault. *Annals of Emergency Medicine*, 14(5):447.

Warner, C. G. (Ed.) (1980). *Rape and sexual assault.* Germantown, MD: Aspen Systems.

Zeitlin, S. B., McNally, R. J., and Cassiday, K. L. (1993). Alexithymia in victims of sexual assault: An effect of repeated traumatization? *American Journal of Psychiatry*, 150(4):661.

SELF-STUDY AND CRITICAL THINKING

Write a brief response in answer to the following:

1. Name four areas that the nurse carefully documents in the victim's chart.

   A. ______________________
   B. ______________________
   C. ______________________
   D. ______________________

2. Name four responsibilities of the nurse working with a victim of rape during physical examination.

   A. ______________________
   B. ______________________
   C. ______________________
   D. ______________________

Multiple choice

3. When a person who has been sexually assaulted is assessed, all of the following are important considerations. Which of the following is not appropriate during the assessment in the emergency room?

   A. Do not touch the person, unless she reaches out for tactile support.
   B. Do not leave the person alone.
   C. If the person is extremely anxious, remove her to the treatment room or private place right away.
   D. The victim should not be seen until the emergency room is almost empty.

4. When helping with the physical part of the assessment, the nurse should be aware of all of the following except:

   A. The victim has the right to refuse a medical examination.
   B. The absence of sperm proves the absence of a rape.
   C. The physical examination should be carefully explained to the victim, and a nurse should stay with the person.
   D. Fresh clothes and a shower should be made available after the examination.

5. Choose the goal that is a long-term goal formulated for rape-trauma syndrome.

   A. The victim will experience reduction of anxiety before leaving the emergency room.
   B. The victim will state a short-term plan for handling the immediate situation.
   C. The victim will begin to express reactions and feelings before leaving the emergency room.
   D. The victim will state that physical symptoms (e.g., sleep disturbances and poor appetite) have subsided.

6. Choose the intervention that is not a therapeutic technique for use with a victim of sexual assault.

   A. Never leave the woman alone.
   B. Allow negative expression and behavioral self-blame.
   C. Emphasize that the person did the right thing in order to save her life.
   D. Initiate touching the victim as a means of emotional support.

7. The main focus of the telephone contact in a rape crisis hotline is to

   A. Get the victim to prosecute her assailant.
   B. Find out where she is and get the police.
   C. Insist that she come to the hospital emergency room for further treatment.
   D. Provide information to facilitate the victim's decision making and help plan the next steps.

8. Which of the following is not a reason many rapes go unreported?

   A. The rape victim goes on trial as well as the rapist.
   B. Men are less likely to report rape because of strong reactions from society.
   C. Fear and anguish prevent people from seeking medical help and reporting the crime.
   D. Rape is not a crime.

Critical thinking

9. Role play, with a classmate, counseling Latisha (in the case example) regarding risks for pregnancy, STDs, and HIV infection.

____
____
____
____

10. How would you evaluate a rape survivor's recovery from the assault? Describe three behaviors you would assess for that would indicate successful recovery, and three behaviors that would necessitate referral for more help. Include time frames.

____
____
____
____

11. Role play responding to (1) a colleague, (2) a friend, (3) a relative, (4) a neighbor, and (5) a classmate who was perpetuating rape myths. Refer to Table 16–2.

12. Compare and contrast counseling interventions that are useful in the emergency department and on the crisis hotline.

13. Draw up a list of primary prevention activities in which nurses can engage in order potentially to decrease the occurrence of rape in our society. Identify prevention activities in your area.

14. Describe how a nurse working in a community health clinic could facilitate case finding for rape survivors who might be experiencing lingering effects that are impairing their physical or emotional health.

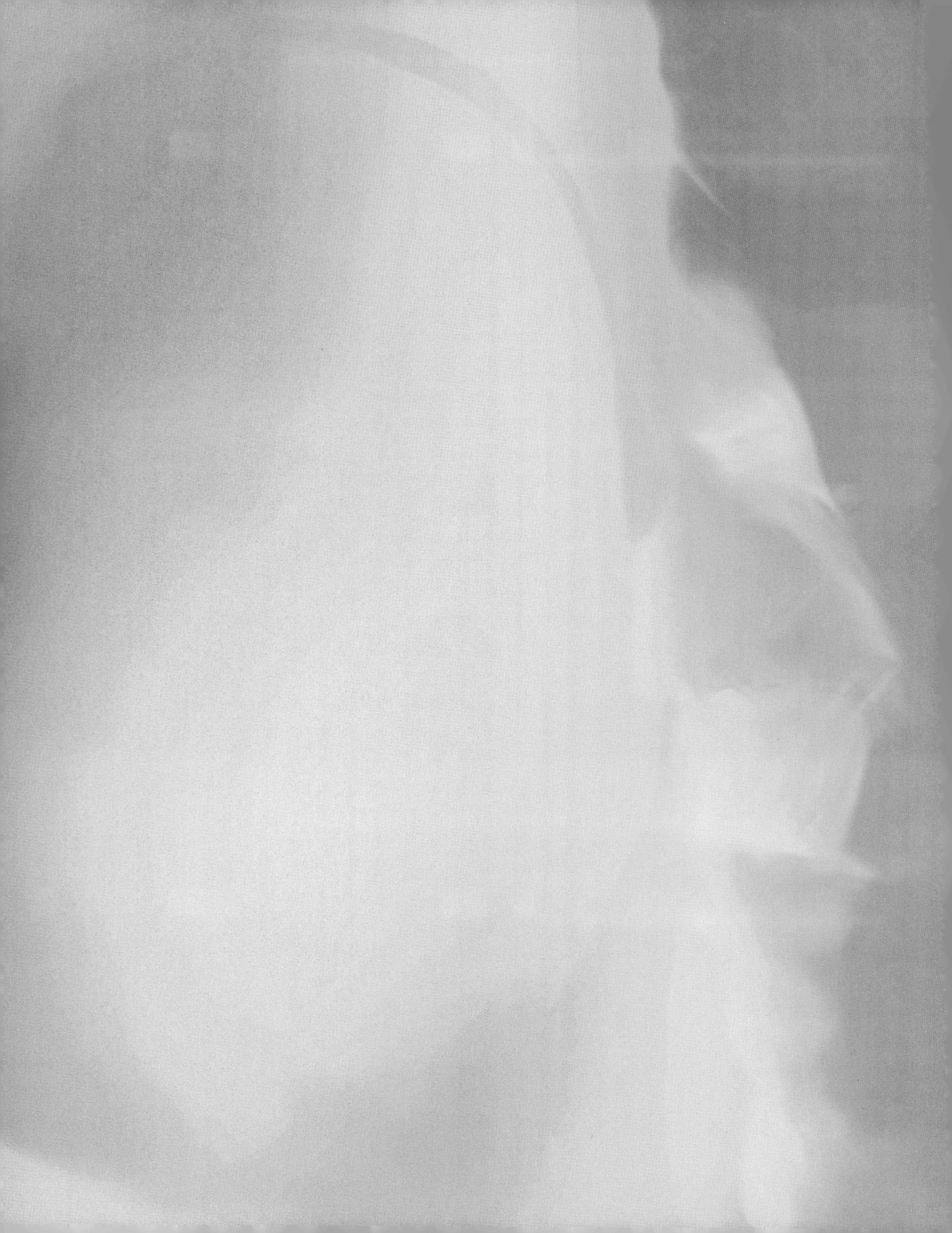

UNIT FOUR

People in the Moderate to Severe Range on the Mental Health Continuum

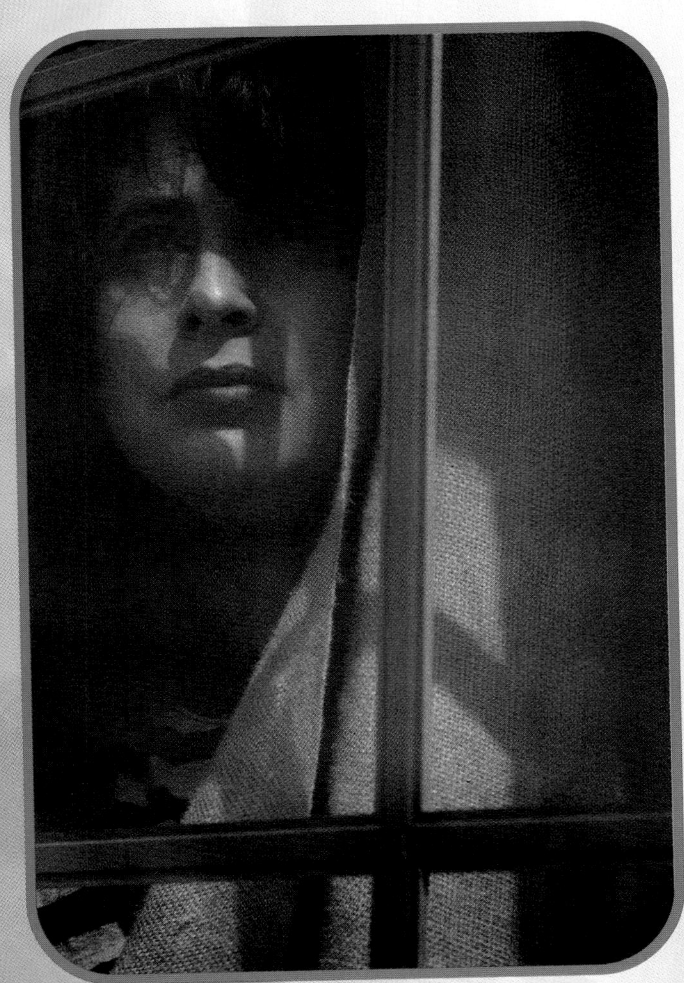

My life has been filled with terrible misfortunes, most of which never happened.

MARK TWAIN

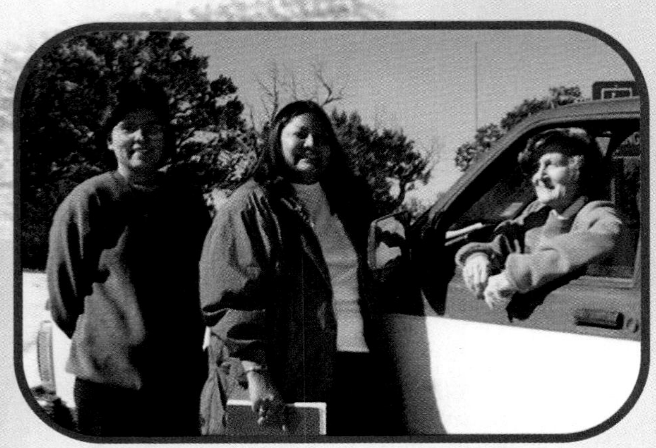

A Nurse Speaks

*Jane Bruker**

The increase in home care poses new challenges for nurses. These challenges include how to adapt technology in the home, how to interact with the family on their own turf, and how to be practical in very unfamiliar situations.

I was asked by the local home health agency to visit an elderly Indian woman. She had been hospitalized for leg ulcers, then placed in a nursing home for about a year. She was a problem in the nursing home and had run away on at least two occasions. She was diagnosed as schizophrenic and discharged to the home health agency.

Annie is in her seventies. She lives in a hogan on the Navajo Indian Reservation in New Mexico. She speaks and understands only Navajo. The Navajo language is unique and there are many variations of it, depending on the area of the reservation in which one lives. I asked one of my Navajo nursing students to accompany me on my visit and serve as interpreter. Although Sarah is fluent in Navajo, she asked another student to join us. Sarah felt she did not know Navajo tradition well enough for Annie to feel comfortable with us.

The three of us started out on a cold Saturday morning. In northern New Mexico one is in the mountains, so there was about a foot of snow on the ground. Our drive took us out Interstate 40 about 12 miles. Then we had to head out onto the reservation. Although we had a map with us, on a snow-covered dirt road one turn looks very much like another, a one-lane bridge is a one-lane bridge, and the vastness of the open terrain with unfamiliar landmarks found us in a small settlement where no one knew who we were looking for. Using four-wheel drive and lots of prayer, we were able to get turned around. We restudied the map and retraced our path, taking a different turn about 10 miles back. This attempt brought us to our destination.

Although there are two hogans and a house in close proximity to where Annie lives, one hogan and the house are deserted. She lives there alone. There is no electricity, no running water, no telephone. Although I say she lives there alone, she has two cats, six dogs, five chickens, and a herd of sheep that live with her. She did not appear to be lonely.

When we arrived, Annie was outside in the sun. She hurried back into the hogan. She greeted the two Navajo students and appeared pleased to have the visit. She ignored me completely, not in an unkind way, more as if I did not exist. She told us she had been told by the nurses to stay inside so she wouldn't fall outside in the snow. She was trying to comply and knew what had been asked of her. The hogan was very cluttered. There were sacks of feed for the chickens and a huge pile of wood for the stove. She had her chair in front of the stove, which is in the middle of the hogan. From her chair she could reach a log to add to the fire. On the stove were three pans. Two of the pans held small amounts of water from which she said she would make cups of instant coffee. The coffee was within a few steps of the stove. The third pan was quite large and was full of snow that would be melted for drinking water.

---

*I thank Sara Lee and Yvonne Stefaniak for sharing this experience with me.

There were indications in the hogan of the presence of Western medicine. There was a walker being used to hang things on. She uses a cane that looked rather "home made," but she gets around quite nimbly with it. The walker could not be used without inviting more danger, as the floor is dirt and bedrock. Since she has lived there for her entire life, it is reasonable to assume she knows every spot of the floor. There was a pill container with the days of the week identified on each box. We were there on Saturday. While we were there, Annie showed us the container and told us the pills were for high blood pressure. She took one. It was in the container marked Monday. Elderly Navajos do not relate to the concept of days of the week or months in the same way we do. The days and weeks and months are related to the seasons and to life activities: what season is the time to take the sheep to a different area for grazing, and how long does it take to accomplish a task? Someone had carefully cut up a banana so she could eat it without difficulty. The problem is that she doesn't like bananas, she doesn't understand bananas. They don't grow on the reservation and they don't look like anything that does grow there. She will leave the banana until it rots. She will not even give it to the chickens. Annie does not intend to be noncompliant, but it doesn't make any sense to her.

The Navajo tribe tries to take care of their elderly. A community health representative visits her on a weekly basis. She has firewood and coal within reach. She appears to be well nourished. She enjoyed visiting with the students and telling them her stories. As I sat listening to the students and Annie, I noticed many things. First, they were having a neighborly visit. She was telling them stories. They were all laughing. There was an element of camaraderie and kinship. I also noticed how many things would be considered dangerous and need to be changed from the textbook standpoint: the clutter, the uneven floor, the open fire, the chickens. But I believe that the next visit should include assisting her to walk out to the corral so that she can see her sheep. Maybe it should include sitting and watching the sun go down over the mountains. Maybe it should not include bananas and pills and diagnoses of schizophrenia.

Students Speak

We are two students in the associate degree nursing program at the University of New Mexico—Gallup Branch. We are both American Indian and full-blooded members of the Navajo tribe. We have spoken Navajo from birth and grew up in traditional families on the Navajo reservation.

Our instructor asked us to accompany her on a home visit to an elderly Navajo woman to assist with a psychosocial assessment based on the assessment tool in our mental health textbook. On our way to the visit, we discussed the assessment tool and how we might best obtain the requested information. To understand a Native American person, one has to know the culture, language, tradition, and history of the person. When you approach an elderly Navajo, you may find it very difficult. You need to understand the sense of humor used, the gestures, and the difference between what is true and what is a story. There is an appropriate way of saying hello, shaking hands, and stating your name, your clan, your profession, where you are from, and finally the reason for your visit. This makes the person feel comfortable and secure with you.

Obtaining the person's name is not difficult. Obtaining the age, however, can be very difficult since a large portion of older Navajos were not born in a hospital and only guess at their age. Many words in Navajo are almost alike in sound, but they can have a very different meaning. It is necessary to know the usage of the glottal stops, high tones, and other sounds.

Many older Navajos may appear dirty and sloppy, but you must realize that they live in a harsh land and learned to exist there without wasting their resources. They have no running water, no indoor bathroom, no kitchen sink, and no regular floor in the hogan, and they often live in very remote areas.

It is very difficult to translate from English to Navajo and vice versa. A simple word in English could be a full sentence in Navajo. It is best to lead into questions. For example, before speaking of depression, you would ask if the parents were still living. Finding the person's family roots may help you understand the strong family ties that most Navajos have. Then you could ask about depression or hopelessness. Some Navajos would laugh or get upset at this question because they believe if they say or feel hopeless they will be cursed. And you must always allow them time to finish their thought no matter how far they may stray from the original question. Questions relating to childhood may be answered in a lifetime story. These are the good times, hilarious events, and tragic events. Older Navajos do not withhold secrets that are embarrassing to them or give simple answers to questions. They are proud of how they were brought up, who raised them, and what they were taught, so their answers are never short.

We visited with Annie for a rather long time. She told us stories about her life. She talked a lot about her sheep. She said that her sheep were her life. She stated that her heart and will are very strong and that this is why she is not upset or sad about her other aches and pains such as some problems with her knees. She believes she will be out walking with her herd again. Most Navajo women are strong inside and nothing stands in their way. This is why some people believe that they are stubborn or uncooperative about suggestions relating to their health. They are brought up to believe that a woman is in control of herself. No one rules you but yourself. During the Womanhood Ceremony we are told that the woman is stronger than the man; the will of a woman is never to quit. From the elderly Navajo woman brought up in a strict home, one can see a lot of strength that we admire.

Annie does not know medical terminology. Explanations are difficult. She told us they showed her an x-ray of her feet at the clinic. She laughed about it and said, "I never realized I had such small bones in my feet. Maybe that is why my knees hurt." We wonder if she has ever had her medications and the treatments adequately explained to her. She believes that her sickness is due to witchcraft. Other than those supposed to be due to witchcraft, there are few illnesses that a Navajo can have. There are things such as that during an eclipse you should not eat, go outside, or look at the eclipse. This will cause weakness. The only way for Annie to recover is through a medicine man. She could then be healed psychologically.

Annie is naturally suspicious of people. She lives alone and in a remote area. She has never married and has no children. She was brought up to always be obedient. But it is difficult for her to be obedient when she doesn't understand what is happening. So in our visit we sat down and listened. We helped each other with the translating. We asked questions in a variety of ways. We enjoyed our visit and believe that Annie enjoyed it as well.

17

Anxiety Disorders

HELENE S. (KAY) CHARRON

OUTLINE

KEY TERMS AND CONCEPTS

The key terms and concepts listed here also appear in bold where they are defined or discussed in this chapter.

primary gain
secondary gain
panic disorder
agoraphobia
phobias
specific phobias

social phobias
obsessions
compulsions
generalized anxiety disorder
posttraumatic stress disorder
flashbacks
cognitive restructuring
systematic desensitization
modeling
graduated exposure
flooding
anxiolytic drugs (antianxiety drugs)
antidepressants

OBJECTIVES

After studying this chapter, the reader will be able to

1. Identify various theories of the causes of anxiety disorders.
2. Formulate appropriate nursing diagnoses that can be used with a person with an anxiety disorder.
3. Propose realistic and measurable outcomes for clients with anxiety disorders.
4. Discuss interventions that (a) reduce anxiety and ego-dystonic symptoms, (b) assist a client to use more effective coping strategies, (c) foster mental health and prevent mental illness and disability, and (d) support the client during ongoing therapy.
5. Evaluate the effectiveness of care based on established outcome criteria.
6. Identify examples of primary and secondary gain.
7. Analyze the value of ego-dystonic symptoms to the client.
8. Describe clinical manifestations of each anxiety disorder.
9. Identify psychiatric treatment modalities useful for each anxiety disorder.
10. Write a medication teaching plan that focuses on the action, side effects, and nursing responsibilities, including client teaching, that are associated with the administration of the anxiolytic medications used in treatment of anxiety disorders.
11. Recognize feelings that are commonly experienced by nurses caring for clients with anxiety disorders.

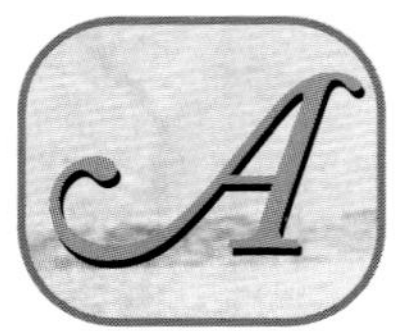

nxiety is a normal response to threatening situations. Anxiety is pathological only when it is excessive and persistent or when it no longer serves to signal danger. This chapter focuses on a group of disorders that result when anxiety is not relieved by usual coping mechanisms. These disorders are classified in the *Diagnostic and statistical manual of mental disorders*, fourth edition (DSM-IV), as anxiety disorders (APA 1994). The individual with an anxiety disorder uses rigid, repetitive, and ineffective behaviors to try to control anxiety. The common element of these disorders is that individuals experience a degree of anxiety that is so high it interferes with personal, occupational, or social functioning. Placement of these disorders on the mental health continuum can be seen in Figure 17–1. According to Noyes and Holt (1994), these disorders have a lifetime prevalence of 10% to 30% in the general population, and they are the most prevalent of all psychiatric disorders (Jenike 1993). Anxiety disorders produce symptoms that range from mild to severe, and they tend to be persistent and often disabling. For example, Billings (1993a) reported that

- 67% of panic clients lost or quit their jobs because of panic disorder.
- 50% were unable to drive more than 3 miles from their homes.
- 43% were completely incapable of working for periods ranging from 1 month to 25 years.

This chapter explores the current theories of anxiety disorders, the manifestations of anxiety disorders that can be found on assessment, and the treatment modalities that are most appropriate for each of the anxiety disorders. Attention to updated biological discoveries and treatment protocols is stressed.

THEORY

Clinical features of anxiety disorders include

1. *Panic attacks*, manifested by symptoms of severe anxiety that involves unpleasant physical, psychological, and cognitive symptoms, as described in Chapter 13 (e.g., palpitations, feelings of impending death, inability to concentrate).

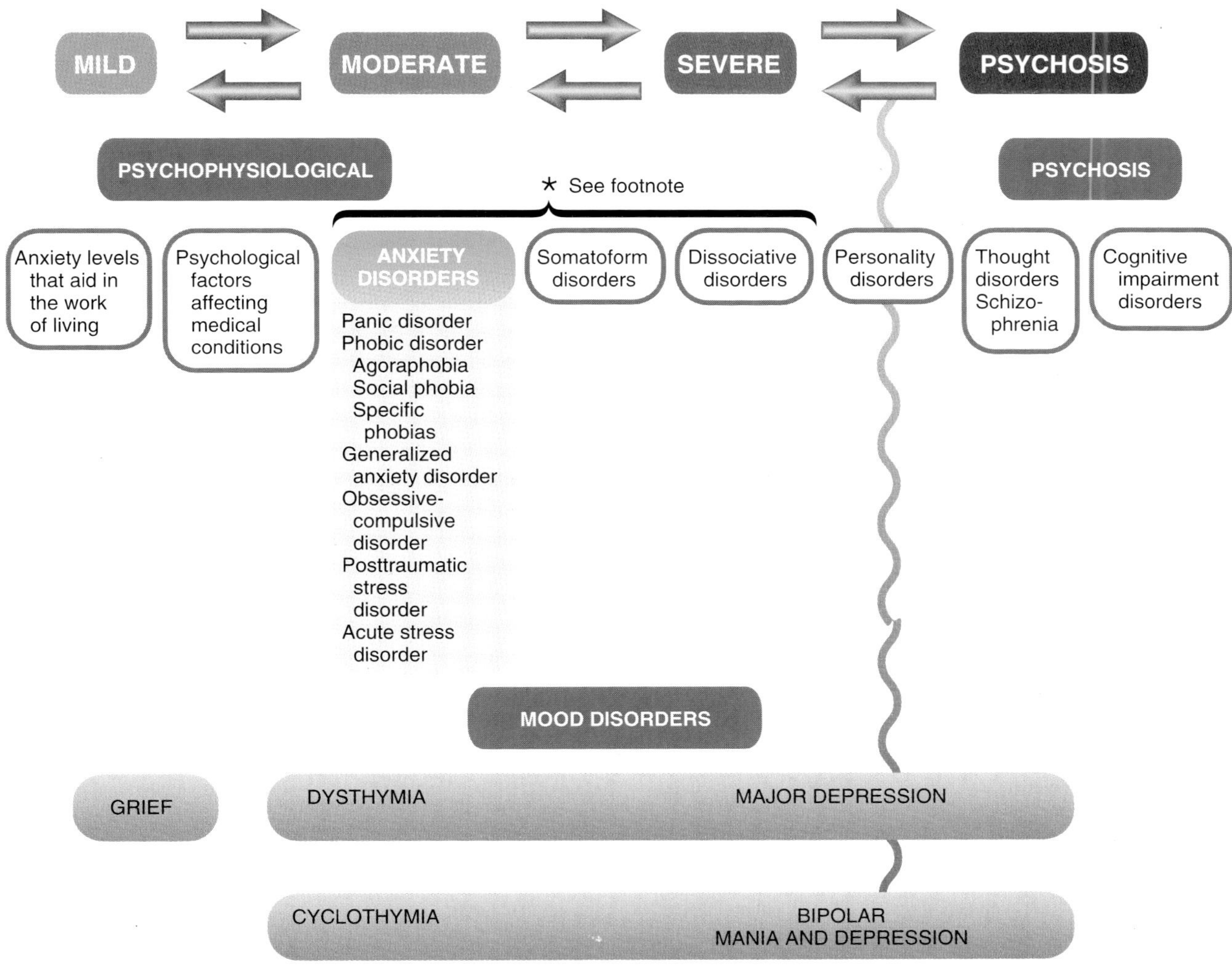

** These disorders are currently classified by presenting clinical symptoms. Previously they were called "neurotic" disorders.*

Figure 17–1 The mental health continuum for anxiety disorders.

2. *Phobias*, which are defined as excessive, irrational fears that cause the individual to avoid the feared object or situation in an attempt to control anxiety.
3. *Obsessions*, defined as persistent, recurrent, and intrusive thoughts, impulses, or images that cannot be dismissed from the mind.
4. *Compulsions*, or ritualistic behaviors that an individual feels driven to perform repetitively in an attempt to reduce anxiety.

Personal phobias, obsessions, and compulsions are often recognized by individuals as being odd, yet they are unable to do anything about the symptom. Such a symptom is called *ego-alien* or *ego-dystonic*. In contrast, *ego-syntonic* symptoms (e.g., delusions, hallucinations) are usually more consistent with the individual's beliefs.

A person with an ego-dystonic symptom, such as a compulsion to check and recheck on-off switches, might state, "It's silly for me to do all this checking—it takes up so much of my time—but I can't help myself. If I don't check, I get so anxious I can't stand it." This individual experiences feelings of dissatisfaction, unhappiness, and low self-esteem as a result of the ego-dystonic symptom.

Why is it that people do not change their behavior when they are able to recognize a personal behavior as "silly" or irrational? Their feeling of powerlessness is reflected in comments like "I can't help myself! I get so anxious!"

When working with a client who has an anxiety disorder, the nurse can often identify both primary and secondary gains achieved by the client. The term **primary gain** refers to anxiety relief resulting from the use of defense mechanisms, or symptom formation, or both. **Secondary gain** is defined as any benefit the individual obtains as a result of the disorders. Gaining attention, being able to avoid responsibility, having dependent needs met, and getting one's own way are examples of secondary gain.

Little is known about the causes of anxiety disorders. Research is being conducted to explore biochemical, genetic, psychosocial, and sociocultural factors.

Biochemical Factors

Current research into anxiety focuses on neurobiology, brain imaging, and neuroanatomy. Two lines of thinking exist. One theory suggests that any biological or anatomical changes that occur in the brains of clients with anxiety disorders result from the presence of the disorders; the other suggests that the biological changes cause the anxiety disorder (i.e., the body's alarm system may be malfunctioning). Research thus far has been able to describe the changes and to suggest treatments but has been unable to pinpoint actual causes. Kaplan and co-workers (1994) offered the following information:

1. Some clients with anxiety disorder, especially those with panic disorder, have an autonomic nervous system that exhibits increased sympathetic tone and responds excessively to moderate stimuli.
2. Clients affected by anxiety disorders may have a poorly regulated noradrenergic system that produces occasional bursts of activity. This theory implicates excess norepinephrine as a cause of anxiety disorders. In clients with panic disorder, beta-adrenergic antagonists, such as isoproterenol (Isuprel), and alpha-adrenergic antagonists, such as yohimbine (Yocon), can *provoke* frequent and severe panic attacks, while clonidine (Catapres), an alpha-adrenergic antagonist, *reduces* symptoms of anxiety.
3. Serotonin may have a role in producing symptoms that are associated with anxiety disorders. We know that drugs that affect brain serotonin level are effective in the treatment of anxiety disorders: the serotonergic antidepressant clomipramine (Anafranil) has therapeutic effects in obsessive-compulsive disorder (OCD), and buspirone (BuSpar), a serotonergic receptor antagonist, is effective in the treatment of other anxiety disorders.
4. Abnormal functioning of GABA (gamma-aminobutyric acid) receptors has also been implicated as a cause of anxiety disorders. The GABA system is believed to exert a "braking effect" on anxiety. Benzodiazepines, which enhance the activity of GABA at the receptor site, are effective in reducing anxiety.
5. Brain imaging studies of clients with anxiety disorders, including studies conducted by computed tomography, magnetic resonance imaging, and positron emission tomography, have variously revealed abnormalities in the frontal cortex, the occipital and temporal areas, and the parahippocampal gyrus.
6. Neuroanatomy suggests possible explanations. For example, the cell bodies of the noradrenergic system are localized in the locus ceruleus and project their axons to the cerebral cortex, the limbic system, the brainstem, and the spinal cord. Serotonergic neurons are located in the raphe nuclei of the brainstem and project to the cerebral cortex, the limbic system, and the hypothalamus. The limbic system receives both noradrenergic and serotonergic innervation. In addition, the limbic system also contains a high concentration of GABA receptors. Two other areas, the septohippocampal pathway and the cingulate gyrus, are currently under study.

Recent findings suggest that clients with OCD have frantic interactions between the orbital cortex, the caudate nucleus, and the cingulate gyrus. An encouraging result of a study by Schwartz and colleagues (1996) found that behavior therapy for clients with OCD changed not only behavior but also brain chemistry, as shown by positron-emission tomography.

In clients with posttraumatic stress disorder (PTSD), some investigators suggest that extreme stress in the form of physical, sexual, or psychological abuse is associated with damaging effects to the brain. Teicher and colleagues (1993) found an association between abuse during childhood and limbic system dysfunction in more than 25% of adult outpatients. Abuse that occurred before 18 years of age was associated with greater limbic system dysfunction than abuse experienced after that age (Teicher et al. 1993). Other studies support the hypothesis that abuse affects brain structure by reduction in hippocampal size in clients with PTSD (Bremner et al 1997).

Genetic Factors

Genetic studies have produced solid data that a genetic component contributes to the development of anxiety disorders. Nearly half of all clients with panic disorder have a relative with the disorder. Twin studies indicate a genetic component to both panic disorder and OCD (APA 1994). First-degree biological relatives of persons with OCD and persons with phobias have a higher frequency of these disorders than exists in the general population (APA 1994).

Psychosocial Factors

Early theories about the development of anxiety disorders center around the idea that unconscious childhood conflicts are the basis for symptom development. Freud taught that anxiety resulted from the threatened breakthrough of repressed ideas or emotions from the unconscious into consciousness. Freud also suggested that ego defense mechanisms are used by the individual to keep anxiety at manageable levels. Table 17–1 defines and gives examples of defense mechanisms commonly used by individuals with anxiety disorders. The use of defense mechanisms results in behavior that is not wholly adaptive, because of its rigidity and repetitive nature. Chapter 2 provides more information on defense mechanisms.

Harry Stack Sullivan placed anxiety in an interpersonal context. He believed that all anxiety is linked either to the emotional distress caused when early needs go unmet or to the anxiety transmitted to the infant from the caregiver

TABLE 17–1 DEFENSES USED IN ANXIETY DISORDERS

PHENOMENON	DEFENSE	PURPOSE	EXAMPLE
Phobia	Displacement	In phobias, anxiety is reduced when strong feelings about the original object are directed at a less threatening object and that object is avoided.	Client has abnormal fear of cats. In therapy, it is discovered that the client unconsciously links cats to a feared and cruel mother.
Compulsions	Undoing	Performing a symbolic act cancels out an unacceptable act or idea.	Symbolic rituals, e.g., handwashing, cleaning, and checking. Handwashing removes guilt. Cleaning removes dirty thoughts. Checking protects against hositle thoughts.
Obsession	Reaction-formation	Anxiety-producing unacceptable thoughts or feelings are kept out of awareness by the opposite feeling or idea.	Clients with strong aggressive feelings toward husband repeatedly thinks the opposite ("I love him with all my heart") to keep hostile feelings out of awareness.
	Intellectualization	Excessive use of reasoning, logic, or words is used to prevent the person from experiencing associated feelings.	Person talks in detail about parents' funeral but is unable to feel the associated pain of loss.
Posttraumatic Stress Disorder	Isolation	Facts associated with an anxiety-laden event remain conscious, but associated painful feelings are separated from the experience.	Client describes feeling "numb and empty inside."
	Repression	Repression unconsciously pushes an idea or feeling out of awareness.	Client is unable to trust authority figures at work after taking orders from commanding officer to kill civilians while in combat.

through the process of empathy. Thus, the anxiety experienced early in life becomes the prototype for that experienced when unpleasant events occur later in life.

Learning theories provide another view. Behavioral psychologists see anxiety as a learned response that can be unlearned. Some individuals may learn to be anxious from the modeling provided by parents or peers. For example, a mother who is fearful of thunder and lightning and who hides in closets during storms may transmit her anxiety to her children, who continue to adopt her behavior even into adult life. Such individuals can unlearn behaviors by observing others who react normally to a storm.

Cognitive theorists take the position that anxiety disorders are caused by distortions in an individual's thinking and perceiving. Ellis (1962) suggested that socially anxious people believe they must be approved of by everyone at all times. Because such individuals believe that any mistake they make will have catastrophic results, they experience acute anxiety.

Sociocultural Factors

Reliable data on the incidence of anxiety disorders and ritualistic behaviors in this and other cultures are sparse. Leff (1988) suggested that traditional or "culture-bound" illnesses must be differentiated from anxiety disorders. Hispanic Americans may suffer a traditional illness called *susto* (fright). Susto is believed to cause a part of the self (the spirit) to separate from the body. As the spirit leaves, cold air rushes in. The victim experiences anxiety, fear, weakness, malaise, and anorexia. A traditional illness identified among African Americans is the "nervous breakdown," characterized by increased anxiety, tension, altered self-care activities, and (in some instances) sadness and the hearing of voices.

Values conflicts created by immigration and assimilation into a new culture may be responsible for increased anxiety. For example, young adult émigrés of certain cultures (e.g., Asian Americans, Puerto Rican Americans, Vietnamese Americans) often experience increased anxiety when they challenge the traditional belief that the father is the authoritarian head of the family. Sociocultural variation in symptoms of anxiety disorders has also been noted (*Science News* 1990). The way in which anxiety is manifested differs from culture to culture. Individuals of some cultures express anxiety through somatic symptoms, while in other cultures, cognitive symptoms of anxiety predominate. In some cultures, panic attacks involve fear of magic or witchcraft. Panic attacks experienced by Latin Americans and Northern Europeans often involve sensations of choking, smothering, numbness, or tingling, as well as fear of dying. Because fear of magic or spirits is considered normal in some cultures, it cannot be diagnosed as phobic unless the fear is excessive *in the con-*

text of the culture. Social phobias manifested by individuals from the Japanese and Korean cultures may involve extreme anxiety centered on a belief that the individual's blushing, eye contact, or body odor is offensive to others. Similarly, one must be aware of the cultural norm before labeling ritualistic behavior as obsessive-compulsive. Nurses must be particularly alert for symptoms of PTSD in individuals who have recently emigrated from areas of social and civil unrest (APA 1994).

ASSESSMENT

DSM-IV and the Clinical Picture of Anxiety Disorders

DSM-IV (1994) lists 11 anxiety disorders, each of which is explored in this section. Figure 17–2 presents the DSM-IV criteria for various anxiety disorders.

Panic Disorder Without Agoraphobia

Panic disorder without agoraphobia is characterized by recurrent unexpected panic attacks, about which the individual is persistently concerned (APA 1994). A *panic attack* involves the sudden onset of extreme apprehension or fear, usually associated with feelings of impending doom. The feelings of terror present during a panic attack are so severe that normal function is suspended, the perceptual field is severely limited, and misinterpretation of reality may occur. Severe personality disorganization is evident. Persons experiencing a panic attack may believe that they are losing their mind or are having a heart attack. The attacks are often accompanied by highly uncomfortable physical symptoms, such as palpitations, chest pain, breathing difficulties, nausea, feelings of choking, chills, and hot flashes. Typically, panic attacks "come out of the blue" (i.e., suddenly and not necessarily provoked by stress), are extremely intense, last a matter of minutes, and then subside (Preston and Johnson 1995).

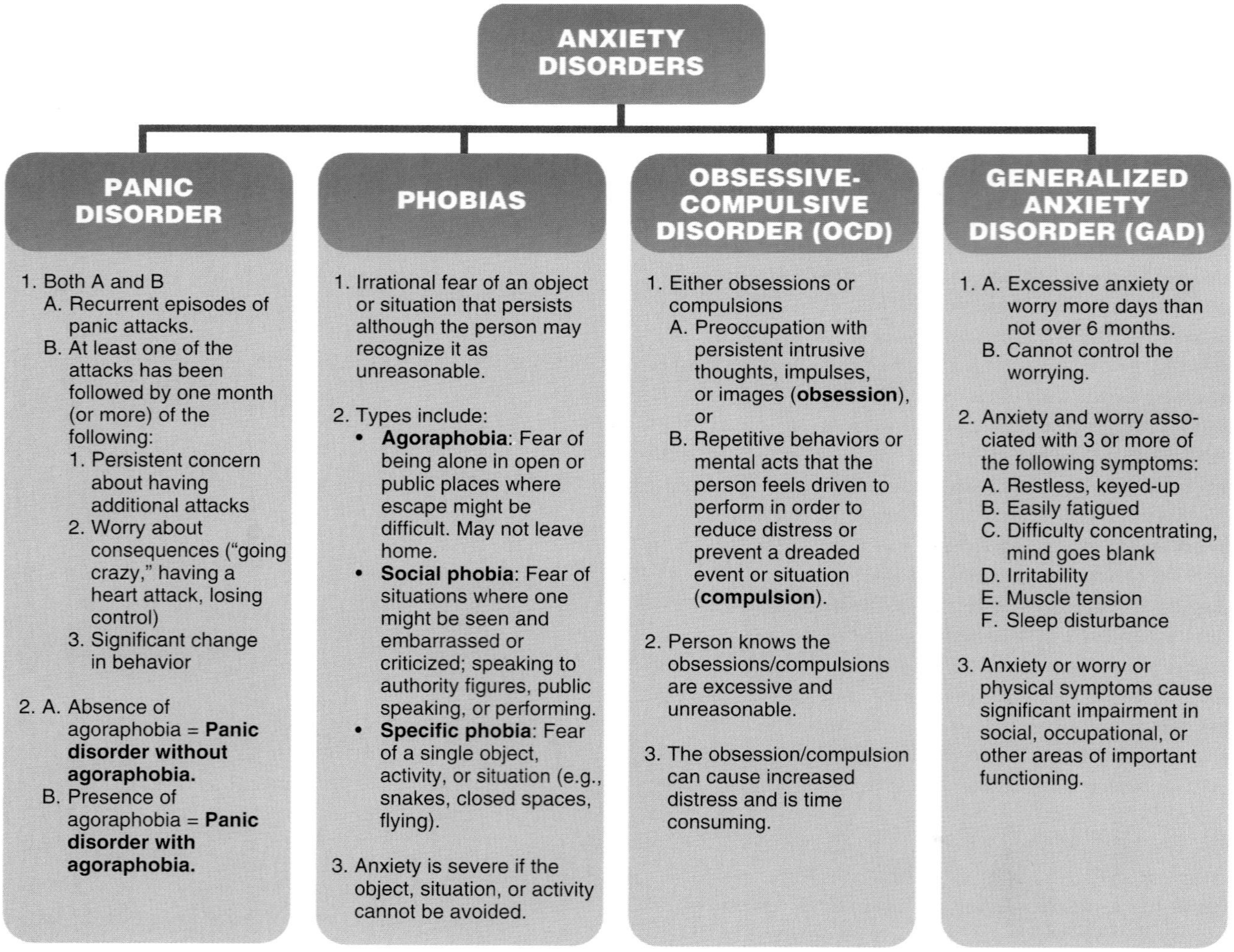

ANXIETY DISORDERS

PANIC DISORDER

1. Both A and B
   A. Recurrent episodes of panic attacks.
   B. At least one of the attacks has been followed by one month (or more) of the following:
      1. Persistent concern about having additional attacks
      2. Worry about consequences ("going crazy," having a heart attack, losing control)
      3. Significant change in behavior
2. A. Absence of agoraphobia = **Panic disorder without agoraphobia.**
   B. Presence of agoraphobia = **Panic disorder with agoraphobia.**

PHOBIAS

1. Irrational fear of an object or situation that persists although the person may recognize it as unreasonable.
2. Types include:
   - **Agoraphobia**: Fear of being alone in open or public places where escape might be difficult. May not leave home.
   - **Social phobia**: Fear of situations where one might be seen and embarrassed or criticized; speaking to authority figures, public speaking, or performing.
   - **Specific phobia**: Fear of a single object, activity, or situation (e.g., snakes, closed spaces, flying).
3. Anxiety is severe if the object, situation, or activity cannot be avoided.

OBSESSIVE-COMPULSIVE DISORDER (OCD)

1. Either obsessions or compulsions
   A. Preoccupation with persistent intrusive thoughts, impulses, or images (**obsession**), or
   B. Repetitive behaviors or mental acts that the person feels driven to perform in order to reduce distress or prevent a dreaded event or situation (**compulsion**).
2. Person knows the obsessions/compulsions are excessive and unreasonable.
3. The obsession/compulsion can cause increased distress and is time consuming.

GENERALIZED ANXIETY DISORDER (GAD)

1. A. Excessive anxiety or worry more days than not over 6 months.
   B. Cannot control the worrying.
2. Anxiety and worry associated with 3 or more of the following symptoms:
   A. Restless, keyed-up
   B. Easily fatigued
   C. Difficulty concentrating, mind goes blank
   D. Irritability
   E. Muscle tension
   F. Sleep disturbance
3. Anxiety or worry or physical symptoms cause significant impairment in social, occupational, or other areas of important functioning.

Figure 17–2 DSM IV diagnostic criteria for anxiety disorders. (Adapted from American Psychiatric Association (1994). *Diagnostic and statistical manual of mental disorders* (4th ed.). Washington, DC: American Psychiatric Association. Reprinted with permission. Copyright 1994 American Psychiatric Association.)

◗ Dora, a 30-year-old pharmacist, lives at home and cares for her mother. After her mother's death from heart disease, Dora begins to experience tension, irritability, and sleep disturbance. On several occasions, Dora awakens gasping for breath. Her heart pounds, and she feels a tight sensation, like a band around her chest. Her pulse typically increases to more than 110 beats per minute, and she experiences dizziness. She fears that she is going to die. On these occasions, Dora telephones a friend. The friend finds her wringing her hands, moaning, and appearing totally disorganized. In each instance, the friend takes Dora to the emergency department, where she remains overnight for observation and tests. All diagnostic test results are normal. The physician suggests that because no apparent organic basis exists for the episodes, they likely are panic attacks.

Beck (1996) emphasized that nurses can best help their clients if they learn to view panic as a separate concept from anxiety, especially in the clinical setting. Panic is not, according to Beck, a continuation of anxiety from moderate to severe; panic itself has an all-or-nothing quality, noted by its sudden and unexpected onset.

Panic Disorder with Agoraphobia

Panic disorder with agoraphobia is characterized by recurrent panic attacks combined with agoraphobia. **Agoraphobia** involves intense, excessive anxiety or fear about being in places or situations from which escape might be difficult or embarrassing, or in which help might not be available if a panic attack occurred (APA 1994). The feared places are avoided by the individual in an effort to control anxiety. Examples of places or situations that are commonly avoided by agoraphobics include being alone outside; being alone at home; traveling in a car, bus, or airplane; being on a bridge; and riding in an elevator. Avoidance behaviors can be debilitating and life constricting. Consider the effect on a father whose avoidance renders him unable to leave home and who thus cannot see his child's high school graduation, or the businesswoman whose avoidance of flying prevents her from attending distant business conferences, or the individual who avoids elevators and has no way to get to the twenty-seventh floor for an appointment.

◗ Jim is a 28-year-old man who suffers from panic attacks with agoraphobia. He once lived a very active life, often participating in thrill-seeking activities, like bungee jumping and skydiving. Jim's father, who had severe cardiovascular disease, died 2 years ago on his way to work. Since that time, Jim has become increasingly fearful of the outdoors. He gradually stopped leaving the family home because he experienced panic attacks; he feared that he would die if he left home.

Simple Agoraphobia

Agoraphobia without a history of panic disorder (i.e., unaccompanied by panic attacks) occurs only rarely, and it occurs early in the client's history. Over time, agoraphobia with panic attacks develops (Billings 1993b). Situations that trigger simple agoraphobia are the same as those listed earlier.

Specific and Social Phobias

A **phobia** is a persistent, irrational fear of a specific object, activity, or situation that leads to a desire for avoidance, or actual avoidance, of the object, activity, or situation (APA 1994). **Specific phobias** are characterized by the experience of high levels of anxiety or fear provoked by a specific object or situation, such as dogs, spiders, heights, storms, water, sight of blood, closed spaces, tunnels, and bridges (APA 1994). Specific phobias are common and usually do not cause much difficulty because people can contrive to avoid the feared object. Clinical names for common phobias are given in Table 17–2.

◗ Tran, who lives and works in Philadelphia, developed a morbid fear of closed spaces, such as elevators, after he read about the bombing of the World Trade Center in New York, even though he was not involved in the bombing. As his fear and anxiety intensified, it became necessary for him to use only stairs or escalators. Tran even became anxious if he had to enter closets or small storage rooms. Claustrophobia (fear of closed spaces) had developed.

Social phobias are characterized by severe anxiety or fear provoked by exposure to a social situation or a performance situation (e.g., saying something that sounds foolish in public, not being able to answer questions in a classroom, eating in public, and performing on stage).

TABLE 17–2 CLINICAL NAMES FOR COMMON PHOBIAS

CLINICAL NAME	FEARED OBJECT OR SITUATION
Acrophobia	Heights
Agoraphobia	Open spaces
Astraphobia	Electrical storms
Claustrophobia	Closed spaces
Glossophobia	Talking
Hematophobia	Blood
Hydrophobia	Water
Monophobia	Being alone
Mysophobia	Germs or dirt
Pyrophobia	Fire
Zoophobia	Animals

Fear of public speaking is the most common social phobia.

Characteristically, phobic individuals experience overwhelming and crippling anxiety when they are faced with the object of the phobia. Phobic people go to great lengths to avoid the feared object or situation. A phobic person may not be able to think about or visualize the object or situation without becoming severely anxious. The life of a phobic person becomes more restricted as activities are given up so that the phobic object is avoided. All too frequently, complications ensue when people try to decrease anxiety through self-medication with alcohol or drugs.

▶ Tim, age 22, a music theater major, develops a fear of performing on stage. He suffers severe anxiety attacks whenever he is scheduled to appear in a student production. Recently, he has become severely anxious when he is faced with classroom readings or singing solo in music class. He is thinking about changing his major.

Obsessive-Compulsive Disorder

Obsessions are defined as thoughts, impulses, or images that persist and recur, so that they cannot be dismissed from the mind. Obsessions often seem senseless to the individual who experiences them (ego-dystonic), while still causing the individual to experience severe anxiety.

Compulsions are ritualistic behaviors that an individual feels driven to perform in an attempt to reduce anxiety. The compulsive act temporarily reduces high levels of anxiety. Primary gain is achieved by compulsive rituals, but because the relief is only temporary, the compulsive act must be repeated again and again.

Although obsessions and compulsions can exist independently of each other, they most often occur together. Examples of common obsessions and compulsions are given in Table 17–3. Obsessive-compulsive behavior exists along a continuum. "Normal" individuals may experience mildly obsessive-compulsive behavior. Nearly everyone has had the experience of having a persistent tune run through the mind, despite attempts to push it

TABLE 17–3 COMMON OBSESSIONS AND COMPULSIONS

TYPE OF OBSESSION	EXAMPLE	ACCOMPANYING COMPULSION
Doubt/need to check	"Did I turn off the stove?" repeatedly intrudes upon the thinking of a woman who has recently gone from housewife to secretary.	Checks to see if appliance is turned off, returning home several times each workday.
Sexual imagery or ideation	Young woman has recurrent thought when in presence of a man, "Pat his buttocks."	Avoids the presence of men if possible; if with men, excuses self to wash hands every 10–15 minutes.
Need for order	"Everything must be in its place" is the recurrent thought.	Arranges and rearranges items.
Violence	Man repeatedly thinks the thought "I should kill her" when he sees blonde women.	Abruptly turns head away from women and squints eyes to try to avoid seeing blondes.
Germs or dirt	Woman ruminates, "Everything is contaminated."	Avoids touching all objects. Scrubs hands if she is forced to touch any object.
Illness or death	Adolescent boy repeatedly thinks, "My teeth are decaying."	Repeats ritual of brushing and flossing up to a dozen times an hour.
TYPE OF COMPULSION	**EXAMPLE**	**ACCOMPANYING OBSESSIONS**
Counting	Man counts aloud each step he takes.	Counting prevents mistakes and often serves to keep troublesome thoughts out of awareness.
Touching	Anorexic girl touches each doorknob she sees.	"Touch the knob or be a blob."
Washing or cleaning	Young woman repeatedly washes hands.	"Wash away my sins." Thought appeared after a sexual encounter with a married man.
Avoidance	Man uses a paper towel to touch objects touched by others.	"Maybe someone with AIDS touched it."
Doing or undoing	Woman walks forward, then backward, sits in a chair, then gets up and sits down again.	"Whatever I do has to be perfect or my husband won't love me."
Symmetry	Secretary lines up objects in rows on her desk, then realigns them repeatedly during the day.	"Secretaries who practice neatness never get fired."

AIDS, acquired immunodeficiency syndrome.

away. Many people have had nagging doubts as to whether a door is locked or the stove is turned off. These doubts require the person to go back to check the door or stove. Minor compulsions, such as touching a lucky charm, knocking on wood, and making the sign of the cross on hearing disturbing news, are not harmful to the individual. Mild compulsions about timeliness, orderliness, and reliability are valued traits in U.S. society.

At the pathological end of the continuum are obsessive-compulsive symptoms that typically involve issues of sexuality, violence, contamination, illness, or death. These obsessions or compulsions cause marked distress to the individual. People often feel humiliation and shame regarding these behaviors. The rituals are time consuming and interfere with normal routine, social activities, and relationships with others. Severe OCD consumes so much of the individual's mental processes that the performance of cognitive tasks may be impaired. Figure 17–3 shows positron-emission tomographic scans of OCD before and after successful pharmacological and behavioral treatment.

◗ Tina, a 32-year-old single parent, has OCD. She was born 12 years after her older sister to parents who were aloof, perfectionistic, and morally strict. Tina related that she often felt she was an unwanted child. Like her sister, she majored in business administration in college, but Tina presently earns considerably less than her sister. During her senior year of college, Tina became pregnant. She did not seek an abortion because she believed it to be morally wrong. The father of the baby left the area. Tina, too embarrassed to return home, quit school to support herself and the child. She works as a clerk and takes courses at night. The senior secretary who was her friend retired recently, and a younger woman was hired as a replacement.

◗ Recently, Tina started to have intrusive thoughts that some harm would come to her 10-year-old daughter. She recognizes the "stupid, irrational" nature of the obsessions and the disproportionate anxiety they cause, but she cannot control them either. She checks on her daughter's safety by calling school hourly. She does not allow her daughter to play sports, screens her daughter's friends, monitors her activities, and generally tries to control her daughter's every move. Tina hardly eats and has given up all social activities. She sleeps little at night because she repeatedly goes to her daughter's room "to check that she is safe."

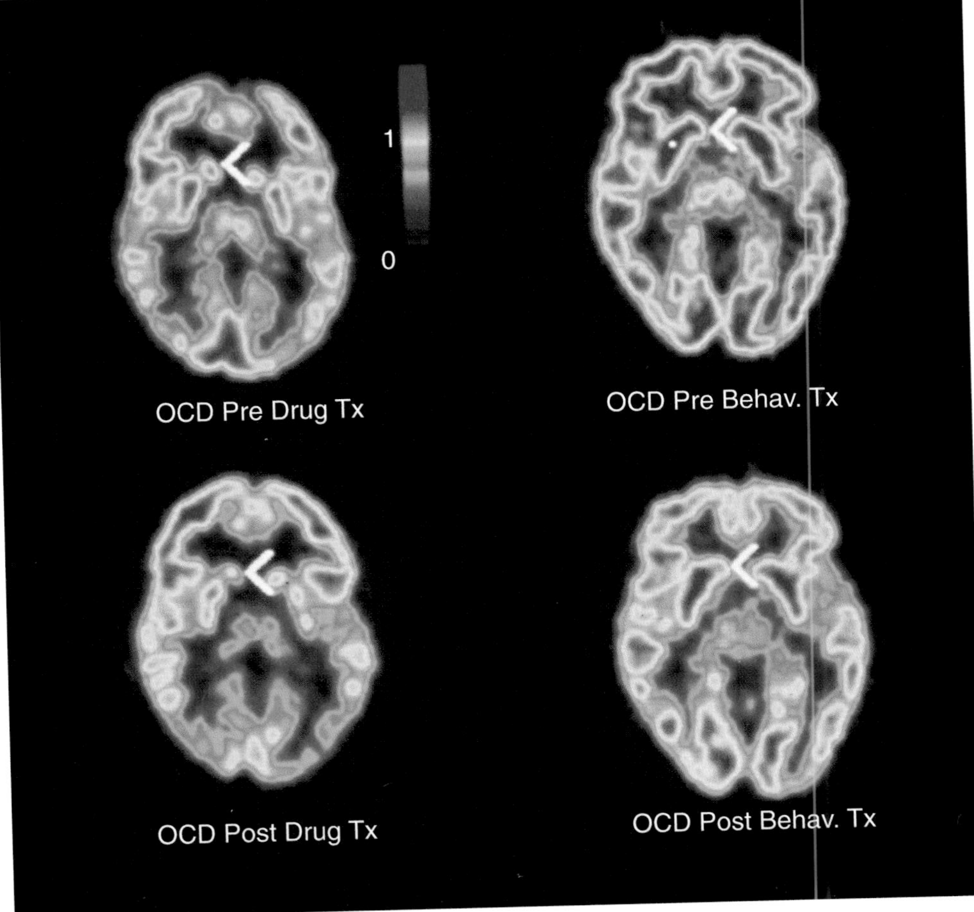

Figure 17–3 PET (positron emission tomography) scans of obsessive-compulsive disorder (OCD) clients show that the same reductions in brain caudate nucleus activity (center of brain) that occur after successful drug treatment with clomipramine are also produced by successful behavior therapy. The scans provide tangible evidence that OCD involves a brain dysfunction that can be corrected by treatment—behavioral or pharmacological. (From Lewis Baxter, MD, University of Alabama. Courtesy of the National Institutes of Mental Health.)

Generalized Anxiety Disorder

Generalized anxiety disorder is characterized by excessive anxiety or worrying about numerous things that lasts for 6 months or longer (APA 1994). The individual with generalized anxiety disorder also displays many of the following symptoms: restlessness, fatigue, poor concentration, irritability, tension, and sleep disturbance. The individual's worry is out of proportion to the true impact of the event or situation about which the individual is worried. Examples of worries typical in generalized anxiety disorder are inadequacy in interpersonal relationships, job responsibilities, finances, health of family members, household chores, and lateness for appointments. Sleep disturbance is common because the individual worries about the day's events and real or imagined mistakes, reviews past problems, and anticipates future difficulties. Decision making is difficult, owing to poor concentration and dread of making a mistake.

- June is a 49-year-old legal secretary. She comes to the clinic complaining of feeling "so anxious I could jump out of my skin." She is shaky and diaphoretic; she has dilated pupils, an elevated pulse, and a quivering voice. She tells the nurse "It was probably foolish to come here. Nobody understands me." June's only daughter is expecting her first child. Although the pregnancy is going well, June worries that something is wrong with the baby. "What if it's premature?" "What if it's deformed?"
- June describes herself as tense and irritable. She has difficulty initiating sleep and cannot concentrate at work. She worries about making mistakes at work, about being fired from her position, and about the financial problems that could result. She often says "I just can't cope." Her daughter has begun calling several times a day to reassure her that all is well with the pregnancy and to try to decrease June's worry over other matters. The daughter has also begun shopping and housecleaning for June "to help her get some rest."

Anxiety Due to Medical Conditions

In this disorder, the individual's symptoms of anxiety are a direct physiological result of a medical condition, such as pheochromocytoma, hyperthyroidism, pulmonary embolism, cardiac dysrhythmias, and chronic obstructive pulmonary disease (APA 1994).

- Edmund is a 67-year-old who has poorly controlled atrial fibrillation. His chief complaint is that he feels anxious most of the time. Edmund often experiences a feeling of impending doom and describes himself as "worrying a lot about my heart."

Substance-induced anxiety disorder is characterized by symptoms of anxiety, panic attacks, obsessions, and compulsions that developed with the use of the substance or within a month of stopping use of the substance (APA 1994).

- Juana is a 46-year-old advertising executive whose physician had prescribed diazepam (Valium) "for nerves" over a period of 2 years. When Juana changes physicians, she stops using diazepam. Three weeks after stopping the benzodiazepine, Juana begins to experience symptoms of severe anxiety and contacts her physician, who makes the diagnosis of substance-induced anxiety disorder arising as a result of diazepam withdrawal.

Anxiety disorder not otherwise specified, including mixed anxiety-depressive disorder, is a diagnostic category used for the coding of disorders in which anxiety or phobic avoidance predominates and which do not meet other diagnostic criteria.

Posttraumatic Stress Disorder

Posttraumatic stress disorder (APA 1994) is characterized by repeated re-experiencing of a highly traumatic event that involved actual or threatened death or serious injury to self or others, to which the individual responded with intense fear, helplessness, or horror. PTSD may occur after any traumatic event that is outside the range of usual experience; examples are military combat; experience as a prisoner of war; natural disasters, such as floods, tornadoes, and earthquakes; man-made disasters, such as plane and train accidents; crime-related events, such as bombings, assaults, muggings, rapes, and hostage taking; or a diagnosis of a life-threatening illness. PTSD symptoms often begin within 3 months after the trauma, but a delay of months or years is not uncommon (Fig. 17–4). The major features of PTSD are

1. Persistent re-experiencing of the trauma through recurrent intrusive recollections of the event, through dreams, and through flashbacks. (**Flashbacks** are dissociative experiences during which the event is relived and the person behaves as though experiencing the event at that time.).
2. Persistent avoidance of stimuli associated with the trauma that results in the individual's avoiding talking about the event or avoiding activities, people, or places that arouse memories of the trauma.
3. After the trauma, experiencing of persistent numbing of general responsiveness, as evidenced by feeling detached or estranged from others, feeling empty inside, feeling "turned off" to others.
4. After the trauma, experiencing of persistent symptoms of increased arousal, as evidenced by irritability, difficulty sleeping, difficulty concentrating, hypervigilance, or exaggerated startle response.

ANXIETY DISORDERS: STRESS RESPONSE

POSTTRAUMATIC STRESS DISORDER

1. The person experienced, witnessed, or was confronted with an event that involved actual, threatened death to self or others, responding in fear, helplessness, or horror.
2. The event is persistently reexperienced by:
   (a) Distressing dreams or images
   (b) Reliving the event through flashbacks, illusions, hallucinations
3. Persistent avoidance of stimuli associated with trauma:
   (a) Avoidance of thoughts, feelings, conversations
   (b) Avoidance of people, places, activities
   (c) Inability to recall aspects of trauma
   (d) Decreased interest in usual activities
   (e) Feelings of detachment, estrangement from others
   (f) Restriction in feelings (love, enthusiasm, joy)
   (g) Sense of shortened feelings
4. Persistent symptoms of increased arousal (two or more):
   (a) Difficulty falling/staying asleep
   (b) Irritability/outbursts of anger
   (c) Difficulty concentrating
5. **Duration more than 1 month:**
   - Acute: Duration less than 3 months
   - Chronic: Duration 3 months or more
   - Delayed: If onset of symptoms is at least 6 months after stress

ACUTE STRESS RESPONSE

1. The person experienced, witnessed, or was confronted with an event that involved actual, threatened death to self or others, responding in fear, helplessness, or horror.
2. Three or more of the following dissociative symptoms:
   (a) Sense of numbing, detachment, or absence of emotional response
   (b) Reduced awareness of surroundings (e.g., "in a daze")
   (c) Derealization
   (d) Depersonalization
   (e) Amnesia for an important aspect of the trauma
3. The event is persistently reexperienced by:
   (a) Distressing dreams or images
   (b) Reliving the event through flashbacks, illusions, hallucinations
4. Marked avoidance of stimuli that arouse memory of trauma (thoughts, feelings, people, places, activities, conversations).
5. Marked symptoms of anxiety:
   (a) Difficulty falling/staying asleep
   (b) Irritability/outbursts of anger
   (c) Difficulty concentrating
6. Causes impairment in social, occupational, and other functioning, or impairs ability to complete some memory tasks.
7. **Lasts from 2 days to 4 weeks, and occurs within 4 weeks of the traumatic event.**

Figure 17–4 DSM-IV diagnostic criteria for acute stress disorder. (Adapted from American Psychiatric Association (1994). *Diagnostic and statistical manual of mental disorders* (4th ed.). Washington, DC: American Psychiatric Association. Reprinted with permission. Copyright 1994 American Psychiatric Association.)

Difficulty with interpersonal, social, or occupational relationships nearly always accompanies PTSD, and trust is a common issue of concern. Child and spousal abuse may accompany hypervigilance and irritability. Chemical abuse may begin as an attempt to self-medicate to relieve anxiety.

▶ While visiting in Mexico, Julio experienced a severe earthquake. He was unhurt except for cuts and bruises, but he was trapped for 2 days in a collapsed building. Six months later, back in the United States, Julio says of himself, "I'm a mess! I can't relate to my friends the way I used to. I feel numb inside, and I can't concentrate on what anyone is saying to me." He re-experiences hearing and seeing the building collapse around him and feels the sense of fear he experienced when he thought that he might not be found in the rubble (flashback). He startles at any crackling, creaking, or rumbling noise. He is awakened at night by nightmares in which he is trapped.

It is important for health care workers to realize that exposure to stimuli that are reminiscent of the original trauma may cause an exacerbation of the trauma. For example, Noyes (1996) stated that the infamous bombing of Oklahoma City caused an exacerbation of symptoms in veterans from World War II, the Korean war, and the Vietnamese conflict.

Acute Stress Disorder

Acute stress disorder occurs within 1 month after exposure to a highly traumatic event, such as those listed in the section on PTSD. To be diagnosed with acute stress disorder, the individual must display three dissociative symptoms either during or after the traumatic event: a subjective sense of numbing, detachment, or absence of emotional responsiveness from the emotional experience; a reduction in awareness of surroundings; derealization (a sense of unreality related to the environment); depersonalization (experiencing a sense of unreality or self estrangement); or dissociative amnesia (loss of memory) (APA 1994).

▸ Barbara, a 22-year-old college student, is sexually assaulted by a family friend. In the emergency department, she describes feeling detached from her body and being unaware of her surroundings during the assault, "as though it took place in a vacuum." She displays virtually no affect (i.e., she does not cry or appear anxious, angry, or sad). Barbara finds it difficult to concentrate on the examiner's questions. Three days later, Barbara still feels as though her mind is detached from her body and reports having difficulty sleeping, poor concentration, and startling whenever anyone touches her. When she sees the nurse 4 weeks after the event, Barbara expresses feelings of anger and sadness over the assault, displays the ability to concentrate, and states that she no longer feels as though her mind and body were detached. She describes being able to "sleep better" and "not being so jittery and easily startled."

Assessing Clients

Anxiety disorders often exist with depressive disorders. For example, in approximately 50% of clients with panic disorders, at least one episode of major depression occurs in their lifetime (Gorman 1995). Likewise, clients with anxiety disorders are frequently diagnosed with addiction disorders. Therefore, systematic clinical assessment is needed to identify and differentiate coexisting or comorbid illnesses (Menninger 1995).

Because clients with anxiety disorders remain in contact with reality, they are usually able to collaborate with the nurse during assessment. Suggestions for questions that the nurse can use to gather assessment data are presented in Table 17–4.

Assessment should focus on collection of physical, psychological, and social data. The nurse should be particularly aware of the fact that major physical symptoms are often associated with autonomic nervous system stimulation. Specific symptoms should be noted, along with statements made by the client about subjective distress. The nurse must use clinical judgment to determine the level of anxiety being experienced by the client. Social data are important because clients with anxiety disorders are consumed by the need to keep anxiety at manageable levels, leaving them little time or energy to devote to personal growth or to develop mutually satisfying relationships.

Clients with anxiety disorders are at risk for suicide. For example, Weissman and colleagues (1989) found that

- 20% of subjects with panic disorder attempted suicide.
- 12% of subjects with panic attacks attempted suicide.
- 1% of subjects with no disorder attempted suicide.

Clinicians may use numerous tools when assessing anxious clients' syndromes. The Maudsley Obsessive-Compulsive Scale (Table 17–5) is useful in identifying various types of OCD symptoms. This tool gives the reader a sense of the anxious person's experience and the behaviors that can cause the anxious person significant distress.

NURSING DIAGNOSIS

Several nursing diagnoses should be considered for clients experiencing anxiety disorders. Causal statements vary with individual clients.

For example, **anxiety** may be related to

- Concern that a panic attack will occur.
- Exposure to phobic object or situation.
- Presence of obsessive thoughts.
- Interference with ability to perform compulsive acts.
- Recurrent memories of traumatic event.

Ineffective individual coping is common. It leads to interference in ability to work, disruptions in relationships, and drastic changes in ability to interact satisfactorily with others. Causes include

- Severe or panic-level anxiety.
- Excessive negative beliefs about self.
- Hypervigilence after a traumatic event.
- Presence of obsessions and compulsions associated with fear of contamination.
- Avoidance behavior associated with phobia (list phobia).

Altered thought processes may be considered as a nursing diagnosis when severe or panic-level anxiety is present. Causes include

- Inability to understand directions.
- Excessive use of reason and logic associated with overcautiousness and fear of making a mistake.
- Preoccupation with obsessive thoughts.
- Disorganization associated with exposure to phobic object or situation.

Self-esteem disturbance is nearly always present and is often related to inability to control ego-dystonic symptoms. **Powerlessness** related to inability to control symptoms may also be an appropriate diagnosis. A diagnosis of **altered role performance** is possible when assessment reveals inability to assume responsibilities associated with usual roles. **Altered health maintenance** may be diagnosed if ritualistic behavior or excessive caution prevents the individual from seeking health care.

TABLE 17–4 NURSING ASSESSMENT: ANXIETY DISORDERS

ASSESSMENT	DATA-GATHERING STRATEGIES
	Physical Parameters
Presence of anxiety	"Tell me what you are presently feeling." "Tell me about the symptoms of anxiety you experience." "Do you worry about feeling anxious or about having a panic attack?"
Potential to flee/fight	Observe appearance, behavior, posture, gait, expression.
Impact of anxiety on physical functioning	Monitor pulse, respirations, sleep patterns, elimination, appetite, energy level.
	Psychological Parameters
Understanding of illness	"What problems bring you here?" "Did this problem occur suddenly or over a period of time?" "Describe how you are feeling." Observe affect.
Mood	"How would you describe the mood you experience most of the time?"
Self-esteem	"What do you like and dislike about yourself?"
Normal coping ability	"When you experience stress, what do you do to decrease it?"
Defense mechanisms used	Observe and listen during interview. Note distractibility, vigilance.
Thought content or process	Note circumstantiality (many digressions before eventually concluding a thought), blocking (sudden stopping of speech because of anxiety). "Are you preoccupied with any idea?" "Does one thought repeatedly force itself into awareness?" "Do you have any especially strong fears?" "Do you try to avoid any situation for fear of embarrassing yourself?" "Do you avoid any object or situation, such as insects, heights, tunnels, water, darkness?" "Do you worry excessively?" "Do you perform rituals?"
Potential for suicide	If a client indicates feeling hopeless, helpless, or worthless, investigate whether he or she has considered suicide.
	Social Parameters
Characteristic patterns of relationships	"Describe your relationship with family/friends/peers."
Identification of stressors or threats to self-concept, role, values, social status, or support system.	"What do you think might be causing this problem?" "What changes occurred in your life this past year?"
Ability to function	"How is this problem interfering with your life?" Investigate effects on work, school, church, hobbies, social activities, sexual functioning.
Degree of strain in relationships	"Describe any strain on relationships with others this problem has caused." "How has this problem changed your relationship with . . . .?
Secondary gains	Note benefits to client as result of symptoms.
Diversional activity	"What do you like to do for fun or recreation?"

PLANNING

Planning Outcome Criteria

When nursing assessment has taken place and nursing diagnoses have been made, reasonable outcomes must be identified for each nursing diagnosis. Desired outcomes are then written in measurable behavioral terms. Table 17–6 lists nursing diagnoses relevant to anxiety disorders and offers examples of outcome criteria. Whenever possible, outcome criteria should be a collaborative process involving the client and members of the health care team. Client satisfaction with outcomes is more likely to occur if the client actually desired the outcome.

Anxiety disorders are encountered in numerous settings. Nurses encounter people with anxiety disorders in medical-surgical units while the people are undergoing treatment for physical illness, in outpatient medical or psychiatric clinics, in home care settings, or in schools,

TABLE 17–5 MAUDSLEY OBSESSIVE-COMPULSIVE INVENTORY

INSTRUCTIONS: Please answer each question by putting a circle around the "TRUE" or the "FALSE" following the question. There are no right or wrong answers and no trick questions. Work quickly and do not think about the exact meaning of the question.

1.	I avoid using public telephones because of possible contamination.	TRUE	FALSE
2.	I frequently get nasty thoughts and have difficulty in getting rid of them.	TRUE	FALSE
3.	I am more concerned than most people about honesty.	TRUE	FALSE
4.	I am often late because I can't seem to get through everything on time.	TRUE	FALSE
5.	I don't worry unduly about contamination if I touch an animal.	TRUE	FALSE
6.	I frequently have to check things (e.g., gas or water taps, doors) several times.	TRUE	FALSE
7.	I have a very strict conscience.	TRUE	FALSE
8.	I find that almost every day I am upset by unpleasant thoughts that come into my mind against my will.	TRUE	FALSE
9.	I do not worry unduly if I accidentally bump into somebody.	TRUE	FALSE
10.	I usually have serious doubts about the simple everyday things I do.	TRUE	FALSE
11.	Neither of my parents was very strict during my childhood.	TRUE	FALSE
12.	I tend to get behind in my work because I repeat things over and over again.	TRUE	FALSE
13.	I use only an average amount of soap.	TRUE	FALSE
14.	Some numbers are extremely unlucky.	TRUE	FALSE
15.	I do not check letters over and over again before mailing them.	TRUE	FALSE
16.	I do not take a long time to dress in the morning.	TRUE	FALSE
17.	I am not excessively concerned about cleanliness.	TRUE	FALSE
18.	One of my major problems is that I pay too much attention to detail.	TRUE	FALSE
19.	I can use well-kept toilets without any hesitation.	TRUE	FALSE
20.	My major problem is repeated checking.	TRUE	FALSE
21.	I am not unduly concerned about germs and diseases.	TRUE	FALSE
22.	I do not tend to check things more than once.	TRUE	FALSE
23.	I do not stick to a very strict routine when doing ordinary things.	TRUE	FALSE
24.	My hands do not feel dirty after touching money.	TRUE	FALSE
25.	I do not usually count when doing a routine task.	TRUE	FALSE
26.	I take rather a long time to complete my washing in the morning.	TRUE	FALSE
27.	I do not use a great deal of antiseptics.	TRUE	FALSE
28.	I spend a lot of time every day checking things over and over.	TRUE	FALSE
29.	Hanging and folding my clothes at night does not take up a lot of time.	TRUE	FALSE
30.	Even when I do something very carefully I often feel that it is not quite right.	TRUE	FALSE

From Hodgson, R., and Rachman, S. (1977), Obsessional-compulsive complaints. *Behavior Research and Therapy*, 15:389–395. Copyright 1977, with kind permission from Elsevier Science Ltd, The Boulevard, Langford Lane, Kidlington, U.K.

day hospitals, nursing homes, and so on. Cost containment measures generally preclude admitting clients with anxiety disorders to inpatient psychiatric units. Therefore, planning for care usually involves selecting interventions that can be implemented in a community setting.

Whenever possible, the client should be encouraged to participate actively in planning. By sharing decision making with the client, the nurse increases the likelihood that positive outcomes will be attained. Shared planning is especially appropriate with a client with mild or moderate anxiety. When the client is experiencing severe levels of anxiety, the client may be unable to participate in planning, requiring the nurse to take a more directive role. Nursing interventions for a client who is experiencing mild to moderate and severe levels of anxiety are discussed more fully in Chapter 13. Nursing care plans at the end of this chapter include nursing diagnoses commonly identified for clients with anxiety disorders, outcomes, key interventions, and rationales for the interventions:

- The plan for June, who has generalized anxiety disorder, can be seen in Nursing Care Plan 17–1. The seven interventions for anxiety listed in this nursing care plan can be used for anxious clients, regardless of the medical diagnosis.
- The plans for Dora, who has panic disorder; for Tran, who has a specific phobia of small spaces; and for Julio, who has PTSD, are shown in Nursing Care Plan 17–2.
- A plan for Tina, who has OCD, is shown in Nursing Care Plan 17– 3. This plan also shows the evaluation of outcomes.

TABLE 17–6 NURSING DIAGNOSES: ANXIETY DISORDERS

NURSING DIAGNOSIS	EXPECTED OUTCOMES
Anxiety related to unexpected panic attacks; related to reexperiencing traumatic events	Client will demonstrate psychological and physiological comfort by (date), as evidenced by ▶ Pulse and respiration within normal parameters. ▶ Absence of symptoms associated with autonomic stimulation. ▶ Statement that anxiety has decreased.
Ineffective individual coping related to excessive anxiety (related to distorted cognitive perception of problem)	Client will use alternative coping resources by (date), as evidenced by ▶ Appropriate balancing of dependence or distancing from others. ▶ Controlled expression of feelings. ▶ Successful use of problem-solving skills. ▶ Verbalization of ability to cope.
Self-esteem disturbance related to shame or guilt	Client will demonstrate improved self-esteem by (date), as evidenced by ▶ Giving accurate nonjudgmental self-assessment. ▶ Identifying personal strengths. ▶ Making positive statements about self. ▶ Reporting decreased shame or guilt.
Self-esteem disturbance related to change in role performance	Client will use ability to perform in usual roles at premorbid level by (date), as evidenced by ▶ Performing usual work and social activities and hobbies. ▶ Interacting with significant others in mutually supportive ways.
Altered thought processes related to severe anxiety	Client will demonstrate ability to concentrate by (date). Client will report absence of obsessive thoughts by (date). Client will report experiencing, and will exhibit, mild to moderate anxiety in presence of phobic object by (date).
Diversional activity deficit related to preoccupation with symptoms	Client will use leisure time constructively by (date), as evidenced by ▶ Listing diversional activities of interest. ▶ Participating in one diversional activity each day.
Social isolation related to avoidance behavior or related to shame associated with symptoms	Client will increase interaction with others by (date), as evidenced by ▶ Interacting with a significant other or peer daily for 20 minutes. ▶ Participating in two group activities each week.
Knowledge deficit related to dysfunctional appraisal of situation	Client will state relationship between anxiety and the developing of symptoms by (date).
Sleep-pattern disturbance related to physiological symptoms of anxiety	Client will express satisfaction with rest-sleep pattern by (date), as evidenced by ▶ Verbalizing, "I slept well." Client will appear rested by (date), as evidenced by ▶ Absence of yawning. ▶ Absence of dark circles under eyes.
Self-care deficit related to ritualistic behavior	Client will independently perform bathing, hygiene, grooming, and dressing tasks by (date), as evidenced by clean, appropriate appearance.
Altered nutrition (less than body requirements) related to inability to stop performance of rituals	Client will maintain ideal body weight ± 10 pounds, as evidenced by weekly weight graph.
Impaired skin integrity related to rituals of excessive washing or excessive picking at the skin	Client's skin will be intact, as evidenced by ▶ Absence of chapping or excoriation. ▶ Absence of scratches or other self-inflicted lesions.

Nurse's Feelings and Self-Assessment

While implementing the interventions set forth in the nursing care plans for clients with anxiety disorders, nurses may experience uncomfortable personal reactions. Self-monitoring is vital to identify feelings that originate in the nurse. Peer supervision is a helpful technique to ensure that both negative and positive countertransference feelings are appropriately resolved.

Often, anxiety originating in the client is experienced by the nurse empathically. To help the nurse who is unable to self-monitor effectively, Figure 17–5 depicts the cyclical nature of anxiety, both experienced and transmitted. The nurse may experience feelings of frustration or anger while implementing the care plans for clients with anxiety disorders. The rituals of the client with OCD may frustrate the nurse's need to accomplish certain tasks within a given time. Communication with the client with

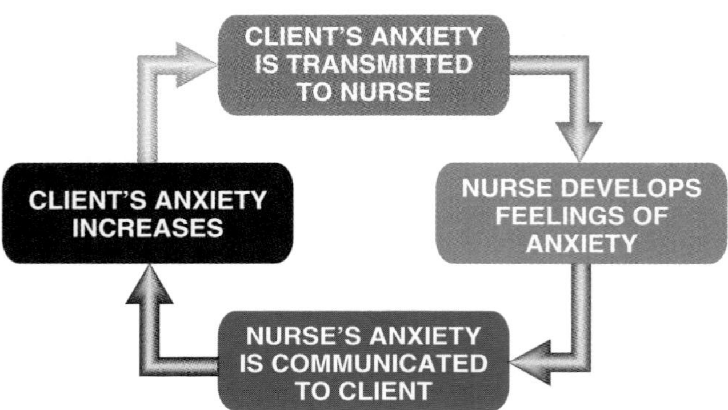

Figure 17–5 The cycle of transmitting anxiety between the nurse and the client.

OCD can also be frustrating. These clients correct and clarify repeatedly, as though they cannot let go of any topic. If the nurse uses therapeutic communication techniques, such as reflecting and paraphrasing, the client takes this opportunity to review material again and again, often angrily implying that the nurse has not understood. The client may introduce detail after detail, although the conversation becomes less and less clear. Communication requires much patience and the ability to provide clear structure.

In caring for the phobic client, the nurse may become frustrated after realizing that both client and nurse regard the fear as exaggerated and unrealistic, but the client is still unable to overcome the avoidant behavior. Behavioral change is often accomplished slowly. The process of recovery is different from that seen in a client with an infection, who is given antibiotics and demonstrates improvement within 24 hours. Nurses tend to become impatient with the anxious client and may feel angry when the client does not make rapid progress. Negative feelings are easily transmitted to the client, who then feels increasingly anxious.

The nurse who feels anger or frustration may withdraw from the client both emotionally and physically. This results in the client's feeling increasingly anxious and also withdrawing. Staging outcomes in small attainable steps can help prevent the nurse from feeling overwhelmed by the client's slow progress and can help the client gain a sense of control.

At the very least, the nurse often experiences increased tension and fatigue from mental strain when working with anxious clients. Because the client's anxiety is controlled for only a short time by his or her ego-dystonic behaviors, the client's anxiety recurs, and the nurse is called on to intervene again and again. Unlike the client whose dressing needs to be changed several times a week, the client with anxiety requires emotional bandaging many times a week.

It may be helpful for the nurse to consider the level of regression displayed by the client. When a client's behavior is viewed as regressive rather than perverse, it can help care providers intervene more effectively. For example, dependence, excessive demands, and frequent reassurance seeking are associated with the unmet needs of infancy and early childhood. Excessive neatness, rituals, obsessions, and pickiness are behaviors that are related to the period of toilet training. These behaviors provide clues to needs that must be met before the client can go on to develop more mature behaviors.

By having a clear understanding of the emotional pitfalls of working with clients who have anxiety disorders, the nurse is more prepared to minimize and avoid guilt associated with strong negative feelings. By examining personal feelings, the nurse is better able to understand their origin and to act objectively and constructively.

IMPLEMENTATION

Counseling/Therapy (Basic Level and Advanced Practice)

Psychiatric nurses use counseling to assist clients to improve or regain coping abilities, to foster mental health, and to prevent mental illness and disability. Treatment approaches that produce positive outcomes for clients with anxiety disorders include cognitive restructuring, relaxation training, and the behavioral techniques of modeling, graduated exposure (systematic desensitization therapy), flooding, and response prevention. Research has shown that combinations of these therapies may be more effective than single therapies (Blumenreich and Lippman 1994; Marks 1995). Advanced practice psychiatric nurses are able to prescribe and conduct the therapies described in this section. While the nurse generalist does not prescribe therapy, he or she is often the health professional who implements the prescribed counseling; thus, the nurse generalist must have a clear understanding of the various therapies.

Cognitive Restructuring

Cognitive therapy, which was introduced in Chapter 2, assumes that cognitive errors made by the client produce mistaken negative beliefs that persist, despite evidence to the contrary. These distortions in thinking result in negative self-talk.

Counseling to promote **cognitive restructuring** calls for the nurse to assist the client to identify automatic negative anxiety-arousing thoughts and negative self-talk, to help the client discover the basis for these thoughts, and to assist the client to appraise the situation realistically and to replace the negative self-talk with supportive and calming self-talk. Cognitive restructuring was used to help June, a client with generalized anxiety disorder.

NURSING CARE PLAN 17–1 A PERSON WITH ANXIETY DISORDER

NURSING DIAGNOSIS

Ineffective individual coping: related to anxiety

Supporting Data

- Increased muscle tension and restlessness.
- Reports feeling apprehensive, jittery, and shaky.
- States, "No one seems to understand."
- Voice quivering, frequently diaphoretic, pulse elevated, skin pale, and pupils dilated.

Outcome Criteria: Client will cope adaptively with anxiety.

CLIENT OUTCOMES	INTERVENTION	RATIONALE
1. Client will state that immediate distress is relieved by end of the session.	1a. Stay with client.	1a. Conveys acceptance and ability to give help.
	1b. Acknowledge the client's anxiety.	1b. Assists client in identifying feelings.
	1c. Speak slowly and calmly.	1c. Conveys calm and promotes security.
	1d. Use short, simple sentences.	1d. Promotes comprehension.
	1e. Assure client that you are in control and can assist him or her.	1e. Severe anxiety gives feeling of loss of control.
	1f. Give brief directions.	1f. Reduces indecision. Conveys belief that client can respond in healthy manner.
	1g. Decrease excessive stimuli; provide quiet environment.	1g. Reduces need to focus on diverse stimuli. Promotes ability to concentrate.
	1h. Walk with pacing client.	1h. Gives support while client uses anxiety-generated energy.
	1i. Increase level of supervision for acutely anxious client.	1i. Minimizes self-injury and loss of control.
	1j. Allow client to use defenses as long as physical well-being is not seriously jeopardized.	1j. Challenging defenses when client is acutely anxious causes further anxiety and may lead to panic.
	1k. After assessing level of anxiety, administer appropriate dose of anxiolytic agent, if warranted.	1k. Reduction of anxiety allows client to use coping skills.
	1l. Monitor and control own feelings.	1l. Anxiety is transmissible. Displays of negative emotion can cause client anxiety.
2. Client will state that he or she feels understood by nurse by end of the session.	2a. Listen.	2a. Conveys interest. Fosters trust. Provides tension relief. Permits data gathering. Identifies defenses.
	2b. Use empathy.	2b. Conveys concern. Helps client identify and accept feelings.
	2c. Focus on reality of present discomfort but not on ego-dystonic symptoms, e.g., rituals.	2c. Acknowledges client's distress but does not reinforce maladaptive behavior.
	2d. Encourage description of feelings.	2d. Facilitates identification of feelings.
	2e. Help client recognize anxiety.	2e. Overcomes denial, resistance.
	2f. Teach signs and symptoms of anxiety.	2f. Factual information promotes accurate perceptions and decreases excessive concern.

Continued on following page

NURSING CARE PLAN 17–1 A PERSON WITH ANXIETY DISORDER *(Continued)*

CLIENT OUTCOMES	INTERVENTION	RATIONALE
3. Client will be able to identify sources of anxiety by (date).	3a. Encourage client to discuss preceding events.	3a. Identification of stressors promotes future change.
	3b. Link client's behavior to feelings.	3b. Promotes self-awareness.
	3c. Teach cognitive therapy principles: ■ Anxiety is the result of a dysfunctional appraisal of a situation. ■ Anxiety is the result of automatic thinking	3c. Provides a basis for behavioral change.
	3d. Ask questions that clarify and promote logical thinking: "What evidence do you have?" "Explain the logic in that." "Are you basing that conclusion on fact or feeling?" "What's the worst thing that could happen?"	3d. Helps promote accurate cognition.
	3e. Have client give alternative interpretation.	3e. Broadens perspective. Helps client think in a new way about problem or symptom.
	3f. Instruct client to refer to self by first name and comment on own anxiety or thoughts, e.g. "June's heart is beating fast." "June thinks everyone is looking at her now."	3f. Increases self-awareness while distancing self from own anxiety.
4. Client will identify strengths and coping skills by (date)	4a. Identify what has provided relief in the past.	4a. Provides awareness of self as individual with some ability to cope.
	4b. Give positive reinforcement for use of healthy behavior.	4b. Positively reinforced behavior tends to be repeated.
	4c. Have client write assessment of strengths.	4c. Increases self-acceptance.
	4d. Have client realistically assess weaknesses and state ways to convert them to strengths.	4d. Weaknesses can become assets with careful work.

- Initially, June is assisted to identify several possible outcomes of making a mistake at work. The next step is to help her test the faulty thinking that making a mistake would automatically result in her being fired. June is able to see that being fired for making a mistake is highly unlikely. The same process is used to help June restructure her thinking about her daughter's pregnancy.
- In addition to working with June, the nurse gets in touch with June's daughter. Often, clients with anxiety disorders have "trained" significant others to act in ways that support their symptoms; this allows the client to receive secondary gains. June's daughter has taken over shopping and housecleaning for her mother. The nurse counsels June's daughter to allow her mother to gradually resume these activities.

Cognitive restructuring was also helpful to Jim:

- Jim is required to monitor and record his automatic thoughts and phobic avoidance behaviors. Whenever

NURSING CARE PLAN 17–1 A PERSON WITH ANXIETY DISORDER *(Continued)*

CLIENT OUTCOMES	INTERVENTION	RATIONALE
5. Client will use new effective coping strategies by (date)	5a. Provide support while new coping measures are learned.	5a. Promotes understanding of universality of feelings.
	5b. Assist client to decrease caffeine intake and increase daily exercise.	5b. Caffeine produces symptoms like those of anxiety. Exercise produces endorphins, which promote a sense of well-being.
	5c. Assist with practice of relaxation technique.	5c. Relaxation response is enhanced by frequent use. Competence in use increases self-esteem and feelings of being able to control symptoms.
	5d. Promote sleep with warm bath, warm milk, or sitting with client.	5d. Provides alternative to, and prevents overuse of, anxiolytics.
	5e. Encourage full schedule of activities, especially familiar ones client has enjoyed in the past.	5e. Expands anxiety-generated energy constructively. Decreases self-preoccupation. Increases self-esteem by providing success experiences.
	5f. Give positive feedback for capabilities and competence.	5f. Enhances self-esteem.
	5g. Have client use positive self-talk, e.g., "I can handle this" or "I can cope."	5g. Increases tolerance to anxiety.
6. Client will apply what is learned during therapy to life situation by (date).	6a. Provide opportunities to engage in normal (healthy) role behaviors.	6a. Strengthens role taking and view of self as having options.
	6b. Provide behavioral rehearsals for anticipated stressful situations.	6b. Predetermination of coping strategy and practice increases potential for success.
	6c. Discuss coping strategies client successfully uses.	6c. Reinforces use of healthy coping strategies.
7. Family will alter behavioral patterns that have been supportive of dysfunctional behavior by (date).	7a. Teach family to give reinforcement for use of healthy behaviors.	7a. Positively reinforced behaviors tend to be repeated.
	7b. Teach family not to take over roles normally reserved for client.	7b,c. Minimizes secondary gain.
	7c. Teach family to give attention to client, not to client's symptoms.	

Jim is faced with the need to leave his home, automatic thinking takes place: "When my father left home to go to work, he died. I'll die if I leave home to go to work." The nurse helps Jim to explore his father's health status in comparison with his own. This understanding helps Jim make a more rational appraisal of the possibility of his death.

Relaxation Training

Muscle groups cannot be both tense and relaxed at the same time; therefore, teaching a client how to relax the body results in tension reduction. Relaxation produces physiological effects that are opposite to those produced by anxiety (e.g., slowed heart rate, neuromuscular relax-

NURSING CARE PLAN 17–2 CLIENTS WITH PANIC DISORDER, PHOBIA, OR POSTTRAUMATIC STRESS DISORDER

PANIC DISORDER

NURSING DIAGNOSIS

Anxiety: panic attacks related to loss of significant other, unmet emotional needs, and negative thoughts about self.

CLIENT OUTCOMES	INTERVENTION	RATIONALE
1. Client's anxiety will decrease to moderate by (date).	1a. If hypercapnia occurs, instruct client to take slow, deep breaths. Breathe with client to obtain cooperation.	1a. Shifts focus from distressing symptoms.
	1b. Keep expectations minimal and simple.	1b. Anxiety limits ability to attend to complex tasks.
2. Client will gain mastery over panic episodes by (date).	2a. Help client connect feelings before attack with onset of attack: "What were you thinking about just before the attack?" "Can you identify what you were feeling just before the attack?"	2a. Physiological symptoms of anxiety usually appear first as the result of a stressor. They are immediately followed by automatic thoughts, e.g., "I'm dying" or "I'm going crazy," which are distorted assessments.
	2b. Help client recognize symptoms as resulting from anxiety, not from a catastrophic physical problem, e.g. ▪ Explain physical symptoms of anxiety. ▪ Discuss the fact that anxiety causes sensations similar to physical events, e.g., heart attack. *See the seven interventions in Nursing Care Plan 17–1.	2b. Factual information and alternative interpretations can help client recognize distortions in thought.
	2c. Teach client abdominal breathing, to be used immediately when anxiety is detected.	2c. Breaks cycle of escalating symptoms of anxiety.
	2d. Teach client to use positive self-talk, e.g., "I can control my anxiety."	2d. Cognitive restructuring is an effective way to replace negative self-talk.

ation, calm state of mind). Anxious clients should be counseled that learning an effective relaxation method can be beneficial. Various relaxation techniques are described later, in the section on health teaching.

Modeling

This technique, explained in Chapter 2, permits a client to see how an individual copes effectively with an object or a situation. In **modeling,** the client is expected to imitate the healthy coping behavior. The nurse often serves as a model of healthy behavior for clients, but family members and friends may also assume the role. Modeling was used by the nurse who, while working with Tran, did not show anxiety as she used elevators and obtained materials from storage.

Systematic Desensitization/Graduated Exposure

The technique of **systematic desensitization** through **graduated exposure** involves gradually introducing

NURSING CARE PLAN 17–2 CLIENTS WITH PANIC DISORDER, PHOBIA, OR POSTTRAUMATIC STRESS DISORDER *(Continued)*

PHOBIA

NURSING DIAGNOSIS

Fear: related to a specific object or situation.

CLIENT OUTCOMES	INTERVENTION	RATIONALE
1. Client will use adaptive coping strategies instead of avoidance	1a. Determine type of phobia and when it first appeared.	1a. Determines whether phobia developed as a result of trauma, childhood experiences, or adult experiences.
	1b. Have client list consequences of contacting feared object.	1b. Isolates a specific fear associated with the object, e.g., a specific fear of flying may be a fear of being hurt in a plane crash. These data can aid the therapist using cognitive therapy.
	1c. Discuss concept that clients may be afraid of own feelings and sensations, not of the object or situation.	1c. Casts doubt on the feared consequence of contact with the phobic object or situation.
	1d. Encourage client to practice techniques to promote relaxation and decrease physiologic sensations associated with fear or anxiety.	1d. Enhances client control over feelings and over level of anxiety.
	1e. Do not force client to face phobic object or situation on own.	1e. The treatment decision to use flooding or implosion must be carefully considered.
	1f. Model unafraid behavior in phobic situation and discuss with client.	1f. Role modeling provides an opportunity to see healthy response to the phobic object or situation.

Continued on following page

the client to a phobic object or situation in a predetermined sequence of least to most frightening. The following strategy might be used for an agoraphobic client like Jim.

At the direction of the therapist, the client may be asked to visualize being in a public place. When anxiety becomes severe, the client may be instructed to use a relaxation technique. When the imagined encounters become tolerable for the client, he or she goes on to work through a hierarchy of live (in vivo) exposures, for example:

1. Opening the door and leaving the house
2. Walking down a street within a block from home
3. Riding in a car with a trusted person more than a block from home
4. Entering a small shop to purchase one item
5. Going to a supermarket to purchase a small list of items
6. Attending a movie or a play

Often, the activity is first undertaken with a trusted supportive person present; then, it is undertaken alone. A psychiatrist, psychologist, or nurse therapist is usually responsible for setting up the hierarchy and for conducting the graduated exposure. However, the nurse generalist is often responsible for reinforcing gains made by the client by providing support as various objects on the continuum are revisited. At the Institute of Psychiatry in London, Marks (1995) reported that self-exposure treatment is being used more often in order to avoid frequent therapy sessions and to contain costs. The clinician's role is to teach the client how to perform the self-exposure.

NURSING CARE PLAN 17–2 CLIENTS WITH PANIC DISORDER, PHOBIA, OR POSTTRAUMATIC STRESS DISORDER *(Continued)*

POSTTRAUMATIC STRESS DISORDER

NURSING DIAGNOSIS

Posttraumatic stress response: related to a specific event.

CLIENT OUTCOMES	INTERVENTION	RATIONALE
1. Client will cope effectively with thoughts and feelings associated with traumatic events.	1a. Be honest, nonjudgmental, and empathetic.	1a. Builds trust.
	1b. Assess the type of trauma, e.g., natural or human induced.	1b. Victims of natural disasters experience less guilt. Victims of man-made disasters experience more humiliation and guilt.
	1c. Assess immediate posttraumatic reaction and later coping.	1c. Numbing and denial are common. Knowing the range of behavior can help assess impact and meaning of trauma.
	1d. Assess functioning before event, including drug and alcohol use.	1d. Knowing premorbid function may suggest additional diagnoses.
	1e. Assess drug and alcohol use since the event.	1e. Attempts to self-medicate are common to reduce anxiety or induce sleep.
	1f. Explore shattered assumptions, e.g., "I'm a good person; why did this happen to me?" "This is a safe world."	1f. Victims need to find meaning in the event. Helplessness and anxiety result from lost feelings of safety.
	1g. Promote discussion of possible meanings of event. Compare this situation with others that are worse.	1g. Helps client see self as less victimized, and his or her world as more understandable.
	1h. Suggest that client was not responsible for traumatic event but is responsible for learning to cope.	1h. Reduces powerlessness.
	1i. Encourage the use of social support system.	1i. Increases feelings of safety and of being understood.

Flooding (Implosion Therapy)

The purpose of flooding is to extinguish anxiety as a conditioned response. **Flooding** involves exposing an individual to large amounts of a stimulus that he or she finds undesirable. This technique may require the client to touch an object that is feared or found revolting or severely anxiety producing. For example, Sam, a client so obsessed with the idea of avoiding contamination that he used a paper towel to touch things, was required to touch objects in the room with his bare hand for an hour. Gradually, the client demonstrated less anxiety over having to touch "dirty" objects.

Response Prevention (Behavior Therapy)

Response prevention therapy is performed by a nurse practitioner or a clinical nurse specialist only on physician's orders. When compulsive individuals feel anxiety, they respond by performing a ritualized behavior with the hope of reducing anxiety; not permitting the individual to perform the compulsive behavior is termed *response prevention*. From response prevention, a form of behavior therapy, the client learns that anxiety can be managed if the compulsion is not carried out. Arlene, a client who engaged in hand-scrubbing after touching any object or person, was helped gradually to lengthen the time before

NURSING CARE PLAN 17–3 A PERSON WITH OBSESSIVE-COMPULSIVE DISORDER

NURSING DIAGNOSIS

Ineffective individual coping: related to unresolved conflict

Supporting Data

- Reported obsessive thoughts that daughter will be harmed
- Compulsive checking designed to ensure daughter's safety

Outcome Criteria: Client will demonstrate ability to cope effectively without the use of obsessive-compulsive behavior.

CLIENT OUTCOMES	INTERVENTION	RATIONALE	EVALUATION
1. By (date) client will experience a decrease in incidence of obsessive thinking and compulsive behavior, as evidenced by ▪ Normal food and fluid intake. ▪ Six hours of sleep per night. ▪ No calls to school.	1a. Anticipate needs, e.g., need for information.	1a. Increases feelings of security.	*GOAL MET* Client states that she likes the idea that the nurse explains things to her; she states that she worries less.
	1b. Focus on client rather than on symptoms.	1b. Reinforces self-worth.	Client is able to adhere to a schedule.
	1c. Permit client to call school six times per day for 2 days, then four times per day for 4 days, twice daily for 2 days, and no calls thereafter.	1c. Allowing performance of ritual prevents panic. Reduction in frequency of rituals leads to extinction.	Client has been able to call school according to schedule and not exceed moderate-level anxiety.
	1d. Firmly encourage client to attend and eat meals. Encourage nutritious snacks between meals.	1d. Limits must be placed on behaviors that threaten health.	Client is able to sit through meals without checking on daughter. Two-pound weight gain in past week.
	1e. Advise client to take sedation if client has not initiated sleep by midnight.	1e. Promotes relaxation and sleep.	Client initiates sleep within 45 minutes but awakens several times nightly. Refuses sedation because she has daytime grogginess.
	1f. Avoid hurrying client.	1f. Hurrying client increases anxiety and performance of rituals.	
2. By (date) client will state that she is able to dismiss obsessive thoughts and will acknowledge that compulsion is not carried out.	2a. Teach to interrupt obsessive thoughts by snapping on rubber band wrist. 2b. Give positive reinforcement for nonritualistic behavior.	2a,b. Gives control over obsessive thinking and compulsive rituals. Positive reinforcement promotes repetition of adaptive behavior.	*GOAL MET* By the sixth day, client states, "It's getting easier to ignore my obsessive thoughts."

Continued on following page

NURSING CARE PLAN 17–3 A PERSON WITH OBSESSIVE-COMPULSIVE DISORDER *(Continued)*

NURSING DIAGNOSIS

Disturbance in self-esteem: related to lack of perceived strengths

Supporting Data

- Verbalization of stupidity associated with not being able to manage life as well as sister can
- Statement that she is "stupid" for not being able to get rid of worrisome ideas

Outcome Criteria: Client will verbalize positive self-perception

CLIENT OUTCOMES	INTERVENTION	RATIONALE	EVALUATION
1. Client will list five good things about self by (date).	1. Encourage client to identify strengths.	1. Fosters realistic self-concept.	*GOAL MET* On seventh day, client talks with nurse about list of strengths.
2. Client will make realistic positive statements about self by (date).	2. Arrange for activities at which she can succeed. Give merited praise.	2. Raises self-esteem.	Client states that she sees that she copes well under difficult conditions as a single parent.
3. Self-deprecatory statements will be absent by (date).	3. Avoid power struggles. Expect cooperation.	3. Power struggles increase anxiety. When client loses power struggle, self-esteem is lowered. When staff loses, anger is generated.	Skilled negotiation by nurse avoids power struggle.

NURSING DIAGNOSIS

Diversional activity deficit: related to preoccupation with performance of rituals

Supporting Data

- Giving up all social activities

Outcome criteria: Client will balance work and pleasurable activity.

CLIENT OUTCOMES	INTERVENTION	RATIONALE	EVALUATION
1. Client will make list of things she used to enjoy by (date).	1. Encourage client to survey activities at which she was proficient and activities she enjoyed.	1. Reduces preoccupation with rituals. Provides anxiety relief. Fosters awareness that enjoyment is deserved.	*GOAL MET* Client lists activities she would enjoy. Attends activities as required but without enjoyment during the first week. Now shows enjoyment. Plans to take ceramics class and to attend single parents social group.
2. Client will engage in scheduled activity as assigned by (date).	2. Expect participation.	2. Relieves guilt over attendance.	
3. Client will choose daily activities and participate in them by (date).	3. Encourage helping of others during activities.	3. Lowers anxiety.	

scrubbing and to shorten the time of scrubbing. Eventually, the urges subsided. Such therapy not only changes behavior but also can change the brain's chemistry (Schwartz et al. 1996). At the beginning of the session, Arlene's anxiety was severe, but by the end, with support from the nurse, her anxiety had decreased to the point that she was able to touch a "clean" object without experiencing the urge to scrub.

NURSING CARE PLAN 17–3 A PERSON WITH OBSESSIVE-COMPULSIVE DISORDER *(Continued)*

NURSING DIAGNOSIS

Altered family process: related to client's domination of daughter

Supporting Data

- Not allowing daughter to play sports
- Screening daughter's friends
- Monitoring daughter's activities to the point of calling school several times daily

Outcome Criteria: Client will verbalize positive self-perception

CLIENT OUTCOME	INTERVENTION	RATIONALE	EVALUATION
1. Client will allow daughter to have appropriate social contacts and school activities by (date).	1. Using cognitive therapy techniques, evaluate the "dangers" she imagines for her daughter.	1. Promotes reality.	*GOAL MET* Client states that she understands that the dangers are more in her own mind than actual. Signs permission for daughter to play intramural sports. Allows daughter to attend peer group party.

Thought Stopping

Thought-stopping techniques have proved helpful to some clients with OCD. One technique calls for the client to shout "Stop!" when the obsession comes to mind. Eventually, the client learns to give the command silently. Another technique is to place a rubber band on the client's wrist with instructions to snap it whenever the obsession comes into awareness. Both techniques serve the purpose of helping the client dismiss the obsessive thought. This technique was helpful in treatment of Tina in the earlier vignette.

Milieu Therapy (Basic Level)

As mentioned earlier, most clients who demonstrate anxiety disorders can be treated successfully as outpatients. Hospital admission is necessary only if prolonged severe anxiety is present, if symptoms that interfere with the individual's health are present, or if the individual is suicidal. When hospitalization is necessary, the following features of the therapeutic milieu can be especially helpful to the client:

1. Structuring the daily routine to offer physical safety and predictability, thus reducing anxiety over the unknown
2. Providing daily activities to prevent constant focus on anxiety or symptoms
3. Providing therapeutic interactions
4. Evaluating and communicating the effects of the environment on the client to facilitate nursing care planning

Self-Care Activities (Basic Level)

Clients with anxiety disorders are usually able to meet their own basic physical needs. Self-care activities that are most likely to be affected are discussed in the following sections.

Nutrition and Fluid Intake

Clients who use ritualistic behaviors may be too involved with their rituals to take time to eat and drink; some phobic clients may be so afraid of germs that they cannot eat. In general, nutritious diets with snacks should be provided. Ade/quate intake should be firmly encouraged, but without entering into a power struggle. Weighing clients frequently (e.g., three times a week) is useful in assessing nutrition.

Personal Hygiene and Grooming

Some clients, especially those with OCD and phobias, may be excessively neat and may engage in time-consuming rituals associated with bathing and dressing. Hygiene, dressing, and grooming may take many hours. Maintenance of skin integrity may become a problem when the rituals involve excessive washing and the skin becomes excoriated and infected.

Some clients are indecisive about bathing or about what clothing should be worn. For the latter, limiting choices to two outfits is helpful. In the event of severe indecisiveness, simply presenting the client with the clothing to be worn may be necessary. The nurse may also need to remain with the client to give simple directions: "Put on your shirt . . . now, put on your slacks." Matter-of-fact support is effective in assisting the client to perform as much of the task as possible. The client should be encouraged to express thoughts and feelings about self-care. This communication can provide a basis for later health teaching or for ongoing dialogue about the client's abilities.

Elimination

Clients with OCD may be so involved with the performance of rituals that they may suppress the urge to void and defecate. Constipation and urinary tract infections may result. Interventions may include creating a regular schedule for taking the client to the bathroom.

Sleep

Anxious clients frequently have difficulty sleeping. Ritualistic clients may perform their rituals to the exclusion of resting and sleeping. Physical exhaustion may occur in highly ritualistic clients. Clients with generalized anxiety disorder, PTSD, and acute stress disorder often experience sleep disturbance from nightmares. Monitoring sleep and keeping a sleep record may be useful in establishing the diagnosis of **sleep pattern disturbance** and evaluating progress.

Psychobiologic Interventions (Basic Level)

Anxiolytics

Anxiolytic drugs (antianxiety drugs) can be used to treat the somatic and psychological symptoms of anxiety disorders. When moderate to severe anxiety is reduced, clients are better able to participate in therapies directed at their underlying problems. Table 17–7 presents the actions, indications for use, and daily doses of drugs commonly used in the treatment of anxiety disorders.

Symptoms of severe anxiety, such as that seen in panic disorder, can be treated with alprazolam (Xanax) and other short-acting benzodiazepines. Benzodiazepines (e.g., diazepam, alprazolam, lorazepam) should be used only on a short-term basis because dependence and addiction can develop quickly. However, Blair and associates (1996) cautioned against fear of addiction and undertreatment of anxiety disorders that could result from withholding a client's as-needed (prn) antianxiety dose. A survey of nurses found that 68% believed that addiction from hospitalized use of prn medication was "likely," whereas only 0.009% of clients (one in 10,096) actually become addicted as a result of hospitalized treatment (Blair et al. 1996). Benzodiazepines have many side effects, making it necessary for the nurse to take care in assessing clients' reactions to the drugs. The more common side effects of the benzodiazepines are listed by body system in Table 17–8.

By contrast, diphenylmethane antihistamines, such as hydroxyzine hydrochloride (Atarax) and hydroxyzine pamoate (Vistaril), relieve symptoms of anxiety but produce no dependence, tolerance, or intoxication. This group of drugs can be used for anxiety relief over an indefinite period.

Buspirone, another nonbenzodiazepine anxiolytic, does not cause dependence. Unlike the benzodiazepines and diphenylmethane antihistamines, buspirone does not produce an immediate calming effect. Thus, it cannot be given as a prn medication. Initial effects are experienced in 2 to 3 weeks, and full effects may take 4 to 6 weeks or even longer. Buspirone is particularly useful for the treatment of generalized anxiety disorder, which tends to be a long-term disorder. Clients taking this drug should be counseled to take the drug regularly for maximal effectiveness. Two to 3 weeks are required before the full antianxiety effect of this drug is achieved.

Antidepressants

Antidepressants also have a place in the treatment of anxiety disorders. Tricyclic antidepressants, such as imipramine (Tofranil), desipramine (Norpramine), and clomipramine (Anafranil), are used to reduce the frequency and intensity of panic attacks with or without agoraphobia. Clomipramine is the tricyclic antidepressant of choice for the treatment of OCD. PTSD is effectively treated with imipramine and amitriptyline (Elavil) (Sutherland and Davidson 1994). Tricyclic antidepressants have anticholinergic side effects that may be annoying enough to cause people to discontinue their use. Clients should be counseled that these side effects often disappear with time. Clients should also be counseled that tricyclic antidepressants may take 2 to 4 weeks to take effect. Monoamine oxidase inhibitors, such as phenelzine (Nardil) and tranylcypromine (Parnate), have also been found to be effective in the treatment of panic attacks and social phobias. An important nursing consideration is that clients taking monoamine oxidase inhibitors must adhere to a tyramine-free diet or risk life-threatening hypertensive crisis (see Chapter 20). Selective serotonin reuptake inhibitors, such as fluoxetine (Prozac), sertraline (Zoloft), paroxetine (Paxil), and fluvoxamine (Luvox), are used to treat panic disorder, agoraphobia, OCD (DeVaugh-Geiss 1994), and general-

TABLE 17–7 DRUG INFORMATION: TREATMENT OF ANXIETY DISORDERS

GENERIC NAME	TRADE NAME	USUAL DAILY DOSE (MG/DAY)	ACTION AND INDICATION
Benzodiazepines (BZDs)			
Alprazolam	Xanax	0.25–4.0	Increase GABA release and receptor binding at synapses. Show preferential effect on limbic system. Useful for short-term treatment of anxiety, dependence and tolerance can develop.
Clonazepam	Klonopin	0.5–20.0	
Diazepam	Valium	4–30	
Lorazepam	Ativan	2–6	
Oxazepam	Serax	30–60	
Antihistamines			
Hydroxyzine hydrochloride	Atarax	200–400	Depress subcortical centers. Produce **no dependence, tolerance, or intoxication.** Can be used for anxiety relief for indefinite periods.
Hydroxyzine pamoate	Vistaril	200–400	
Nonbenzodiozepine antianxiety agents			
Buspirone hydrochloride	BuSpar	15–30	Alleviates anxiety. Less sedating than the benzodiazepines. **Does not appear to produce physical or psychological dependence.** Requires 3 weeks or more to be effective.
Beta blockers			
Propranolol	Inderal	30–80	Used to relieve physical symptoms of anxiety, as in stage fright. Acts by attaching to sensors that detect arousal messages.
Tricyclics			
Amitriptyline	Elavil	150–300	Used to prevent panic attacks, phobias, and PTSD. Acts by regulating brain's reactions to serotonin. Clomipramine helpful for some in lowering obsessions in OCD.
Clomipramine	Anafranil	25–250	
Imipramine	Tofranil	150–300	
Nortriptyline	Aventyl, Pamelor	75–125	
Desipramine	Norpramin	100–300	
MAOIs			
Phenelzine	Nardil	45–90	Used to treat panic disorders, phobias, and PTSD. Acts by blocking reuptake of norepinephrine and serotonin in central nervous system.
SSRIs			
Sertraline	Zoloft	50–200	Used to treat OCD, panic, agoraphobia, generalized anxiety disorder. **Few anticholinergic effects.**
Fluoxetine	Prozac	10–40	
Paroxetine	Paxil	20–50	
Fluvoxamine	Luvox	100–300	

OCD, obsessive-compulsive disorder; PTSD, posttraumatic stress disorder; MAOI, monoamine oxidase inhibitor; GABA, gamma-aminobutyric acid; SSRI, selective serotonin reuptake inhibitor.

TABLE 17–8 SIDE EFFECTS OF BENZODIAZEPINES

CENTRAL NERVOUS SYSTEM	CARDIOVASCULAR	BLOOD	GASTRO INTESTINAL	OTHER
Drowsiness	Hypotension	Agranulocytosis, sore throat, fever	Dry mouth	Skin rash
Clumsiness	Palpitations	Thrombocytopenia, unusual bruising	Nausea, vomiting	Pain at injection site
Blurred vision	Tachycardia		Abdominal discomfort	Urinary retention
Slurred speech	Dizziness			Aggravation of narrow-angle glaucoma
Headache	Fainting			Menstrual irregularity
Mental confusion				
Disorientation				
Nystagmus				
Ataxia				
Agitation				
Sleep disturbance				
Psychological dependence				
Physical tolerance				

ized anxiety disorder. Selective serotonin reuptake inhibitors are less likely than tricyclic antidepressants to produce anticholinergic side effects but may cause agitation, headaches, gastrointestinal disturbances, or sexual dysfunction.

Beta blockers, such as propranolol (Inderal) and atenolol (Tenormin), can be helpful with anxiety disorders that are characterized by marked physical symptoms of anxiety, such as social phobia. Beta blockers are often given in a single dose in order to relieve severe physical symptoms of anxiety before a theatrical or concert performance, a public speaking engagement, or a job interview. Box 17–1 summarizes nursing implications and important client teaching as they relate to antianxiety drug therapy.

The nurse generalist is responsible for administering medications; evaluating client response; educating clients and families about the medications, their side effects, and

BOX 17–1 CLIENT TEACHING IN ANTIANXIETY DRUG THERAPY

ASSESSMENT

1. Identify other medications or drugs the client is taking.
2. Assess frequency of client requests for medication (many anxiolytics are schedule IV controlled substances).
3. Observe for indications that client is exceeding recommended dosage (e.g., ataxia, mental confusion, dizziness, slurred speech, and other symptoms of intoxication).
4. Observe for paradoxical excitation (e.g., restlessness, rage, and agitation); more common in elderly.
5. Observe for sleep disturbance: nightmares and vivid dreams may occur related to stage IV sleep suppression.
6. Assess change in urinary frequency, odor, or color because urinary retention may occur.
7. Before initiating medication, record presence or absence of skin rash, flulike symptoms, or bruising.
8. Obtain information about baseline sexual functioning because changes in libido or functioning may occur, causing client to discontinue medication without discussing with therapist.
9. Obtain information about menstrual regularity because irregularity may occur.

CLIENT TEACHING

1. Caution client not to increase dose or frequency of ingestion without prior approval of therapist.
2. Caution client that these medications reduce ability to handle mechanical equipment, e.g., cars, saws, and machinery.
3. Caution client not to drink alcoholic beverages or take other antianxiety drugs because depressant effects of both would be potentiated.
4. Caution client to avoid drinking beverages containing caffeine because it decreases the desired effects of the drug.
5. Caution women to avoid becoming pregnant because taking benzodiazepines increases the risk of congenital anomalies.
6. Caution new mothers taking benzodiazepines not to breast-feed because the drug is excreted in the milk and would have adverse effects on the infant.
7. Teach clients taking monoamine oxidase inhibitors and the details of tyramine-restricted diet. (see Chapter 20).

OTHER NURSING MEASURES

1. Abrupt stoppage of benzodiazepines after 3 to 4 months of daily use may cause withdrawal symptoms, e.g., insomnia, irritability, nervousness, dry mouth, tremors, convulsions, and confusion.
2. Remain with the client until medication is swallowed.
3. Medications should be taken with, or shortly after, meals or snacks to reduce gastrointestinal discomfort.
4. Be alert for possible drug interactions:
   - Antacids may delay absorption.
   - Cimetidine interferes with metabolism of benzodiazepines, causing increased sedation.
   - Central nervous system depressants, e.g., alcohol and barbiturates, cause increased sedation
   - Phenytoin serum concentration may build up because of decreased metabolism.
5. Lower doses should be considered for elderly clients.
6. Read drug literature carefully regarding reconstitution, storage, and administration of parenteral drugs:
   - Some drugs, e.g., hydroxine pamoate and diazepam, produce irritation at intramuscular injection sites.
   - Diazepam and chlordiazepoxide require slow intravenous injection.
   - Do not use if solution is cloudy or discolored.
   - Some drugs must be stored away from light.
7. When intramuscular injection is ordered, administer deeply and slowly into large muscle to minimize irritation and discomfort.
8. After intramuscular or intravenous administration, the client should remain recumbent to minimize orthostatic hypotension.
9. Note contraindications of administration of individual drugs, e.g., many benzodiazepines should not be given to clients in shock, clients with narrow-angle glaucoma, or clients with hepatic or renal disease.
10. Investigate complaints of sore throat or fever as possible symptoms of agranulocytosis.
11. Adopt a positive attitude that medication will be effective.

ways to diminish them; and educating about when to call the physician. The advanced practice nurse may have prescriptive privileges to treat anxiety disorders with pharmacologic agents, in addition to determining other aspects of the treatment plan. Table 17–9 summarizes accepted pharmacological therapy and effective therapeutic modalities for selected anxiety disorders.

Health Teaching (Basic Level)

Clients often lack accurate knowledge about symptoms of anxiety, effects of stress on the body, and healthful methods for coping with stress and anxiety. The nurse generalist has the expertise to teach clients about many important health practices.

Nutrition

Clients with anxiety disorders should be taught that caffeine can intensify symptoms of anxiety by keeping a person in a chronically tense and aroused state. Such clients are encouraged to assess caffeine intake and set goals to consume less than 100 mg/day, the amount found in one cup of coffee or two diet cola beverages. The nurse needs

TABLE 17–9 ACCEPTED TREATMENT FOR SELECTED ANXIETY DISORDERS

DISORDER	PHARMACOTHERAPY	THERAPEUTIC MODALITY	COMMENTS
Panic disorder	**Antidepressants** a. TCAs (imipramine) b. SSRIs c. MAOIs (second-line therapy because of dietary restrictions) **Benzodiazepines** a. Alprazolam (Xanax) Lorazepam (Ativan) Clonazepam (Klonopin)	Cognitive behavioral therapy (CBT) Behavioral Relaxation Breathing techniques	Current CBT emphasizes a. Information on anxiety and the panic cycle. b. Symptom management (relaxation breathing). c. Cognitive restructuring. d. Systematic desensitization. e. In vivo exposure aimed at elementary avoidance behavior.
Agoraphobia	a. Treatment of panic attacks (above) if present b. Phenelzine (Nardil), an MAOI, may have anti-agoraphobic effects	Behavioral	Systematic desensitization. Deep muscle relaxation. Rebreathing techniques. Self-hypnosis. Biofeedback.
		Cognitive therapy	Recognition of irrational beliefs. Stopping of irrational thoughts. Replacing of irrational thoughts with new thoughts or activities.
		Insight-oriented psychotherapy	Especially for agoraphobia without history of panic disorder.
Generalized anxiety disorder	a. Benzodiazepines b. Buspirone c. TCAs, especially imipramine	Cognitive therapy Behavioral therapy	
Posttraumatic stress disorder	a. MAOIs (especially phenelzine) may diminish nightmares and flashbacks b. TCAs (imipramine and amitriptyline) and SSRIs for depressive symptoms	Psychotherapy Family therapy Vocational rehabilitation Group therapy Relaxation techniques	More than one treatment modality should be used:* a. Establish support. b. Focus on abreaction, survivor guilt or shame, anger, and helplessness.
Obsessive compulsive disorder	a. SSRIs (fluvoxamine [Luvox] and fluoxetine [Prozac]) b. Clomipramine (Anafranil) (TCA)	Behavioral therapy	Effective and necessary in addition to serotonergic medications. Exposure in vivo plus response prevention are the crucial essential factors.

Data from Billings, C. K. (1993). An update on panic disorder, agoraphobia and social phobia. Workshop sponsored by U. S. Psychiatric and Mental Health Congress, New Orleans, LA, December 3 1993; Menninger W. W. (1995). Coping with anxiety: Integrated approaches to treatment. *Bulletin of the Menninger Clinic*, 59(2):A4–A26.

TCA, tricyclic antidepressant; MAOI, monoamine oxidase inhibitor; SSRI, selective serotonin reuptake inhibitor.

*The sooner treatment begins, the more successful recovery is likely to be.

to teach about the sources of caffeine in the diet and about ways to reduce caffeine intake. Vitamins of the B complex and vitamin C are considered by some clinicians to be antistress vitamins. Teaching clients about natural sources of these vitamins can promote general well-being. Based on knowledge that an adequate level of serotonin is necessary for proper brain function, teaching the importance of including tryptophan-rich foods, such as turkey, tuna, milk, and eggs, in the diet may be helpful. (Tryptophan is a precursor of serotonin.)

Relaxation Techniques

Learning to achieve a deep state of relaxation and practicing relaxation for 20 to 30 minutes daily has the effect of reducing generalized anxiety. Some of the common methods of achieving a state of deep relaxation include abdominal breathing, progressive muscle relaxation, visualizing a peaceful scene, and meditation (refer to Chapter 13).

People who are anxiety ridden often have ineffective breathing patterns (e.g., breathing in a shallow fashion from the top of the chest, hyperventilating). Abdominal breathing promotes relaxation and can easily be taught to clients (Box 17–2).

Progressive Muscle Relaxation

Progressive muscle relaxation is helpful for people whose anxiety is associated with muscle tension. The client should be taught the following:

1. Practice the technique at least 20 minutes twice a day, at regular times.
2. Select a quiet location that is undisturbed by telephones or other interruptions.
3. Assume a comfortable position lying on a bed or sitting in a reclining chair.
4. Loosen tight clothing.
5. Adopt a detached “let it happen” attitude rather than worrying about the need to relax.
6. Take three deep abdominal breaths, imagining that the tension is flowing out of your body with each breath.
7. Then, using a predetermined sequence, perhaps beginning with the toes and moving upward (toes, calves, thighs, buttocks, lower back, stomach, chest, fingers, forearms, upper arms, shoulders, neck, chin/mouth, eyes, forehead), tighten the muscles of the selected area. Hold, then relax.

The nurse can direct the sequence for tensing and relaxing the muscles, or an audiotape can be used. Eventually, the client should be able to perform the tensing and relaxing without external direction.

Visualization

Visualizing a peaceful scene is a technique that can initially be used after progressive muscle relaxation or any other relaxation technique. The client must be able to identify the peaceful scene that he or she wishes to visualize and describe it in detail to the nurse or write it down. The written script can be taped and played after the progressive muscle relaxation instructions. A typical script is shown in Box 17–3.

Meditation

Meditation may be a skill that some clients have already learned. It allows an individual to focus only on “being”

BOX 17–2 TEACHING ABDOMINAL BREATHING

Instruct the client to do the following:

1. Place one hand on your abdomen beneath your rib cage.
2. Inhale slowly and deeply through your nose, sending the air as far down into your lungs as you can. Your hand should rise.
3. After taking the full breath, pause for a moment, then exhale slowly and fully.
4. As you exhale, allow your whole body to go limp.
5. Count each breath up to 10 by saying the appropriate number after each exhalation.
6. Do two or three sets of 10 abdominal breaths; this produces a state of considerable relaxation.

BOX 17–3 SCRIPT FOR VISUALIZING A PEACEFUL SCENE

Imagine releasing all the tension in your body . . . letting it go.

Now with every breath you take, feel your body drifting down deeper and deeper into relaxation . . . floating down . . . deeper and deeper.

Imagine your peaceful scene. You are sitting beside a clear blue mountain stream. You are barefoot, and you feel the sun-warmed rock under your feet. You hear the sound of the stream tumbling over the rocks. The sound is hypnotic, and you relax more and more. You see the tall pine trees on the opposite shore bending in the gentle breeze. Breathe the clean, pine-scented air, each breath moving you deeper and deeper into relaxation. The sun warms your face.

You are very comfortable. There is nothing to disturb you. You experience a feeling of well-being.

You can return to this peaceful scene by taking time to relax. The positive feelings can grow stronger and stronger each time you choose to relax.

You can return to your activities now, feeling relaxed and refreshed.

rather than doing. It requires that a person stop, let go of thoughts about the past or the future, and focus on being in the here and now. A *mantra* (a sound or word) is repeated mentally while the person sits in a quiet place. All other distractions just pass through the mind. Although meditation takes persistent, disciplined effort and is often easier to learn in a class or group, a nurse generalist who practices meditation can teach clients.

Value of Regular Physical Exercise

An excellent method for reducing generalized anxiety and combating panic attacks and phobic anxiety is regular exercise. Exercise fosters metabolism of adrenaline, the chemical responsible for the "fight or fight" arousal experienced by clients with anxiety disorders. Exercise also stimulates the production of endorphins, which are natural substances that increase the sense of well-being. Before a client undertakes an exercise program, the nurse should help the client assess personal fitness level and consider what type of exercise the client prefers. Realistic goals must be established to prevent both physical harm and "dropout." Walking is often the best choice for someone beginning an exercise program.

Social Skills

Nurse generalists are in an excellent position to identify teaching needs that will allow the client to develop effective social skills. One method is role playing, which allows clients to gain confidence by rehearsing approaches to difficult situations. Assertiveness training can heighten self-awareness and should include methods for expressing feelings, asking for what is desired, and saying no to something that is not wanted. Being unable to do these things creates tension and anxiety. Being able to behave assertively gives confidence and increased self-esteem. Nurse generalists can teach and role model assertive behavior for clients.

Case Management (Basic Level)

Case management aims to provide continuity of care, cost-effective use of resources, and reduced readmissions. Case management for clients with anxiety disorders is usually provided in an outpatient setting. For most clients with anxiety disorders, case management involves the components of resource linkage, consultation, advocacy, crisis intervention, and psychiatric rehabilitation.

Two distinct schools of thought exist regarding who may be a case manager. In psychiatric nursing, the advanced practice nurse is the preferred case manager; this type of nurse is able to provide comprehensive therapy services in addition to performing case management tasks. Nurse generalists can be called on by the case manager to provide education, advocacy, linkage, and so on, under the direction of the case manager. In areas where a shortage of advanced practice nurses exists, nurse generalists may assume the case manager position.

The case manager for Dora was a psychiatric nurse clinical specialist. She prescribed the following program for Dora:

1. Imipramine, 300 mg daily.
2. Training in abdominal breathing to be used at the first sign of rising anxiety.
3. Use of positive self-talk when experiencing anxiety: "I can control my anxiety. My breathing and my heart will slow. I will feel calm."
4. Reduction in caffeine intake to 1 cup of coffee per day.

In addition, Dora was encouraged to engage in an hour of vigorous physical exercise at least three times weekly and had clinic appointments at weekly intervals. When the case manager took her to a community-based, self-help group meeting for individuals with anxiety disorders, Dora decided to join the group. In the event of an impending panic attack, Dora was instructed to call her case manager, who would provide crisis intervention in an effort to avoid an expensive ED visit.

Health Promotion and Health Maintenance (Basic Level)

Clients with anxiety disorders may ignore basic rules of health maintenance, such as having physical and dental examinations. Many are too embarrassed by their symptoms or too involved with the symptoms to make and keep health care appointments. Caregivers need to remember to focus on the health of the whole person as opposed to treating only the presenting symptoms.

EVALUATION

Identified outcomes serve as the basis for evaluation. In general, evaluation of outcomes for clients with anxiety disorders deals with questions such as the following:

- Is the client experiencing a reduced level of anxiety?
- Does the client recognize symptoms as anxiety related?
- Does the client continue to display obsessions, compulsions, phobias, worry, or other symptoms of anxiety disorders?
- Is the client able to use newly learned behaviors to manage anxiety?
- Can the client adequately perform self-care activities?
- Can the client maintain satisfying interpersonal relations?
- Can the client assume usual roles?

SUMMARY

Individuals with anxiety disorders experience high levels of anxiety or use ritualistic behaviors. Clients who have panic disorder and generalized anxiety disorder experience diffuse symptoms of anxiety.

Clients with phobias experience extreme fear of certain objects or situations and go to great lengths to avoid the feared object or situation.

Clients who have obsessions and compulsions experience the presence of repetitive, intrusive thoughts and the repetitive need to perform ritualized actions designed to relieve anxiety. Clients with acute stress disorder and PTSD experience the symptoms of acute anxiety, in addition to re-experiencing the traumatic event via nightmares, flashbacks, and illusions.

Clients with anxiety disorders have the ability to stay in touch with reality, while not being in touch with their true feelings. Individuals with anxiety disorders expend great amounts of psychological energy and use multiple ego defense mechanisms to cope with anxiety, only to find that the defenses are inadequate for long-term anxiety reduction. These individuals recognize that the symptoms being experienced are odd or strange (ego-dystonic).

Issues of primary and secondary gain are present with anxiety disorders. Primary gain relieves discomfort, while secondary gain reinforces the sick role. Individuals with anxiety disorders share the common experience of low self-esteem associated with powerlessness to control ego-dystonic symptoms.

The presence of negative self-talk is nearly universal among clients with anxiety disorder; in clients who use it, cognitive restructuring may be helpful. Research has demonstrated positive responses to combined therapies involving cognitive, behavioral, educative, and psychobiological approaches.

Clients with anxiety disorders seem to have the ability to incite predictable negative feelings in health care workers, making it necessary for nurses to practice self-assessment and use supervision to resolve uncomfortable reactions. Clients with anxiety disorders usually have positive responses to staff who demonstrate a nonjudgmental, calm demeanor.

Nurses are challenged to use the nursing process to provide effective treatment for clients with anxiety disorders. Nurses are called on to educate both clients and significant others regarding the need for active participation in the treatment process in order to produce desired outcomes.

REFERENCES

American Psychiatric Association. (1994). *Diagnostic and statistical manual of mental disorders* (4th ed.). Washington, DC: American Psychiatric Association.

Beck, C. T. (1996). A concept analysis of panic. *Archives of Psychiatric Nursing*, 10(5):165.

Bille, D. A. (1993). Road to recovery, post traumatic stress disorder: The hidden victim. *Journal of Psychosocial Nursing Mental Health Services*, 31(9):19.

Billings, C. K. (1993b). An update on panic disorder, agoraphobia and social phobia. Workshop sponsored by U. S. Psychiatric & Mental Health Congress, New Orleans, December 3, 1993.

Blair, D., et al. (1996). The undertreatment of anxiety: Overcoming the confusion and stigma. *Journal of Psychosocial Nursing and Mental Health Services*, 24(6):9.

Blumenreich, P. E., and Lippman, S. B. (1994). Phobias: How to help patients overcome irrational fears. *Postgraduate Medicine*, 96(1):125.

Bremner, J.D. et al. (1997). Magnetic resonance imaging-based measurement of hippocampal volume in posttraumatic stress disorder related to childhood sexual abuse. *Biological Psychiatry*, 41(1):23–32.

DeVaugh-Geiss, J. (1994). Pharmacologic therapy of obsessive compulsive disorder. *Advanced Pharmacology*, 30:35.

Ellis, A. (1962). *Reason and emotion in psychotherapy*. New York: Lyle Stuart.

Gorman, J. (1995). Depression and comorbid panic. Workshop sponsored by U.S. Psychiatric & Mental Health Congress, New York, November 16, 1995.

Jenike, M. (1993). Neurobiology of anxiety disorders. Workshop sponsored by U. S. Psychiatric & Mental Health Congress, New Orleans, December 3, 1993.

Jenike, M., and Rauch, S. (1994). Managing the patient with treatment-resistant obsessive compulsive disorder: Current strategies. *Journal of Clinical Psychiatry*, 55(Suppl. 3):11.

Kaplan, H., et al. (1994). *Kaplan and Sadock's synopsis of psychiatry*. Baltimore: Williams & Wilkins.

Leff, J. (1988). *Psychiatry around the globe: A transcultural view* (2nd ed.). London: Royal College of Psychiatrists.

Marks, I. (1995). Advances in behavioral-cognitive therapy of social phobia. *Journal of Clinical Psychiatry*, 56(Suppl. 5):25.

Menninger, W. W. (1995). Coping with anxiety: Integrated approaches to treatment. *Bulletin of the Menninger Clinic*, 59(2):A4.

Noyes, F. (1996). Oklahoma city bombing: Evaluation of symptoms in veterans with PTSD. *Archives of Psychiatric Nursing*, 10(1):55.

Noyes, R., and Holt, C. (1994). Anxiety disorders. In G. Winokur and P. Clayton (Eds.), *The medical book of psychiatry* (pp 139–160). Philadelphia: W. B. Saunders.

Preston, J., and Johnson, J. (1995). *Clinical pharmacology made ridiculously simple*. Miami: MedMaster.

Schwartz, J. M., et al. (1996). Systematic changes in cerebral glucose metabolic rate after successful behavior modification treatments of obsessive-compulsive disorder. *Archives of General Psychiatry*, 53(2):109.

Sutherland, S., and Davidson, J.R. (1994). Pharmacotherapy for post-traumatic stress disorder. *Psychiatric Clinics of North America*, 17(2):409.

Teicher, M. H., Glod, C.A., Surray, J., and Swett, C. (1993). Effects of childhood abuse on brain development. *Journal of Neuropsychiatry and Clinical Neuroscience*, 5(3):301–306.

Weissman, M. M., et al. (1989). Suicidal ideation and suicide attempts in panic disorder and attacks. *New England Journal of Medicine*, 321:1209.

Further Reading

Billings, C. K. (1993a). Consequences of untreated anxiety. Workshop sponsored by U. S. Psychiatric & Mental Health Congress, New Orleans, December 4, 1993.

Billings, C. K. (1993c). Anxiety, depression and the heart. Workshop sponsored by U. S. Psychiatric & Mental Health Congress, New Orleans, December 3, 1993.

Dahl, J., and O'Neal, J. (1993). Stress and coping behaviors of nurses in Desert Storm. *Journal of Psychosocial Nursing Mental Health Services*, 31(2):29.

Jefferson, J. W. (1995). Social phobia: A pharmacologic treatment overview. *Journal of Clinical Psychiatry*, 56(Suppl. 5):18.

Lepine, J. P., et al. (1993). Suicide attempts in patients with panic disorder. *Archives of General Psychiatry*, 50(2):144.

Lipinski, J., and Pope, H. (1994). Do "flashbacks" represent obsessional imagery? *Comprehensive Psychiatry*, 35(4):245.

Mackenzie, T. (1994). Obsessive compulsive neurosis. In G. Winokur and P. Clayton (Eds.), *The medical book of psychiatry* (pp. 161–168). Philadelphia: W. B. Saunders.

Menninger, W. W. (1994). Psychotherapy and integrated treatment of social phobia and comorbid conditions. *Bulletin of the Menninger Clinic*, 58(2 Suppl, A):84.

Ost, I. G., and Westling, B. E. (1995). Applied relaxation vs cognitive behavior therapy in the treatment of panic disorder. *Behaviour Research and Therapy*, 33(2):145.

Rasmussen, S. A., and Eisen, J. L. (1994). The epidemiology and differential diagnosis of obsessive compulsive disorder. *Journal of Clinical Psychiatry*, 55(Suppl. 5).

Rosenbaum, J. F., et al. (1994). The etiology of social phobia. *Journal of Clinical Psychiatry*, 55(Suppl.):10.

Shueman, S., et al. (Eds). (1994). *Managed behavioral care*. Springfield, IL: Charles C Thomas.

Swinson, R. P., et al. (1995). Efficacy of telephone-administered behavioral therapy for panic disorder with agoraphobia. *Behaviour Research and Therapy*, 33(4):465.

Walker, M. (1994). Principles of a therapeutic milieu: An overview. *Perspectives Psychiatric Care*, 30(3):5.

SELF-STUDY AND CRITICAL THINKING

Multiple choice

1. Which of the following is one possible cause of obsessive-compulsive disorder?
   A. Dopamine deficiency
   B. Secondary gain
   C. Faulty learning
   D. Clomipramine excess

2. The plan of care for a client with obsessive-compulsive disorder who has elaborate washing rituals specifies that response prevention is to be used. Which scenario is an example of response prevention?
   A. Not allowing the client to wash hands after touching a "dirty" object
   B. Not allowing the client to seek reassurance from staff
   C. Telling the client that the client must relax whenever he or she seems tense
   D. Having the client repeatedly touch dirty objects

3. A client is experiencing a panic attack. The nurse can be most therapeutic by
   A. Telling the client to take slow, deep breaths.
   B. Asking the client what he means when he says "I'm dying."
   C. Verbalizing mild disapproval of his anxious behavior.
   D. Offering explanations about the sympathetic nervous system's role in symptom production.

4. The nurse caring for a client with panic attacks might anticipate that the psychiatrist would order
   A. Standard antipsychotic medication.
   B. Anticholinergic medication.
   C. Tricyclic antidepressant medication.
   D. Antihistamine medication.

5. Mr. Thomas is a combat veteran who is being treated for posttraumatic stress disorder. An important nursing task shortly after admission is to
   A. Ascertain how long ago the trauma occurred.
   B. Establish whether the client has chronically elevated blood pressure related to high anxiety.
   C. Set firm limits on acting out behaviors.
   D. Assess use of chemical substances for anxiety relief.

6. The psychiatrist orders lorazepam, 1 mg by mouth four times a day. The nurse caring for the client should
   A. Question the physician's order, as the dose is excessive.
   B. Teach the client to limit caffeine intake.
   C. Expect to observe mild ataxia and slurred speech.
   D. Explain the long-term nature of anxiolytic therapy.

Place a Y before the diagnoses that are commonly seen in clients with anxiety disorders and an N before those that are seldom seen.

7. ________ Fluid volume excess

8. ________ Impaired social interaction

9. ________ Altered role performance
10. ________ Risk for infection
11. ________ Dressing/grooming self-care deficit
12. ________ Body image disturbance
13. ________ Personal identity disturbance

Match the ego defense mechanism and the anxiety disorder with which it is associated.

14. ________ Displacement
15. ________ Isolation
16. ________ Undoing

A. Posttraumatic stress disorder
B. Phobia
C. Obsessive-compulsive disorder

Place a Y before the interventions that would be helpful in caring for clients with anxiety disorders and an N before those that are not helpful.

17. ________ Leave anxious clients strictly alone.
18. ________ Insist that anxious clients sit down.
19. ________ Help link client behavior and feelings.
20. ________ Provide a schedule of daily activities.
21. ________ Laugh at the performance of rituals.
22. ________ When a client mentions that his or her obsessive thoughts are "silly," say, "Knowing your unwanted thoughts are irrational and that you are unable to control them seems upsetting to you."
23. ________ Teach clients the importance of maintaining caffeine intake at 750 mg or more, daily.
24. ________ Reinforce client using positive self-talk to change negative assumptions.
25. ________ Advise client to minimize daily exercise to conserve endorphins.

Critical thinking

26. Ms. Smith, a client with obsessive-compulsive disorder, washes her hands until they are cracked and bleeding. Your nursing goal is to promote healing of her hands. What interventions will you plan?
27. This is Mr. Olivetti's third emergency department visit in a week. He is experiencing severe anxiety accompanied by many physical symptoms. He clings to you, desperately crying, "Help me! Help me! Don't let me die!" Diagnostic tests have ruled out physical disorder. The client outcome has been identified as "Client anxiety level will be reduced to moderate/mild within 1 hour." What interventions should you use?

    Mr. Olivetti is given an appointment at the anxiety disorders clinic. How will you explain the importance of keeping the clinic appointment?

    At the clinic, Mr. Olivetti is assigned a case manager. If you were the case manager, what outcomes would you identify? What interventions would you plan?
28. Mr. Zeamans is a client with posttraumatic stress disorder. He has a history of substance abuse and is now a recovering alcoholic. During a clinic visit, he tells you he plans to ask his psychiatrist to prescribe diazepam (Valium) to use when he's

feeling anxious. He asks whether you think this is a good idea. How would you respond? What action could you take?

29. You are to perform a nursing assessment for Miss Lee, a Chinese American client with generalized anxiety disorder. What cultural considerations might play a role in conducting the assessment?

18

Somatoform and Dissociative Disorders

HELENE S. (KAY) CHARRON

OUTLINE

Assessing Mood
Assessing Use of Alcohol and Other Drugs
Assessing Impact on Client and Family
Assessing Suicide Risk

NURSING DIAGNOSIS

PLANNING

Planning Outcome Criteria
Nurses' Feelings and Self-Assessment
Establishing a Relationship
Meeting Safety and Security Needs
Communication
Addressing Memory and Identity Alterations

IMPLEMENTATION

Counseling (Basic Level)
Psychotherapy (Advanced Practice)
Hypnotherapy
Behavioral Therapy
Cognitive Restructuring
Family Therapy
Milieu Therapy (Basic Level)
Self-Care Activities (Basic Level)
Psychobiological Interventions (Basic Level)
Medication Administration
Narcotherapy
Health Teaching (Basic Level)
Case Management (Basic Level)
Health Promotion and Health Maintenance (Basic Level)

EVALUATION

KEY TERMS AND CONCEPTS

The key terms and concepts listed here also appear in bold where they are defined or discussed in this chapter.

somatization
malingering
factitious disorder
somatization disorder
hypochondriasis
pain disorder
body dysmorphic disorder
conversion disorder
secondary gains
dissociative disorders
depersonalization disorder
dissociative amnesia
dissociative fugue
dissociative identity disorder
alternate personality or subpersonality
hypnotherapy
narcotherapy

OBJECTIVES

After studying this chapter, the reader will be able to

1. Distinguish between somatoform disorder and dissociative disorder.
2. Discuss theories of the causes of somatoform and dissociative disorders.
3. Identify characteristics of somatoform and dissociative disorders according to *Diagnostic and statistical manual of mental disorders, fourth edition* (DSM-IV) (1994).
4. Identify assessment data that should be gathered regarding clients with somatoform and clients with dissociative disorders.
5. Formulate nursing diagnoses for clients with somatoform disorders and clients with dissociative disorders.
6. Discuss some common reactions that health care workers experience when they work with clients with somatoform disorders and clients with dissociative disorders.
7. Develop realistic and measurable outcomes for clients with somatoform disorders and clients with dissociative disorders.
8. Plan interventions for clients with somatization disorders and those with dissociative disorders.
9. Evaluate effectiveness of care based on established outcomes.

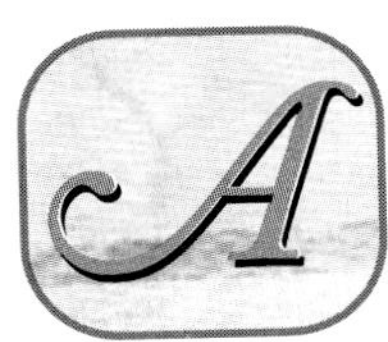

Anxiety exerts a powerful influence on the lives of individuals. People vary a great deal in their ability to cope with anxiety successfully. The ways in which anxiety is manifested dysfunctionally also differ considerably. In this chapter, the nurse will learn about the nursing care of clients who experience somatoform disorders and clients with dissociative disorders. The placement of these disorders on the mental health continuum can be seen in Figure 18–1.

SOMATOFORM DISORDERS

Soma is the Greek word for body. **Somatization** can be defined as the expression of psychological stress through physical symptoms. Somatoform disorders are a group of conditions in which somatization is present. They are characterized by the following elements:

1. Complaints of physical symptoms that cannot be explained by physiological tests
2. Strong possibility that the physical symptoms have been precipitated by psychological factors (e.g., stress, unmet psychological needs)
3. Client's inability to control the symptom voluntarily
4. Symptoms not intentionally produced, as in **malingering** (making a conscious attempt to deceive others by pretending to have a false or exaggerated symptom) or **factitious disorder** (Munchausen's syndrome, in which physical signs of illness are produced through voluntary physiological tampering)

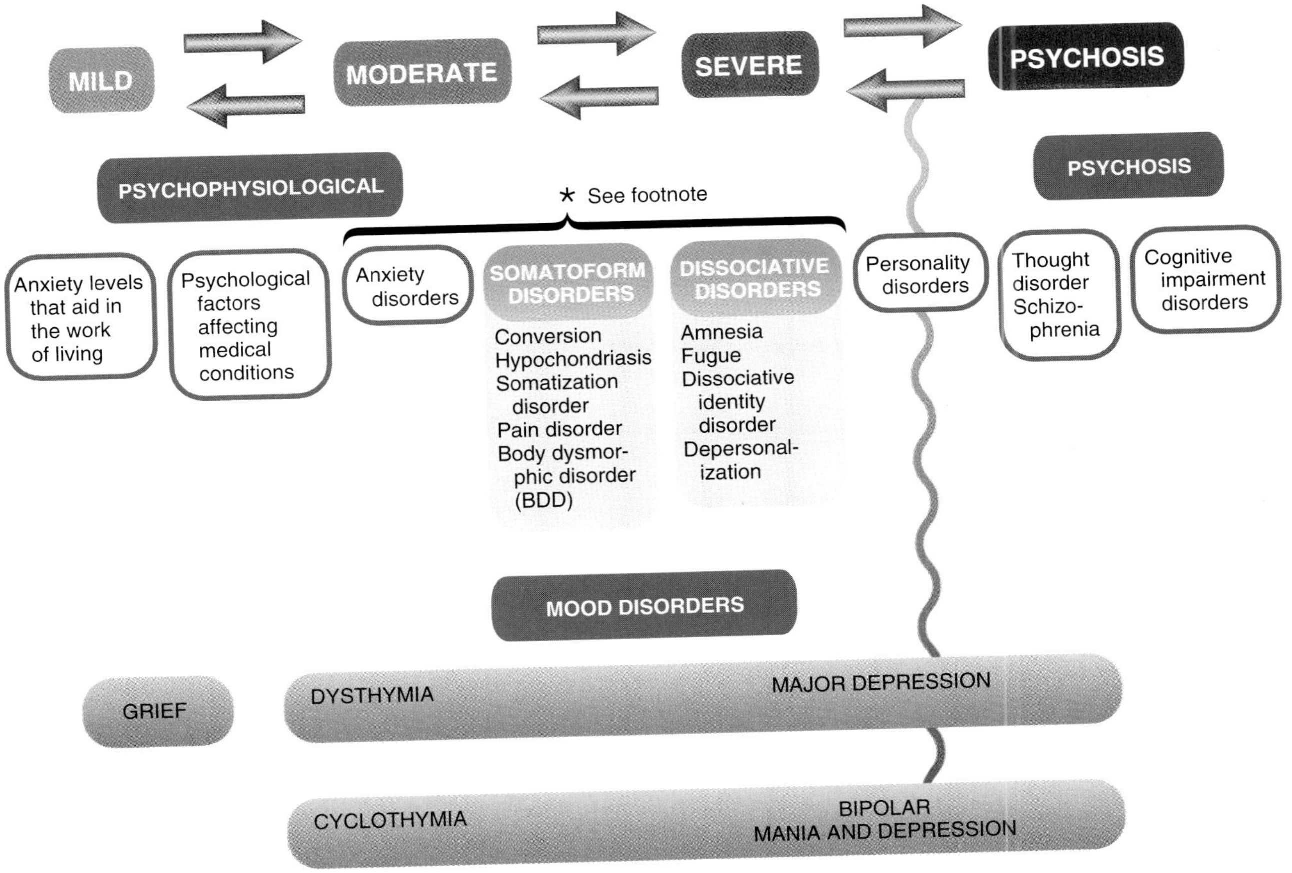

* *These disorders are currently classified by presenting clinical symptoms. Previously they were called "neurotic" disorders.*

Figure 18–1 The mental health continuum for somatoform and dissociative disorders.

THEORY

Because no clear cause exists for somatoform disorders, various theoretical positions are reviewed in this chapter.

Biological Factors

Studies reported by Kaplan and associates (1994) provide information about the possible neurophysiological basis for somatoform disorders. Research suggests that the physical symptoms that are unexplained by medical disease can arise from faulty perceptions and incorrect assessments of body sensations associated with attention deficits and cognitive impairments (e.g., increased distractibility, impressionistic tendencies, partial and circumstantial associations). Symptoms seen in **somatization disorder** (a condition in which an individual experiences numerous unexplainable physical symptoms) and **hypochondriasis** (an intense preoccupation with fear of disease) may develop this way.

Clients who experience somatoform **pain disorder** (pain unrelated to a medical disease) may be predisposed to the experience of severe pain because of abnormalities in brain chemical balance or because of structural abnormalities of the sensory or limbic systems. Serotonin and endorphin deficiency in an individual may cause the individual to perceive incoming pain stimuli as being more intense than others do. Serotonin deficiency is also being considered as a causal factor in the development of misperceptions about one's body **(body dysmorphic disorder).**

Biological factors related to central nervous system arousal disturbances are implicated in the development of pseudoneurological symptoms, such as loss of sensory abilities and loss of voluntary motor function **(conversion disorder).** Abnormal regulation of the cytokine system is also being considered to result in some somatoform disorder symptoms, such as fatigue and anorexia. Cytokines are the messenger molecules the immune system uses to communicate among its parts and to communicate with the brain and nervous system.

Genetic Factors

Studies show that somatoform disorders may have a genetic component. Somatization disorder tends to run in families, occurring in 10% to 20% of first-degree female relatives of clients with somatization disorder (Kaplan et al. 1994). One study reported a concordance rate for somatization disorder of 29% in monozygotic twins and 10% in dizygotic twins. Other researchers showed an increased likelihood that first-degree relatives of individuals with pain disorder would be diagnosed with the disorder, and twin studies have shown an increased prevalence of hypochondriasis among identical twins.

Cultural Factors

Diagnostic and statistical manual, fourth edition (DSM-IV) (1994) provides information about the role of culture in somatoform disorders and states that the type and the frequency of somatic symptoms vary across cultures. Burning hands and feet or the experience of worms in the head or ants under the skin is more common in Africa and southern Asia than in North America. Alteration of consciousness with falling is a symptom commonly associated with culture-specific religious and healing rituals. Somatization disorder, which is rarely seen in males in the United States, is more often reported in Greek and Puerto Rican men, suggesting that cultural mores may permit these men to use somatization as an acceptable approach to dealing with life stress.

Symptoms related to male reproductive function are more prevalent in Eastern cultures. For example, Leff, in his work *Psychiatry around the globe: A transcultural view* (1988), discusses syndromes or illnesses that are confined to a particular culture. *Koro* is an illness seen in Chinese males. The affected individual becomes convinced that his genitals are withdrawing into his abdomen, and that when the last of the genitals disappears, he will die. Panic-level anxiety ensues.

Conversion disorder is reported to be more common in individuals in low socioeconomic groups, those in rural settings, and those with little education. The incidence is higher in developing regions.

In some cultures, certain physical symptoms are thought to result from spells having been cast on the individual. Spellbound individuals often seek the help of traditional healers in addition to modern medical help. The modern medical diagnostician may point to the presence of a non–life-threatening somatoform disorder, while the traditional healer may offer an entirely different explanation and prognosis. The individual may not show improvement until the traditional healer removes the spell.

Psychosocial Factors

Psychoanalytical Theory

Psychoanalytical theorists believe that psychogenic complaints of pain, illness, or loss of physical function are related to repression of a conflict (usually of an aggressive or sexual nature), and transformation of anxiety into a physical symptom that is symbolically related to the conflict. In conversion disorder, the ego defense mechanisms involved are repression and conversion. According to Freudian theory, conversion symptoms allow a forbidden wish or urge to be partly expressed but sufficiently disguised so that the individual does not have to face the unacceptable wish. Therefore, the symptom is said to be symbolic of the conflict.

Freudian theory suggests that conversion symptoms also permit the individual to communicate a need for special treatment or consideration from others. The following vignette is an example of how a symptom can be both symbolic of, and a solution to, a conflict.

▶ Anita, aged 18 years, lives with her mother and stepfather. The stepfather has been physically abusive to Anita for many years. Anita hates him but is dependent on him for financial support. One day, as the family steps off the curb to cross a busy street, the father is hit by a speeding automobile. Anita attempts to shout at her stepfather to warn him, but no sound comes out. She suffers aphonia (loss of voice) that lasts until psychotherapy helps her regain her ability to speak. It is obvious that the conflict was whether to warn her physically abusive and hated stepfather. The loss of her voice solved the problem and made it impossible to save him.

Hypochondriasis is considered by many clinicians to have psychodynamic origins. These clinicians suggest that anger, aggression, or hostility that had its origins in past losses or disappointments is expressed as a need for help and concern from others. Other clinicians suggest that hypochondriasis is a defense against guilt or low self-esteem. In this hypothesis, the somatic symptoms that the individual has are experienced as deserved punishment. In pain disorder, the individual's pain may serve an unconscious function, such as atonement, a way to obtain the love and concern of others, and punishment for real or imagined wrongdoing. The defense mechanisms responsible are repression and displacement.

In cases of body dysmorphic disorder, some theorists believe that the individual invests a part of the body with special meaning that may be traceable to some event occurring at an earlier stage of psychosexual development. The original event is repressed, and the attachment of special meaning to a part of the body comes about through symbolization. Projection is used when the individual makes statements such as "It makes everyone look at me with horror" and "I know my husband hates it." Table 18–1 provides clinical examples of each of the somatoform disorders and their defenses.

Behavioral Theory

Behaviorists suggest that somatoform symptoms are learned ways of communicating helplessness and that they allow the individual to manipulate others. The symptoms become more intense when they are reinforced by attention from others. In the United States, most individuals are concerned about others who have pain, and physicians and nurses are taught to be attentive and responsive to a client's reports of pain. Other reinforcers include avoiding activities that the individual considers distasteful, obtaining financial gain from the pain, and gaining some advantage in interpersonal relationships as a result of the pain.

Cognitive Theory

Cognitive theorists believe that the client with hypochondriasis focuses on body sensations, misinterprets their meaning, and then becomes excessively alarmed by them.

DSM-IV and the Clinical Picture of Somatoform Disorders

DSM-IV lists five somatoform disorders that are reviewed in this section. Clinical vignettes accompany the criteria for each disorder.

Somatization Disorder

The diagnosis of somatization disorder requires that the client have a history of many physical complaints, beginning before the age of 30 years, that occur over a period of years and result in treatment being sought or in significant impairment in social, occupational, or other areas of functioning. The symptoms are displayed in Figure 18–2. In addition, the symptoms experienced by the client cannot be explained by a medical condition, or if it is explained by a medical condition, the complaints or social and occupational impairment that results is in excess of what would be expected.

▶ Susanne, a 26-year-old beautician, is admitted to the hospital after an overdose of sedatives. She states that she is sick of not being able to get help from anyone. In describing herself, she mentions being unwell since the age of 14, shortly after her father died of valvular heart disease. She describes having seizures, fainting spells, and occasional weakness of the left leg. One year ago, she began having abdominal pain, nausea, and diarrhea. Exploratory surgery revealed no pathology. The symptoms still recur "sometimes." She mentions experiencing painful menstruation and excessive bleeding over a period of several years. Recently, she has experienced palpitations and tightness of her chest after emotionally trying events.

▶ Susanne lived at home with her mother until 6 months ago, when she married a man 15 years her senior. She says that she is "turned off by sex," and she reveals that her husband is upset by her constant illness. He is considering divorce. She has attempted suicide, and a short admission is advised.

Hypochondriasis

Nondelusional preoccupation with having a serious disease or the fear of having a serious disease marks hypochondriasis. The preoccupation or fear is based on

TABLE 18–1 SOMATOFORM DISORDERS: DEFENSE AND EXAMPLES

DEFENSE MECHANISMS	EXAMPLE*
	Conversion Disorder
Conversion	Jan, a 28-year-old former secretary, awakens one morning to find that she has a tingling in both hands and cannot move her fingers. Two days earlier, her husband had told her that he wanted a separation and that she would have to go back to work to support herself. The conversion of anxiety relates the separation and increase in dependency needs to "paralysis of her fingers" so that she is unable to work.
	Pain Disorder
Displacement	Henry, 47, a laborer, "pulled a muscle" in his back a year ago. Two weeks before this, his wife, a waitress, told him that she wanted to go back to school to get her bachelor's degree. He suffers severe, constant pain, despite negative results from myelography, computed tomography, magnetic resonance imaging, and neurological exams. He watches television all day and collects disability. His wife, unable now to go back to school, waits on him and has assumed his home responsibilities. Henry displaces his anxiety over the threat to his own self-esteem by his wife's potential change of status onto "pain in his back." The focus of his anxiety is now on his back and not on his threatened self-esteem.
	Body Dysmorphic Disorder
Symbolism and projection	Michele, a young, attractive woman, is preoccupied that her nose is too long and "ugly." She is preoccupied and distressed over her perception. Two plastic surgeons she consulted are hesitant to reshape her nose but have not altered her thinking that her nose makes her ugly.
	Somatization Disorder
Somatization	Deanna, 27, presents at the doctor's office with excessive, heavy menstruation. She tells the nurse that recently she experienced pain "first in my back and then going to every part of my body." She states that she is often bothered with constipation and frequent vomiting when she "eats the wrong food." She states she was "unwell" and had suffered from seizures and still has them occasionally. The nurse becomes confused, not knowing what symptoms she wants the doctor to evaluate. Deanna tells the nurse that she lives at home with her parents because her poor health makes it hard for her to hold a job.
	Hypochondriasis
Denial and somatization	Julio, 52, lost his wife to colon cancer 5 months ago, which he "took very well." Recently, he saw the sixth physician with the same complaint. He believes that he has liver cancer, despite repeated and extensive diagnostic tests, which are all negative. He has ceased seeing his friends, has dropped his hobbies, and spends much of his time checking his sclera and "resting his liver." His son finally demands that he see a doctor.

*All entail somatization.

the client's misinterpretation of bodily symptoms, despite medical evaluation and reassurance, and has lasted more than 6 months, causing the client significant distress or impaired social or occupational function (Fig. 18–2).

- Anthony, aged 54 years, is referred to the mental health center outpatient clinic from the sexually transmitted disease (STD) clinic. Anthony has visited the clinic almost weekly for 2 years, asking for diagnostic tests for various STDs. He is always told that the test results are negative and that he has no illness. Most recently, his preoccupation has centered on AIDS.
- Anthony, a widower whose wife died of uterine cancer 3 years ago, is a self-employed plumber. Since the onset of his wife's illness and his own preoccupation with illness, his two daughters have visited at least weekly. He has no other social contacts, having given up attendance at an ethnic social club he once enjoyed.
- The client was brought up in a strict religious environment, joined the Navy at age 17, and married shortly after discharge. Anthony reveals that despite his religious upbringing, he had several encounters with prostitutes while he was in the Navy. When his wife's illness was diagnosed, he began to wonder if he had acquired a "disease" and passed it on to her. He appears worried as he discusses with the nurse therapist his concern about having an STD and shares the story of his unsuccessful search for accurate diagnosis and treatment.

SOMATOFORM DISORDERS

SOMATIZATION DISORDER

1. History of many physical complaints beginning before 30 years of age, occurring over a period of years and resulting in impairment in social, occupational, or other important areas of functioning.
2. Complaints must include *all* of the following:
   - History of pain in at least four different sites or functions
   - History of at least two gastrointestinal symptoms other than pain
   - History of at least one sexual or reproduction symptom
   - History of at least one symptom defined as or suggesting a neurological disorder

CONVERSION DISORDER

1. Development of a symptom or deficit suggesting:
   - Neurologic disorder (blindness, deafness, loss of touch)

   or
   - Voluntary motor function (aphonia, impaired coordination, paralysis, seizures, and more)
2. Not due to malingering or factitious disorder and not culturally sanctioned.
3. Causes impairment in social or occupational functioning, causes marked distress, or requires medical attention.

HYPOCHONDRIASIS

For at least 6 months:

1. Preoccupation with fears of having, or the idea that one has, a serious disease.
2. Preoccupation persists despite appropriate medical tests and reassurances.
3. Other disorders are ruled out (e.g., somatic delusional disorders).
4. Preoccupation causes significant impairment in social or occupational functioning or causes marked distress.

PAIN DISORDER

1. Pain in one or more anatomical sites is a major part of the clinical picture.
2. Causes significant impairment in occupational or social functioning or causes marked distress.
3. Psychological factors thought to cause onset, severity, or exacerbation. **Pain associated with psychological factors.**
4. If medical condition present, it plays minor role in accounting for pain. **Pain associated with both psychological and medical conditions.** Both factors are judged to be important in onset, severity, exacerbation, and maintenance of pain.

BODY DYSMORPHIC DISORDER (BDD)

1. Preoccupation with some imagined defect in appearance. If the defect is present, concern is excessive.
2. Preoccupation causes significant impairment in social or occupational functioning or causes marked distress.

Figure 18–2 DSM-IV diagnostic criteria for somatoform disorders. (Adapted from American Psychiatric Association (1994). *Diagnostic and statistical manual of mental disorders* (4th ed.). Washington, DC: American Psychiatric Association. Reprinted with permission. Copyright 1994 American Psychiatric Association.)

Pain Disorder

Diagnostic criteria for pain disorder cite pain in one or more anatomical sites as the predominant feature of this disorder. The pain must be of sufficient severity to cause significant distress, deserve clinical attention, and cause impaired social or occupational functioning. Psychological factors must be judged to play an important role in the onset, severity, exacerbation, or maintenance of the pain (Fig. 18–2).

▶ Robert, aged 36 years, is referred to the outpatient mental health clinic by his private physician. He has suffered from chronic back pain for 2 years, during which he has been unable to work as a longshoreman. He leans heavily on a cane and moves slowly and deliberately when he walks. Robert states that he has had myelography, computed tomography (CT), and magnetic resonance imaging (MRI) that have shown no cause for his pain. He has used diazepam (Valium) and a variety of analgesics that afford him little relief. He states that he is never free of severe pain.

▶ His back pain began after he played baseball at a picnic celebrating his wife's graduation from a community college nursing program. She had returned to school against his wishes when their youngest child entered high school. When his wife completed the program, he grudgingly agreed to her acceptance of a part-time position, but she instead chose a full-time position. He now states, "It's a good thing she went against me, because she's the breadwinner and has to take care of me, now that I can't work."

Body Dysmorphic Disorder

Body dysmorphic disorder involves preoccupation with an imagined defect in appearance that causes significant distress or impairment in social or occupational functioning (Fig. 18–2).

▶ Anna, a 32-year-old office worker, is referred to the mental health center clinic by a plastic surgeon. She has been preoccupied with the size of her breasts for several years. Initially, she sought breast augmentation from the referring surgeon. After augmentation surgery, she reported seeing another plastic surgeon in hopes of having her breast size increased still further. Two years later, she returned to the first surgeon, seeking breast reduction. She was persuaded not to have surgery at that time. Two months ago, she again returned to the surgeon, expressing dissatisfaction with the size and shape of her breasts.

Conversion Disorder

Conversion disorder is characterized by the presence of one or more symptoms that suggest the presence of a neurological disorder that cannot be explained by a known neurological or medical disorder or a culturally bound symptom. Psychological factors, such as stress and conflicts, are present that are associated with the onset or exacerbation of the symptom (Fig. 18–2).

▶ Pat, a fashion model, is admitted to the neurological unit on the eve of her thirtieth birthday, after the sudden onset of convulsions during a modeling assignment. She is an attractive woman whose manner with female nursing staff is indifferent and with male nursing staff and physicians is coy and flirtatious.

▶ The first seizure recorded after hospitalization happens during morning rounds. As staff enter her room, Pat arches her back and begins pelvic thrusting motions while thrashing her arms and legs about on the bed. No loss of consciousness occurs. She is not incontinent, nor does she bite her tongue. Afterward, she is alert and well oriented. The second "seizure" occurs in the afternoon during a visit from her mother and father. This episode lasts 5 minutes. It begins with an outcry that brings nurses running. This time, she exhibits a period of generalized muscular rigidity, followed by pelvic thrusting and thrashing of her limbs. Again, no biting of the tongue or incontinence occurs during the seizure, nor was there a period of lethargy or confusion after the seizure.

▶ During her hospital stay for a neurological work-up, Pat remains relatively unconcerned about her convulsions (la belle indifférence) and their potential impact on her career. She seems to enjoy the attention of the male staff, who respond to her attractiveness and vivacious interactions by seeking her out. When she is told that her electroencephalogram and other test results are normal, she shrugs and agrees to transfer to the mental health unit for a few days for further work-up "if all the boys [medical staff] could come over" to see her.

▶ On the mental health unit, her seizures continue once or twice daily but always occur in the presence of others, never occur with incontinence or self-injury, and always include sensual body movements. Initially, Pat refuses to come out of her room for fear of "an attack." During this time, helpless, dependent behavior is noticeable. Visits from her parents seem to support this, as her father calls her his "little girl" or "princess," and her mother frequently pleads with the nurses to take good care of her daughter.

ASSESSMENT

Assessment of clients with somatoform disorders is a complex process that requires careful and complete documentation. This section outlines several areas that are not normally included in a nursing assessment but are of considerable importance in the assessment of a client with suspected somatoform disorder.

Assessment of Symptoms and Unmet Needs

Assessment should begin with data collection about the nature, location, onset, character, and duration of the symptom or symptoms. Often, clients with conversion disorder report having a sudden loss in function of a body part. "I woke up this morning and couldn't move my arm" or "Suddenly, my legs were paralyzed" or "I tried to speak but I'd lost my voice." Other common "losses" associated with conversion disorder are vision and hearing. Some clients with conversion disorder describe their symptoms with an inappropriate lack of concern (la belle indifférence). Clients with somatization disorder, hypochondriasis, or somatoform pain disorder usually discuss their symptoms dramatically. They often use colorful metaphors and exaggerations: "The pain was searing, like a hot sword drawn across my forehead" or "My symptoms are so rare that I've stumped hundreds of doctors." Individuals with body dysmorphic disorder are concerned about only one part of the body and seek cosmetic surgery; their affective display is that of disgust with the offending body part.

Assessment should also include the client's ideas about personal symptoms and the diagnostic work-ups that have been performed. When somatization disorders are confirmed, laboratory findings and other diagnostic tests reveal no pathology. Medical histories, however, show that the client has sought repeated tests and treatments, often from a series of physicians and hospitals. Clients with somatoform disorders are not content to learn that they have no organic basis for their symptoms and repeatedly seek confirmation of physical illness from a variety of health care professionals. When it is suggested that clients with somatoform disorders seek help from a psychiatrist, psychologist, or psychiatric nurse, they are uniformly resistant to the suggestion.

Information should be sought about clients' ability to meet their own basic needs. Common problems associated with the need for oxygen include tachypnea and tachycardia associated with anxiety. Nutrition, fluid balance, and elimination needs should be evaluated because clients with somatization disorders often complain of gastrointestinal distress, diarrhea, constipation, and anorexia. The physiological need for sex may be altered by client experiences of painful intercourse, pain in another part of the body, or lack of interest in sex.

Rest, comfort, activity, and hygiene needs may be altered as the result of client problems such as fatigue, weakness, insomnia, muscle tension, pain, and avoidance of diversional activity. Safety and security needs may be threatened by client experiences of blindness, deafness, inability to speak, convulsive movements, gait disturbances, loss of balance and falling, and anesthesia of various parts of the body.

Assessing Voluntary Control of Symptoms

During assessment, it is important to determine if the symptoms are under the client's voluntary control. Somatoform symptoms are not under the individual's voluntary control; however, symptoms associated with malingering and factitious disorder are under voluntary control. Low back pain is frequently chosen as the malingerer's symptom because it is difficult to disprove. Clients with factitious disorder (Munchausen's syndrome) produce physical signs of illness through voluntary physiological tampering, such as ingesting substances that cause diarrhea and injecting themselves with material to cause inflammatory reactions. Heating thermometers to give a high reading is common practice among such clients. Individuals who use malingering or who display factitious symptoms deceive others, but not themselves, about the symptoms. By contrast, individuals with somatoform disorders are deceived by their symptoms. They cannot see relationships between symptoms and conflicts that are obvious to others.

Assessing Secondary Gains

Self-care and role performance may be compromised, depending on the symptoms experienced by the client. Ability to perform the usual family, work, and social roles is nearly always diminished. The physical symptoms may make it difficult, if not impossible, to continue employment. Family roles and processes are altered when one member takes on a sick role. Preoccupation with illness or pain may produce observable emotional and social isolation, inattention to the needs of others, manipulation of others, and excessively demanding behaviors. Powerlessness may be noted as a theme, with clients citing numerous self-care activities and roles they can no longer perform and responsibilities they have surrendered to others.

Therefore, the nurse might identify **secondary gains** the client may be receiving from the symptoms. These can include getting out of usual responsibilities, getting extra attention, and manipulating others. One approach to identifying the presence of secondary gains is to ask the client questions such as

- What can't you do now that you used to be able to do?
- How has this problem affected your life?

Assessing Cognitive Style

In general, these clients misinterpret physical stimuli and distort reality regarding their symptoms. For example, sensations a normal individual might interpret as a headache might suggest a brain tumor to a client with somatoform disorder, or indigestion might be interpreted as cancer. Exploring the client's cognitive style may be helpful in distinguishing between hypochondriasis and somatization disorder. The client with hypochondriasis exhibits more anxiety and an obsessive attention to detail, along with a preoccupation with the fear of serious illness, while the client with somatization disorder is often rambling and vague about the details of his or her many symptoms and may give a poor or vague history.

Assessing Ability to Communicate Feelings and Emotional Needs

Often, clients with somatoform disorders have difficulty communicating their emotional needs. Although able to describe their symptoms, they have difficulty verbalizing feelings, especially those related to anger, guilt, and dependence. The somatic symptom may be the client's chief means of communicating emotional needs. Psychogenic blindness or hearing loss may represent the symbolic statement "I can't face this knowledge." Consider the wife who overheard friends discussing her husband's sexual infidelity and developed total deafness.

Assessing Client's Self-Esteem and Perceived Strengths

Low self-esteem is often present in clients with somatoform disorders. An assessment of the client's self-esteem should include perceived strengths, since the client normally focuses on the things that can no longer be performed. During treatment, strengths can be reinforced to help the client see himself or herself as someone with coping ability.

Assessment of Dependence on Medication

Individuals experiencing many somatic complaints often become dependent on medication to relieve pain or anxiety or to induce sleep. Physicians often prescribe diazepam or other anxiolytic agents for clients who seem highly anxious and concerned about their symptoms. Clients often return to the physician, seeking prescription renewal. If the client has sought treatment from numerous physicians, the possibility of medication misuse increases. Dependence on anxiolytics develops quickly; thus, it is important that the nurse assess the types and the amounts of medications being used.

NURSING DIAGNOSIS

Clients with a somatoform disorder present various nursing problems. **Ineffective individual coping** is frequently diagnosed. Causal statements might include

- Distorted perceptions of body functions and symptoms.
- Chronic pain of psychological origin.
- Dependence on pain relievers or anxiolytics.

Impaired social interaction may be related to preoccupation with illness when clients focus their psychic and physical energy on somatic symptoms, leaving little energy to expend on others or on diversional activities. This tendency to isolate themselves may be due to an unconscious awareness that they may receive little attention in busy social situations or to an unconscious realization that participating in many social activities might imply wellness rather than illness.

Altered family process related to adoption of the sick role is nearly always present. Secondary gains derived by the client nearly always signal the presence of compromised family functioning. Adoption of the sick role by a family member causes alterations in family roles (e.g., a parent's illness is likely to require children to assume increased responsibility at an early age). The assumption of the illness role by an adolescent may cause the mother to become overinvolved with that child, giving less attention to other siblings or the father.

Altered sexuality patterns related to preoccupation with physical symptoms or pain or altered sexual patterns related to adoption of sick role is another possible nursing diagnosis. When an individual perceives himself or herself to be ill and is perceived as ill by others, sexual expression is invariably altered. The sexual partner's role shifts to caregiver/parent, and the client's role, to recipient of care/child.

Self-esteem disturbance or **chronic low self-esteem** may be a useful diagnosis if the client has expressed a negative self-evaluation related to losing body function, feeling useless, or not feeling valued by significant others.

Other possible diagnoses include

Powerlessness related to somatic symptoms of psychogenic origin.
Self-care deficit related to pain associated with somatoform pain disorder or related to a specific conversion symptom, such as paralysis, seizures, and loss of voice.
Sleep pattern disturbance related to psychogenic pain.

PLANNING

Planning Outcome Criteria

Identifying client outcomes should be a process in which the client participates; shared decision making promotes goal attainment. Outcome criteria must be realistic and attainable. Structuring outcomes in small steps helps the client see concrete evidence of progress. The following are possible goals and outcomes for nursing diagnoses that are frequently established for clients with somatoform diagnoses.

Ineffective individual coping related to distorted perceptions of bodily functions and symptoms.

By (date) the client will cope adaptively, as evidenced by

- Appropriately interpreting physical symptoms: "The bruises on my leg resulted from bumping the chair, not from leukemia."

- Verbalizing relationship of conflicts and feeling to somatic symptoms: "I was so angry with him, but I was afraid he'd leave me if I showed it. Being sick punished him."
- Replacing reliance on anxiolytics through the use of alternative coping strategies, such as assertive communication and relaxation techniques.
- Replacing demanding, manipulative, attention-seeking behaviors with behaviors that respect others' rights.
- Expressing feelings verbally rather than somatically.

Impaired social interaction related to preoccupation with somatic symptoms or pain.

By (date) client will demonstrate improved social interaction, as evidenced by

- Establishing and completing a contract to attend a specified number of social or diversional activities daily.
- Verbalizing satisfaction with improved level of social interaction.
- Sustaining conversations for 5 or more minutes at a time without mentioning somatic symptoms or their effects.

Low self-esteem related to feelings of shame.

By (date) client will demonstrate improved self-esteem, as evidenced by

- Making a realistic appraisal of strengths and weaknesses.
- Reporting absence of feelings of shame or guilt.

Altered family coping related to client's adoption of sick role.

By (date) the family will demonstrate interactions that maximize optimal functioning of client, as evidenced by

- Reports of increased client independence.
- Client resumption of pre-illness roles, including work.
- Family reports of absence of manipulative behaviors or excessive dependence.

Because clients with somatoform disorders are seldom admitted to psychiatric units, and then only for short stays, interventions must be planned that can be implemented on an outpatient or home care basis. Planning may also be initiated by a psychiatric liaison nurse called to consult about a client with somatoform disorder who has been admitted to a medical-surgical unit. Such a stay would be short, and discharge would occur as soon as diagnostic tests are completed and negative results are received.

Nursing interventions should focus initially on establishing a helping relationship with the client. The therapeutic relationship is vital to the success of the care plan, given the client's resistance to the concept that no physical cause for the symptom exists and the client's tendency to go from caregiver to caregiver.

Other interventions should focus on assisting the client to recognize the somatic symptoms as a coping strategy and helping the client learn more effective coping strategies. To be successful, therapeutic interventions must address ways to assist the client to get needs met without resorting to somatization. The secondary gains the client has derived from illness behaviors become less important to the client when underlying needs can be met directly. Collaboration with significant others is essential for success.

Table 18–2 shows key nursing interventions and rationales for planning care for clients with somatoform disorders. Nursing Care Plan 18–1 gives the plan of care for Pat, the earlier client with conversion disorder.

Nurse's Feelings and Self-Assessment

Nurses and other health care workers often find working with clients with somatoform disorders to be difficult and unsatisfying. The nurse notes objective data that indicate a lack of physiological basis for the client's symptoms. The nurse then wonders why this client who is "not sick" is taking up valuable time that might better be spent on a "sick" client. The tendency, at times, is for nurses to feel resentment or anger toward these clients. These negative feelings occur whether the client is being cared for by medical-surgical staff, who tend to prefer working with clients who have physical illnesses, or by psychiatric staff, who often prefer to work with psychotic clients. It is helpful to remember that the symptom the client is experiencing is real to him or her, even though the objective data do not substantiate a physiological basis.

Anger may also rise when staff find themselves dealing with a client who uses somatic symptoms to manipulate the environment and the people in the environment. In addition, health care workers may experience feelings of helplessness over not being able to make the client realize that his or her symptom has no organic basis. Clients who use somatization exhibit remarkable resistance to change. They cling to their unrealistic beliefs about the origin of the somatic symptoms, despite objective evidence to the contrary. Setting goals that have staged outcomes (i.e., outcomes occurring in small, attainable steps) helps the nurse avoid feelings of helplessness.

Clients with somatoform disorders should be discussed in conferences with other health care members to allow for expression of feelings and consistency of care.

◗ From the first day of admission, the staff discuss having negative feelings about Pat. Female staff report that Pat makes them feel as though they were her personal maids. Many of the staff admit wanting to avoid her. Male staff report feeling uncomfortable with her seductive behaviors, and all staff feel annoyed with her flirting and dependence. A psychiatric liaison nurse directs all staff to provide a safe environment during "seizures" in which as few staff as possible are used so

TABLE 18–2 INTERVENTIONS AND RATIONALES: SOMATOFORM DISORDERS

INTERVENTION	RATIONALE
Nursing Diagnosis:	
Ineffective individual coping **related to inadequate coping skills, as evidenced by total focus on self and on physical symptoms**	
1. Offer explanations and support during diagnostic testing.	1. Reduces anxiety while ruling out organic illness.
2. After physical complaints have been investigated, avoid further reinforcement, e.g., do not take vital signs each time client complains of palpitations.	2. Directs focus away from physical symptoms.
3. Spend time with client at times other than when client summons nurse to offer physical complaint.	3. Rewards non–illness-related behaviors and encourages repetition of desired behavior.
4. Observe and record frequency and intensity of somatic symptoms. (Client or family can give information.)	4. Establishes a baseline and later evaluation of effectiveness of interventions.
5. Do not imply that symptoms are not real.	5. Acknowledges that psychogenic symptoms are real to the client.
6. Shift focus from somatic complaints to feelings or to neutral topics.	6. Conveys interest in client as a person rather than in client's symptoms. Reduces need to gain attention via symptoms.
7. Assess secondary gains that "physical illness" provides for client, e.g., attention, increased dependency, and distraction from another problem.	7. Allows these needs to be met in healthier ways and thus minimizes secondary gains.
8. Use matter-of-fact approach to clients exhibiting resistance or covert anger.	8. Avoids power struggles. Demonstrates acceptance of anger and permits discussion of angry feelings.
9. Have client direct all requests to case manager.	9. Reduces manipulation.
10. Help client look at effect of illness behavior on others.	10. Encourages insight. Can help improve intrafamily relationships.
11. Show concern for client while avoiding fostering dependency needs.	11. Shows respect for client's feelings while minimizing secondary gains from "illness."
12. Reinforce client's strengths and problem-solving abilities.	12. Contributes to positive self-esteem. Helps client realize that needs can be met without resorting to somatic symptoms.
13. Teach assertive communication.	13. Provides client with a positive means of getting needs met. Reduces feelings of helplessness and need for manipulation.
14. Teach client stress-reduction techniques, such as mediation, relaxation, and mild physical exercise.	14. Provides alternate coping strategies. Reduces need for medication.
Nursing Diagnosis:	
Self-care deficit **related to "physical inability," as evidenced by inability to perform usual ADLs***	
1. Encourage client to perform normal ADLs to highest level of ability.	1. Enhances self-esteem and minimizes secondary gains.
2. Teach client alternative ways to perform ADLs if "physical disability" interferes, assisting only when necessary.	2. Gives client support while minimizing secondary gains.
3. Maintain nonjudgmental approach when assisting client with ADLs.	3. Decreases anxiety and need for defenses.
4. Feed, bathe, and assist with hygiene, if necessary, while encouraging client participation.	4. May increase client's sense of security.
Nursing Diagnosis:	
Diversional activity deficit **related to preoccupation with self and symptoms, as evidenced by complete absorption with self**	
1. Help client establish a minimum of one daily goal, e.g., attend one activity daily. Gradually increase the number of goals.	1. Ensures success and reinforces client's new behaviors.
2. Explore uses of community resources for social or diversional activities.	2. Often provides inexpensive opportunities for social interactions. Gives client a sense of control.

ADL, activity of daily living.

NURSING CARE PLAN 18–1 A PERSON WITH CONVERSION DISORDER: PAT

NURSING DIAGNOSIS

Ineffective Individual Coping: (use of conversion symptoms [seizures]) related to low self-esteem and unmet needs for recognition and attention

Supporting Data

- No incontinence. No injury. Seizures vary and occur only in the presence of others.
- Relates with seductive behavior toward males.
- Relates with superiority and contempt toward friends.
- Bland affect regarding personal problems (la belle indifférence).

Outcome Criteria: Client will cope effectively with life stress without using conversion.

SHORT-TERM GOAL	INTERVENTION	RATIONALE	EVALUATION
1. Client will adjust to unit routine by (date).	1. Explain routine. Establish expectations regarding unit routines, e.g., do not allow special privileges. Expect client to eat in dining room, perform ADLs, attend activities.	1. Reduces anxiety. Reduces secondary gain and manipulation.	*GOAL MET* Client initially refuses to leave room for meals. Misses one meal. Goes to dining room thereafter. Performs all ADLs, with special attention to applying make-up.
2. Client will remain safe.	2. Provide safety measures during seizures but limit attention and discussion about seizures afterwards. Monitor physical condition unobtrusively.	2. Prevents harm. Reduces secondary gain. Minimizes secondary gain while condition is assessed.	Client does not sustain injury during seizures. States, "I guess my seizures don't interest staff. No one will talk to me about them." Client has no seizures after day 3 on psychiatric unit.
3. Client will identify stressor by (date).	3. Encourage client to discuss life, work, significant others, and goals.	3. Uncovers stress, conflict, and strengths.	Client repeatedly mentions that 30th birthday means she is over the hill as a model.
4. Client will express feelings about the conflict by (date).	4. Encourage exploration of feelings.	4. Conveys interest.	Client states she is scared of losing her glamorous appearance and her job. Demonstrates appropriate affect.
5. Client will evaluate possible solutions to the problem by (date).	5. Focus on alternatives available to her to earn a living when modeling is no longer an option.	5. Encourages problem solving.	Client shows fashion sketches to nurse and reveals that she had once thought that she might be a good designer. With encouragement, decides to explore evening classes in illustration and design to prepare for second career.
6. Client will discuss alternative ways to cope with stress by (date).	6. Encourage use of alternative anxiety reduction techniques. Encourage client to select and learn such a method.	6. Develops skill in use of a healthy technique.	Client chooses to use jogging and progressive muscle relaxation and attends teaching sessions upon discharge.

Continued on following page

NURSING CARE PLAN 18–1 A PERSON WITH CONVERSION DISORDER: PAT *(Continued)*

NURSING DIAGNOSIS

Chronic Low Self-Esteem: related to not seeing self as a capable adult

Supporting Data

- Helpless, dependent behavior
- Seductive, flirtatious behavior
- Manipulative behavior, such as playing one staff member against another and seeking special privileges

Outcome Criteria: Client will demonstrate adequate self-esteem by relating in age-appropriate ways.

SHORT-TERM GOAL	INTERVENTION	RATIONALE	EVALUATION
1. Client will identify maladaptive behaviors of excessive dependence, seductiveness, and manipulation by (date).	1a. Set limits. Use consistent team approach.	1a. Minimizes maladaptive behavior.	*GOAL PARTIALLY MET* Client has not named any of the cited interpersonal problems, but incidence of behaviors has decreased to less than one per day.
	1b. Be nonjudgmental and accepting.	1b. Fosters self-acceptance.	
	1c. When negative countertransference occurs, seek supervision.	1c. Helps keep relationship in perspective.	
	1d. Affirm to client that symptoms can improve.	1d. Conveys hope.	
	1e. Reflect on father's choice of nickname ("princess"). Assist client in assessing role behaviors that might perpetuate the infantile image.	1e. Fosters mature role-taking.	Client admits that it is nice to be pampered by her parents but decides that this might not be congruent with a mature role.
	2a. Encourage client to attend assertiveness training to learn to ask directly for what she needs.	2a. Decreases manipulation	Client reports that she never realized people would meet her requests when she asked in an assertive way. Client expresses desire to learn more.
	2b. Encourage client to consider needs of others as an alternative to self-absorption.	2b. Gains satisfaction and increased self-esteem.	Client organizes a make-up class for female clients. Client states she might start a "make-over" business.

ADL, activity of daily living.

that attention giving is reduced. Staff are directed not to discuss seizures with Pat, but to give positive reinforcement for all appropriate interactions, including discussion of feelings. Matter-of-fact limit setting is used to help Pat become compliant with the unit routine. Pat's time with the staff is directed toward helping her see herself as a capable person with talents and options. Pat is discharged after a few days of hospitalization. She continues in therapy with a nurse psychotherapist for 6 months, then moves to another city.

IMPLEMENTATION

Generally, implementation of plans takes place in the home or clinic setting.

Counseling (Basic Level)

Psychiatric nurses use counseling to help the client improve overall functioning through the development of effective coping strategies. Often, a blend of therapeutic approaches is considered for a client for whom behavioral methods and alternative therapies are being combined in the treatment plan (Table 18–2).

Psychotherapy (Advanced Practice)

Insight-Oriented Therapy

Individual and group counseling designed to foster development of insight is usually conducted by an advanced practice nurse. The nurse therapist with advanced training assists the client to explore feelings and the way feelings are expressed via physical symptoms. The nurse generalist often continues the therapeutic process by supporting and encouraging the client to identify and express feelings and needs. Direct verbalization of troubling feelings and thoughts can help diminish the need to use somatization.

◗ Insight-oriented counseling is chosen as the primary form of therapy for Susanne. Susanne is able to relate her physical symptoms to her parents' concern with health and illness themes. Her father, an invalid as a result of mitral valve disease, receives all her mother's attention. Susanne shares this attention only when she too is ill. In group therapy, Susanne is able to gain an understanding of how she used her symptoms to ensure that her emotional needs were met, and how her use of physical symptoms controlled others. Her nurse psychotherapist teaches her assertive communication techniques and encourages her to use them to ask directly for what she needs, rather than resort to manipulation. Marital therapy is arranged to explore the negative effects of Susanne's coping via somatization, and Susanne's husband is counseled not to reinforce illness behaviors. He is told to ignore somatic complaints and helpless behaviors and to reinforce "well" behaviors.

Family Therapy

Family involvement is recommended as an important part of treatment for somatoform disorders by many therapists. At a minimum, family therapy can help family members place the client's illness in perspective, teach ways of supporting each other, and provide anticipatory strategies for coping with predictable problems. The role of the family in maintaining somatoform symptoms should be considered, along with the importance of their collaboration in the treatment of the client.

Behavioral Therapy

The nurse generalist is often responsible for overseeing behavioral treatment plans established by a nurse therapist or other staff trained in behavioral therapy. Exposure and response prevention have been helpful in the treatment of clients with hypochondriasis. The client is forced to confront personal fears by reading about the feared disease, writing extensive information about the illness, and visiting hospitals. During this time, the client is not allowed to seek reassurance. Relatives and associates are instructed to ignore statements about somatic symptoms or bids for reassurance.

Cognitive Restructuring

With guidance, clients with somatization disorders explore their thoughts about their illnesses and correct their misconceptions through logical questioning and reasoning. The client who concludes that the presence of an insect bite on an ankle means that he has Lyme disease would be helped to explore other possibilities. The client who experiences back pain and uses negative self-talk ("I can't stand the pain when I do stretching exercises") can be taught to use positive self-talk ("The stretching exercises may relieve my discomfort"). The client with body dysmorphic disorder who thinks everyone is looking at her pointed chin can be helped to re-evaluate this thinking. Both advanced practice nurses and nurse generalists can assist clients with cognitive restructuring.

◗ The advanced practice psychiatric nurse who is Anthony's therapist decides to use a cognitive-behavioral approach. Cognitive therapy helps Anthony gain an intellectual understanding that his fear of having contracted AIDS more than 30 years ago is unrealistic. Anthony is given homework assignments to read literature about AIDS. His daughters are taught to change the subject whenever their father mentions STDs or AIDS. He contracts with the nurse therapist not to visit the STD clinic unless he is referred by the therapist. He also agrees to resume attendance at his social club at least once each week. After 3 months of therapy, Anthony is evaluated as being considerably less preoccupied with the possibility of illness.

Milieu Therapy (Basic Level)

Most clients with somatoform disorders are seen in medical, rather than psychiatric, settings. Hospitalizations and frequent visits to medical clinics may allow suggestible clients to witness the symptoms of others and later incorporate them into their own symptom repertoires. Because these clients are often rejected by medical-surgical staff, their anxiety levels may rise, causing an intensification of their somatic complaints. Nurses can teach family and significant others how to minimize secondary gains while providing respect and attention to "realistic" thoughts and feelings.

Self-Care Activities (Basic Level)

When somatization is present, the client's ability to perform self-care activities may be impaired, and nursing intervention may be necessary. In general, interventions involve the use of a matter-of-fact approach to support the highest level of self-care of which the client is capable.

For clients manifesting paralysis, blindness, or severe fatigue, an effective nursing approach is to matter-of-factly support clients while expecting them to feed, bathe, or groom themselves. For example, the client who demonstrates paralysis of an arm can be expected to eat using the other arm. The client who is experiencing blindness can be told at what numbers on an imaginary clock the food is located on the plate and encouraged to feed himself or herself. These strategies are effective in reducing secondary gain.

Psychobiological Interventions (Basic Level)

Clients with somatoform disorders rarely profit from antianxiety medication. Benzodiazepine use should be monitored carefully because clients with somatoform disorders may use them unreliably. Clients with somatoform pain disorder rarely benefit from the use of anxiolytics, analgesics, or sedatives. Presently, the antidepressants, specifically the selective serotonin reuptake inhibitors, show the greatest promise for helping clients with somatoform disorder.

Health Teaching (Basic Level)

Some clients who use somatization as a way of coping with anxiety have little formal education. Therefore, teaching these clients basic information about body functions is often warranted. Pictures and charts can be helpful. It is useful to review with the family the information that the client has been given because their information may also be lacking or in error.

Relaxation techniques (Chapter 17) and assertiveness training (Chapter 13) are often identified as appropriate skills to teach clients with somatoform disorders. Learning relaxation techniques gives the client a means of controlling symptoms. Assertiveness techniques give clients a direct means of getting needs met so that clients have less need to resort to somatic symptoms.

Biofeedback can be used as a means of teaching a client awareness and control of physiological processes associated with anxiety. By monitoring gauges or lights that signal the intensity of tension, the client learns to produce greater relaxation.

Case Management (Basic Level)

"Doctor shopping" is common among clients with somatoform disorder. The client goes from physician to physician, clinic to clinic, or hospital to hospital, hoping to establish a physical basis for distress. Repeated computed tomographic scans, magnetic resonance imaging, and other diagnostic tests are often seen as part of the assembled medical record for a given client. Case management can help limit health care costs associated with such visits. The case manager can recommend to the medical doctor that the client be scheduled for brief appointments every 4 to 6 weeks at set times rather than on demand and that laboratory tests, surgery, and hospitalization be avoided unless they are absolutely necessary. The client who establishes a relationship with the case manager often feels less anxiety because the client has someone to contact and knows that someone is "in charge."

▶ Robert, who has pain disorder, benefited from case management. His case manager arranges an outpatient clinic withdrawal from analgesic medication. Visits to the anxiety clinic are arranged. There, Robert is taught relaxation techniques, and biofeedback is used to help him develop awareness of muscle tension and other physiological processes associated with anxiety. Last, he is taught self-hypnosis. He states that being in control of his pain helps him feel like a man rather than a whimpering baby. The case manager works with his wife and family, teaching them to reinforce wellness behaviors and ignore comments about pain. The case manager arranges for job counseling that enables him to obtain a position as a dispatcher for a taxi company and resume his former breadwinner role.

Health Promotion and Health Maintenance (Basic Level)

Although clients with somatoform disorders make many contacts with physicians, these contacts are illness oriented. Such clients should be encouraged to pursue regular physical examinations and routine screening tests.

Most clients with somatoform disorders avoid physical exercise. After consulting with a physician, the client may experience an increased sense of well-being by undertaking a program of mild physical exercise.

▶ In the case of Anna, who has body dysmorphic disorder, health promotion and support of strengths are the treatment of choice. Anna is enrolled in an aerobic exercise program designed to help her feel more comfortable with her body, and the nurse undertakes interventions designed to enhance Anna's self-esteem and to support her perceived strengths. She is encouraged to talk with a department-store fashion consultant for assistance in choosing clothing that is becoming.

EVALUATION

Evaluation is a simple process when measurable behavioral outcomes have been clearly and realistically written. For clients with somatoform disorders, nurses often find the goals and outcomes are only partially met. This should be considered a positive finding because these clients often exhibit remarkable resistance to change. Clients are likely to report the continuing presence of somatic symptoms, but they often say that they are less concerned about the symptoms. Families are likely to report relatively high satisfaction with outcomes, even without total eradication of the client's symptoms.

DISSOCIATIVE DISORDERS

THEORY

Dissociative disorders involve disruption in the usually integrated mental functions of consciousness, memory, identity, or perception of the environment. Kopelman (1987) hypothesized that dissociative disorders involve attempts to use repression to block a traumatic event from awareness and to avoid the anxiety its memory would cause. When complete repression proves impossible because of the strength of the traumatic experience, dissociation of certain mental processes takes place to protect the individual

A common dissociative experience is **depersonalization disorder,** which is an elusive sensation of being not quite human, not fully alive, or disconnected from parts of one's body. Mild, fleeting dissociative experiences are relatively common. One study on dissociation (Grinspoon 1992a) suggested that about one third of people have occasionally felt as though they are watching themselves in a movie. Up to 70% of young adults may have brief episodes in which they feel that they are not themselves, or as though the world has a dreamlike quality. The incidence of these experiences steadily declines after 20 years of age.

When the ability to integrate consciousness is impaired, the individual is unable to remember (**dissociative amnesia** and **dissociative fugue**). When the ability to integrate identity is affected, fragmented aspects of the self may emerge as distinct personalities (**dissociative identity disorder** [DID]) and the individual loses the sense of who he or she is. DID is also known as multiple personality disorder.

Because the unconscious mind contains learned behaviors, clients with dissociative disorders continue to be able to read, write, and perform skills such as driving a car. This use of automatic behaviors is similar to what goes on in our everyday lives when we say we have been operating on "automatic pilot," performing an act or skill without concentrating on it.

The cause of dissociative disorders is unknown. Childhood sexual abuse has been associated with adult dissociation symptomatology (Zlotnick et al. 1994). Several theories are reviewed in the following sections.

Biological Factors

Current research suggests that the limbic system may be involved in the development of dissociative disorders. Traumatic memories are processed in the limbic system, and the hippocampus stores this information. Animal studies show that early prolonged detachment from the caretaker negatively affects the development of the limbic system. If this is true in humans, early trauma could remain detached from memory, and stress could precipitate dissociation. Significant early trauma and lack of attachment have also been demonstrated to have effects on neurotransmitters (specifically, serotonin).

Depersonalization disorder has a possible neurological link. The perception of change in one's own reality has been associated with neurological diseases, such as epilepsy and brain tumors, and psychiatric disorders, such as schizophrenia. Depersonalization is also experienced by individuals under the influence of certain drugs (e.g., alcohol, barbiturates, benzodiazepines, hallucinogens, and beta-adrenergic antagonists).

Genetic Factors

Several studies suggest that DID is more common among first-degree biological relatives of individuals with the disorder than in the population at large.

Cultural Factors

Certain culturally bound disorders exist in which there is a high level of activity, a trancelike state, and running or fleeing, followed by exhaustion, sleep, and amnesia regarding the episode. These syndromes include *piblokto*, seen in native people of the Arctic, Navajo "frenzy" witchcraft, and *amok* in Western Pacific natives. These syndromes, if seen in individuals native to these geographical areas, must be differentiated from dissociative disorders.

DSM-IV lists dissociative trance disorder, which may involve a possession state, among diagnoses in need of further study. Possession is a concept that is often culturally determined. In the possession state, the individual believes the self to be controlled by a force, demon, deity, or other person. Clients and families profess little faith in conventional psychiatric treatment and instead seek rituals of atonement and exorcism.

Psychosocial Factors

Learning theory suggests that dissociative disorders can be explained as learned methods for avoiding stress and anxiety. The pattern of avoidance occurs when an individual deals with an unpleasant event by consciously deciding not to think about it (i.e., "tuning out"). The more anxiety-provoking the event, the greater the need not to think about it. Some individuals practice tuning out and become good at it, as evidenced by students' "tuning out" what goes on in lectures, or marriage partners' seeming oblivious to the nagging of a spouse. It seems that the more dissociation is used, the more likely it is to become automatic. When stress is intolerable and ego disintegration becomes a possibility, the individual may unconsciously use dissociation to force the offending memory out of awareness. Abused individuals may learn to use dissociation to defend against feeling pain and to avoid remembering.

DSM-IV and the Clinical Picture of Dissociative Disorders

DSM-IV lists four major dissociative disorders: (1) depersonalization disorder, (2) dissociative amnesia, (3) dissociative fugue, and (4) DID.

Depersonalization Disorder

DSM-IV describes depersonalization disorder as a persistent or recurrent alteration in the perception of the self to the extent that the sense of one's own reality is temporarily lost while reality testing ability remains intact. The person experiencing depersonalization may feel mechanical, dreamy, or detached from the body. These experiences of feeling a sense of deadness of the body, of seeing self from a distance, or of perceiving the limbs to be larger or smaller than normal are described by clients as being very disturbing (ego-dystonic) (Fig. 18–3).

▶ Margaret describes becoming very distressed at perceiving changes in her appearance when she looks in a mirror. She thinks that her image looks wavy and indistinct. Soon after, she describes feeling as though she is floating in a fog with her feet not actually touching the ground. Questioning reveals that Margaret's son has recently revealed to her that he is HIV positive.

Dissociative Amnesia

Dissociative amnesia is marked by an inability to recall important personal information, often of a traumatic or stressful nature, that is too pervasive to be explained by ordinary forgetfulness (Fig. 18–3).

The client with generalized amnesia is unable to recall information about one's entire lifetime.

▶ A young woman, found wandering in a Florida park, is partly dressed and poorly nourished. She has no knowledge of who she is. Her parents identify her 2 weeks later when she appears in an interview on a national television show.

The client with localized amnesia is unable to remember all events of a circumscribed period of time from a few hours to a few days (e.g., the hours following the death of a loved one).

▶ Ann, a college student, is found walking along a major highway by a police road patrol. She can give her name and address but is not able to account for how she came to be walking along the highway. She is able to remember going to a party off campus but has no recall of the party or events after. Hospital examination reveals the probability of recent rape.

Selective amnesia involves the ability to remember some events, but not others, during a short period (e.g., remembering an automobile accident, but not remembering the death of someone involved in the accident).

Dissociative Fugue

Dissociative fugue is characterized by sudden, unexpected travel away from the customary locale and inability to recall identity and information about some or all of the past; in rare cases, a fugue has involved the assumption of a new identity. If a new identity is assumed, the new personality may be somewhat more outgoing. During a fugue state, individuals tend to lead rather simple lives, rarely calling attention to themselves. After a few weeks to a few months, they may remember their former

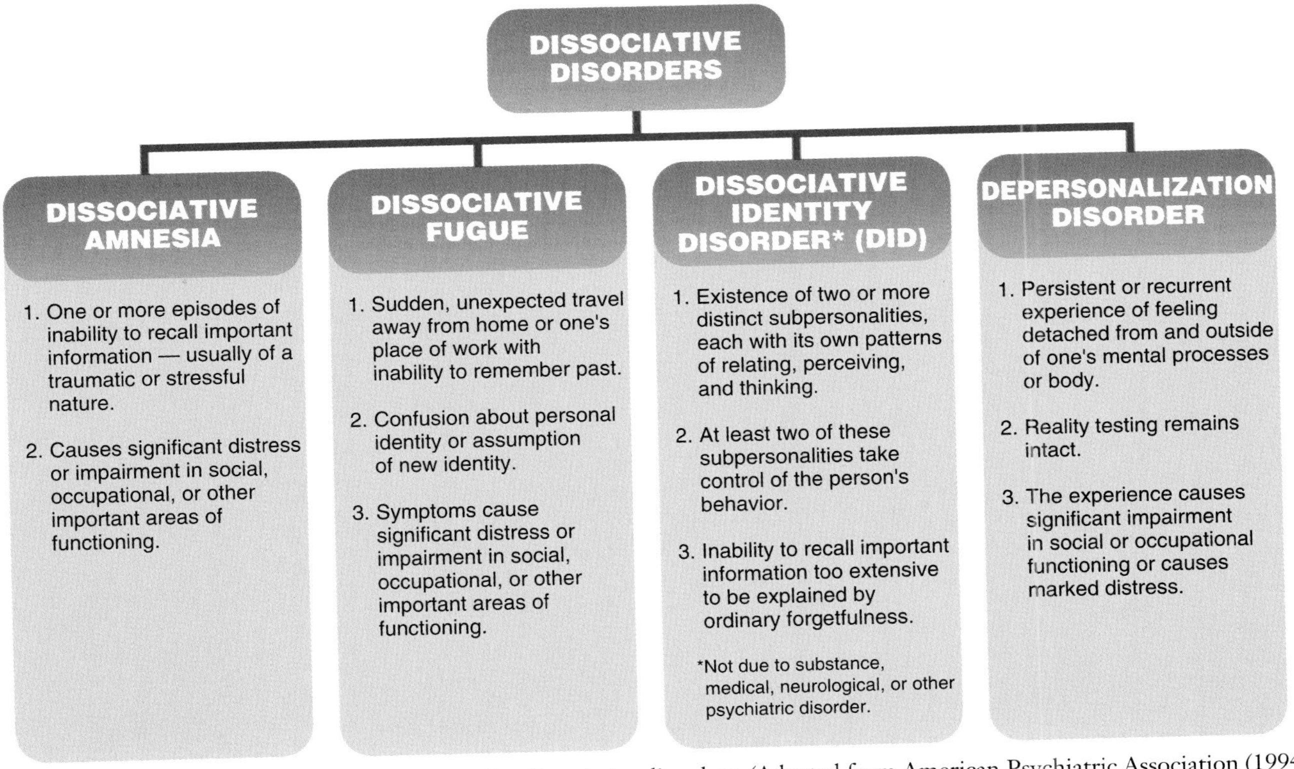

Figure 18–3 DSM-IV diagnostic criteria for dissociative disorders. (Adapted from American Psychiatric Association (1994). *Diagnostic and statistical manual of mental disorders* (4th ed.). Washington, DC: American Psychiatric Association. Reprinted with permission. Copyright 1994 American Psychiatric Association.)

identities and become amnesic for the time spent in the fugue (see Fig. 18–3 for DSM-IV criteria).

▸ A middle-aged woman awakens one morning and notices snow outside the window, swirling around unfamiliar buildings and streets. The radio tells her it is December. She is perplexed to find herself in a residential hotel in Chicago with no idea of how she got there. She feels confused and shaken. As she leaves the hotel, she is surprised to have strangers recognize her and say "Good morning, Sally." The name Sally does not seem right, but she cannot remember her true identity. She finds her way to a hospital, where she is evaluated and referred to the psychiatric nurse in the emergency department. A day later, "Sally" is able to remember her true identity, Mary Hunt. She tells the nurse tearfully that she can now recall that her husband came home one day and "out of the blue" told her he wanted a divorce to marry a younger woman. Mary calls her sister in New York, who comes to Chicago to take her home.

Most theorists agree that spontaneous loss of memory, as in amnesia and fugue, has been preceded by a severely traumatic event. Amnesia or fugue is most likely to occur during a time of great disorganization, such as a war or a disaster in which the threat of physical injury or death exists. Other stressors severe enough to produce psychogenic amnesia or fugue include the loss of a loved one and the stress of having to face the unacceptability of certain impulses or acts, such as an extramarital affair.

Dissociative Identity Disorder

The essential feature of DID is the presence of two or more distinct **alternate personality** or **subpersonality** states that recurrently take control of behavior. Each alternate or subpersonality has its own pattern of perceiving, relating to, and thinking about the self and the environment. It is believed that severe sexual, physical, or psychological trauma in childhood predisposes an individual to the development of DID. The steps in the development of dissociated personalities are thought to be as follows (Greenberg 1982):

1. A young child is confronted with an intolerable terror-producing event at a time when defenses are inadequate to handle the intense anxiety.
2. The child dissociates the event and the feelings associated with the event. The dissociated processes are split off from the memory of the primary personality.
3. The dissociated part of the personality takes on an existence of its own, becoming a subpersonality.
4. The subpersonality learns to deal with feelings and emotions that could overwhelm the primary personality.

This process may occur several times, creating one or several subpersonalities. When the individual is faced with an anxiety-producing situation, one of the subpersonalities takes over to protect the primary personality from disorganization and disintegration.

Each alternate personality or subpersonality is a complex unit with its own memories, behavior patterns, and social relationships that dictate how the person acts when that personality is dominant. Often, the original or primary personality is religious and moralistic, and the subpersonalities are quite different: aggressive, pleasure seeking, nonconforming, or sexually promiscuous. They may think of themselves as being a different sex, race, religion, or sexual orientation. Sometimes, the dominant hand is different, and the voice may sound different; intelligence and electroencephalographic findings may also be different. Alternate or subpersonalities may exhibit signs of emotional disturbance. A common alternate personality is a fearful, insecure child. Some subpersonalities have names for themselves. Some may be identified by roles they play: *host,* who provides the social front for interacting with the world; *protector,* who defends against harm; and *persecutor,* who attempts to harm other personalities.

The primary personality is usually not aware of the alternate or subpersonalities but may be aware of, and perplexed by, lost time and unexplained events. Experiences such as finding unfamiliar clothing in the closet, being called a different name by a stranger, waking up or coming out of a "blank spell" in strange surroundings, or not having childhood memories are characteristic of DID. Subpersonalities are often aware of the existence of each other to some degree. Some may even interact with each other. Occasionally, one alternate personality may attempt to harm another. Alternate personalities may "listen in" on whatever personality is dominant at the time. Transition from one personality to another often occurs during times of stress and may range from a dramatic to a barely noticeable event. Some clients experience the transition when awakening. Shifts from personality to personality last from minutes to months, although shorter periods are more common.

- Andrea, a conservative, 28-year-old electrical engineer, is the primary personality. Three alternate personalities coexist and vie for supremacy.
- *Michele* is a 5-year-old who is sometimes playful and sometimes angry. She speaks with a slight lisp and with the facial expressions, voice inflections, and vocabulary of a precocious child. She likes to play on swings, draw with a crayon, and eat ice cream. She likes to cuddle a teddy bear and occasionally sucks her thumb. Her favorite outfit is jeans and a Mickey Mouse sweatshirt.
- *Ann* is an accomplished ballet dancer. She is shy but firm about needing time to practice. When she is dominant, she likes to wear white and fixes her hair in a severe, pulled-back style. She does little but dance when she is in control.
- *Bridget* is near Andrea's age, although she says a lady never tells her age. She dresses seductively in bright colors, wears her hair tousled, and likes to frequent bars and stay out late. She often drinks to excess and has several male admirers. Bridget has many moods. She states that she would like to get rid of Ann and Andrea because they're such "goody-goodies."
- *Andrea* does not drink, hates ice cream, and sees herself as somewhat awkward. She does not dance. Instead, she is a paid soloist in a church choir. Andrea takes public transportation, but Ann and Bridget have driver's licenses. Andrea goes to bed and arises early, but Bridget and Michele like to stay up late.
- Andrea seeks treatment when she finds herself behind the wheel of a moving car and realizes that she does not know how to drive. She has been concerned for some time because she has found strange clothes in her closet. She has also received phone calls from men who insist that she has flirted with them in bars. She sometimes misses appointments and cannot account for periods of time. Although she goes to bed early, she is often unaccountably tired in the morning.

ASSESSMENT

For a diagnosis of dissociative disorder to be made, medical and neurological status, substance use, and coexistence of other psychiatric disorders need to be ruled out. Therefore, medical personnel collect objective data from physical examination, electroencephalography, CT, or MRI in order to rule out organic or other medical or psychiatric disorders. A client with DID is admitted to a psychiatric unit when suicidal. At that time, nursing assessment takes place through observation over a period of time as the nurse gathers information about identity, memory, consciousness, life events, mood, suicide risk, and impact of the disorder on the client and the family.

Assessing Identity and Memory

Assessing a client's ability to identify himself or herself requires more than asking the client to state his or her name. In addition, inability to identify self, or changes in client behavior, voice, and dress, might signal the presence of an alternate personality. Referring to self by another name or in the third person, using the word "we" instead of "I," are indications that the client may have assumed a new identity, as occurs in some fugue states. The nurse should consider the following when assessing memory:

Can the client remember recent and past events?
Is the client's memory clear and complete or partial and fuzzy?
Is the client aware of gaps in memory, such as lack of memory for events such as a graduation or a wedding?

Do the client's memories place the self with a family, in schools, in an occupation?

Clients with amnesia and fugue may be disoriented for time and place as well as person. Relevant assessment questions include the following:

- Do you ever lose time or have blackouts?
- Do you find yourself in places with no idea how you got there?

Assessing Client History

The nurse must gather information about events in the person's life. Has the client sustained a recent injury, such as a concussion? Does the client have a history of epilepsy, especially temporal lobe epilepsy? Does the client have a history of early trauma, such as physical, mental, and sexual abuse? If DID is suspected, pertinent questions include the following:

- Have you ever found yourself wearing clothes you don't remember?
- Have you ever found strange clothing in your closet?
- Have you ever found among your belongings new items that you can't remember buying?
- Have you ever had strange people greet and talk to you as though they were old friends?
- Have you ever found writing or drawing that you can't remember doing?
- Does your ability to do things such as athletics, artistic activities, or mechanical tasks seem to change?
- Do you have differing sets of memories about childhood? (This is often an indicator of DID.)

Assessing Mood

Is the individual depressed, anxious, or unconcerned? Many clients with DID seek help when the primary personality is depressed. The nurse also observes for mood shifts. When subpersonalities of DID take control, their predominant moods may be different from that of the principal personality. If the subpersonalities shift frequently, marked mood swings may be noted. Clients with DID or fugue may seem indifferent and unconcerned or may be uneasy or perplexed. A client with DID is likely to exhibit moderate to severe anxiety. This client often seeks help because of fear of "going crazy."

Assessing Use of Alcohol and Other Drugs

Specific questions should be asked to identify drug or alcohol use or abuse. Dissociative episodes may be associated with recent alcohol use. Marijuana is known to produce symptoms of depersonalization. Some clients with dissociative disorders turn to alcohol in an attempt to cope with the disorder itself.

Assessing Impact on Client and Family

Has the client's ability to function been impaired? Have disruptions in family functioning occurred? Is secondary gain evident? In fugue states, individuals often function adequately in their new identities by choosing simple, undemanding occupations and having few intimate social interactions. The families of clients in fugue states report being highly distressed over the client's disappearance. Clients with amnesia may be more dysfunctional. Their perplexity often renders them unable to work, and their memory loss impairs normal family relationships. Families often direct considerable attention and solicitude toward the client but may exhibit concern over having to assume roles that were once assigned to the client. Clients with DID often have both family and work problems. Families find it difficult to accept the seemingly erratic behaviors of the client. Employers dislike the lost time that may accompany subpersonalities' being in control. Clients with depersonalization disorder are often fearful that others may perceive their appearance as distorted and may avoid being seen in public. If they exhibit high anxiety, the family is likely to find it difficult to keep relationships stable.

Assessing Suicide Risk

Whenever a client's life has been substantially disrupted, the client may have thoughts of suicide. The nurse gathering data should be alert for expressions of hopelessness, helplessness, or worthlessness and for verbalization or other behavior of a subpersonality that indicates the intent to engage in self-destructive or self-mutilating behaviors.

NURSING DIAGNOSIS

Nursing diagnoses for clients with dissociative disorders include those discussed in this section. For example, the nurse needs to remember that nursing diagnoses may be required for subpersonalities as well as for the primary personality.

Personal identity disturbance (amnesia or fugue) related to a traumatic event would be an appropriate diagnosis for a client who is unable to recall his or her identity. This diagnosis would also be appropriate for a client experiencing symptoms of depersonalization disorder and feelings of unreality and body image distortions. The diagnosis of personal identity disturbance related to childhood abuse could be used when evidence of a traumatic childhood exists.

Ineffective individual coping related to alterations in consciousness, memory, or identity may be the diagnosis if the individual has thought about, or attempted, suicide or abuses chemicals as a way of dealing with having a dissociative disorder.

Anxiety related to alterations in memory or identity would be an appropriate diagnosis if the client demonstrates symptoms of anxiety that are attributable to not being in control of behavior, feelings, awareness, or memory. A client with depersonalization disorder would be a likely candidate for this diagnosis.

The diagnosis **altered role performance** related to disturbances in identity or memory and altered family processes related to amnesia or erratic and changing behaviors related to subpersonalities may be appropriate. Assessment data would verify disorganization or dysfunction, such as unexplained absences from work, social inappropriateness, withdrawal from relationships, and other phenomena that are unusual for the person.

The nursing diagnosis **risk for violence:** self-directed related to suicidal ideation associated with dissociative disorder, or related to lack of impulse control over subpersonalities, may also be warranted.

Other diagnoses that may be considered include **social isolation, body image disturbance, self-esteem disturbance, powerlessness,** and **sleep pattern disturbance.**

PLANNING

Planning Outcome Criteria

Outcomes must be established for each nursing diagnosis. Because each client presents an individual set of circumstances, outcomes must be highly individualized and consistent with each client's assessment. Examples of outcomes for selected nursing diagnoses follow.

Personal identity disturbanc*e* (specify amnesia, fugue, depersonalization, DID).

By (date) client will demonstrate ability to integrate identity and memory, as evidenced by

- Describing who he or she is.
- Identifying significant others.
- Describing feelings about events in the past.
- Being able to recognize the environment.
- Having absence of appearance of subpersonalities.
- Reporting absence of depersonalization episodes.

Anxiety related to alteration in identity or memory, related to severe stress.

By (date) client will demonstrate reduction in anxiety, as evidenced by

- Verbalizing feelings of comfort and safety.
- Verbalizing ability to control awareness.
- Using orderly logical thought process.

Altered role performance related to loss of memory, presence of multiple identities, or depersonalization episodes.

By (date) client will resume preillness roles, as evidenced by

- Resuming occupation.
- Expressing satisfaction with interactions with family, friends, and co-workers.
- Making decisions about daily living.

Social isolation related to inability to remember or fear of depersonalization episode.

By (date) client will interact appropriately on a social level with family and peers, as evidenced by

- Attending a specified number of social or diversional activities weekly.
- Verbalizing satisfaction with ability to interact with others.

Altered family coping related to having a family member with a dissociative disorder.

By (date) family will demonstrate interactions that promote optimal functioning of client, as evidenced by

- Absence of behaviors that promote secondary gain.
- Reports of client's ability to function independently.
- Resumption of preillness roles.

Self-directed violence related to presence of multiple identities, one of whom wishes to harm another.

By (date) client will refrain from attempts at self-harm.

Nurses' Feelings and Self-Assessment

Nurses may experience feelings of skepticism while caring for clients with dissociative disorders. They may find it difficult to believe in the authenticity of the symptoms the client is displaying.

The nurse caring for a client with amnesia or fugue may experience feelings of frustration in any of the following situations:

- If the client's confusion and bewilderment persist even after identity has been established.
- If the client seems helpless and needs assistance with activities of daily living, such as grooming and nutrition.
- If the client seems to be receiving many secondary gains, such as attention, media sensationalism, and avoidance of responsibility.

Feeling confused and bewildered by the presence of multiple identities is not unusual. Anger is commonly experienced as a reaction toward a subpersonality of a client with DID, if one personality is perceived as immature, challenging, or unpleasant. Some nurses experience feelings of fascination and are caught up in the intrigue of caring for a client with multiple identities. A sense of inadequacy may accompany the need to be ready to interact in a therapeutic way with whatever personality is in control at the moment.

Similarly, the nurse may feel inadequate when establishment of a trusting relationship occurs slowly. It is important for the nurse to remember that the client with a dissociative disorder has often experienced relationships in which trust was betrayed. When subpersonalities vie for control and attempt to embarrass or harm each other, crises are common. The nurse must be alert and ready to intervene and must always be prepared for the unexpected, including the possibility of a client's suicide attempt. Continuing hypervigilence by staff can eventually lead to feelings of fatigue. Anxiety may also be experienced by the nurse caring for a client with dissociative disorder in any of the following situations:

- When a client who has regained memory develops panic-level anxiety related to guilt feelings
- When a client becomes assaultive because of extreme confusion or panic-level anxiety
- When a client attempts self-harm by acting out against the primary personality or other personalities
- When a client develops panic-level anxiety during a depersonalization experience

If the client manifesting symptoms of a dissociative disorder has been involved in the commission of a crime, the nurse may experience concern over the fact that the medical record is likely to be a court exhibit. Nurses may feel anger in this situation if they believe that the client is faking illness to avoid being found guilty of the crime.

Supervision should always be available for staff caring for a client with a dissociative disorder in all settings. By discussing feelings as well as the plan for care with a competent peer or peers, the nurse can better ensure objective and appropriate care for the client.

Hospitalization of clients with dissociative disorders is brief and crisis centered, if it is required at all. Most therapy is conducted at the outpatient level. Planning should involve the client. Opportunities to participate in the care of the self combat feelings of helplessness and powerlessness.

Establishing a Relationship

The establishment of a trusting relationship is a primary task, although nurses on the inpatient unit have the opportunity for only a short-term relationship. Establishing trust is likely to be difficult because most clients with dissociative disorders have experienced a lifetime of poor relationships, beginning with childhood abuse. Giving simple explanations of what is expected of the client and being consistent are helpful strategies for establishing the relationship.

Meeting Safety and Security Needs

During the first 24 to 48 hours after admission, the nurse should be prepared to manage a variety of crises. Suicide attempts are common. It may be necessary to institute suicide precautions, one-to-one supervision, and a no-suicide contract as safety measures.

High levels of anxiety may accompany depersonalization episodes or may follow memory return in amnesia or fugue. An alternate personality or subpersonality may also appear and may become severely anxious. The appearance of subpersonalities may be a dramatic occurrence that requires the nurse to obtain as much information as possible about the new personality. The nurse may need to intervene spontaneously, with little opportunity to plan strategies. If a subpersonality has a violent agenda (e.g., to destroy another personality or to act out against staff), the nurse may need to institute emergency measures, such as seclusion and restraints, to prevent violence (see Chapter 12 for protocol).

Communication

Since the appearance of a client with a dissociative disorder is often considered a sensational event, the nurse may be required to deal with reporters seeking information. *The need for confidentiality cannot be overstressed.* Nurses should not comment to the media but should adhere to agency policy, which usually involves referring all requests for information to the hospital's public relations department. Communication among unit staff should be fostered, however, because knowing the plan of care is essential to reducing chaos and promoting effective care.

Addressing Memory and Identity Alterations

Memory loss deprives the individual of information necessary to solve even simple problems. Absence of family because of distance or estrangement deprives the client of support. The nurse may be the client's chief source of information and guidance as well as the major support-giving figure. However, the nurse should never try to force clients to accept information they are not ready to know. Memory loss and identity disturbance serve protective functions.

IMPLEMENTATION

Because nurses see relatively few clients with dissociative disorders, they are often anxious and unsure about the clinical decisions they are called on to make.

Counseling (Basic Level)

Counseling strategies are aimed at offering emotional presence during the recalling of painful experiences, to provide a sense of safety and encourage an optimal level of functioning (Table 18–3).

Psychotherapy (Advanced Practice)

The advanced practice psychiatric nurse may assume the role of primary therapist for clients with depersonalization disorder, amnesia, fugue, or DID. Nurse generalists usually have supportive roles.

Individual counseling for clients with amnesia, fugue, and depersonalization disorder focuses on creating a therapeutic alliance in which the client trusts the therapist and feels safe and relaxed. Feelings, conflicts, and situations that the client experienced before the onset of the dissociative disorder can then be explored. It is important to identify, as early as possible, triggers in the environment that lead to dissociation.

Hypnotherapy

Hypnotherapy may be used as an adjunct to counseling. Hypnotherapy allows the client's conscious control to relax so the therapist and the client can access material from the unconscious or make contact with subpersonalities. Counseling for clients with DID is of much longer duration and moves through several phases.

The first phase involves establishing communication with all subpersonalities and mapping names, roles, attitudes, behaviors, and relationships. The therapist informs each personality that acting out against each other is unacceptable and that each will be held accountable for his or her actions. Contracts with the personalities that gain agreement not to inflict harm or embarrassment are helpful.

The working stage extends over several years. The therapist, the primary personalities, and the alternate personalities or subpersonalities explore relevant issues, such as anger, sexuality, depression, and dependence, as well as the client's traumatic experiences. Compromises among personalities are negotiated during this phase.

The goal of the *final phase* is integration of the personalities. In addition, the therapist works with the newly in-

TABLE 18–3 INTERVENTIONS AND RATIONALES: DISSOCIATIVE DISORDERS

INTERVENTION	RATIONALE
Nursing Diagnosis: **Personal identity disturbance related to a traumatic event, as evidenced by an inability to remember past events**	
1. Ensure client safety by providing safe, protected environment and frequent observation.	1. Sense of bewilderment may lead to inattention to safety needs. Some subpersonalities may be thrill seeking, violent, or careless.
2. Provide nondemanding, simple routine.	2. Reduces anxiety.
3. Confirm identity of client and orientation to time and place.	3. Supports reality and promotes ego integrity.
4. Encourage client to do things for himself or herself and make decisions about routine tasks.	4. Builds ego strength, enhances self-esteem by reducing sense of powerlessness, and reduces secondary gain associated with dependence.
5. Assist with other decision making until memory returns.	5. Lowers stress and prevents client from having to live with the consequences of unwise decisions.
6. Support client during exploration of feelings surrounding the stressful event.	6. Helps lower the defense of dissociation used by the client to block awareness of the stressful event.
7. Do not flood the client with data regarding past events.	7. Memory loss serves the purpose of preventing severe to panic levels of anxiety to overtake and disorganize the individual.
8. Allow client to progress at own pace as memory is recovered.	8. Prevents undue anxiety and resistance.
9. Provide support during disclosure of painful experiences.	9. Can be healing while minimizing feelings of isolation.
10. Help client see consequences of using dissociation to cope with stress.	10. Increases insight and helps client understand own role in choosing behaviors.
11. Accept client's expression of negative feelings.	11. Conveys permission to have negative or unacceptable feelings.
12. Teach stress-reduction methods.	12. Provides alternatives for anxiety relief.
13. If client does not remember significant others, work with involved parties to reestablish relationships.	13. Helps client experience satisfaction and relieves sense of isolation.

tegrated personality to promote self-acceptance and use of new coping strategies.

Behavioral Therapy

When triggers in the environment that lead to dissociation have been identified, behavioral methods can be used by the client to interrupt the stimulus to dissociate by focusing on the present. The nurse generalist is often the person who helps the client learn to use these techniques and who guides and supports the client in their use.

WRAPPING SELF IN A BLANKET. Dissociation often begins with a feeling that one is "coming apart." Wrapping oneself in a blanket can help reinforce external boundaries.

HOLDING ICE IN THE HANDS. When dissociation threatens, holding an ice cube in each hand helps the client focus on a real, tangible sensation. This is calming and often prevents dissociation.

GOING TO A SAFE PLACE. Designating a particular room or a piece of furniture provides a client with a safe haven where nothing harmful will take place.

COUNTING. Counting backward or forward can be calming and can help the client focus on the present, rather than slipping into dissociation.

Cognitive Restructuring

Because of the relative newness of cognitive therapy and the rarity of dissociative disorder, little information is available about its usefulness. Cognitive counseling teaches the client about the process of dissociation and how it is used as a protective mechanism. It explores the cognitive distortions held by the client and fosters more accurate perceptions.

Family Therapy

Family counseling may assist in exploring and reducing role strain and family dysfunction. Often, the family member who has been physically absent because of fugue, mentally absent because of amnesia, or socially absent because of self-imposed isolation associated with depersonalization episodes must be reassimilated into the family. Families with members who are being treated for multiple identities need support to cope with the chaotic behaviors and to accept the integrated personality at the conclusion of therapy.

Milieu Therapy (Basic Level)

Providing a safe environment is fundamental. Other desirable characteristics of the environment are that it is quiet, simple, structured, and supportive. Confusion and noise increase anxiety and the potential for depersonalization, delayed memory return, or shifts among subpersonalities. Group therapy has not proved to be helpful, but task-oriented groups, such as occupational and art therapy, give an opportunity for self-expression. Attendance at community or unit milieu meetings relieves feelings of isolation.

Self-Care Activities (Basic Level)

Although a client with dissociative disorder may appear "healthier" than other clients, disruptions in self-care activities are often noted. The nurse may need to give simple directions to assist the client to complete grooming or to ensure nutrition if the client displays confusion, disorientation, severe anxiety, or immobilizing grief. Sleep patterns should be observed and documented because sleep loss and fatigue seem to increase the incidence of depersonalization episodes and may delay memory return.

Psychobiological Interventions (Basic Level)

Medication Administration

Antianxiety medication, such as clonazepam (Klonopin) and lorazepam (Ativan), may be prescribed as needed or as maintenance doses for short periods of time to treat severe anxiety states. Selective serotonin reuptake inhibitors, tricyclic antidepressants, or antipsychotics, such as haloperidol (Haldol), may be prescribed in order to treat severe psychiatric symptoms displayed by a subpersonality.

Antidepressants that work through monoamine oxidase inhibition should be used with great caution with clients who have DID because one of the subpersonalities may violate diet restrictions.

Narcotherapy

Narcotherapy, or interviewing under the relaxing influence of thiopental sodium (Pentothal) given intravenously, gives the therapist access to the client's repressed memories and conflicts. When the client has experienced psychogenic amnesia or fugue, the therapist may explore dissociated events. When the client being treated has multiple identities, the barbiturate interview may be used to access other personalities. The therapist is often able to learn the names, personalities, and roles played by alternate or subpersonalities, as well as how much each knows about the others. The nursing care of the client before and after the interview is similar to that of a client undergoing general anesthesia.

Health Teaching (Basic Level)

Preventing dissociative episodes is a skill the nurse can help the client learn. It involves becoming aware of triggers to dissociation and developing a plan to interrupt the dissociative episode. Some clients choose to use the behavioral methods described earlier in the chapter. Others choose to play an instrument or sing, engage in a specific physical activity, or interact with another person. Staff and significant others are made aware of the plan in order to foster their cooperation.

Clients should also be taught to write a daily journal. The journal puts the client in touch with feelings and provides concrete examples of overcoming triggers to dissociation. The journal should be shared with the nurse on a periodic basis. If a client has never written a journal, the nurse should suggest beginning with a 5- to 10-minute daily writing exercise.

Case Management (Basic Level)

Clients with dissociative disorders may require long-term case management. It may be necessary for the case manager to interact with numerous health professionals and health care agencies to facilitate the client's access to services and to maintain psychosocial functioning.

Health Promotion and Health Maintenance (Basic Level)

Clients with dissociative disorders should be encouraged to follow basic rules of health promotion and health maintenance, such as having regular physical examinations and screenings and regular dental care.

EVALUATION

Treatment is considered successful when outcomes are met. In the final analysis, the evaluation is positive when

- Client safety has been maintained.
- Anxiety has been alleviated and the client has returned to a state of comfort.
- Conflicts have been explored.
- New coping strategies permit the client to function at his or her optimal level.
- Stress is handled adaptively, without the use of dissociation.

SUMMARY

Somatoform disorders involve client complaints of physical symptoms that closely resemble actual medical conditions. Physical examination and diagnostic testing reveal no organic basis for the symptoms. Dissociative disorders make up a group of relatively rare conditions involving alteration in consciousness, memory, or identity. The cause of somatoform and dissociative disorders is assumed to be psychological (i.e., the appearance of symptoms provides relief of anxiety associated with a conflict or a traumatic event). Secondary gain is often present and must be minimized if treatment is to be successful.

Common nursing diagnoses are

- Anxiety.
- Ineffective individual coping.
- Impaired social interaction.
- Altered family coping.
- Self-esteem disturbance.
- Self-care deficit.

Discussions of planning and intervention for clients with these disorders included the need to provide for client safety, to reduce secondary gain, to encourage performance of self-care activities, to promote effective communication, and to provide a therapeutic milieu.

Psychotherapy is the treatment of choice for clients with somatoform and dissociative disorders. The nurse's roles include providing counseling, developing and implementing plans for behavioral change, assisting with cognitive restructuring, teaching anxiety-reducing strategies, and engaging in health promotion and maintenance activities.

REFERENCES

American Psychiatric Association (1994). *Diagnostic and statistical manual of mental disorders* (4th ed.)Washington, DC: American Psychiatric Association.

Greenberg, W. C. (1982). The multiple personality. *Perspectives in Psychiatric Care*, 20(3):100.

Grinspoon, I. (Ed.) (1992a). Dissociation and dissociative disorders (part 1). *Harvard Mental Health Letter*, 8(9):1.

Kaplan, H., et al. (1994). *Kaplan and Sadock's synopsis of psychiatry*. Baltimore: Williams & Wilkins.

Kopelman, J. D. (1987). Amnesia: Organic and psychogenic. *British Journal of Psychiatry*, 144:293.

Leff, J. (1988). *Psychiatry around the globe: A transcultural view* (2nd ed.). London: Royal College of Physicians.

Zlotnick, C., et al. (1994). The relationship between characteristics of sexual abuse and dissociative experiences. *Comprehensive Psychiatry*, 35(6):465.

Further Reading

Anderson, G., and Ross, C. (1988). Strategies for working with a patient who has multiple personality disorder. *Archives of Psychiatric Nursing*, 2:236.

Barstow, D. G. (1995). Self-injury and self-mutilation: Nursing approaches. *Journal of Psychosocial Nursing and Mental Health Services*, 33(2):19.

Cloninger, C. R. (1994). Somatoform and dissociative disorders. In G. Winokur and P. Clayton (Eds.), *The medical basis of psychiatry* (2nd ed., pp. 169–192). Philadelphia: W. B. Saunders.

Coons, P. M., and Milstein, V. (1992). Psychogenic amnesia: A clinical investigation of 25 cases. *Dissociation*, 5(6):2.

Curtin, S. (1993). Recognizing multiple personality disorder. *Journal of Psychosocial Nursing and Mental Health Services*, 31(2):29.

Fallon, B., et al. (1993). Hypochondriasis: Treatment strategies. *Psychiatric Annals*, 23(57):374.
Kellner, R. (1994). Psychosomatic syndromes, somatization and somatoform disorders. *Psychotherapy and Psychosomatics*, 61(1–2):4.
Lim, L. E. (1994). Psychogenic pain. *Singapore Medical Journal*, 35(5):519.
McCahill, M. E. (1995). Focus on the somatoform disorders. *Hospital Practice (Office Edition)*, 30(2):59.
Putnam, F. (1991). Recent research on multiple personality disorders. *Psychiatric Clinics of North America*, 14(3):489.
Ross, C. (1992). Epidemiology of multiple personality disorder and dissociation. *Psychiatric Clinics of North America*, 14:503.
Smith, G. R., et al. (1995). A trial of the effect of a standardized psychiatric consultation on health outcomes and costs in somatizing patients. *Archives of General Psychiatry*, 52:238.

SELF-STUDY AND CRITICAL THINKING

Multiple choice

1. Somatization and dissociative disorders fit on the anxiety continuum at the
   A. Mild level.
   B. Moderate level.
   C. Severe level.
   D. Panic level.
   E. They do not belong on the continuum, as anxiety has been reduced by ego defense mechanisms.
2. Which nursing diagnosis would be appropriate for a client with a somatoform disorder?
   A. Self-care deficit
   B. Personal identity disturbance
   C. Fluid volume deficit
   D. Altered growth and development
3. Which nursing diagnosis would be appropriate for a client with a dissociative disorder?
   A. Altered growth and development
   B. Pain
   C. Personal identity disturbance
   D. Noncompliance
4. Which of the following conditions involves assumption of a new identity in a distant locale?
   A. Hypochondriasis
   B. Conversion disorder
   C. Fugue
   D. Depersonalization disorder
5. Which statement about somatoform and dissociative disorders is true?
   A. There is no relationship between these disorders and early childhood trauma or loss.
   B. Clients with these disorders are perceived by nurses as being easy to care for.
   C. Clients with these disorders lack awareness of the relationship between symptoms and their anxiety and unconscious conflicts.
   D. An organic basis exists for each of these disorders.

Place a Y (for yes) next to necessary assessment data and an N (for nice to know but not essential) next to the others.

6. ________ Voluntary control of symptoms
7. ________ Description of symptoms, including onset

8. ________ Level of self-esteem
9. ________ Results of diagnostic work-ups
10. ________ Dependence on medication
11. ________ Limitations in activities of daily living
12. Which data should be routinely gathered during the assessment of a client with a dissociative disorder?

    A. ________ Potential for violence
    B. ________ Level of confusion
    C. ________ History of alcohol or drug abuse
    D. ________ Ability to remember
    E. ________ State of nutrition and fluid balance

Identify the helpful interventions with an H and those not helpful with an N.

13. Which of the following interventions would be helpful for a client with a somatoform disorder?

    A. ________ Focusing on client's physical symptoms
    B. ________ Offering sympathy
    C. ________ Encouraging activity
    D. ________ Offering advice

14. Which of the following interventions would be helpful for a client with a dissociative disorder?

    A. ________ Exposing to information about traumatic precipitating event
    B. ________ Scheduling client for a full range of activities: volleyball, community meeting, unit picnic, and carnival
    C. ________ Developing a no-suicide contract
    D. ________ Observing for mood or behavioral changes

Critical thinking

15. A client with dissociative identity disorder has been admitted to the crisis unit for a short-term stay after a suicide threat. On the unit, the client has repeated the statement that she will kill herself to get rid of "all the others," meaning her subpersonalities. The client refuses to sign a "no harm" contract. Design a care plan to meet her safety and security needs.
16. A client with suspected somatization disorder has been admitted to the medical-surgical unit after an episode of chest pain with possible electrocardiographic changes. While on the unit, she frequently complains of palpitations, asks the nurse to check her vital signs, and begs staff to stay with her. Some nurses take her pulse and blood pressure when she requests it. Others evade her requests. Most staff try to avoid spending time with her. Consider why staff wish to avoid her. Design interventions to cope with the client's behaviors. Give rationales for your interventions.
17. A client who has pain disorder complains of sleep pattern disturbance. Design a plan to teach this client ways of improving his sleep pattern.
18. A client with body dysmorphic disorder talks incessantly about how big her nose is, the way those around her are offended by her appearance, and how her appearance has negatively affected her employment and her social life. What interventions could you take to promote cognitive restructuring?

19

Personality Disorders

FRANCESCA PROFIRI

OUTLINE

KEY TERMS AND CONCEPTS

The key terms and concepts listed here also appear in bold where they are defined or discussed in this chapter.

splitting
self-mutilation
histrionics
narcissism

OBJECTIVES

After studying this chapter, the reader will be able to

1. Analyze the interrelatedness of biological determinants, chronic trauma, and psychodynamic issues in the cause of personality disorders.
2. Compare and contrast the main characteristics of each of the three clusters of personality disorders.

3. Describe the *Diagnostic and statistical manual of mental disorders,* fourth edition (1994) characteristics as seen on assessment of one personality disorder from each cluster and give a clinical example.
4. Formulate at least three nursing diagnoses for a person with a specific personality disorder.
5. Discuss the nature and the importance of crisis intervention for people with personality disorders.
6. Become aware of how the nurse would react to the personal feelings that may be aroused when the nurse works with a person who has a personality disorder.
7. Explain to a colleague the steps in countering manipulative behaviors in the hospital setting.
8. Explain the importance of keeping clear boundaries when working with a person with a personality disorder.
9. Role play with a classmate two useful counseling techniques for clients with personality disorder.

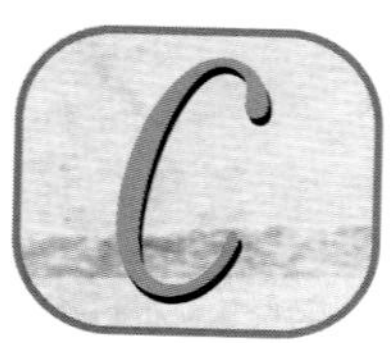

Clients diagnosed as having personality disorders (PDs) have multiple needs that pose many challenges to nurses and other health care providers. The client with PD requires that the nurse (1) have an understanding of the presenting problem, (2) be able to make an objective needs assessment, (3) be able to offer skills instruction and assistance in problem solving with follow-through, and (4) evaluate their nursing interventions. Most important, clients with PD require that the nurse possess a psychodynamic, cultural, and biological understanding of their maladaptive internal world. Underlying the PD is a developmental paralysis that results in clients' identifying and solving problems in an immature manner. Despite this, people with PDs are not always in extreme distress or even emotional discomfort. Often, it is the people who live or work with these individuals who are the most distressed (Maxmen and Ward 1996).

The hallmark of a person with PD is a lack of ability to implement change. Long-standing inability to tolerate frustration and pain, combined with overreaction to stimuli, can lead the client with PD to choose maladaptive responses to the ordinary problems of daily living. These behaviors, which reflect both disorganization of personality and intrapsychic imbalance, create ongoing patterns of learned helplessness and hopelessness. Clients with PD are then unable to identify their feelings and the needs that they represent and thus cannot understand how to meet their own needs successfully within community norms and without harm to themselves and others. Effective treatment of a client with PD calls on the nurse's behavioral and cognitive skills, which are aimed at soothing the inner pain that often overwhelms and disables the client. Psychopharmaceutical agents need to be used with caution; however, for some clients with PD, medication may promote the ability to learn adaptive coping skills and reveal the strength to initiate change.

Personality disorders occur in about 10% of the population; they are often overdiagnosed in clients who are ethnically and culturally different from the health care practitioner (Kaplan and Sadock 1991). It is important that assessment be performed in the context of the client's national, cultural, and ethnic background (see Chapter 5).

Personality disorders are a major source of long-term disability and frequently occur in conjunction with other psychiatric disorders or with general medical conditions. A study by Oldham and associates (1995) found that when any PD was present, it was likely that a mood, anxiety, psychotic, or eating disorder was also present. In people with borderline PD (BPD) or histrionic PD (HPD), psychoactive substance abuse was common. All of the PDs have four characteristics in common:

1. Inflexible and maladaptive responses to stress
2. Disability in working and loving
3. Ability to evoke interpersonal conflict
4. Capacity to have an intense effect on others (this process is often unconscious and generally produces undesirable results)

Often, people with PDs seek help from primary care physicians for physical complaints, rather than seeking psychiatric help (Oldham et al. 1995). Box 19–1 presents the DSM-IV criteria for a person with a PD. Under stress, some people with PD may become psychotic; therefore, the diagnosis of PD borders *severe* and *psychosis* on the mental health continuum (Fig. 19–1).

THEORY

Theorists who study PDs place emphasis on biological determinants, chronic trauma, and psychodynamic issues. Social and family issues interface with these different yet overlapping theories.

Biological Determinants

The most recent advances in psychobiology show some fascinating discoveries. A study by Cloninger and associ-

BOX 19-1 GENERAL DIAGNOSTIC CRITERIA FOR A PERSONALITY DISORDER

1. An enduring pattern of inner experience and behavior that deviates markedly from the expectations of the individual's culture. This pattern is manifested in two (or more) of the following areas:
   - Cognition (i.e., ways of perceiving and interpreting self, other people, and events)
   - Affect (i.e., range, intensity, lability, and appropriateness of emotional response)
   - Interpersonal functioning
   - Impulse control
2. The enduring pattern is inflexible and pervasive across a broad range of personal and social situations.
3. The enduring pattern leads to clinically significant distress or impairment in social, occupational, or other important areas of functioning.
4. The pattern is stable and of long duration, and its onset can be traced back at least to adolescence or early adulthood.
5. The enduring pattern is not better accounted for as a manifestation or consequence of another mental disorder.
6. The enduring pattern is not due to the direct physiological effects of a substance (e.g., a drug of abuse, a medication) or a general medical condition (e.g., head trauma).

Adapted from American Psychiatric Association (1994). *Diagnostic and statistical manual of mental disorders* (4th ed.) Washington, DC: American Psychiatric Association. Reprinted with permission. Copyright 1994 American Psychiatric Association.

ates (1993) measured the preexisting temperament and personality determinants inherent at birth as seen in infant studies. Four inheritable traits were identified:

1. Novelty seeking
2. Harm avoidance
3. Reward dependence
4. Persistence

This research revealed that people are born with an individual tolerance to stimulation or stress. This tolerance varies across a continuum, from stress avoidance to stimulation seeking. Living in a family with similar personality styles is likely to result in feelings of familiarity, empathy, and being understood; however, being born into a family whose personality styles differ may predispose a person to feeling isolated and misunderstood. Such a person might even become a target or scapegoat of the other family members' aggressions.

A study by Maier and associates (1994) found that schizotypal PD occurred more frequently in the nonpsychotic relatives of schizophrenics than in control families. Paranoid PD occurred much more frequently in relatives with major depression than in control subjects. A study by Lyons and associates (1995) of adult antisocial behavior or criminality found that genetic factors were more important than environment. In studies of delinquency, however, environment seemed to play a larger role.

Recent data on the social origins of personality demonstrate that from 2 years of age, children recognize conflict between a parent and an older sibling, that they take sides in the dispute, and that they often comfort the party they perceive as injured. Children develop skills to draw positive attention to themselves and to deflect negative attention by parents and siblings (Dunn and McGuire 1993). As children mature, they become able to differentiate clearly between themselves and siblings as to how they were treated by their mother and father and begin to parent themselves in a like manner (Baker and Daniels 1990). As an extension of this, children in large families think of themselves in terms of birth order. However, this has major impact on personality development only in cultures that emphasize birth-order privileges (e.g., primogeniture) or in families in which a parent has a stigmatizing condition, such as alcoholism, in which the oldest is more likely to become an active alcoholic than the siblings that follow (Bennett et al. 1987).

Chronic Trauma

Theorists who study the effects of long-term, persistent trauma have identified numerous stress response syndromes. Field studies of survivors of military combat, concentration camps, bereavement, natural disasters, long-term illness, rape, and mental illness show that many common elements exist among responses to a broad spectrum of traumatic events. First, the client has a compulsion to deny the impact of the event simultaneously with a need to compulsively act out the traumatic events. For example, an incest survivor may engage in sexual conduct that repeats the sense of powerlessness and exploitation (e.g., bondage, discipline, shaming, physical pain); however, the person might also feel empowered on completion of the eroticized ritual or rituals (Lewis-Herman 1992).

After a single traumatic event, each of us experiences conscious fear of its repetition, fear of being victimized or being powerless to prevent it, shame and rage over the vulnerability, rage at the cause of the event, fear of losing the power to respond aggressively to that rage, guilt or shame over the aggressive impulses themselves, guilt or shame for surviving, and sadness over the losses experienced, ranging from a previous sense of naive safety to the diminished ability to cope with the daily stress of adult living (Horowitz 1992).

Chronic trauma repeats this cycle over and over, reorganizing the brain's cortical map, the individual's cognitive and behavioral development, and the unconscious

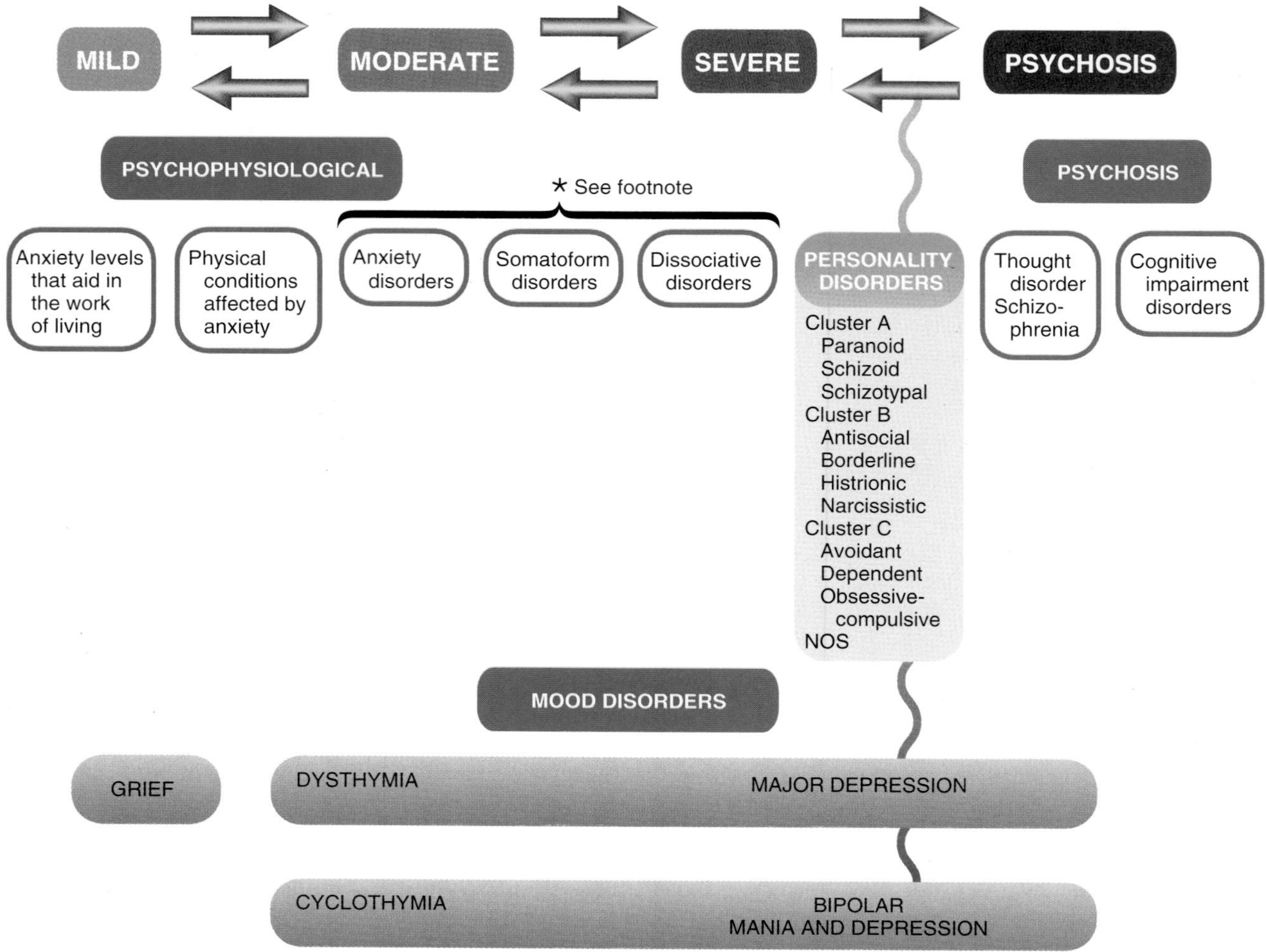

Figure 19–1 The mental health continuum for personality disorders.

(Dawson and Fischer 1994). The aftermath of such trauma for the client with PD can be seen more in their behavior than in their words. Clients with PD act out a forgotten history, or a past that has gone unquestioned—it being the only reality that they have ever experienced. They also project that everyone else has experienced what they have and thinks and feels as they do.

Along with the forgotten history, clients with PD experience an everyday, continuing terror that is the raw resource from which all their perceptions and self-regard are built. They disconnect unconsciously from their emotions, and at the same time, they have an inability or unwillingness to attach adaptively to others, including a failure to perceive cues others give them about how to do so. Manipulation and power struggles are thus the norm in all relationships of a person with PD. Fear of closeness results, and a precarious dance ensues, in which chronically traumatized clients attempt to work systems, personal relationships, and themselves to get their needs met from those they perceive to be at a safe distance. In this context, intimacy can feel like captivity (Lewis-Herman 1992).

One could view chronic mental illness, specifically PDs, as resulting from long-term stressors or chronic trauma. New data arising from recent discoveries in neurobiology show how electrical and chemical stimulation caused by psychosocial stressors influences gene expression and thus presents a way in which acute events can cause a subsequent overreactive response in a person's nervous system. That is, new cortical pathways specifically and selectively respond with rapidly increasing intensity of the neurotransmitters to stress.

This means that neurobiological encoding through memory-like functioning could provide a long-term vulnerability to subsequent episodes, some of which may arise in situations of relatively lower psychosocial stress. In other words, stress begets a more efficient neurochemical system for begetting stress. Eventually, activities that were once performed with ease may trigger or "rekindle" neurotransmitters via chemical and electrical transduction that induces an inner experience of crisis, which is in no way equivalent to the triggering event. Intrapsychic flashbacks become, through forgotten history and denial, disconnected from the primary traumatic event over time. Instead, these traumatic memories become translated into chemical and behavioral patterns of response to normal adult daily living (Post 1992).

Psychodynamic Issues

Psychodynamic theorists use a different clinical language. Kernberg (1985) gave the following examples:

- Repression and suppression (unconscious and conscious actions that exhibit a forgotten history)
- Undoing (unconscious repetition of a primary traumatic event)
- Regression (neurochemical flashbacks)
- Consolidation and recognition (integrating cognition, emotion, and behavior with acceptance of the past events and conscious awareness of their inner responsiveness to their past)

Psychodynamic theorists continue to point out the healing qualities of a corrective relationship, in which the client with PD is understood from a near-experience (Kohut 1984). Kohut's "near-experience" means understanding from the client's perspective and not through the distorting lens of theory or of a caregiver's personality. This understanding helps the therapist better identify the core conflict. The therapist then works to establish clear boundaries, provide emotional constancy (empathetic, respectful, helpful), and contribute developmental information. Through this process, clients with PD are enabled to interpret themselves and others from a more pragmatic and realistic perspective. The goal of psychodynamic therapy is to form a relationship that can correct and readjust maladaptive learning from the past.

These divergent theories share some common perspectives: first, chronic trauma can create social, familial, individual, and eventually biochemical, imbalances; second, a healing relationship can intervene to reconstruct the personality chemically, cognitively, and experientially.

ASSESSMENT

Taking a full medical history can help determine if this is a psychiatric problem, a medical problem, or both. Medical illness should never be ruled out as the cause until the data support this conclusion. Questions regarding a history of suicidal or homicidal ideation, intent, gestures, or attempts and current use of medicines, illegal substances, food, and money elicit information about the client's current level of crisis as well as dysfunctional coping styles. These are important data regarding clients who have PDs.

Important areas to explore are elicited through questions that detail involvement with the courts; current or past physical, sexual, or emotional abuse; and level of current endangerment from self or others. At times, immediate interventions may be needed to ensure the client's or others' safety. Information regarding prior use of any medication, including psychopharmacological agents, is important. This information gives evidence of other contacts the client has made for help and indicates how the health care provider found the client at that time.

From the data, the nurse identifies whether immediate action needs to be taken (e.g., medicate, arrange hospitalization). The nurse's plan may also include referrals (e.g., consultation with team psychiatrist, provisions for day treatment, need for disability, family conference). In consultation with the *Diagnostic and statistical manual*, fourth edition (DSM-IV) (1994), to establish criteria for each disorder—and with the orderly accumulation of observed data, history, and assessment—the diagnosis is made. From this diagnosis and its stated problem to be solved, a plan of action is indicated.

This chapter groups the PDs into three clusters, based on descriptive similarities. Cluster A includes paranoid, schizoid, and schizotypal disorders. Individuals with these disorders often appear odd or eccentric. Figure 19–2 presents the DSM-IV criteria for the disorders in cluster A.

Clinical Picture of Cluster A Disorders (Odd or Eccentric)

Paranoid Personality Disorder

Individuals with paranoid PD (PPD) greatly fear that others will exploit, harm, or deceive them, to the point of endangering their lives. Even when no evidence exists, clients with PPD interpret all experience from the perspective that they have been done irreversible damage by others; therefore, people with PPD are extremely reluctant to share information about themselves. Compliments or loyalty are misread as manipulation or attempts to disempower them. These individuals are hypervigilant, anticipate hostility, and can actually create hostile responses by *initiating* a "counterattack." Jealousy, controlling behaviors, avoidance of others, and unwillingness to forgive are all characteristics of PPD. Because of their excessive suspiciousness and fear of attack, people with PPD are usually argumentative, sarcastic, and complaining, or they are quietly hostile and aloof (Gunderson and Phillips 1995). The best approach with paranoid individuals is neutral, matter of fact, and respectful. A warm, enthusiastic approach is perceived as being intrusive, phony, and threatening.

Psychotic episodes can occur with these individuals, especially during times of stress (e.g., mourning, illness, change). Experiences that overwhelm them with frustration and anger aggravate their preexisting high level of fear, increase their need for solitude, and exacerbate their poor peer relationships and social anxiety. As people with

CLUSTER A (Odd or Eccentric)

PARANOID PERSONALITY DISORDER

A. A pervasive distrust and suspiciousness of others such that their motives are interpreted as malevolent, beginning by early adulthood and present in a variety of contexts, as indicated by four (or more) of the following:

(1) Suspects, without sufficient basis, that others are exploiting, harming, or deceiving self
(2) Is preoccupied with unjustified doubts about the loyalty or trustworthiness of friends or associates
(3) Is reluctant to confide in others because of unwarranted fear that the information will be used maliciously against self
(4) Reads hidden demeaning or threatening meanings into benign remarks or events
(5) Persistently bears grudges (i.e., is unforgiving of insults, injuries, or slights)
(6) Perceives attacks on his or her character or reputation that are not apparent to others and is quick to react angrily or to counterattack
(7) Has recurrent suspicions, without justification, regarding fidelity of spouse or sexual partner

SCHIZOID PERSONALITY DISORDER

A. A pervasive pattern of detachment from social relationships and a restricted range of expression in interpersonal settings, beginning by early adulthood and present in a variety of contexts, as indicated by four (or more) of the following:

(1) Neither desires nor enjoys close relationships, including being part of a family
(2) Almost always chooses solitary activities
(3) Has little, if any, interest in having sexual experiences with another person
(4) Takes pleasure in few, if any, activities
(5) Lacks close friends or confidants other than first-degree relatives
(6) Appears indifferent to the praise or criticism of others
(7) Shows emotional coldness, detachment, or flattened affect

SCHIZOTYPAL PERSONALITY DISORDER

A. A pervasive pattern of social and interpersonal deficits marked by acute discomfort with, and reduced capacity for, close relationships as well as by cognitive or perceptual distortions and eccentricities of behavior, beginning by early adulthood and present in a variety of contexts, as indicated by five (or more) of the following:

(1) Ideas of reference (excluding delusions of reference)
(2) Odd beliefs or magical thinking that influence behavior and are inconsistent with subcultural norms (e.g., superstitiousness, belief in clairvoyance, telepathy, or "sixth sense"; in children or adolescents, bizarre fantasies or preoccupations)
(3) Unusual perceptual experiences, including bodily illusions
(4) Odd thinking and speech (e.g., vague, circumstantial, metaphorical, overelaborate, or stereotyped)
(5) Suspiciousness or paranoid ideation
(6) Inappropriate or constricted affect
(7) Behavior or appearance that is odd, eccentric, or peculiar
(8) Lack of close friends or confidants other than first-degree relatives
9) Excessive social anxiety that does not diminish with familiarity and tends to be associated with paranoid fears rather than negative judgments about self

Figure 19–2 DSM-IV diagnostic criteria for cluster A personality disorders. (Adapted from American Psychiatric Association (1994). *Diagnostic and statistical manual of mental disorders* (4th ed.). Washington, DC: American Psychiatric Association. Reprinted with permission. Copyright 1994 American Psychiatric Association.)

PPD age, their isolation, underachievement, and hypersensitivity give them a more idiosyncratic and eccentric presentation. They may even develop peculiar habits in dress, language, and thoughts that further set them apart.

Individuals with PPD rarely initiate contact with a medical system and are usually in contact with health care professionals against the client's will or in an emergency situation in which they have no choice. Once in the system, people with PPD may suddenly flee or sign out against medical advice because of suspicion and fear (Goldberg 1995). To counteract fear, straightforward explanations of tests, history taking, and procedures are helpful. The person with PPD should be warned about the side effects of drugs, any changes in the treatment plan, and the possibility of further procedures.

Paranoid PD is most commonly diagnosed in males and is more prevalent in families with a history of schizophrenia. However, paranoid ideation is common. Paranoid ideation is expected when found in populations where harm, betrayal, and isolation have occurred, e.g., refugees, POWs, the elderly, and the hearing impaired (Gunderson and Phillips 1995). Cocaine-related disorders can look similar to PPD (APA 1994, pp. 634–638).

◗ Mr. Cortez, a 50-year-old employed factory worker, is seen in the emergency department after complaining of heart palpitations and chest pain. He refuses to have his blood drawn, to have lab tests done, or to answer questions. He also refuses to give his address and telephone number, stating that there are no relatives he wishes to have contacted, and begins a long and complicated diatribe against the medical system. The nurse explains calmly, and in reassuring detail, why all these questions need to be answered and the tests need to be done.

Obtaining Mr. Cortez's permission to complete each task would facilitate his cooperation and compliance. Increasing his sense of power over what is happening to him by giving him control and information can measurably decrease his paranoia.

Schizoid Personality Disorder

The client with schizoid PD has difficulty expressing any emotion, whether it be anger at being abused or joy in a fine meal. Usually, people with schizoid PD are seen as drifters on the periphery of society, avoiding relationships of even the most superficial type. Their lack of desire for companionship or sexual relationships produces social isolation. People who have schizoid PD infrequently marry, but when they do, the marriage is impaired by their lack of affect and flat experience of emotions. Occupational functioning is poor, especially if they must relate interpersonally, but they tend to do well if they can be the "lone wolf." In response to stress, they may become delusional. People with this disorder appear cold and aloof, indifferent to the approval or criticism of others. However, in rare instances, people with schizoid PD reveal having painful feelings, especially related to social interaction (APA 1994).

Schizoid PD can be a precursor to schizophrenia or delusional disorder; the prevalence is increased if a family history of schizophrenia or schizotypal PD exists. If persistent psychotic symptoms (e.g., delusions, hallucinations) exist, schizoid disorder is ruled out. Sometimes, it is difficult to differentiate schizoid PD from autistic disorder, especially in the presence of long-term substance abuse.

Onset begins in early adulthood and is wide reaching in its effects on the client's life and family. Because schizoid individuals lack social awareness and insight into other people's behaviors, their relationship skills become rigid, maladaptive, and distressing to themselves; hence, they increasingly avoid others. This fear of others is fed by the confusion in other people's responses to them. In dealing with others, the schizoid client's most common experience is failure.

It is dangerous to assume that street people, hermits, and shut-ins may be diagnosed with schizoid PD, as other medical and psychiatric problems have a schizoid appearance. For example, speaking only a foreign language, being a new immigrant to this country, or being extremely agoraphobic or obsessive-compulsive can all present a picture similar to that of schizoid PD (APA 1994, pp. 638–641).

◗ Mr. Wong, a 28-year-old homeless man, is admitted to the hospital after a physical assault. Although compliant with his treatment, he spends most of his time in the smoking area of the hospital, sitting cross-legged and staring at the floor. He does not respond verbally when spoken to. He avoids eye contact and remains a passive recipient in his treatment and discharge planning. At night, Mr. Wong is often found in the darkest and most secluded area of the unit, sleeping on the floor in a fetal position with all his possessions around him. When spoken to, he gets up and walks away. All nursing interventions for socialization are rejected, although he continues to be outwardly compliant.

Mr. Wong is likely to be most responsive when the nurse tells him what he can expect, and what is expected from him, on a task-by-task basis. Simplification and clarity can decrease his anxiety.

Schizotypal Personality Disorder

The history of a client with schizotypal PD shows eccentricity from early childhood, with strong although uncommon beliefs that display perceptual and cognitive distortions. Many cultures have beliefs that may appear eccentric outside of that culture but within it are adaptive and enhancing (see Chapter 5). This is not the case with clients with schizotypal PD. Their behavior, which is far outside cultural norms, is maladaptive. Such clients broadcast their beliefs, calling attention to themselves even though they do not seek attention. Their eccentric ideas stem from incorrect interpretations of internal and external events; the clients then spiritualize or concretize these distortions, convinced of their reality, and present them with significant conviction (which seems superstitious, magical, or grandiose to other members of the culture).

Clients with schizotypal PD may have magical rituals or a belief that they can control the actions of others; perceptually, they may hear murmuring voices or the presence of another person when no one is there. Their speech is idiosyncratic in phrasing and syntax. Their conversation is loose, in that they easily digress, are vague, or may become incoherent. They can be concrete and abstract, sometimes on the same topic; while it all makes sense to them, to others it may appear illogical. As a consequence, these clients become suspicious of others who do not share their reality. They may perceive others as dense or crazy, and likely to undermine them.

Because people with schizotypal PD cannot pick up on interpersonal cues, they relate stiffly, apprehensively, and inappropriately. Their range of affect can be constricted, even though their beliefs may be fantastical. Their eccentric and unkempt behaviors and inattention to social conventions make it impossible for them to have a give-and-take conversation. Consequently, they can be frightened and paranoid in social situations. Ideas of reference, odd communication, social isolation, and transient psychosis may be ameliorated by neuroleptics (e.g., haloperidol [Haldol], 1 to 10 mg) (Maxmen and Ward 1995).

Unlike those with schizoid PD, whose behavior suggests that they want diminished social contact, people with schizotypal PD are unhappy about having no functional relationships. Their social anxiety does not abate over time, and tension and unhappiness increase; their life is plagued by social and interpersonal deficits. This disorder is most prevalent in first-degree relatives of schizophrenics. Schizotypal PD occurs in 3% of the population, and only a small portion of those with the disorder develops a psychotic disorder (APA 1994, pp. 641–645).

▶ Ms. Carol, a 36-year-old unemployed woman receiving permanent psychiatric disability, enters day treatment after her fifth psychiatric hospitalization. She is appropriately dressed except for opera-length gloves and a lace scarf that is wrapped as a turban around her head. She is quiet and sits separately in a corner of the community room during most of her time there, appearing to be deep in thought and occasionally talking to herself. However, during group meetings, she suddenly begins to speak very loudly (but with flat affect) about how she is going to become an independent movie producer, director, and writer, to prove once and for all that the unidentified foreign objects visiting us are really angels from heaven and that 21st-century space ships have taken the place of 14th-century wings.

▶ She follows her nurse therapist wherever he goes and has difficulty understanding the limits placed on her regarding this behavior. The nursing strategy is to calm Ms. Carol's apparent anxiety about being in a group setting by introducing her to each individual in day treatment and identifying their reason for being there. For example, Ms. Carol is told that the case manager will be helpful with housing and disability, and the nurse with therapy and medications. Other clients are introduced by their goals: "Mr. Tom wants to learn how to stay out of the hospital."

Clinical Picture of Cluster B Disorders (Dramatic, Emotional, or Erratic)

The cluster B PDs include antisocial, borderline, histrionic, and narcissistic PDs (NPDs). Individuals in cluster B often appear dramatic, emotional, or erratic. Figure 19–3 presents the DSM-IV criteria for cluster B disorders.

Antisocial Personality Disorder

In the past, this PD has been called psychopathy, sociopathy, or dyssocial PD because it is characterized by deceit, manipulation, revenge, and harm to others with an absence of guilt or anxiety. People with antisocial PD have a sense of entitlement (i.e., they believe they have the right to hurt others). This disorder may be underdiagnosed in females and overdiagnosed in clients in lower socioeconomic areas of cities. Currently, 3% of males and 1% of females in the population are diagnosed as having antisocial PD. These traits may become less evident as the client ages, especially in the early forties or fifties, when antisocial criminal behavior—and, often, associated substance abuse—tend to decline.

Usually, first contact with this client occurs because of court-ordered treatment; the norm is a long history of illegal activity. The presentation of clients with antisocial PD is one of intent to deceive, along with impulsivity in action, so that the combination of reckless disregard for others and themselves is evident. They neglect responsibilities to others, lie, and repeatedly perform destructive acts—which may include vandalism, unsafe sex, driving under the influence, and assault—without developing any insight as to the predictable consequences. It is difficult for them to hold a job, to parent or relate to others, or to pay their bills because of their consistently defaulting on responsibility. Indifference to their own pain or the pain they inflict on others is defended by clients with antisocial PD by their presumed right to hold themselves above others; their assumption is that if they do not do these things to others first, then others will do these things to them. They accept no traditional value or moral as a boundary for their actions.

This lack of empathy combines with a contemptuous attitude toward others and an arrogant or grandiose opinion of self. Verbally, these clients can be adept, charming, and self-assured. This superficial charm engages others in their web of intrigue, which is designed for exploitation. They have difficulty tolerating boredom, seek out high stimulation to avoid depression, and can become tense if they do not feel in control of others. Frustration is familiar to them, as is compulsive behavior regarding food, alcohol, sex, and gambling.

Research among non–blood-related families (e.g., in cases of adoption) indicates that both genetic and environmental factors contribute to the risk of developing antisocial PD. Adopted children resemble their biological parents more than their adoptive ones, but the environment of the adoptive family highly influences the risk of this pathology (APA 1994, pp. 645–650). These clients rarely seek help but may be hospitalized when they are remanded by the courts or found to be a danger to others or even to themselves.

▶ Mr. James, a 23-year-old unemployed truck driver, is admitted to the unit after an episode of drunken driving.

CLUSTER B (Dramatic, Emotional, or Erratic)

ANTISOCIAL PERSONALITY DISORDER

A. A pervasive pattern of disregard for and violation of the rights of others occurring since age 15, as indicated by three (or more) of the following:

(1) Failure to conform to social norms with respect to lawful behaviors as indicated by repeatedly performing acts that are grounds for arrest
(2) Deceitfulness, as indicated by repeatedly lying, use of aliases, or conning others for personal profit or pleasure
(3) Impulsivity or failure to plan ahead
(4) Irritability and aggressiveness, as indicated by repeated physical fights or assaults
(5) Reckless disregard for safety of self or others
(6) Consistent irresponsibility, as indicated by repeated failure to sustain consistent work behavior or honor financial obligations
(7) Lack of remorse, as indicated by being indifferent to, or rationalizing, having hurt, mistreated, or stolen from another

B. The individual is at least 18 years of age.

C. There is evidence of conduct disorder with onset before age 15 years.

BORDERLINE PERSONALITY DISORDER

A. A pervasive pattern of instability of interpersonal relationships, self-image, and affects, and marked impulsivity beginning in early adulthood and present in a variety of contexts, as indicated by five (or more) of the following:

(1) Frantic efforts to avoid real or imagined abandonment. *Note:* Do not include suicidal or self-mutilating behavior covered in criterion 5.
(2) A pattern of unstable and intense interpersonal relationships characterized by alternating between extremes of idealization and devaluation
(3) Identity disturbance: markedly and persistently unstable self-image or sense of self
(4) Impulsivity in at least two areas that are potentially self-damaging (e.g., spending, sex, substance abuse, reckless driving, binge eating). *Note:* Do not include suicidal or self-mutilating behavior covered in criterion 5.
(5) Recurrent suicidal behavior, gestures, or threats, or self-mutilating behavior
(6) Affective instability due to a marked reactivity of mood (e.g., intense episodic dysphoria, irritability, or anxiety, usually lasting a few hours and rarely more than a few days)
(7) Chronic feelings of emptiness
(8) Inappropriate intense anger or difficulty controlling anger (e.g., frequent displays of temper, constant anger, recurrent physical fights)
(9) Transient, stress-related paranoid ideation or severe dissociative symptoms

NARCISSISTIC PERSONALITY DISORDER

A. A pervasive pattern of grandiosity (in fantasy and behavior), need for admiration, and lack of empathy, beginning in early adulthood and present in a variety of contexts, as indicated by five (or more) of the following:

(1) Has a grandiose sense of self-importance (e.g., exaggerates achievements and talents, expects to be recognized as superior without commensurate achievements)
(2) Is preoccupied with fantasies of unlimited success, power, brilliance, beauty, or ideal love
(3) Believes that he or she is "special" and unique and can only be understood by, or should associate with, other special or high-status people (or institutions)
(4) Requires excessive admiration
(5) Has sense of entitlement (i.e., unreasonable expectations of especially favorable treatment or automatic compliance with personal expectations)
(6) Is interpersonally exploitative (i.e., takes advantage of others to achieve personal ends)
(7) Lacks empathy: is unwilling to recognize or identify with the feelings and needs of others
(8) Is often envious of others or believes that others are envious of self
(9) Shows arrogant, haughty behaviors or attitudes

HISTRIONIC PERSONALITY DISORDER

A. A pervasive pattern of excessive emotionality and attention seeking, beginning in early adulthood and present in a variety of contexts, as indicated by five (or more) of the following:

(1) Is uncomfortable in situations in which self is not the center of attention
(2) Interaction with others is often characterized by inappropriate sexually seductive or provocative behavior
(3) Displays rapidly shifting and shallow expression of emotions
(4) Consistently uses physical appearance to draw attention to self
(5) Has a style of speech that is excessively impressionistic and lacking in detail
(6) Shows self-dramatization, theatricality, and exaggerated expression of emotion
(7) Is suggestible (i.e., easily influenced by others or circumstances)
(8) Considers relationships to be more intimate than they actually are

Figure 19–3 DSM-IV diagnostic criteria for cluster B personality disorders. (Adapted from American Psychiatric Association (1994). *Diagnostic and statistical manual of mental disorders* (4th ed.). Washington, DC: American Psychiatric Association. Reprinted with permission. Copyright 1994 American Psychiatric Association.)

He is on bed rest and traction, owing to a broken pelvis. In his admission work-up, he denies any active drug or alcohol use. When bathed by the nursing staff, he requests sexual contact. He complains loudly and angrily that his pain medication regimen is not adequate. When his requests are not met immediately, he begins to scream and throw objects around the room. His constant demanding behavior overwhelms the staff. His call light is always on, and the nursing staff begin to avoid answering it. On his third day of hospitalization, his temperature and blood pressure begin to rise, and he begins pharmacological treatment for drug and alcohol withdrawal.

- To promote optimal client care and avoid staff burnout, the staff formulate a written plan of care that is posted in his room, detailing Mr. James' daily regimen: when his bath is to be given, what his meds are and when they are to be given, when he is to receive his meals, when the doctor can be expected to visit, when as-needed nursing contacts are to be made, and so on. Clarification of boundaries and consistent adherence to the routine in the nursing care plan are designed to minimize Mr. James' acting out behaviors, especially when his opportunities for manipulation are drastically reduced.

Borderline Personality Disorder

People with BPD experience overwhelming needs, both internal and external, which they seek to have met in relationships. A major defense of the client with BPD is **splitting,** or alternating between idealizing and devaluation. Splitting is a failure to integrate the positive and negative qualities of self or others. For example, on first meeting, they idealize others (lovers, health care providers), imagining that at last they have found someone to give them what they need. But, at the first disappointment, frustration, or denied request, they dramatically shift to devaluing and despising the other person. They threaten abandonment and may actually abandon the other person, but internally they are frantically searching to reattach; alternately, they try to find someone new to attach to as quickly and as intensely as before. Splitting is a primitive defense in which people see themselves or others as either all good or all bad and are unable to integrate the positive and negative qualities of the self or others into an integrated whole. The person may alternately idealize and devalue the same person (APA 1994). This behavior results in unstable and difficult interpersonal relationships; this situation, in turn, diminishes self-esteem.

Internally, people with BPD exist in a state of intense fear of abandonment. Just as they experience others as either perfect or worthless, they experience themselves in similarly dramatic terms. A continuous cycle of failure with themselves and others produces great internal despair. A repetitive pattern of despair leads to feelings of deadness, panic, and fury. Self-mutilation and suicide-prone behaviors are responses to their sensitivity to present or anticipated stress and loss. **Self-mutilation** is the "deliberate alteration or destruction of body tissue without conscious suicidal intent" (Favazza and Rosenthal 1993). Self-mutilation is usually not meant to be lethal. It generally occurs sporadically or repetitively. Examples include skin cutting, head banging, scratching, burning, eyeball pressing, and self-punching (Bonnivier 1996).

Completed suicide occurs in 8% to 10% of people with BPD. Self-mutilation is more common and usually occurs during a dissociative period. Paradoxically, self-mutilation may be used as a self-soothing behavior, which can become a ritualized part of the attempt to gain boundaries and clarity. People who have BPD also display impulsive self-destructive behaviors. For example, they may spend money irresponsibly, gamble, abuse substances, engage in unsafe sex, drive recklessly, or binge eat. These self-destructive acts are usually precipitated by threats of separation or rejection or by expectations that they assume increased responsibility (APA 1994). Without adequate nurturing, support, and provision of clarity and boundaries, people with BPD can lose the feeling of existing at all. Frantically, they act as victim, then rescuer, then perpetrator, trying to fill their inner emptiness.

Dysphoria, irritability, or anxiety can be intense, although short-lived. Clients with BPD rarely experience feelings of satisfaction or well-being. Clients with BPD are extremely angry, and intervention needs to target their anger. Anger management is difficult but crucial in helping the client with BPD to regulate emotions. These clients often direct extreme sarcasm, enduring bitterness, or angry outbursts toward others. The need to destroy is an expression of intense and primitive rage, and it can undermine any treatment, especially if the destructive impulse is experienced by the client as filling a need. Treatment is often complicated by the client's self-destructive tendencies and instability. Goldberg (1995) states that when behavioral problems emerge, the therapeutic goals and boundaries must be calmly reviewed. Setting limits is definitely necessary but in the short run may lead to hostility, noncompliance, termination of treatment, or suicide attempt.

Sadly, people with BPD may have a history of leaving functional relationships, quitting jobs that are going well, or leaving school just before graduating. It may be no surprise, in light of this, that the occurrence of physical or sexual abuse, neglect, hostile conflict, and early parental loss or separation is common in clients' early childhood.

About 2% of the population is estimated to have BPD. Borderline PD is thought to occur in 30% to 60% of all of the clinical populations with PD and accounts for about 20% of the inpatient population. Common co-occurring disorders include mood disorder (depression), substance abuse, eating disorders (bulimia), and posttraumatic stress disorder; it may also occur with other PDs (APA, 1994). Clearly, people with BPD are high users of all health and mental health resources, chronically traveling from one crisis to another and from one caretaker to another. In families with a history of BPD, the offspring are five times more likely to be diagnosed. Females are about 75% more likely than males to be diagnosed with BPD; males are more likely to be diagnosed with a psychosis-related disorder.

Maxmen and Ward (1995) stated that no drug treats BPD effectively. The best use of medications is to target symptoms: antipsychotics are used for cognitive problems; valproic acid (Depakene), for mood swings; carbamazepine (Tegretol), to decrease behavioral outbursts and mood swings; and antidepressants, for depression.

▶ Mrs. Suez, a 35-year-old mother of two with a history of psychiatric hospitalizations, has come for her usual clinic appointment. Her hand bears razor marks spelling adios, her most recent self-mutilation. This is her last session before her nurse therapist leaves for a 2-week vacation. Mrs. Suez begins the session by saying that she wants to terminate therapy. She tells her nurse therapist "I know you don't like me and I hope you have a really wonderful vacation with that sexy boyfriend of yours. Don't worry about me. No one else does."

▶ The nurse therapist helps Mrs. Suez understand that she is angry at her for going on vacation. She asks Mrs. Suez if she is thinking about or planning suicide. The nurse therapist again clarifies the resources available to Mrs. Suez during the vacation (e.g., who will be seeing her while the nurse therapist is gone, exactly when she will return) and reassures her that no matter what happens during the vacation, the two of them will continue to meet and work together on Mrs. Suez's problems afterward.

The nurse uses this strategy to help create a safety net for Mrs. Suez, so that if she decompensates during the vacation, the mental health system will be quickly and protectively responsive. The goal of the reassurance is to identify that the nurse therapist will not abandon Mrs. Suez.

Histrionic Personality Disorder

Hysteria (from the Greek *hyster*, for uterus) was historically seen as a female disease. However, stereotypes have given way to clinical investigation and education, and the new diagnosis of HPD reflects the change. Hysteria and histrionics differ significantly. Hysteria is usually the last resort of a greatly distressed individual in an attempt to convey a need or information that has been ignored, neglected, or denied by others. On the other hand, **histrionics** is a dramatic presentation of oneself with pervasive and excessive emotionality in order to seek attention, love, and admiration. People with HPD may appear flamboyant, seductive, charming, and confident. They need to be the center of attention, the "life of the party," and when they are not, they often do something dramatic to regain attention.

Clients with HPD are overly concerned with impressing others and are preoccupied with their appearance. Their dramatic and intense emotional expressions are frequently shallow, with rapid shifts from person to person or idea to idea. These people seductively draw others to them in relationships or work projects, but the attraction is usually short lived. Soon, they begin to embarrass these new friends and co-workers through their theatrical and exaggerated expression of emotion. They also begin to get caught in stories they have made up to aggrandize themselves. Thus, others experience their intense and short-term ardor as shallow, with no enduring substance.

Clients with HPD effusively embrace their new health care practitioner, endowing instantaneous trust, and assume that the caregiver experiences the same intimacy. They have elaborate fantasies about those whom they instantly idealize, especially those in authority over them, imagining that they are involved in a great meeting of mind and heart with their caregiver. When they are disappointed, these clients plummet from exaggerated loyalty to suspected betrayal; their need to control, manipulate, and idolize is an attempt to prevent this "fall from grace."

Understandably, others experience people with HPD as smothering, destructive, and unable to understand anyone else's experience. Highly impaired relationships result. Without the instant gratification from others' admiration, clients with HPD can experience significant to major depression. During this time, they are most likely to be seen in a health care setting. All suicidal ideation and gestures must be taken seriously by the health care practitioner, but doing so is difficult with this type of client.

The behavior of the client with HPD can be interpreted as coercive and attention seeking. However, underresponding in such situations may put the caregiver in the role of enabling a potential suicide. When clients with HPD receive the "appropriate responsiveness," they are likely to be on to the next novelty—all life being a stage with them as the playwright, director, and star. Although they initiate activities with great enthusiasm, when real obstacles and limitations set in, they lose interest and search anew for something that will be more immediately gratifying (APA 1994).

▶ Mrs. Mahoney, a 61-year-old widow, initiates psychotherapy after the death of her husband. Unaccustomed to being alone and no longer having her mate to take care of her, she seeks out a nurse therapist, whom she immediately views as nurturing and caring. Mrs. Mahoney describes herself in grandiose terms as she outlines her ideas for success now that she is "free."

- However, she has a history of never completing her schooling, a job, or any of her many other projects. She indicates that she richly deserved the adoration of her late husband and implies that the nurse therapist is not giving her enough "praise and celebration" for doing as well as she is doing—that is, writing checks for the first time in her life.
- Mrs. Mahoney makes frequent phone calls to the nurse, soliciting help with everyday tasks, such as balancing her check book and knowing when to schedule her car for a tune-up. When it becomes clear that the nurse therapist will not respond to her demands for adoration and enabling caretaking, Mrs. Mahoney becomes insulting to her therapist. She devalues and berates her, while dramatizing her own suffering, finally threatening to kill herself if her therapist is not more accommodating.
- The nurse therapist initially assesses Mrs. Mahoney's degree of lethality and offers support in the form of clear parameters of psychotherapy. She encourages Mrs. Mahoney to discuss her everyday problems in the session, where new skills can be taught.

Approaching the client's dependence as a strength and refusing to identify with the client's devaluation are essential to working with clients with HPD.

Narcissistic Personality Disorder

The primary feature in NPD is a pervasive pattern of grandiosity, a need for admiration, and a lack of empathy for others (APA 1994). Clients who have NPD exploit others to meet their own needs and desires; when they are successful, they experience a sense of superiority and omnipotence. Often, they are admired and envied by others for what appears to be a rich and talented life. Eventually, they require this admiration in greater and greater quantity because they believe that if they are not admired, they are "bad." Conversely, they may begrudge others their success or possessions, feeling that they deserve the admiration and privileges more (APA 1994).

A sense of shame compels clients with NPD never to make a mistake and never to tolerate the mistakes of others. This shame defends against the fear that if they are "bad," they will be abandoned or annihilated. Internally, a great pendulum exists, swinging from a grandiose position to one of intense feelings of inferiority, danger, and shame. During the grandiose cycle, clients with NPD feel invulnerable and perfect; during the shame cycle, their fear causes them intense anxiety, and they frantically search for what they have done wrong and exhaust themselves correcting others' opinions of them. They fear that if they do not carry out these acts, great harm will come to them. Having human limitations and disappointing or frustrating others can feel like a life-or-death situation. Conversely, disappointment or frustration regarding others' limitations can also feel like life or death, and they are as intolerant of that in others as they are in themselves.

Internally, therefore, clients with NPD do not have the ability to recognize realistic limitations. Frequently, they feel that others do not give them the rewards they deserve. In overestimating themselves and underestimating others, they find that what others give them never seems enough, and they frequently have fantasies of unlimited success, power, brilliance, and beauty.

When seen in a health care setting, these clients can demand the "the best of everything," including practitioners. They measure their self-worth by surrounding themselves with what they project as being the "crème de la crème." This feeling of entitlement has significant impact. Clients with NPD, who demonstrate lack of sensitivity, envy, demands, and disparagement of others, are seen as arrogant, highly critical, patronizing, and rude. However, this constant need for admiration, overevaluation of their own ability, and devaluation of others covers a fragile sense of self.

When these clients are corrected, when their boundaries are defined, or when limits are set on their behavior, they are left feeling humiliated, degraded, and empty. To reestablish internal balance, they may launch a counterattack. Sometimes, vocational endeavors are minimal, reflecting an attempt to avoid injury in competitive or risky situations. Social withdrawal, depression, and mood disorders may result.

Narcissism is essentially a maladaptive social response characterized by egocentric attitude, fragile self-esteem, constant seeking of praise or admiration, and envy. At about 4 years of age, narcissism is normal. During adolescence, many narcissistic traits are seen as being culturally normal, and, after a period of adjustment, this narcissism usually evolves into a greater scope of understanding of self and others. In the mental health care setting, those diagnosed with NPD are predominantly male (APA 1994).

- Mr. Varick is a 43-year-old gay man who has lived with his partner for 15 years. He thinks of himself as a successful salesman, going into debt to drive a sports car and live on the "right" street. In his belief, being seen with the "right" people is more important than liking them. As his partner has grown older, Mr. Varick's sexual attention has focused outside their relationship on handsome younger men. These encounters help Mr. Varick believe that he himself is still young and handsome. However, Mr. Varick's sexual encounters are usually in the bushes of a park or in public bathrooms, and he has twice been arrested for indecent exposure, which has led to his initiating psychotherapy.
- Once in therapy, he regales his nurse therapist with stories that he hopes will amuse and impress her, but her response is a neutral one, listening but not displaying the hoped-for responses. Mr. Varick escalates his attempts to amuse and impress, until he finally expresses anger at his therapist for not being worldly enough to appreciate him. He wonders aloud whether another therapist might be better for him.

▸ The nurse therapist compassionately identifies his attempts to seek and become perfect, his grandiosity, and his sense of entitlement. The therapist shows how this thinking ends up hurting his partner, in addition to placing both of them at great risk through his sexual acting out. Because his actions are making him feel more inadequate rather than fulfilled, he despairs that he is beyond help; his shaming of his nurse therapist expresses the fear that she cannot help him either.

Over time, clients with NPD can use such confrontation to begin to have compassion for themselves and, eventually, others.

Clinical Picture of Cluster C Disorders (Anxious or Fearful)

Cluster C includes the avoidant, dependent, and obsessive-compulsive PDs (OCPDs). Individuals with cluster C PDs often appear anxious or fearful. Figure 19–4 presents the DSM-IV criteria for the cluster C disorders.

Avoidant Personality Disorder

Shyness and avoidance of conflict, risk, and new situations are common in early childhood and are expected to diminish by the end of adolescence. Attainment and mastery of psychomotor skills, as well as skill development that becomes transferable to new situations, ordinarily make avoidance behaviors diminish with age. When avoidance instead grows into a pervasive pattern of social inhibition, with accompanying feelings of inadequacy and hypersensitivity to criticism, then avoidant PD (APD) is a possible diagnosis. Preoccupation with fear of rejection and criticism is the hallmark of this disorder.

Clients with APD have little tolerance for normal group process and perceive that they are receiving the rejection they most fear. Because their social presentation appears shy, timid, and socially inept, with low self-esteem and poor self-care, they can become objects of derision in any group. Although they can emphasize only the negative perceptions they receive, clients with APD often exaggerate the dangers of these experiences. Internally, they are fearful that the self-doubts they have of themselves will be seen by others, and they attempt to hide from others, which leaves them emotionally and physically isolated.

Restricted interpersonal contacts diminish the likelihood that they will learn how to interact with others and reinforces shame over such things as blushing or crying in the presence of others. Their low self-esteem and hypersensitivity increase as support networks decrease. Demands in the workplace and in normal adult daily living can begin to overwhelm them, and they may retreat to an inner world of fantasy where their desires for ideal love and acceptance can be met.

Clients with APD may long to feel part of a group or family, but hypersensitivity to the slightest hint of disapproval prevents them from joining in, even if they are given repeated reassurances and generous offers of support and nurturance. Building a therapeutic relationship with these clients is difficult. They enter the relationship with the projection that their caregiver will harm them through disapproval, and they perceive rejection where it does not exist. They have great difficulty trusting a correction of their interpretations, and they are unwilling to trust unless they are certain they will be liked. Because they have so often experienced shame and ridicule in social situations, even when trust is built, they restrain themselves from the intimacy that they desire in order to avoid the anticipated pain of rejection. These inhibitions, their conviction that they are inferior and unable to learn how to be with people, and their reluctance to take risks hinder the caregiver at every turn.

A friendly, gentle, reassuring approach is the best way to treat clients with APD. Virtually all people with APD have social phobias. Monoamine oxidase inhibitors have been found to be effective, as have cognitive-behavioral therapies that focus on assertiveness, desensitization, and cognitive change. Group therapy is also useful for people with APD (Maxmen and Ward 1996).

▸ Ms. Knight is a 48-year-old single woman who is retired from a career in the army and now works for an electronics firm. She has never been involved in an intimate relationship with another adult but was able to make superficial contacts while in the military because of the clear social structure. Since she moved 3 years ago, Ms. Knight has met many people but has not made friends. She rarely speaks with her co-workers and faithfully returns to her mobile home each evening after work. Her sense of loneliness has become unbearable, and she finally seeks psychotherapy because she does not know where else to turn.

▸ The nurse-therapist's strategy is to teach and facilitate Ms. Knight's socialization skills, while providing positive feedback from which Ms. Knight can build her self-esteem.

Dependent Personality Disorder

Self-sacrifice, or toleration of physical, sexual, or emotional abuse when alternatives for self-care and escape exist, is the most startling aspect of dependent PD (DPD). The person with DPD has a poignant sense of being incapable of survival if left alone; this may be expressed in lack of ability even to pick out the day's wardrobe without considerable reassurance and guidance. Clients with DPD experience a deep foreboding about personal incompetence; consequently, they solicit caretaking by clinging and being pervasively and excessively submissive. By early adulthood, these people perceive themselves as being unable to

CLUSTER C (Anxious or Fearful)

DEPENDENT PERSONALITY DISORDER

A. A pervasive and excessive need to be taken care of that leads to submissive and clinging behavior and fear of separation, beginning by early adulthood and present in a variety of contexts, as indicated by five (or more) of the following:

(1) Has difficulty making everyday decisions without an excessive amount of advice and reassurance from others
(2) Needs others to assume responsibility for most major areas of life
(3) Has difficulty expressing disagreement with others because of fear of loss of support or approval. *Note*: Does not include realistic fears of retribution.
(4) Has difficulty initiating projects or doing things on own (because of a lack of self-confidence in judgment or abilities rather than a lack of motivation or energy)
(5) Goes to excessive lengths to obtain nurturance and support from others, to the point of volunteering to do things that are unpleasant
(6) Feels uncomfortable or helpless when alone because of exaggerated fears of being unable to care for self
(7) Urgently seeks another relationship as a source of care and support when a close relationship ends
(8) Is unrealistically preoccupied with fears of being left to take care of self

OBSESSIVE-COMPULSIVE PERSONALITY DISORDER

A. A pervasive pattern of preoccupation with orderliness, perfectionism, and mental and interpersonal control, at the expense of flexibility, openness, and efficiency, beginning by early adulthood and present in a variety of contexts, as indicated by four (or more) of the following:

(1) Is preoccupied with details, rules, lists, order, organization, or schedules to the extent that the major point of the activity is lost
(2) Shows perfectionism that interferes with task completion (e.g., is unable to complete a project because overly strict personal standards are not met)
(3) Is excessively devoted to work and productivity to the exclusion of leisure activities and friendships (not accounted for by obvious economic necessity)
(4) Is overconscientious, scrupulous, and inflexible about matters of morality, ethics, or values (not accounted for by cultural or religious identification)
(5) Is unable to discard worn-out or worthless objects even when they have no sentimental value
(6) Is reluctant to delegate tasks or to work with others unless they submit exactly to own way of doing things
(7) Adopts a miserly spending style toward both self and others; money is viewed as something to be hoarded for future catastrophes
(8) Shows rigidity and stubbornness

AVOIDANT PERSONALITY DISORDER

A. A pervasive pattern of social inhibition, feelings of inadequacy, and hypersensitivity to negative evaluation, beginning by early adulthood and present in a variety of contexts, as indicated by four (or more) of the following:

(1) Avoids occupational activities that involve significant interpersonal contact, because of fears of criticism, disapproval, or rejection
(2) Is unwilling to get involved with people unless certain of being liked
(3) Shows restraint within intimate relationships because of fear of being shamed or ridiculed
(4) Is preoccupied with being criticized or rejected in social situations
(5) Is inhibited in new interpersonal situations because of feelings of inadequacy
(6) Views self as socially inept, personally unappealing, or inferior to others
(7) Is unusually reluctant to take personal risks or to engage in any new activities because they may prove embarrassing

Figure 19–4 DSM-IV diagnostic criteria for cluster C personality disorders. (Adapted from American Psychiatric Association (1994). *Diagnostic and statistical manual of mental disorders* (4th ed.). Washington, DC: American Psychiatric Association. Reprinted with permission. Copyright 1994 American Psychiatric Association.)

separate from others and to work independently. They believe that it is necessary to be dependent on others in order to function at all. They are passive and follow other people's preferences or advice, even when they know it to be inaccurate and potentially harmful to themselves or others. If others do not initiate or take responsibility for them, then their needs remain neglected.

In clients with DPD, anger and assertiveness are suppressed by a passivity that masks a fear of others' retaliation or alienation. When they are able to maintain a dependent position in a stable relationship, they can function adequately; however, they may still fear appearing too competent, which could lead to abandonment. Thus, they often avoid skill-enhancing learning, instead mastering dependency-perpetuating behaviors.

Submissive behaviors intended to strengthen attachment to their partner, spouse, or family often result in unbalanced and distorted relationships. When a close relationship ends—whether because of children leaving home, death, or divorce—clients with DPD may become anxious, and this is the time they are most likely to seek a health care practitioner. They become intensely and prematurely attached to another person without pausing to evaluate the consequences. This inability to discriminate and discern stems from the fearfully held certainty that they will not survive on their own. These clients see themselves as so dependent that even the thought of loss is anxiety provoking. Their fears are excessive, extreme, persistent, and not amenable to logic.

The pessimism of clients with DPD pervades any logical cognitive intervention. Their self-doubt is projected on others, and they devalue others' helpfulness unless it is the idealized, self-sacrificial caretaking they perceive as being "just good enough." Any setting of realistic expectations can deflate their self-esteem, and they then devalue themselves. This perpetual cycle of losing faith in themselves reinforces their belief in the necessity of self-sacrifice, making them willing to endure anything to remain attached. This can appear as *masochism* (soliciting dominance from others), but they feel it is what they must do to get the protection they need from others.

When a decision is left up to them, clients who have DPD experience painful levels of anxiety that derive from the belief that they will make a horrible mistake, and then not only will they suffer the sadism of others but they will also be abandoned in their misery. They can obsessively ruminate and fantasize about abandonment, even when it is not threatened.

The client with DPD is at greater risk for anxiety and mood disorders, and DPD can occur with borderline, avoidant, and histrionic PDs. This disorder commonly occurs in individuals who have a general medical condition or a disability that requires them to be dependent on others. Long-term inability to care independently for the self erodes confidence, autonomy, and personal integrity. Fear of losing support can be life threatening for this population (APA 1994, pp. 665–669). More insightful clients often benefit from psychodynamic psychotherapy that targets the client's low self-esteem, fears regarding autonomy, and relationship with the therapist. Others may benefit from supportive group therapy and/or assertiveness training (Maxmen and Ward 1996).

▶ Mrs. Patterson, a 70-year-old widow of an abusive spouse, is seen for the first time at a mental health clinic. She presents with suicide ideation arising from intractable pain of osteoarthritis. She has been a widow for 15 years, but her most recent loss is that of her 50-year-old son, who is leaving his childhood home after returning to it periodically during his adulthood, never having fully emancipated himself from his family. This last extended return was of 3 years' duration. Mrs. Patterson says she could not live without her son to take care of her.

▶ Nursing strategies include finding solutions to Mrs. Patterson's chronic pain. In this instance, a transcutaneous electrical nerve stimulation (TENS) unit is successful. She is given antidepressants to quell her anxiety, and workers are assigned to assist her with adult daily living chores that will increase her sense of adequacy. Supportive therapy is encouraged in order to teach her new skills of problem solving, and it has the desired outcome of increasing her self-confidence.

Obsessive-Compulsive Personality Disorder

Pack ratting, endlessly repeating tasks until perfection is achieved, rigid and literal enforcement of rules or laws designed to avoid disorder—all are essential features of OCPD. On presentation, clients with OCPD stubbornly insist that their way of doing things is the only right way. Gathering a history can be inordinately time consuming as the client offers endless irrelevant details.

Although excessive in verbosity, these clients are miserly with material goods, emotions, and behaviors. Their rationale is that catastrophe is imminent and that they must prepare by hoarding and protecting their resources. "You never know when you'll need it" is a frequently heard refrain from the individual with OCPD about the tidy stacks of old newspapers, magazines, and appliances that cause havoc for families or roommates. Their resistance to help arises partly from this fear of catastrophe and partly from the belief that no one can perform these acts better. They tend to take firm control of everything in their lives and refuse to delegate tasks, even when they are unable to keep deadlines that could endanger their work life.

Although they may appear devoted to their work or occupation, in reality, the work behaviors of individuals with OCPD cause much friction with others. If they do turn over some task, it is with high expectations, along with minutely detailed instructions, and they are angry if any deviation from their directions occurs. Highly critical of others, they hold themselves to a scrupulous moral code that allows little room for the ambiguities of normal adult life. Thus, they are also merciless with themselves when they make a mistake, and they almost never forgive what they see as a wrong; for them, the world is black and white.

In relationships, individuals with OCPD can be taskmasters, turning even the most leisurely activity into a lesson or an opportunity to perfect oneself. They often believe that they cannot afford to rest, take time off, or go on vacation. There may be such a great emphasis on cleanliness, making lists, and refining that attempted projects never reach a stage of completion, causing considerable stress for themselves and those around them. Insight regarding the impact that their actions have on others is slight, if present at all.

Individuals with OCPD experience a loss of control when they are called on to make decisions, prioritize, or streamline; they find these processes time consuming, difficult, and painful. When such activities are called for, the person with OCPD is likely to respond defensively (although not with anger). Although they ruminate endlessly about what has displeased them, this activity serves only to make them more anxious about what is the "right thing to do."

Intimacy in relationships is superficial and rigidly controlled, even though clients with OCPD may feel deep and genuine affection for friends and family. Their everyday interactions have a formal and serious quality. Internally, they rehearse over and over again how they will react or what they will say in social situations. Emotional displays by others seem childish to them, and they have great difficulty trying to convey tender feelings of their own. When confronted with situations that demand flexibility or compromise, they are unable to compromise and often lose many opportunities in relationships and in the workplace (APA 1994, pp. 669–673).

- Mr. Lopez, a 48-year-old married man who is a middle manager for a microchip company, keeps canceling the appointment for his yearly health check-up by the company nurse. His reason is that he has to do so much of his unit's job himself because his staff is incompetent. When he finally keeps an appointment, he is 30 minutes late and begins to give directions to the nurse: she should take his blood pressure on his right arm instead of his left, her name tag is on crooked, and the scale is 2¾ pounds off his scale at home.
- Mr. Lopez's blood pressure is high, and he complains of not sleeping well and of trouble at home with his teenaged children about their curfew. He also complains of severe heartburn and an 80-hour work week. He has been passed over for promotion for the past 5 years and has received poor job reviews for high employee turnover in his work unit. The nurse refers Mr. Lopez to a primary care provider for a cardiac and gastrointestinal work-up. She asks him if he feels he would like some help from someone who specializes in teaching relaxation techniques and problem-solving skills. Mr. Lopez declines these, saying that he does not have time, and besides, he knows all he needs to know about such things.

NURSING DIAGNOSIS

People with PDs are usually admitted to psychiatric institutions for reasons other than their disorder (e.g., for substance abuse, suicide attempts, or self-mutilation or by court order).

Personality disorders seen most often in the health care system are BPD and antisocial PD. Because the behaviors central to these disorders often cause upheaval and disruption on psychiatric units, as well as on medical-surgical wards and clinics, nursing diagnoses and interventions for these two disorders are emphasized.

Data collected from the client provide the nurse with information about the presenting problem or behaviors, emotional state, precipitating situations, and maladaptive coping behaviors. The client with PD may exhibit any number of problematic behaviors. These behaviors are not in themselves pathological or maladaptive. Behaviors that are repetitive or rigid, or those that present an obstacle to meaningful relationships or functioning, are considered in the management and care of the client.

Nursing diagnoses may be numerous. The person with a diagnosis of PD often presents with gross behavioral problems. These behaviors usually cause a great deal of difficulty in interpersonal relationships. For example, for a client with antisocial PD, **ineffective individual coping** may be diagnosed. Ineffective coping may be evidenced by overt hostility, manipulation of others, egocentricity, habitual disregard of social norms, impulsive acts, or dependence on drugs or alcohol.

People with BPD use manipulative tactics to get needs met. As with clients with antisocial PD, the manipulations of clients with BPD may result in harm to others. At other times, clients with BPD act out anxiety in the form of impulsive acts, which may include promiscuity, gambling, shoplifting, binge eating, excessive spending, and drug use. Therefore, ineffective individual coping for this population may be evidenced by manipulation of others, inability to solve problems, impulsive acts, or long-term use of maladaptive behaviors.

Many people with antisocial PD end up in jail, juvenile courts, and houses of detention because of unlawful behavior and physical aggression toward others. Therefore, the nursing diagnosis of **risk for violence directed at others** is often applicable; it may be evidenced by lack of impulse control, overt aggression and hostility, or emotional immaturity.

The behavior of a person with BPD is also punctuated with angry outbursts, impulsive acts, and manipulation. However, these clients are more apt to carry out physically self-damaging acts, such as suicidal and self-mutilating behaviors. Because these acts are usually impulsive, hospitalization may be necessary to ensure a safe environment. When this happens, an appropriate nursing diagnosis may be **risk for violence to self** or **risk for self-mutilation.** Violence to self or others may be evidenced by behaviors such as anxiety, self-mutilation, frequent displays of temper, and poor impulse control.

A person with antisocial PD may be a parent. Because, by definition, a person with an antisocial PD is unable to empathize, cherish, or support the needs of another human being, children suffer emotionally from such a parent. Therefore the nursing diagnosis of **altered parenting,** as evidenced by abuse, rejection, inadequate resources, or impaired judgment, is possible.

Almost all individuals with PD have serious **impaired social interaction** because of their defensive styles. For example, the schizoid person is indifferent to being with others and prefers to be alone. Clients with schizotypal PD and PPD, on the other hand, are suspicious of others and thus lack close relationships; they deal with others in a stiff and aloof fashion. Individuals with histrionic PD or NPD are totally involved with themselves and lack genuine concern for others. People with DPD need others to take care of them in their daily life and thus are unable to form close and loving, give-and-take, adult relationships.

Unfortunately, most people with PD do not seek treatment unless a crisis occurs, and they often leave treatment once the crisis is over.

PLANNING

Planning Outcome Criteria

A therapeutic plan for the client with a PD is created by identifying short-term and long-term outcome criteria. Short-term goals are defined as those that can be and need to be accomplished as soon as possible, especially when a person is in crisis. As stated earlier, people with PD are generally seen in a health care setting because of a crisis. Because many leave the system after the crisis is over, attention to short-term goals is especially important.

Short-term goals are usually related to the clients' safety and comfort and are pertinent to their physical and mental well-being. For the client with PD, affect management is necessary; internal emotional states need to be balanced so that these clients are not compelled into using destructive behaviors to avoid the overwhelming flood of feeling and shaming thoughts they experience in a crisis. Often, the first goals for the management of an acute crisis are to evaluate the need for medication and to identify appropriate verbal interventions to decrease the client's immediate emotional distress. Frequently, clients with PD require medication management to soothe the pain, rage, and paranoia they experience in crisis. Evaluation of their need for decreased stimulation, which hospitalization can provide, is an important part of ensuring their safety.

Verbal interventions in a crisis are focused on relieving the pressure of emotion rather than on gaining insight. Instead of "You think you did something bad and you deserve to be punished so that's why you ate the glass," the gentler "Maybe you're being very hard on yourself right now" may give relief. Alternatively, the problem can be repeated in their own words; this strategy helps some clients take a more understanding view of their distress. Sometimes, tactful reconstruction of the events leading to the crisis can neutralize histrionic or grandiose perceptions.

When health care workers express irritation, frustration, or anger, it reactivates the original trauma for the client. Clients who have PD have been frequent targets of these emotions all their lives, and they interpret them fearfully as aggression directed toward them by their caregiver. Any therapeutic alliance previously attained is lost, and in its place are even greater paranoia, rage, and panic than before. The nurse's most effective approach is to exhibit respect and patience and to make a genuine attempt to understand the client's experience. Solving the immediate crisis is the first step in long-term goal setting with clients with PDs. Therefore, outcome criteria for the acute phase include the client's appearing calmer, as evidenced by being able to identify options for personal comfort and safety in behavioral terms: "If I feel like killing myself I'll call the crisis line, and I'll keep my appointment with my therapist tomorrow."

Long-term outcomes deal with the cause of the persistent state of crisis. Because the client with a PD tends not to plan ahead and thus repeats dysfunctional behaviors, long-term goals usually center on skill attainment in the areas of

- Linking consequences to both functional and dysfunctional behaviors.
- Learning and mastering skills that facilitate functional behaviors.
- Practicing the substitution of functional alternatives during crisis.
- Initiating functional alternatives to prevent a crisis.
- Ongoing management of anger, anxiety, shame, and happiness.
- Creating a life style that prevents regressing (e.g., HALT, never getting too **h**ungry, too **a**ngry, too **l**onely, too **t**ired).

Realistic goal setting with individuals with PDs comes from the perspective that personality change happens one behavioral solution and one learned skill at a time. This can be expected to take much time and repetition. No matter how intelligent they may appear or how insightful they can be about themselves and others, these clients find that change is slow and occurs via trial and error, with the support of affect management and much interpersonal reinforcement. No short-cuts occur with the client with a PD; in permanent change, the learning can literally be integrated at the cellular level. In practical terms, this means that by the time they come to the nurse for help, these clients may have already seen several caregivers and are likely to take whatever the nurse can give and then move on to the next caregiver. Theirs is a long and circuitous road, and the nurse is their most recent attempt to find healing.

Nurse's Feelings and Self-Assessment

Finding an approach for helping clients with PDs who have overwhelming needs can be overwhelming for caregivers as well. These individuals can evoke intense feelings in the nurse (often the same feelings being experienced by the client). Being in the role of caregiver can result in feeling chronically confused, helpless, angry, and frustrated; these clients tell the nurse that the nurse is inadequate, incompetent, and abusive of authority. Clients with PD can be manipulative and may disparage the nurse to peers in such a way that the peers begin to believe the client; usually, this is the peers' attempt to defend against their own feelings of frustration and powerlessness, but the result is that substantial conflict can ensue in the workplace, with teams splitting or factions forming. Therefore, the interventions discussed next can be used on behalf of both clients and staff.

INTERVENTION

It is often difficult to create a therapeutic relationship with clients with PD. Because most have experienced a series of interrupted therapeutic alliances, their suspiciousness, aloofness, and hostility can be a set-up for failure. The guarded and secretive style of these clients tends to produce an atmosphere of combat. When clients blame and attack others, the nurse needs to understand the context of their complaints; these attacks spring from feeling threatened and, the more intense the complaints, the greater the fear of potential harm or loss.

Lacking the ability to trust, clients with PD require a sense of control over what is happening to them. Giving them choices—whether to come to a clinic appointment in the morning or afternoon, for example—may enhance compliance with treatment. Because clients with PD are hypersensitive to criticism yet have no strong sense of autonomy, the most effective teaching of new behaviors builds on their own existing skills.

When people with PDs exhibit fantasies that attribute malevolent intentions to the nurse or others, it is important to orient them to reality. They need to know that even though they have insulted or threatened their caregiver, they will still be helped and protected from being hurt. When they are hurt by others, as naturally happens in everyday life, the nurse takes time to dissect the situation with them, asking when, where, and how it happened, and honestly maps out for them how people, systems, families, and relationships work. It is important to be honest about their limitations and assets. The client with a PD may already be aware of them, but acknowledging them demonstrates trustworthiness.

Clients with PDs do not know how they participate in getting hurt, and gaining this understanding is helpful to them. When they come to understand, often they try to use the knowledge. However, much correction and assistance are needed because their experiences can become distorted when they begin to act on new insights. It is important for these clients to learn that being hurt does not always mean that they are in danger. It is necessary to map out for them where the dangers do lie and where they do not. The nurse can help them understand what their rights are and where their safety zones are. This understanding gives these individuals some relief from the fear, anger, and shame that are their most common inner experiences.

Counseling (Basic Level)

Everyone has his or her own communication style. This style not only conveys what people have to say but also represents who people see themselves to be. Nurses greatly enhance their ability to be therapeutic when they combine the following qualities with their own natural style. Many nurse clinicians work with clients who have personality disorders as therapists in clinics, health care centers, private practice, and institutes. These nurses are prepared at the advanced practice level and have had special training in conducting therapy. The following approaches and/or skills are needed by all nurses at all levels when working with a client with a PD.

Authenticity

Simply defined, *authenticity* is achieved when words match actions. When nurses model emotional honesty, they teach that they can be conscious of their own needs and express them verbally in a way that does no harm to others and sometimes (but not always) gets a "good enough" response. This modeling also includes nonverbal communication, which must be congruent with stated needs or experience in order to be viewed as authentic. This is a powerful therapeutic tool. The client with PD, like most people, experiences nonverbal content as more genuine than the words people say.

Trustworthiness

Trustworthiness is demonstrated by being constant, but not rigid and inflexible. When the nurse is predictable, clients with PD can begin to incorporate therapeutic ideas; they may even hear the nurse's voice inside their head, instructing them about the consequences of their behavior, and may come to understand (perhaps for the first time) that they have choices in responding to stressful life events. Constancy also means being flexible, not rigid or dogmatic, and recognizing personal limitations. Frequently, life can be so overwhelming and problems can be so vast that a sympathetic nurse clinician is moved to say "I don't know right now what to say that would be helpful, but we will keep working on this together." This lets the client use aspects of the nurse's personality and lets the nurse be genuine. It is never a mistake for a nurse to be open about his or her limitations to a client. Denying personal limitations can lead to many problems.

Setting Limits

When to say no is as important as how to say no. At the first opportunity, the nurse needs to educate clients with PD about what the nurse's job is and what caregivers can and cannot do. The nurse initiates a detailed conversation explaining the nurse-client relationship and what responsibilities each has in the relationship. Clients do not already know this, even if they have had a lot of experience in the mental health setting.

In the instruction, the nurse focuses on the cause-and-effect nature of responsibilities; for example, if the nurse has responsibility for medications, then if clients have any issues about medications, they must talk with the nurse to resolve them. This sets boundaries clearly and cognitively, with the additional information of what will happen (resolution) if the client adheres to them. When the client does not adhere to the boundaries, repetition is useful for reinforcement. However, the most helpful strategy is focusing again on the consequences of not adhering to boundaries. For example, if the client complains about medication to another staff person but not to the responsible nurse, the complaint is never addressed, and the problem may escalate. The established boundary is that the nurse is the one to talk to about medication. When the client respects the boundary, the client gets results. Specific guidelines for setting limits are discussed in the next section.

Dealing with Manipulation

Through a combination of dependency and lack of skills, clients with PD experience vulnerability as danger and have learned to empower themselves through manipulation. The solution, therefore, is to teach clients how to empower themselves less destructively. Within a safe relationship or environment, clients with PD can be confronted with the idea that they must be feeling powerless when they are manipulating caregivers, friends and family, or themselves.

An important step in decreasing manipulative behaviors is to set clear and realistic limits on specific behaviors. A manipulative client may react to the limit setting with resentment and resistance; however, some manipulative clients really want limits placed on their behaviors. Following are six steps in the setting of limits (Chitty and Maynard 1986):

1. Set limits only in those areas in which a clear need to protect the client or others exists.
2. Establish realistic and enforceable consequences of exceeding limits.
3. Make the client aware of the limits and the consequences of not adhering to the limits before incidents occur. The client should be told in a clear, polite, and firm manner what the limits and consequences are and should be given the opportunity to discuss any feelings or reactions to them.
4. All limits should be supported by the entire staff. The limits should be written in the care plan, if the client is hospitalized, and should also be communicated verbally to all those involved.
5. When the limits are consistently adhered to, a decision to discontinue the limits should be made by the staff and should be noted on the nursing care plan. The decision should be based on consistent behavior, not on promises or sporadic efforts.
6. The staff should formulate a plan to address their own difficulty in maintaining consistent limits.

Table 19–1 outlines some goals and interventions aimed at decreasing manipulative behaviors.

When the nurse is able to point out the manipulative behaviors of the client with PD in a nonjudgmental way, this fosters conscious problem identification and encourages the individual to maintain new functional attachments and relationships. When clients who have PD understand their manipulations and the feelings behind them, they may think about what they are doing that makes functional relationships maladaptive. Pointing out the client's manipulative behavior with humor, gently and in private, any shame can be neutralized. Not all clients want to change their manipulative behavior (e.g., the client who has antisocial PD). Appropriate and firm limit setting, as discussed earlier, may be the only useful interventions.

Milieu Therapy (Basic Level)

The primary therapeutic goal of milieu therapy is affect management in a group context. Through desensitiza-

TABLE 19–1 GOALS AND INTERVENTIONS FOR MANIPULATIVE BEHAVIOR

GOAL	INTERVENTION
Client will demonstrate limiting setting on own for manipulative behavior by (date).	◗ Identify manipulative behaviors by client. ◗ Set limits on manipulative behaviors by communicating expected behaviors. ◗ Convey to the team consistency of approach in setting limits. ◗ Be realistic as to which behaviors can be limited. ◗ Be clear with client about the consequences of exceeding limits. ◗ Assist client in developing means of setting limits on own behavior. ◗ Assess degree of insight into manipulative behavior and motivation to change. ◗ Avoid getting into power struggles by accusing and arguing with client.
Client will develop two alternative nonmanipulative behaviors by (date).	◗ Discuss client's behaviors in nonjudgmental and nonthreatening manner. ◗ Assist client in identifying personal strengths and effective communication skills. ◗ Assist client in testing out alternative behaviors for obtaining needs or fulfilling expectations. ◗ Support client and provide feedback in trying new behaviors.

tion via social group experience, overwhelming and painful internal states can be felt and endured, even while the task of the group is accomplished. Viewing acting out as unconscious communication that needs to be made conscious and verbal, so that it is possible to understand the need that it communicates, enables the group and the individual to decide how to meet that need.

To make the unknown known eases pain and focuses the client with PD on thoughts, words, and actions that can reduce the painful internal state. This balances the inner chaos as well as the outer chaos that the group may be experiencing.

Psychobiological Therapy (Basic Level)

Clients with PD may be supported by a broad array of psychotropics, all geared toward maintaining cognitive function and managing affect. However, with clients who have PD, it is important to remember that medications are both a curse and a blessing; they can be simultaneously intrusive, untrustworthy, and soothing. Enhancing medication compliance with these clients requires that they understand their experiences consciously. Clients with PD usually do not like taking medicine unless it calms them down. They worry if they do not have an adequate supply but have difficulty organizing themselves to fill the prescription. Sometimes, they panic, somatocize about side effects, and stop taking the medication, while still demanding more tranquilizing drugs. As these complaints demonstrate, clients with PD are fearful about taking something over which they have no control.

Despite these cautions about prescribing drugs, antipsychotics may be useful for brief periods to control agitation, rage, and brief psychotic episodes. Pimozide (Orap) has been helpful in reducing paranoid ideation in some clients, and antidepressants may be useful at times, particularly for clients with BPD.

Case Management (Basic Level)

Case management is usually required for clients with PD who are persistently and severely impaired, have been hospitalized previously, have been unable to maintain work or personal relationships, and are relatively alone in their attempts to care for themselves. Most clients with PD are high functioning, but a significant number still meet the requirements of needing assistance in order to stay out of the hospital. Case management of a client, therefore, is geared toward reducing the necessity for hospitalization by creating a homeostasis that is based on the client's highest functioning level. Very little change is expected with most clients who have PD, and the primary focus is on health promotion and maintenance through stress reduction and crisis intervention. Refer to this chapter's case study for an example of how staff deal with manipulative and aggressive behaviors.

EVALUATION

Evaluating effectiveness with this population is difficult. Nurse clinicians might never know the real measure of their interventions. Clients with PD generally find long-term relationship too intimate an experience to remain long enough for useful evaluation; if they do, they probably no longer have PD. In these circumstances, self-care for the nurse clinician becomes important. Perhaps effectiveness can be measured by how successfully the nurse was able to be genuine with the client, to maintain a helpful posture, to offer substantial instruction, and to still care for himself or herself. The mixed therapeutic picture of effectiveness and lack of effectiveness with clients is a given. This means that it is important that the caregiver not measure personal effectiveness on the basis of the client's ability to change. Learning to find meaning and peace in the process, rather than "proof" of personal effectiveness, is the reward that is possible with these clients.

Text continued on page 533

CASE STUDY: WORKING WITH A PERSON WHO HAS AN ANTISOCIAL PERSONALITY DISORDER

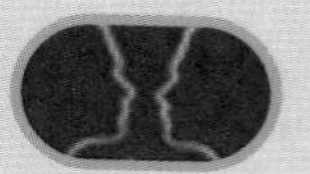

Donald Mann, a 32-year-old divorcé, is hospitalized for uncontrollable aggressive impulses. On admission, there is no indication of thought disorders, hallucinations, or depressed affect. Mr. Mann is angry because he feels "forced" to admit himself voluntarily to the hospital. His boss stated that if he did not admit himself, Mr. Mann would be fired from his job. Mr. Mann had threatened a fellow history teacher and later assaulted him. The client states, "I was only arguing a historical point and got carried away." He smiles and winks his eye as he is relating the course of events to the nurse, Ms. Burke.

Mr. Mann states that he is unable to finish writing a book because his third wife divorced him. When asked about his childhood, he comments, "Fighting is

CASE STUDY: WORKING WITH A PERSON WHO HAS AN ANTISOCIAL PERSONALITY DISORDER *(Continued)*

synonymous with being a street kid." He has a history of wife abuse and frequent barroom fights. For the past year, he has been employed as a teacher of history in a private college. Previously, he held numerous teaching positions in several states. Mr. Mann states that he enjoys teaching and especially likes the students.

On the unit, Mr. Mann is generally cooperative. However, on two occasions, he violates the rules of the unit. Once, he is found with a bottle of alcohol ("I was celebrating one of our famous presidents"). In the second incident, he threatens to harm another client on the unit. On both occasions, his response is a glib "I'm sorry." The female staff usually have no difficulty dealing with him, but the male staff generally complain about him.

On the third day after admission, Mr. Mann threatens another client. His infractions of the rules and his aggressiveness are disrupting the unit. The unit coordinator asks Ms. Burke to write a comprehensive care plan for him. Ms. Burke, who admitted him to the unit, has spent time with him over the past few days. She often feels flattered by his attention. He has told her that he finds her "the best nurse on the unit." That afternoon, his case is to be presented at a staff conference.

During the meeting, each female member reports that Mr. Mann has stated that she is his favorite. He would also "tell tales" to each staff member about the other staff members. The female staff would often do special favors for Mr. Mann (e.g., getting him cigarettes, the newspaper, or candy). The male staff members find him argumentative, infuriating, and contemptuous of them. They try to avoid him as much as possible. It is clear that almost everyone has strong positive or negative reactions to Mr. Mann. During the meeting, many of the female staff feel annoyed and angry at being manipulated. The staff together decide on goals and a plan of approach.

ASSESSMENT

Ms. Burke divides her data into objective and subjective components:

OBJECTIVE DATA

1. Had two incidents of infractions of the rules.
2. Has history of spousal abuse.
3. Assaulted co-worker before admission.
4. Has had three marriages.
5. Is argumentative with male staff.
6. Rationalizes improper and aggressive behaviors—sees nothing wrong.
7. Has difficulty with interpersonal relationships at work.
8. Has physically threatened another client.
9. Is verbally aggressive with male staff.
10. Has made sexual advances toward female staff.
11. Manipulates special favors from female staff.

SUBJECTIVE DATA

1. Sets one staff member against another: "Nurse Y said this about you . . ."
2. States he was "forced into coming to the hospital."
3. Tells each female nurse that she is his favorite.

NURSING DIAGNOSIS

Staff think two nursing diagnoses are the most important initially.

1. **Ineffective individual coping** related to inadequate psychological resources, as evidenced by verbal manipulation
   - Tells each female nurse that she is his favorite.
   - Sets one staff member against another.
   - Manipulates special favors from female nurses.
   - Makes sexual advances toward female staff.
   - Is insincere and superficial.
2. **Risk for violence directed at others** related to antisocial character, as evidenced by history of overtly aggressive acts
   - Is verbally aggressive with male staff.
   - Has threatened physical assault on another client.
   - Has history of spousal abuse.
   - Rationalizes violent behavior; does not see behavior as undesirable.
   - Has had two episodes of infraction of rules.
   - Assaulted a co-worker before admission.

Continued on following page

CASE STUDY: WORKING WITH A PERSON WHO HAS AN ANTISOCIAL PERSONALITY DISORDER (Continued)

PLANNING

PLANNING OUTCOME CRITERIA

Ms. Burke and the rest of the staff decide on strategies designed to reduce Mr. Mann's manipulation and aggressiveness, then sets long-term outcome criteria and short-term goals. The aim of the goals is to alter Mr. Mann's behavior while he is on the unit and to elicit more appropriate behaviors for meeting needs and responding to frustration.

NURSING DIAGNOSIS	LONG-TERM OUTCOME	SHORT-TERM GOALS
1. **Ineffective individual coping** related to inadequate psychological resources, as evidenced by verbal manipulation	Client will ask directly for basic needs.	1a. Client will state awareness of manipulative behavior by (date). 1b. Client will state awareness of thoughts and expectations surrounding two situations of manipulation by (date).
2. **High risk for violence** directed at others related to antisocial character, as evidenced by history of overt, aggressive acts	Client will demonstrate appropriate behaviors in response to frustration, without violence, most of the time.	2a. Client will talk about his anger and frustration rather than acting out by (date). 2b. By (date) client will develop two appropriate alternative behaviors to relieve frustration.

NURSE'S FEELINGS AND SELF-ASSESSMENT

During the planning, it is decided that Ms. Burke would be the primary nurse during the day, and Ms. Hubb, during the evening shift. Ms. Burke is to get supervision from the advanced practice psychiatric nurse on the unit. The nursing coordinator suggests that communication regarding Mr. Mann be given in some detail during shift reports until modification of his aggressive and manipulative behavior is evident.

INTERVENTION

The nursing care plan involves input from all staff members. It is anticipated that Mr. Mann would become easily frustrated and angry when limits were set on his manipulative and aggressive behavior. Ms. Burke (days) and Ms. Hubb (evenings) would be the primary staff members working with Mr. Mann. All requests, favors, and sharing of personal information would be channeled through these two nurses. Setting limits was an important aspect of the care plan. Both Ms. Burke and Mrs. Hubb were to set the limits on flattery, gifts, and compliments. When such behavior occurred, interaction would be refocused back to Mr. Mann.

Clear limits were set regarding aggressive behavior. Mr. Mann was told that angry and inappropriate verbal aggressiveness would result in loss of a privilege on the unit for that day (e.g., telephone calls, television at night). Physical acting out would have more severe consequences. For any physical assault, weekend passes would be withheld, and any other appropriate precautions would be taken (e.g., time in the quiet room, use of medication).

Expected client behaviors were clearly explained, and when elicited, would meet with recognition and positive feedback. The following is an interview between the nurse and Mr. Mann after his threat to strike another client.

CASE STUDY: *WORKING WITH A PERSON WHO HAS AN ANTISOCIAL PERSONALITY DISORDER* (*Continued*)

DIALOGUE		THERAPEUTIC TOOL/COMMENT
Nurse:	I would like to talk with you about what happened this morning.	Be clear as to purpose of interview.
Mr. Mann:	OK, shoot.	
Nurse:	Tell me what started the incident.	Use open-ended statements. Maintain a nonjudgmental attitude.
Mr. Mann:	Well, as I told you before, I always had to fight to get what I wanted in life. My father and mother abandoned me emotionally when I was a child.	
Nurse:	Yes, but tell me about this morning.	Redirect client to present problem or situation.
Mr. Mann:	OK. I disliked Richard from the first. He has it in for me, I just know it. He doesn't get along with anyone here. Just 2 days ago, he almost had a fight.	
Nurse:	Donald, what do you mean, Richard has it in for you?	Explore situation.
Mr. Mann:	When I'm talking to one of the nurses, he stares and makes comments under his breath.	
Nurse:	What does he say?	Encourage description.
Mr. Mann:	How I'm "in" with the nurses. I'm just trying to do what is expected of me here.	
Nurse:	You mean that Richard is envious of your relationship with the nurses?	Validate client's meaning.
Mr. Mann:	Right. He really doesn't want to be here. He doesn't care about all that therapeutic junk.	
Nurse:	You seem to know a lot about how Richard thinks. I wonder how that is?	Assist client to make association to present situation.
Mr. Mann	He reminds me of someone I knew when I was young. His name was Joe. We called him "Bones."	
Nurse:	Tell me more about Bones.	Explore situation further.
Mr. Mann:	We called him Bones because he was skinny. He was into drugs and never ate. He was also called Bones because he was selfish. He never shared anything. He never even had a girl that I knew about.	

Continued on following page

CASE STUDY: WORKING WITH A PERSON WHO HAS AN ANTISOCIAL PERSONALITY DISORDER *(Continued)*

Nurse:	So Richard reminds you of someone who is selfish and lonely?	Make interpretation of information. Note increasing anxiety.
Mr. Mann:	That's right. I've had three marriages and girlfriends on the side. No one can take them away from me. *(angrily)* Just let them try!	
Nurse:	What makes you so angry now?	Identify feelings and explore threat or anxiety.
Mr. Mann:	Richard! I know he wants to be like me, but he can't. I'll hurt him if he makes any more comments about me.	
Nurse:	Donald, you will *not* hurt anyone here on the unit.	Set limits on, and expectations of, client's behavior.
Mr. Mann:	I'm sorry, I didn't mean that.	
Nurse:	It's important that we examine your part in the incident this morning and how to cope without threats or violence.	Focus on client's responsibility and suggest alternative methods of coping with situation.
Mr. Mann:	Listen, I know I've gotten into trouble because I can't control my temper, but that's because I won't get any respect until I can show them I don't fear them.	Exhibits rationalization.
Nurse:	Who are "they"?	Clarify pronoun.
Mr. Mann:	People like Richard.	
Nurse:	You've told me that fighting was a way of survival as a child, but as an adult, there are other ways of handling situations that make you angry.	Shows understanding and suggests other means of coping.
Mr. Mann:	You're right. I've thought about this. Do you think it would help if you gave me some meds to control my anger?	Exhibits superficial and concrete thinking—possible manipulation.
Nurse:	I wasn't thinking of medications but of a plan for being aware of your anger and talking it out instead of fighting it out.	Clarify meaning toward behavioral change.
Mr. Mann:	I told you before, I have to fight.	
Nurse:	Have you thought about the consequences of your fighting?	Identify results of impulsive behavior.
Mr. Mann:	I feel bad afterwards. Sometimes I wish it hadn't happened.	

CASE STUDY: WORKING WITH A PERSON WHO HAS AN ANTISOCIAL PERSONALITY DISORDER (Continued)

Nurse:	Tell me about a time when you felt this way.	Explore previous situations of impulsiveness.
Mr. Mann:	I really loved my third wife, but she made me mad. I didn't want to hurt her, but I couldn't help myself.	
Nurse:	Couldn't help yourself?	Use reflection to get client to further describe situation.
Mr. Mann:	She wanted me to stay home and not go out with the guys, but I didn't want her to tell me what to do.	
Nurse:	And then what happened?	Continue to explore situation.

EVALUATION

As expected, Mr. Mann becomes outraged when limits are set. He starts to shout at the doctor and calls him names. The staff calmly tell him that because of his inappropriate shouting, he is unable to use the telephone for the rest of the day, as outlined in his plan. Over the next few days, he does some more testing (e.g., yelling and throwing a can of soda at one of the evening staff). He is taken to the seclusion room for 1 hour. That weekend, he is refused a pass. By the end of the third week, his behavior on the unit shows marked modification. His pitting of staff against staff is thwarted. By discharge, his verbal aggressiveness has flared up once in a while, but much less often than on previous occasions. Refer to Mr. Mann's written care plan (Nursing Care Plan 19–1).

The editor would like to acknowledge and thank Kem B. Louie, Ph.D., for this case study prepared for the first and second editions of this text.

NURSING CARE PLAN 19–1 A PERSON WITH ANTISOCIAL PERSONALITY DISORDER: MR MANN

NURSING DIAGNOSIS

Ineffective individual coping: related to inadequate psychological resources, as evidenced by verbal manipulation

Supporting Data

- Sexual advances toward female staff.
- Infraction of the rules on unit.
- Attempts to set staff at odds with each other.
- Insincere and superficial interactions.
- Manipulation of special favors from nurses

Outcome Criteria: Mr Mann will ask directly for basic needs.

SHORT-TERM GOAL	INTERVENTION	RATIONALE	EVALUATION
1. Mr. Mann will state awareness of manipulative behavior by (date).	1a. One nurse assigned to Mr. Mann on both evening and day shifts. 1b. One-to-one interaction with primary care staff on a day-to-day basis.	1a, b. Limits chance of mixed communication. Decreases ability to manipulate.	*GOAL PARTIALLY MET* After 2 weeks, client acknowledged some manipulative behaviors and stated that he understood the consequences of continuing some of his manipulative behaviors.

Continued on following page

NURSING CARE PLAN 19–1 A PERSON WITH ANTISOCIAL PERSONALITY DISORDER: MR MANN *(Continued)*

SHORT-TERM GOAL	INTERVENTION	RATIONALE	EVALUATION
	1c. Communicate clear limits on manipulative behavior. 1d. Communicate expected behavior. 1e. Spell out the consequences of manipulation. 1f. Share limits, expected behavior, and consequences of manipulation with all other staff daily at report time and at team conferences.	1c–f. Clear expectations for behavior and consequences provide sound framework for intervention.	
	1g. Avoid power struggles; do not be defensive.	1g. Arguments take focus away from client and issue.	
	1h. Offer positive reinforcement and feedback when expected behavior is evident.	1h. Can increase expected behavior.	
2. Mr. Mann will state awareness of thoughts and expectations surrounding two situations of manipulation by (date).	2a. Identify situations in which client is manipulative. 2b. Explore needs or expectations in each manipulative situation. 2c. Discuss impact of manipulative behavior on self and others.	2a–c. Change in behavior facilitated when client is aware of each manipulation.	*GOAL PARTIALLY MET* Client was able to discuss one incident with primary nurse in terms of expectations and thoughts.

NURSING DIAGNOSIS

Risk of violence directed at others: related to antisocial character, as evidenced by history of overtly aggressive acts

Supporting Data

- Past history of spousal abuse.
- Past history of fighting.
- Assault of a co-worker before admission.
- Threats to another client on the unit.
- Rationalization of behavior—does not see anything wrong.
- Infraction of rules (two episodes).
- Verbally aggressive with male staff.

Outcome Criteria: Mr. Mann will demonstrate appropriate behaviors in response to frustration, without violence, most of the time.

NURSING CARE PLAN 19–1 A PERSON WITH ANTISOCIAL PERSONALITY DISORDER: MR MANN *(Continued)*

SHORT-TERM GOAL	INTERVENTION	RATIONALE	EVALUATION
1. Mr. Mann will verbalize anger and frustration rather than act out by (date).	1a. Identify feelings of anxiety, anger, and frustration. 1b. Encourage appropriate verbalization of these feelings with the nurse.	1a,b. Client learns to talk it out instead of act it out.	*GOAL MET* Client initiated discussions twice with nurse when he "felt like wasting" another client.
	1c. Discuss events that lead to aggressive behavior.	1c. Client learns to acknowledge and anticipate feelings of frustration that can lead to aggression.	Physical acting out had decreased in incidence by the end of the third week.
2. By (date) Mr. Mann will develop two appropriate alternative behaviors to relieve frustration.	2a. Explore relief felt when aggression is used by client. 2b. Discuss impact or consequences of behavior on self and others. 2c. Explore alternative behaviors in coping with anger and frustration. 2d. Assist client in developing effective communication skills.	2a–d. Learning to deal appropriately with aggression allows client to take responsibility for his own behavior.	*GOAL PARTIALLY MET* Initially, the client continued to test staff by throwing things and name calling. On (date), the client sought out nurse two times when he was angry to discuss thoughts and feelings.
	2e. Provide feedback to client on behaviors. 2f. Reward client when he is not using aggressive behaviors.	2e, f. Positive feedback and rewards help elicit desired behaviors.	By the third week, the incidence of verbal and physical acting out had sharply declined.

SUMMARY

The special needs of the client with PD project from an inner core of terror, rage, and confusion, around which neurochemical pathways have formed to create thoughts, feelings, and actions that are rigid and maladaptive. The role of the nurse with such clients is to understand the theoretical underpinnings of their disorder, along with its many diagnostic expressions, and to be able to intervene to change the crisis-oriented client into the client who is consciously aware of the consequences of his or her behavior and can soothe inner painful states while still accomplishing the tasks of adult daily living.

REFERENCES

American Psychiatric Association (1994). *Diagnostic and statistical manual of mental disorders* (4th ed.). Washington, DC: American Psychiatric Association.

Baker, L. A., and Daniels, D. (1990). Nonshared environmental influences and personality differences in adult twins. *Journal Personality and Social Psychology*, 58:103–110.

Bennett, L. A., Wolin, S. J., Reiss, D., and Teitelbaum, M. A. (1987). Couples at risk for transmission of alcoholism: Protective influences. *Family Process*, 26:111–129.

Bonnivier, J. F. (1996). Management of self-destructive behaviors in an open inpatient setting. *Journal of Psychosocial Nursing and Mental Health Services*, 34(2):38–42.

Chitty, K. K., and Maynard, C. K. (1986). Managing manipulation. *Journal of Psychosocial Nursing and Mental Health Services*, 24(6):9.

Cloninger, C. R., Svrakic, D.M., and Przybeck, T.R. (1993). A psychobiological model of temperament and character. *Archives of General Psychiatry*, 50:975–990.

Dawson, G., and Fischer, K. W. (Eds.) (1994). *Human behavior and the developing brain*. New York: Guilford Press.

Dunn, J., and McGuire, S. (1993). Young children's non-shared experiences: A summary of studies in Cambridge and Colorado. In E. M. Hetherington, D. Reiss and R. Plomin (Eds.), *Nonshared environments* (pp. 111-128). Hillsdale, NJ: Lawrence Eribaum.

Favazza, A. R., and Rosenthal, R. J. (1993). Diagnostic issues in self-mutilation. *Hospital and Community Psychiatry*, 44:134–140.

Goldberg, R. J. (1995). *Practical guide to the care of the psychiatric patient.* St. Louis, MO: C. V. Mosby.

Gunderson, J. G., and Phillips, K. A. (1995). Personality disorders. In H. I. Kaplan and B. J. Sadock (Eds.), *Comprehensive textbook of psychiatry-VI* (6th ed., Vol. 2, pp. 1425–1462). Baltimore: William & Wilkins.

Horowitz, M. J. (1992). *Stress response syndromes.* Northvale, NJ: Jason-Aronson.

Kaplan, H. I., and Sadock, B. J. (1991). *Synopsis of psychiatry.* Baltimore: Williams & Wilkins.

Kernberg O. (1985). *Internal world and external reality.* London: Aronson.

Kohut, H. (1984). *How does analysis cure.* Chicago: University of Chicago Press.

Lewis-Herman, J. (1992). *Trauma and recovery.* New York: Harper-Collins.

Lyons, M. J., et al. (1995). Differential heritability of adult and juvenile antisocial traits. *Archives of General Psychiatry*, 52(11):906–915.

Maier, W., Lichtermann, D., Minges, J., and Heun, R. (1994). Personality disorders among the relatives of schizophrenia patients. *Schizophrenia Bulletin*, 20(3):481–493.

Maxmen, J. S., and Ward, N. G. (1995). *Psychotropic drugs fast facts* (2nd ed.). New York: W. W. Norton.

Maxmen, J. S., and Ward, N. G. (1996). *Essential psychopathology and its treatment* (2nd ed.). New York: W. W. Norton.

Oldham, J. M., et al. (1995). Comorbidity of axis I and axis II disorders. *American Journal of Psychiatry*, 152(4):571–578.

Post, R. M. (1992). Transduction of psychosocial stress into the neurobiology of recurrent affective disorder. *American Journal of Psychiatry*, 149:999–1007.

SELF-STUDY AND CRITICAL THINKING

Multiple choice

1. Which of the following *least* describes people with personality disorders? They
   A. Are very resistant to change.
   B. Have an inability to tolerate frustration and pain.
   C. Have serious difficulty forming satisfying and intimate relationships.
   D. Often seek out help to change their maladaptive behaviors.
2. Choose the statement that is *not* true. People with personality disorders have
   A. The ability to evoke interpersonal conflict.
   B. The capacity to have an intense negative effect on others.
   C. Usually just one DSM-IV diagnosis.
   D. The potential for psychotic behaviors under stress.

True or false

Put a T for true or an F for false next to each statement.

3. ______ Tendencies to develop personality disorders may be influenced by genetics.
4. ______ Personality disorders are easy to treat and are best treated in the hospital setting.
5. ______ Early traumatic trauma may contribute to an inability to form satisfying interpersonal relationships.
6. ______ Theoretically healing relationships may intervene to reconstruct the personality chemically, cognitively, and experientially.
7. ______ Initial interventions with this population often involve crisis interventions.
8. ______ The backgrounds of these clients are often trouble free and their homes are loving and supportive.

Multiple choice

9. Mr. Rogers is undergoing surgery for a broken leg. He is very suspicious of the staff and believes that everyone is trying to harm him and "do him in." He scans his environment constantly for danger (hypervigilant) and speaks very little to the nurses or the other clients. The best approach with Mr. Rogers for the nurses to adopt would be

   A. Friendly and outgoing, showing him that people care.
   B. To explain how the staff want to help him, not harm him.
   C. To be matter of fact and neutral sticking to the facts of situations.
   D. To alternate among being friendly, aloof, business-like, and reticent.

10. Other approaches with a person who is very paranoid would include (circle all that apply)

    A. Giving him as much control over the situation as possible.
    B. Answering all of his questions about the tests, procedures, and policies, giving clear explanations.
    C. Telling him as little as possible so as not to frighten him.
    D. Responding to sarcasm and hostility with information and a neutral stance.

11. Ms. Lind, a 32-year-old woman, is brought into the emergency department after having been raped and badly beaten while living on the street. She is delusional and thinks the hospital is the gateway to hell. She is very withdrawn and does not seem to want to talk to anyone. She is thought to have a schizoid personality disorder. Which approach would be the most useful for Ms. Lind?

    A. Give detailed information on what is going on, what has happened to her, the protocol for a rape trauma victim, and so on.
    B. Simply and clearly inform her of what is going on. For example, "I am going to examine your sores and put something on them to keep them from becoming infected. First, I will look at those on your face."

12. Which of the following is the *least accurate* description of a person with schizotypal personality disorder?

    A. They are viewed as eccentric and may believe that they have magical powers.
    B. Their speech is often difficult to follow and often illogical to others.
    C. They are often frightened and become very suspicious of others' motivations.
    D. They do not want contact or relationships with others and are content in isolation.

13. Mr. Stowe is a 29-year-old man who has been in and out of jail several times for stealing and selling drugs. He is HIV positive and often works as a prostitute to get money, never using a condom: "Let them get what I have, why should I be the only one?" When he wants something, he can be very charming and tells people anything to get what he wants from them. What other behaviors would you assess for in a person with an antisocial personality disorder?

    A. Shows lack of caring for others, arrogant and callous of others' feelings.
    B. Feels shame when he has done something wrong.
    C. Rarely takes drugs or engages in other thrill-seeking behaviors.
    D. Carefully plans for his future.

14. Mr. Stowe is brought into court for selling drugs (cocaine laced with PCP) outside a grade school. He tells his lawyer that he was framed and that the police planted the drugs on him. He later tells the police that his lawyer said that the police are all corrupt and cannot be trusted. Mr. Stowe is using a form of

A. Splitting.
B. Hypervigilance.
C. Manipulation.
D. Storytelling.

15. While waiting for his lawyer to get him out of jail, Mr. Stowe makes frequent requests of the guards and feigns a stomachache to get attention and favors. The best approach with someone like this client would be to

A. Set clear limits on behavior and have everyone know what the limits are.
B. Give him some privileges, but only a few.
C. Ignore his behavior.
D. Explain to him why what he is doing is wrong.

16. Ms. Pemrose is brought into the emergency department (ED) after slashing her wrists with a razor. She has previously been in the ED for drug overdose and has a history of addictions. She is avoided by the ED staff because they find her behavior trying and exhausting. Ms. Pemrose can be sarcastic, belittling, and aggressive to those who try to care for her. She has a history of difficulty with interpersonal relationships at her job. When a new doctor comes in to examine her, she is at first adoring and compliant, telling him "You are the best doctor I have ever seen, and I truly want to change." When he refuses to order diazepam (Valium) for her and refuses to give her meperidine (Demerol) for "pain," she yells at him that he is "a stupid excuse for a man, and I want another doctor immediately." Her behavior could be termed

A. Projecting.
B. Splitting.
C. Denying.
D. Rationalizing.

17. The best response for the doctor to make to Ms. Pemrose when she says she wants to change doctors would be

A. In a matter-of-fact but clear way: "You cannot change doctors or have control substances, but discussing what was going on before slashing your wrists would be helpful."
B. In a caring way: "I cannot give you controlled substances because you have a history of addictions."
C. In a serious way: "I do not like to be talked to in such a rude manner. If you can't talk more respectfully, I cannot help you."
D. In a placating way: "OK, if you promise to keep your clinic appointment this time, I will give you a Valium to help you relax."

18. Ms. Stacks, a 23-year-old woman, is diagnosed with a histrionic personality disorder. The nurse would most likely find on assessment a woman who is

A. Dramatic, attention seeking, seductive and superficial in relationships with others.
B. Aloof and withdrawn, not seeking out others, preferring to be alone.
C. Confused and disorganized, with hallucinations of voices telling her she is a queen.
D. Clear minded, caring in close relationships, and concerned for others' well-being.

19. Mr. Jordan, a 41-year-old man, believes he is the most important man at his job. He fantasizes that one day he will be the boss and will receive world recognition for his brilliance and unique contributions. He is demanding, contemptuous, and belittling of those around him. He is to be worked up at his HMO for evaluation for a possible bleeding ulcer. Which of the following behaviors would be the most in character for a person diagnosed with a narcissistic personality disorder?

    A. Arriving late for his appointment, very apologetic, saying that the cab driver didn't know the way and that he hoped the doctor would still see him even if he was late.
    B. Arriving late, telling the nurse that he had to first check out the building and that he didn't want to go into one of those back rooms, and that if the doctor wanted to see him he would have to come to the front desk.
    C. Arriving late for his appointment dressed in brightly colored clothes and greeting everyone in the waiting room. He gets angry when he is asked to keep his voice down.
    D. Arriving late for his clinic appointment, blaming the "stupid cab driver," and telling the nurse that he will only see the head physician, not some little guy in training, and to get him right away.

20. Knowing how to deal with manipulation is crucial for working with clients with personality disorders, especially clients with antisocial, borderline, and histrionic personality disorders. Which of the following steps would you *omit* when you set limits on behaviors?

    A. Set limits only on behaviors that protect the client or others.
    B. Establish realistic and enforceable consequences of exceeding the limits.
    C. Make sure the client is aware of both the limits and the consequences of exceeding the limits.
    D. All health care workers who come into contact with the client can use their best judgment on how they want to handle clients exceeding the limits.

UNIT FIVE

People in Severe to Psychotic Range on the Mental Health Continuum

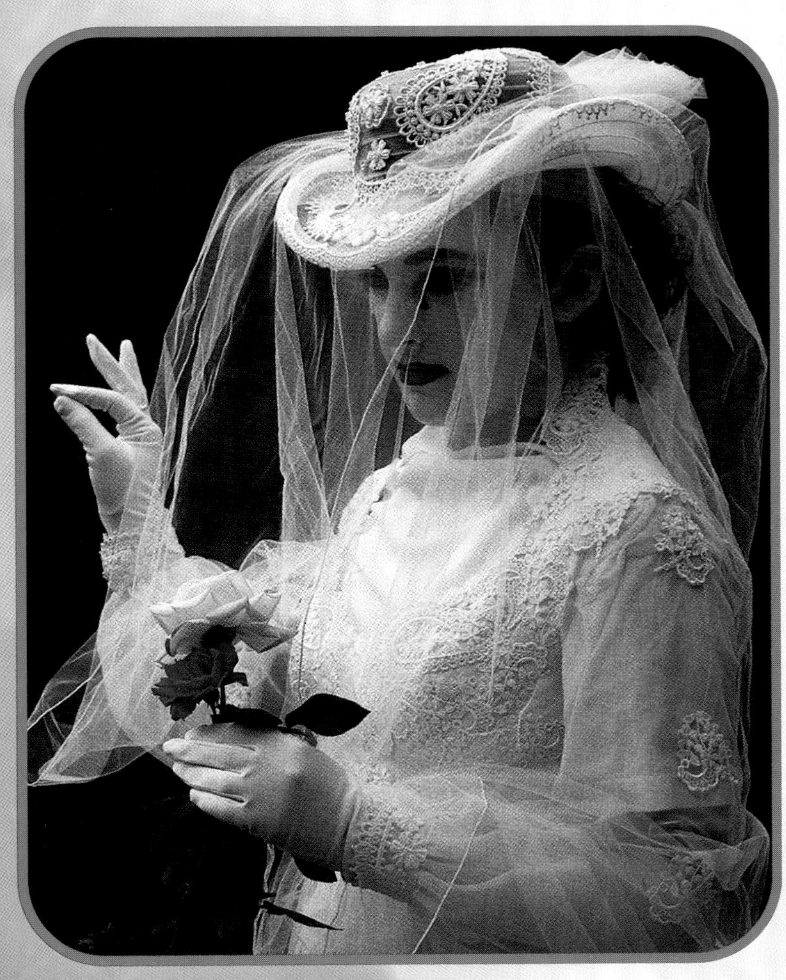

We don't see things as they are, we see them as we are.

ANAÏS NIN

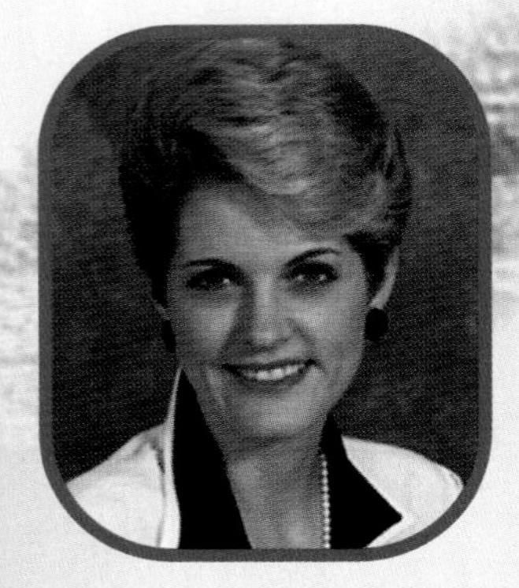

A Nurse Speaks

Mary D. Moller

People with schizophrenia are victims of fluctuating brain chemistry. Caring for people who are psychotic entails making the effort to understand another person's experience whose reality is distorted, frightening, and filled with terror of the unknown. People with schizophrenia are talking a foreign language, and we have to struggle to find the meanings of their words and phrases. The story I relate is a story of that struggle to translate a young man's experience—a story with a very happy ending.

"I'm controlled by God and my roommates are trying to hurt me. I'm at the apostrophe point—the other thought hasn't erupted yet—it makes me nervous. The TV is reading my alpha waves and my entropy is all used up. I am looking for the sublime but I end up with bifurcations." Brad, a 27-year-old single white male, was extremely disheveled and unkempt when he came to our clinic in May of 1995. His hair was unwashed and wild. His fingers were orange from chronic cigarette smoking. He was very pleasant and cooperative, however, and was able to establish and maintain eye contact for short periods. Initially he needed to take cigarette breaks about every 30 minutes. Brad had been diagnosed with schizophrenia 6 years earlier. He was in the last semester of his senior year of college studying to be a conservation biologist when he had his first psychotic break. His parents are both teachers and there is no history of mental illness in the family. Brad is now a guitarist with a rock band. He had been hospitalized several times in the 6 years before our meeting. He was taking 30 mg of thiothixene (Navane) and was somewhat sedated. He was not interested in switching medications because he thought it meant going back to the hospital.

He seemed to demonstrate classic symptoms of formal thought disorder and ideas of reference, but careful scrutiny of the content of his responses revealed thoughtful and eloquent answers to each question. He would strum an invisible guitar as he sang the answers to most questions with lyrics from heavy metal rock music. As his anxiety increased, the strumming motions would become more rapid and forceful and his singing became quite loud. He frequently sang "dangerous this game we play," "get outta here," "changes in you," "I wonder how you do, your troubles run deeper, broke the rule," and "pins and needles." When he was not singing, his speech was soft, yet pressured. As his anxiety decreased, the rate, rhythm, and pitch of his speech were within normal limits. Brad's answers were frequently preceded by loud bursts of laughter that appeared to be in response to almost constant auditory hallucinations, but he rarely made reference to these voices. He reported that he almost had a heart attack once from laughing at what the voices told him. (It would be several weeks before he shared the content of his hallucinations with me.) He exhibited frequent akathisic movements but was always able to return to a seated position.

He used numerous neologisms but would readily interpret them when asked for the meaning; i.e., *Fletus* is a beast that will bear you to perfection and *Undos* means playing on Saturday night. Persons with schizophrenia typically assign personalized meanings to common words and speak in what is referred to as metaphoric speech. Brad would often refer to the *apostrophe point*, which he used to describe blank spots in his ability to think, *reaching the sublime*, which meant experiencing peace and quiet in his brain, *bifurcate*, which meant he lost touch with reality, and *steal away*, which referred to having sex with other people's friends.

These communication abnormalities can be likened to the speech patterns of individuals who have experienced a cerebrovascular accident. In fact, I would encourage new students to evaluate the patient with schizophrenia in terms of a person with both expressive and receptive aphasia. Adopting that type of mind set allows the caregiver to assume primary responsibility for communication until the patient's patterns of speech are understood.

Brad was very unhealthy. Every day he would drink at least 15 cups of coffee, two to six beers, and smoke three or four packs of cigarettes, and occasionally he would use marijuana. He would frequently stay up all night on the weekends, particularly if he had been performing. The ultimate treatment outcome was for him to complete his college degree. Long-term goals included eliminating caffeine over a 6-week period, decreasing his daily number of cigarettes to 15, eliminating alcohol completely, beginning an intensive AA (Alcoholics Anonymous) program, and for him and his family to enroll in our summer series of classes entitled "Recovering From Psychosis: A Wellness Approach," which were starting in July.

My initial interventions focused on understanding Brad's form of speech with the eventual goal of also understanding the content of his hallucinations. I observed that he had major gaps in his ability to execute a thought and complete a sentence. He literally "spaced out" with anxiety and would begin strumming his guitar when asked a question either he couldn't or the voices wouldn't let him answer. In evaluating his street drug use, I learned he had used PCP and LSD. I showed him color brain scans of the effects of drugs on the brain, and he was most willing to work on getting "his brain cleaned out." I was very straightforward, open, and honest in my approach to patient teaching. Brad was very receptive to learning. He remarked, "No one has ever taken this kind of time with me before, I like you." He became enthusiastic when I invited him to share his use of language at our upcoming class series.

He attended the classes, shared with the group, and brought a tape of his music. He began the caffeine, alcohol, and nicotine withdrawal and noticed that the thiothixene had a much stronger effect (just as I had told him it would). He then became interested in beginning a full-fledged medication change. During August, September, and October of 1995 we engaged in a 12-week crossover and he successfully switched to 6 mg of risperidone. He re-enrolled at the university (against my advice, as I knew it was too soon, but he was thrilled with his early response to risperidone) and started in AA. He was beginning to correlate symptom intensification with use of alcohol, caffeine, and nicotine. He was totally abstinent from street drugs. His affect and eye contact brightened. His speech became noticeably clearer and thoughts were articulated more clearly. He still experienced *exploding thoughts*, several *null and voids*, and *apostrophe points*. He continued to emphasize every thought with a guitar chord and song.

School became too much and he had to withdraw at midterm. He described the episode that occurred before dropping out in this way: "I saw angels and demons and they went to school with me. I had stayed up all night studying and drinking coffee. It lasted about a day and a half. They talked to me and went to school with me, it was kinda cool. It's really mellow in my head since I dropped out of school. I've reached the *sublime* and the *apostrophe points* have stopped. It's weird having it quiet in my head but it helps me think." After he dropped out of school his case manager encouraged him to enroll in a local clubhouse, to which Brad replied, "I really don't want to go to the clubhouse because I don't like the people there. I'm not one of them. I don't want to do janitorial work." I convinced him to go and see if he could handle the routine and discipline of having to get up in the mornings. I suggested that if he was successful there he would have a good chance of success at returning to school. He agreed. During that fall he focused on improving his personal appearance and implementing his wellness plan.

Chart notes from that period include the following quotes: "I looked better yesterday than I do today." "Last night I had some non-alcohol beer, and even the little bit of alcohol in it and the chemicals made my wig tight." "Yeah, I'm in this awakenings you talked about, I don't have anymore voices and I don't *bifurcate* with the television anymore." "I am trying to quit the cigarettes because they bring me to the *apostrophe point.* Coffee is bad, it also makes my wig tighten." "Things are really quiet in my head, my thoughts don't twist back on themselves anymore. I used to think I could read people's minds and it was kind of fun to think I could send them messages, but I can't do that anymore. It's much better this way." "I'm wearing my sobriety shoes, though. I go to AA every noon and it's really helping. I'm doing mental health now, not mental illness. I'm no longer frustrated incorporated. That relapse is full of hot air." "When I drink I get the null hypothesis and my mind goes wild. When I go to the bars, I just drink that non-alcohol beer, the bartenders downtown know not to serve me alcohol."

Brad tried to re-enroll for second semester, but his counselor was against it. I intervened and he was allowed to sign up for one course. He passed that course with a C− and took a summer school course in conservation and natural resources, which he also passed. His comments in August of 1996 included "I am high on life, things are really improving. My head is much more peaceful. I have energy and am motivated to finish school. I didn't get quite the grades I wanted, but I passed. I only have two classes left and I'll graduate." He was animated and had expression and enthusiasm. His basic creativity was starting to emerge. His mother shared her excitement at his "coming out." There were no longer any psychotic symptoms. I was, however, concerned about him taking two classes with the ultimate pressure of graduation, but he did.

In December of 1996 he came to see me and began the session with "I'm going to graduate in 2 weeks. I'm getting pretty good grades. My degree will be in biology and ecology. I'll go where the jobs are, but I would like to do something with writing environment impact statements. I turn 29 next Friday. I'm doing so good. My mind is quiet and at peace. There is none of the former stuff. I really think it was all the alcohol and caffeine. Now if I could just quit smoking I could get really healthy. I'm still smoking at least ½ pack a day. I'm completely off the booze. I've even lost a few pounds this semester. You have really helped me."

Brad is now neatly groomed and his fingers are no longer yellow. However, we weren't out of the woods yet! Two weeks later I got an emergency page—he had passed one of the classes and relapsed before the final for the second class. I faxed a letter to his professor explaining Brad's disability. Brad was able to get an "incomplete" for that course instead of an F.

So where are we in January of 1997? Brad has taken the final, has passed the course, and will receive his degree in May. The world now has one more college graduate and one less person on welfare. Together we will continue to monitor symptoms and response to medications. Brad realizes he has a severe and persistent mental illness that will remit and exacerbate throughout his life. He is determined never to be admitted to a psychiatric hospital again.

I will always treasure and build upon the lessons he taught me. What is the greatest lesson he taught me? Never give up hope because of the severity of presenting symptoms—a mind is a terrible thing to waste. Brad knows that what he taught me will benefit countless others.

20

Alterations in Mood: GRIEF AND DEPRESSION

ELIZABETH M. VARCAROLIS

OUTLINE

KEY TERMS AND CONCEPTS

The key terms and concepts listed here also appear in bold where they are defined or discussed in this chapter.

grief
mourning
phenomena experienced during mourning
anticipatory grief
mood
major depression
dysthymia
anhedonia
anergia
psychomotor agitation
psychomotor retardation
vegetative signs of depression
hypersomnia
selective serotonin inhibitors
tricyclic antidepressants

GRIEF

OBJECTIVES

After studying this section on grief, the reader will be able to

1. Describe the process of mourning.
2. Give examples of phenomena people may experience during the course of mourning (1 to 2 years).
3. Role play and demonstrate five interventions helpful to a family that is grieving.
4. Explain how a task-based model of death, dying, and bereavement can help health care workers.
5. Identify when the work of mourning has been successful.
6. List six factors that can negatively affect the successful work of mourning.

Change is a part of life, and every change involves both loss and gain. People come and go in everyone's lives. As individuals gain experience, they lose their youth—dreams are realized or hopes are abandoned. People are constantly faced with giving up one mode of life for another.

Loss is part of the human experience, and grief is the normal response to loss. The loss may be of a relationship (divorce, separation, death, abortion), of health (a body function or part, mental or physical capacity), of status or prestige, of security (occupational, financial, social, cultural), of self-confidence, of a dream, or of self-concept, or loss can be of a symbolic nature. Other losses include changes in circumstances, such as retirement, promotion, marriage, and aging. All losses affect a person's self-concept. People undergoing therapy may grieve as they give up old and familiar—even if maladaptive—ways of viewing the world. A loss can be real or perceived. Although grief and loss are universal experiences, loss through death is a major life crisis (Davis et al. 1992; Parker 1992).

In this chapter, **grief** refers to the subjective feelings and affect that are precipitated by a loss. The term **mourning** refers to the processes (grief work) by which grief is resolved.

Grief is not a mood disorder, although a depressive syndrome is often part of the grieving process. Grief is the normal response to a significant loss. Although it is a normal phenomenon, it may at times be the focus of treatment.

Zisook and Shuchter's (1992) study of 350 widows and widowers found that

1. A depressive episode, as defined by the *Diagnostic and statistical manual of mental disorders*, fourth edition (1994) (DSM-IV), frequently occurs within the first year after the death of a spouse.
2. The depressive episode may occur not only in the early months of bereavement but also many month after the death.
3. Among the individuals at highest risk for depressive episodes 13 months *after* their loss were those who
    - Were younger widows and widowers.
    - Had past histories of depression.
    - Perceived themselves to be in poor health.

Mourning is a distinct psychological process that involves disengaging strong emotional ties from a significant relationship and reinvesting those ties in a new and productive direction. This reinvestment of emotional energy into new relationships or creative activities is necessary for a person's mental health and functioning in society. When the mourning process is successfully completed, the griever is released from one interpersonal relationship and is able to form new relationships. The entire process of mourning may take a year or more to complete.

Many theorists have studied the grief process. Some of the most widely known are George Engel, Colin Parkes, Elizabeth Kübler-Ross, Erich Lindemann (1944), John Bowlby, and Edgar Jackson. Although each theorist uses different terminology, the process they outline is fundamentally the same. Each describes commonly experienced psychological and behavioral characteristics. These characteristics follow a pattern of response:

1. Shock and disbelief
2. Sensation of somatic distress
3. Preoccupation with image of the deceased
4. Guilt
5. Anger
6. Change in behavior (e.g., depression, disorganization, or restlessness)
7. Reorganization of behavior directed toward a new object or activity

A person may demonstrate a different clinical picture at each stage of mourning. Each stage of mourning has its own characteristics, and the duration and form of each stage may vary considerably from person to person. People react within their own value and personality structure, as well as within their social environment and cultural patterns. Most people are preprogrammed in their response to death. Distinct characteristics, however, can be identified throughout the grieving process.

The process of mourning is often divided into stages. The stages have been identified by Engel (1964) as (1) acute and (2) long term.

ACUTE STAGE

The acute state (4 to 8 weeks after the death) involves shock and disbelief, developing awareness, and restitution.

Shock and Disbelief

The bereaved's first response is that of *denial.* The person is emotionally unable to accept his or her painful loss. Denial functions as a buffer against intolerable pain and slowly allows the person to acknowledge the reality of death. The mourner may appear to be functioning like a robot. Often, the bereaved person feels numb. A death may be "accepted" intellectually during this stage—"It's just as well, she was suffering"—although the emotional responses are still repressed. Denial is a needed defense that lasts for a few hours to a few days. *Denial that persists for longer than a few days could indicate difficulty in progressing through the process of mourning.*

Development of Awareness

As denial fades, painful feelings begin to surface. The finality of the loved one's death becomes more of a reality. Waves of anguish and pain are experienced and may be localized in the chest or the epigastric area. *Anger* often surfaces at this time. Doctors and nurses are often the subject of blame. Awareness by staff that anger is often displaced onto people in the hospital environment may decrease defensive staff behaviors. *Guilt* is often experienced, and the bereaved blames himself or herself for taking or for failing to take specific actions. Impulsive and self-destructive acts by the mourner, such as smashing a hand through a window or beating the head against a wall, may be seen. *Crying* is a common phenomenon during this stage. "It is during this time that the greatest degree of anguish or despair, within the limits imposed by cultural patterns, is experienced or expressed" (Engel 1964). Crying can afford a welcome release from pent-up anguish and tension. Assessment of cultural patterns is important for making clinical judgments about the appropriateness of the bereaved's behavior. Not crying can be the result of cultural influences or environmental restraints. The person may cry in private. Inability to cry, however, may be the result of a high degree of ambivalence toward the deceased. *A person who is unable to cry may have difficulty in successfully completing the work of mourning.*

Restitution (different than Kübler-Ross)

Restitution is the formal, "ritualistic" phase of mourning during the acute stage. It is the institutionalization of mourning: it brings friends and family together in the rites of the funeral service, and serves to emphasize the finality of death. The viewing of the body, the lowering of the casket, and the various religious and cultural rituals all help the bereaved shed any residual denial in an atmosphere of support. Every human society has its own moral and cultural standards, according to which the rituals of mourning take place. The gathering in ritualistic farewell for the deceased provides support and sustenance for the family.

LONG-TERM STAGE

After the acute stage has been completed, the main work of mourning goes on intrapsychically for 1 to 2 years or longer. The various **phenomena experienced during mourning** by the bereaved are described in Table 20–1.

TABLE 20–1 PHENOMENA EXPERIENCED DURING MOURNING

SYMPTOMS	EXAMPLES
Sensation of Somatic Distress	
Tightness in throat, shortness of breath, sighing, "mental pain," exhaustion. Food tastes like sand; things feel unreal. Pain or discomfort may be identical to the symptoms experienced by the dead person. Normally symptoms are brief.	A woman whose husband died of a stroke complains of weakness and numbness on her left side.
Preoccupation with the Image of the Deceased	
The bereaved brings up and thinks and talks about numerous memories of the deceased. The memories are positive. This process goes on with great sadness. The idealization of the deceased lets the bereaved relive the gratifications associated with the deceased and helps resolve any guilt the bereaved has toward the deceased. The bereaved may also take on many of the mannerisms of the deceased through identification. Identification serves the purpose of holding onto the deceased. Preoccupation with the dead person takes many months before it lessens.	A man whose wife just died states, "I just can't stop thinking about my wife. Everything I see reminds me of her. We picked up this seashell on our honeymoon. I remember every wonderful moment we had together. The pain is so great, but the memories just keep coming." His friends notice that when he talks, his hand gestures and expressions are very like those of his recently deceased wife.
Guilt	
The bereaved reproaches himself or herself for real or fancied acts of negligence or omissions in the relationship with the deceased.	"I should have made him go to the doctor sooner." "I should have paid more attention to her, been more thoughtful."
Anger	
The anger the bereaved experiences may not be toward the object that gives rise to it. Often, the anger is displaced onto the medical or nursing staff. Often, it is directed toward the deceased. The anger is at its height during the first month but is often intermittent throughout the first year. The overflow of hostility disturbs the bereaved, resulting in the feeling that he or she is going "insane."	"The doctor didn't operate in time. If he had, Mary would be alive today." "How could he leave me like this . . . how could he?"
Change in Behavior (Depression, Disorganization, Restlessness)	
A person may exhibit marked restlessness and an inability to organize his or her behavior. Routine activities take a long time to do. Depressive mood is common as the year passes and as the intensity of the grief declines. Absence of depression is more abnormal than its presence. Loneliness and aimlessness are most pronounced 6 to 9 months after the death.	Six months after her husband died, Mrs. Faye stated, "I just can't seem to function, I have a hard time doing the simplest tasks. I can't be bothered with socializing." "I feel so down . . . so, so empty."
Reorganization of Behavior Directed Toward a New Object or Activity	
Gradually, the person renews his or her interest in people and activities. The grieving thus releases the bereaved from one interpersonal relationship, and new ones are free to take its place.	Twenty months after her husband's death, Mrs. Faye tells a friend, "I'll be away this weekend. I am going fishing with my brother and his friend. This is the first time I've felt like doing anything since Harry died."

THE TASKS OF MOURNING

Worden (1991) identified a task-based model that attempted to describe tasks that are involved in the process of mourning. Worden's tools are (Corr and Doka 1994):

- Task I, to accept the reality of the loss
- Task II, to share in the process of working through the pain of grief
- Task III, to adjust to an environment in which the deceased is missing

- Task IV, to restructure the family's relationship with the deceased and to reinvest in other relationships and life pursuits.

Many writers believe that task-based models permit a framework that incorporates diverse coping skills that can be identified and taught. Corr (1993) believes that task-based models in the field of dying and bereavement meet four requirements that are desirable for theoretical models in this field:

1. Help improve our understanding of the complex processes involved in coping with dying and bereavement
2. Foster empowerment on the part of those who are coping with death-related experiences
3. Enhance appreciation of interactive participation among all of those who are coping with a shared death-related experience
4. Provide guidelines for persons who are helping those who are coping with death-related experiences

UNRESOLVED GRIEF REACTION

Most bereaved persons resolve their loss with support from family and friends. However, more than 30% may require professional support (Lloyd-Williams 1995). Unresolved grief reactions have been called "the hidden disease" and may account for many of the physical symptoms seen in doctors' offices and hospital units. The "broken heart syndrome" is supported by statistics that show that surviving spouses die within a year at a much higher rate than do members of control groups (Carr 1985). Suicide is higher among people who have had a significant loss, especially if loses are multiple and grieving mechanisms are limited (Gregory 1994).

In some cases, bereaved persons become disorganized, neglect themselves, do not eat, use alcohol or drugs, and are susceptible to physical disease. Several studies have shown that the health of widows and close relatives declines within 1 year of bereavement, and medical and psychiatric problems increase (Bowlby and Parkes 1970; Carr 1985).

Health care workers are not immune to grief reactions. A study by Feldstein and Gemma (1995) found that oncology nurses scored higher than the norm in despair, social isolation, and somatization.

Reactions to loss may occur throughout life. However, two specific atypical reactions to grief have been identified: prolonged grief and delayed grief.

In *prolonged grief*, the bereaved remains intensely preoccupied with the memories of the deceased many years after the person has died.

▸ Mrs. Green has lived by herself since her husband died 5 years ago. When her nephew comes to visit, he finds everything as it was at the time of her husband's death. Mr. Green's coat is still on the hook in the front hall, and his slippers are by the daybed where he used to nap. Mrs. Green talks tearfully of how much she misses him and mentions many incidents in their life together.

In *delayed grief*, a person may not experience the pain of loss; however, that pain is altered by chronic depression into intense preoccupation with body functioning (hypochondriasis), phobic reactions, or acute insomnia. Suicidal thinking should always be assessed in a person experiencing a pathological grief response, especially if depression is the presenting symptom. Hallucinations, delusions, or obsessions may be assessed. These symptoms may not surface for months or years after the death.

▸ Mr. Bolla's wife died of cancer 3 years ago. Everyone remarked how well he handled himself and how well he did after the funeral was over. He was always a quiet man and kept to himself. Mr. Bolla has a severe anxiety attack one day while in the supermarket. As time progresses, he becomes fearful of going out and experiences severe insomnia. A neighbor brings him to the hospital when he develops pneumonia and is too fearful to leave his house to seek medical attention.

REACTIONS TO DEATH AND DYING

Culture plays an important part in our responses to death and dying. Our capacity to grieve stems from our view of death. In contemporary American society, a strong denial of becoming sick, growing old, and dying exists (Benton 1978). Rakoff (1973) stated

> America conjured into its superficial stereotype, is a country of the eternal now, of the young, face lifting, good teeth into the seventies, old ladies in Bermuda shorts, hair colored at will, endless euphemisms for chronic disease, affliction and death.

It is important for nurses to understand that cultural influences may dictate how people experience death and dying. For example, a study by Alford and Catlin (1993) found that after the death of a loved one, Americans experienced a lowering of both self-esteem and their liking and trusting of others. Spaniards reported a greater negative effect on self-esteem and a positive effect on the liking and trusting of others. Denial and fear of death are strong in the American culture. This denial and fear affect the behavioral responses of the bereaved, the family, and those who support the family in the face of death. Nurses are affected by cultural myths in the same way as the rest of society; when they are faced with a person who is dying, nurses remember their own losses. Difficult memories and unresolved feelings are often awakened. When staff members have not been able to resolve their own conflicts with death, their ability to help others is minimized. Psychological support needs to be available to help staff better understand the grieving process. When nurses examine their own feelings and their personal experience of loss, verbal and nonverbal clues to the needs of a grieving family member of a dying client become more apparent (Marks 1976).

Sometimes, nurses grieve with family members at the death of a person they have cared for and become fond of. Sometimes, an entire staff may mourn the death of a client. After clients die, nurses manage bereavement tasks, such as making sense of the death, managing mild to intense emotions, and realigning relationships. When multiple deaths are encountered, these tasks become more difficult. Understanding theories, models, tasks, and other factors can help nurses facilitate their own grief and reduce bereavement overload (Saunders and Valente 1995).

HELPING PEOPLE GRIEVE

Prolonged and serious alterations in social adjustment, as well as medical diseases, may develop if the phases of mourning are interrupted or if needed support is not available. Talking and listening are most important for acute grief. The helping person should keep his or her own talking to a minimum. Banal advice and philosophical statements are useless. Unhelpful responses by others, such as "He's no longer suffering" or "You can always have another child" or "It's better this way," can lead the bereaved to believe that others do not understand the acute pain being suffered and that the personal impact of the loss is being minimized. Such statements can compound feelings of isolation.

More helpful responses are "His death will be a terrible loss" or "No one can replace her" or "He will be

TABLE 20–2 NURSING INTERVENTIONS FOR GRIEVING FAMILIES

INTERVENTION	RATIONALE
Nursing Diagnosis: Family grieving related to loss of family member or significant other	
1. At the death or imminent death of a family member:	
▶ Communicate the news to the family in an area of privacy.	▶ Family members can support each other in an atmosphere in which they can behave naturally.
▶ If only one family member is available, stay with that member until clergy, a family member, or a friend arrives.	▶ The presence and comfort of the nurse during the initial stage of shock can help minimize feelings of acute isolation and anxiety.
▶ If the nurse feels unable to handle the situation, the aid of another who can support the family should be enlisted.	▶ The individual or family needs support, answers to questions, and guidance as to immediate tasks and information.
2. If the family requests to see and take leave of the dying or dead person:	
▶ Always grant this request.	▶ The need to take leave can be of overwhelming importance for some—to kiss good-bye, ask for forgiveness, or take a lock of hair. This helps people face the reality of death.
3. If angry family members accuse the nurse or doctor of abusing or mismanaging the care of the deceased:	
▶ Continue to provide the best care for the dying or final care to the dead. Avoid becoming involved in angry and painful arguments and power struggles.	▶ Complaints are not directed toward the nurse personally. The anger may serve the purpose of keeping grieving relatives from falling apart. Projected anger may be an attempt to deal with aggression and guilt toward the dying person.
4. If relatives behave in a grossly disturbed manner (e.g., refuse to acknowledge the truth, collapse, or lose control):	
▶ Show patience and tact, and offer sympathy and warmth.	▶ Shock and disbelief are the first responses to the news of death, and people need ways to protect themselves from the overwhelming reality of loss.
▶ Encourage the person to cry.	▶ Crying helps provide relief from feelings of acute pain and tension.
▶ Provide a place of privacy for grieving.	▶ Privacy facilitates the natural expression of grief.
5. If the family requests specific religious, cultural, or social customs that are strange or unknown to the nurse:	
▶ Help facilitate steps necessary for the family to carry out the desired arrangements.	▶ Institutional mourning rituals of various cultures provide important external supports for the grief-stricken person.

Data from Engel, G. L. (1964). Grief and grieving. *American Journal of Nursing*, 64(9):93.

missed for a long time." Statements such as these validate the bereaved's experience of loss and communicate the message that the bereaved is understood and supported.

Talking by the bereaved person can release negative emotions. When a person is faced with an unwanted loss, strong feelings of anger, guilt, and hate are normal reactions that need to be expressed in order to facilitate the process of mourning. It is important that someone listen and encourage the expression of feelings surrounding the person's loss or anticipated loss.

Six to ten sessions of psychotherapy have been found to be helpful during the crisis period. At a later stage, the use of 15 sessions or more has been found to have a good outcome. More complicated or pathological patterns of grief may require special techniques, such as "regrief work" (Middleton and Raphael 1992). One study demonstrated that highly religious clients with grief and bereavement issues tended to improve faster when religious psychotherapy was added to a cognitive-behavioral approach (Azhar and Varma 1995).

Nurses frequently encounter people faced with loss. For example, on maternity and pediatric units, parents may be anticipating the loss of a terminally ill child **(anticipatory grief)** or experiencing the loss of a stillborn baby. In these cases, the focus of intervention is on facilitating the family's mourning. Specific guidelines that the nurse can use in the general hospital setting with families of dying or deceased clients are described in Table 20–2.

RESOLUTION OF GRIEF

The work of mourning is over when the bereaved can remember realistically both the pleasures and the disappointments of the lost loved one. If, after a normal period of time (12 to 24 months), a person has not completed the grieving process, reassessment and re-evaluation are indicated. Some of the factors that can affect the successful completion of the mourning process are

1. *The level of dependency in the relationship.* The more dependent the mourner was on the deceased, the more difficult is the resolution of the loss.
2. *The degree of ambivalence in the relationship.* Persistent, unresolved conflicts interfere with successful grief work.
3. *The age of the deceased.* The death of a child may have a more profound effect than the death of an older person.
4. *The bereaved person's support system.* A person with few meaningful relationships would have more difficulty letting go of ties with the deceased.
5. *The number of previous losses.* Present losses can trigger the pain of past losses. Unresolved feelings from past losses can complicate the present grief process.
6. *The physical and psychological health of the person grieving.* Physical well-being and good coping skills can greatly affect a person's capacity for grief work.

SUMMARY

The process of mourning is a distinct psychological process and is the normal reaction to a loss. A loss can be real or perceived. Types of losses include loss of a person, loss of security, loss of self-confidence, and loss of a dream. Essentially, the loss results in loss of self-concept.

The stage of acute grief may last from 4 to 8 weeks; the complete process of mourning *(long-term stage)* may take a year or two, or longer (see Table 20–1).

Culture greatly affects patterns of response to death and dying in both clients and nurses. Grief can reactivate distressing feelings of previous losses in health care workers. If a nurse has unresolved issues of grief and depression, the nurse's ability to help others is greatly minimized. Staff members need psychological support when they work with people who are grieving. Two specific atypical grief reactions are prolonged grief and delayed grief.

Grief work is successful when specific phenomena identified with the process have been experienced. A person in mourning should be given time to talk and relive memories in the presence of a caring person who can share the pain. Guidelines for nursing interventions in a family that is grieving are outlined in Table 20–2.

The work of mourning is complete when the bereaved can remember realistically both the pleasures and the disappointments of the lost relationship. A number of factors can affect the normal process of mourning.

Self-study exercises 1 to 21 at the end of this chapter help the reader review material outlines in this section.

DEPRESSIVE DISORDERS

OBJECTIVES

After studying this section on depressive disorders, the reader will be able to

1. Compare and contrast major depression and dysthymia.
2. Explain four theories of the cause of depression.
3. Identify possible behaviors for each of the following areas in the assessment of a depressed client: (a) affect, (b) thought processes, (c) feelings, (d) physical behavior, (e) communication, and (f) indications of masked depression.
4. Formulate five nursing diagnoses for a client who is depressed, and include outcome criteria.
5. Name three unrealistic expectations that a nurse may have while working with a depressed person that can result in increased feelings of anxiety in the nurse.
6. Role play at least six principles of communication that are appropriate for a depressed client.
7. Plan three interventions with rationales targeting the self-care needs of depressed clients in each of the following categories: nutrition, elimination, rest and sleep, hygiene, and activities and recreation.
8. Develop a medication teaching plan for clients on the tricyclic antidepressants, including (a) common side effects, (b) adverse side effects, and (c) drugs that can trigger an adverse reaction.
9. Evaluate the advantages of using the selective serotonin reuptake inhibitors rather than the tricyclic antidepressants.
10. Discuss two common side effects of the monoamine oxidase inhibitors, and state one serious adverse reaction and the appropriate medical intervention.
11. Identify five foods and four drugs that are contraindicated with the use of the monoamine oxidase inhibitors.
12. Describe the procedure used in electroconvulsive therapy, and state two important nursing actions to be implemented before, during, and after treatment.

Mood refers to a prolonged emotion that colors a person's whole psychic life (APA 1994). *Joy, grief, elation,* and *sadness* are all terms used to describe a particular mood.

Normal moods are universal experiences. Happiness and unhappiness are appropriate responses to life events. When sadness, grief, or elation is extremely intense and the mood unduly prolonged, a mood disorder results.

A depressed mood is the most common presenting problem encountered by mental health professionals. Indeed, about 10% of all people seeking medical advice from their family doctor have mild to moderate degrees of depression. Unfortunately, doctors often fail to recognize these conditions (Bech 1992). *Depression* is a term that can be used in many ways; it can refer to a symptom, a syndrome, a disorder, or an illness (Zisook and Shuchter 1992).

A depressive illness is painful and can be debilitating. Many well-known and highly creative people have had severe depressions (e.g., Sigmund Freud, Winston Churchill, Ernest Hemingway, Marilyn Monroe, Sylvia Plath, Albert Camus, and William James). The author William Styron, in his book *Darkness visible: A memoir of madness* (1990), described his depression as a "howling tempest in the brain." He wrote further:

> Rational thought was usually absent from my mind at those times, . . . this state of being, a condition of helpless stupor in which cognition was replaced by that "positive and active anguish". . . . The libido made an early exit. . . . Many people lose all appetite. . . . My few hours of sleep were usually terminated at 3 or 4 in the morning, when I stared up into yawning darkness, wondering and writhing at the devastation taking place in my mind.

Most people experience a normal lowering of mood in response to various stressful life events. However, about 15% of people in the general population experience a depressive episode during their lifetime. About one in 20 people have a major depressive disorder each year (U. S. Department of Health 1993). Women have a greater risk of developing depression than do men; the lifetime prevalence of major depression for women is 10% to 25% and for men is 5% to 12%, according to several studies (Wyeth-Ayerst Laboratories 1995). A depressive episode usually warrants treatment. However, only one of four people actually receives treatment for depression

(Abraham et al. 1991). Figure 20–1 identifies depression on a continuum from the clinical depression often experienced in a normal grief reaction to an actual mood disorder, dysthymia, or major depression.

When moods become severe or prolonged or when they affect a person's occupational or interpersonal functioning, the alteration in mood may constitute a mood disorder. The mood disorders in DSM-IV include depressive disorders and bipolar disorders. This chapter discusses the depressive disorders; Chapter 21 discusses the bipolar disorders.

A depressive illness may be precipitated by various factors. For example, some environmental events are more likely than others to trigger the onset of depression. Death in the family is the most common precipitator of depression. The anniversary of the death of a loved one can precipitate depression. The second most common precipitators are separation and divorce. The third is physical illness, followed by sexual identity threat, work failures, and disappointment in a child (Goodwin 1982). Other depressions that are predominantly biologically based may not be precipitated by environmental events. Many people state that they have no reason to be depressed, and they cannot identify any problems or environmental stressors in their lives.

Depression and fatigue can be important indications of various medical disorders, such as hepatitis, mononucleosis, multiple sclerosis, and cancer. Ten percent or more of major depressive conditions are caused by general medical illness or other conditions (U. S. Department of Health and Human Services 1993). DSM-IV refers to this disorder as *mood disorder due to general medical conditions.*

A depressive syndrome frequently accompanies other psychiatric disorders, such as schizophrenia, substance dependence disorder, and eating disorders. A depressive syndrome can occur as part of a physical illness, another psychiatric disorder, or a cognitive impairment disorder. A depressive disorder can co-exist with other psychiatric

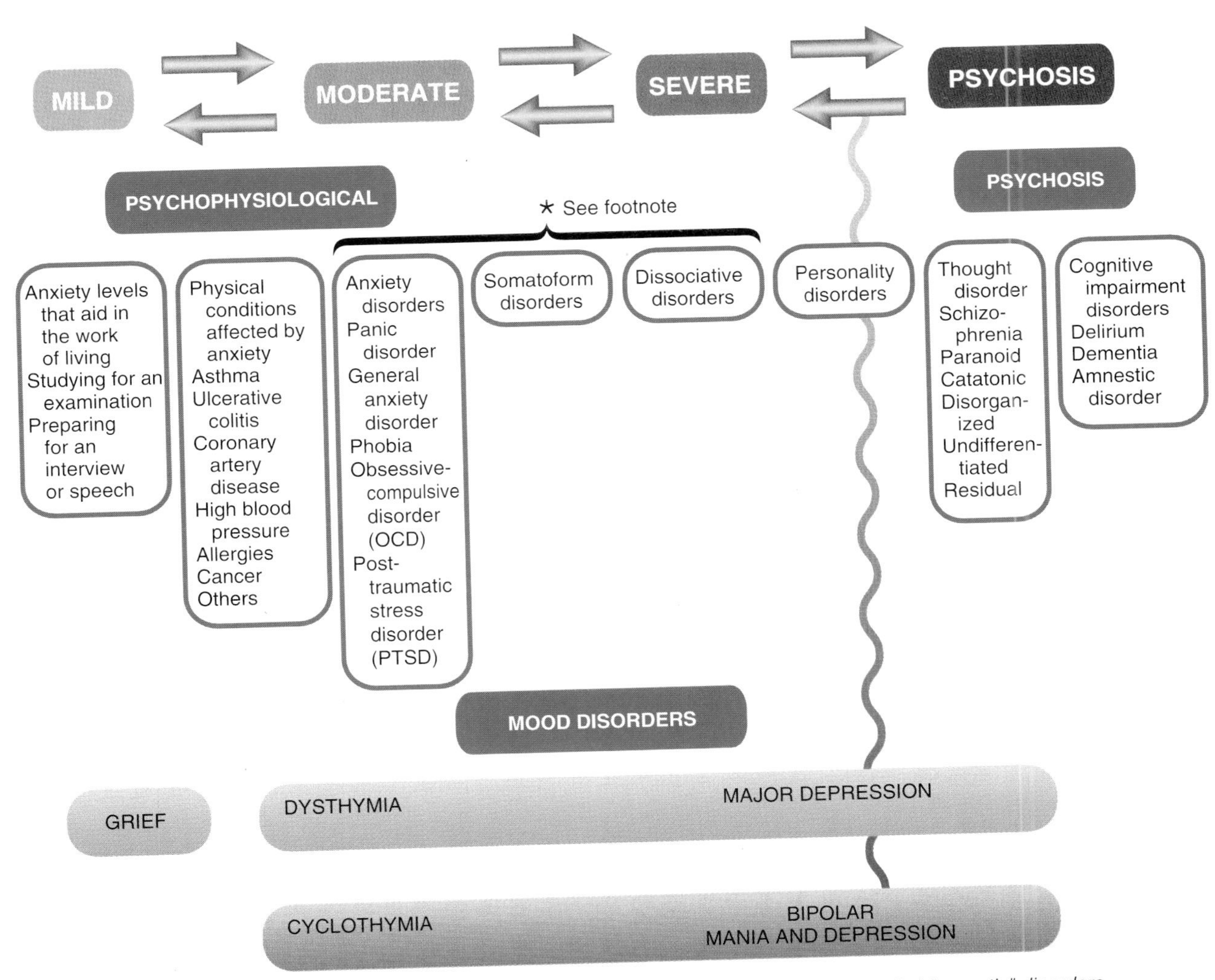

Figure 20–1 The mental health continuum for anxiety disorders.

disorders (e.g., anxiety disorder) or can be caused by use of drugs or by intoxication or withdrawal of other substances. This disorder is referred to as *substance-induced mood disorder* (APA 1994). Depression and anxiety disorders seem to coexist frequently (Zajecka 1995a):

- 33% to 85% of people with depression have anxiety disorder.
- 21% to 91% of clients with anxiety disorder have a minor depression.

When a depressive disorder coexists with an anxiety disorder, complications occur (Zajecka 1995a):

- Increased risk for suicide
- Increased social and vocational impairment
- Poorer prognosis and treatment response
- Increased chronic illness

PRIMARY DEPRESSIVE DISORDERS

The two most common primary depressive disorders are (1) major depressive disorder and (2) dysthymia disorder.

Major Depressive Disorder

Clients with major depression experience substantial pain and suffering, as well as psychological, social, and occupational disability during the depression. A client with **major depression** has a history of one or more major depressive episodes and no history of manic or hypomanic episodes. In a major depression, the symptoms often interfere with the person's social or occupational functioning and in some cases may include psychotic features. Delusional or psychotic major depression is a severe form of mood disorder that is characterized by delusions or hallucinations. For example, clients might have delusional thoughts that interfere with their nutritional status (e.g., "God put snakes in my stomach and told me not to eat").

The emotional, cognitive, physical, and behavioral symptoms an individual exhibits during a major depressive episode represent a change in the person's usual functioning. When the symptoms of a major depressive episode have subsided, most people experience complete remission and return to their premorbid functioning (APA 1994).

Dysthymia

Dysthymia (depressive neurosis) is mild to moderate in degree and is characterized by a chronic depressive syndrome that is usually present for most of the day, more days than not, for at least 2 years (APA 1994). The depressive mood disturbance, because of its chronic nature, cannot be distinguished from the person's usual pattern of functioning (APA 1994). Because the individual has minimal social and occupational impairment, hospitalization is rarely necessary unless the person becomes suicidal. The age of onset varies from the early to middle teens to late in life. Clients with dysthymia are at risk for developing major depressive episodes as well as other psychiatric disorders. Figure 20–2 shows the diagnostic criteria for both depressive disorders.

Differentiating a major depression from dysthymia can be difficult because the disorders have similar symptoms. The main differences are in the duration and the severity of the symptoms (APA 1994).

Related Phenomena

The diagnosis of major depressions may include a specifier in clients with specific symptoms. Specifiers include

- Psychotic features.
- Catatonic features.
- Melancholic features.
- Postpartum onset.
- Seasonal affective patterns (generally related to fall or winter and remitting in the spring).

This chapter deals with the phenomena of depression; however, specific treatments are geared toward adults. For issues regarding depression in the child and adolescent, see Chapter 29. For issues and treatments for depression addressed to the elderly population, refer to Chapter 31.

THEORY

Although many theories attempt to explain the cause of depression, many psychological, biological, and cultural variables make identification of any one cause difficult. Four common theories of depression are discussed here: (1) biological, (2) cognitive, (3) psychoanalytic, and (4) learned helplessness.

Biological Theories

Genetic Theories

Twin studies consistently show that genetic factors play a role in the development of depressive disorders (Nurnberger and Gershon 1992). Various studies reveal that the average concordance rate for mood disorders among monozygotic twins (twins sharing the same genetic structure) is 60%. The percentage for dizygotic twins (separate genetic structure) is 12%. Thus, identical twins (monozygotic) have a fivefold greater concordance rate than dizygotic twins (Merikangas and Kupfer 1995).

Biochemical Factors

It is currently believed that depression is a biologically heterogeneous disorder; that is, many central nervous

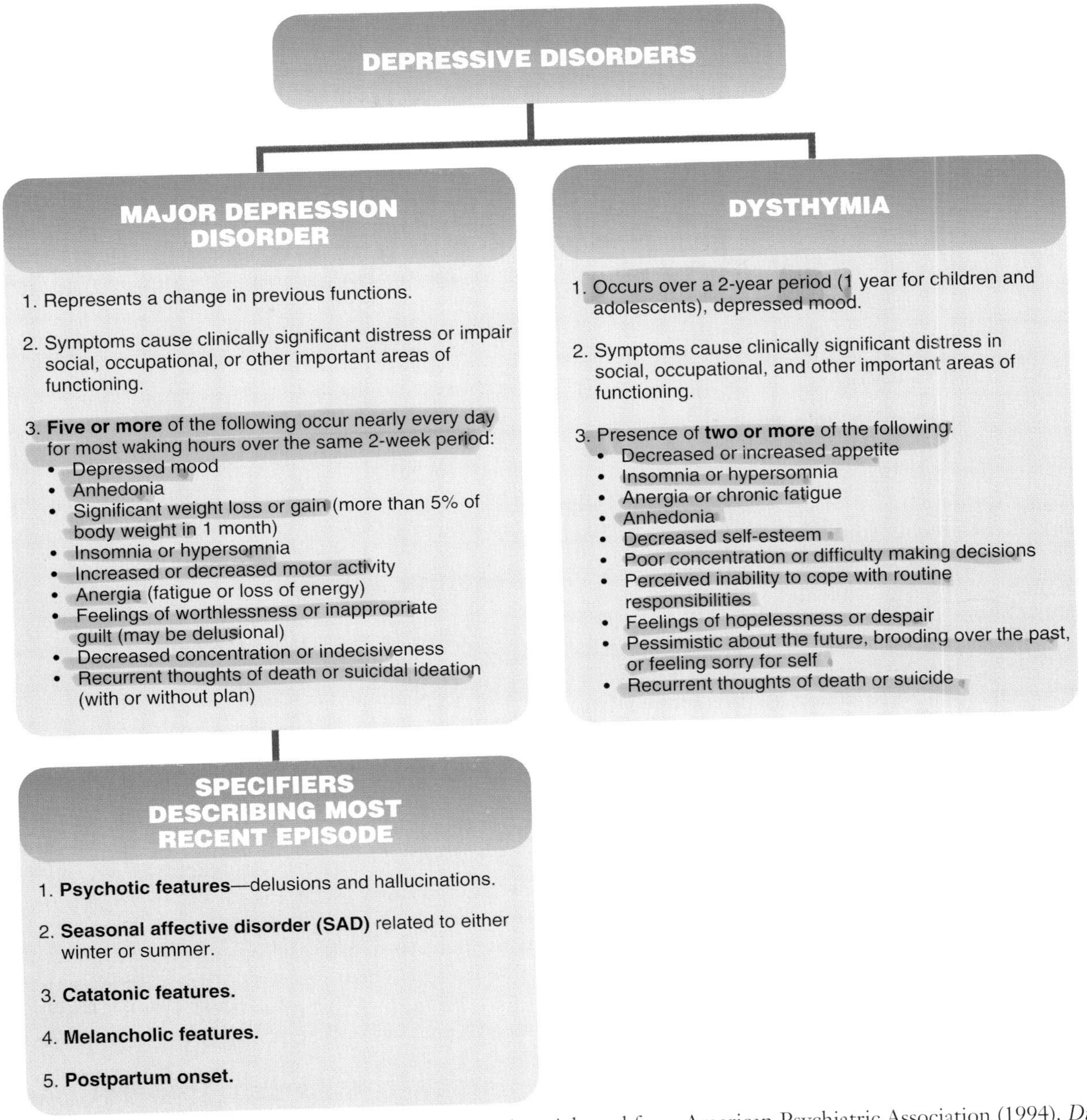

DEPRESSIVE DISORDERS

MAJOR DEPRESSION DISORDER

1. Represents a change in previous functions.
2. Symptoms cause clinically significant distress or impair social, occupational, or other important areas of functioning.
3. **Five or more** of the following occur nearly every day for most waking hours over the same 2-week period:
   - Depressed mood
   - Anhedonia
   - Significant weight loss or gain (more than 5% of body weight in 1 month)
   - Insomnia or hypersomnia
   - Increased or decreased motor activity
   - Anergia (fatigue or loss of energy)
   - Feelings of worthlessness or inappropriate guilt (may be delusional)
   - Decreased concentration or indecisiveness
   - Recurrent thoughts of death or suicidal ideation (with or without plan)

DYSTHYMIA

1. Occurs over a 2-year period (1 year for children and adolescents), depressed mood.
2. Symptoms cause clinically significant distress in social, occupational, and other important areas of functioning.
3. Presence of **two or more** of the following:
   - Decreased or increased appetite
   - Insomnia or hypersomnia
   - Anergia or chronic fatigue
   - Anhedonia
   - Decreased self-esteem
   - Poor concentration or difficulty making decisions
   - Perceived inability to cope with routine responsibilities
   - Feelings of hopelessness or despair
   - Pessimistic about the future, brooding over the past, or feeling sorry for self
   - Recurrent thoughts of death or suicide

SPECIFIERS DESCRIBING MOST RECENT EPISODE

1. **Psychotic features**—delusions and hallucinations.
2. **Seasonal affective disorder (SAD)** related to either winter or summer.
3. **Catatonic features.**
4. **Melancholic features.**
5. **Postpartum onset.**

Figure 20–2 DSM-IV diagnostic criteria for depression. Adapted from American Psychiatric Association (1994). *Diagnostic and statistical manual of mental disorders (DSM-IV)*. Washington, DC: American Psychiatric Association. Reprinted with permission. Copyright 1994 American Psychiatric Association.

system (CNS) neurotransmitter abnormalities that can probably cause clinical depression. These neurotransmitter abnormalities may be the result of inherited or environmental factors, or even other medical conditions, such as cerebral infarction, hypothyroidism, acquired immunodeficiency syndrome, and drug use (Delgado et al. 1992). Therefore, specific neurotransmitters in the brain are believed to be related to altered mood states. The two main neurotransmitters are *serotonin* and *norepinephrine*, both of which are catecholamines.

For many years, the belief was that low levels of serotonin and norepinephrine at the synaptic receptor sites in the brain cause depression and that high levels trigger mania. The use of antidepressant drugs supported this biological theory because all antidepressant drugs inhibit the reuptake of serotonin and norepinephrine, increasing the amount of time these neurotransmitters are available to the postsynaptic receptors in the CNS (see Boxes 3–6 to 3–8 in Chapter 3). However, it is now considered unlikely that a catecholamine deficiency alone is the actual cause of depression (Delgado et al. 1992).

Present research is investigating the complex interactions of norepinephrine, serotonin, and acetylcholine, and changes in receptor numbers and sensitivity are being examined (Calarcro and Krone 1991). Norepinephrine, serotonin, and acetylcholine also play a role in stress regulation. When these neurotransmitters become overtaxed through stressful events, neurotransmitter depletion may occur. This connection to stress regulation and alteration of mood continues to be evaluated.

At this stage, no unitary mechanism of antidepressant action has been found. The relationships between the serotonin, norepinephrine, dopamine, and acetylcholine systems are complex and need further assessment and research (Delgado et al. 1992). However, treatment with medication has proved empirically successful for many clients. Figure 20–3 shows a positron-emission tomographic scan of the brain of a woman before and after taking medication. Refer to Chapter 3 (Fig. 3–9) for comparison of a PET scan of an individual when depressed and nondepressed.

Neuroendocrine Findings

Although neuroendocrine findings are as yet inconclusive, the neuroendocrine symptom most widely studied in relation to depression has been hyperactivity of the limbic-hypothalamic-pituitary-adrenal axis. Approximately half of depressed individuals studied demonstrate a hypersecretion of cortisol (Green et al 1995). Dexamethasone, an exogenous steroid that suppresses cortisol, is used in the dexamethasone suppression test for depression. Results of the dexamethasone suppression test are abnormal in about 50% of depressed clients, indicating hyperactivity of the limbic-hypothalamic-pituitary-adrenal axis. However, the findings of this test may also be abnormal in people with obsessive-compulsive disorders and other medical conditions. Significantly, clients with psychotic major depression are among those with the highest rates of nonsuppression of cortisol on the dexamethasone suppression test (Schatzberg and Rothschild 1992).

Sleep Abnormalities

Studies show that sleep holds promise as a biological marker for depression. The rapid eye movement (REM) phase of sleep associated with dreaming occurs earlier in two thirds of clients with bipolar and major depressive illnesses. This sign is referred to as *REM latency*, as Cartwright et al. (1991) reported in a study of people who met the DSM criteria for major depression. Although subjects with REM latency still had the sign a year later, when they were no longer depressed, they had both higher rates of recovery from depression and better life adjustment than did the depressed clients who did not have REM latency. Data also suggest that depressed clients without this sign are not likely to respond to tricyclic antidepressant (TCA) therapy, which suppresses early REM sleep. A study by Lauer and associates (1995) demonstrated that about 20% of nondepressed individuals who had at least one first-degree relative with a mood disorder had "depression-like" sleep patterns. Further follow-up studies may determine if specific sleep abnormalities do, indeed, represent a biological marker for vulnerability to depression.

Cognitive Theory

Albert Ellis, a well-known cognitive behavior therapist, views emotional disturbance as the product of irrational or illogical thinking. Ellis's rational emotive behavioral therapy has had success with people who are shy, are nonassertive in social situations, are experiencing marital problems, or have fears surrounding sexual situations, as well as a great deal of other problematic behaviors. Expanding on Ellis's work, Aaron T. Beck applied the cognitive behavior theory to depression. Beck proposed that people acquire a psychological predisposition to depression through early life experiences. These experiences contribute to negative, illogical, and irrational thought processes that may remain dormant until they are activated during times of stress (Beck and Rush 1995). Beck found that depressed persons process information in neg-

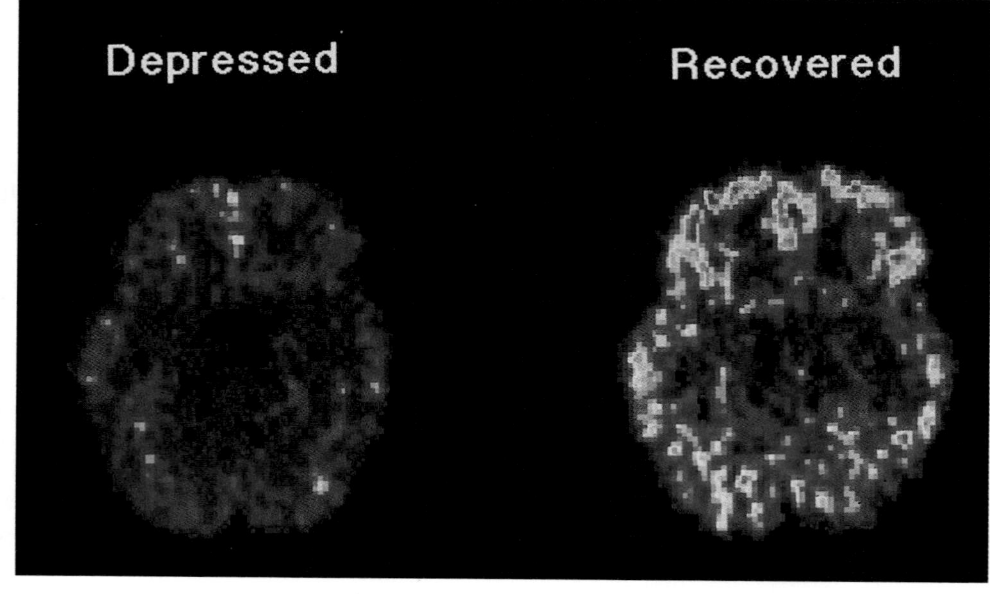

Figure 20–3 Positron-emission tomography (PET) scans of a 45-year-old woman with recurrent depression. The scan on the left was taken when she was on no medication and very depressed. The scan on the right was taken several months later when she was well, after medication had treated her depression. Note that her entire brain is more active when well, particularly the left prefrontal cortex. (From Mark George, MD, Biological Psychiatry Branch, National Institutes of Mental Health.)

ative ways, even in the midst of positive factors that affect the person's life. Beck believes three automatic negative thoughts are responsible for people's becoming depressed. These three thoughts are called *Beck's cognitive triad.* They are

1. A negative, self-deprecating view of self.
2. A pessimistic view of the world.
3. The belief that negative reinforcement (or no validation for the self) will continue in the future.

Automatic negative thoughts refer to thoughts that are repetitive, unintended, and not readily controllable (Haaga and Beck 1992). This cognitive triad seems to be consistent in all depressions, regardless of clinical subtype.

The goal of cognitive behavior therapy is to change the way clients think and thus relieve the depressive syndrome. This is accomplished by assisting the client in the following:

1. Identifying and testing negative cognition
2. Developing alternative thinking patterns
3. Rehearsing new cognitive and behavioral responses

Cognitive therapy has been remarkably successful with acutely depressed individuals and is associated with a significantly lower rate of relapse (Hallon and Fawcett 1995).

Psychoanalytic Theory

Freud believed that after the loss of a significant person for whom the individual harbored extreme ambivalence, hostility toward this person is directed toward the self through the process of introjection. Therefore, two themes central to the psychoanalytic theory of depression are *loss* and *aggression.* According to psychoanalytic theory, depression is triggered by a loss, and the depressive mood is the result of aggression turned inward toward the self.

Loss

Freud, in his classic, *Mourning and melancholia* (1917), identified both grief and depression as reactions to a real or a symbolic loss. When people lose a crucial source of security, they may become depressed. A sense of helplessness and hopelessness is central to the experience of depression.

When an infant between the ages of 6 and 36 months experiences the physical or emotional loss of the mothering figure, the biological response is a depressive affect. The loss of the mother's love can be a physical loss (e.g., death or divorce) or an emotional loss (e.g., withdrawal of affection because of depression, alcohol, or narcissism). The loss of the mother disrupts the normal development of the child. This early loss leaves the child extremely vulnerable to losses later in life. The young child interprets the withdrawal of affection (loss) as rejection of self and feels unworthy of love and approval. Earlier studies supported the relationship between the early loss of a parent (death or divorce) and the increased incidence and severity of depressive illness in an individual's later life (Ripley 1977; Bowlby 1961). However, an analysis of studies of adult depression as resulting from childhood parental loss found little evidence to support a link between parental death and depression (Parker 1992).

Aggression

Psychoanalytic theory states that depression is the result of anger turned inward against the self. However, in the past 15 years, the focus of studies of mood disorders has shifted from psychoanalytic aspects to inherited biological aspects of these disorders (Mendelson 1992).

Learned Helplessness

One of the most popular theories of the cause of depression is Martin Seligman's theory of learned helplessness. Seligman (1973) stated that although anxiety is the initial response to a stressful situation, anxiety is replaced by depression if the person feels that the self has no control over the outcome of a situation. A person who believes that an undesired event is his or her fault and that nothing can be done to change it is prone to depression. The theory of learned helplessness has been used to help explain the development of depression in certain social groups, such as the aged, people living in ghettos, and women.

A study by Gulesserian and Warren (1987) found data supporting the theory that "depression is linked with poor adaptational/coping abilities that may lead to learned helplessness, panic and depression." The lack of the following specific coping skills appeared to increase the likelihood of depression: social supports, tension reduction skills, and effective problem-solving skills. The behavioral therapeutic approach includes teaching depressed individuals new and more effective coping skills and ways to increase their self-confidence.

ASSESSMENT

A depressed mood and **anhedonia** (an inability to find meaning or pleasure in existence) are the key symptoms in depression. Almost 97% of people with depression have **anergia** (reduction in or lack of energy). *Anxiety,* a common symptom in depression, is seen in about 60% of clients (Zajecka 1995a).

When people are depressed, their thinking is slow, and their memory and concentration are usually affected. Depressed people dwell on and exaggerate their perceived faults and failures and are unable to focus on their strengths and successes. A person with major depression may experience delusions of being punished for "doing bad deeds" or "being a terrible person." Feelings of worthlessness, guilt, anger, and helplessness are common. **Psychomotor agitation** may be evidenced by constant pacing and wringing of hands. The slowed movements of **psychomotor retardation,** however, are more common. Somatic complaints (headaches, malaise, backaches) are also common. **Vegetative signs of depression** (change in bowel movements and eating habits, sleep disturbances, and disinterest in sex) are usually present. Dryman and Eaton (1991) reported on a study examining the relationship of depressive symptoms and the subsequent onset of a major depression. Significant symptoms included diminished sexual drive, feelings of worthlessness or excessive guilt, and trouble concentrating or thinking. Sleeping disturbances in women and fatigue in men were also significant symptoms.

Although individual variations in depression occur, commonalties are revealed through the assessment of affect, thought processes, feelings, physical behavior, and communication. Sometimes, the symptoms of depression are not so obvious and are masked by other kinds of complaints, as is discussed later. Therefore, assessing symptoms that mask depression is useful in all hospital settings.

Affect

A person who is depressed sees the world through "gray-colored" glasses. Posture is poor, and clients may look older than their stated age. Facial expressions convey sadness and dejection, and the client may have frequent bouts of weeping. Conversely, the client may say that he or she is unable to cry. Feelings of hopelessness and despair are readily reflected in the person's affect.

Thought Processes

Identifying the presence of suicidal thoughts and suicide potential has the highest priority in the initial assessment. Approximately two thirds of depressed people contemplate suicide, and up to 15% of untreated or inadequately treated clients give up hope and kill themselves (Akiskal 1995). Asking a depressed person openly "Have you thought about killing yourself?" can encourage the expression of painful, pent-up feelings (see Chapter 24). The risk of suicide is not necessarily correlated with the severity of the symptoms. Although depressed persons can attempt suicide at any time, the highest mortality exists within a year of discharge from a psychiatric hospital (Litman 1992), with the suicide rate decreasing but notable thereafter.

During the time a person is depressed, the person's ability to solve problems and think clearly is negatively affected. Judgment is poor, and indecisiveness is common. People claim that their mind is slowing down. Memory and concentration are poor. Evidence of delusional thinking may be seen in a major depression. Common statements of delusional thinking are "I have committed unpardonable sins" or "God wants me dead" or "I am wicked and should die."

Feelings

Feelings frequently reported by depressed people include anxiety, worthlessness, guilt, helplessness and hopelessness, and anger. As previously mentioned, *anxiety* is present in about 60% of depressed persons. Feelings of *worthlessness* range from feeling inadequate to having an unrealistic evaluation of self-worth. These feelings reflect the low self-esteem that is a painful partner to depression. Statements such as "I am no good; I'll never amount to anything" are common. Themes of one's inadequacy and incompetence are repeated relentlessly.

Guilt is a common accompaniment to depression. A person may ruminate over present or past failings. Extreme guilt can assume psychotic proportions: "I have committed terrible sins. God is punishing me for my evil ways."

Helplessness is evidenced by the inability to carry out the simplest tasks. Everything is too difficult to accomplish (e.g., grooming, doing housework, working, caring for children). With feelings of helplessness come feelings of *hopelessness.* Even though most depressive states are usually time limited, during a depressed period, people believe that things will never change. This feeling of utter hopelessness can lead people to look at suicide as a way out of constant mental pain. An analysis of the concept of hopelessness by Campbell (1987) cited findings in the literature that identified hopelessness as one of the core characteristics of depression and suicide, as well as a characteristic of schizophrenia, alcoholism, and physical illness. Campbell identified the common cognitive and emotional components of hopelessness as having the following attributes:

- Negative expectations for the future
- Loss of control over future outcomes
- Passive acceptance of the futility of planning to achieve goals
- Emotional negativism, as expressed in despair, despondency, or depression

Anger and irritability are natural outcomes of profound feelings of helplessness. Anger in depression is often expressed inappropriately. For example, anger may be expressed in destruction of property, hurtful verbal attacks, or physical aggression toward others. However, in people who are depressed, anger may be directed toward the self, resulting in feelings of low self-esteem and worthlessness. An extreme example of turning aggression against the self is suicide. The psychoanalytic view is that the impulse to commit suicide is related to an impulse to murder someone else. The biological view links low levels of serotonin with an increase in suicidal behavior.

Physical Behavior

Lethargy and fatigue can result in psychomotor retardation. Movements are extremely slow, facial expressions are decreased, and gaze is fixed. The continuum in psychomotor retardation may range from slowed and difficult movements to complete inactivity and incontinence. At other times, the nurse may note psychomotor agitation. For example, clients may constantly pace, bite their nails, smoke, tap their fingers, or engage in some other tension-relieving activity. At these times, clients commonly feel "fidgety" and unable to relax.

Grooming, dress, and personal hygiene are markedly neglected. People who usually take pride in their appearance and dress may be poorly groomed, allowing themselves to look shabby and unkempt.

Vegetative signs of depression are universal. Vegetative signs refer to alterations in those activities necessary to support physical life and growth (eating, sleeping, elimination, sex). For example, *changes in eating patterns* are common. About 60% to 70% of people who are depressed report having anorexia; overeating occurs more often in dysthymia. *Changes in sleep patterns* vary. Often, people have insomnia, waking at 3 or 4 AM and staying awake, or sleeping only for short periods. For some, sleep is increased **(hypersomnia)** and provides an escape from painful feelings. In any event, sleep is rarely restful or refreshing. *Changes in bowel habits* are common. Constipation is seen most frequently in clients with psychomotor retardation. Diarrhea occurs less frequently, often in conjunction with psychomotor agitation. *Interest in sex declines* (loss of libido) during depression. Some men experience impotence, which can further complicate marital and social relationships.

Communication

A person who is depressed may speak very slowly. Their comprehension is slow. The lack of an immediate response by the client to a remark does not mean that the client has not heard or chooses not to reply: the client just needs a little more time to compose a reply. In extreme depression, however, a person may be mute.

Indications of Masked Depression

Masked depressions are depressions that are not recognized in the familiar form. The manner in which depression is masked depends on the depressed person's cultural background, age and sex, socioeconomic background, and heredity.

In children, truancy, school phobias, underachievement, hyperactivity, learning disorders, and antisocial behaviors may be the dominant characteristics of underlying depression.

In adolescents, underachievement, dropping out of school, compulsive use of drugs and sex, delinquent behavior, and hostile outbursts may indicate masked depression.

Adults in the United States may mask depression behind hypochondriasis and psychosomatic disorders, as well as compulsive gambling and work habits. Other behaviors associated with underlying depression include accident proneness, anorexia, bulimia, and substance-dependence disorders.

The symptoms of depression are experienced by people on a continuum from mild to severe. Table 20–3 organizes the symptoms of depression on a continuum.

NURSING DIAGNOSIS

During the initial assessment, a high priority for the nurse is identification of the presence of suicide potential. Therefore, the nursing diagnosis of **risk for self-directed violence** should always be considered. The diagnosis of risk for self-directed violence may be related to a pathophysiological condition (e.g., terminal illness), a medical treatment (e.g., dialysis), a situation (e.g., divorce and child abuse), or a maturational issue (e.g., social isolation in the elderly). Suicide rates are high in adolescents, elderly persons, and other specific populations. The risk for self-directed violence needs to be explored when data support this possibility (see Chapter 24 for significant risk factors).

Because concentration, judgment, and memory are usually poor and psychotic behavior may be evidenced, **altered thought processes** are often present. Feelings of worthlessness, guilt, helplessness, anger, and hopelessness all increase feelings of low self-esteem. Therefore, **self-esteem disturbance, chronic low self-esteem,** or **powerlessness** are often present. Feelings of hopelessness and despair may be interpreted as **spiritual distress,** which may be the most appropriate diagnosis.

Many people experiencing a major depressive episode are withdrawn and demonstrate psychomotor retardation, so the focus of care may be **impaired social interaction** or **activity intolerance.**

Most depressed clients exhibit some of the vegetative signs of depression. For example, the nurse may identify **altered nutrition, constipation, diarrhea,** or **sleep pattern disturbance.**

Disturbance in the ability to function in usual occupational and interpersonal roles suggests **ineffective individual coping. Altered family processes** often surface. The nurse is frequently in a key position to alert other members of the health care team to support the family and to mobilize additional financial and psychological supports.

TABLE 20–3 DEPRESSION ON A CONTINUUM

MILD TO MODERATE	SEVERE
Communication	
Slow speech, long pauses before answering; monotone.	Slow in extreme; may be mute and not talk at all
Affect	
Crying and weeping, slumping in chair, drooping shoulders, look of gloom and pessimism Anxiety may or may not be manifested. **Anhedonia**—inability to experience pleasure	May appear without affect; may be experiencing "nothingness"; can sit for hours staring into space **Anhedonia**
Thinking	
No impairment in reality testing. Thinking is slow, concentration and memory are poor, interest narrows; perspective in situations is lost, e.g. ▸ "Every one always lets me down." ▸ "No one cares." Thoughts reflect doubts and indecisions. Thinking is often repetitive in negative cycle: ▸ "Why was I born? What's life all about?" Mild feelings of guilt and worthlessness. **May have suicidal ideation.**	Grasp of reality may be tenuous. Thoughts may indicate delusional thinking, reflecting feelings of ▸ Low self-esteem. ▸ Worthlessness. ▸ Helplessness. ▸ "I'm no good." ▸ "God is punishing me for my terrible sins." ▸ "My insides are rotting." ▸ "My heart has stopped beating." Concentration is extremely poor. Preoccupation with bodily symptoms. **May have suicidal ideation.**
Physical Behavior	
Fatigue and lethargy are hallmark symptoms. They do not prevent the person from working, although the person often works below potential. Initiative and creativity are impaired. Grooming and hygiene are usually neglected.	Severe and extreme chronic fatigue and lethargy markedly interfere with occupational functioning, social activities, or relationships with others Client may show extreme neglect of personal grooming and hygiene.
Vegetative Signs	
Sleep—middle or late insomnia, hypersomnia; EEG studies show shortened REM latency. Energy is often highest in AM, lowest in PM. Eating—may have anorexia or overeat. Sexual appetitie is diminished. Bowels—constipation if psychomotor retardation is present; may have diarrhea if psychomotor agitation is present. Psychomotor retardation (slow motor movements)—everything is an effort. *or* Psychomotor agitation (agitated depression)—pacing up and down halls, wringing hands.	Sleep—usually insomnia; early morning waking at 3:00 or 4:00 AM often occurs. Energy is often lowest in AM, highest in PM. Eating—usually has anorexia; weight loss of more than 5% in 1 month. Loss of libido. Bowels—usually constipation. Psychomotor retardation (most common). *or* Psychomotor agitation.

EEG, electroencephalographic; REM, rapid eye movement.

PLANNING

Planning Outcome Criteria

Outcome criteria and short-term goals are formulated for each nursing diagnosis. Each client is different, and goals are devised according to each person's individual needs. When possible, the nurse and client discuss desired outcomes of health care interventions. Outcome criteria are identified, and concrete measurable steps are formulated as short-term goals. For the following diagnoses, some outcome criteria and short-term goals are presented. When a person is severely depressed, the planning of goals with the client may start in the hospital setting, especially if the client is suicidal or unable to take care of basic needs. For the most part, however, nurses and therapists plan goals and work with depressed individuals in community-based settings (home care, partial hospital settings, mental health clinics, institutes).

For the nursing diagnosis **risk for self-directed violence,** as evidenced by suicidal ideation, the following outcome criteria and short-term goals may be formulated.

OUTCOME CRITERIA

- Client will remain free of self-directed injury.
- Client will verbalize reasons for living.
- By (date), client will name three places or people he or she can turn to if suicidal thoughts or impulses arise in the future.

SHORT-TERM GOALS

- Client will make a suicide contract.
- By (date), client will discuss feelings (anger, frustration, helplessness, hopelessness)
- By (date), client will explore thoughts, feelings, and circumstances that precede impulses to harm self.
- By (date), client will demonstrate two alternative actions he or she can take when experiencing impulses to harm self.

For the nursing diagnosis **altered thought processes,** the following outcome criteria and short-term goals might be considered.

OUTCOME CRITERIA

- Client will state that memory has improved.
- Client will demonstrate an increased ability to make appropriate decisions.
- Client will accurately interpret events happening in the environment.
- Client will state that he or she was able to participate in an activity that takes moderate concentration (e.g., reading, card games, Scrabble).

SHORT-TERM GOALS

- Client will keep appointments, attend activities, and attend to grooming with the aid of medication and nursing interventions if in the hospital.
- Client will make two decisions about the future with aid of medications and nursing counseling by (date).
- Client will discuss with nurse three irrational thoughts about self and others by (date).
- Client will demonstrate the ability to concentrate on two 5-minute activities (e.g., grooming or recreation) with the aid of medication and nursing interventions by (date).

Goals for a nursing diagnosis of **self-esteem disturbance** should reflect an increase in the client's sense of self-worth.

OUTCOME CRITERIA

- By (date), client will name two or three positive attributes of self.
- Client will demonstrate an increased interest in personal appearance (grooming, hygiene, and dress) by (date).

Goals concerning **powerlessness** might include the following.

OUTCOME CRITERIA

- By (date), client will discuss one new coping skill.
- By (date), client will name three alternative solutions to a particular problem.
- By (date), client will demonstrate ability to cope adaptively with ongoing stressors.

When people feel hopeless and isolated, they are no longer able to find strength or sustenance from previous religious or spiritual beliefs. General goals for people in **spiritual distress** follow.

OUTCOME CRITERIA

- Client will state that he or she once again finds strength and meaning in life through personal spiritual beliefs.
- Client will resume usual spiritual activities by (date).

Clients who are depressed are often withdrawn and unwilling or unable to participate in usual activities. Outcome criteria and short-term goals for **impaired social interaction** or **activity intolerance** may include the following.

OUTCOME CRITERIA

- Client will resume sustaining relationships with friends and family members.
- Client will initiate attendance at one or two group activities a week.

SHORT-TERM GOALS

- By (date), client will discuss three alternative actions to take when feeling the need to withdraw.
- Client will participate in one activity by the end of each day.
- By (date), client will identify two personal behaviors that might discourage others from seeking contact.

Goals for any of the vegetative or physical signs of depression should be formulated such that they show evidence of weight gain, return to normal bowel activity, duration of sleep of 6 to 8 hours per night, or return of sexual desire.

For an individual whose work and interpersonal relationships have been negatively affected during the depressive episode, the ability to use previous adaptive coping skills would be an important outcome criteria. For a family in which altered family processes have occurred, the outcome criteria would be resumption of previously satisfying and desired family coping behaviors.

Nurse's Feelings and Self-Assessment

Depressed clients often reject the overtures of the nurse and others. People when they are depressed do not appear to respond to nursing interventions and appear resistant to change. When this occurs, nurses can experience feelings of frustration, hopelessness, and annoyance. Nurses can alter these problematic responses by

- Recognizing any unrealistic expectations they have of themselves or the client.
- Identifying feelings they are experiencing that originate in the client.
- Understanding the part that neurotransmitters play in the precipitation and maintenance of a depressed mood.

Unrealistic Expectations of Self

Health care workers new to working with depressed individuals may have expectations of themselves and their clients that are not realistic, and problems result when these expectations are not met. Unmet expectations usually result in the client's feeling anxious, hurt, angry, helpless, or incompetent. Unrealistic expectations of oneself and others may be held even by experienced health care workers, and this phenomenon contributes to staff burnout. Many of the nurse's expectations may not be conscious. However, when these expectations are made conscious and worked through with peers and more experienced clinicians (supervisors), more realistic expectations can be formed and attainable goals can be set. Realistic expectations of oneself and the client can decrease feelings of helplessness and can increase the nurse's self-esteem and therapeutic potential.

Unrealistic expectations are common, especially for nursing students and nurses who are new to the psychiatric setting. Common expectations and reactions are outlined in Table 20–4.

Client Feelings Experienced by the Nurse

Intense feelings of anxiety, frustration, annoyance, and helplessness may be experienced by the nurse, although the feelings may originate in the client. These feelings can be important diagnostic clues to the client's experience. Often, the nurse senses what the client is feeling through empathy. Sometimes, the client has pushed these feelings out of awareness, and the feelings are manifested behaviorally in psychosomatic complaints, substance abuse, or destructive behaviors. Helping clients recognize these intense negative unconscious feelings is part of the therapeutic process.

When the nurse's feelings of annoyance, hopelessness, and anxiety are the result of empathetic communications with the client, the nurse can discuss these feelings with peers and supervisors in order to separate personal feelings from those originating in the client. If personal feelings are not recognized, named, and examined, with-

TABLE 20–4 UNREALISTIC EXPECTATIONS OF DEPRESSED CLIENTS

EXPECTATION	POSSIBLE RESULTS	POSSIBLE OUTCOMES
Nurse expects to feel needed and helpful to the client.	Client does not respond, shows lack of interest.	Nurse feels useless and ineffectual.
	Client tells the nurse to leave him or her alone and may show hostility.	Nurse feels hurt and avoids the client to avoid arousing these feelings.
Nurse expects to form "therapeutic relationship" with the client.	Client acts aloof and cold.	Nurse feels rejected by the client and may withdraw from the client to avoid these feelings of rejection.
Nurse expects the client to show signs of improvement after the nurse spends a lot of time with the client.	Client does not improve or slips back to being withdrawn and depressed.	Nurse feels impatient and loses interest in such a "hopeless case."
	Client shows contempt for the nurse after the nurse has worked with the client.	Nurse's self-esteem is lowered. Nurse interprets the client's behavior as a sign of the nurse's incompetence.
	Client's feeling of hopelessness and helplessness are sensed empathetically by the nurse.	Nurse feels helpless and anxious around the client. Nurse withdraws from the client to get away from feeling helpless. *or* Nurse becomes angry at the client: "Why can't you shape up?" or "Stop acting like a baby." Anger may also trigger withdrawal.

drawal by the nurse is likely to occur. People naturally stay away from situations and persons that arouse feelings of frustration, annoyance, or intimidation. If the nurse has unresolved feelings of anger and depression, the complexity of the situation is compounded. There is no substitute for competent and supportive supervision to facilitate growth, both professionally and personally. Supervision by a more experienced clinician and sharing with peers help minimize feelings of confusion, frustration, and isolation and can increase therapeutic potential and self-esteem in the nurse. The nurse is then free to intervene more directly with the client, and more direct communication can result in increased opportunities for the client to learn new coping skills.

IMPLEMENTATION

Recovery from depression can be conceptualized as a process. Kupfer (1991) has identified three phases in the treatment of and recovery from a major depression:

1. Acute phase (6 to 12 weeks)
2. Continuation phase (4 to 9 months)
3. Maintenance phase (1 or more years)

During the acute phase, hospitalization may be necessary. With the advent of managed care, hospital stays have been greatly decreased. Clinical Pathway 20–1 includes staff interventions that cover 20 or more days. In most

CLINICAL PATHWAY 20–1 Major Depression

Initiation Date: Expected LOS: 20 days Actual LOS: ________ Exclusions: Patients refusing all TX: Pending

Court Hearing: Major Medical Comorbidity Date Reviewed with PT/SO: ________ Signature: ________

	DAYS 1–3 Dates ________	DAYS 4–10 Dates ________	DAYS 11–19 Dates ________	DAYS 20–ONWARD Dates ________
Medical Interventions Physician: ________	H&P, MSE Lab studies Review old records and med history. Admission orders. RX medications. Complete initial assessment and discharge plan. Determine status of advance directives.	Monitor mental status, labs, therapeutic and adverse reactions to medications. Educate patient about depressive illness and medication. RMS consultation. Substance abuse consultation. Complete treatment plan. Complete advance directive, if appropriate.	Evaluate patient's response to treatment. Monitor for adverse actions to medication. Reinforce education. Assist with discharge plan.	Complete discharge instruction form. Complete discharge orders. Reinforce education about depressive illness and medication RX.
Nursing Interventions Primary Nurse: ________	Initial nursing assessment within 8 hours. Complete form within 24 hr. VS and weights. Complete initial plan of care within 8 hr. Orient to ward. Assign primary nurse.	VS and weights. Monitor safety, sleep, nutrition, mental status, ADLs, socialization. Complete plan of care. Educate patient about depressive illness, sleep hygiene, medications, and nutrition. Conduct nursing therapies/ groups (specify): ________ ________	VS and weights. Monitor safety, sleep, nutrition, mental status, ADLs, socialization. Teach coping skills, reinforce education about depressive illness, meds, sleep, hygiene practices, and adequate nutrition. Evaluate patient's response to interventions. Assist with discharge plan.	Continue interventions from phase 3. Educate patient about how to manage adverse reactions to medication while in community. Evaluate response to interventions. Provide discharge instructions, meds, diet, follow-up plan.
Nutrition and Food Service Dietitian: ________	Provide well-balanced diet. Nutritional screening, including IBW, height, weight, diet order, risk status, consistency, food/drug interactions, IPC. Educate patient about diet.	Evaluate patient's response to diet. Complete nutrition assessment, if indicated. Complete treatment plan. Educate patient about diet.	Continue to evaluate patient's response to diet.	Follow-up assessment according to criteria. Respond to concerns about diet as needed. Educate patient/caregiver about discharge plan for diet.
Psychology Interventions Psychologist: ________	Initial evaluation.	Complete IPA 1:1 therapy (specify): ________ Conduct therapy groups (specify) ________ ________	Consultation with ancillary psychological services. Psychological testing.	Arrange for psychological services aftercare.

Continued on following page

CLINICAL PATHWAY 20–1 Major Depression *(Continued)*

Initiation Date: Expected LOS: 20 days Actual LOS: ________ Exclusions: patients refusing all TX: Pending
Court Hearing: Major Medical Comorbidity Date Reviewed with PT/SO: ________ Signature: ________

	DAYS 1–3 Dates ________	DAYS 4–10 Dates ________	DAYS 11–19 Dates ________	DAYS 20–ONWARD Dates ________
Social Work Social worker: ________	Initial evaluation. Begin planning appropriate community discharge placements.	Complete social work database within 7 days. Establish contact with family/SO. Identify legal/financial issues. Determine placement options. Obtain funds and clothing. Complete treatment plan. Complete advance directives. Conduct therapy groups (specify): ________	Have ongoing contact with family/SO. Schedule meeting with family/SO. Monitor legal/financial status/ Complete referrals for aftercare.	Ongoing contact with family/SO. Evaluate status of patient regarding privileges, social interactions, competence, continence, self-care level, legal/financial status in regard to aftercare plan. Complete discharge note.
RMS OT: ________ KT: ________ RT: ________		Complete RMS evaluation. Complete OT initial database Complete RT initial database. Complete treatment plan. Conduct groups (specify): ________ ________	Evaluate patient's response to RMS therapies. Revise treatment plan. Assist with discharge plan.	Reinforce patient's aftercare plan. RT: assist patient to identify at least 2 leisure/recreational activities that can be done after discharge.

Adapted from Veterans Affairs Maryland Health Care System, Perry Point Division.
LOS, length of stay; PT/SO, patient/significant other; TX, treatment; RX, prescription; RMS, rehabilitative medicine service; VS, vital signs; ADL, activity of daily living; IBW, ideal body weight; IPA, initial psychiatric assessment; IPC, interdisciplinary plan of care; OT, occupational therapy; RT, recreation therapy; H&P, history and physical; MSE, mental status examination; KT, kinesiotherapy.

hospitals today, the length of stay is shorter. Therefore, in hospitals that have adopted clinical pathways, modified versions of this pathway are used. The clinical pathway for major depression identifies specific responsibilities of members of the health care team during a client's hospital stay for a major depressive disorder. Please note that this clinical pathway is adopted from one used at a Veterans Administration Hospital. Hospital stays are usually a lot shorter and clients, if hospitalized, are generally sent home during phase one, the acute phase. The continuation and maintenance phases refer to medication and/or group or individual, short-term or supportive therapy. The continuation and maintenance phases occur in outpatient settings, such as clinics, home visits, partial hospitalization, and other community-based sites.

Counseling/Communication Strategies (Basic Level)

Nurses often have great difficulty communicating with a client without talking. However, some depressed clients are so withdrawn that they are unwilling or unable to speak. Just sitting with a client in silence may seem like a waste of time to the nurse. Often, the nurse becomes uncomfortable not "doing something," and, as anxiety increases, the nurse may start daydreaming, feel bored, remember something that "must be done now," and so on. It is important to be aware that this time spent together can be meaningful to the depressed person, especially if the nurse has a genuine interest in learning about the depressed individual.

▶ Doris, a senior nursing student, is working with a depressed, suicidal, withdrawn woman. The instructor notices in the second week that Doris spends a lot of time talking with other students and their clients and little time with her own client. In postconference, Doris acknowledges feeling threatened and useless and says that she wants a client who will interact with her. After reviewing the symptoms of depression, its behavioral manifestations, and the needs of depressed persons, Doris turns her attention back to her client and spends time rethinking her plan of care. After 4 weeks of sharing her feelings in postconferences, working with her instructor, and trying a variety of approaches with her client, Doris is rewarded. On the day of discharge, the client tells Doris how important their time together was for her: "I actually felt someone cared."

It is difficult to say when a withdrawn or depressed person will be able to respond. However, certain techniques are known to be useful in guiding effective nursing interventions. Some communication guidelines are listed in Table 20–5.

Health Teaching (Basic Level)

Health teaching is best started in the hospital setting and is continued in the community setting both with clients and with their families. It is important for both clients and their families to understand that depression is a legitimate medical illness over which the client has no voluntary control. Depressed clients and their families need to learn about the biological symptoms of depression, as well as about the psychosocial and cognitive changes in depression. Review of the medications, side effects, and toxic effects helps families evaluate clinical change and stay alert for reactions that might affect client compliance. The section "Psychobiological Interventions" provides information on the side effects of antidepressants

TABLE 20–5 COMMUNICATION GUIDELINES FOR A PERSON WHO IS DEPRESSED

INTERVENTION	RATIONALE
Nursing Diagnosis: Altered thought process related to hopelessness, as evidenced by extreme withdrawal and low verbalization	
1. Spend short periods of time (5–10 minutes) with the client frequently throughout the day.	1. Frequent short periods minimize anxiety for both the nurse and the client.
2. Let the client know beforehand when, and for how long, the visits will be.	2. Clear expectations minimize anxiety. Scheduled times bring structure and purpose to empty periods of time.
3. Be on time and stay the full time contracted, even when the client does not acknowledge your presence.	3. Consistency and reliability lay the foundations for trust. The client experiences attention without having to earn it. When the nurse does not come on time or stay the stated time, a depressed person may personalize the nurse experience: "I'm not worthy of attention."
4. When the client is not speaking, sit with the person in silence for short periods.	4. Even if the client does not acknowledge the nurse, the client knows that the nurse is there. The nurse's presence and interest over time can reinforce that the nurse views the client as worthwhile.
5. When a client is mute, use the technique "making observations": "There are many new pictures on the wall" or "You are wearing your new shoes."	5. When a client is not ready to talk, direct questions can raise the client's anxiety level and frustrate the nurse. Pointing to commonalties in the environment draws the client into, and reinforces, reality.
6. Use simple, concrete words.	6. Slowed thinking and difficulty concentrating impair comprehension.
7. Allow time for the client to respond.	7. Slowed thinking necessitates time to formulate a response.
8. Listen for covert messages and ask about suicide plans.	8. People often experience relief and decrease in feelings of isolation when they share thoughts of suicide.
9. Spend time listening and sharing feelings.	9. Feeling understood can help diminish feelings of alienation and isolation and can facilitate the sharing of painful feelings necessary for healing.
10. *Avoid* laughing, joking, and "acting cheerful."	10. The nurse's cheerful attitude increases feelings of alientation and isolation in the client by contrasting the nurse's "up" feelings with the client's own feelings of low worth.
11. *Avoid* platitudes, such as "Things will look up" or "Everyone gets down once in a while."	11. Platitudes tend to minimize the client's feelings and can increase feelings of guilt and worthlessness because the client cannot "look up" or "snap out of it."
12. Accept expressions of anger without becoming defensive.	12. Argumentative or self-righteous responses serve to diminish both the client's and nurse's self-esteem.
13. *Avoid* the use of value judgments:	13. When depressed, a person sees the negative side of everything, e.g.
"You look nice this morning."	◗ Can be interpreted as "I didn't look nice yesterday morning"
"I like the way you did your hair."	◗ Can be thought of as being done to please the nurse: "If I do my hair another way, maybe he or she will not like it."
Say instead, "You are wearing a new dress this morning" or "You've changed your hairstyle."	Neutral comments avoid negative interpretations.

and specific areas to be covered in client and family teaching.

When a client has been hospitalized and is leaving the hospital, predischarge counseling should be performed with the client and the client's relatives. One purpose of this counseling is to clarify the interpersonal stresses and discuss steps that can alleviate tension for the family system. Predischarge counseling can be performed by the psychiatrist, the psychiatric nurse clinician, or the psychiatric social worker. Including families in discharge planning can bring about the following results:

- Increase the family's understanding and acceptance of the depressed family member during the aftercare period
- Increase the client's use of aftercare facilities in the community
- Contribute to higher overall adjustment in the client after discharge

Self-Care Activities (Basic Level)

A depressed person may report having many physical complaints. Because depressed clients often view themselves as worthless, it is the nurse's responsibility to notice signs and symptoms of physical neglect. Nursing measures for improving physical well-being and promoting adequate self-care are then initiated. Some effective interventions targeting the physical needs of the depressed client are listed in Table 20–6. Nurses in the community can work with family members to encourage a depressed family member to perform and maintain his or her health care needs.

TABLE 20–6 SELF-CARE GUIDELINES FOR A DEPRESSED PERSON

INTERVENTION	RATIONALE
Nursing Diagnosis: Activity intolerance related to poor concentration and motivation, as evidenced by withdrawal from others	
1. While the client is most severely depressed, involve the client in one-to-one activities.	1. Because concentration is impaired, this strategy maximizes the potential for interacting and may minimize anxiety levels.
2. Engage the client in activities involving gross motor activity and calling for minimal concentration (e.g., taking a walk, making beds with the nurse, setting up chairs.)	2. Physical activities are thought to help temporarily mobilize aggression and relieve tension.
3. Provide activities that require very little concentration (e.g., walking, playing simple card games, looking through a magazine, drawing, playing with clay).	3. Concentration and memory are poor in depression. Activities that have no "right" or "wrong" minimize opportunities for the client to put himself or herself down.
4. Eventually bring the client into contact with one other person and then into a group of three.	4. Contact with others distracts the client from self-preoccupations and provides the client with opportunity to spend more time with people and activities that are based in reality.
5. Eventually involve the client in group activities (e.g., dance therapy, art therapy, group discussions).	5. Socialization can decrease feelings of isolation. Genuine regard from others can increase feelings of self-worth.
6. In *psychomotor agitation,* provide activities that involve the use of the hands and gross motor movements (e.g., ping-pong, volleyball, finger painting, drawing, working with clay).	6. These activities give the client a more appropriate way of discharging motor tension than pacing and wringing hands.
Nursing Diagnosis: Altered nutrition, less than body requirements related to anorexia, as evidenced by refusal to eat and/or weight loss	
1. Offer small high-calorie and high-protein snacks frequently throughout the day and evening.	1. Low weight and poor nutrition render the client susceptible to illness. Small, frequent snacks are more easily tolerated than large plates of food when the client is anorexic.
2. Offer high-protein and high-calorie fluids frequently throughout the day and evening.	2. These fluids prevent dehydration and can minimize constipation.
3. When possible, remain with the client during meals.	3. This strategy reinforces the idea that someone cares, can raise the client's self-esteem, and can serve as an incentive to eat.
4. Ask the client which foods or drinks he or she likes. Offer choices. Involve the dietitian.	4. The client is more likely to eat the foods provided.
5. Weigh the client weekly and observe the client's eating patterns.	5. Monitoring the client's status gives the information needed for revision of the intervention.

TABLE 20–6 SELF-CARE GUIDELINES FOR A DEPRESSED PERSON *(Continued)*

INTERVENTION	RATIONALE
Nursing Diagnosis: Sleep-pattern disturbance related to insomnia as evidenced by frequent awakenings, difficulty going to sleep, and persistent fatigue	
1. Provide rest periods after activities.	1. Fatigue can intensify feelings of depression.
2. Encourage the client to get up and dress and to stay out of bed during the day.	2. Minimizing sleep during the day increases the likelihood of sleep at night.
3. Provide relaxation measures in the evening (e.g., back rub, tepid bath, or warm milk).	3. These measures induce relaxation and sleep.
4. Reduce environmental and physical stimulants in the evening—provide decaffeinated coffee, soft lights, soft music, and quiet activities.	4. Decreasing caffeine and epinephrine levels increases the possibility of sleep.
5. Spend more time with the client before bedtime.	5. This strategy helps allay anxiety and increases feelings of security.
Nursing Diagnosis: Self-care deficit related to poor concentration and lack of motivation, as evidenced by poor grooming and dress	
1. Encourage the use of toothbrush, washcloth, soap, make-up, shaving equipment, and so forth.	1. Being clean and well groomed can temporarily raise self-esteem.
2. Give step-by-step reminders, such as "Wash the right side of your face, now the left . . ."	2. Slowed thinking and difficulty concentrating make organizing simple tasks difficult.
Nursing Diagnosis: Constipation related to inadequate daily intake	
1. Monitor intake and output, especially bowel movements.	1. Many depressed clients are constipated. If the condition is not checked, fecal impaction can occur.
2. Offer foods high in fiber and provide periods of exercise.	2. Roughage and exercise stimulate peristalsis and help evacuation of fecal material.
3. Encourage the intake of fluids.	3. Fluids help prevent constipation.
4. Evaluate the need for laxatives and enemas.	4. These measures prevent fecal impaction.

Psychobiological Interventions (Basic Level)

Depression is a recurring disorder. About 75% to 95% of depressed individuals have multiple episodes. However, the discovery of effective antidepressant modalities has resulted in depression's being one of the most "treatable" disorders encountered in medicine (Zajecka 1995b). Keller (1995) noted that

- 65% to 75% of depressed clients "respond" to antidepressant treatment.
- 25% to 35% of clients with a major depression fail to respond meaningfully to presently available treatment.

However, waiting too long to start treatment leads to (Greden 1995):

- Greater morbidity.
- Greater disability.
- Greater expense.
- Treatment refractoriness.

All depressed persons should be evaluated for suicidal risk whether they are in the hospital or the community. When a depressed person is hospitalized, staff members need to check to make sure that all medications are swallowed (not placed in the cheek or under the tongue). If a client is being treated in an outpatient setting, only a week's supply should be given to a severely depressed person. Ten to 15 times the prescribed dose of any antidepressant can prove fatal.

Antidepressant drugs can positively alter poor self-concept, degree of withdrawal, vegetative signs of depression, and activity level. Target symptoms include

1. Sleep disturbance.
   - Early morning awakening.
   - Frequent awakening.
   - Hypersomnia (excessive sleeping).
2. Appetite disturbance (decreased or increased).
3. Fatigue.
4. Decreased sex drive.
5. Psychomotor retardation or agitation.
6. Diurnal variations in mood (often worse in the morning).
7. Impaired concentration or forgetfulness.
8. Anhedonia.

One drawback to the use of antidepressant medication is that the client may have to take antidepressant agents for 1 to 3 weeks before improvement is noticed. However, if a client is acutely suicidal, 2 to 3 weeks may be too long to wait. At these times, electroconvulsive therapy (ECT) may be the treatment of choice. The major types of antidepressant drugs are the **selective serotonin reuptake inhibitors** (SSRIs) or selective serotonin/norepinephrine reuptake inhibitors (SSNRIs), the **tricyclic antidepressants** (TCAs), the atypical antidepressants, and the monoamine oxidase inhibitors (MAOIs).

Selective Serotonin Reuptake Inhibitors

The **SSRIs** represent an important advance in pharmacotherapy. They are neither TCAs nor MAOIs. Essentially, the SSRIs selectively block the neuronal uptake of serotonin. Therefore, through blockade of the reuptake process, serotonergic neurotransmission is enhanced, thereby permitting serotonin to act for an extended period of time at the synaptic binding sites in the brain. Chapter 3 provides more information on how the SSRIs work.

Selective serotonin reuptake inhibitors are recommended as first-line therapy in all depressions *except* severe inpatient depression (in which ECT may be the first choice) or melancholic depression or mild outpatient depression (Maxmen and Ward 1995).

Selective serotonin reuptake inhibitor antidepressant drugs have a lower incidence of anticholinergic side effects (dry mouth, blurred vision, urinary retention), less cardiotoxicity, and faster onset of action than TCAs. The SSRIs seem to be effective in depressions with anxious features as well as in clients with psychomotor agitation (Tollefson 1995). Since its introduction, fluoxetine (Prozac), the first of the SSRI antidepressant drugs on the market, is still one of the most widely prescribed antidepressant in the United States (Lehne et al. 1994).

For most clients, the SSRIs are better tolerated than the TCAs. Tollefson (1995) cited a study with the following percentages of discontinuation of the drug because of adverse effects:

- 5% to 10% for placebo
- 10% to 20% for SSRIs
- 30% to 35% for TCAs

This increased degree of tolerance translates into superior client acceptance and compliance for most depressed individuals. The SSRIs cause fewer side effects and, because of their low cardiotoxicity, they are less dangerous when they are taken in overdose. The SSRIs, selective serotonin/norepinephrine reuptake inhibitors, and atypical antidepressants have a low lethality risk for suicide attempts compared with the TCAs, which have a very high potential for lethality with overdose (Maxmen and Ward 1995).

TYPES AND INDICATIONS. The SSRIs appear to have a broad base for clinical use. In addition to their use in depressive disorders, the SSRIs have been prescribed with success in some of the anxiety disorders, in particular, obsessive-compulsive disorder and panic disorder (see Chapter 17). The SSRIs have also been a successful part of treatment for many individuals with eating disorders. They are useful in the treatment of bulimia nervosa and in the suppression of appetite in obese individuals (see Chapter 26).

Many SSRIs are on the market. Some of the major ones in current use are fluoxetine, sertraline (Zoloft), paroxetine (Paxil), and fluoxamine (Luvox).

COMMON SIDE EFFECTS. Agents that selectively enhance synaptic serotonin within the CNS may induce agitation, anxiety, sleep disturbance, tremor, sexual dysfunction (primarily anorgasmia), or headache. Autonomic reactions (e.g., dry mouth, sweating, weight change, nausea, altered gastrointestinal motility) may also be experienced with the SSRIs.

SERIOUS SIDE EFFECTS. One rare and life-threatening event associated with the SSRIs is the *central serotonin syndrome*. This is thought to be related to overactivation of the central serotonin receptors. Symptoms include abdominal pain, diarrhea, sweating, fever, tachycardia, elevated blood pressure, altered mental state (delirium), myoclonus, increased motor activity, irritability, hostility, and mood change. Severe manifestation can induce hyperpyrexia, cardiovascular shock, or death. The risk of this syndrome seems to be the greatest when an SSRI is administered temporally with a second serotonin-enhancing agent, such as an MAOI. For example, a person taking fluoxetine would have to be medication-free for a full 5 weeks before being switched to an MAOI (5 weeks is the half-life for fluoxetine). If clients are already taking an MAOI, they should wait at least 2 weeks before starting fluoxetine therapy. Other SSRIs have shorter lives; for example, sertraline and paroxetine have half-lives of 2 weeks, so there would need to be a 2-week gap between medications. Box 20–1 lists the signs and symptoms of central serotonin syndrome. Box 20–2 offers emergency treatment guidelines. This serotonin syndrome closely resembles neuroleptic malignant syndrome and malignant hyperthermia (Beasley et al 1993; Gabbard 1995).

Selective Serotonin/Norepinephrine Reuptake Inhibitors

Nefazodone (Serzone) and venlafaxine (Effexor) are two antidepressants with pharmacological actions and side-effect profiles that differ from those of the SSRIs. These drugs enrich the synapse with serotonin while inhibiting the reuptake of selective serotonin/norepinephrine reuptake inhibitors.

NAFAZODONE (SERZONE). Nafazodone inhibits serotonin, is a potent antagonist of serotonin (5-HT2) receptors, and binds to the serotonin transmitter.

BOX 20–1 CLINICAL MANIFESTATIONS OF THE CENTRAL SEROTONIN SYNDROME

Neuropsychiatric
- Hyperactivity/restlessness
- Elevated or dysphoric mood
- Racing thoughts
- Pressured speech
- Apprehension
- Anxiety/agitation
- Hallucinations
- Confusion
- Altered level of consciousness

Neurological
- Myoclonus
- Increased deep tendon reflexes
- Dysarthria
- Tremulousness
- Incoordination
- Dilated pupils (minimally or unreactive)
- Tonic rigidity
- Trismus/opisthotonus
- Rigors
- Seizures
- Status epilepticus

Gastrointestinal
- Diarrhea
- Hyperactive bowel sounds
- Cramping
- Bloating

Cardiovascular
- Tachycardia
- Hypertension
- Cardiovascular collapse

Other
- Hyperthermia
- Diaphoresis
- Hyperlacrimation
- Increased creatine phosphokinase level
- Apnea
- Disseminated vascular necrosis
- Death

From Zajecka, J. (1995). Treatment strategies for depression complicated by anxiety disorders. Presented at the U. S. Psychiatric and Mental Health Congress, Marriott Marquis, New York, November 16, 1995.

BOX 20–2 CENTRAL SEROTONIN SYNDROME TREATMENT

Remove offending agent(s)
Symptomatic treatments
- Block serotonin receptors
  - Cyproheptadine, methysergide, propranolol
- Hyperthermia
  - Cooling blankets, chlorpromazine
- Muscle rigidity/rigors
  - Dantrolene, diazepam
- Anticonvulsants
- Artificial ventilation
- Paralysis
  - Pancuronium, succinylcholine

From Zajecka, J. (1995). Treatment strategies for depression complicated by anxiety disorders. Presented at the U. S. Psychiatric and Mental Health Congress, Marriott Marquis, New York, November 16, 1995.

Nefazodone also binds to the norepinephrine transporter. It is different from other antidepressants because of its two actions in the serotonin system: moderate serotonin selective reuptake blocking and direct 5-HT2 antagonisms that may be more anxiolytic than other antidepressants. It appears to be a safe and well-tolerated drug after both short-term and long-term use. The most common adverse effects of nefazodone are nausea, somnolence, dry mouth, dizziness, constipation, asthenia, lightheadedness, and blurred vision. Much to its credit, the drug causes a low incidence of sexual dysfunction, weight change, sleep dysfunction, and cardiotoxicity.

VENLAFAXINE (EFFEXOR). Venlafaxine is chemically unrelated to any of the currently available antidepressants. It is a potent inhibitor of serotonin as well as norepinephrine in the CNS. This drug has demonstrated effective antidepressant properties with a good side effect profile. The main side effects are nausea, somnolence, dry mouth, dizziness, constipation, nervousness, sweating, asthenia, abnormal ejaculation/orgasm, and anorexia (Wyeth-Ayerst Laboratories 1995). A 40% response rate to venlafaxine has been reported in clients who have not improved with adequate trials of other treatments (Post 1995).

Tricyclic Antidepressants

The **TCAs** inhibit the reuptake of norepinephrine and serotonin by the presynaptic neurons in the CNS. Therefore, the amount of time that norepinephrine and serotonin are available to the postsynaptic receptors is increased. This increase in norepinephrine and serotonin in the brain is thought by many to be responsible for mood elevations when TCAs are given to depressed persons (see Chapter 3).

Tricyclic antidepressants benefit about 65% to 80% of people with nondelusional depressive disorders, but only about 33% of those with delusional depression (Maxmen and Ward 1995). Clients with delusional depression respond well to ECT (75% to 85%). Antipsychotic agents, given along with an antidepressant, are also effective for some depressed clients who have psychotic symptoms (65% to 70%) (Maxmen and Ward 1995).

TABLE 20–7 ANTIDEPRESSANTS: ADVERSE EFFECTS AND EFFECTS ON NEUROTRANSMITTERS

	Transmitter Reuptake Antagonism		Anti-cholin-ergic Activity*	Seda-tion	Hypo-tension	Seizure Risk	Cardio-toxicity	Comments
	NE	5-HT						
Tricyclic Antidepressants (TCAs)								
Amitriptyline (Elavil)	++	++++	++++	++++	+++	+++	++++	The sedating and anticholinergic effects are difficult for some patients to tolerate; frequent cause of cardiac arrhythmias.
Desipramine (Norpramin)	++++	+	++	++	++	++	+++	More energizing TCA. Also has fewer anticholinergic side effects.
Doxepin (Sinequan)	++	++	+++	++++	++	+++	++	Helps lower anxiety and agitation; sedating.
Imipramine (Tofranil)	+++	+++	+++	+++	+++	+++	++++	Useful in agoraphobia with panic attacks. High incidence of hypotension.
Nortriptyline (Aventyl, Pamelor)	+++	++	++	+++	+	++	+++	Fewest cardiac problems of TCAs, especially postural hypotension; useful for the elderly.
Protriptyline (Vivactil)	++++	++	+++	+	++	++	++++	More energizing; useful for lethargy and psychomotor retardation.
Trimipramine (Surmontil)	+	+	+++	++++	+++	+++	++++	Good choice for the elderly: low side-effect profile and promotes sleep.
Monoamine Oxidase Inhibitors (MAOIs)								
Isocarboxazid (Marplan)	a	a	0	+	++	0	0	Hypertensive crisis from tyramine in foods.
Phenelzine (Nardil)	a	a	0	+	++	0	0	Hypertensive crisis from tyramine in foods.
Tranylcypromine (Parnate)	a	a	0	b	++	0	0	Hypertensive crisis from tyramine in foods.
Selective Serotonin Reuptake Inhibitors (SSRIs)								
Fluoxetine (Prozac)	0	+++++	0	b	0	+	0	Associated with fewer cardiac problems. Wait 5 to 6 weeks before changing to an MAOI.
Paroxetine HCl (Paxil)	0	++++	0	0	0		0	Studies show a beneficial effect on symptoms of anxiety and agitation in depressed clients.
Sertraline (Zoloft)	0	++++	0	b	0	+	0	Good side effect profile (similar to that of fluoxetine) and also useful for obsessive-compulsive disorder

Selective Serotonin/ Norepinephrine Reuptake Inhibitors (RF)								
Venlafaxine (Effexor)	++	+++	+	+	e	0	+	SSRI-like side effects (anorexia, sexual dysfunction, nervousness). ↑ in BP dictate BP monitoring.
Nafazodone (Serzone)	++	+++	+	++	+	0	0	More anxiolytic than most antidepressants; low incidence of sexual dysfunction, sleep disturbance, and cardiotoxicity.
Atypical Antidepressants								
Amoxapine (Asendin)	+++c	++c	+++	++	+	+++	+	EPS reported—Akathisia, even dyskinesia in some. Drug should be tapered or discontinued when this occurs. Parkinsonism and TD. It has a high frequency of seizures.
Bupropion[d] (Wellbutrin)	+	0	++	b	+	+++++	+	Fewer cardiac problems than TCAs. Seizures reported in 0.4% of patients treated
Maprotiline (Ludiomil)	+++	+	+++	+++	++	++++	+++	Seizures reported at high doses.
Trazodone (Desyrel)	0	++	0	+++	+++	++	+	Fewer cardiac problems than TCAs. Has antianxiety properties. Priapism is a rare adverse reaction.

\+ = the least; +++++ = the most.
*Anticholinergic side effects include dry mouth, constipation, difficulty in urinating and blurred vision. Can cause confusion and memory disturbance in the elderly.
a = MAOIs do not block transmitter reuptake. Rather, they increase intraneurona stores at NE, 5-HT, and DA.
b = Produces moderate stimulation, not sedation.
c = In addition to blocking NE and 5-HT reuptake, amoxapine blocks receptors for DA.
d = Bupropion primarily inhibits reuptake of DA rather than NE or 5-HT.
E = Effexor may cause hypertension in some
– = unknown
NE, norepinephrine; 5-HT, serotonin; DA, dopamine; EPS, extrapyramidal side effects; TD, tardive dyskinesia; BP, blood pressure.
Data from Lehne, R. A., et al. (1994). *Pharmacology for nursing* (2nd ed.). Philadelphia: W. B. Saunders; U. S. Department of Human Services, Public Health Service, Agency for Health Care and Research (1993). *Depression in primary care: Detection, diagnosis, and treatment.* Washington, DC: U. S. Department of Human Services; Lader, M. H. (1996). Tolerability and safety: Essentials in antidepressant pharmacology. *Journal of Clinical Psychiatry*, 57(2):39–44; Robinson, D. S., et al. (1996). The safety of nefazodone. *Journal of Clinical Psychiatry*, 57(2):31–38.

Clients must take therapeutic doses of TCAs for 10 to 14 days or longer before these agents start to work. The full effects may take from 4 to 8 weeks to be seen. An effect on some symptoms of depression, such as insomnia and anorexia, may be noted earlier. Currently, a person who has had a positive response to TCA therapy would probably be maintained on that medication from 6 to 12 months in order to prevent an early relapse. Choice of TCA is based on

1. What has worked for the client or a family member in the past.
2. The drug's side effects.

For example, for a client who is lethargic and fatigued, a more stimulating TCA, such as desipramine (Norpramin) and protriptyline (Vivactil) may be best. If a more sedating effect is needed for agitation or restlessness, drugs such as amitriptyline (Elavil) and doxepin (Sinequan) may be more appropriate choices. *No matter which TCA is given, the dose should always be low initially and gradually increased.* Caution should be used, especially in elderly persons, in whom slow drug metabolism may be a problem. Schatzberg and Cole (1991) found trimipramine (Surmontil) to be a good choice for the elderly because of its low side-effect profile and its rapid effects on promoting sleep.

COMMON SIDE EFFECTS. The chemical structure of the TCAs is similar to that of the antipsychotic medications. Therefore, the *anticholinergic* actions are similar (e.g., dry mouth, blurred vision, tachycardia, postural hypotension, constipation, urinary retention, and esophageal reflux). These side effects are both more common and more severe in clients taking antidepressants. These side effects are usually not serious and are often transitory, but *urinary retention and severe constipation warrant immediate medical attention.*

Administering the total daily dose of TCA at night is beneficial for two reasons. First, most TCAs have sedative effects, thereby aiding sleep. Second, the minor side effects occur during sleep, thereby increasing compliance with drug therapy. Table 20–7 lists commonly used TCAs, effects on neurotransmitters, and adverse effects, and Table 20–8 identifies dose ranges. Information for the SSRIs, MAOIs, and atypical drugs is found in these tables also.

SERIOUS SIDE EFFECTS. The most serious side effects of the TCAs are cardiovascular. Dysrhythmias, tachycardia, myocardial infarction, and heart block have been reported. Because the cardiac side effects are so serious, the TCAs are considered a risk in clients with cardiac disease and in the elderly. Clients should have a thorough cardiac work-up before beginning TCA therapy.

ADVERSE DRUG INTERACTIONS. Individuals taking TCAs can have adverse reactions to numerous other medications. For example, use of a MAOI along with a TCA is contraindicated. A few of the more common medications usually *not* given while the TCAs are being administered are listed in Box 20–3. Any client who is taking any of these medications along with the TCAs should have medical clearance because some of the reactions can be fatal. Table 20–9 identifies the common and most troublesome side and adverse effects of the TCAs.

Antidepressants may precipitate a psychotic episode in a person with schizophrenia. An antidepressant can pre-

BOX 20–3 DRUGS USED WITH CAUTION IN CLIENTS TAKING A TRICYCLIC ANTIDEPRESSANT

- Phenothiazines
- Barbiturates
- Monoamine oxidase inhibitors
- Disulfiram (Antabuse)
- Oral contraceptives (or other estrogen preparations)
- Anticoagulants
- Some antihypertensives (clonidine, guanethidine, reserpine)
- Benzodiazepines
- Alcohol
- Nicotine

BOX 20–4 TEACHING CLIENTS AND THEIR FAMILIES ABOUT TRICYCLIC ANTIDEPRESSANTS

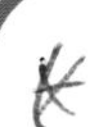

1. Tell the client and the client's family that mood elevation may take from 7 to 28 days. It may take up to 6–8 weeks for the full effect to take place and for major depression symptoms to subside.
2. Have the family reinforce this frequently to the depressed family member because depressed people have trouble remembering and respond to ongoing reassurance.
3. Reassure the client that drowsiness, dizziness, and hypotension usually subside after the first few weeks.
4. When the client starts taking tricyclic antidepressants (TCAs), caution the client to be careful working around machines, driving cars, and crossing streets because of possible altered reflexes, drowsiness, or dizziness.
5. Alcohol can block the effects of antidepressants. Tell the client to refrain from drinking.
6. If possible, the client should take full dose at bedtime to reduce the experience of side effects during the day.
7. If the client forgets the bedtime dose (or the once-a-day dose), the client should take the dose within 3 hours; otherwise the client should wait for the next day. The client should *not* double the dose.
8. Suddenly stopping TCAs can cause nausea, altered heartbeat, nightmares, and cold sweats in 2 to 4 days. The client should call the doctor or take one dose of TCA until the physician can be contacted.

TABLE 20–8 ADULT DOSAGES FOR ANTIDEPRESSANTS

GENERIC NAME	TRADE NAME	INITIAL DOSE*† (MG/DAY)	DOSE AFTER 4–8 WEEKS* (MG/DAY)	MAXIMUM DOSE‡ (MG/DAY)
Tricyclic Antidepressants (TCAs)				
Amitriptyline	Elavil, Endep	50–150	100–200	300
Desipramine	Norpramin, Pertofrane	50–150	75–200	300
Doxepin	Adapin, Sinequan	50–150	100–200	300
Imipramine	Tofranil	50–150	100–200	300
Nortriptyline	Aventyl, Pamelor	25–100	75–150	150
Protriptyline	Vivactil	10–40	15–40	60
Trimipramine	Surmontil	50–150	75–250	250
Monoamine Oxidase Inhibitors (MAOIs)				
Isocarboxazid	Marplan	20–30	20–30	30
Phenelzine	Nardil	45–75	45–75	75
Tranylcypromine	Parnate	20–30	20–30	30
Selective Serotonin Reuptake Inhibitors (SSRIs)				
Fluoxetine	Prozac	20	20–40	80
Fluvoxamine§	Floxyfral	50–100	50–300	300
Paroxetine	Paxil	20	20–50	50
Sertraline‡	Zoloft	50	50–200	200
Selective Serotonin/Norepinephrine Reuptake Inhibitors (SSNRIs)				
Venlafaxine	Effexor	50	75–225	375
Nefazodone	Serzone	200	300–600	600
Atypical Antidepressants				
Amoxapine	Asendin	50–150	200–300	400
Bupropion	Wellbutrin	200	225–450	450
Maprotiline	Ludiomil	50–150	100–150	225
Trazodone	Desyrel	150	150–200	400–600

Adapted from Lehne, R. A., et al. (1994). *Pharmacology of Nursing* (2nd ed.). Philadelphia: W. B. Saunders; Robinson, D. S., et al. (1996). Therapeutic range of nefazodone in the treatment of depression. *Journal of Clinical Psychiatry*, 57(2):6–9.

*Doses listed are total daily doses. Depending on the drug and the patient, the total dose may be given in a single dose or in divided doses.

†Initial doses are for 4–8 weeks, the time required for most symptoms to respond. The smaller dose within the range listed is used initially. Dosage is gradually increased as required.

‡Doses higher than these may be needed for some persons with severe depression.

§Investigational agent.

cipitate a manic episode in a client with bipolar disorder. Depressed clients with bipolar disorder should receive lithium along with the antidepressant.

CONTRAINDICATIONS. People who have recently had a myocardial infarction (or other cardiovascular problems), those with narrow-angle glaucoma or a history of seizures, and pregnant women should not be treated with TCAs, except with extreme caution and careful monitoring.

CLIENT TEACHING. Teaching clients and their family members about medications is an expected nursing responsibility. Medication teaching should be started in the hospital when a client is hospitalized. The nurse or another qualified health care provider needs to review with the client and, whenever possible, one or more family members, the client's medications, expected side effects, and necessary client precautions. Areas for the nurse to discuss when teaching a client about TCA therapy are presented in Box 20–4. Clients and family members need to have written information to refer to when at home. Written information should be provided for all medications people will be taking at home.

Atypical/Miscellaneous Antidepressants

Several important antidepressants are often classified as "atypical" since they do not fit into the category of TCAs, SSRIs, or MAOIs. Examples of such drugs are trazodone hydrochloride (Desyrel), bupropion hydrochloride (Wellbutrin), and alprazolam (Xanax); these are briefly discussed in this section. Others are available now, and many others are currently in clinical trials and are soon to be released.

TRAZODONE HYDROCHLORIDE (DESYREL). Trazodone hydrochloride has been found to be effective in outpatients who have mild to moderate depres-

TABLE 20–9 SIDE EFFECTS AND TOXIC EFFECTS OF TRICYCLIC ANTIDEPRESSANTS

PHENOMENA	COMMENTS
Anticholinergic Effects	
1. Dry mouth, blurred vision, postural hypotension, dry eyes, photophobia, nasal congestion.	1. Most side effects are not serious and are transitory (1–2 weeks). For people with orthostatic hypotension, nortriptyline may be a good alternative.
2. **Urinary retention and severe constipation.**	2. Bethanechol, 10–25 mg tid or tid–qid, may help urinary retention. Both urinary retention and severe constipation need immediate medical attention. Check for fecal impaction.
Cardiac Effects	
All patients should be checked for TCA-cardiac interactions before starting a TCA therapy.	
1. Low blood pressure (hypotension with dizziness).	1a. Take blood pressure with patient lying and standing. 1b. Instruct the client to rise slowly and hang onto objects. 1c. Instruct the client to use support hose. 1d. Have the doctor change the TCA. 1e. Occurs with greater frequency in patients with cardiac conditions. 1f. Protect the client against falls, especially the elderly client.
2. Tachycardia and arrhythmias.	2. Use TCAs with caution in people with cardiac conditions and the elderly.
3. Cardiac ECG changes.	3. TCAs are fatal in people with second-degree and third-degree heart block.
4. Heart failure.	4. Use with caution. Monitor the client's vital signs regularly.
Central Nervous System Responses	
1. Sedation (especially during the first 2 weeks).	1. Have the doctor prescribe a less sedating TCA and give full dose at bedtime.
2. Delirium (in high doses).	2. Withhold further doses of the drug and contact the doctor immediately.
3. Memory impairment (especially in elderly clients).	3. Evaluate change in the status of the client's memory.
4. Seizures (with maprotiline).	4. Most seizures reported for maprotiline result from the administration of high doses.
5. "Spaciness," depersonalization.	5. Increase the drug dose more slowly or switch the TCA.
6. Tremors.	6. Lower the dose. The doctor may prescribe propranolol.
Endocrine and Sexual Effects	
1. Decreased or increased libido.	1. Have the doctor evaluate; may change to another TCA.
2. Priapism (trazodone).	2. Medical intervention is crucial within 4 to 6 hours to maintain sexual ability.
3. Breast enlargement in women and men.	3. Doctor may try an alternative drug if this effect causes embarrassment (men or women).
4. Appetite stimulation—carbohydrate cravings.	4. Weight gain can be a problem.

Data from Maxmen, J. S., and Ward, N. G. (1995). *Psychotropic drugs fast facts* (2nd ed.). New York: W. W. Norton; Preston, J., and Johnson, J. (1995). *Clinical psychopharmacology made ridiculously simple*. Miami, FL: Medmaster; Schatzberg, A. F., and Cole, J. O. (1991). *Manual of clinical psychopharmacology* (2nd ed.). Washington, DC: American Psychiatric Press.
ECG, electrocardiographic; TCA, tricyclic antidepressant; bid, twice a day; tid, three times a day; qid, four times a day.

sion and anxiety, especially depressed individuals who have difficulty falling asleep (Golden et al. 1995). The main side effects of this drug are sedation, acute dizziness, and fainting (particularly if the drug is taken on an empty stomach). Priapism is a relatively rare but dramatic side effect that usually occurs in the first month of treatment. Priapism is a persistent erection of the penis that results from organic causes, not sexual desire. This condition is serious and may require surgical intervention. If it is not treated within a few hours, priapism can result in impotence (Schatzberg and Cole 1991).

BUPROPION HYDROCHLORIDE (WELLBUTRIN). Bupropion is effective in depressed clients, especially those who are refractory or intolerant to the TCAs. It has had some success with individuals with rapid-cycling bipolar II disorder (see Chapter 21). It has also been used successfully with children with attention-deficit hyperactivity disorder and in some clients with chronic fatigue syndrome (Golden et al. 1995). Bupropion has a favorable side-effect profile, although nausea can occur in some clients. It does not induce orthostatic hypotension or stimulate appetite, but it may cause seizures. For this reason, the drug is contraindicated in people with epilepsy, major head injury, bulimia, and anorexia nervosa (Schatzberg and Cole 1991).

ALPRAZOLAM (XANAX). Alprazolam is a benzodiazepine anxiolytic (see Chapter 17). Although this is an effective drug for anxiety disorders (e.g., panic disorders, agoraphobia), it is also as effective as the TCAs for the treatment of mild to moderate depression with anxious features. Its side-effect profile (sedation, minimal cardiovascular effects, lack of anticholinergic activity) can be advantageous for some individuals (Golden et al. 1995). The downside is that the benzodiazepines can cause potentially severe withdrawal reactions after abrupt discontinuation. Refer to Tables 20–7 and 20–8 for adverse effects and dosages.

Monoamine Oxidase Inhibitors

The **MAOIs** are being rediscovered by American medicine. A serious side effect of these drugs is that they interact with foods containing tyramine, a natural product of bacterial fermentation found in many cheeses, some wines, chopped liver (Box 20–5), and certain medications, including the sympathomimetic amines (Box 20–6). The interaction results in a hypertensive crisis that can be fatal. Chapter 3 provides more information on the action of the MAOIs.

The MAOIs are therefore usually contraindicated for people who are debilitated, elderly, or hypertensive; those who have cardiac or cerebrovascular disease; and those who have severe renal and hepatic disease. The MAOIs were traditionally given when the TCAs were ineffective. At present, MAOI administration is the preferred treatment for "atypical" depression. Atypical depression that responds well to MAOIs is characterized by clinical features such as

- Overeating.
- Hypersomnia.
- Phobic anxiety.
- Panic attacks.
- Masked depression (hypochondriasis).
- Feeling better in the morning and worse in the evening.
- Rejection sensitivity (feeling rejection for the slightest reason or no observable reason at all).
- Chronic pain.

The most common MAOIs are phenelzine (Nardil) and tranylcypromine sulfate (Parnate). MAOIs are also effective (Davidson 1992) in some people with

- Panic disorder.
- Social phobia.
- Generalized anxiety disorder.
- Obsessive-compulsive disorder.
- Posttraumatic stress disorder.
- Bulimia nervosa.
- Parkinson's disease.

Renewed interest in the MAOIs is related to the findings of Preston and Johnson (1995):

- When dietary restrictions are observed, the MAOIs are actively safer than the TCAs and have fewer side effects.
- They work in many clients who do not respond to the TCAs.

Clients should be carefully selected for MAOI therapy. Periodic reminders of dietary restrictions are advised. Even a clear-thinking person can have difficulty keeping the list of forbidden foods constantly in mind in restaurants and in the homes of friends. It is easy to understand why prescribing a MAOI for a client who is having cognitive difficulty with memory and concentration could be a problem if the client's diet is not supervised. Meperidine hydrochloride (Demerol), epinephrine, and decongestants can be particularly dangerous.

COMMON SIDE EFFECTS. Some common and troublesome long-term side effects of the MAOIs are orthostatic hypotension, weight gain, edema, change in cardiac rate and rhythm, constipation, urinary hesitancy, sexual dysfunction, vertigo, overactivity, muscle twitching, hypomanic and manic behavior, insomnia, weakness, and fatigue.

ADVERSE REACTIONS. The most serious reactions to these agents involve an increase in blood pressure, with the possible development of intracranial hemorrhage, hyperpyrexia, convulsions, coma, and death. Therefore, routine monitoring of blood pressure, especially during the first 6 weeks of treatment, is necessary.

Because so many other drugs, foods, and beverages can have adverse interactions with the MAOIs, increase in blood pressure is a constant concern. The beginning of a hypertensive crisis usually occurs within a few hours of ingestion of the contraindicated substance. The crisis may begin with headaches; stiff or sore neck; palpitations; increase or decrease in heart rate, often associated with chest pain; nausea; vomiting; or increase in temperature (pyrexia). When a hypertensive crisis is suspected, immediate medical attention is crucial. Antihypertensive medications, such as phentolamine (Regitine), are slowly administered intravenously. Pyrexia is treated with

BOX 20–5 FOODS THAT CAN INTERACT WITH MONOAMINE OXIDASE INHIBITORS

FOODS THAT CONTAIN TYRAMINE

Category	Unsafe Foods (High Tyramine Content)	Safe Foods (Little or No Tyramine)
Vegetables	Avocados, especially if overripe; fermented bean curd; fermented soybean; soybean paste; sauerkraut	Most vegetables
Fruits	Figs, especially if overripe; bananas, in large amounts	Most fruits
Meats	Meats that are fermented, smoked, or otherwise aged; spoiled meats; liver, unless very fresh; beef and chicken liver	Meats that are known to be fresh (exercise caution in restaurants; meat may not be fresh)
Sausages	Fermented varieties; bologna, pepperoni, salami, others	Nonfermented varieties
Fish	Dried, pickled or cured fish; fish that is fermented, smoked, or otherwise aged; spoiled fish	Fish that is known to be fresh; vacuum-packed fish, if eaten promptly or refrigerated only briefly after opening
Milk, milk products	Practically all cheeses	Milk, yogurt, cottage cheese, cream cheese
Foods with yeast	Yeast extract (e.g., Marmite, Bovril)	Baked goods that contain yeast
Beer, wine	Some imported beers, Chianti	Major domestic brands of beer; most wines
Other foods	Protein dietary supplements; soups (may contain protein extract); shrimp paste; soy sauce	

FOODS THAT CONTAIN OTHER VASOPRESSORS

Food	Comments
Chocolate	Contains phenylethylamine, a pressor agent; large amounts can cause a reaction.
Fava beans	Contain dopamine, a pressor agent; reactions are most likely with overripe beans.
Ginseng	Headache, tremulousness, and manic-like reactions have occurred.
Caffeinated beverages	Caffeine is a weak pressor agent; large amounts may cause a reaction.

From Lehne, R. A., et al. (1994). *Pharmacology for nursing* (2nd ed.). Philadelphia: W. B. Saunders.

BOX 20–6 DRUGS THAT CAN INTERACT WITH MONOAMINE OXIDASE INHIBITORS

Drug restrictions

- Over-the-counter medications for colds, allergies, or congestion (any product containing ephedrine, phenylephrine hydrochloride, or phenylpropanolamine)
- Tricyclic antidepressants (imipramine, amitriptyline)
- Narcotics
- Antihypertensives (methyldopa, guanethidine, reserpine)
- Amine precursors (levodopa, L-tryptophan)
- Sedatives (alcohol, barbiturates, benzodiazepines)
- General anesthetics
- Stimulants (amphetamines, cocaine)

hypothermia blankets or ice packs. Box 20–7 identified common side effects and toxic effects. Box 20–8 reviews information for clients and their families relating to the MAOIs.

CONTRAINDICATIONS. MAOIs may be contraindicated in

- Cerebrovascular disease.
- Hypertension and congestive heart failure.
- Liver disease.
- Foods containing tyramine, tryptophan, and dopamine (see Box 20–5).
- Medications (see Box 20–6).
- Recurrent or severe headaches.
- People having surgery in 10 to 14 days.
- Children younger than 16 years of age.

Some people do not respond to MAOIs or TCAs. For others, side effects of these agents prohibit their use. The advent of the SSRIs and some of the more atypical antidepressants has greatly enhanced the ability of the medical profession to decrease the suffering of people with

BOX 20–7 COMMON SIDE EFFECTS AND TOXIC EFFECTS OF MONOAMINE OXIDASE INHIBITORS

SIDE EFFECTS	COMMENTS
▸ Hypotension ▸ Sedation, weakness, fatigue ▸ Insomnia ▸ Changes in cardiac rhythm ▸ Muscle cramps ▸ Anorgasmia or sexual impotence ▸ Urinary hesitancy or constipation ▸ Weight gain	Hypotension is the most critical side effect (10%); the elderly especially may sustain injuries from it.
TOXIC EFFECTS	**COMMENTS**
Hypertensive crisis* ▸ Severe headache ▸ Stiff, sore neck ▸ Flushing, cold, clammy skin ▸ Tachycardia ▸ Severe nosebleeds, dilated pupils ▸ Chest pains, stroke, coma, death ▸ Nausea and vomiting	1. Client should go to local emergency department immediately—blood pressure should be checked. 2. May receive one of the following to lower blood pressure ▸ Intravenous phentolamine (Regitine) *or* ▸ Oral chlorpromazine *or* ▸ Nifedipine (calcium channel blocker), 10 mg every hour intravenously until relief occurs (one to two doses)

*Related to interaction with foodstuffs and cold medication.

depression, and the SSRIs and atypical antidepressants are often used as first-line treatments.

In summary, many medications can be used to treat depression: TCAs, SSRIs, atypical antidepressants, and MAOIs. Each group of antidepressants seems to be the first choice for specific situations (Table 20–10).

Electroconvulsive Therapy

Electroconvulsive therapy is indicated when antidepressant drugs have no effect; however, in some situations, ECT may be considered a primary treatment and may be given before a trial of antidepressant medication. ECT is indicated when (Dubovsky 1995)

1. There is a need for a rapid, definitive response when a client is suicidal or homicidal.
2. A client is in extreme agitation or stupor.
3. The risks of other treatments outweigh the risks of ECT.
4. The client has a history of poor drug response, a history of good ECT response, or both.
5. The client prefers it.

Electroconvulsive therapy is useful in clients with major depressive and bipolar depressive disorders, especially when psychotic symptoms are present (delusions of guilt, somatic delusions, or delusions of infidelity). Clients who have depressions with marked psychomotor retardation and stupor also respond well (Fink 1992). Depressed clients with a major depressive disorder who have responded to medication have a 80% to 90% response rate to bilateral ECT. In depressed, medication-resistant clients, the rate is closer to 50% (Devanand et al. 1991).

Electroconvulsive therapy is also indicated in manic clients whose conditions are resistant to lithium and an-

BOX 20–8 TEACHING CLIENTS AND THEIR FAMILIES ABOUT MONOAMINE OXIDASE INHIBITORS

- Tell the client and the client's family to avoid certain foods and all medications (especially cold remedies) unless prescribed by and discussed with the client's doctor (see Boxes 20–5 and 20–6 for specific food and drug restrictions).
- Give the client a wallet card describing the monoamine oxidase inhibitor (MAOI) regimen (Parke-Davis will supply them if contacted at 1-800-223-6432).
- Instruct the client to avoid Chinese restaurants (sherry, brewer's yeast, and other products may be used).
- Tell the client to go to the emergency department right away if he or she has a severe headache.
- Ideally, blood pressure should be monitored during the first 6 weeks of treatment (for both hypotensive and hypertensive effects).
- After stopping the MAOI, the client should maintain dietary and drug restrictions for 14 days.

TABLE 20–10 SPECIAL PROBLEMS AND MEDICATIONS OF CHOICE

THE PROBLEM	DRUGS OF CHOICE
1. High suicide risk	1. Trazodone, fluoxetine, sertraline, paroxetine, bupropion, venlafaxine
2. Concurrent depression and panic attacks	2. Phenelzine, imipramine, fluoxetine
3. Delusional depression	3. Antidepressant and antipsychotic (electroconvulsive therapy probably the most effective treatment)
4. Atypical depression	4. Monoamine oxidase inhibitors
5. Weight gain on other antidepressants	5. Fluoxetine, bupropion, sertraline, paroxetine
6. Sensitivity to anticholinergic side effects	6. Trazodone, fluoxetine, phenelzine, tranylcypromine, bupropion, sertraline, paroxetine
7. Orthostatic hypotension	7. Nortriptyline, bupropion, sertraline

From Preston, J., and Johnson, J. (1995). *Clinical psychopharmacology made ridiculously simple.* Miami, FL: MedMaster.

Note: Most antidepressants are quite toxic when taken in an overdose. Extreme caution should be taken in prescribing to high-risk suicidal patients. Of the existing antidepressants, trazodone appears to have the lowest degree of cardiotoxicity.

tipsychotic drugs and in clients who are rapid *cyclers.* A rapid cycler is a client with bipolar disorder who has many episodes of mood swings close together (four or more in 1 year) (see Chapter 21). People with schizophrenia (especially catatonia), those with schizoaffective syndromes, psychotic clients who are pregnant, and clients with Parkinson's disease can also benefit from ECT.

However, ECT is not necessarily effective in clients with dysthymic depressions or those with depression and personality disorders, those with drug dependence, or those with depression secondary to situational or social difficulties.

A usual course of ECT for a depressed client is 6 to 12 treatments given two or three times per week. Although no absolute contraindications to ECT exist, according to Fink (1992), several conditions have special risks that demand special attention and skill; these include clients with recent myocardial infarction, cerebrovascular accident, and cerebrovascular malformation or intracranial mass lesion. Clients with these high-risk conditions are usually not treated with ECT unless the need is compelling (Fink 1992).

THE PROCEDURE. The procedure is explained to the client, and informed consent must be obtained when voluntary clients are being treated. For involuntary clients, when informed consent cannot be obtained, permission may be obtained from the next of kin, although in some states treatment must be court ordered.

The client receives nothing by mouth after midnight, or at least 4 hours before treatment. Vital signs are taken, and the client is requested to void. Hairpins, contact lenses, and dentures are removed. Table 20–11 describes nursing care with clients before, during, and after ECT treatment.

POTENTIAL SIDE EFFECTS. The major side effects with bilateral treatments are confusion, disorientation, and short-term memory loss. On awakening, the client may be confused and disoriented. The nurse needs to orient the client frequently: "Mr. Taylor, you are in Mercy Hospital. It's 9 AM, and I will take you back to your room, where you will have breakfast." The client needs to be oriented frequently during the course of the treatments. Many people state that they have memory deficits for the first few weeks before and after the course of treatment. Memory usually recovers completely, although some clients have memory loss lasting up to 6 months (Burns and Stuart 1991). ECT is not a permanent cure for depression, and maintenance treatment with TCAs or lithium decreases the relapse rate. Maintenance ECT (once a month) may also help to decrease relapse rates for clients with recurrent depression.

Milieu Therapy (Basic Level)

When a person is acutely and severely depressed, hospitalization may be indicated. The depressed person needs protection from suicidal acts, a supervised environment for regulating antidepressant medications, and (when indicated) a course of ECT. Often, being removed from a stressful interpersonal situation in itself has therapeutic value. Hospitals have protocols regarding the care and protection of the suicidal client. Chapter 24 discusses the nurse's responsibility for providing a therapeutic environment that is structured to protect the client against self-inflicted harm. Table 20–12 provides nursing guidelines for a suicidal hospitalized client.

During the continuation phase of depression (4 to 9 months) and maintenance phase (≥1 years), people find that various short-term therapies—individual and group—are useful for dealing with the presence and aftermath of a major depressive episode. Numerous sup-

TABLE 20–11 NURSING CARE IN ELECTROCONVULSIVE THERAPY

1. Emotional and educational support to the client and family.	1a. Encourage the client to discuss feelings, including myths regarding ECT. 1b. Teach the client and the family what to expect with ECT.
2. Pretreatment protocol.	2a. Ascertain if the client and the family have received a full explanation, including the option to withdraw the consent at any time. 2b. **Pretreatment care:** ▸ Withhold food and fluids for 6 to 8 hours before treatment (cardiac medication is given with sips of water). ▸ Remove dentures, glasses, hearing aids, contact lenses, hairpins, and so on. ▸ Have client void before treatment. 2c. **Preoperative medications: (if ordered)** ▸ Give either glycopyrrolate (Robinul) or atropine to prevent potential for aspiration and to help minimize bradyarrhythmias in response to electrical stimulants.
3. Nursing care during the procedure.	3a. Place a blood pressure cuff on one of the client's arms. 3b. As the intravenous line is inserted and EEG and ECG electrodes are attached, give a brief explanation to the client. 3c. Clip the pulse oximeter to the client's finger. 3d. Monitor blood pressure throughout treatment. 3e. Medications given: ▸ Short-acting anesthetic (methohexital sodium [Brevital], thiopental [Pentothal]) ▸ Muscle relaxant (succinylcholine [Anectine]) ▸ 100% oxygen by mask via positive pressure throughout 3f. Check that the bite block is in place to prevent biting of the tongue. 3g. Electrical stimulus given (seizure should last 30–60 seconds).
4. Posttreatment nursing care	4a. Have the client go to a properly staffed recovery room (with blood pressure cuff and oximeter in place) where oxygen, suction, and other emergency equipment is available. 4b. Once the client is awake, talk to the client and check vital signs. 4c. Often the client is confused; give frequent orientation reassurance; orientation statements are brief, distinct, and simple. 4d. Return the client to the unit after he or she has maintained a 90% oxygen saturation level, vital signs are stable, and mental status is satisfactory. 4e. Check the gag reflex before giving the client fluids, medicine, or breakfast.

Data from Burns, C. M., and Stuart, G. W. (1991). Nursing care in electroconvulsive therapy. *Psychiatric Clinics of North America*, 14(4):971.
ECG, electrocardiographic; ECT, electroconvulsive therapy; EEG, electroencephalographic.

port groups may also prove extremely valuable; these include groups sponsored by the National Alliance for the Mentally Ill (NAMI) or bipolar support groups.

Psychotherapy (Advanced Practice)

No need!

Many modalities have been applied in the treatment of depression. However, studies have demonstrated that traditional psychotherapies (e.g., psychoanalytic psychotherapy) are only slightly more effective than placebos in reducing depressive symptoms (Beck and Young 1985). Most recently, there has been an increased emphasis on short-term therapies. Therapies that have received the most attention in outcome research include behavioral therapy, interpersonal psychotherapy, brief psychodynamic therapy, and cognitive therapy.

Interpersonal psychotherapy is a short-term psychological treatment of depression. It focuses on the role of the dysfunctional interpersonal relationships in the onset and perpetuation of depression. A study by Elkin and colleagues (1989), sponsored by the National Institute of Mental Health, found interpersonal psychotherapy to be highly effective in reducing depressive symptoms in depressed persons (Luby and Yalom 1992).

Cognitive therapy has been gaining momentum. The use of specific cognitive interventions has proved successful in individual therapy with depressed persons. Cognitive therapy for depression is brief, structured, and directive treatment designed to alter dysfunctional beliefs and the negative automatic thoughts that are typical of depression (Haaga and Beck 1992). Essentially, the depressed person learns

1. The connection between thoughts and feelings.
2. The negative thoughts typical of depression.
3. How different feelings can emerge when he or she is taught to think differently in the same circumstance (reframing).

A review of several studies (Haaga and Beck 1992) shows apparent prophylactic effects with cognitive therapy in depressed clients, especially those with unipolar depression, that is, people seem to learn something in cognitive therapy that is helpful after the acute phase of treatment, and this knowledge may help minimize a relapse.

TABLE 20–12 MILIEU INTERVENTION: ACUTELY DEPRESSED/SUICIDAL CLIENT

INTERVENTION	RATIONALE
Nursing Diagnosis: High risk for self-harm related to hopelessness and inability to find solution for overwhelming psychic pain, as evidenced by covert or overt clues	
1. Assess the client for overt and covert suicide clues.	1. A high percentage of depressed people have suicidal thoughts.
2. Ask the client directly, "Have you thought of killing yourself?"	2. Often, the client is relieved to talk to someone else about these thoughts. Talking about this can minimize painful feelings of isolation and loneliness.
3. Assess the lethality of the suicide plan.	3. If the method is highly lethal (e.g., gun or hanging) and readily available and if the plan is well thought out, the risk is extremely high.
4. Assess the high-risk factors.	4. Assessing risk factors can help determine suicidal risk.
5. Remove all potentially harmful objects from the environment (e.g., belts, straps, ties, sharp objects, glass).	5. Client safety is a nursing priority.
6. If the client is suicidal, place the client on a one-to-one suicide precaution, following hospital protocol.	6. Constant one-to-one observation of the suicidal client can maximize client safety. *Always follow hospital protocol.*
7. Form a written no-suicide contract with the client, such as "I will not kill myself during the next 8 hours." Then renegotiate the contract at that time.	7. Because suicide is often an ambivalent solution, the nurse stresses life-affirming considerations.
8. Secure the promise that the client will seek out a staff member if or when suicidal thoughts emerge or become overpowering.	8. Because people who are suicidal have "tunnel vision," discussing feelings, fears, and any alternatives can lower anxiety and may help the client put events in a more favorable perspective.

Behavioral therapy has also gained some recognition for success in the treatment of depression. Behavioral therapy attempts to teach depressed people effective social and coping skills that increase positive reinforcements from other people and the environment; behavioral therapy also attempts to decrease the number of negative interactions. The treatment program is highly structured and is generally short term. Behaviorists believe that altering personal behavior is the most effective way to change depressed thoughts and feelings (Hirschfeld and Shea 1995).

The cognitive and behavioral approaches to therapy are thought to be at least as effective as TCA therapy, although pharmacological treatment remains the standard against which all other treatments are judged (Beck and Young 1985). The National Institute of Mental Health has research showing that the combination of drug therapy and psychotherapy is more effective than either treatment alone.

Group treatment is a widespread modality for the treatment of depression. One advantage of group treatment is that it increases the number of people who can receive treatment at a decreased individual cost. A second advantage is that groups increase clients' socialization and offer people an opportunity to share common feelings and concerns, thereby decreasing feelings of isolation. Support from other group members can lessen feelings of hopelessness and helplessness. A widely used model for outpatient group treatment is fashioned after Beck's cognitive theory of depression (Luby and Yalom 1992).

Another popular group approach is *interactional group therapy*. In this type of therapy, groups consist of clients with different types of disorders. The therapist in this setting focuses on the here and now. Maladaptive behaviors displayed within the group are interpreted as the kinds of psychopathology the person displays in his or her outside relationships. Therefore, the target of treatment is not the depression itself but rather the interpersonal manifestations of the disorder (Luby and Yalom 1992).

EVALUATION

The short-term and long-term goals are frequently evaluated. For example, if the client comes into the unit with suicidal thoughts, the nurse evaluates whether suicidal thoughts are still present, whether the depressed person is able to state alternatives to suicidal impulses in the future, whether he or she is able to explore thoughts and feelings that precede suicidal impulses, and so forth. Goals relating to thought processes, self-esteem, and social interactions are frequently formulated because these areas are often problematic in people who are depressed. Physical needs warrant nursing or medical attention. If a person has lost weight because of anorexia, is the appetite returning? If a person was constipated, are the bowels now functioning normally? If the person was suffering from insomnia, is he or she now getting 6 to 8 hours of sleep per night?

If the goals have not been met, an analysis of the data, nursing diagnoses, goals, and planned nursing interventions is made. The care plan is reassessed and reformulated when necessary.

Text continued on page 586

CASE STUDY: WORKING WITH A PERSON WHO IS DEPRESSED

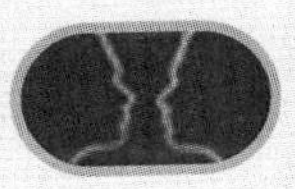

Mrs. Olston is a 35-year-old executive secretary. She has been divorced for 3 years and has two sons, 11 and 13 years of age. She is brought into the emergency department (ED) by her neighbor. She has some superficial slashes on her wrists and is bleeding. The neighbor states that both of Mrs. Olston's sons are visiting their father for the summer. Mrs. Olston has become more and more despondent after terminating a 2-year relationship with a married man 4 weeks ago. According to the neighbor, for 3 years after her divorce, Mrs. Olston talked constantly about not being pretty or good enough and doubted that anyone could really love her. The neighbor states that Mrs. Olston has been withdrawn for at least 3 years. After the relationship with her boyfriend ended, she became even more withdrawn and sullen. Mrs. Olston is about 20 pounds overweight, and her neighbor states that Mrs. Olston often stays awake late into the night, drinking by herself and watching television. She sleeps through most of the day on the weekends.

After receiving treatment in the ED, Mrs. Olston is seen by a psychiatrist. The initial diagnosis is dysthymia with suicidal ideation. Although the physician does not think that Mrs. Olston is acutely suicidal at this time, a decision is made to hospitalize her briefly for suicide observation and evaluation for appropriate treatment.

The nurse, Mrs. Weston, admits Mrs. Olston to the unit from the ED.

Nurse: Hello, Mrs. Olston, I'm Marcia Weston. I will be your primary nurse.
Mrs. Olston: Yeah . . . I don't need a nurse, a doctor, or anyone else. I just want to get away from this pain.
Nurse: You want to get away from your pain?
Mrs. Olston: I just said that, didn't I? Oh, what's the use. No one understands.
Nurse: I would like to understand, Mrs. Olston.
Mrs. Olston: Look at me. I'm fat . . . ugly . . . and no good to anyone. No one wants me.
Nurse: Who doesn't want you?
Mrs. Olston: My husband didn't want me . . . and now Jerry left me to go back to his wife.
Nurse: You think because Jerry went back to his wife that no one else could care for you?
Mrs. Olston: Well . . . he doesn't anyway.
Nurse: Because he doesn't care, you believe that no one else cares about you?
Mrs. Olston: Yes . . .
Nurse: Who do you care about?
Mrs. Olston: No one . . . except my sons . . . I do love my sons, even though I don't often show it.
Nurse: Tell me more about your sons.

Mrs. Weston continues to speak with Mrs. Olston. Mrs. Olston talks about her sons with some affect and apparent affection; however, she continues to state that she does not think of herself as worthwhile.

ASSESSMENT

The nurse divides the data into objective and subjective components.

OBJECTIVE DATA

1. Slashed her wrists.
2. Recently broke off with boyfriend.
3. Has thought poorly of herself for 3 years, since divorce.
4. Has two sons she cares about.
5. Is 20 pounds overweight.
6. Stays awake late at night, drinking by herself.
7. Has been withdrawn since divorce.

Continued on following page

CASE STUDY: WORKING WITH A PERSON WHO IS DEPRESSED *(Continued)*

SUBJECTIVE DATA

1. "No one could ever love me."
2. "I'm not good enough."
3. "I just want to get rid of this pain."
4. "I'm fat and ugly . . . no good to anyone."
5. "I do love my sons, although I don't always show it."

NURSING DIAGNOSIS

The nurse evaluates Mrs. Olston's strengths and weaknesses, and decides to concentrate on two initial nursing diagnoses that seem to have the highest priority.

1. **Risk for self-directed violence** related to separation from 2-year relationship, as evidenced by actual suicide attempt
   - Slashed her wrists.
   - Recently broke off with boyfriend.
   - Drinks at night by herself.
   - Withdrawn for 3 years, since divorce.
2. **Disturbance in self-esteem** related to divorce and recent termination of love relationship, as evidenced by derogatory statements about self
   - "I'm not good enough."
   - "No one could ever love me."
   - "I'm fat and ugly . . . no good to anyone."
   - "I do love my sons, although I don't always show it."

PLANNING

PLANNING OUTCOME CRITERIA

Because Mrs. Olston is acutely suicidal, she is put on suicide precautions (see Chapter 24 for suicide precaution protocol). The nurse devises the following outcome criteria and short-term goals with some input from Mrs. Olston.

NURSING DIAGNOSIS	OUTCOME CRITERIA	SHORT-TERM GOALS
1. **Risk for self-directed violence** related to separation from 2-year relationship, as evidenced by actual suicide attempt	1. Client will remain safe.	1a. Client will state she has a reason to live by (date). 1b. Client will state two alternative actions she can take when feeling suicidal in the future.
2. **Disturbance in self-esteem** related to divorce and recent termination of love relationship, as evidenced by derogatory statements about self	2. By discharge, client will identify a plan to deal with her poor self-esteem.	2. By (date), client will name two things she would like to change about herself.

Because Mrs. Olston was discharged after 48 hours, the *disturbance in self-esteem* issue is continued in her therapy after discharge. Mrs. Weston later reviews the goals for her work with Mrs. Olston in the community. See Nursing Care Plan 20–1.

NURSE'S FEELINGS AND SELF-ASSESSMENT

Ms. Weston is aware that when clients are depressed, they can be negative, think life is hopeless, and be hostile toward those who want to help. When Ms. Weston was new to the unit, she withdrew from depressed clients and sought out clients who appeared more hopeful and appreciative of her efforts. The unit coordinator was very supportive of Ms. Weston when she was first on the unit. Ms. Weston, along with other staff, was sent to in-service education sessions on working with depressed clients, and was encouraged to speak up in staff meetings about the feelings that many of these depressed clients evoke in her. As a primary nurse, she was

CASE STUDY: WORKING WITH A PERSON WHO IS DEPRESSED *(Continued)*

now assigned a variety of clients. She found that as time went on, with the support of her peers and the opportunity to speak up at staff meetings, she was able to take what clients said less personally and not feel so responsible when clients did not respond as fast as she would like. After 2 years, she had had the experience of seeing many clients who seemed hopeless and despondent on admission respond well to nursing and medical interventions, and go on to lead full and satisfying lives. This also made it easier for Ms. Weston to understand that even though the client may think that life is hopeless and may believe that there is nothing in life to live for, change is always possible.

INTERVENTION

Mrs. Olston is put on 24-hour suicide precautions. She appears to respond positively to the attention from the nurses, as well as to that from some of the other clients on the unit. She tells the nurse that since her divorce, she has become more withdrawn and has stopped socializing with others and participating in her usual outside activities. Her married boyfriend never took her out, and together they did not share any social activities. Just being around people who seemed interested in her made her feel better. After 2 days, Mrs. Olston says that she really did not want to kill herself.

Mrs. Olston agrees that she will try therapy when she is discharged, because she wants her life to change.

The following Monday, she starts therapy with Mr. Wiley, a nurse clinical specialist at the community health center near Mrs. Olston's home.

During therapy sessions, Mr. Wiley uses various cognitive therapy approaches with Mrs. Olston. She is encouraged to look at her life and herself differently, to assess her strengths, and to identify those things she values. The therapist assists Mrs. Olston in questioning and changing inaccurate thoughts and beliefs she holds toward herself and her future. He first assists Mrs. Olston in learning new behaviors to cope with her loneliness, lack of motivation, and negative thinking. Mr. Wiley also works with Mrs. Olston to help her get her needs met through more assertive behavior.

With the encouragement of Mr. Wiley, Mrs. Olston schedules activities throughout her day. A record of these activities will be kept by the client and discussed with Mr. Wiley at the following session. The nurse also role plays with Mrs. Olston some of the new behaviors she is learning in her therapy sessions (see Nursing Care Plan 20–1).

EVALUATION

During the course of her work with Mr. Wiley, Mrs. Olston decides to go to some meetings of Parents Without Partners. She states that she is looking forward to getting back to work and feels much more hopeful about her life. She has also lost 3 pounds while attending Weight Watchers. She states, "I need to get back into the world."

Although Mrs. Olston still has negative thoughts about herself, she admits to feeling much better about herself, and she has learned important tools to deal with her negative cognitions.

NURSING CARE PLAN 20–1 A PERSON WITH DEPRESSION: MRS. OLSTON

NURSING DIAGNOSIS (Hospital Focus)

Risk for self-violence: related to separation from two-year relationship, as evidenced by suicide attempt

Supporting Data

- Slashed her wrists.
- Recently broke off with boyfriend.
- Withdrawn for 3 years since divorce.
- Drinks at night by herself.
- "I just want to die."

Outcome Criteria: Client will remain safe while in the hospital

SHORT-TERM GOAL	INTERVENTION	RATIONALE	EVALUATION
1. Client will state she has a reason to live by (date).	1a. Observe the client every 15 minutes while she is suicidal. 1b. Remove all dangerous objects from the client.	1a,b. Ensures client safety. Minimizes impulsive self-harmful behavior.	GOAL MET By the end of the second day, Mrs. Olsten states she really did not want to die, she just couldn't stand the loneliness in her life.
	1c. Spend regularly scheduled periods of time with the client throughout the day.	1c. Reinforces that she is worth-while; builds up experience to begin to better relate to nurse on one-to-one basis.	
	1d. Assist the client in evaluating the positive as well as the negative aspects of her life.	1d. A depressed person is often unable to acknowledge any positive aspects of her life unless they are pointed out by others.	
	1e. Encourage the appropriate expression of angry feelings.	1e. Providing for expression of pent-up hostility in a safe environment can reinforce more adaptive methods of releasing tension and may minimize the need to act out self-directed anger.	
	1f. Accept the client's negativism.	1f. Acceptance enhances feelings of self-worth.	
2. Client will state two alternative actions she can take when feeling suicidal in the future.	2a. Explore usual coping behaviors.	2a. Identifies behaviors that need reinforcing and new coping skills that need to be introduced.	GOAL MET By discharge, Mrs. Olsten states that she is definitely going to try cognitive-behavior therapy. She also discusses joining a women's support group that meets once a week in a neighboring town.
	2b. Assist the client in identifying members of her support system.	2b. Evaluate strengths and weaknesses in the support available.	

NURSING CARE PLAN 20–1 A PERSON WITH DEPRESSION: MRS. OLSTON *(Continued)*

SHORT-TERM GOAL	INTERVENTION	RATIONALE	EVALUATION
	2c. Suggest a number of community-based support groups she might wish to discuss or visit (e.g., hotlines, support groups, women's groups).	2c. The client needs to be aware of community supports in order to use them.	
	2d. Assist the client in identifying realistic alternatives that she is willing to use.	2d. Unless the client is in agreement with any plan, she will be unable or unwilling to follow through in a crisis.	

NURSING DIAGNOSIS (Goals revised by Mr. Wiley for community treatment)

Disturbance in self-esteem: related to divorce and recent termination of love relationship, as evidenced by derogatory statements about self

Supporting Data

- "I'm not good enough."
- "No one could ever love me."
- "I'm fat and ugly . . . no good to anyone."
- "I do love my sons, although I don't always show it."

Outcome Criteria: At the end of therapy, patient will learn coping skills do deal with depression.

SHORT-TERM GOAL	INTERVENTION	RATIONALE	EVALUATION
1. Client will evidence two positive changes in her thinking and behavior.	1a. Assist the client in identifying two realistic things about herself that she would like to change.	1a. Helps the client to problem-solve in two important areas of her life that are amenable to change.	GOAL MET By the end of treatment, Mrs. Olsten demonstrates ■ Ability to reform negative thoughts ■ Involvement with two community groups ■ Increased assertiveness in getting her needs met.
	1b. Work with the client to identify the various steps needed to help make these changes come about.	1b. Depressed clients often have difficulty solving problems because of poor concentration and faulty judgment.	
	1c. Identify specific skills the client might need to attain her goals, e.g. ■ Assertiveness training. ■ More effective communication skills. ■ Tension-reducing activities.	1c. Identifying and teaching more effective coping skills can increase perception of control and decrease feelings of hopelessness.	
	1d. Role-play new coping skills with client.	1d. Aids in incorporating new skills into more automatic behavior.	

Continued on following page

NURSING CARE PLAN 20–1 A PERSON WITH DEPRESSION: MRS. OLSTON *(Continued)*

SHORT-TERM GOAL	INTERVENTION	RATIONALE	EVALUATION
	1e. Encourage participation in community group activities.	1e. Increases arena in which client can gain positive reinforcement.	
	1f. Assist client in planning a structured daily routine.	1f. Reduces time spent in negative rumination and helps client in thinking more in terms of goal directedness.	

SUMMARY

Depression is probably the most commonly seen mental disorder in the health care system. The two primary depressive disorders are *major depressive disorder* and *dysthymia*. The symptoms in a major depression are usually severe enough to interfere with a person's social or occupational functioning. A person with major depressive disorder may or may not have psychotic symptoms, and the symptoms a person usually exhibits during a major depression are different from the characteristics of the normal premorbid personality.

In dysthymia, the symptoms are often chronic (lasting ≥2 years) and are considered mild to moderate. Usually, a person's social or occupational functioning is not greatly impaired. The symptoms in a dysthymic depression are often congruent with the person's usual pattern of functioning.

Many theories about the cause of depression exist. Four common theories are psychophysiological theory, cognitive theory, learned helplessness theory, and psychoanalytic theory.

Nursing assessment includes the assessment of affect, thought processes, feelings, physical behavior, and communication. The nurse also needs to be aware of the symptoms that mask depression.

Nursing diagnoses can be numerous. Depressed individuals are always evaluated for risk for self-directed violence. Some other common nursing diagnoses are altered thought processes, self-esteem disturbance, altered nutrition, bowel elimination, sleep pattern disturbance, ineffective individual coping, and ineffective family coping.

Working with people who are depressed can evoke intense feelings of hopelessness and frustration in health care workers. Initially, nurses need support and guidance to clarify realistic expectations of themselves and their clients and to sort out personal feelings from those communicated by the client via empathy. Peer supervision and individual supervision with an experienced nurse clinician or a psychiatric social worker or psychologist is useful in increasing therapeutic potential.

Interventions with clients who are depressed involve several approaches. The nurse intervenes therapeutically, using specific principles of communication, planning activities of daily living, administering or participating in somatic therapies, maintaining a therapeutic environment, and teaching clients about the biochemical aspects of depression.

Many short-term therapies have been found to be effective in the treatment of depression:

1. Interpersonal therapies
2. Cognitive therapy
3. Behavioral therapy
4. Some forms of group therapy

Evaluation is ongoing throughout the nursing process, and the client's outcomes are compared with the stated outcome criteria and short-term goals. The care plan is revised throughout the client's hospital stay by use of the evaluation process.

Self-study exercises 22–58 help the student review the material discussed in this section.

REFERENCES

Abraham I. L., Neese J. B., and Westerman, P. S. (1991). Nursing implications of a clinical and social problem. *Nursing Clinics of North America*, 26(3):527.

Akiskal, H. S. (1995). Mood disorders: Introduction and overview. In H. I. Kaplan and B. J. Sadock (Eds.), *Comprehensive textbook of psychiatry IV* (Vol. 1, pp. 1067–1078). Baltimore: Williams & Wilkins.

Alford, J. W., and Catlin, G. (1993). The role of culture in grief. *Journal of Social Psychology*, 133(2):173.

American Psychiatric Association (1990). *The practice of electroconvulsive therapy: Recommendations for treatment, training and privileges*. Washington, DC: American Psychiatric Association.

Azhar, M. Z. , and Varma, S. L. (1995). The religious psychotherapy as management of bereavement. *Acta Psychiatrica Scandinavica*, 91(4):233.

Beasley, C. M., et al. (1993). Possible monoamine oxidase inhibitor-serotonin uptake inhibitor interaction: Fluoxetine clinical data and preclinical findings. *Journal of Clinical Psychopharmacology*, 13:312.

Bech, P. (1992). Symptoms and assessment of depression. In E. S. Paykel (Ed.), *Handbook of affective disorders* (2nd ed.). New York: Guilford Press.

Beck, A. T., and Ruch, A. J. (1995). Cognitive therapy. In H. I. Kaplan and B. J. Sadock (Eds.), *Comprehensive textbook of psychiatry IV* (Vol. 2, pp. 1847–1856). Baltimore: Williams & Wilkins.

Beck, A. T., and Young, J. E. (1985). Depression. In D. H. Barlow (Ed.), *Clinical handbook of psychological disorders*. New York: Guilford Press.

Benton, R. G. (1978). *Death and dying: Principles and practices in patient care.* New York: Van Nostrand.

Bowlby, J. (1961). Separation anxiety: A critical review of the literature. *Journal of Child Psychology and Psychiatry*, 1:251.

Bowlby, J., and Parkes, C. (1970). Separation and loss within the family. In E. J. Anthony and C. Koupernik (Eds.), Child in his family. New York: John Wiley.

Burns, C. M., and Stuart, G. W. (1991). Nursing care in electroconvulsive therapy. *Psychiatric Clinics of North America*, 14(4):971.

Calarco, M. M., and Krone, K. P. (1991). An integrated nursing model of depressive behavior in adults: Theory and implementation. *Nursing Clinics of North America*, 26(3):573.

Campbell, L. (1987). Hopelessness. *Journal of Psychosocial Nursing*, 25(2):18.

Carr, A. L. (1985). Grief, mourning, and bereavement. In H. I. Kaplan and B. J. Sadock (Eds.), *Comprehensive textbook of psychiatry* (4th ed.). Baltimore: Williams & Wilkins.

Cartwright, R. D., et al. (1991). REM latency and the recovery from depression: Getting over divorce. *American Journal of Psychiatry*, 148(11):1530.

Corr, C. A., and Doka, K. J. (1994). Current models of death, dying and bereavement. *Critical Care Nursing Clinics of North America*, 6(3):545.

Corr, C. A. (1993). Coping with dying: Lessons that we should and should not learn from the work of Elizabeth Kübler-Ross. *Death Studies*, 17:69.

Davidson, J. R. T. (1992). Monoamine oxidase inhibitors. In E. S. Paykel (Ed.), *Handbook of affective disorders* (2nd ed.) (pp. 345–358). New York: Guilford Press.

Davis, J. M., et al. (1992). The effects of a support group on grieving individuals' level of perceived support and stress. *Archives of Psychiatric Nursing*, 6(1):35.

Delgado, P. L., et al. (1992). Neurochemistry. In E. S. Paykel (Ed.), *Handbook of affective disorders* (2nd ed.) (pp. 219–254). New York: Guilford Press.

Devanand, D. P., et al. (1991). Electroconvulsive therapy in the treatment-resistant patient. *Psychiatric Clinics of North America*, 14(4):905.

Dryman, A., and Eaton, W. W. (1991). Affective symptoms associated with the onset of major depression in the community: Findings from the US National Institute of Mental Health. *Acta Psychiatrica Scandinavica*, 84(1):1.

Dubovsky, S. L. (1995). Electroconvulsive therapy. In H. I. Kaplan and B. J. Sadock (Eds.), *Comprehensive textbook of psychiatry IV* (Vol. 2, pp. 2129–2139). Baltimore: Williams & Wilkins.

Elkin, I., et al. (1989). 1989 National Institute of Mental Health treatment of depression collaborative research program. *Archives of General Psychiatry*, 46:971.

Engel, G. L. (1964). Grief and grieving. *American Journal of Nursing*, 64(9):93.

Feldstein, M. A., and Gemma, P. B. (1995). Oncology nurses and chronic compounded grief. *Cancer Nursing*, 18(3):228.

Fink, M. (1992). Electroconvulsive therapy. In E. S. Paykel (Ed.), *Handbook of affective disorders* (2nd ed.) (pp. 359–368). New York: Guilford Press.

Gabbard, G. O. (1995). Mood disorders: Psychodynamic etiology. In H. I. Kaplan and B. J. Sadock (Eds.), *Comprehensive textbook of psychiatry IV* (Vol. 1, pp. 1116–1123). Baltimore: Williams & Wilkins.

Golden, R. N., et al. (1995). Trazodone and other antidepressants. In A. F. Schatzberg and C. B. Nemeroff (Eds.), *The American psychiatric press textbook of psychopharmacology* (pp. 195–214). Washington, DC: American Psychiatric Press.

Goodwin, F. K. (1982). *Depression and manic-depressive illness.* Bethesda, MD: U. S. Department of Health and Human Services, National Institute of Mental Health.

Greden, J. (1995). *Better outcomes with difficult cases.* Presented at U. S. Psychiatric and Mental Health Congress, Marriot Marquis, New York, November 17, 1995.

Green, A. G., et al. (1995). Mood disorders: Biochemical aspects. In H. I. Kaplan and B. J. Sadock (Eds.), *Comprehensive textbook of psychiatry IV* (Vol. 1, pp. 1089–1102). Baltimore: Williams & Wilkins.

Gregory, R. J. (1994). Grief and loss among Eskimos attempting suicide in western Alaska. *American Journal of Psychiatry*, 15(12):1815.

Gulesserian, B., and Warren, C. J. (1987). Coping resources of depressed patients. *Archives of Psychiatric Nursing*, 1(6):392.

Haaga, D. F, and Beck, A. T. (1992). Cognitive therapy. In E. S. Paykel (Ed.), *Handbook of affective disorders* (2nd ed.) (pp. 511–524). New York: Guilford Press.

Hallon, S. D., and Fawcett, J. (1995). Combined medication and psychotherapy. In G. O. Gabbard (Ed.), *Treatment of psychiatric disorders* (2nd ed., Vol. 1, pp. 1221–1263). Washington, DC: American Psychiatric Press.

Hirschfeld, R. M. A., and Shea, M. (1995). Mood disorders: Psychological treatment. In H. I. Kaplan and B. J. Sadock (Eds.), *Comprehensive textbook of psychiatry IV* (Vol. 1, pp. 1178–1190). Baltimore: Williams & Wilkins.

Keller, M. (1995). Depression in adults. Presented at the U. S. Psychiatric and Mental Health Congress, Marriot Marquis, New York, November 18, 1995.

Kupfer, D. J. (1991). Long-term treatment in depression. *Journal of Clinical Psychiatry*, 32:(Suppl.)28–34.

Lader, M. H. (1996). Tolerability and safety: Essentials in antidepressant pharmacology. *Journal of Clinical Psychiatry*, 57(2):39.

Lauer, C. J., et al. (1995). In the quest of identifying vulnerability markers for psychiatric disorders by all-night polysomnography. *Archives of General Psychiatry*, 52(2):145.

Lehne, R. A., et al. (1994). *Pharmacology of nursing* (2nd ed.). Philadelphia: W. B. Saunders.

Lindemann, E. (1944). Symptomatology and management of acute grief. *The American Journal of Psychiatry*, 101:141.

Litman, R. E. (1992) Predicting and preventing hospital suicides. In R. W. Maris, et al. (Eds.), *Assessment and prediction of suicide.* New York: Guilford Press.

Lloyd-Williams, M. (1995). Bereavement referrals to a psychiatric service: An audit. *European Journal of Cancer Care*, 4(1):17.

Luby, J. L., and Yalom, I. D. (1992). Group therapy. In E. S. Paykel (Ed.), *Handbook of affective disorders* (2nd ed.) (pp. 475–486). New York: Guilford Press.

Marks, M. J. (1976). The grieving patient and family. *American Journal of Nursing*, 76:1488.

Maxmen, J. S., and Ward, N. G. (1995). *Psychotropic drugs fast facts* (2nd ed.). New York: W. W. Norton.

Mendelson, M. (1992). Psychodynamics. In E. S. Paykel (Ed.), *Handbook of affective disorders* (2nd ed.) (pp. 195–208). New York: Guilford Press.

Merikangas, K. R., and Kupfer, D. J. (1995) Mood disorders: Genetic aspects. In H. I. Kaplan and B. J. Sadock (Eds.), *Comprehensive textbook of psychiatry IV* (Vol. 1, pp. 1102–1116). Baltimore: Williams & Wilkins.

Middleton, W., and Raphael, B. (1992). Bereavement. In E. S. Paykel (Ed.), *Handbook of affective disorders* (2nd ed.) (pp. 619–634). New York: Guilford Press.

Nurnberger, J. I., Jr, and Gershon, E. S. (1992). Genetics. In E. S. Paykel (Ed.), *Handbook of affective disorders* (2nd ed.) (pp. 131–148). New York: Guilford Press.

Parker, G. (1992). Early environment. In E. S. Paykel (Ed.), *Handbook of affective disorders* (2nd ed.) (pp. 171–184). New York: Guilford Press.

Post, R. (1995). Mood disorders: Somatic treatment. In H. I. Kaplan and B. J. Sadock (Eds.), *Comprehensive textbook of psychiatry IV* (Vol. 1, pp. 1152–1177). Baltimore: Williams & Wilkins.

Preston, J., and Johnson, J. (1995). *Clinical psychopharmacology made ridiculously simple.* Miami: MedMaster.

Rakoff, V. M. (1973). Psychiatric aspects of death in America. In A. Mack (Ed.), *Death in American experience.* New York: Schocken Books.

Ripley, H. S. (1977). Depression and the life span epidemiology. In D. Usdin (Ed.), *Depression: Clinical, biological and psychological perspectives*. New York: Brunner-Mazel.

Robinson, D. S., et al. (1996a). The safety of nefazodone. *Journal of Clinical Psychiatry*, 57(2):31.

Robinson, D. S., et al. (1996b). Therapeutic drug range of nefazodone in the treatment of depression. *Journal of Clinical Psychiatry*, 57(2):6.

Saunders, J. M., and Valente, S. M. (1994). Nurse' grief. *Cancer Nursing*, 17(4):318.

Schatzberg, A. F., and Cole, J. O. (1991). *Manual of clinical psychopharmacology* (2nd ed.). Washington, DC: American Psychiatric Press.

Schatzberg, A. F, and Rothschild, A. J. (1992). Psychiatric (delusional) major depression: Should it be included as a distinct syndrome in DSM-IV? *American Jorrnal of Psychiatry*, 149(6):733.

Seligman, M. E. (1973). Fall into hopelessness. *Psychology Today*, 7:43.

Styron, W. (1990). *Darkness visible: A memoir of madness.* New York: Random House.

Tollefson, G. D. (1995). Selective serotonin reuptake inhibitors. In A. F. Schatzberg and C. B. Nemeroff (Eds.), *The American psychiatric press textbook of psychopharmacology* (pp. 161–182). Washington, DC: American Psychiatric Press.

U. S. Department of Health and Human Services, Public Health Service, Agency for Health Care and Research (1993). *Depression in primary care: Detection, diagnosis, and treatment.* Washington, DC: U. S. Department of Health and Human Services.

Wyeth-Ayerst Laboratories (1995). *Effexor: Venlafaxine HCL.* Pearl River, NY: Wyeth-Ayerst Laboratories.

Worden, J. W. (1991). *Grief counseling and grief therapy: A handbook for the mental health practitioner* (2nd ed.). New York: Springer.

Zajecka, J. (1995a). *Treatment strategies for depression complicated by anxiety disorder.* Presented at the U. S. Psychiatric and Mental Health Congress, Marriot Marquis, New York, November 16, 1995.

Zisook, S., and Shuchter. (1992). Depression through the first year after the death of a spouse. *American Journal of Psychiatry*, 148(10):1346.

Further Reading

American Psychiatric Association (1994). *Diagnostic and statistical manual of mental disorders* (4th ed.). Washington, DC: American Psychiatric Association.

Buckwalter, K. C., and Abraham, I. L. (1987). Alleviating the discharge crisis: The effects of cognitive-behavioral nursing intervention for depressed patients and their families. *Archives of Psychiatric Nursing*, 1(5):350.

Charney, D. S., et al. (1995). Treatment of depression. In A. F. Schatzberg and C. B. Nemeroff (Eds.), *The American psychiatric press textbook of psychopharmacology* (pp. 575–602). Washington, DC: American Psychiatric Press.

Delgado, P. L., and Gelenberg, A. J. (1995). Antidepressant and antimanic medications. In G. O. Gabbard (Ed.), *Treatment of psychiatric disorders* (2nd ed., Vol. 1, pp. 1131–1168). Washington, DC: American Psychiatric Press.

Hirschfeld, R. M. A., and Goodwin, F. K. (1988). Mood disorders. In J. A. Talbott, R. E. Hales and S. C. Yudofsky (Eds.), *Textbook of psychiatry*. Washington, DC: American Psychiatric Press.

Kaplan, H. I, and Sadock, B. J. (1991). *Synopsis of psychiatry: Behavioral sciences and clinical psychiatry* (6th ed.). Baltimore: Williams & Wilkins.

Krishman, K. R. R. (1995). Monoamine oxidase inhibitors. In A. F. Schatzberg and C. B. Nemeroff (Eds.), *The American psychiatric press textbook of psychopharmacology* (pp. 183–194). Washington, DC: American Psychiatric Press.

Krupnick, S. L. W. (1996). Antidepressant medications. In S. Lego (Ed.), *Psychiatric Nursing* (2nd ed.) (pp. 525–531). Philadelphia: J. B. Lippincott.

Lesse, S. (1983). The masked depression syndrome: Results of a seventeen year clinical study. *American Journal of Psychotherapy*, 37:456.

Oren, D. A., and Rosenthal, N. E. (1992). Seasonal affective disorder. In E. S. Paykel (Ed.), *Handbook of affective disorders* (2nd ed.) (pp. 551–568). New York: Guilford Press.

Potter, W. Z., et al. (1995). Tricyclics and tetracyclics. In A. F. Schatzberg and C. B. Nemeroff (Eds.), *The American psychiatric press textbook of psychopharmacology* (pp. 141–160). Washington, DC: American Psychiatric Press.

Rush, J. R., and Kanthol, R. (1995). Strategies and tactics in the treatment of depression. In G. O. Gabbard (Ed.), *Treatment of psychiatric disorders* (2nd ed., Vol. 1, pp. 1349–1411). Washington, DC: American Psychiatric Press.

Zajecka, J. (1995b). *Emergency problems in managing mood disorders*. Presented at the U. S. Psychiatric and Mental Health Congress, Marriot Marquis, New York, November 16, 1995.

SELF-STUDY AND CRITICAL THINKING

GRIEF

Identify the phase of grief (shock, developing awareness, restitution) occurring in the acute stage of mourning.

1. ________ A person begins to feel intense feelings of anguish and despair. Anger, guilt, and crying are common at this phase.
2. ________ A person gathers together with family and friends in rituals of saying good-bye and ending the last remnants of denial.
3. ________ A person is not capable of emotionally accepting the intense feelings of pain and may have difficulty accepting the fact of death or may intellectualize feelings instead of feeling them.

True or false

Correct the false statements.

4. ________ Completing the work of mourning takes 4 to 8 weeks.
5. ________ Being with a person who is grieving can bring up one's own feelings of loss and sadness.
6. ________ Nurses have minimal difficulties dealing with people who are grieving and dying because they are around death so often.

The following are examples of the normal phenomena experienced during the mourning process. Match the example from the left column with the expected phenomenon from the right column.

7. ________ "If his brother had not been so hard on him, he would not have had the heart attack."

8. ________ There were so many things I wanted to tell him . . . how much he meant to me. I should have said more kind things."

9. ________ "It sounds silly, but I am having difficulty swallowing, just the way John did before he died."

10. ________ "I just can't do anything . . . everything is so confusing. I don't even feel like eating or dressing."

11. ________ "Thoughts and memories just keep popping into my head . . . everything I see or do reminds me of the things we used to do together, everything."

12. ________ "I am thinking of resuming typing lessons . . . last night was the first night in a long time that I went to bingo at church."

A. Sensations of somatic distress
B. Preoccupation with the deceased
C. Guilt
D. Anger
E. Disorganization and depression
F. Reorganization behavior

Evaluate the work of mourning as successful (S) or unsuccessful (U).

13. ________ "She was so strong. Why, I don't even think she cried the whole time—went through the whole process with a 'stiff upper lip.'"

14. ________ "She was a wreck when her sister died. Cried and carried on . . . why, it took her a year or more before she returned to church duties with any zest and started doing things again."

15. ________ "You know, Sid still talks about his mother as if she were alive today—weeps every time he talks about her. Well . . . she's been dead for 4 years."

16. ________ "I remember the good times we had together, but we had our rough times too before she died."

Multiple choice

17. Regina, a 24-year-old woman whose mother has just died a painful death from cancer, tells the nurse tearfully she does not think she will ever get over her mother's death. Which of the following would be the most appropriate response for the nurse to make?

    A. "Time heals all wounds, and yours will heal in time also."
    B. "It was the best thing that could happen to her; she was in so much pain."
    C. "The loss must be very painful for you."
    D. "The hardest part will be the next couple of months. In a year you will feel fine again."

18. Three of the following are factors that could interfere with Regina's successful resolution of the grief process. Which factor would facilitate the mourning process?
    A. Regina said that she loved her mother but that so often their relationship was stormy; at other times she stated that she hated her mother.
    B. Regina had lost her job 2 months before, and she and her husband had recently separated.
    C. Regina had always been a good problem solver, and she had many friends whom she counted on as a sounding board and for support.
    D. Regina was always complaining of physical illnesses, and 2 months ago, she was hospitalized with hepatitis.

List three nursing actions that can facilitate a family's grieving process (see Table 20–2).

19. ______________________________

20. ______________________________

21. ______________________________

DEPRESSIVE DISORDERS

Indicate whether the following are most likely characteristic of a major depression (MD) or a dysthymic depression (D).

22. ________ May have psychotic symptoms.

23. ________ Usually has a chronic course of 2 years or more.

24. ________ The symptoms are *not* congruent with the person's premorbid personality.

25. ________ Usually considered mild to moderate. The symptoms do not greatly interfere with the person's occupational or interpersonal functioning.

Identify the corresponding theoretical approach: P (psychoanalytic), C (cognitive), B (biological), or L (learned helplessness).

26. ________ The success of the tricyclic antidepressants (TCAs) and the monoamine oxidase inhibitors (MAOIs) helps to support this theory.

27. ________ Thoughts can affect a person's mood.

28. ________ Loss and aggression turned against the self are two of the basic components of this theory.

29. ________ If a person believes that he or she has no power to change a situation, and the situation is hopeless, the person can become depressed.

Name two pieces of data one might find with a depressed person on assessment for each of the following:

30. Affect

    1. ______________________________
    2. ______________________________

31. Thinking
    1. ______________________________
    2. ______________________________

32. Feelings
    1. ______________________________
    2. ______________________________

33. Physical behavior
    1. ______________________________
    2. ______________________________

34. Communication
    1. ______________________________
    2. ______________________________

35. Indications of masked depression
    1. ______________________________
    2. ______________________________

For each of the following possible nursing diagnoses formulated for the depressed client, write one outcome criterion and one short-term goal:

36. High risk for self-directed violence:
    Outcome criterion:
    Short-term goal:

37. Altered thought processes:
    Outcome criterion:
    Short-term goal:

38. Social isolation:
    Outcome criterion:
    Short-term goal:

Feelings of frustration, anger, and worthlessness may originate in the depressed client and be experienced by the nurse. Which of the following actions by the nurse would be productive (P) and which would be nonproductive (NP)?

39. __________ Say little and realize that these feelings will go away.

40. __________ Discuss these feelings in team meetings and validate feelings, perceptions, and ways to handle these feelings when with the client.

41. __________ Ask for supervision by an experienced nurse clinician, social worker, or psychologist in order to increase self-awareness and therapeutic skills.

Label the following responses made by a nurse as H (helpful) or NH (not helpful) with a depressed client.

42. __________ "Don't worry, we all get down once in a while."

43. __________ Don't talk of suicide, the person might get ideas.

44. __________ "Debra, I like your new dress."

45. ________ "I will stay with you for 5 minutes at 10 AM, 1 PM, and 3:30 PM today."

46. ________ Try to cheer the person up with a personal story or joke.

47. ________ If a client says an angry word, help him or her control the anger.

State a common self-care need a depressed person may have for each of the following areas, and offer two suggestions for intervention:

48. Nutrition
    Need:
    Interventions:
    1. ________
    2. ________

49. Elimination
    Need:
    Interventions:
    1. ________
    2. ________

50. Rest and sleep
    Need:
    Interventions:
    1. ________
    2. ________

51. Physical activity
    Need:
    Interventions:
    1. ________
    2. ________

Multiple choice

52. Amitriptyline (Elavil) has been prescribed for Mr. Smith. The intern asks the nurse how often and when the best time might be to give this drug. Which of the following would be the nurse's best response?

    A. Every morning, since it has a stimulant effect.
    B. With meals, since it is irritating to the gastric mucosa.
    C. At night—the full dose—to aid sleep and to minimize side effects when the client is awake.
    D. In four divided doses throughout the day.

53. Serious side effects can occur in people with heart conditions when they are given a TCA. Adverse drug reactions can also occur with all the following drugs *except*

    A. Insulin.
    B. MAOIs.
    C. Alcohol.
    D. Oral contraceptives, e.g., estrogen preparations.

54. When Mr. Smith did not respond to the TCAs, phenelzine (Nardil), an MAOI, was ordered. Which of the following would be the *least* important nursing consideration for Mr. Smith?

    A. Wait 10 to 14 days after the amitriptyline therapy has been stopped.
    B. Monitor blood pressure closely after the MAOI therapy is started.
    C. Stop the medication if the client complains of fatigue and constipation.
    D. Carefully teach the client and family about certain foods and drugs that may *not* be taken with an MAOI.

55. Which of the following is an important nursing consideration with electroconvulsive therapy (ECT)?

    A. Permanent brain damage occurs with several treatments.
    B. ECT has had good results in clients with paranoid schizophrenia and "neurotic" depressions.
    C. Virtually no physical contraindications to ECT exist.
    D. During the course of treatment, a client needs frequent orientation to time, place, and person.

56. Mr. Green has been on fluoxetine (Prozac), a selective serotonin reuptake inhibitor (SSRI) for 3 weeks. Your teaching includes telling Mr. Green that he might experience which of the following common side effects?

    A. Severe hypertension and neck pain
    B. Cardiac dysrhythmias
    C. Sleep disturbance and weight changes
    D. Urinary retention and constipation

57. Which of the following types of therapy for depressed clients is highly effective?

    A. Psychoanalytic
    B. Cognitive
    C. Drug therapy
    D. Ego psychology

Critical thinking

58. When you are teaching Mr. Mac about his SSRI, sertraline (Zoloft), he asks you "What makes this such a good drug?" What are some of the positive attributes of the SSRIs? What is one of the most serious, although rare, side effects of the SSRI?

21

Alterations in Mood:
ELATION IN BIPOLAR DISORDERS

ELIZABETH M. VARCAROLIS

OUTLINE

KEY TERMS AND CONCEPTS

The key terms and concepts listed here also appear in bold where they are defined or discussed in this chapter.

bipolar disorders
mania
hypomania
cyclothymia
flight of ideas
clang associations
lithium carbonate
anticonvulsant drugs

OBJECTIVES

After studying this chapter, the reader will be able to

1. Make an assessment of a manic client's (a) mood, (b) behavior, and (c) thought processes.
2. Formulate three nursing diagnoses appropriate for a manic client, including supporting data.
3. Identify one long-term outcome and two short-term goals for each of the three nursing diagnoses.
4. Explain the rationale for five principles of communication that may be used with a manic client.
5. Role play two interventions that a nurse may use when caring for the physical needs of the manic client for each of these areas: nutrition, rest and sleep, elimination, dress and hygiene, and physical activities.
6. Identify four (a) expected side effects for a person on lithium therapy, (b) early signs of lithium toxicity, (c) advanced signs of lithium toxicity, and (d) indications of severe toxic effects of lithium.
7. Write a medication care plan specifying five areas of client teaching regarding lithium carbonate.
8. Discuss two clinical conditions that often respond better to anticonvulsant therapy than to lithium therapy.
9. Evaluate specific indications for the use of seclusion with a manic client.
10. Distinguish between the focus of treatment for a person in the acute manic phase and that of a person in the continuation or maintenance phase of a bipolar I disorder.

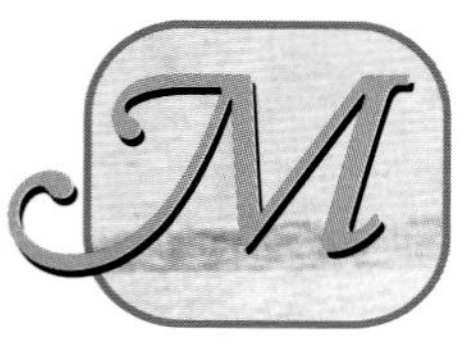

ood disorders, also referred to as affective disorders, are divided into the bipolar and depressive disorders. The depressive disorders were addressed in Chapter 20. This chapter discusses the bipolar disorders. The **bipolar disorders** include the occurrence of depressive mood episodes and one or more elated mood episodes. Bipolar disorders are chronic disorders that require supportive therapy and education for clients and family. These measures can effectively discourage relapse and increase the client's quality of life. Medications, however, are crucial in reducing mania and minimizing future episodes.

ALTERATIONS IN MOOD

An elated mood can range from normal elevated mood to hypomania to mania. In extreme mania, thought processes become incoherent, and delusions may be bizarre. Figure 21–1 places hypomania and mania along the mental health continuum.

In **mania,** a person's elevated mood may be described as euphoric, and for those who know the person, it may be viewed as excessive. Inflated self-esteem is typically present, ranging from uncritical self-confidence to marked grandiosity, and it may reach delusional proportions (APA 1994, p. 328). Although elevated mood is most often associated with mania, irritability may be the predominant mood disturbance. During a manic episode, a person has marked impairment in judgment, often leading to serious legal, social, occupational, or interpersonal consequences. When symptoms of mania or hypomania are observed, treatment should be initiated (Delgado and Gelenberg 1995). Hospitalization is usually indicated for a person with acute mania.

In mania, frenetic behavior is evidenced by constant physical activity, pressured speech, and racing thought patterns. Although outwardly the person may act elated, arrogant, and superior, there is almost always a strong depressive force behind the unstable and "upbeat" facade. Mania can escalate to psychotic proportions. The next section discusses bipolar I disorder, bipolar II disorder, cyclothymia disorder, and bipolar disorders not otherwise specified.

The symptoms of **hypomania** are less severe than those of mania. A hypomanic person does *not* experience impairment in reality testing, nor do the symptoms markedly impair the person's social, occupational, or interpersonal functioning. Figure 21–2 presents the diagnostic criteria for hypomania and mania. Hypomania is often treated in an outpatient setting.

Bipolar Disorders

Bipolar disorders are mood disorders that include one or more manic or hypomanic episodes (elevated, expansive, or irritable mood) and usually one or more depressive episodes. Between the elevated and depressed mood episodes, the person may experience long periods of a normal stable mood. (Refer to Chapter 20 for the depressive component of a bipolar disorder.) The symptoms observed in bipolar I and bipolar II disorders are more severe than those seen in cyclothymia.

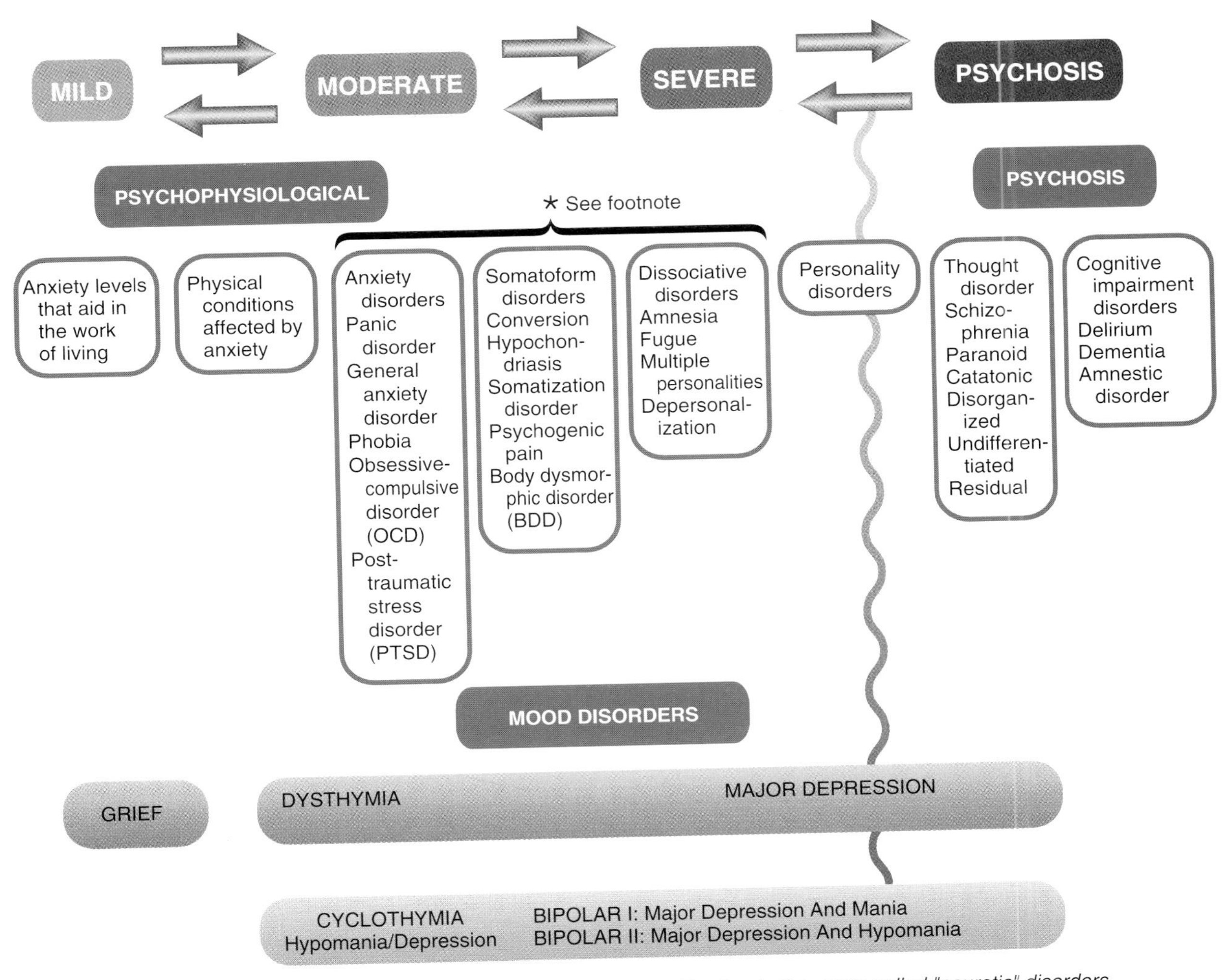

Figure 21–1 The mental health continuum for elation.

The manic episode in bipolar disorder may begin suddenly and last a few days to months. Impairment in reality testing may take the form of grandiose or persecutory delusions. Considerable impairment in social, occupational, and interpersonal functioning exists. Hospitalization is often warranted to protect the person from the consequences of poor judgment and hyperactivity.

Bipolar disorder has been further divided into two types (American Psychiatric Association 1994):

1. Bipolar I consists of one or more periods of major depression plus one or more periods of clear-cut mania.
2. Bipolar II consists of one or more periods of major depression plus periods of hypomania.

In *bipolar I disorders* (alternating mania with a major depressive episode), more than 90% of people who have a single manic episode go on to have future episodes. Most people with bipolar I disorder return to a fully functional level between episodes. Unfortunately, 20% to 30% continue to experience more erratic behavior (lability) and interpersonal or occupational difficulties (American Psychiatric Association 1994). When a person has manic episodes with psychotic features, subsequent manic episodes usually include psychotic phenomena (e.g., paranoid or grandiose delusions). The prevalence of bipolar I disorder in the general population is 0.4% to 1.6%.

In bipolar II disorders (alternating major depression with hypomania), individuals often do not find hypomania to be problematic, although others may find the individual's chronic episodes of unpredictable mood and fluctuating, unreliable interpersonal or occupational behavior annoying and disturbing. When people with bipolar II disorder are depressed, they do not remember the periods of hypomania, and information from friends and relatives is critical in establishing the diagnosis of bipolar II disorder (American Psychiatric Association 1994). The lifetime prevalence for bipolar II disorder in the general population is about 0.5%.

1. A distinct period of abnormality and persistently elevated, expansive, or irritable mood for at least:
   - 4 days for hypomania
   - 1 week for mania
2. During the period of mood disturbance, **at least three (or more)** of the following symptoms have persisted (four if the mood is only irritable) and have been present to a significant degree:
   - Inflated self-esteem or grandiosity
   - Decreased need for sleep (e.g., the person feels rested after only 3 hours of sleep)
   - Increased talkativeness or pressure to keep talking
   - Flight of ideas or subjective experience that thoughts are racing
   - Distractibility (i.e., the person's attention is too easily drawn to unimportant or irrelevant external stimuli)
   - Increase in goal-directed activity (either socially, at work or school, or sexually) or psychomotor agitation
   - Excessive involvement in pleasurable activities that have a high potential for painful consequences (e.g., the person engages in unrestrained buying sprees, sexual indiscretions, or foolish business investments)

HYPOMANIA

1. The episode is associated with an unequivocal change in functioning that is uncharacteristic of the person when not symptomatic.
2. Absence of marked impairment in social or occupational functioning.
3. Delusions are never present.
4. Hospitalization is not indicated.

MANIA

1. Severe enough to cause marked impairment in occupational activities, usual social activities, or relationships
   or
2. Hospitalization is needed to protect client and others from irresponsible or aggressive behavior
   or
3. There are psychotic features (e.g., grandiose and/or paranoid delusions).

Figure 21–2 Diagnostic criteria for manic symptoms. (Adapted from American Psychiatric Association (1994). *Diagnostic and statistical manual of mental disorders (DSM-IV)*, 4th ed. Washington, DC: American Psychiatric Association. Reprinted with permission. Copyright 1994 American Psychiatric Association.)

Cyclothymia

Cyclothymia is a chronic mood disturbance of at least 2 years' duration. Cyclothymia denotes the recurrent experience of some of the symptoms of hypomania and depression that do not meet the full *Diagnostic and statistical manual of mental disorders*, fourth edition (DSM-IV) criteria for a major depressive episode (APA 1994). Essentially, the symptoms of cyclothymia consist of alternating periods of dysthymia and hypomania. Periods of normal mood, if present at all, are short (not longer than 2 months).

The episodes of hypomania or depression are not usually severe enough to warrant hospitalization. Delusions are never present, and the person's social, occupational, and interpersonal functioning are not grossly impaired. Hospitalization is rarely necessary unless the person is thought to be suicidal.

Cyclothymia disorder usually begins in adolescence or early adult life. There is a 15% to 50% risk that an individual will subsequently develop bipolar I or bipolar II disorder.

Bipolar Disorders Not Otherwise Specified

Bipolar disorders include disorders with bipolar features that do not meet any of the above criteria. DSM-IV gives the following examples:

1. Rapid alternating mania and depressive symptoms
2. Recurrent hypomania episodes without depressive episodes
3. A mania or mixed (mania and depression) superimposed on delusional disorder, residual schizophrenia, or psychotic disorder not otherwise specified

THEORY

Bipolar disorders (one or more episodes of both elated and depressed moods) are thought to be distinctly different from nonbipolar depressive disorders, such as a major depressive episode or dysthymia. Table 21–1 lists the differences between bipolar and depressive disorders. A vast

TABLE 21–1 CHARACTERISTIC DIFFERENCES BETWEEN BIPOLAR AND DEPRESSIVE DISORDERS

	BIPOLAR DISORDER	DEPRESSIVE DISORDER
Age of onset	Earlier: 19–30 years (mean, 21 years).	Later: 40–44 years (mean, 40 years).
Sex	Equally frequent in men and women.	Twice as frequent in women than in men.
Family environment	Higher rate of divorce and marital conflict.	Divorce rate same as in general population.
Stressful life events	Contributory in the occurrence of both.	Contributory in the occurrence of both.
Personality traits	Dominance, exhibition, and autonomy needs higher in bipolar disorder. More hypomanic drive toward success and achievement.	Defense of status and guilt feeling higher in depressive disorder. Tendency toward a lack of autonomy.
Symptoms in a depressed phase	*More likely to show* Psychomotor retardation. Hypersomnia. Fewer somatic complaints. Less anxiety.	*More likely to show* Increased motor activity. Insomnia. Somatic complaints. Hypochondriasis.
Course and outcome	Higher frequency of relapse than in a major depressive disorder.	Lower frequency of relapse than in bipolar disorder.

Adapted from Perris, C. (1992). Bipolar-unipolar disorder. In E. S. Paykel (Ed.), *Handbook of affective disorders* (2nd ed.). New York: Guilford Press.

amount of research is now being conducted to identify causes for the mood disorders. Most of this research is being performed in the biological sphere. Some theoretical data pertaining specifically to the cause of the bipolar disorders are genetic, interactive transmitter system (biogenic amines), social, and psychosocial.

Genetic

Significant evidence exists to support the theory that bipolar disorders are a result of genetic transmission. For example, the rate of bipolar disorder is higher in relatives of people with bipolar disorders than in those of the general population (Merikangas and Kupfer 1995). A study at the National Institutes of Mental Health found that 25% of relatives of bipolar clients had a bipolar or a major depressive disorder. For clients with a depressive disorder, 20% of relatives had a bipolar or major depressive disorder, compared with 7% of relatives of control clients (Nurnberger and Gershon 1992). Twin studies bear out a genetic marker for both the bipolar disorders and the depressive disorders; however, the incidence of illness is significantly higher in the bipolar disorders. Identical twins are 78% to 80% more concordant than fraternal twins (14% to 19%) for bipolar disorder (Merikangas and Kupfer 1995; Nurnberger and Gershon 1992). Twin, family, and adoption studies provide evidence for a partial genetic cause, but the modes of inheritance have not been identified (Ginns et al. 1996).

Biogenic Amines

The neurotransmitters (norepinephrine, dopamine, and serotonin) have been studied since the 1960s as causal factors in mania and depression. For example, during a manic episode, clients with bipolar disorder demonstrate significantly higher norepinephrine and epinephrine plasma levels than they do when they are depressed or euthymic (have normal mood) (Nathan et al. 1995). Other research has found that the interrelationships within the neurotransmitter system are complex. More complex hypotheses have developed since the amine hypotheses were originally proposed. Mood disorders are most likely a result of complex interactions between various chemicals, including neurotransmitters and hormones.

The hypothalamic-pituitary-thyroid axis has been closely scrutinized in people with mood disorders. Hypothyroidism is known to be associated with depressed moods, and hypothyroidism is seen in some clients who are experiencing rapid cycling. Some clients with rapid cycling respond to thyroid hormone treatment (Nathan et al. 1995).

Social Status

Some evidence suggests that the bipolar disorders may be more prevalent in the upper socioeconomic classes. The exact reason for this is unclear; however, people with bipolar disorders appear to achieve higher levels of education and occupational status than nonbipolar depressed individuals. However, no difference exists in education across various socioeconomic classes with the nonbipolar depressions. Also, a high proportion of bipolar clients has been found among creative writers, artists, highly educated men and women, and professional people.

Psychosocial

Although there is increasing evidence for genetic and biological vulnerabilities in the cause of the mood disorders, psychological factors may play a role in the precipitation of manic episodes for many individuals. Two studies of family atmosphere suggest an association between high expressed emotion and relapse. However, the relationship between psychosocial stress and bipolar disorder requires further and more detailed research (Ramaka and Bebbington 1995).

Once a manic client has been stabilized through medication, psychotherapy can play an important role in preventing subsequent episodes and in dealing with shame and guilt associated with behaviors during the manic episodes (Gabbard 1995). From a psychodynamic point of view, the manic defense can be conceptualized as a reaction-formation to, or a denial of, an underlying depression.

ASSESSMENT

The three most common initial symptoms in the onset of mania are (1) elated mood, (2) increased activity, and (3) reduced sleep. Not all people in the manic state experience euphoria; some people become extremely irritable, especially when limits are set on their behavior. The nurse evaluates these characteristics when assessing a manic client's mood, behavior, and thought processes.

Assessing Mood

The euphoric mood associated with a bipolar illness is unstable and inconstant. During euphoria, clients may state that they are experiencing an intense feeling of well-being, are "cheerful in a beautiful world," or are becoming "one with God" (Silverstone and Hunt 1992). This mood may change to irritation and quick anger when the elated person is thwarted. The irritability and belligerence may be short-lived, or it may become the prominent feature of a person's manic illness. When elated, the person's overjoyous mood may seem out of proportion to what is going on, and a cheerful mood may be inappropriate to the circumstances.

The person in a manic state may laugh, joke, and talk in a continuous stream, with uninhibited familiarity. Manic people demonstrate boundless enthusiasm, treat everyone with confidential friendliness, and incorporate everyone into their plans and activities. They know no strangers. Energy and self-confidence seem boundless.

Elaborate schemes to get rich and famous and acquire unlimited power are frantically pursued, despite objections and realistic constraints. Excessive phone calls and e-mails are made, and telegrams may be sent to famous and influential people all over the world. People in the manic phase are busy all hours of the day and night furthering their grandiose plans and wild schemes. To the manic person, no aspirations are too high and no distances are too far. No boundaries exist in reality to curtail the elaborate schemes.

In the manic state, a person often gives away money, prized possessions, and expensive gifts. The manic person throws lavish parties, frequents expensive nightclubs and restaurants, and spends money freely on friends and strangers alike. This spending, excessive use of credit cards, and high living continues, even in the face of bankruptcy. Intervention is often needed to prevent financial ruin.

As the clinical course progresses, sociability and euphoria are replaced by a stage of hostility, irritability, and paranoia. The following is a client description of the painful transition from hypomania to mania (Jamison 1995).

Hypomania

▶ At first when I'm high, it's tremendous . . . ideas are fast . . . like shooting stars you follow until brighter ones appear . . . all shyness disappears, the right words and gestures are suddenly there . . . uninteresting people, things become intensely interesting. Sensuality is pervasive, the desire to seduce and be seduced is irresistible. Your marrow is infused with unbelievable feelings of ease, power, well-being, omnipotence, euphoria . . . you can do anything . . . but somewhere this changes. . . .

Mania

▶ The fast ideas become too fast and there are far too many . . . overwhelming confusion replaces clarity . . . you stop keeping up with it—memory goes. Infectious humor ceases to amuse—your friends become frightened . . . everything now is against the grain . . . you are irritable, angry, frightened, uncontrollable, and trapped in the blackest caves of the mind—caves you never knew were there. It will never end. Madness carves its own reality.

Table 21–2 displays the symptoms of mania along a continuum from moderate to severe.

Assessing Behavior

During Mania

When in full-blown mania, a person constantly goes from one activity to another, one place to another, and one project to another. Many projects may be started, but few, if any, are completed. Inactivity is impossible, even for the shortest period of time. Hyperactivity may range from mild, constant motion to frenetic, wild activity. Writing flowery and lengthy letters and making numerous and excessive long-distance telephone calls are common. Individuals become involved in pleasurable activities that can have painful consequences. For example, spending large sums of money on frivolous items, giving money away indiscriminately, or making foolish business investments can leave a family penniless. Sexual indiscretion can dissolve relationships and marriages.

Bipolar individuals can be manipulative, profane, fault finding, and adept at exploiting other's vulnerabilities. They constantly push limits. These behaviors often alienate family, friends, employers, health care providers, and others.

When people are hypomanic, they have voracious appetites for food as well for indiscriminate sex. Although the constant activity of the hypomanic prevents proper sleep, short periods of sleep are possible. However, a reduced need for sleep is experienced by all manic clients, and some clients may not sleep for several days in a row. The manic person is too busy to eat, sleep, or engage in sexual activity. *This nonstop physical activity and the lack of sleep and food can lead to physical exhaustion and even death.*

Modes of dress often reflect the person's grandiose yet tenuous grasp on reality. Dress may be described as outlandish, bizarre, colorful, and noticeably inappropriate. Make-up may be garish or overdone. Manic people are highly distractible. Concentration is poor, and manic individuals go from one activity to another without completing anything. Judgment is poor. Impulsive marriages and divorces take place. People often emerge from a manic state startled and confused by the shambles of their lives. The following description conveys one client's experience (Jamison 1995).

TABLE 21–2 MANIA ON A CONTINUUM

MODERATE Hypomanic	SEVERE Acute Mania	PANIC Severe Mania
	Communication	
1. Talks and jokes incessantly, is the "life of the party," gets irritated when not center of attention.	1. May go suddenly from laughing to anger or depression. *Mode is labile.*	1. Totally out of touch with reality.
2. Treats everyone with familiarity and confidentiality; often borders on crude.	2. Becomes inappropriately demanding of people's attention, and intrusive nature repels others.	—
3. Talk is often sexual—can reach obscene, inappropriate propositions to total strangers.	3. Speech may be marked by profanities and crude sexual remarks to everyone (nursing staff in particular).	—
4. Talk is fresh; flits from one topic to the next. Marked by *pressure of speech.*	4. Speech marked by *flight of ideas,* in which thoughts race and fly from topic to topic. May have *clang association.*	4. Most likely has *clang associations.*
	Affect and Thinking	
1. Full of pep and good humor, feelings of euphoria and sociability; may show inappropriate intimacy with strangers.	1. Good humor gives way to increased irritability and hostility, short-lived period of rage, especially when not getting his or her way or controls are set on behavior. May have quick shifts of mood from hostility to docility.	1. May become destructive or aggressive—totally out of control.
2. Feels boundless self-confidence and enthusiasm. Has elaborate schemes for becoming rich and famous. Initially, schemes may seem plausible.	2. Grandiose plans are totally out of contact with reality. Thinks he or she is musician, prominent businessman, great politician, or religious figure, without any basis in fact.	2. May experience undefined hallucinations and delirium.
3. Judgment often poor. Gets involved with schemes in which job, marriage, or financial status may be destroyed.	3. Judgment is extremely poor.	—
4. May get involved with writing large quantities of letters to rich and famous people regarding schemes or may make numerous world-wide telephone calls.	—	—
5. Decreased attention span to both internal and external cues.	5. Decreased attention span and distractibility are intensified.	—

Continued on following page

TABLE 21–2 MANIA ON A CONTINUUM *(Continued)*

MODERATE	SEVERE	PANIC
	Physical Behavior	
1. Overactive, distractible, buoyant, and busily occupied with grandiose plans (not delusions); goes from one action to the next.	1. Extremely restless, disorganized, and chaotic. Physical behavior may be difficult to control. May have outbursts, e.g., throwing things or becoming briefly assaultive when crossed.	1. *Dangerous state.* Incoherent, extremely restless, disoriented, and agitated. Hyperactive. Motor activity is totally aimless (must have physical or chemical restraints to prevent exhaustion and death).
2. Increased sexual appetite; sexually irresponsible and indiscreet. Illegitimate pregnancies in hypomanic women and venereal disease in both men and women are common. Sex used for escape, not for relating to another human being.	2. Too busy—no time for sex. Poor concentration, distractibility, and restlessness are severe.	2. Same as in acute mania but in the extreme.
3. May have voracious appetite, eat on the run, or gobble food during brief periods.	3. No time to eat—too distracted and disorganized.	3. Same as acute mania but in the extreme.
4. May go without sleeping; unaware of fatigue. However, may be able to take short naps.	4. No time for sleep—psychomotor activity too high; if unchecked, can lead to exhaustion and death.	—
5. Financially extravagant, goes on buying sprees, gives money and gifts away freely, can easily go into debt.	5. Same as in hypomania but in the extreme.	5. Too disorganized to do anything.

Data from Klerman, G. L. (1978). Affective disorders. In A. M. Nicholi, Jr. (Ed.), *The Harvard guide to modern psychiatry*. Cambridge, MA: Belknap Press of Harvard University Press; Silverstone, T., and Hunt, N. (1992). Symptoms and assessment of mania. In E. S. Paykel (Ed.), *Handbook of affective disorders* (2nd ed.). New York: Guilford Press.

After Mania

▶ Now there are only others' recollections of your behavior—your bizarre, frenetic, aimless behavior—at least mania has the grace to dim memories of itself . . . now it's over, but is it? . . . Incredible feelings to sort through . . . Who is being too polite? Who knows what? What did I do? Why? And most hauntingly, will it, when will it, happen again? Medication to take, to resist, to resent, to forget . . . but always to take. Credit cards revoked . . . explanations at work . . . bad checks and apologies overdue . . . memory flashes of vague men (what did I do?) . . . friendships gone, a marriage ruined.

Assessing Thought Processes

Flight of ideas is a nearly continuous flow of accelerated speech with abrupt changes from topic to topic that are usually based on understandable associations or plays on words. At times, the attentive listener can keep up with the changes, even though direction changes from moment to moment. Speech is rapid, verbose, and circumstantial (including minute and unnecessary details). When the condition is severe, speech may be disorganized and incoherent. The incessant talking often includes joking, puns, and teasing:

▶ How are you doing, kid, no kidding around, I'm going home . . . home sweet home . . . home is where the heart is, the heart of the matter is I want out and that ain't hay, . . . hey, Doc . . . get me out of this place. . . .

The content of speech is often sexually explicit and ranges from grossly inappropriate to vulgar. Themes in the communication of the manic may revolve around extraordinary sexual prowess, brilliant business ability, or unparalleled artistic talents (e.g., writing, painting, and dancing). The person may actually have only average ability in these areas.

Speech is not only profuse, but also loud, bellowing, or even screaming. One can hear the force and energy behind the rapid words. As mania escalates, flight of ideas may give way to clang associations. **Clang associations** is the stringing together of words because of their rhyming sounds, without regard to their meaning (Shiller and Bennett 1994):

▶ Cinema I and II, last row. Row, row, row your boat. Don't be a cutthroat. Cut your throat. Get your goat. Go out and vote. And so I wrote . . .

Grandiosity (inflated self-regard) is apparent in either the ideas expressed or the person's behavior. Manic people may exaggerate their achievements or importance, state that they know famous people, or believe that they have great powers (Silverstone and Hunt 1992). The boast of exceptional powers and status can take delusional proportions in mania. Grandiose persecutory delusions are common. For example, manic people may think that God is speaking to them or that the Federal Bureau of Investigation is out to stop them from saving the world. Sensory perceptions may become altered as the mania escalates, and hallucinations may occur. However, in *hypomania*, no evidence of delusions or hallucinations is present.

NURSING DIAGNOSIS

Nursing diagnoses vary for the manic client. When an acutely manic client comes into the hospital, the primary consideration is the prevention of exhaustion and death from cardiac collapse. Because of the client's poor judgment, excessive and constant motor activity, probable dehydration, and difficulty evaluating reality, **risk for injury** is a likely and appropriate diagnosis if the client's activity level is dangerous to his or her health. Immediate medical and nursing interventions are often vital to prevent physical exhaustion. Bruises or wounds, resulting from falling or bumping into objects, or secondary infections, resulting from lack of nutrition, lack of sleep, and personal neglect, indicate that the client is at risk for injury.

Risk for violence directed at self or others related to rage reaction, as evidenced by inability to control behavior, occurs frequently when excitation becomes so severe that the client may be destructive, hostile, and aggressive. Aggression is a common feature in mania. At times, intrusive and taunting behavior can induce others to strike out against these clients.

Grandiosity, poor judgment, and giving away of possessions can result in bankruptcy, neglect of family, and impulsive major life changes (e.g., divorce, marriage, or career changes). These behaviors suggest **altered thought processes.** Getting involved in impossible schemes, shady legal deals, and questionable business ventures may be a result of **ineffective individual coping** related to altered affect, caused by changes in body chemistry or inadequate psychological resources.

Defensive coping may be evidenced by the client's manipulative, angry, or hostile verbal and physical behaviors, which are an attempt to gain a sense of control when the manic client is unable to control racing thoughts or erratic behavior.

The client in the acutely manic state may have numerous unmet physical needs. The manic client is too busy to eat and sleep and is often constipated and poorly groomed. The client's dress may be flamboyant and bizarre. **Fluid volume deficit, altered nutrition** (less than body requirements), **constipation, sleep-pattern disturbance,** and **self-care deficit** are all possible diagnoses.

Because of the manic client's rapid speech (flight of ideas), poor attention span, and difficulty concentrating, **altered family process** related to an ill family member should always be assessed. The family as well as the client need to have their questions answered and need understanding, support, and interventions.

PLANNING

Planning Outcome Criteria

After the assessment has been made and the nursing diagnoses have been prioritized, short-term and long-term goals are formulated. Goals are made for each nursing diagnosis according to the client's unmet needs. Listed subsequently are possible desired outcomes or goals for the following diagnoses:

1. **Risk for injury:**
   - The client's cardiac status will remain stable during hospitalization.
   - While in an acutely manic state, the client will drink 8 ounces of fluid every hour throughout the day.
   - The client will spend time with the nurse in a quiet environment 3 or 4 times a day between 7 AM and 11 PM.
   - The client's skin will be free from abrasions and scrapes every day while in the hospital.
2. **Risk for violence directed at others:**
   - By (date) the client will display nonviolent behavior toward others in the hospital, with the aid of medication and nursing interventions.
   - With the aid of seclusion or nursing interventions, the client will refrain from provoking others to physically harm themselves.
   - The client will respond to external controls (medication, seclusion, nursing interventions) when potential or actual loss of control occurs.
3. **Ineffective coping or altered thought process:**
   - Client will retain valuables or other possessions while in the hospital.
   - Client will make a limited number (one to three) of 5-minute telephone calls per hour.
   - Client will have competent medical assistance and legal protection when signing any legal documents regarding personal or financial matters.
4. **Fluid volume deficit, altered nutrition (less than body requirements), constipation, sleep pattern disturbance, and self-care deficit:**
   - Client will have good skin turgor by (time).
   - Client will have normal bowel movements within 2 days with the aid of high-fiber foods and fluids.

- Client will take a 10-minute rest period every 2 hours during the day (8:00 AM to 10:00 PM).
- Client will sleep 6 hours in 24 hours with the aid of medication and nursing measures within 3 days.
- Client will be appropriately groomed each day while in the hospital.
- Client will wear appropriate attire each day while in the hospital.
- Client will bathe at least every other day while in the hospital.

5. **Altered family process.** Usually, when an episode of mania ceases (a few days to a few months), people return to normal functioning. Often, however, during a manic flight, an individual may unknowingly violently overthrow what was once a "normal" life. People may come out of their manic sprees startled to find themselves broke, without a job, without friends, and without a spouse. Families need to understand what is happening and need support and counseling for themselves. The goals a nurse sets depend on the complexity of the situation. Members of the health team need to become involved with supporting the families. For example, social workers, psychologists, psychiatrists, psychiatric nurse clinicians, and staff nurses can give important information and realistic reassurances and can make appropriate referrals. Goals may include
   - Family or spouse will meet with the nurse to assess family needs by the end of the week.
   - Family or spouse will discuss prognosis, use of medications, and how to recognize prodromal signs of mania before discharge.
   - Family or spouse will be given information on family and/or family group counseling.

Nurse's Feelings and Self-Assessment

A nurse working with a manic client for the first time needs guidance and support and needs to become aware of possible client behaviors. The manic client poses problems and requires interventions that are different from those of the withdrawn and depressed individual.

First, the manic client, unlike most all other clients on the psychiatric unit, needs to be directed *away* from active environmental stimuli (e.g., upbeat music, activity groups, games, or large meetings) to minimize the escalation of the mania.

A quiet, dimly lit, and calm atmosphere is ideal for the manic client. Getting a client to stay in such an environment is a formidable task. A firm and neutral approach usually works best. *Because manic clients are so distractible, the nurse can use this distractibility to move them from potentially problematic situations to more productive activities.* Often, activities that involve motor activity requiring the use of large muscle groups (e.g., ping-pong or punching bag) as well as writing provide constructive outlets for energy. A few hours of keeping up with a person who is manic can deplete the nurse's energy. Often, nurses take turns monitoring a manic client's behavior while the client is still extremely hyperactive.

Second, the manic client can elicit numerous intense emotions in the nurse. A manic client is out of control and resists being controlled. The client may use humor, manipulation, power struggles, or demanding behavior to prevent or minimize the staff's ability to set limits on and control dangerous behavior.

When the manic is joking, punning, and being the life of the party, the mood can be infectious. A manic client can be genuinely funny and entertaining. The nurse needs to remain uninvolved or neutral and needs to take measures to prevent further escalation of the mania. Joking with or encouraging the manic client's humor is meeting the health care worker's needs at the client's expense.

The behavior of a manic client is often aimed at decreasing the effectiveness of staff control. He or she might accomplish this by getting involved with power plays. For example, the client might taunt the staff by pointing out faults or oversights, drawing negative attention to one or more staff. Usually, this is done in a loud and disruptive manner, which serves to get staff defensive, thereby escalating the environmental tension and the client's degree of mania.

Another unconscious tactic is to divide staff as a ploy to keep the environment unsettled. The manic client is sensitive to the vulnerabilities and conflicts within a group. Often, a manic client manipulates staff by turning one group of staff against another in an unconscious attempt to discourage outside controls. For example, a client might tell the day shift, "You are the only nurse who listens. On evenings, they hardly look at you. You could drop dead, and the nurses wouldn't even know it." To the evening shift the client might say, "Thank God you're here. At last, someone who cares. All the day people do is push pills and drink coffee."

The client can become aggressively demanding. This behavior often triggers frustration and exasperation from the staff. Again, the manic distracts the staff into a defensive position and sets up an environment that allows the manic defense to go unchecked. Setting limits is an important skill for staff to develop. Adequate administration and medications (anxiolytic, antipsychotic) are essential.

When the staff start to feel confused and angry at each other, it is often an indication that a client is splitting the staff. Frequent staff meetings dealing with the behaviors of the client and the nurses' responses to these behaviors can help minimize staff splitting and feelings of anger and isolation by the staff. The consistent setting of limits is the main theme with a person in mania.

Consistency among staff is imperative if the limits are to be carried out effectively.

INTERVENTION

Counseling (Basic Level)

Table 21–3 suggests basic principles of communication for use with the client who is manic. The table suggests approaches that can be effective in speaking to clients who are in a hyperactive state. It also suggests approaches for structuring the milieu to decrease risk for injury and for structuring the client's social interactions in order to minimize aggressive acting out and disruption on the unit.

Self-Care Activities (Basic Level)

A person in mania has great difficulty meeting personal physical needs. Thus, the nurse finds that much attention is directed toward interventions associated with activities of daily living. Table 21–4 suggests interventions that are appropriate for safeguarding the physical health of the manic client. Basic physical needs of a manic client revolve around deficits in eating and sleeping, problems with constipation, and deficit in caring for basic hygiene. Approaches for these issues are presented in Table 21–4.

Psychobiological Interventions (Basic Level)

Lithium, valproate, and carbamazepine are all effective treatments for acute mania.

Lithium Carbonate

Lithium carbonate is the drug of choice for treating the manic phase of a bipolar disorder. Lithium is a mood stabilizer and is the prototypical *antimanic* drug. Often, it can calm manic clients, prevent or modify future manic episodes, and protect against future depressive episodes. Lithium is most effective in up to 90% of clients with pure manic symptoms (elation and grandiosity); of that 90%, 70% experience a full initial response and 20% experience a partial initial response (Maxmen and Ward 1995). Lithium is less effective in people with mixed mania (elation and depression) or in those with rapid cycling (Bowden 1995).

Lithium is particularly effective (Maxmen and Ward 1995) in reducing

- Elation, grandiosity, and expansiveness.
- Flights of ideas.
- Irritability and manipulativeness.
- Anxiety.

To a lesser extent, lithium controls

- Insomnia.
- Psychomotor agitation.
- Threatening or assaultive behavior.
- Distractibility.

When a client comes into the hospital in severe mania, an antipsychotic drug is given. Antipsychotics act promptly to slow speech, inhibit aggression, and decrease psychomotor activity. The immediate action of the antipsychotic medication is to prevent exhaustion, coronary collapse, and death. (See Chapter 22 for a discussion of the antipsychotic drugs.) Electroconvulsive therapy may also be used to subdue severe manic behavior, especially in treatment-resistant manic clients and clients with rapid cycling, (i.e., those who suffer four or more episodes of illness a year). In bipolar clients, clients with rapid cycling and those with paranoid-destructive features often respond poorly to lithium therapy (Abou-Saleh 1992).

Lithium must reach therapeutic levels in the client's blood to be effective (Table 21–5). This usually takes from 7 to 14 days, or longer for some. As lithium levels become effective in reducing manic behavior, the antipsychotics are usually discontinued. Lithium is 70% to 90% effective in treating the manic phase of a bipolar disorder; however, it is not a cure. Many clients receive indefinite lithium maintenance and experience manic and depressive episodes if the drug is discontinued.

Trade names for lithium carbonate include Lithane, Eskalith, and Lithonate. During the *active phase*, 300 to 600 mg by mouth is given two to three times a day, to reach a clear therapeutic result or a lithium level of 0.8 to 1.4 mEq/L. The actual maintenance blood levels should range between 0.4 to 1.0 mEq/L. To avoid serious toxicity, lithium levels should *not* exceed 1.5 mEq/L (Lehne et al. 1994).

A small range exists between the therapeutic dose and the toxic dose of lithium. Initially, blood levels are drawn weekly or biweekly until the therapeutic level has been reached. After therapeutic levels have been reached, blood levels are drawn every month. After 6 months to a year of stability, blood levels every 3 months may suffice (Schatzberg and Cole 1991). Blood should be drawn 8 to 12 hours after the last dose of lithium is taken.

Toxic effects are usually associated with levels of 2.0 mEq/L or more, although they can occur at much lower levels (even within a therapeutic range).

Maintenance Therapy

According to Maxmen and Ward (1995), bipolar relapses occur within 2 years of onset in 20% to 40% of people taking lithium and in 65% to 90% of people not taking lithium. When clients stop taking lithium, relapse usually occurs within several weeks.

Some suggest that clients with bipolar disorder need to be given lithium from 9 to 12 months, and some clients may need lifelong lithium maintenance in order to prevent further relapses. Many clients respond well

TABLE 21–3 COUNSELING/MILIEU NEEDS OF MANIC CLIENTS

INTERVENTION	RATIONALE
Nursing Diagnosis: Altered thought processes related to biological changes, as evidenced by hyperactivity and inability to concentrate	
1. Use firm and calm approach, "John. Come with me. Eat this sandwich."	1. Provides structure and control for a client who is out of control. Can result in feelings of security: "Someone is in control."
2. Use short and concise explanations or statements.	2. Short attention span limits comprehension to small bits of information.
3. Remain neutral; avoid power struggles and value judgments.	3. Client can use inconsistencies and value judgments as justification for arguing and escalating mania.
4. Be consistent in approach and expectations.	4. Consistent limits and expectations minimize potential for client's manipulation of staff.
5. Avoid getting caught up in joking and repartee. Maintain calm and neutral manner.	5. Minimizes the manic spiral. Joking and laughing with the manic client is disrespectful of the client's needs.
6. Have frequent staff meetings to plan consistent approaches and to set agreed-on limits.	6. Consistency of all staff is needed to maintain controls and minimize manipulation by client.
7. When limits are decided by staff, they need to be told to the client in simple, concrete terms, including the consequences, e.g., "John, do not yell at or hit Peter. If you cannot control yourself, we will help you," or "The seclusion room will help you feel less out of control and prevent harm to yourself and others."	7. Clear expectations help client experience outside controls as well as understand reasons for medication, seclusion, or restraints (if he or she is not able to control behaviors).
8. Legitimate complaints should be heard and acted on.	8. Reduces underlying feelings of helplessness and can raise self-esteem.
9. Accept acting-out behavior (e.g., obscene remarks, crude jokes, and gestures) calmly.	9. Acceptance thwarts unconscious attempt to trigger anger and get the nurse to act irrationally (out of control), thus maintaining the manic defense.
10. Firmly redirect energy into more appropriate and constructive channels.	10. Distractibility is the nurse's most effective tool with the manic client.
Nursing Diagnosis: Risk for injury related to extreme hyperactivity, as evidenced by increased agitation and poor impulse control	
1. Maintain low level of stimuli in client's environment (e.g., away from bright lights, loud noises, and people).	1. Helps decrease escalation of anxiety.
2. Provide structured solitary activities with nurse or aide.	2. Structure provides security and focus.
3. Provide frequent high-calorie fluids.	3. Prevents serious dehydration.
4. Provide frequent rest periods.	4. Prevents exhaustion.
5. Redirect violent behavior.	5. Physical exercise can decrease tension and provide focus.
6. Acute mania may warrant the use of phenothiazines and seclusion to minimize physical harm.	6. Exhaustion and death can result from dehydration, lack of sleep, and constant physical activity.
7. Observe for signs of lithium toxicity.	7. There is a small margin of safety between therapeutic and toxic doses.
8. Protect client from giving away money and possessions. Hold valuables in hospital safe until rational judgment returns.	8. Client's "generosity" is a manic defense that is consistent with irrational, grandiose thinking.
Nursing Diagnosis: Impaired social interaction related to altered thought processes, as evidenced by intrusive and aggressive social behavior	
1. When possible, provide an environment with minimal stimuli, e.g., quiet, soft music, dim lighting.	1. Reduction in stimuli lessens distractibility.
2. Solitary activities requiring short attention span with mild physical exertion are best initially, e.g., writing, painting (finger painting, murals), woodworking, or walks with staff.	2. Solitary activities minimize stimuli; mild physical activities release tension constructively.
3. When less manic, client may join one or two other clients in quiet, nonstimulating activities, e.g., board games, drawing, cards. *Avoid competitive games.*	3. As mania subsides, involvement in activities that provide a focus and social contact becomes more appropriate. Competitive games can stimulate aggression and can increase psychomotor activity.

TABLE 21–4 SELF-CARE NEEDS OF MANIC CLIENTS

INTERVENTION	RATIONALE
Nursing Diagnosis: Altered nutrition less than body requirements related to excessive physical agitation, as evidenced by inadequate food and fluid intake	
1. Monitor intake, output, and vital signs.	1. Ensures adequate fluid and caloric intake; minimizes dehydration and cardiac collapse.
2. Offer frequent high-calorie protein drinks and finger foods (e.g., sandwiches, fruit, milkshakes).	2. Constant fluid and calorie replacement are needed. Client may be too active to sit at meals. Finger foods allow "eating on the run."
3. Frequently remind client to eat. "Tom, finish your milkshake." "Sally, eat this banana."	3. The manic client is unaware of bodily needs and is easily distracted. Needs supervision to eat.
Nursing Diagnosis: Sleep-pattern disturbance related to biochemical alteration, as evidenced by frequent wakening episodes during the night	
1. Encourage frequent rest periods during the day.	1. Lack of sleep can lead to exhaustion and death.
2. Keep client in areas of low stimulation.	2. Promotes relaxation and minimizes manic behavior.
3. At night, provide warm baths, soothing music, and medication when indicated. Avoid giving client caffeine.	3. Promotes relaxation, rest, and sleep.
Nursing Diagnosis: Self-care deficit related to excessive hyperactivity, as evidenced by poor hygiene	
1. Supervise choice of clothes, minimize flamboyant and bizarre dress, e.g., garish stripes, plaids, and loud, unmatching colors.	1. Lessens the potential for ridicule, which lowers self-esteem and increases the need for manic defense. Assists client in maintaining dignity.
2. Give simple step-by-step reminders for hygiene and dress. "Here is your razor. Shave the left side . . . now the right side. Here is your toothbrush. Put the toothpaste on the brush."	2. Distractibility and poor concentration are countered by simple, concrete instructions.
Nursing Diagnosis: Constipation related to inadequate dietary intake and fluids	
1. Monitor bowel habits; offer fluids and food that is high in fiber. Evaluate need for laxative. Encourage client to go to the bathroom.	1. Prevents fecal impaction resulting from dehydration and decreased peristalsis.

to lower doses during maintenance or "prophylactic" lithium therapy.

Lithium is unquestionably effective in preventing both manic and depressive episodes in clients with bipolar disorder. However, complete suppression may occur in only 50% of clients or fewer, even with compliance to maintenance therapy. Therefore, both the person with a bipolar disorder and his or her spouse need careful instructions about (1) the purpose and requirements of lithium therapy, (2) its side effects, (3) its toxic effects and complications, and (4) situations in which the physician should be contacted. Box 21–1 elaborates client and family teaching.

Indications for Lithium Use

Lithium use can be divided into four general clinical situations (Schatzberg and Cole 1991):

1. To control rapidly acute, overt psychopathology, as in mania or psychotic agitation
2. To attempt to modify milder ongoing or frequent but episodic clinical symptoms, such as chronic depression or episodic irritability
3. To establish a prophylactic maintenance regimen to avert future affective or psychotic episodes
4. To enhance the effect of antidepressants in clients with a major depressive disorder

Lithium has also been used with success in the following.

SCHIZOAFFECTIVE DISORDER. Lithium used in combination with antipsychotic therapy can be useful in clients who demonstrate overactivity, insomnia, irritability, or other manic symptoms during an excited episode.

SCHIZOPHRENIA. For some treatment-resistant clients, a combination of lithium and antipsychotic drug therapy may prove helpful. It can also be useful in decreasing angry outbursts.

IMPULSE CONTROL DISORDERS. Impulse disorders include episodic violence and rage. People who have unpremeditated outbursts of violence, and those in whom rage reactions are seemingly unprovoked by happenings in the environment, often respond well to lithium. Violence that is premeditated, however, is not responsive to lithium.

TABLE 21–5 DRUG INFORMATION: SIDE EFFECTS AND SIGNS OF LITHIUM TOXICITY

LEVEL	SIGNS*	INTERVENTIONS
	Expected Side Effects	
≤0.4–1.0 mEq/L (therapeutic levels)	Fine hand tremors, polyuria, and mild thirst. Mild nausea and general discomfort. Weight gain.	Symptoms may persist throughout therapy. Symptoms often subside during treatment. Weight gain may be helped with diet, exercise, and nutritional management.
	Early Signs of Toxicity	
<1.5 mEq/L	Nausea, vomiting, diarrhea, thirst, polyuria, slurred speech, muscle weakness.	Medication should be withheld, blood lithium levels drawn, and dose re-evaluated.
	Advanced Signs of Toxicity	
1.5–2.0 mEq/L	Coarse hand tremor, persistent gastrointestinal upset, mental confusion, muscle hyperirritability, electroencephalographic changes, incoordination.	Use interventions outlined above or below, depending on severity of circumstances.
	Severe Toxicity	
2.0–2.5 mEq/L	Ataxia, serious electroencephalographic changes, blurred vision, clonic movements, large output of dilute urine, seizures, stupor, severe hypotension, coma. Death is usually secondary to pulmonary complications.	There is no known antidote for lithium poisoning. The drug is stopped, and excretion is hastened. Gastric lavage and treatment with urea, mannitol, and aminophylline all hasten lithium excretion.
>2.5 mEq/L	Confusion, incontinence of urine or feces, coma, cardiac arrhythmia, peripheral circulatory collapse, abdominal pain, proteinuria, oliguria, and death.	Hemodialysis may also be used in severe cases.

Data from Scherer, J. C. (1985). *Nurses' drug manual* (pp. 631–632). Philadelphia: J. B. Lippincott; Lehne, R. A., et al. (1994). *Pharmacology for nursing care* (2nd ed., pp. 269–299). W. B. Saunders.
*Careful monitoring is needed because the toxic levels of lithium are close to the therapeutic levels.

Contraindications for Lithium Use

Before the administration of lithium, a medical evaluation is performed to assess a client's ability to tolerate the drug. In particular, baseline physical and laboratory examinations should include renal function; thyroid status, including thyroxine and thyroid-stimulating hormone; and evaluation for dementia or neurological disorders, which signal a poor response to lithium.

Other clinical and laboratory assessments, including an electrocardiogram, are done as needed, depending on the individual's physical condition.

Lithium is not given to people who are pregnant, have brain damage, or have cardiovascular, renal, or thyroid disease. Both the fear of and the wish to become pregnant are a major concern for many bipolar women taking lithium. Lithium is also contraindicated in mothers who are breast-feeding or have myasthenia gravis and in children younger than 12 years of age.

Expected Side Effects

Mild hand tremors, polyuria, and mild thirst often occur and may persist throughout therapy. Mild nausea and general discomfort may occur initially, and the client can be reassured that these side effects usually subside with treatment. Weight gain is sometimes an undesirable side effect of long-term use. Table 21–5 identifies early, advanced, and severe signs of toxic poisoning with lithium. Two major long-term risks of lithium therapy are hypothyroidism and impairment of the kidney's ability to concentrate urine. Therefore, a person on lithium therapy needs to have periodic thyroid and renal follow-up.

Other Antimanic Drugs

Although lithium is the drug of choice for bipolar clients, up to 40% of bipolar clients may not respond or respond

BOX 21–1 TEACHING CLIENTS AND THEIR FAMILIES ABOUT LITHIUM

The client and the client's family should be instructed about the following, encouraged to ask questions, and given the material in written form as well.

1. Lithium can treat your current emotional problem and also helps prevent relapse. Therefore, it is important to continue taking the drug after the current episode is resolved.
2. Because therapeutic and toxic dosage ranges are so close, lithium blood levels must be monitored very closely, more frequently at first, then once every several months after that.
3. Lithium is not addictive.
4. A normal diet and normal salt and fluid intake (1500–3000 ml/day or six 12-ounce glasses) should be maintained. Lithium decreases sodium reabsorption by the renal tubules, which could cause sodium depletion. A low sodium intake causes a relative increase in lithium retention, which could lead to toxicity.
5. Stop taking drug if excessive diarrhea, vomiting, or diaphoresis occurs. Dehydration can raise lithium levels in the blood to toxic levels. **Inform your physician if you have any of these problems.**
6. Diuretics (water pills) are contraindicated with lithium.
7. Lithium is irritating to the gastric mucosa. Therefore, take lithium with meals.
8. Periodic monitoring of renal functioning and thyroid function is indicated with long-term use. Discuss follow-up with the doctor.
9. Avoid taking any over-the-counter medications without checking first with the doctor.
10. If weight gain is significant, client may need to see a physician or nutritionist.
11. Many self-help groups have been developed to provide support for people with bipolar disorder and their families. The local self-help group is (give name and telephone number).
12. You can find out more information by calling (give name and telephone number).

Data from Maxmen, J. S., and Ward, N. G. (1995). *Psychotropic drugs: Fast facts* (2nd ed.). New York: W. W. Norton; Schatzberg, A. F., and Cole, J. O. (1991). *Manual of clinical psychopharmacology.* Washington, DC: American Psychiatric Press; Preston, J., and Johnson, J. (1995). *Clinical psychopharmacology made ridiculously simple.* Miami: MedMaster.

insufficiently to, or tolerate, lithium (Post 1992). Some subtypes of bipolar clients who may not respond well to lithium (Post 1992) include

- Those with dysphoric mania (depressive thoughts and feelings during manic episodes).
- Those with rapid cycling (four or more episodes a year).
- Those whose initial mood episode consists of a depression, then mania, and then an interval of wellness (D-M-I); they are often nonresponders. Those whose initial episode consists of mania, then depression, and then an interval of wellness (M-D-I) often do respond more readily to lithium.

Another population in which a positive lithium response may occur is clients who have a family history of bipolar disorder in first-degree relatives. Those with no family history of first-degree relatives with bipolar disorder often have a poorer response to lithium but may respond to the anticonvulsants carbamazepine (Tegretol) or valproic acid (Depakene).

Anticonvulsants

Although many **anticonvulsant drugs** may eventually prove useful in treating mood disorders, carbamazepine and valproic acid have been most frequently studied as long-term maintenance therapies. According to Maxmen and Ward (1995), anticonvulsants have been found to

- Clearly control acute mania (with or without lithium).
- Often prevent mania.
- Occasionally treat and prevent major depression or bipolar depression.
- Aid more rapid-cycling clients than does lithium.
- Relieve psychotic symptoms secondary to complex partial seizures.
- Infrequently reduce schizophrenia.
- Dampen affective swings in schizoaffective clients.
- Diminish impulsive and aggressive behavior in some nonpsychotic clients.
- Facilitate alcohol and benzodiazepine withdrawal.

Clinical benefits include the ability to control mania (within 2 weeks) and depression (within 3 weeks) or more).

CARBAMAZEPINE (TEGRETOL). In 25% to 50% of clients with treatment-resistant bipolar disorder, carbamazepine has clear clinical benefits (Table 21–6). Some treatment-resistant clients with bipolar disorder improve after taking carbamazepine and lithium or carbamazepine and an antipsychotic. Carbamazepine seems to work better in 60% of clients with rapid cycling and better in severely paranoid, angry, manic clients than in euphoric, overactive, overfriendly manic clients (Schatzberg and Cole 1991). It is also thought to be more effective in dysphoric manic clients. Table 21–6 presents clinical profiles of lithium and carbamazepine.

For acute mania, the combination of lithium and an antipsychotic agent are more effective than the combination of lithium and carbamazepine; however, carbamazepine does not induce tardive dyskinesia and has

TABLE 21–6 DRUG INFORMATION: CLINICAL PROFILES OF LITHIUM AND CARBAMAZEPINE/VALPROIC ACID

CLINICAL PROFILE	LITHIUM	VALPROIC ACID OR CARBAMAZEPINE (CBZ)
Mania	++	+
Dysphoria (mixed)	+	++
Rapid cycling	+	++
Continuous cycling	+	++
Negative family history	+	++
Neurological history or findings (head trauma or nonparoxysmal EEG abnormalities)	+	++
Depression	+	+ (CBZ)
Prophylaxis of mania and depression	++	− (Valproic acid)

From Maxmen, J. S., and Ward, N. G. (1995). *Psychotropic drugs: Fast facts* (2nd ed.) New York: W. W. Norton. Copyright © 1995 by Nicholas J. Ward and the Estate of Jerrold S. Maxmen. Copyright © 1991 by Jerrold S. Maxmen. Reprinted by permission of W. W. Norton & Company, Inc.

+, effective; ++, very effective

fewer side effects. Table 21–7 lists side effects and toxic effects of other antimanic (mood-stabilizing) medications. Blood levels of carbamazepine should be monitored at least weekly through the first 8 weeks of treatment because the drug can increase liver enzymes, which then speed its own metabolism (Schatzberg and Cole 1991).

VALPROIC ACID (DEPAKENE, DEPAKOTE). Valproic acid has been found helpful for lithium nonresponders in initial studies. It can be useful in treating lithium nonresponders who are in acute mania, who are in rapid cycles, who are in dysphoric mania, or who have not responded to carbamazepine. It has also been helpful in preventing future manic episodes.

Anxiolytics

CLONAZEPAM AND LORAZEPAM. Clonazepam (Klonopin) and lorazepam (Ativan) have been found to be useful in the treatment of acute mania in some treatment-resistant manic clients. These drugs are also effective in managing psychomoter agitation seen in mania. Further studies are needed to provide conclusive evidence for its universal use. Table 21–7 listed the major concerns of these other mood stabilizers.

Health Teaching (Basic Level)

Ongoing encouragement and support are needed after a person receives treatment because it may take a while to discover what therapeutic regimen is best for that particular person. The effects of a bipolar illness can cause severe problems in peoples' lives. Some of the issues that clients need to deal with are

- Actions performed in the manic phase.
- Actions not performed in the depressed phase.
- When to tell others about the illness.
- Role of therapy.
- Need for long-term medication.

Clients and families need information about bipolar illness, and the chronic and highly recurrent nature of the illness needs to be emphasized and reemphasized to both clients and families. Charts can be used to illustrate the high relapse rate and worsening course in untreated illness, as well as the dramatic effect of the mood stabilizers on the course of manic-depressive illness (Jamison 1995).

Clients and their families also need to be taught the symptoms of impending episodes. For example, changes in sleep patterns are particularly important, since they usually precede, accompany, or precipitate mania. Even a single night of unexplainable sleep loss can be taken for an early warning of impending mania. The regularization of sleep patterns, meals, exercise, and other activities should be stressed to clients (Jamison 1995).

TABLE 21–7 DRUG INFORMATION: OTHER ANTIMANIC (MOOD STABILIZING) MEDICATIONS

DRUG	TYPE	MAJOR CONCERN/SIDE EFFECT
Carbamazepine (Tegretol)	Anticonvulsant	Agranulocytosis or aplastic anemia are most serious side effects. Blood levels should be monitored through first 8 weeks because drug induces liver enzymes that speed its own metabolism. Dose may need to be adjusted to maintain serum level of 6–8 mg/L. Sedation is most common problem; tolerance usually develops. Diplopia, incoordination, and sedation can signal excessive levels.
Valproic acid (Depakane)	Anticonvulsant	Baseline liver function tests should be performed and monitored at regular intervals. Hepatitis, although rare, has been reported, with fatalities in children. Signs and symptoms to watch for: fever, chills, right upper-quadrant pain, dark-colored urine, malaise, and jaundice. Common side effects: tremors, gastrointestinal upset, weight gain, and rarely, alopecia.
Clonazepam (Klonopin)	Benzodiazepine	Same as those of all benzodiazepines, e.g., sedation, ataxia, and incoordination (see Chapter 17, Table 17–8).

Milieu Therapy (Basic Level)

Acute Phase

Hospitalization is indicated for people in the acute manic state. Hospitalization helps the client gain control over extremely hyperactive behavior and allows for medication stabilization. Within the confines of the managed care environment, people in the manic phase of a bipolar disorder have a shorter hospital stay than previously. Important aspects of clients' care are addressed in community-based health care centers at times when clients may still be having difficulty controlling their behavior and following medical guidelines. Therefore, the client must perform specific tasks and sound discharge planning must be in place during the client's hospital stay. An important part of discharge planning is finding support for clients' families and locating community resources.

A popular way to structure tasks for health care workers is through a clinical pathway. Clinical Pathway 21–1

CLINICAL PATHWAY 21–1 Diagnosis: Bipolar Manic Disorder

Initiation Date:

	DAY 1	DAYS 2–4	DAYS 5–7	DAYS 8–12*
Medical Interventions	H&P, MSE, thought process and content, psychomotor agitation, judgment, SI/HI. Substance abuse. Order laboratory studies: toxicology screen, ECG 40+, lithium, carbamazepine level. Admission orders. Drug screen. Restrict for 24 hr.	Complete treatment plan. Monitor side effects of medications and lithium level. Review laboratory results and any previous records. Re-evaluate restriction.	Update treatment plan. Monitor symptoms, medications, and side effects. Initiate D/C plans for F/U.	Discharge instruction form. Discharge orders. Prescriptions and F/U appointment. Terminate therapy.
Nursing Interventions	Admission, assessment, documentation. Provide safety. Orient to ward, schedule and give ITP. Check VS and weight; monitor intake.	Assess adaptation to ward, monitor activity level, agitation, mood, sleep, appetite, and side effects of medications. Assess VS. Assist with grooming. Educate PT/family illness about medications.	Continue monitoring (see previous). Evaluate ability to participate in small group. Evaluate ADLs. Evaluate medication/ illness teaching.	Continue monitoring/ evaluation (see previous). Complete D/C summary. Reinforce medication/ illness teaching.
Social Work Interventions	Emergency intervention	Assessment by third workday. Identify living situation, financial status, and support systems. Initiate D/C planning and family counseling.	Continue counseling PT/family. Review with PT/family available support systems.	Terminate counseling. Make outpatient appointments.
Psychology Interventions		Initial psychological testing	Review findings	
Recreation Therapy Interventions	Initial contact	Initial RT assessment completed. Begin attendance to specified groups.	Begin or continue leisure plan, including activities for energy release.	Complete leisure D/C plan(s).
Key Patient Outcomes	Accepts staffs' verbal redirection and limits @ ____	Abides by ward rules @ ____ PT verbalizes feeling of safety @ ____ Maintains control @ ____ Attends assigned groups @ ____ Identifies current medications @ ____	Sleeps >5 hr @ ____ Eats 75% of meals @ ____ Participates in assigned groups @ ____ Reports improved mood @ ____	Decreased or cessation of symptoms of altered thought process; content, misperceptions, grandiosity, agitation @ ____ Improved behavioral control @ ____ Identifies D/C plan and F/U care with medications @ ____

Adapted from Veterans' Administration Medical Center, 10 North Green Street, Baltimore, MD 21201.
Circle = variance (see back); # = Date-progress note regarding specific evaluation/intervention goal; @ = achievement data.
H&P, history and physical; MSE, mental status examination; F/U, follow-up; D/C, discharge; PT, patient; VS, vital signs; ECG, electrocardiogram; RT, recreational therapy; ADL, activities of daily living. SI/HI, suicidal ideation/homocidal ideation; ITP, interdisciplinary treatment plan.
*Most often the client is discharged at or before this time.

shows a diagnosis for a bipolar-manic client. The clinical pathway identifies the responsibility of various health care personnel and identifies outcome criteria.

Control during the acute phase of hyperactive behavior almost always includes immediate treatment with an antipsychotic, such as haloperidol (Haldol) or chlorpromazine (Thorazine). However, when a client is dangerously out of control, use of the seclusion room or restraints may also be indicated. The seclusion room can provide comfort and relief to many clients who can no longer control their own behavior.

Seclusion serves the following purposes:

1. Reduces overwhelming environmental stimuli
2. Protects a client from injuring self, others, or staff
3. Prevents destruction of personal property or property of others

Seclusion is warranted when documented data by the nursing and medical staff reflect the following points:

1. Substantial risk of harm to others or self is clear.
2. Client is unable to control his or her actions.
3. Behavior has been sustained (continues or escalates despite other measures).
4. Other measures have failed (e.g., setting limits or using chemical restraints).

The use of seclusion or restraints involves complex therapeutic, ethical, and legal issues. Most state laws prohibit the use of unnecessary physical restraint or isolation. Barring an emergency, the use of seclusion and restraints warrants the client's consent. Therefore, most hospitals have well-defined protocols for treatment with seclusion. Protocols include a proper reporting procedure through the chain of command when a client is to be secluded. For example, the use of seclusion and restraint is permitted only on the written order of a physician, which must be reviewed and rewritten every 24 hours. The order should also include the type of restraint to be used. As-necessary (prn) orders are updated.

Only in an emergency may the charge nurse place a client in seclusion or restraint; under these circumstances, a written physician's order needs to be obtained within a specified period of time (15 to 30 minutes).

Seclusion protocols also identify specific nursing responsibilities, such as how often the client's behavior is to be observed and documented (e.g., every 15 minutes), how often the client is to be offered food and fluids (e.g., every 30 to 60 minutes), and how often the client is to be toileted (e.g., every 1 to 2 hours). Because phenothiazines are often used with clients in seclusion, vital signs should be taken frequently (e.g., every 1 to 2 hours).

Careful and precise documentation is a legal necessity. The nurse documents

1. The behavior leading up to the seclusion/restraint.
2. What actions were taken to provide the least restrictive alternative.
3. The time the client was placed in seclusion.
4. Every 15 minutes, the client's behavior, needs, nursing care, and vital signs.
5. The time and type of medications given and their effects on the client.

When a client does require seclusion to prevent harm to himself or herself or others, it is ideal to have one nurse on each shift work with the client on a continuous basis. Communication with a client in seclusion should be concrete and direct but should be kind and limited to brief instructions. Clients should be reassured that the seclusion is only a temporary measure, and that they will be returned to the unit when their behavior is safer and quieter.

Frequent staff meetings regarding personal feelings about seclusion are necessary to prevent possible dangers. Dangers include using seclusion as a form of punishment and leaving a client in seclusion for long periods of time without proper supervision. Restraints and seclusion should never be used as punishment or for the convenience of the staff. Chapter 4 discusses the legal implications of seclusion and restraints, and Chapter 12 provides more discussion and guidelines.

Continuation of Treatment Phase

This phase is a crucial one for clients and families. The goal of this phase is to prevent relapse. This phase usually lasts 4 to 9 months. People with bipolar illness and their families can find support in most communities. A client may attend a mental health center for medication follow-up. Other clients may attend day hospitals if they are not too excitable and are able to tolerate a certain amount of stimuli. Day hospitals can offer structure, encourage medication compliance, decrease social isolation, and help clients channel their time and energy. Other clients and families may find that home visits are most appropriate for monitoring medications and side effects, supervising health care needs, and evaluating family needs. Community resources are chosen based on the needs of the client, the appropriateness of the referral, and the availability of community resources. Frequently, it is a case manager who evaluates appropriate follow-up care for clients and their families. Medication compliance during this phase is perhaps the most important goal of treatment. Clients and families need support and a place to go for health education when needed.

Maintenance Treatment Phase

Maintenance therapy is aimed at preventing the recurrence of an episode of a bipolar illness. Along with some of the community resources cited earlier, clients and families often greatly benefit from mutual support and self-help groups mentioned later in this chapter.

Psychotherapy (Advanced Practice)

Psychotherapy is important in the treatment of bipolar illness, specifically in encouraging lithium compliance (Jamison 1995b). Often, the clients receiving medication and therapy place more value on psychotherapy than do clinicians. Moreover, clients treated with cognitive therapy more often took their medication as prescribed than did clients who were not in therapy (Jamison 1995).

A client describes her feelings about drug therapy and psychotherapy (Jamison 1995a):

> I cannot imagine leading a normal life without lithium. From startings and stoppings of it, I now know it is an essential part of my sanity. Lithium prevents my seductive but disastrous highs, diminishes my depressions, clears out the weaving of my disordered thinking, slows me, gentles me out, keeps me in my relationships, in my career, out of a hospital, and in psychotherapy. It keeps me alive, too. But psychotherapy heals, it makes some sense of the confusion, it reins in the terrifying thoughts and feelings, it brings back hope, and the possibility of learning from it all. Pills cannot, do not, ease one back into reality. They bring you back headlong, careening, and faster than can be endured at times. Psychotherapy is a sanctuary, it is a battleground, it is where I have come to believe that someday I may be able to contend with all of this. No pill can help me deal with the problem of not wanting to take pills, but no amount of therapy alone can prevent my manias and depressions. I need both.

The belief that bipolar clients are not suitable candidates for group therapy has become well accepted among therapists (Luby and Yalom 1992). Bipolar clients have generally been considered poor psychotherapeutic candidates because of their difficult defensive styles. However, two studies have demonstrated that a long-term homogeneous group of bipolar clients focusing on interpersonal issues can be successful for this population (Luby and Yalom 1992).

Support Groups

People with bipolar disorders who are receiving treatment benefit from forming mutual support groups, such as those sponsored by the National Depression and Manic Depressive Association (NDMDA), the National Alliances for the Mentally Ill (NAMI), the National Mental Health Association, and the Manic Depressive Association. Friends and families of people with bipolar disorders can also benefit from mutual support and self-help groups such as those sponsored by NDMDA and NAMI. See Appendix E for more information.

EVALUATION

The outcome criteria often dictate the frequency of evaluation of the short-term goals. For example, are the client's vital signs stable, and is he or she well hydrated? Is the client able to control his or her own behavior or respond to external controls? Is the client able to sleep for 4 or 5 hours per night or take frequent short rest periods during the day? Does the family have a clear understanding of the client's disease and need for medication? Do they know which community agencies may be able to help them?

If goals are not met, the preventing factors are analyzed. Were the data incorrect or insufficient? Were nursing diagnoses inappropriate or goals unrealistic? Was the intervention poorly planned? After the goals and care plan are reassessed, the plan is revised, if indicated.

CASE STUDY: WORKING WITH A PERSON WHO IS MANIC

Ms. Horowitz is brought into the emergency department after being found on the highway shortly after her car breaks down. When the police come to her aid, she tells them that she is "driving herself to fame and fortune." She appears overly cheerful, constantly talking, laughing, and making jokes. At the same time, she walks up and down beside the car, sometimes tweaking the cheek of one of the policemen. She is coy and flirtatious with the police officers, saying at one point, "Boys in blue are fun to do."

She is dressed in a long red dress, a blue-and-orange scarf, many long chains, and a yellow-and-green turban. When she reaches into the car and starts drinking from an open bottle of bourbon, the police decide that her behavior and general condition might result in harm to herself or others. When they explain to Ms. Horowitz that they want to take her to the hospital for a general check-up, her jovial mood turns to anger and rage, yet 2 minutes after getting into the police car, she is singing "Carry Me Back to Old Virginny."

On admission to the emergency department, she is seen by a psychiatrist, and her sister is called. The sister states that Ms. Horowitz stopped taking her lithium about 5 weeks ago and is becoming more and

Continued on following page

CASE STUDY: WORKING WITH A PERSON WHO IS MANIC *(Continued)*

more agitated and out of control. She states that Ms. Horowitz has not eaten in 2 days, has stayed up all night calling friends and strangers all over the country, and finally fled the house when the sister called an ambulance to take her to the hospital. The psychiatrist contacts Ms. Horowitz's physician, and previous history and medical management are discussed. It is decided to hospitalize her during the acute manic phase and restart her lithium therapy. It is hoped that medications and a controlled environment will prevent further escalation of the manic state and prevent possible exhaustion and cardiac collapse.

ASSESSMENT

On Ms. Horowitz's admission to the unit, Mr. Atkins is assigned as her primary nurse. Ms. Horowitz is unable to sit down. She strides ceaselessly up and down the halls, talking loudly, pointing to other clients, and making loud sexual or hostile comments. Some of the other clients laugh at her actions and her dress. Others become angry and defensive.

Mr. Atkins suggests that they go to a quieter part of the unit. Ms. Horowitz turns to him angrily and says, "Let me be . . . set me free, lover . . . I am untouchable . . . I'll get the FBI to set me free."

Mr. Atkins divides the data into subjective and objective components.

OBJECTIVE DATA

- Little if anything to eat for days.
- Little if any sleep for days.
- History of mania.
- History of lithium maintenance.
- Constant physical activity—unable to sit.
- Very loud and distracting to others.
- Anger when wishes are curtailed.
- Flight of ideas.
- Dress loud and inappropriate.
- Remarks suggestive of sexual themes—calls nurse "lover."
- Some clients find her behavior amusing.
- Remarks suggest grandiose thinking.
- Poor judgment.

SUBJECTIVE DATA

- "Driving myself to fame and fortune."
- "I'm untouchable . . . I'll get the FBI to set me free."
- "Let me be . . . set me free, lover."

NURSING DIAGNOSIS

Mr. Atkins discusses Ms. Horowitz's immediate needs with the admitting psychiatrist. The psychiatrist orders 5 mg of intramuscular haloperidol (Haldol), to be given immediately. Then, he prescribes 5 mg intramuscularly every 8 hours until she can take the medication by mouth. Thereafter, Ms. Horowitz is to receive an extra 5 mg every other day. If dystonia occurs, she is to be given an anticholinergic agent (benztropine [Cogentin], trihexyphenidyl [Artane]) (see Chapter 22). She is to be observed for behaviors that might indicate harm to herself or others. The medical staff state that if medication and nursing interventions do not reduce her activity level, the nurses should allow for possible periods of rest and ingestion of fluids. Failing that, the use of seclusion would have to be considered. It is agreed that her physical safety is greatly jeopardized.

Mr. Atkins's initial diagnoses reflect the nursing and medical staffs' main concern: Ms. Horowitz's physical condition. Although she present many possible nursing diagnoses and needs at the time, the following two nursing diagnoses are formulated because they focus on her physical safety.

1. **Risk for injury** related to dehydration and faulty judgment, as evidenced by inability to meet own physiological needs and set limits on own behavior
   - Has not slept for days
   - Has not consumed food or fluids for days
   - Constant physical activity; unable to sit
2. **Defensive coping** related to biochemical changes, as evidenced by change in usual communication patterns
   - Very loud and distracting to others.
   - Remarks suggested sexual themes.
   - Some clients found her behavior amusing.
   - Remarks suggested grandiose thinking.
   - Flight of ideas.
   - Loud, hostile, and sexual remarks to other clients.

CASE STUDY: WORKING WITH A PERSON WHO IS MANIC *(Continued)*

PLANNING

PLANNING OUTCOME CRITERIA

Mr. Atkins formulates the following goals.

NURSING DIAGNOSIS	LONG-TERM OUTCOME	SHORT-TERM GOALS
1. **Risk for injury** related to dehydration and faulty judgment, as evidenced by inability to meet own physiological needs and set limits on own behavior.	1. Client's cardiac status will remain stable during manic phase.	1a. Client will be well hydrated, as evidenced by good skin turgor and normal urinary output within 24 hours. 1b. Client will sleep or rest 3 hours during first night in hospital, with aid of medication and nursing intervention. 1c. Client's blood pressure and pulse will be within normal limits within 24 hours, with aid of medication and nursing measures.
2. **Defensive coping** related to inadequate psychological resources, as evidenced by change in usual communication patterns.	2. Within 3 days, client will respond to verbal external controls when aggression escalates.	2a. Client will engage in safe activities aimed at reducing aggressive energy within 24–48 hours.

NURSE'S FEELINGS AND SELF-ASSESSMENT

Mr. Atkins has worked on the psychiatric unit for 2 years. He has learned to deal with many of the challenging behaviors associated with the manic defense. For example, he no longer takes most of the verbal insults personally, although many of the remarks could be cutting and could hit "close to home." He is also better able to recognize and set limits on some of the tactics used by the manic client to split the staff. The staff on this unit work closely with each other, which makes the atmosphere positive and supportive; therefore, communication is good among staff. Frequent and effective communication is needed among those working with clients who try to divide staff. Clear staff communication is vital to maximize external controls and maintain consistency in nursing care.

The only aspect of Ms. Horowitz's behavior that Mr. Atkins thought he might have some difficulty with is the sexual assaults and loud sexual comments she might make toward him. He knew that this could make him anxious, and his concern is that his anxiety might be picked up by the client.

When discussing this with the unit coordinator, they both decide that two nurses should provide care for Ms. Horowitz. A female nurse would spend time with her in her room, and Mr. Atkins would spend time with her in quiet areas on the unit. It is decided that neither Mr. Atkins nor any male staff member would be alone with Ms. Horowitz in her room at any time. Mr. Atkins should ask for relief if Ms. Horowitz's sexual remarks and acting-out behaviors make him anxious.

INTERVENTION

Because the most immediate concerns for Ms. Horowitz on admission are those of physical safety, 5 mg of intramuscular haloperidol (Haldol) is given intramuscularly. Other clients are moved so that Ms. Horowitz can have a single room. She does not allow vital signs to be taken at first; however, vital signs are eventually

Continued on following page

CASE STUDY: WORKING WITH A PERSON WHO IS MANIC *(Continued)*

taken and recorded at regular intervals. After the nurse spends 2 hours of pacing with Ms. Horowitz and coaxing her into less stimulating areas of the unit, Ms. Horowitz starts taking some fluids. Within 5 hours, she is drinking 8 ounces of high-caloric fluids per hour, after much reminding and encouragement.

By the next day, Ms. Horowitz's behaviors are much less hyperactive, and although her verbal sexual and aggressive assaults are less intense, she continues to provoke other clients. At this time, Mr. Atkins begins to assist her to channel some of her physical energy into less disruptive activities. He and Ms. Horowitz perform some slow exercises to relaxing music in a quiet part of the unit; he provides writing paper for her, and she spends 5 to 10 minutes writing furiously. She continues to pace and yell out to other clients, but with continued medication and nursing intervention, Mr. Atkins sees that this behavior is decreasing.

When Ms. Horowitz's sister comes to visit, she brings clothes, and Mr. Atkins spends some time with the sister finding out more about Ms. Horowitz. He learns that she is a schoolteacher, was depressed for 3 months before her first manic episode 2 years before, and is recently coming out of her second depressive episode. Although the second depressive episode is less severe than the first, the sister is concerned that Ms. Horowitz will "do something foolish," meaning suicide. Ms. Horowitz is separated from her husband and is having a difficult time adjusting to being back at work.

Mr. Atkins and the female nurse encourage Ms. Horowitz to dress and groom herself more appropriately because some of the other clients are beginning to laugh at her appearance. Mr. Atkins is aware that ridicule could further lower Ms. Horowitz's self-esteem, thus increasing her anxiety and need for the manic defense.

Ms. Horowitz's behavior is beginning to be controlled by the lithium about 10 days later, and she is being weaned off the haloperidol. At this time, she is able to talk to Mr. Atkins about how upset and depressed she is about her life (job and separation) and the fact that she must take medication for the "rest of my life." See Nursing Care Plan 21–1.

Mr. Atkins discusses with her some of the side effects of lithium that contributed to her noncompliance. He works with her to reduce and control some of her reactions to lithium. He then reviews other possible side effects and toxic effects of lithium and dietary and other precautions. At the end of her hospital stay, Ms. Horowitz states that she is resigned to continuing her lithium. After talking to Mr. Atkins, she decides to re-enter therapy to "help me get back into life."

EVALUATION

After 2 days, the medical staff think that Ms. Horowitz's cardiac status is stable. Her vital signs are within normal limits, she is consuming sufficient fluids, and her urinary output is normal. Although her hyperactivity persists, it does so to a lesser degree, and she is able to get periods of rest during the day and is sleeping 3 to 4 hours during the night.

Ms. Horowitz's hyperactivity continues to be a challenge to the nurses; however, she is able to attend to some activities that require gross motor movement. These activities are useful in channeling some of her aggressive energy. Shortly after her arrival on the unit, Ms. Horowitz starts a fight with another client, but seclusion is avoided because she is able to refrain from further violent episodes as a result of medication and nursing interventions. She could be directed toward solitary activities, which channel some of her energies, at least for short periods.

As the effectiveness of the drugs progresses, Ms. Horowitz's activity level decreases, and by discharge, she is able to discuss issues of concern with the nurse and make some useful decisions about her future. She is to be followed up at the community center and agrees to join a family psychoeducational group with her sister and other families with a bipolar member.

NURSING CARE PLAN 21–1 A PERSON WITH MANIA: MS. HOROWITZ

NURSING DIAGNOSIS

High Risk for Injury: related to dehydration and faulty judgment, as evidenced by inability to meet own physiological needs and set limits on own behavior.

Supporting Data

- Has not slept for days.
- Has not taken in food or fluids for days.
- Constant physical activity—is unable to rest.

Outcome Criteria: Client's cardiac status will remain stable during manic phase.

SHORT-TERM GOAL	INTERVENTION	RATIONALE	EVALUATION
1. Client will be well hydrated, as evidenced by good skin turgor and normal urinary output and specific gravity within 24 hours.	1a. Give haloperidol intramuscularly immediately and as ordered.	1a. Continuous physical activity and lack of fluids can eventually lead to cardiac collapse and death.	*GOAL MET* After 3 hours, client takes small amounts of fluids (2–4 ounces per hour).
	1b. Check vital signs frequently (every 1–2 hours).	1b. Monitor cardiac status.	
	1c. Place client in private or quiet room (whenever possible).	1c. Reduce environmental stimuli—minimize escalation of mania and distractibility.	
	1d. Stay with client and divert client away from stimulating situations.	1d. Nurse's presence provides support. Ability to interact with others is temporarily impaired.	
	1e. Offer high-calorie, high-protein drink (8 ounces) every hour in quiet area.	1e. Proper hydration is mandatory for maintenance of cardiac status.	After 5 hours, client starts taking 8 ounces per hour with a lot of reminding and encouragement.
	1f. Frequently remind client to drink: "Take two more sips."	1f. Client's concentration is poor; she is easily distracted.	
	1g. Offer finger food frequently in quiet area.	1g. Client is unable to sit; snacks she can eat while pacing are more likely to be consumed.	
	1h. Maintain record of intake and output.	1h. Enables staff to make accurate nutritional assessment for client's safety.	
	1i. Weigh client daily.	1i. Monitoring nutritional status is necessary.	*GOAL MET* After 24 hours, specific gravity is within normal limits.
2. Client will sleep or rest 3 hours during the first night in the hospital with aid of medication and nursing interventions	2a. Continue to direct client to areas of minimal activity.	2a. Lower levels of stimulation can decrease excitability.	Client is awake most of the first night. Sleeps for 2 hours from 4 AM to 6 AM.

Continued on following page

NURSING CARE PLAN 21–1 A PERSON WITH MANIA: MS. HOROWITZ *(Continued)*

SHORT-TERM GOAL	INTERVENTION	RATIONALE	EVALUATION
	2b. When possible, try to direct energy into productive and calming activities (e.g., pacing to slow, soft music; slow exercise; drawing alone; or writing in quiet area).	2b. Directing client to paced, nonstimulating activities can help minimize excitability.	Client is able to rest on the second day for short periods and engage in quiet activities for short periods (5–10 minutes).
	2c. Encourage short rest periods throughout the day (e.g., 3–5 minutes every hour) when possible.	2c. Client may be unaware of feelings of fatigue. Can collapse from exhaustion if hyperactivity continues without periods of rest.	
	2d. Client should drink decaffeinated drinks only—decaffeinated coffee, teas, or colas.	2d. Caffeine is a central nervous system stimulant that inhibits needed rest or sleep.	
	2e. Provide nursing measures at bedtime that promote sleep—warm milk, soft music, or backrubs.	2e. Promotes nonstimulating and relaxing mood.	
3. Client's blood pressure (BP) and pulse (P) will be within normal limits within 24 hours with the aid of medication and nursing interventions.	3a. Continue to monitor blood pressure and pulse frequently throughout the day (every 30 minutes).	3a. Physical condition is presently a great strain on client's heart.	Baseline measure on unit is not obtained because of hyperactive behavior. Information from family physician states BP 130/90 and P 88 base line.
	3b. Keep staff informed by verbal and written reports of baseline vital signs and client progress.	3b. Alerting all staff regarding client status can increase medical intervention if a change in status occurs.	BP at end of 24 hours is 130/70; P is 80.

NURSING DIAGNOSIS

Defensive Coping: related to inadequate psychological resources, as evidenced by change in usual communication patterns

Supporting Data

- Remarks suggest sexual themes.
- Some clients find her behavior amusing.
- Remarks suggest grandiose thinking.
- Has flight of ideas.
- Makes loud hostile and sexual remarks to other clients.

NURSING CARE PLAN 21–1 A PERSON WITH MANIA: MS. HOROWITZ

Outcome Criteria: Within 3 days, client will respond to external controls when aggression escalates.

SHORT-TERM GOAL	INTERVENTION	RATIONALE	EVALUATION
1. Client will engage in safe activities to express hostile and aggressive energy within 24–48 hours with the aid of medication and nursing interventions.	1a. Maintain a calm and matter-of-fact (neutral) attitude. 1b. Avoid power struggles and defensive postures when client is verbally abusive.	1a. Anxiety can be transmitted from staff to client. 1b. Client does not mean abuse personally; it is part of manic defense. Power struggles and defensive remarks by staff can escalate mania and potentiate violent acting out.	*GOAL PARTIALLY MET* Six hours after admission, client starts fight with another client. Staff explains that seclusion might be needed to help her gain control over her behavior.
	1c. Set limits and provide controls when necessary, e.g., "You are not to hit George. Come with me now," or "If you have trouble controlling yourself, we will help you."	1c. When client is out of control, external controls are needed to prevent client from acting out violently.	
	1d. Engage client in solitary activities that use large muscle groups (e.g., punching bag, ping-pong, or pacing with nurse).	1d. Activities client can do alone or with nurse that require large muscle groups can help drain physical tension.	On second day, client is able to participate with nurse in solitary activities using large muscle groups for short periods of time (5–10 minutes).

SUMMARY

Genetic factors appear to play a role in the etiology of the bipolar disorder. In addition, little doubt exists that an excess of, and an imbalance in, neurotransmitters are also related to bipolar mood swings. The outward gaiety and expansive, self-confident facade of a manic client often mask feelings of depression. Mania can be observed on a continuum from hypomania to acute mania.

The three main features of mania are (1) euphoria, (2) hyperactivity, and (3) flight of ideas. The nurse assesses the client's mood, behavior, and thought processes to plan the appropriate nursing interventions.

The analysis of the data helps the nurse choose appropriate nursing diagnoses. Some of the nursing diagnoses appropriate for a client who is manic are risk for violence, defensive coping, ineffective individual coping, altered thought processes, and self-esteem disturbance. Physical needs often take priority and demand nursing interventions. Therefore, fluid volume deficit and altered nutrition or elimination, as well as sleep-pattern disturbance, are usually part of the nursing plan. Altered family process is also an important consideration. Support, information, and guidance for the family can greatly affect the client's eventual recovery from his or her manic episode.

Planning nursing care involves setting realistic and measurable short-term and long-term outcomes for each of the nursing diagnoses. It is helpful for the nurse to understand that the manic symptoms help keep painful feelings out of awareness. Therefore, the client goes to great lengths to prevent outside controls from limiting his or her manic behavior. The manic client has numerous unconscious tactics to keep the nursing staff defensive, divided, and confused. When these tactics are successful, staff are less able to set consistent limits and monitor erratic behaviors. Unconscious tactics include pitting members of the staff against each other through manipulation, loudly and persistently pointing to faults and shortcomings in staff, constantly demanding attention and favors of the staff, and provoking clients as well as staff with profane and lewd remarks. The manic client constantly interrupts activities and distracts groups with his or her continuous physical motion and incessant joking and talking. The feelings aroused in such situations are usually anger and frustration toward the client. When these feelings are not examined and shared, the therapeutic potential of the staff is reduced, and feelings of confusion and helplessness remain.

Working with a manic client can be challenging. Interventions involve the use of specific principles of therapeutic communication, assistance with activities of daily living and somatic therapies, maintenance of a therapeutic environment, and when certified, intervention as a nurse therapist.

Evaluation includes examining the effectiveness of the nursing interventions, changing the goals as needed, and reassessing the nursing diagnoses. Evaluation is an ongoing process and is part of each of the other steps in the nursing process.

REFERENCES

American Psychiatric Association (1994). *Diagnostic and statistical manual of mental disorders* (4th ed.). Washington, DC: American Psychiatric Association.

Bowden, C. L. (1995). Treatment of bipolar disorder. In A. F. Schatzberg and C. B. Nemeroff (Eds.), *The American psychiatric press textbook of psychopharmacology* (pp. 603–614). Washington, DC: American Psychiatric Press.

Delgado, P. L., and Gelenberg, A. J. (1995). Antidepressant and antimanic medications. In G. O. Gabbard (Ed.), *Treatment of psychiatric disorders* (2nd ed., Vol. 1, pp. 1131–1168). Washington, DC: American Psychiatric Press.

Gabbard, G. O. (1995). Mood disorders: Psychodynamic etiology. In H. I. Kaplan and B. J. Sadock (Eds.), *Comprehensive textbook of psychiatry IV* (Vol. 1, pp. 1116–1123). Baltimore: Williams & Wilkins.

Ginns, E. I., Ott, J., Egeland, J. M., Allen, C. R., et al. (1996). A genome-wide search for chromosomal loci linked to bipolar affective disorder in the Old Order Amish. *National Genetics*, 12(4):431.

Goldstein, M. J., Baker, B. L., and Jamison, K. R. (1980). *Abnormal psychology: Experiences, origins and interventions.* Boston: Little, Brown.

Jamison, K. R. (1995a). *An unquiet mind.* New York, A. A. Knopf.

Jamison, K. R. (1995b). Psychotherapy of bipolar patients. Presented at the U. S. Psychiatric and Mental Health Congress, Marriot Marquis, New York, November 18, 1995.

Klerman, G. L. (1978). Affective disorders. In A. M. Nicholi, Jr. (Ed.), *The Harvard guide to modern psychiatry*. Cambridge, MA: Belknap Press of Harvard University Press.

Lehne, R. A., et al. (1994). *Pharmacology of nursing* (2nd ed.). Philadelphia: W. B. Saunders.

Luby, J. L., and Yalom, I. D. (1992). Group therapy. In E. S. Paykel (Ed.), *Handbook of affective disorders* (2nd ed.), pp. 475–486. New York: Guilford Press.

Maxmen, J. S., and Ward, N. G. (1995). *Psychotropic drugs: Fast facts* (2nd ed.). New York: W. W. Norton.

Merikangas, K. R., and Kupfer, D. J. (1995) Mood disorders: Genetic aspects. In H. I. Kaplan and B. J. Sadock (Eds.), *Comprehensive textbook of psychiatry IV* (Vol. 1, pp. 1102–1115). Baltimore: Williams & Wilkins.

Nathan, K. I., et al. (1995). Biology of mood disorders. In A. F. Schatzberg and C. B. Nemeroff (Eds.), *The American psychiatric press textbook of psychopharmacology* (pp. 439–477) Washington, DC: American Psychiatric Press.

Nurnberger, J. I., Jr., and Gershon, E. S. (1992). Genetics. In E. S. Paykel (Ed.), *Handbook of affective disorders* (2nd ed.), pp. 131–148. New York: Guilford Press.

Perris, C. (1992). Bipolar-unipolar distinction. In E. S. Paykel (Ed.), *Handbook of affective disorders* (2nd ed.), pp. 57–76. New York: Guilford Press.

Post, R. M. (1992). Anticonvulsants and novel drugs. In E. S. Paykel (Ed.), *Handbook of affective disorders* (2nd ed.), pp. 387–418. New York: Guilford Press.

Preston, J., and Johnson, J. (1995). *Clinical psychopharmacology made ridiculously simple.* Miami: MedMaster.

Ramaka, R., and Babbington, P. (1995). Social influences on bipolar affective disorders. *Social Psychiatry—Psychiatric Epidemiology*, 30(4):152.

Schatzberg, A. F., and Cole, J. O. (1991). *Manual of clinical psychopharmacology.* Washington, DC: American Psychiatric Press.

Scherer, J. S. (1985). *Nurses' drug manual.* Philadelphia: J. B. Lippincott.

Schiller, L., and Bennett, A. (1994). *The quiet room.* New York: Warner Books.

Silverstone, T., and Hunt, N. (1992). Symptoms and assessment of mania. In E. S. Paykel (Ed.), *Handbook of affective disorders* (2nd ed.), pp. 15–24. New York: Guilford Press.

Further Readings

Abou-Saleh, M. T. (1992). Lithium. In E. S. Paykel (Ed.), *Handbook of affective disorders* (2nd ed.), pp. 369–386. New York: Guilford Press.

Baradell, J. C. (1985). Humanistic care of the patient in seclusion. *Journal of Psychosocial Nursing*, 23(2):9.

Coryll, W., and Winokur, G. (1992). Course and outcomes. In E. S. Paykel (Ed.), *Handbook of affective disorders* (2nd ed.), pp. 89–110. New York: Guilford Press.

DePaulo, J. R. (1984). Lithium. *Psychiatric Clinics of North America*, 7(3):587.

Gershon, E. S., et al. (1985). Affective disorder genetics. In H. I. Kaplan and B. J. Sadock (Eds). *Comprehensive textbook of psychiatry* (4th ed.). Baltimore: Williams & Wilkins.

Gitlin, M. J., and Jamison, K. R. (1984). Lithium clinics: Theory and practice. *Hospital and Community Psychiatry*, 35:363.

Goodwin, F. K., and Jamison, K. R. (1990). *Manic-depressive illness.* New York: Oxford Press.

Hirschfeld, R. M. A., and Goodwin, F. K. (1988). Mood disorders. In J. A. Talbott, R. E. Hales and S. C. Yudofsky (Eds.), *Textbook of psychiatry.* Washington, DC: American Psychiatric Press.

Jamison, K. R., and Goodwin, F. K. (1983). Psychotherapeutic treatment of manic-depressive patients on lithium. In M. Greenhill and A. Granlick (Eds.). New York: Macmillan.

Roper, J. M., et al. (1985). Restraint and seclusion. *Journal of Psychosocial Nursing*, 23(6):18.

Weissman, M. M, and Boyd, J. H. (1985). Affective disorders: Epidemiology. In H. I. Kaplan, and B. J. Sadock (Eds.), *Comprehensive textbook of psychiatry* (4th ed.). Baltimore: Williams & Wilkins.

SELF-STUDY AND CRITICAL THINKING

Multiple choice

Choose the most appropriate answer.

1. All of the following may be observed in a person who is manic **except**

   A. "Hey baby, don't baby me . . . me and you can have some fun, fun and games and sugar and spice . . ."

   B. Quick, short periods of anger, quickly changing to another euphoria or depression.

   C. Splitting staff members against each other to prevent control of his or her manic defense.

D. Although thoughts may be fast, thoughts are never illogical or irrational.

2. Mrs. Jack has been taking lithium for months. Her most recent blood level was 2.2 mEq/L. What reactions might the nurse expect to see?

   A. Fine hand tremors, mild thirst, polyuria
   B. Diarrhea, vomiting, and slurred speech
   C. Electroencephalographic changes, ataxia, and seizures
   D. No untoward effects because her blood level is within normal limits

Completion

Complete the nursing diagnosis by filling in the related factor(s). For the nursing diagnosis presented, give two pieces of data that would support the diagnosis for a manic client.

3. **Risk for injury** related to ______________, as evidenced by
   1. ______________
   2. ______________

4. **Impaired verbal communication** related to ______________, as evidenced by
   1. ______________
   2. ______________

5. **Altered family process** related to ______________, as evidenced by
   1. ______________
   2. ______________

For each of these nursing diagnoses, state one long-term and two short-term goals.

6. **Risk for injury:** ______________

   Long-term outcome: ______________
   Short-term goal: ______________
   Short-term goal: ______________

7. **Impaired verbal communication:** ______________

   Long-term outcome: ______________
   Short-term goal: ______________
   Short-term goal: ______________

8. **Altered family process:** ______________

   Long-term outcome: ______________
   Short-term goal: ______________
   Short-term goal: ______________

Name two interventions for each of the following areas and give the rationale for the action.

9. Nutrition:
   1. ______________
   2. ______________

Rationales: ____

____

10. Rest and sleep:

   1. ____
   2. ____

   Rationales: ____

   ____

11. Dress and hygiene:

   1. ____
   2. ____

   Rationales: ____

   ____

12. Activities and recreation:

   1. ____
   2. ____

   Rationales: ____

   ____

List at least three cautions a person on lithium should know.

13. ____
14. ____
15. ____

Name three indications for seclusion.

16. ____
17. ____
18. ____

Place an H (helpful) or NH (not helpful) for each of the statements made by the nurse to a manic client. Explain why.

19. ___H___ "Tom, come with me to the quiet room."
20. ___NH___ "Comb the left side of your head . . . now the right side."
21. ___NH___ "That's a funny joke, Tom . . . have you heard this one?"
22. ___NH___ "I know the other nurses don't want you to join this group, but I'll let you."
23. ___NH___ "I don't like those remarks. They aren't true, and that kind of behavior is disgusting."
24. ___H___ "Come away from this group. Let's write instead."

Critical thinking

25. Donald has been taking lithium for 4 months. During his clinic visit, he tells you, his caseworker, that he does not think he will be taking his lithium anymore because he feels great and he is able to function well at his job and at home with his family. He tells you his wife agrees that "he has this thing licked."

    A. What are Donald's needs in terms of teaching?
    B. What are the needs of the family?
    C. Write out a teaching plan, or use an already constructed plan.
    D. Role play with a classmate how you could teach this family about bipolar illness and approach effective medication teaching, stressing the need for compliance and emphasizing those things that may threaten compliance.

22

Schizophrenic Disorders

ELIZABETH M. VARCAROLIS

OUTLINE

KEY TERMS AND CONCEPTS

The key terms and concepts listed here also appear in bold where they are defined or discussed in this chapter.

affect
associative looseness (looseness of association)
autism
ambivalence
positive symptoms
negative symptoms
delusions
thought broadcasting
thought insertion
thought withdrawal
delusions of being controlled
neologisms
concrete thinking
echolalia
echopraxia
clang association
word salad
hallucinations
illusions
depersonalization
derealization
loss of ego boundaries
extreme motor agitation
stereotyped behaviors
automatic obedience
waxy flexibility
stupor
negativism
water intoxication
extrapyramidal side effects
acute dystonia
akathisia
pseudoparkinsonism
tardive dyskinesia
neuroleptic malignant syndrome
paranoia
ideas of reference
blocking

OBJECTIVES

After studying this chapter, the reader will be able to

1. Describe the progression of symptoms from the prodromal to the acute phase of schizophrenia.
2. Discuss at least three of the neurobiological/anatomical/viral research findings that indicate that schizophrenia is a neurological disease.
3. Differentiate between the positive symptoms of schizophrenia and negative symptoms of schizophrenia as to (a) their response to standard antipsychotic medications, (b) their effect on quality of life, and (c) their influence on the prognosis of the disease.
4. Formulate at least three nursing diagnoses that are appropriate for a person with schizophrenia.
5. Identify common reactions a nurse may experience while working with a schizophrenic client.
6. Role play with a classmate interventions for a client who is hallucinating, delusional, and exhibiting looseness of associations.
7. Develop a teaching plan for a schizophrenic client who is taking an antipsychotic drug, such as haloperidol (Haldol).
8. Compare and contrast the properties of the standard and the atypical antipsychotic drugs in the following areas: (a) target symptoms, (b) indications for use, (c) side effects and toxic effects, and (d) needs for client and family teaching and follow-up.
9. Identify the kinds of individual, group, and family therapies that are most useful for schizophrenic clients and their families.
10. Differentiate among the three phases of schizophrenia as to symptoms, focus of care, and needs for intervention.
11. Explain how frequent evaluation of a schizophrenic client's nursing care plan can improve nursing skills and client progress.
12. Plan nursing intervention for a client with paranoid, agitated, withdrawn, and disorganized symptoms in the following areas: (a) counseling techniques, (b) self-care needs, and (c) milieu needs.

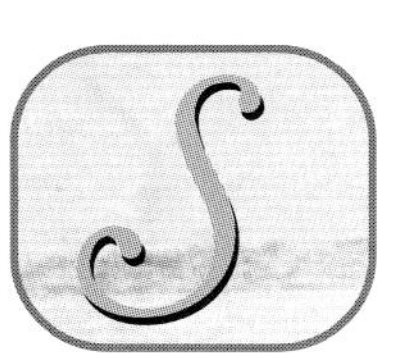

chizophrenia is a tragic, persistent neurological disease that affects a person's perceptions, thinking, language, emotion, volition, and social behavior (Andreasen and Munich 1995). Schizophrenia seriously interferes with people's ability to interpret reality and the world around them, to communicate with others and form relationships, to perform simple tasks or follow simple instructions, and to care for basic needs.

Data from the National Institute of Mental Health show that 1% of the general population have, or will have, the symptoms of schizophrenia. People with schizophrenia occupy approximately 50% of all hospital beds for the mentally ill and 25% of all available hospital beds (Berkow et al. 1992).

There seems to be a high prevalence of schizophrenia in the lower socioeconomic classes. This has been attributed to social disorganization and social stresses as well as to evidence that some people in a prepsychotic phase drift down the social scale (Berkow et al. 1992). People with schizophrenia account for between 35% and 50% of the homeless population in America (Carpenter and Buchanan 1995).

Schizophrenia is a psychotic disorder, which means that a person has impairment in reality testing. Major symptoms identified in psychotic disorders are hallucinations, delusions, and loss of ego boundaries. These terms are defined and discussed later in the chapter.

The symptoms of schizophrenia usually become apparent during adolescence or early childhood (15 to 25 years of age for men, 25 to 35 years of age for women). Paranoid schizophrenia has a later onset.

Schizophrenia has been divided into three phases, or epochs (Carpenter and Buchanan 1995):

1. *Onset.* This phase is slow and insidious (except in the case of catatonia) and may go on for a long time before the onset of hallucinations, delusions, or disorganized thinking. The first part of phase I is often called the *prodromal phase*, which is discussed in more detail in the "Assessment" section. During the second part of phase I, the acute psychotic symptoms are evident, and a high degree of disorganization and poor reality testing (hallucinations, delusions) exists.

2. *Those years immediately following the onset of psychotic symptoms.* The two patterns that characterize this phase are (a) the psychotic process progresses, with ebb and flow of intensity of the disruptive symptoms, and for some, (b) the episodic flow of psychotic symptoms may be followed by complete or relatively complete recovery.

3. *Long-term course and outcome.* Recently, it has been documented that for many severely and persistently mentally ill clients with schizophrenia, the intensity of the psychosis diminishes with age. For many clients, the illness seems to become less disruptive and easier to manage over time. Unfortunately, the long-term dysfunctional effects of the disorder are not so amenable to change (Carpenter and Buchanan, 1995).

Specific interventions are different for each of these phases and are discussed later in this chapter.

THEORY

Early explorations of schizophrenia focused on psychodynamic and family theories to explain how schizophrenia developed. Later, the advances of neuroscience, aided by the use of current neuroimaging techniques, expanded the knowledge of the chemical anatomy and neural circuitry of the brain, the mechanisms of neurotransmission, and the way brain chemicals affect the working of the brain (Andreasen and Munich 1995). Because most advances in neurobiological research offer compelling evidence that symptoms of schizophrenia are associated with abnormalities of the brain, psychoanalytic formulations are no longer adequate for an of understanding schizophrenia (Willick 1993).

Current theories of schizophrenia involve neuroanatomical and neurochemical abnormalities, which may be induced either genetically or environmentally (virus, birth defects). These neurobiological abnormalities may also produce certain vulnerabilities in individuals; the vulnerabilities can result in heightened sensitivity to psychosocial or environmental stressors (Andreasen and Munich 1995).

It has long been demonstrated that stressful life events are associated with the onset of schizophrenia or the exacerbation of schizophrenic symptoms. Stressful events can be categorized as chronic life stressors (family, work, poverty, physical disability) or acute stressors (unanticipated, undesired, and uncontrollable changes e.g., loss, moves, and acute illness) (McGlashan and Hoffman 1995). This is not to say that stress *causes* schizophrenia, but that people with certain neurobiological abnormalities are thought to be extremely vulnerable to stressful life events.

Since there is no scientific basis for the older psychosocial and family theories of schizophrenia, they are not discussed here, although basic psychosocial theories are addressed in Chapter 2, and family theories are presented in Chapter 11. Although these earlier theories are no longer considered valid in a causative sense, psychodynamic and family treatment modalities can be crucial in helping clients optimize and increase their social skills, maximize their ability at self-care and independent living, maintain medical compliance, and—most important of all—increase the quality of their lives.

Numerous theories relating to neurochemical and neuroanatomical findings exist. However, specific causes remain unclear, in part because schizophrenia is not a single disease. Moller (1989) defined schizophrenia as a syndrome that involves cerebral blood flow, neuroelectrophysiology, neuroanatomy, and neurobiochemistry. Neurochemical, genetic, and neuroanatomical findings, as well as other findings, are presented here.

Biological Models

Neurochemical Hypotheses

DOPAMINE HYPOTHESES. Bioamines (brain enzymes) are neurotransmitters to the areas of the brain that mediate emotions, feelings of pleasure and pain, awareness, and levels of consciousness. These bioamines divide into two categories: catecholamines (epinephrine, dopamine, and norepinephrine) and indolamine (serotonin) (see Chapter 3).

High levels of metabolites (products of metabolism) of the brain bioamines can be found in the urine of clients who are frankly psychotic. When the symptoms worsen, the level of metabolites of catecholamines and indolamine increases in the client's urine.

The dopamine theory of schizophrenia is derived from the study of the action of the antipsychotic drugs that have dopamine blocking agents (D_2). These antipsychotics block some of the dopamine receptors in the brain (D_2), which thereby limits the activity of dopamine and reduces some of the symptoms of schizophrenia. *Amphetamines*, *cocaine*, *methylphenidate (Ritalin)*, and *levodopa* are drugs that increase the activity of dopamine in the brain. These drugs produce an excess of dopamine in the brain and, in large doses, can exacerbate the symptoms of schizophrenia in psychotic clients. Amphetamines, cocaine, and other drugs can simulate symptoms of paranoid schizophrenia in a nonschizophrenic person.

The dopamine hypothesis is not considered conclusive, however. Other neurotransmitters that indirectly affect dopamine pathways are thought to be involved in schizophrenia. The efficacy of the newer antipsychotics (clozapine [Clozaril], risperidone [Risperdal], olanzapine [(Zyprexa]) provide strong evidence that mechanisms other than dopamine antagonists alone must be considered (Yamamoto and Meltzer 1995).

PHENCYCLIDINE PIPERIDINE (GLUCOMATE) HYPOTHESIS. It has long been noted that phencyclidine piperidine (PCP) induces a state that closely resembles schizophrenia. Unlike the amphetamine-induced psychosis in the dopamine hypothesis, PCP psychosis incorporates both the positive symptoms (hallucinations and paranoia) and the negative symptoms (emotional withdrawal and motor retardation) of schizophrenia.

Interest has been renewed in the PCP model of schizophrenia because of growing understanding of mechanisms by which PCP affects behavior at the neuroceptor level. However, the development of the hypothesis is still in its early stages.

N-methyl-D-aspartate (NMDA) is a type of gluconate receptor in the brain. PCP, when ingested, inhibits NMDA receptor–mediated neurotransmission. Therefore, one possibility is that problems of regulation of receptor-mediated transmission of NMDA might occur in schizophrenia. Thus, PCP-induced psychosis provides a neurochemical hypothesis of schizophrenia that is different from the dopamine hypothesis. Research in this area continues to hold promise for a better understanding of the neurochemical abnormalities that underlie schizophrenia (Wyatt et al. 1995).

Genetic Hypotheses

There is unquestionable evidence of a genetic contribution to some, and perhaps all, of the diseases classified as schizophrenic (Carpenter and Buchanan 1995). It has long been observed that schizophrenia and schizophrenic-like symptoms occur at an increased rate in relatives with schizophrenia. For example:

- Concordance rate (co-twin similarly affected) for schizophrenia in identical twins is 40% to 50% greater than that of the general population.
- Identical twin concordance is four to five times that of fraternal twins.
- Children of people with schizophrenia who are placed early for nonfamilial adoption have schizophrenia as adults at a higher rate than that in the general population.
- Children of "normal" parents who are placed in foster homes in which a foster parent later had schizophrenia do not show an increased rate of schizophrenia.

Although no individual schizophrenia gene has yet been identified, researchers are able to locate numerous markers that are linked to a gene that produces vulnerability to schizophrenia.

Neuroanatomical Studies

There is a shift from the concept of schizophrenia as a disorder of discrete areas of the brain to that of a disorder of brain circuits (communication pathways). Therefore, structural cerebral abnormalities could cause disruption to the entire circuit in the brain.

New brain-imaging techniques, such as computed tomography, magnetic resonance imaging, and positron-emission tomography, provide substantial evidence that some schizophrenic people have structural brain abnormalities. Computed tomographic and magnetic resonance imaging studies provide evidence for structural cerebral abnormalities. Some findings include

- Enlargement of the lateral cerebral ventricles.
- Cortical atrophy.
- Third ventricular dilation.
- Ventricular asymmetry.
- Cerebellar atrophy.

Some schizophrenic clients may also have changes in the cerebral cortex, the region of the brain that governs higher mental functions. During neurological testing, positron emission tomographic scans also show a low rate of blood flow and glucose metabolism in the frontal lobes of the cerebral cortex, which govern planning, abstract thinking, and social adjustment. Refer to Chapter 3 for a positron-emission tomographic scan that demonstrates reduced brain activity in the frontal lobe of a person with schizophrenia.

Other Considerations

Many other biological hypotheses and findings relating to the cause of schizophrenia exist and are discussed in the following sections (Carpenter and Buchanan 1995).

VIRAL HYPOTHESIS. Six viral theories of schizophrenia exist that are derived from the fact that many birth dates of schizophrenic clients show a modest peak during the late winter and early spring months. However, there is little evidence to give strong support to any of these theories. Wright and associates (1993) contended that exposure to the influenza virus in the second trimester of gestation increases the risk of later schizophrenia.

BIRTH AND PREGNANCY COMPLICATIONS. Theories in this area arise from the fact that infants born with a history of pregnancy or birth complications are at increased risk for developing schizophrenia as adults.

STRESS-RELATED THEORIES. Developmental and family stress, as well as other social, physiological, or physical stress, may play a significant role in the severity and course of the disease, as well as the person's quality of life. There is no evidence that stress causes schizophrenia, although it may precipitate it in a vulnerable individual.

Tollefson (1995) summarized possible causes of schizophrenia:

1. A multifactorial cause is likely but unknown.
2. Neurological structural and functional abnormalities have been identified.
3. Neuropsychological evidence suggests a subcortical cognitive focus; the NMDA receptor complex has been implicated.
4. No single region or transmitter abnormality explains the disease.
5. Abnormal circuitry ("wiring") may best explain schizophrenia.

ASSESSMENT

In 1950, Eugen Bleuler, building on the observations of Emil Kraepelin, coined the term *schizophrenia*. Bleuler's fundamental signs of schizophrenia, referred to as the four As, are still used today for help in the diagnosis of schizophrenia. The four As include

1. **Affect,** the outward manifestation of a person's feelings and emotions. In schizophrenia, one can observe flat, blunted, inappropriate, or bizarre affect.
2. **Associative looseness,** which refers to haphazard and confused thinking that is manifested in jumbled and illogical speech and reasoning. People also use the term ***looseness of association.***
3. **Autism,** thinking that is not bound to reality but reflects the private perceptual world of the individual. Delusions, hallucinations, and neologisms are examples of autistic thinking in a person with schizophrenia.
4. **Ambivalence,** simultaneously holding two opposing emotions, attitudes, ideas, or wishes toward the same person, situation, or object. Ambivalence occurs normally in all relationships. Pathological ambivalence is paralyzing.

▸ Sam, a 25-year-old man soon to be discharged from the hospital, constantly tells the social worker he wants his own apartment. When Sam is told that an apartment has been found for him, he states, "But who will take care of me?" Sam is acting out his ambivalence between his desire to be independent and his desire to be taken care of.

In 1959, Kurt Schneider developed a system of diagnosing a person with schizophrenia by classifying ongoing symptoms as first rank and second rank. In 1975, the World Health Organization (WHO) identified a standard set of symptoms specific to the diagnosis of schizophrenia; this set is common to people in numerous countries. Figure 22–1 presents the *Diagnostic and statistical manual of mental disorders*, fourth edition (DSM-IV) criteria for the diagnosis of schizophrenia developed in 1994 (APA 1994).

Renewed interest has been kindled in the study of the positive and negative symptoms of schizophrenia. The **positive symptoms** (e.g., hallucinations, delusions, bizarre behavior, and paranoia) are the attention-getting symptoms referred to as *florid psychotic symptoms*. Three decades of analysis of treatment and study findings indicate that perhaps these florid psychotic symptoms may not be the core deficiency after all. Actually, the crippling **negative symptoms** (e.g., apathy, lack of motivation, anhedonia, and poor thought processes) persist and seem more fundamental (Talbott et al. 1994). Another reason for renewed interest is that it appears that the positive-negative approach may correlate with prognosis as well as biological variables.

Positive symptoms, such as hallucinations, delusions, bizarre behavior, and paranoia, are associated with

1. Acute onset.
2. Normal premorbid functioning.

DSM-IV Diagnostic Criteria for Schizophrenia

A. Characteristic Symptoms
Two or more of the following during a 1-month period:
1. Delusions
2. Hallucinations
3. Disorganized speech (e.g., LOA)
4. Grossly disorganized or catatonic behavior
5. Negative symptoms (apathy, anhedonia, avolition, alogia)

If delusions bizarre or auditory hallucinations and
a. voices keep a running commentary about person's thoughts/behaviors **or**
b. two or more voices converse with each other

Then only one criterion is needed.

B. Social/Occupational Dysfunction
If one or more major areas of the person's life are markedly below premorbid functioning (work, interpersonal relationships or self-care) **or**
If childhood or adolescence failure to achieve expected level of interpersonal, academic, or occupational achievement
Then meets criteria of **B**.

C. Duration
Continuous signs persist for at least 6 months with at least 1 month that meets criteria of **A** (Active Phase) and may include prodromal or residual symptoms.

D.
1. **All other mental diseases** (e.g., schizoaffective/mood disorder) have been ruled out.
2. **All other medical conditions** (substance use/medications or general medical conditions) have been ruled out.
3. **If history of pervasive developmental disorders**, then prominent hallucinations or delusions for 1 month are needed to make the diagnosis of schizophrenia.

Figure 22–1 DSM-IV diagnostic criteria for schizophrenia. LOA, looseness of association. (Adapted from American Psychiatric Association (1994). *Diagnostic and statistical manual of mental disorders*, 4th ed. Washington, DC: American Psychiatric Association. Reprinted with permission. Copyright 1994 American Psychiatric Association.)

3. Normal social functioning during remissions.
4. Normal computed tomographic findings.
5. Normal neuropsychological test results.
6. Favorable response to antipsychotic medication.

Negative symptoms, such as apathy, anhedonia, poor social functioning, and poverty of thought, are associated with

1. Insidious onset.
2. Premorbid history of emotional problems.
3. Chronic deterioration.
4. Demonstration of atrophy on computed tomographic scans.
5. Abnormalities on neuropsychological testing.
6. Poor response to antipsychotic therapy.

Many researchers feel that the positive-negative dichotomy is an oversimplification, and many see a three-dimensional syndrome of schizophrenia as a better explanation for the symptoms. The three-dimensional model proposed by many (Roy and DeVrient 1994; Brekke et al 1994; Peralta-Martin and Cuesta-Zokita 1994) consists of

1. Positive symptoms.
2. Negative symptoms.
3. Disorganized symptoms.

However, the positive and negative dichotomy is useful in theory for educational purposes. Table 22–1 expands on the discrete attributes of the positive and negative symptoms.

Prodromal Symptoms

Many people who have schizophrenia experience prodromal symptoms a month to a year before their first psychotic break. These symptoms represent a clear deterioration in previous functioning. Often, a person who has schizophrenia was withdrawn from others, lonely, and perhaps depressed as an adolescent. Plans for the future may appear vague or unrealistic to others.

A transitional "preschizophrenic" phase may occur a year or two before the disorder is diagnosed. This phase may include such neurotic symptoms as acute or chronic anxiety, phobias, obsessions, and compulsions, or they may have dissociative features. As anxiety mounts, indications of a thought disorder may be present. An adolescent may have difficulty with concentration and with the ability to complete school work or job-related work. Eventually, severe deterioration of work and deterioration of ability to cope with the environment occur. Patients report having "mind wandering," inability to concentrate, and need to devote more time to maintaining one's thoughts. Finally, the ability to keep out unwanted intrusions into one's thoughts becomes impossible. Eventually, the person finds that his or her mind becomes so distracted that the ability to have ordinary conversations with others is lost (Kolb and Brodie 1982).

The person may initially feel that something strange or wrong is going on. The person misinterprets things going on in the environment and may give mystical or symbolic meanings to ordinary events. For example, the person may think that certain colors hold special powers or that a thunderstorm is a message from God. The person often mistakes other people's actions or words as signs of hostility or evidence of harmful intent (Kolb and Brodie 1982).

As the disease develops, the person has strong feelings of rejection, lack of self-respect, loneliness, and hopelessness. Emotional and physical withdrawal increase feelings of isolation, as does an inability to trust or relate to others. The withdrawal may become severe, and withdrawal from reality may become evident in hallucinations, delusions,

TABLE 22–1 DIFFERENCES BETWEEN POSITIVE AND NEGATIVE SYMPTOMS

EXAMPLES	ASSOCIATED FINDINGS	INTERVENTION
Positive (Florid)		
Delusions Looseness of associations Hallucinations Agitated or bizarre behaviors	Acute onset Least important prognostically History of exacerbations and remissions Normal premorbid functioning No family history of schizophrenia Normal computed tomographic findings Normal neuropsychological findings Good response to antipsychotics	Neuroleptic (antipsychotic medication). Medical assessment to rule out physiological process that may be contributing to symptoms.
Negative (Deficit)		
Apathy Poverty of speech or content of speech Poor social functioning Anhedonia Social withdrawal	Slow onset Interferes with a person's life Positive premorbid history Chronic deterioration Family history of schizophrenia Cerebellar atrophy and lateral and third ventricular enlargement on computed tomographic scan Abnormalities on neuropsychological testing Poor response to antipsychotics	The newer atypical antipsychotics may target some of the negative symptoms. The most use interventions include Skill training interventions: ▸ Identify areas of skill deficit person is willing to work on. ▸ Prioritize skills important to the person. Working with person to identify stressors: ▸ Identify which stressors contribute to maladaptive behaviors. Work with person on increasing appropriate coping skills.

and odd mannerisms. Some persons think their thoughts are being controlled by others or that their thoughts are being broadcast to the world. Others may think that people are out to harm them or are spreading rumors about them. Voices are sometimes heard in the form of commands or derogatory statements about their character. The voices may seem to come from outside the room, from electrical appliances, or from other sources.

Early in the disease the person may be preoccupied with religion, matters of mysticism, or metaphysical causes of creation. Speech may be characterized by obscure symbolisms.

Later, words and phases may become indecipherable, and these can be understood only as part of the person's private world. Sometimes, the person makes up words. People who have been ill with schizophrenia for a long time often have speech patterns that are incoherent, rambling, and devoid of meaning to the casual observer.

Sexual activity is frequently altered in mental disorders. Preoccupation with homosexual themes may be associated with all psychoses but is most prominent in people with paranoid schizophrenia. Doubts regarding sexual identity, exaggerated sexual needs, altered sexual performance, and fears of intimacy are prominent in schizophrenia. The process of regression in schizophrenia is accompanied by increased self-preoccupation, isolation, and masturbatory behavior.

An abrupt onset with good premorbid functioning is usually a favorable prognostic sign. A slow, insidious onset over a period of 2 or 3 years is more ominous. Those whose prepsychotic personalities show good social, sexual, and occupational functioning have greater chances for a good remission or a complete recovery. Childhood histories of withdrawn, seclusive, eccentric, and tense behavior are unfavorable diagnostic signs. The younger the client is at the onset of schizophrenia, the more discouraging the prognosis. Because schizophrenia is a psychotic disorder, it is placed on the high end of the mental health continuum (Fig. 22–2).

Early psychiatric and medical treatment helps secure a more favorable eventual outcome. A delay of months or years allows the psychotic process to become more entrenched. No single symptom is always present in all cases of schizophrenia or occurs only in schizophrenia alone. Figure 22–1 identifies the DSM-IV criteria for schizophrenia. The various subtypes of schizophrenia, with symptoms, are outlined in Figure 22–3. Assessment is organized into positive, negative, and associated symptoms.

Assessing Positive Symptoms

The positive symptoms appear early in the first phase of the illness. These are the symptoms that get people's attention and often precipitate hospitalization. They are, however, the least important prognostically and usually respond to antipsychotic medication. The positive symptoms are presented here in terms of alterations in thinking, perceiving, and behavior.

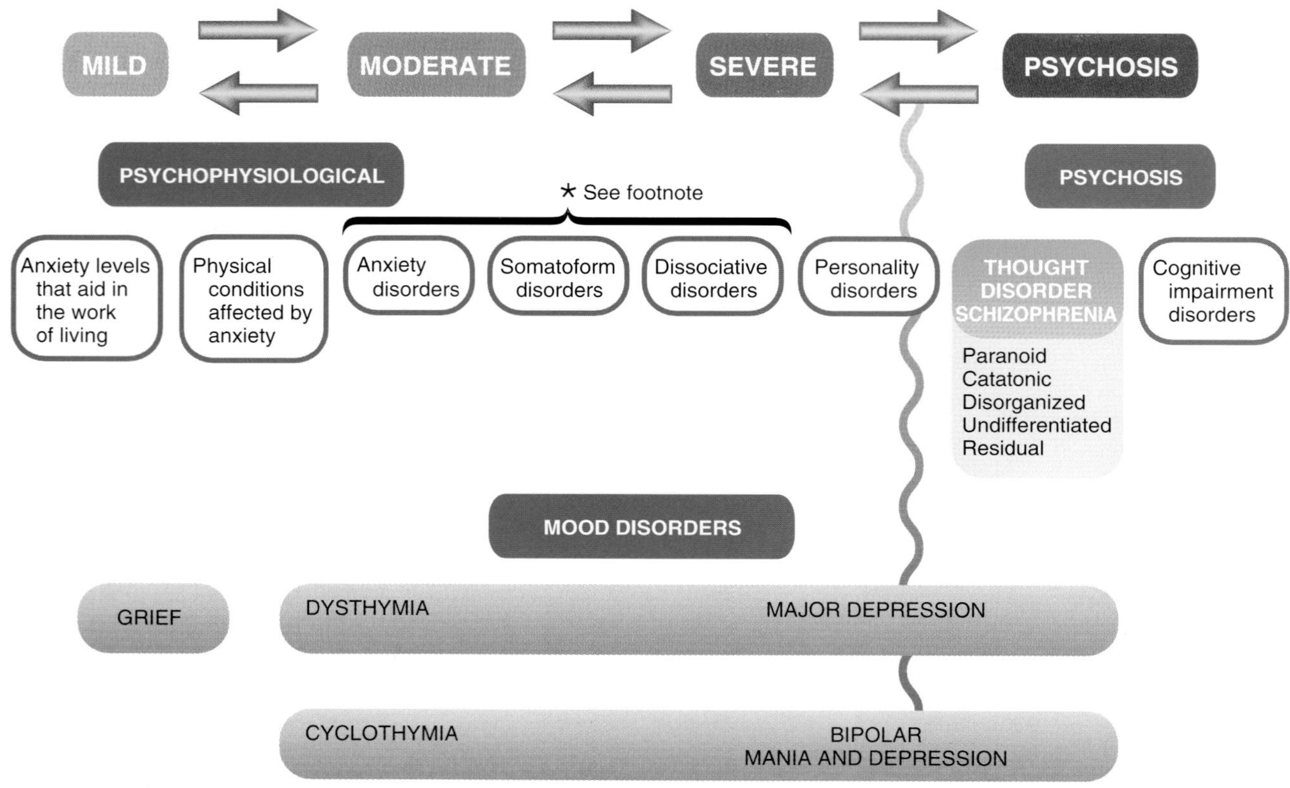

Figure 22–2 The mental health continuum for schizophrenia.

Alterations in Thinking

Alterations in thinking can take many forms. **Delusions** are most often defined as false fixed beliefs that cannot be corrected by reasoning. They may be simple beliefs or part of a complex delusional system. In schizophrenia, delusions are often loosely organized and may be grotesque. Most common delusional thinking involves the following themes:

1. Ideas of reference
2. Persecution
3. Grandiosity
4. Bodily functions
5. Jealousy
6. Control

Table 22–2 provides definitions and examples of delusions.

About 75% of schizophrenic people experience delusions at some time during their illness. In schizophrenia, persecutory and grandiose delusions are the most common, as are those involving religious or hypochondriacal ideas.

In the acute phase of schizophrenia, the person is overwhelmed by anxiety and is not able to distinguish what is inside (thoughts) from what is outside (reality). Therefore, a delusion may stimulate behavior for dealing with confusion and the resulting anxiety.

When delusional, a person truly believes what he or she thinks to be real *is* real. The person's thinking often reflects feelings of great fear and aloneness: "I know the doctor talks to the CIA about getting rid of me" or "Everyone wants me dead." Delusions may reflect the person's feelings of low self-worth through the use of reaction-formation (observed as grandiosity). "I'm the only one who can save the world, but they won't let me."

At times, delusions hold a kernel of truth. One client came into the hospital acutely psychotic. He kept saying that the Mafia was out to kill him. Later, the staff learned that he had been selling drugs, that he had not paid his contacts, and that gang members were out trying to find him and hurt him or even kill him.

Other common delusions observed in schizophrenia are the following:

1. **Thought broadcasting,** the belief that one's thoughts can be heard by others (e.g., "My brain is connected to the world mind. I can control all heads of state through my thoughts.").
2. **Thought insertion,** the belief that thoughts of others are being inserted into one's mind (e.g., "They make me think bad thoughts and are rotting my brain.").
3. **Thought withdrawal,** the belief that thoughts have been removed from one's mind by an outside agency (e.g., "The devil takes my thoughts away and leaves me empty.").

TABLE 22–2 SUMMARY OF DELUSIONS*

DEFINITION	EXAMPLE
Ideas of Reference	
Misconstruing trivial events and remarks and giving them personal significance	When Maria saw the doctor and nurse talking together, she believed they were talking against her. When she heard on the radio that a hurricane was coming, she believed this to be a message that harm was going to befall her.
Persecution	
The false belief that one is being singled out for harm by others; this belief often takes the form of a plot by people in power against the person	Same believed that the secret service was planning to kill him. He became wary of the food he ate, since he believed that the secret service was poisoning his food.
Grandeur	
The false belief that one is a very powerful and important person	Sally believed that she was Mary Magdalene and that Jesus controlled her thoughts and was telling her how to save the world.
Somatic Delusions	
The false belief that the body is changing in an unusual way, e.g., rotting inside	David told the doctor that his brain was rotting away.
Jealousy	
The false belief that one's mate is unfaithful. May have so-called proof.	Harry accused his girlfriend of going out with other men, even though this was not the case. His "proof" was that she came home from work late twice that week. He persisted in his belief, even when the girlfriend's boss explained that everyone had worked late.

*A false belief held and maintained as true, even with evidence to the contrary. This does not include unusual beliefs maintained by one's culture or subculture.

4. **Delusions of being controlled**, beliefs that one's body or mind is controlled by an outside agency (e.g., "There is a man from darkness who controls my thoughts with electrical waves.").

ASSOCIATIVE LOOSENESS. Zelda Fitzgerald wrote her husband, the writer F. Scott Fitzgerald, an account of going mad:

> Then the world became embryonic in Africa—and there was no need for communication. . . . I have been living in vaporous places peopled with one-dimensional figures and tremulous buildings until I can no longer tell an optical illusion from a reality . . . head and ears incessantly throb and roads disappear (Vidal 1982).

Associations are the threads that tie one thought to another and one concept to another. In schizophrenia, these threads are missing, and connections are interrupted. In looseness of association, thinking becomes haphazard, illogical, and confused:

Nurse: Are you going to the picnic today?
Client: Only five dollars at the top.

This client's response initially seems not to be in keeping with the question asked by the nurse. To the client, however, the response has meaning. This young man always referred to his emotional security in dollars and cents. When he was feeling secure and confident, he spoke of himself as having plenty of money: "I have $500 at the top." At times, the nurse may be able to decipher, or decode, the client's messages and begin to understand the client's feelings and needs. Any exchange in which a person feels understood is useful. Therefore, the nurse might respond to the client in this way:

Nurse: Are you saying, Tony, that you don't feel secure enough to go out with the others today?
Client: Yeah . . . not much at the top today.

Often, decoding is not possible because the client's verbalizations are too fragmented. For example:

Client: I sang out for my mother . . . for this to hell I went. How long is road? This little said three hills, hop aboard, share the appetite of the Christmas mice spread . . . within three round moons the devil will be washed away.

If the nurse does not understand what the client is saying, it is important to let the client know this. Clear messages and complete honesty are an important part of working with schizophrenic persons. Letting the person know that the nurse does not understand but would like to understand or will try to understand is honest.

NEOLOGISMS. Neologisms are words a person makes up that have special meaning for the person. ("I was going to tell him the *mannerologies* of his hospitality won't do." "I want all the *vetchkisses* to leave the room and leave me be.")

Children and creative writers often make up their own words. Their creation of neologisms is imaginative, constructive, and adaptive. Neologisms in the schizophrenic reaction represent a disruption in thought processes.

CONCRETE THINKING. In psychiatry, the term **concrete thinking** usually implies overemphasis on specific details and an impairment in the ability to use abstract concepts. For example, during an assessment, the nurse might ask what brought the client to the hospital. The client might answer "a cab" rather than explaining the need for seeking medical or psychiatric aid. When asked to give the meaning of the proverb "people in glass houses shouldn't throw stones," the person might answer, "Don't throw stones or the windows will break." The answer is literal; the ability to use abstract reasoning is absent.

ECHOLALIA. Echolalia is the pathological repeating of another's word by imitation and is often seen in people with catatonia.

Nurse: Mary, come for your medication.
Mary: Mary, come for your medication.

Echolalia is the counterpart of **echopraxia,** mimicking the *movements* of another, and is also seen in catatonia.

CLANG ASSOCIATION. Clang association is the meaningless rhyming of words, often in a forceful manner, "On the track . . . have a Big Mac . . . or get the sack," in which the rhyming is often more important than the context of the word. This form of speech pattern may be seen in schizophrenia; however, it may also be seen in the manic phase of a bipolar disorder or in a person with a cognitive disorder, such as Alzheimer's disease or acquired immunodeficiency syndrome–related dementia.

WORD SALAD. Word salad is a term used to identify a mixture of phrases that is meaningless to the listener and perhaps to the speaker as well. It may include a string of neologisms, as in the following example: "Birds and fishes . . . framewoes . . . mud and stars and thump-bump going."

Alterations in Perceiving

Hallucinations, especially auditory hallucinations, are the major example of alterations in perception in schizophrenia. The following alterations in perceptions are discussed in this section: hallucinations and loss of ego boundaries (depersonalization and derealization).

HALLUCINATIONS. Hallucinations can be defined as sensory perceptions to which there is *no external stimulus exists.* The most common types of hallucinations include

- Auditory—hearing voices or sounds.
- Visual—seeing persons or things.
- Olfactory—smelling odors.
- Gustatory—experiencing tastes.
- Tactile—feeling body sensations.

Table 22–3 provides examples of common hallucinations. Table 22–3 also describes the difference between hallucinations and **illusions.**

It is estimated that 90% of people with schizophrenia experience hallucinations at some time during their illness. Although manifestations of hallucinations are varied, auditory hallucinations are most common in schizophrenia. Voices may seem to come from outside or inside the person's head. The voices may be familiar or strange, single or multiple. Voices speaking directly to the person or commenting on the person's behavior are most common in schizophrenia. A person may believe that the voices are from God, the devil, deceased relatives, or strangers. The auditory hallucinations may occasionally take the form of sounds rather than voices. *Command hallucinations* must be assessed for, because the "voices" may command the person to hurt himself or others. For example, a client might state that "the voices" are telling him to "jump out the window" or "take a knife and kill my child." Command hallucinations are often terrifying for the individual. Command hallucinations may signal a psychiatric emergency. Clients who can give an identity to the hallucinated voice are at somewhat greater risk of compliance with the hallucinated command than are those who can not (Junginger 1995).

Evidence of possible auditory hallucinatory behavior may be the turning or tilting of the head, as if the client is talking to someone, or frequent blinking of the eyes and grimacing. Sometimes, clients verbally respond to "their voices."

Visual hallucinations are less often reported in schizophrenia (about 20%) and are more often noted in organic disorders. Olfactory, tactile, or gustatory hallucinations account for about 10% of hallucinations in people with schizophrenia (Moller 1989).

Grebb and Cancro (1989) pointed out that the frequency of hallucinations may vary among cultures. There is some indication that hallucinations are more common in African, West Indian, and Asian cultures than in American and European cultures.

LOSS OF EGO BOUNDARIES. People with schizophrenia often lack a sense of their body in relationship to the rest of the world—where they leave off and others begin. For this reason, many schizophrenics are confused about their own sexual identity. Clients might say that they are merging with others or are part of inanimate objects.

1. **Depersonalization** is a nonspecific feeling that a person has lost his or her identity, that the self is different or unreal. People may be concerned that body parts do not belong to them. People may have an acute sensation that their body has drastically

TABLE 22–3 SUMMARY OF HALLUCINATIONS*

DEFINITION	EXAMPLE
Auditory	
Hearing voices or sounds that do not exist in the environment but are projections of inner thought or feelings	Anna "hears" the voice of her dead mother call her a whore and a tramp.
Visual	
Seeing a person, object, or animal that does not exist in the environment	Charles, who is experiencing alcohol withdrawal delirium, "sees" hungry rats coming toward him.
Olfactory	
Smelling odors that are not present in the environment	Theresa "smells" her insides rotting.
Gustatory	
Tasting sensations that have no stimulus in reality	Sal will not eat his food because he "tastes" the poison the FBI is putting in his food.
Tactile	
Feeling strange sensations where no external objects stimulate such feelings; common in delirium tremens	Jack, a paranoid schizophrenic "feels" electrical impulses controlling his mind. Susan, experiencing alcohol withdrawal delirium, "feels" snakes crawling on her body.

*A hallucination is a false sensory perception for which no external stimulus exists. They are different from illusions in that illusions are misperceptions or misinterpretations of a real experience. For example, a man saw his coat hanging on a coat rack and believed it to be a bear about to attack him. He did see something real but misinterpreted what it was.
FBI, Federal Bureau of Investigation.

changed. For example, a woman may see her fingers as snakes or her arms as rotting wood. A man may look in a mirror and state that his face is that of an animal.

2. **Derealization** is the false perception by a person that the environment has changed. For example, everything seems bigger or smaller, or familiar surroundings have become somehow strange and unfamiliar.

Both depersonalization and derealization can be interpreted as **loss of ego boundaries,** sometimes referred to as loose ego boundaries.

Alterations in Behavior

Bizarre and agitated behavior are associated with schizophrenia and may take a variety of forms.

BIZARRE BEHAVIOR. Bizarre behaviors may take the form of a stilted rigid demeanor, eccentric dress or grooming, and rituals. The following behaviors are often seen in catatonia:

1. **Extreme motor agitation.** Extreme motor agitation is agitated physical behavior, such as running about, in response to inner and outer stimuli. The person may become dangerous to others or may have exhaustion or collapse and die if not stopped.

2. **Stereotyped behaviors.** Stereotyped behaviors are motor patterns that originally had meaning to the person (e.g., sweeping the floor, washing windows) but have become mechanical and lack purpose.

3. **Automatic obedience.** A catatonic client may perform, without hesitation, all simple commands in a robot-like fashion.

4. **Waxy flexibility.** Waxy flexibility consists of excessive maintenance of posture, evidenced when a person's arms or legs can be placed in any position and the position is held for long periods.

- **Stupor.** The person who is in a stupor may sit motionless for long periods and may be motionless to the point of apparent coma.
- **Negativism.** Negativism is equivalent to resistance. In *active negativism,* the people do the opposite of what they are told to do. When people do not do things they are expected to do (e.g., do not get out of bed, do not dress, do not eat), such behavior is termed *passive negativism.*

Waxy flexibility, stupor, and negativism can be considered negative symptoms.

AGITATED BEHAVIOR. Clients with schizophrenia may have difficulty with impulse control when they are acutely ill. Because of cognitive deterioration, clients lack social sensitivity and may act out impulsively with others (e.g., grab another's cigarette, throw food on the floor, and get the television remote control and change channels abruptly).

Assessing Negative Symptoms

The negative symptoms of schizophrenia develop over a long time. These are the symptoms that most interfere with the individual's adjustment and ability to survive. The presence of negative symptoms interferes with the person's ability to

- Initiate and maintain relationships.
- Initiate and maintain conversations.
- Hold a job.
- Make decisions.
- Maintain adequate hygiene and grooming.

The presence of negative symptoms contributes to the person's poor social functioning and social withdrawal.

On assessment, specific phenomena are noted. During an acute psychotic episode, negative symptoms may be difficult to assess because the positive and more florid symptoms, such as delusions and hallucinations, may dominate. Some of the negative phenomena, which are outlined in Table 22–4, include poverty of speech content, poverty of speech, thought blocking, anergia, anhedonia, affective blunting, and lack of volition.

Affect is the observable behavior that expresses a person's emotions. The affect of a schizophrenic person can usually be categorized in three ways: flat or blunted, inappropriate, or bizarre.

A *flat* (immobile facial expressions or a blank look) or *blunted affect* (minimal emotional response) is commonly seen in schizophrenia. In schizophrenia, people's outward affect may not coincide with their inner emotions.

Inappropriate affect refers to an emotional response to a situation that is not congruent with the tone of the situation. For example, a young man, told that his father is ill, breaks into laughter.

Bizarre affect is especially prominent in the disorganized form of schizophrenia. Grimacing, giggling, and mumbling to oneself come under this heading. Bizarre affect is marked when the client is unable to relate logically to the environment.

A study suggests that cognitive deficits are more likely to be associated with high negative symptom ratings than with positive symptom ratings. Furthermore, improved cognitive abilities are related to improvement in positive symptoms but not negative symptoms (Addington et al. 1991).

Assessing Associated Symptoms

Other symptoms are associated with schizophrenia. Presented in this section are depression and suicide, water intoxication, substance abuse, and violent behavior. These phenomena are not peculiar to schizophrenia but may be found on assessment.

DEPRESSION AND SUICIDE. Depression is often seen in people with schizophrenia. Attempted suicide is a frequent event in the lives of people with schizophrenia, and actual death from suicide occurs in at least 10% to 13%, 20 times higher than in the general population (Lipton and Cancro 1995). Actually, suicide is the leading cause of premature death among people with schizophrenia (APA 1997). People with schizophrenia often feel confused, helpless, and isolated and have fewer personal resources for support and comfort.

Fenton and Cole (1995) suggested specific recommendations for suicide prevention, including the following:

1. Define the high-risk client (male, young, concurrent depression, recent loss or rejection, history of past suicidal attempts, and limited external supports).

TABLE 22–4 NEGATIVE PHENOMENA

PHENOMENON	EXPLANATION
AFFECTIVE BLUNTING	In *affective blunting,* severe reduction in the expression and range and intensity of affects occurs; in *flat affect* no facial expression of emotion exists.
ANERGIA	Lack of energy: passivity, impersistence at work or school.
ANHEDONIA	Inability to experience any pleasure in activities that usually produce pleasurable feelings; result of profound emotional barrenness.
AVOLITION	Lack of motivation: unable to initiate tasks, e.g., social contacts, grooming, and other aspects of activities of daily living.
POVERTY OF CONTENT OF SPEECH	Speech that is adequate in amount but conveys little information because of vagueness, empty repetitions, or use of stereotypes or obscure phases.
POVERTY OF SPEECH	Restriction in the amount of speech—answers range from brief to monosyllabic one-word answers.
THOUGHT BLOCKING	A client may stop talking in the middle of a sentence and remain silent. After a client stops abruptly: Nurse: "What just happened now?" Client: "I forgot what I was saying. Something took my thoughts away."

2. Provide additional support during high-stress periods, such as immediately after discharge.
3. Use appropriate psychopharmacological and psychosocial interventions for comorbid depression and substance abuse.

People with schizophrenia who attempt suicide are more likely to meet criteria for major depression than nonattempters (Jones 1994).

WATER INTOXICATION. Excessive water consumption by psychiatric clients is receiving much attention. **Water intoxication,** or psychosis-induced polydipsia, is thought to occur in 3% to 6% of hospitalized psychiatric clients (Bugle et al. 1992). A high percentage of these psychiatric clients have schizophrenia. Clients may ingest more than 10 to 15 L of fluid per day. When this disorder is not treated, it can lead to cerebral edema, seizures, brainstem herniation, and even death. Water-intoxicated clients are seen constantly carrying a cup or a soda can and making frequent trips to the water fountain or rest room. Clients have also been observed drinking from a toilet, sink, and shower. These clients are often highly agitated and vigorous in their pursuit of fluids (Bugle et al. 1992).

A high percentage of water imbalance in schizophrenic clients is thought to be medication induced. Inappropriate secretion of antidiuretic hormone can be caused by antipsychotics as well as by carbamazepine (Tegretol), lithium, and other drugs.

Initial management of psychosis-induced polydipsia consists of ruling out possible medical causes; acute management involves water restriction and sodium replacement to prevent seizures and other consequences of severe hyponatrenia (APA 1997). Long-term management includes the use of various medications, e.g., lithium, phenytoin, and demeclocycline (APA 1997).

SUBSTANCE ABUSE. Psychoactive drug abuse occurs in about 50% of schizophrenic clients in urban hospitals (Lipton and Cancro 1995) and the lifetime incidence is even higher at 60% (APA 1997). Cannabis, alcohol, and cocaine are the drugs used most frequently by people with schizophrenia. These clients report that all three drugs acutely increase their experience of happiness and decrease their feelings of depression. Most clients report that they use drugs to relieve depression and relax. Others state that they use drugs to counteract their negative symptoms (to help them increase feelings and emotions, talk more, and increase energy). One study suggested that clients may use alcohol to alleviate the symptoms of agitation and dysphoria associated with their medications or treatment (Duke 1994).

Unfortunately, stimulants in particular increase the intensity of delusions and hallucinations as well as the underlying emotional state (Lipton and Cancro 1995). It has also been reported that drug-abusing schizophrenic clients require more hospitalization, have lower compliance with treatment regimens, and are at greater risk for suicide as well as homelessness, violence, incarceration, and human immunodeficiency virus (HIV). The use of these psychoactive substances appears to have a significantly adverse effect on the global outcome of these clients. An unfortunate effect of alcohol ingestion is that it may mask the early symptoms of schizophrenia, leading to a delay in diagnosis (Duke 1994).

VIOLENT BEHAVIOR. Threats of violence and even minor aggressive outbursts are common in acute schizophrenic states and relapses (Berkow et al. 1992). General risk factors for violence in schizophrenia include previous arrests; the presence of substance abuse; and the presence of hallucinations, delusions, or bizarre behavior (APA 1997). Effective management of aggressive behavior may be achieved through behavioral treatment and limit setting. Antipsychoic medication is the mainstay of management. Other drugs for management with schizophrenic clients include anticonvulsants, lithium, and high-dose propranolol (APA 1997). (See Chapter 12 for guidelines for communicating with violent clients.)

NURSING DIAGNOSIS

As indicated by the assessment, a person with schizophrenia may have a variety of symptoms. Schizophrenic clients may be on a unit or in a community setting, but each individual with schizophrenia may present with different symptoms, personal needs, and defensive behaviors. Each client requires nursing care that reflects his or her individual needs and strategies that are appropriate to the client's behaviors and level of functioning.

During the course of schizophrenia, a client is likely to experience positive (hallucinations, delusions) and negative (withdrawal, poor social functioning) symptoms. During this time, impairment in thought processes may be evident in the client's ability to reason, solve problems, make decisions, and concentrate. These distortions alter the client's ability to perceive reality accurately (hallucinations or delusions) and usually impair the client's judgment. A nursing diagnosis of **sensory-perceptual alterations** is appropriate. Sensory-perceptual alterations may be related to alteration in biochemical compounds, stress, and emotional trauma.

With alteration in thought process come changes in language and speech. Therefore, **impaired verbal communication** may be a problem to varying degrees. When looseness of associations is severe, the person is unable to communicate needs or feelings. The nurse interacts in various ways to try to understand and help reduce the client's anxiety. Use of neologisms, echolalia, clang associations, and word salad contribute to the client's impaired verbal communication.

When a person is unable to interpret the world accurately, his or her ability to cope with the environment is also impaired. Therefore, **ineffective individual coping** is almost always present. A person's ineffective individual coping may be evidenced by inappropriate use of defense mechanisms and inability to meet role expectations. Symptoms may include withdrawal or excitability, disorganized or regressive behaviors, paranoid or disorganized thinking, and inability to meet basic needs.

A person who is extremely paranoid may have special problems. For example, if the person is refusing to eat because he or she thinks the food is poisoned, then **altered nutrition: less than body requirements** is diagnosed.

Voices that tell the person to harm others or self can result in bodily harm or even death to the client or others. **Risk for violence directed at self or others** would take priority (refer to section on paranoia).

During the excited phase of catatonia, clients may be highly agitated and can exhaust themselves to a dangerous level if rest and high-calorie fluid replacement are not immediately provided. Extreme hyperactivity can lead to cardiac or respiratory collapse and indicates a nursing diagnosis of **activity intolerance.**

During extreme withdrawal, attention to physical care is vital. Some useful nursing diagnoses might be (1) **constipation** or **incontinence,** (2) **impaired physical mobility,** or (3) **self-care deficit: feeding, bathing, dressing/grooming, and toileting.**

When the disease becomes chronic, clients may be admitted to a hospital many times. Problems with compliance regarding medications is thought to be a major factor. Families with schizophrenic members may have their own confused patterns of communication and insufficient knowledge of the client's problems, or they may feel powerless in coping with the client at home. **Ineffective family coping: compromised or disabling** may be an important area for intervention by members of the health care team, especially in relation to discharge planning.

Most people with schizophrenia have a low self-concept. Clients are often confused about their sexual identity, and they may have an unrealistic and distorted perception of themselves. Depersonalization further confuses the person's perception of body image. **Self-esteem disturbance** is usually present, as is **risk for loneliness.**

PLANNING

Planning involves more than the identification of measurable and attainable goals. Identification of personal reactions and feelings regarding the client is necessary if the interventions in the nursing care plan are to be carried out effectively. Therefore, planning involves identifying realistic outcomes and planning goals and being aware of common nurses' reactions and feelings.

Planning Outcome Criteria

It is important that the outcome (goal) be both meaningful and attainable by nursing action. The goals are related to the first half of the diagnostic statement and provide a blueprint for the evaluation. The "related to" components are the focus of nursing action. The goals listed subsequently are offered as examples and guidelines for nursing actions.

1. **Altered thought processes** related to psychosis, as evidenced by threatening hallucinations/delusions.

OUTCOME CRITERION

- Client will state that the voices are not threatening, nor do they interfere with his or her life.

LONG-TERM AND SHORT-TERM GOALS

- By (date), client will take medications as prescribed and state three benefits.
- Client will meet with nurse once a day for 15 minutes in an activity in which client feels comfortable.
- By (date), client will state that "the voices" or "the thoughts" are less frequent, with the aid of medication and nursing intervention.
- By (date), client will engage in one unit activity per day that provides reality testing.
- By (date), client will identify personal interventions that lower hallucinations.
- By (date), client will talk about concrete happenings without talking about delusions or hallucinations for short periods.
- By (date), client will make needs and wants clearer with the aid of medication and nursing interventions.

2. **Social isolation** related to lack of motivation to respond, as evidenced by feelings of rejection by others.

OUTCOME CRITERION

- Client will demonstrate a willingness to socialize with others.

LONG-TERM AND SHORT-TERM GOALS

- By (date), client will meet with nurse for 10 minutes twice a day in an activity in which client feels safe.
- By (date), client will meet with nurse and one other client in a simple activity.
- Client will state that he or she feels more comfortable with nurse by (date).
- Client will state that he or she feels more comfortable with one other client or staff member by (date).
- Client will attend one simple group activity each day by (date).
- Client will attend one community group meeting a week.
- Client will engage one other person in a social event (shopping, movies, dining out) each week.

3. **Risk for violence directed at others** related to misperceived messages from others, as evidenced by persecutory delusions and hallucinations.

OUTCOME CRITERION

- Client and others will remain safe.

LONG-TERM AND SHORT-TERM GOALS

- By (date), client will state that the voices are less angry, with the aid of medication.
- By (date), client will identify helping behaviors of nurses, staff, family, or case manager.
- Client will join nurse for one activity per day in which client states that he or she feels safe.
- By (date), client will state that he or she feels safe on the unit or in community activities with the staff or others.
- Client will identify increase in agitation and go to staff or designated person(s) in the community.

4. **Self-care deficit** related to perceptual impairment, as evidenced by inability to wash body parts, to carry out toileting procedures, to select appropriate clothes to wear, to feed self adequately.

OUTCOME CRITERION

- Client will perform activities of daily living in an independent manner.

LONG-TERM AND SHORT-TERM GOALS

- Client will bathe self at least every other day with minimum of supervision or prodding by (date).
- Client will maintain adequate hygiene (teeth, hair, grooming) by (date).
- Client will dress self appropriately by (date).
- Client will take in adequate nutrition and be within 5% of normal body weight range by (date).

Nurse's Feelings and Self-Assessment

Working with individuals diagnosed as schizophrenic is bound to bring up strong emotional reactions from health care workers. The psychotic client is intensely anxious, lonely, dependent, and distrustful. The intensity of these emotions can stir up similarly intense, uncomfortable, and frightening emotions in all health care workers. Identification of one's feelings and responses is an important part of working with all clients.

If personal feelings and reactions are ignored by the nurse, feelings of helplessness may follow. Increased feelings of helplessness can increase anxiety. Without the support, opportunity, and willingness to explore these reactions with more experienced nursing staff, defensive behaviors emerge. Defensive behaviors in the nurse (e.g., denial, withdrawal, avoidance) thwart the client's progress and undermine the nurse's self-esteem. These behaviors are associated with staff burnout. Statements such as "These clients are hopeless," "You can't understand these people," and "You waste your time with them" are examples of unexamined or unrecognized emotional reactions to client's behaviors or feelings.

For nurses new to the psychiatric setting, especially for student nurses, the availability of supportive supervision is necessary if learning is to take place. The student's part in the supervisory process is a willingness to discuss and identify personal feelings and to identify problem behaviors. This can be, and often is, accomplished in group supervision. Experienced psychiatric nurses call this process *peer group supervision.*

Feelings that arise when nurses are working with a schizophrenic client on a one-to-one basis include discouragement, fear, worthlessness, rage, and envy. However, the nurse's personal feelings are often an important source of information about the client's state of mind, particularly in clients who are unable to talk (Fenton and McGlashan 1995).

Individual supervision provides the greatest opportunity for a better understanding of the interpersonal issues involved in establishing a working relationship with the client. Individual supervision can increase the learner's understanding of the client and the client's situation, competence with therapeutic skills, and self-confidence.

Menninger (1984) discussed the extreme frustration that staff have with the slow progress of schizophrenic clients. This sense of frustration and feelings of helplessness can lead to burnout. Periodic reassessment of treatment goals and scaling down of expectations can benefit both the nurse and the client. Periodic review of frustrating clients can lead to a better understanding of the client's strengths and weaknesses. A team approach to reevaluating and establishing realistic, obtainable outcomes for clients can help energize staff, reduce helplessness, and benefit the client.

Clinical practice with adequate supervision can increase the nurse's skills, lower personal anxiety, increase confidence, and improve the quality of interpersonal relationships with clients, as well as relationships with others.

INTERVENTION

Interventions are geared to the client's phase of schizophrenia. For example, during *phase I,* the acute phase, the clinical focus is on crisis intervention, acute symptom stabilization, and safety. Interventions are often hospital-based; however, more and more community-based settings and home care agencies are treating acute clients in the community.

A number of factors that affect the choice of treatment setting are based on the following (APA 1997):

- Protection of the person from harm to self or others.
- Client's needs for external structure and support.
- Client's ability to cooperate with treatment.
- Client's need for a particular treatment that may be available only in one setting.
- Client's need for a comorbid general medical or psychiatric condition.

- Availability of psychosocial support to facilitate receipt of treatment and give critical information to staff about clinical status and response to treatment.
- Client and family preferences.

Interventions during the acute phase include

1. Acute psychopharmacological treatment.
2. Supportive and directive communications.
3. Limit setting.
4. Psychiatric, medical and neurological evaluation.

When clients are hospitalized during the acute phase, the length of hospitalization is often determined by hospital policy in the form of clinical pathways. Clinical Pathway 22–1 presents a pathway for schizophrenia. This clinical pathway takes the client through 16 days. Most clients in the acute phase are hospitalized for shorter periods before being discharged to community support, e.g., 7 to 11 days or so. Once the acute symptoms are being treated, the client is discharged to the community, where appropriate treatment can be carried out during phases II and III of the disease.

Phase II and III interventions include

- Client and family teaching about the disease.
- Medication teaching and side-effect management.
- Cognitive and social skills enhancement.
- Identifying signs of relapse.
- Attention to deficit in self-care, social and work functioning.

Table 22–5 provides an overview of the clinical focus, intervention, and professional collaboration that are best suited to each phase.

Throughout the work with schizophrenic clients, the nurse and others attempt to minimize stress and anxiety levels. Lowered anxiety levels can decrease the intensity of schizophrenic symptoms and make the client more amenable to engaging in activities and relationships with others, improving family interactions, and becoming involved in nonthreatening activities. Lowered anxiety levels make it possible for all people, including people with schizophrenia, to define problems and focus on issues.

When planning interventions, it is important that the nurse not overlook the adaptive skills of a psychotic client. *Attention should be given to the client's strengths and healthy functioning as well as to areas of deficiencies.*

Counseling (Basic Level)

Therapeutic strategies for working with schizophrenic clients often involve interventions that address specific behaviors. Interventions are aimed at lowering the client's anxiety, decreasing defensive patterns, encouraging participation in the environment, and raising level of self-worth. Refer to the appropriate sections for specific counseling techniques in paranoid, withdrawn, excitable, and regressed behaviors.

All nurses should be familiar with the principles used in dealing with phenomena that are certain to arise with most schizophrenic clients: hallucinations, delusions, and looseness of association.

HALLUCINATIONS. As previously stated, voices are the most common hallucinatory experience reported by schizophrenic clients. It is important initially to understand what the voices are saying or telling the person to do. Suicidal or homicidal messages necessitate priority measures for all members of the health care team.

Hallucinations are real to the person who is experiencing them. A hallucinating client should be approached in a nonthreatening and nonjudgmental manner (Lipton and Cancro 1995). Moller (1989) emphasized that when a person is hallucinating, the individual is experiencing anxiety, fear, loneliness, and low self-esteem, and the brain is not processing stimuli accurately.

During the acute phase of the illness, it is helpful to maintain eye contact, speak simply in a louder voice than usual, and call the person by name. Moller (1989) outlined 12 steps that nurses can take when working with a hallucinating client after the acute phase has passed (Table 22–6). Moller cautioned that the nurse can be expected to become frustrated at times. When the nurse is feeling frustrated, it helps to remember that progress often follows an uneven course and to reframe the experience in a more positive light. The nurse should focus on reality-based happenings, explanations, and conversations.

DELUSIONS. Delusions are a result of misperception of cognitive stimuli. It is best when the nurse attempts to see the world as it appears through the eyes of the client. In that way, the nurse can better understand the client's delusional experience. For example:

Client: You people are all alike . . . all in on the CIA plot to destroy me.

Nurse: I don't want to hurt you, Tom. Thinking that people are out to destroy you must be very frightening.

First, the nurse clarifies the reality of the client's intent. Second, the nurse empathizes with the client's apparent experience, the feelings of fear. The nurse does not get drawn into the conversation regarding the content of the delusion (CIA and plot to destroy) but looks for the feelings that the person may be experiencing. Talking about the client's feelings can be useful for the client; talking about delusional material is not.

It is *not* useful to argue with the client regarding the content of the delusion. Doing so can intensify the client's retention of irrational beliefs. Although the nurse does not argue with the client's delusions, clarifying misinterpretations of the environment is useful. For example:

Client: I see the doctor is here, and he is out to get me and destroy me.

Nurse: It is true the doctor wants to see you, but he wants to talk to you about your treatment. Would you feel more comfortable talking to him in the day room?

CLINICAL PATHWAY 22–1 Diagnosis: Schizophrenia

Initiation Date:

	DAY 1	#	DAYS 2–6	#	DAYS 7–11	#	DAYS 12–16	#
Medical Interventions	H&P, MSE, thought process and content, misperceptions, SI/HI. Evaluate for substance abuse. Order labs, ECG 40+. Admission orders. Drug screen. Restrict for 24 hr.		Complete treatment plan. Establish antipsychotic dose. Assess for changes in MSE. Review labs and old record. Re-evaluate restriction.		Update treatment plan. Monitor symptoms, meds, and side effects. Continue group/individual therapy. Initiate D/C plans for F/U.		D/C Instruction form. D/C orders. Prescriptions and F/U appt. Terminate therapy.	
Nursing Interventions	Admission Assessment Documentation. Assess for command hallucinations, paranoid delusions, thoughts of self-harm. Monitor intake. Orient to ward, schedule and give ITP. Vital signs and wt.		Assess adaptation to ward. Provide structured environment, ↓ stimulation, ↑contact with reality. Introduce to small group activity. Monitor hallucinations, delusions, thoughts of harm (SI, HI). level of anxiety, response to meds. Assist with grooming. Educate PT/family illness/meds.		Continue monitoring (see previous). Evaluate participation in reality-oriented activities. Evaluate independence in ADLs. Evaluate med/illness teaching.		Continue monitoring/evaluation. (see previous). Complete D/C summary. AMI referral. Reinforce need for continued after care and meds.	
Social Work Interventions	Emergency intervention		Assessment by third workday. Identify living situation, financial status, support systems. Initiate D/C planning.		Continue counseling PT/family. Review with PT/family available support systems.		Coordinate pass with caregiver to evaluate reintegration into community. Terminate counseling. Make outpatient appts.	
Psychology Interventions			Initial psychological testing		Review findings.			
Recreation Therapy Interventions	Initial contact		Initial RT assessment completed. Introduce PT to socialization group.		Begin/continue leisure/D/C plan. Evaluate reality orientation/relatedness.		Complete leisure D/C plan(s). Terminate therapy.	
Key Patient Outcomes	PT verbalizes feelings of safety @ ______		Visible during meals @ ______ Attends ward/team activities @ ______ Maintains control @ ______ Identifies current meds @ ______		Visible on ward 50% of time @ ______ Independent ADLs @ ______ Improved personal hygiene @ ______		↓ or cessation of SXs of altered thought process/ content, misperceptions, self-harm @ ______ Cessation of agitation @ ______ Improved judgment @ ______ Improved relatedness @ ______ F/U and meds @ ______	

Adapted from VA Medical Center, 10 North Green Street, Baltimore, MD 21201.
Patient Identification
PT, patient; D/C, discharge; RT, recreation therapy; ADL, activity of daily living; F/U, follow-up; appt, appointment; SX, symptom; MSE, mental status examination; H & P, history and physical; SI, suicidal ideation; HI, homicidal ideation; ITP, interdisciplinary treatment plan.
KEY: Circle = variance (see back); # = date-progress note re: Specific evaluation/intervention goal; @ = achievement date.

Interacting with the client on concrete realities in the environment can be help minimize the client's time spent thinking delusional thoughts. Specific manual tasks within the scope of the client's abilities can often be useful as distractions from delusional thinking. The more time the client spends with reality-based activities or people, the more opportunity the client has to become comfortable with reality.

LOOSENESS OF ASSOCIATION. Looseness of association often mirrors the client's autistic thoughts. The client's autistic and disorganized ramblings may leave the nurse confused and frustrated. An increase in

TABLE 22–5 TREATMENT FOCUS AT DIFFERENT PHASES OF SCHIZOPHRENIA

	Phase I		Phase II	Phase III
	Acute: Onset, Exacerbation, or Relapse	**Subacute and Convalescent**	**Adaptive Plateau**	**Stable Plateau**
Clinical Focus	Crisis intervention Safety Acute symptom stabilization	Social supports Stress and vulnerability assessment Living arrangements Daily activities Economic resources	Understanding and acceptance of illness Mistrust, isolation, denial, suspiciousness Damage to self-esteem	Social, vocational, and self-care skills Learning or relearning Identifying realistic expectations Adaptation to deficits
Intervention	Acute psychopharmacological treatment Limit setting Supportive and directive Psychiatric, medical, neurological evaluation Meet with family	Psychosocial evaluation Evaluation of human services Linkage with ▸ Social services ▸ Human services ▸ Community treatment agencies Psychoeducational interventions with families	Support and teaching Medication teaching and side effect management Direct assistance with situational problems Identification of prodromal and acute symptoms and signs of relapse Continued psychoeducational work with families as needed.	Attention to detail of self-care, social, and work functioning Direct intervention with family/employers Cognitive/social skills enhancement Medication maintenance Continued psychoeducational intervention with families as needed
Professional Collaboration	Inpatient treatment team Residential alternative to hospitalization Community crisis intervention Internist Neurologist	Social work department Health and human services Day treatment or community support	Community support staff Family support groups Group therapies and self-help groups Behavior therapies using educational models	Group therapists Social, vocational and self-care providers Family, employer, community support staff

Adapted from Fenton, W. S., and Cole, S. A. (1995). Psychosocial therapies of schizophrenia: Individual, group and family. In G. O. Gabbard (Ed.), *Treatment of psychiatric disorders* (2nd ed., Vol. 1, pp. 1006–1007). Washington, DC: American Psychiatric Press.

the client's autistic speech patterns can indicate increased anxiety on the part of the client and can reflect his or her difficulty in responding to internal and external stimuli.

Decoding is a term used for interpreting the meaning of autistic communications. Decoding is not always possible, but when it is possible, it can help the nurse understand the client's experience and needs.

The following guidelines may be useful for spending time with a client whose speech is confused and disorganized.

1. Do not pretend that you understand the client's communications when you are confused by the client's words or meanings.
2. Tell the client that you are having difficulty understanding the communications.
3. Place the difficulty in understanding on yourself, *not* on the client. For example, say "I am having trouble following what you are saying," *not* "You are not making any sense."
4. Look for recurring topics and themes in the client's communications. For example, "You've mentioned trouble with your brother several times. I guess your relationship with your brother is on your mind."
5. When understanding the client's autistic communications is not possible, just listening to, and being accepting of, the client can be meaningful.
6. Emphasize what is going on in the client's immediate environment (here and now) and involve the client in simple reality-based activities. These measures can help the client better focus thoughts.
7. Tell the client what you do understand and reinforce clear communication and accurate expression of needs, feelings, and thoughts.

TABLE 22–6 MOLLER'S INTERVENTIONS WITH HALLUCINATIONS

STEPS	COMMENTS
1. Establish a relationship where the client feels safe.	1. Trust can grow when ◗ The nurse is consistent. ◗ The nurse asks permission to talk about hallucinations. ◗ The nurse is not hurried—the nurse gives the person time to respond and allows the person time to stare into space.
2. Assess for symptoms of auditory hallucinations.	2. Cues include ◗ Eyes looking around the room. ◗ Tilting head to one side. ◗ Mumbling to oneself. ◗ Curling up on the bed and withdrawing (experience of hallucinations can be exhausting).
3. Focus on hallucination symptoms and ask the person to describe what is happening.	3. The goal is to empower the person to help them understand their symptoms: ◗ "What are you experiencing?" ◗ "I'll be here if you want me." ◗ "I see your eyes moving back and forth. Are you anxious?" Give the person time to answer.
4. Identify if drugs or alcohol is currently being used.	4. The nurse asks the client directly whether he or she has taken drugs or alcohol; what was taken; how much, and when? Drugs do not cause schizophrenia but may exacerbate symptoms.
5. If asked, point out simply that you are not experiencing the hallucinations	5. For the person it is real; the goal is to guide the person through the experience: ◗ "What do you feel you need to do?" ◗ "What are you hearing?"
6. Help the person describe present hallucinations.	6. This may be the first time a person has been allowed to discuss the hallucination. ◗ Gives the person the power to manage hallucinated voices ◗ Provides a quiet environment; gives the person permission to share the content of the hallucinations.
7. Encourage the person to describe past experience.	7. The nurse encourages the person to discuss when he or she began experiencing hallucinations. It is essential to understand the past in order to manage the present.
8. Encourage the person to observe and describe feelings, thoughts, and actions, both present and past, as they relate to hallucination.	8. The goal is to connect the cognitive, emotional, and behavioral components of hallucinations. ◗ Identify what person was feeling during the hallucination: "Tell me what you think happened." ◗ The person may have developed skill in covering up hallucinations—this frees up energy to manage the symptoms instead.
9. Help the person identify the needs that may underlie the hallucination	9. Often, hallucinations reflect needs for ◗ Power and self control. ◗ Self-esteem. ◗ Anger. ◗ Sexuality.
10. Help make connection between the hallucination and the need it represents.	10. The nurse focuses on the loneliness the individual may be feeling. ◗ Encourage the person to identify when hallucinations occur and what triggers them.
11. Suggest and reinforce the person's use of interpersonal relationships in meeting needs.	11. The client needs one person who can be trusted to accept him or her. ◗ People often are reluctant to "give up" their voices because they have no close friends.
12. Focus on other related aspects of the person's psychopathological behavior.	12. The nurse talks openly and honestly with the client about concerns other than hallucinations. ◗ Eventually, other aspects of the person's life can be explored.

Adapted from Moller, M. D. (1989). *Understanding and communicating with an individual who is hallucinating* (video). Omaha, NE: NurScience.

Health Teaching: Client and Family (Basic Level)

Teaching methods of health management to clients, families, and other caregivers can be important in stabilizing the schizophrenic person's future adjustment. It is not just the level or source of stress in the client's environment that is crucial; also important are the manner in which people deal with the stress and how effectively stressful issues are resolved. Psychological strategies aimed at reducing exacerbation of the psychotic symptoms follow:

1. Educate the client and the client's family about the illness. Emphasize how stress and medication affect the illness. Such knowledge may increase medication compliance and motivate involvement in psychosocial activities.
2. Assist the client to increase his or her ability to solve problems related to environmental stress.
3. Teach the client coping strategies to deal with the source of symptoms of schizophrenia and the stresses in the social environment.
4. Assist family and client to identify sources for ongoing support in dealing with illness.

Some of these steps may be implemented during the acute phase of the illness (e.g., educating family, identifying sources of support), while others may be implemented or continued once the client is discharged through community-based resources (see Table 22–5).

Studies have indicated the importance of the family environment for a schizophrenic client. When a schizophrenic client is returned to a family environment that consists of warmth, concern, and supportive behavior, a relapse is less likely to occur. An environment that is highly critical of the client's behavior or consists of intrusive involvement into the client's life has a higher correlation with recurrent episodes of schizophrenia.

Some of the critical attitudes toward people with schizophrenia result in a lack of understanding of the symptoms of schizophrenia, especially the negative symptoms. For example, the client's apathy, lack of drive, and motivation may be wrongly interpreted as laziness. This erroneous assumption can encourage hostility on the part of family members, caregivers, or people in the community. Therefore, further teaching of the disease process of schizophrenia can reduce tensions in families and communities. Educating the client, families, and others is most effective when it is carried out over time. Table 22–7 can be used as a guide for client and family teaching. Later in this chapter, the pivotal role of family psychoeducation in enhancing a schizophrenic person's integration into society, decreasing relapse, and increasing the quality of life for schizophrenic persons and their families is discussed.

Self-Care Activities (Basic Level)

Clients who have the most difficulty with the rudiments of self-care generally include those with disorganized or catatonic schizophrenia, and who are in the acute phase of the illness. The paranoid client usually manages basic activities of daily living with relative competence. Interventions regarding basic activities of daily living and nutritional and sleep factors for clients with paranoia, catatonia, and disorganized thinking are discussed later in this chapter.

Psychobiological Intervention (Basic Level)

Until the 1960s, a client who had even one schizophrenic episode spent months to years in a state or private psychiatric hospital acting bizarrely and experiencing a great deal of emotional pain. Additionally, these episodes resulted in great emotional and financial burdens to the families. Only with the advent of antipsychotic drugs could symptoms be controlled and clients managed in the community. Although these drugs can alleviate many of the symptoms of schizophrenia, they cannot cure the underlying psychotic processes. Therefore, when clients stop taking their medications, psychotic symptoms usually return. Although each client is unique, a general rule exists regarding how long a client needs to take medication. A client who has experienced one psychotic break should take medications for at least 1 year. After two psychotic episodes, medications should be continued for a least 2 years. If a client has experienced three or more psychotic episodes, medications may have to be continued throughout the person's life (Slately 1994). A 1997 study by Meltzer and associates confirms previous data that indicated that people with an early onset of schizophrenia are often resistant to antipsychotic medication.

Drugs used to treat psychotic disorders are called antipsychotic medications. Two groups of antipsychotic drugs exist: *standard* (traditional) and *atypical.* In addition, some drugs are used in conjunction with the antipsychotic agents for treatment-resistant clients; they are discussed later in this chapter.

The standard, or traditional, clinically active antipsychotic drugs are able to block postsynaptic dopamine receptors in the central nervous system and are effective in the treatment of schizophrenia. The choice of drug is often based on:

1. Desired side effects (e.g., an agitated client may be given a more sedating antipsychotic).
2. Avoiding adverse side effects (e.g., haloperidol [Haldol] may be used in a person with cardiac problems because of its reduced anticholinergic effects).
3. Client response (what drug worked well for a specific individual in the past).

TABLE 22–7 TEACHING CLIENTS AND THEIR FAMILIES ABOUT SCHIZOPHRENIA

CONTENT	RATIONALE
Medications*	
What the medication can do to help client. **Medication needs to be taken regularly.** Schizophrenia is a relapsing disorder. It is extremely important to keep taking the drug even though things seem fine. **Side effects.** What to do to lessen severity if the effects are not harmful to client. **Side effects.** If effects are not harmful to client but may cause noncompliance (e.g., akathisia, impotence): "You may notice inner feelings of restlessness and nervousness" or "Your may have difficulty during sex." Client should not stop taking the drug; most side effects can be treated. Client should call (give name). **Toxic effects.** Medication should be discontinued. Client should call (give name) and take appropriate action until medical help is available. **Stopping medications.** Tolerance does not develop, but some clients report a rebound effect (e.g., nausea, vomiting, sleep disturbances) if drugs are stopped suddenly. **Risk factors of tardive dyskinesia.** Prolonged exposure to the sun should be avoided and client should wear sunscreen, sun glasses, long sleeves, and hats. These drugs (neuroleptics) are not addicting.	Client compliance may be helped if ▸ Family is supportive and involved. ▸ Client knows what to expect. ▸ Client knows medication can be changed to decrease undesirable side effects.
Signs of Potential Relapse	
Client and family need to be able to identify symptoms that come before frank psychotic symptoms (unique to each client), e.g. ▸ Feeling of tension ▸ Difficulty concentrating ▸ Trouble sleeping ▸ Increased withdrawal ▸ Increased bizarre/magical thinking	Early warning signs recognized by both family and client may ward off psychotic relapse if immediate medical attention is sought.
Substances that Can Exacerbate a Psychotic Relapse	
Marijuana Alcohol Psychomotor stimulants ▸ Amphetamine ▸ Crack cocaine ▸ Cocaine	Family support may influence client to minimize intake if client uses substances.

*Should be written down for client and family.

The antipsychotic drugs are effective for most acute exacerbations of schizophrenia and for the prevention or mitigation of relapse. The standard antipsychotic drugs target the positive symptoms of schizophrenia (e.g., hallucinations, delusions, disordered thinking, and paranoia). The newer atypical antipsychotics (e.g., clozapine, risperidone, and olanzapine) can diminish the negative symptoms as well (deficits in social interaction, blunted or inappropriate emotional expression, and lack of motivation). Antipsychotic drugs can cause

1. Reduction in disruptive and violent behavior.
2. Increase in activity, speech, and sociability in withdrawn or mute clients.
3. Improvement in self-care.
4. Improvement in sleep patterns.
5. Reduction in the disturbing quality of hallucinations and delusions.
6. Improvement in thought processes.
7. Decreased resistance to activity therapies and supportive psychotherapy.
8. Reduced rate of relapse (about 2.5 times less).
9. Decrease in the intensity of paranoid reactions.

Antipsychotic agents are usually effective 3 to 6 weeks after the regimen is started. Only about 10% of schizophrenic clients fail to respond to antipsychotic drug therapy. These clients should not continue to take medication that, for them, holds only risks and no benefit.

Schizophrenia is the most common indication for antipsychotic medication. People in acute mania or psychotic depression may respond to a short course of antipsychotic drugs. These agents are also frequently effective in the treatment of the behavioral disorders associated with cognitive disorders such as dementia.

Standard (Traditional) Antipsychotics

In the phenothiazine group, the five standard chemical classes of antipsychotic medications are the phenothiazines, thioxanthenes, butyrophenones, dibenzoxazepines, and dihydroindolones. The properties and side effects of agents in the five classes are similar. The phenothiazines are usually considered the prototype for assessing the action and side effects of these medications.

The choice of specific drugs is often made on the basis of major side effects, which include **extrapyramidal side effects** (EPSs), anticholinergic side effects, and sedation. Other side effects include orthostatic hypotension and lowered seizure threshold. For example, chlorpromazine (Thorazine) is the most sedating agent and has fewer EPS than do other antipsychotic agents, but it causes hypotension in large doses. Haloperidol (Haldol) is least sedating and is often used in large doses to reduce assaultive behavior but has a high incidence of EPS. The value of haloperidol for treating violent behaviors is its effectiveness in controlling hallucinatory phenomena with a low incidence of hypotension. People who are functioning at work or at home may prefer less sedating drugs; clients who are agitated or excitable may do better with a more sedating medication.

The antipsychotics are often divided into *low potency* and *high potency* on the basis of their anticholinergic side effects (ACH), EPS, and sedation:

Low Potency = High Sedation + High ACH + Low EPS
High Potency = Low Sedation + Low ACH + High EPS

However, all the standard antipsychotic drugs can cause tardive dyskinesia. The newer atypical antipsychotic drugs have drastically fewer reports of tardive dyskinesia. Table 22–8 provides the side-effect profiles of many commonly used antipsychotic drugs.

The phenothiazine-like drugs have some positive attributes. It is difficult to take a lethal overdose. Neither tolerance nor potential for abuse develops. Many of the side effects are minor or temporary, although a few are more serious. These drugs are used with caution in people who have seizure disorders because they can lower the seizure threshold. Table 22–9 identifies some standard antipsychotic drugs, doses for acute symptoms, usual maintenance doses, and other considerations.

Some of the more disturbing side effects caused by the dopamine blockade properties of the standard antipsychotics are the EPSs. Three of the more common EPS are **acute dystonia** (muscle cramps of the head and neck), **akathisia** (internal and external restless pacing or fidgeting), and **pseudoparkinsonism** (stiffening of muscular activity in the face, body, arms, and legs). These side effects often appear early in therapy, can be treated, and are reversible. Treatment usually consists of lowering the dosage or prescribing antiparkinsonian drugs, especially centrally acting anticholinergic drugs. Commonly

TABLE 22–8 DRUG INFORMATION: SIDE EFFECTS PROFILE OF ANTIPSYCHOTIC DRUGS

Drug	Anti-cholinergic	Sedation	Orthostatic Hypotension	Lowered Seizure Threshold	Extra-pyramidal Side Effects
Low Potency					
Chlorpromazine (Thorazine)	++	+++	+++	+++	++
Thioridazine (Mellaril)	+++	+++	+++	+	+
Clozapine (Clozaril)	+++	++	+++	+	0
High Potency					
Trifluoperazine (Stelazine)	+	+	+	+	+++
Perphenazine (Trilafon)	++	+	+	+	+++
Fluphenazine (Prolixin)	+	+	+	+	+++
Thiothixene (Navane)	+	+	+	++	+++
Chlorprothixene (Taractan)	++	+++	+++	+++	++
Haloperidol (Haldol)	0	+	+	++	+++
Loxapine (Loxitane)	+	++	+	++	+++
Molindone (Moban)	++	++	+	0/+	++
Risperidone (Risperdal)		++	+		+

Adapted from Swonger, A., and Matejski, M. P. (1991). *Nursing pharmacology: An integrated approach to drug therapy and nursing practice* (2nd ed.). Philadelphia: J. B. Lippincott.
0, none; +, least; ++, moderate; +++, most.

TABLE 22–9 DRUG INFORMATION: STANDARD ANTIPSYCHOTIC MEDICATIONS

DRUG	ROUTES	ACUTE (MG/DAY)*	MAINTENANCE (MG/DAY)*	SPECIAL CONSIDERATIONS
Chlorpromazine (Thorazine)	PO, IM, R	200–1600	50–800	Frequently prescribed. Increases sensitivity to sun (as with other phenothiazines). Highest sedation and hypotension effects; least potent.
Thioridazine (Mellaril)	PO	200–600	50–800	Known to cause retinitis pigmentosa in large doses; any diminished vision should be investigated. Low incidence of extra-pyramidal side effects. High incidence of low blood pressure and cardiac effects. High incidence of decreased sexuality and retrograde ejaculation in men.
Trifluoperazine (Stelazine)	PO, IM	10–60	2–80	Low sedation—good for withdrawn or paranoid symptoms. High incidence of extra-pyramidal side effects. Neuroleptic malignant syndrome may occur.
Perphenazine (Trilafon)	PO, IM, IV	12–32	8–64	Can help control severe vomiting and intractable hiccups
Mesoridazine (Serentil)	PO, IM	75–300	25–400	Among the most sedative; severe nausea and vomiting may occur in adults.
Fluphenazine (Prolixin)	PO, IM, SC	2.5–20	2–40	Among the least sedative.
		Thioxanthenes		
Thiothixene (Navane)	PO, IM	6–30	6–60	High incidence of akathisia.
Chlorprothixene (Taractan)	PO, IM	50–600	50–400	Weight gain common.
		Butyrophenones		
Haloperidol (Haldol)	PO, IM	5–50	1–15	Has low sedative properties; is used in large doses for assaultive patients, thus avoiding the severe side effect of hypotension. Appropriate for the elderly for the same reason as above; lessens the chance of falls from dizziness or hypotension. High incidence of extra-pyramidal side effects.
		Dibenzoxazepines		
Loxapine (Loxitane)	PO, IM	60–100	20–250	Possibly associated with weight reduction.
		Dihydroindolones		
Molindone (Moban)	PO	50–100	15–225	Possibly associated with weight reduction.
		Decanoate: Long-acting		
Haloperidol decanoate (Haldol)	IM	0	50–100	Given deep muscle Z-track IM. Given every 4 weeks.
Fluphenazine decanoate (Prolixin)	IM	0	25	Given deep muscle Z-track IM. Effective 1–2 weeks.
Fluphenazine enanthate (Prolixin)	IM	0	25–75	Given deep muscle Z-track IM. Effective 3–4 weeks. Can cause acute dystonic reactions.

Data from Kaplan, H. I., and Sadock, B. J. (1995). *Synopsis of psychiatry* (6th ed.). Baltimore: Williams & Wilkins; Maxmen, J. S., and Ward, N.G. (1995). *Psychotrophic drugs: Fast facts.* (2nd Ed.). New York: W. W. Norton; Berkow, R., et al. (Eds.) (1992). *Merck manual* (6th ed.). Rahway, NJ: Merck Research Laboratories.

*Dosages vary with individual responses to antipsychotic agent used.

IM, intramuscular; PO, oral; R, rectal; SC, subcutaneous; IV, intravenous

TABLE 22–10 DRUG INFORMATION: NURSING MEASURES FOR SIDE EFFECTS OF ANTIPSYCHOTIC MEDICATIONS

Side Effects	Onset	Nursing Measures
	Anticholinergic Symptoms	
1. **Dry mouth**		1. Frequent sips of water and sugarless candy or gum. If severe, provide Xero-Lube, a saliva substitute.
2. **Urinary retention and hesitancy**		2. Check voiding; consider catheterization. If severe, bethanechol, 10–25 mg three to four times daily, may be ordered.
3. **Constipation**		3. Encourage high-fiber diet, evaluate need for mild laxative. May need stool softener. Assess for adequate water intake.
4. **Blurred vision**		4. Usually abates in 1 to 2 weeks. If patient is taking thioridazine, do not give it and check with physician.
5. **Nasal congestion**		5. Provide nasal decongestants; body will adjust in a few weeks.
6. **Photophobia**		6. Encourage client to wear sunglasses.
7. **Dry eyes**		7. Use artificial tears.
8. **Inhibition of ejaculation or impotence in men**		8. Alert physician; client may need alternative medication.
	Extrapyramidal Side Effects	
1. **Pseudoparkinsonism:** masklike faces, stiff and stooped posture, shuffling gait, drooling, tremor, "pill-rolling" phenomena	5–30 days	1. Alert medical staff. Physician may lower dosage or switch to another phenothiazine. An anticholinergic agent (e.g., trihexyphenidyl [Artane] or benztropine [Cogentin] may be used. Trihexyphenidyl and benztropine are used with caution since a "high" may result; benztropine has become a popular abused drug. Amantadine (Symmetrel) may also be prescribed.
2. **Acute dystonic reactions:** acute contractions of tongue, face, neck, and back (tongue and jaw first) ▶ **Opisthotonos:** tetanic heightening of entire body, head and belly up ▶ **Orulogyric crisis:** eyes locked upward	1–5 days	2. **First choice:** Diphenhydramine hydrochloride (Benadryl) 25–50 mg IM/IV. Relief occurs in minutes. **Second choice:** Benztropine, 1–2 mg IM/IV. **Prevent further dystonias** with any anticholinergic agent (see Table 22–11). Experience is very frightening. Take patient to quiet area, and stay with him or her until medicated.
3. **Akathisia:** motor inner-driven restlessness (e.g., tapping foot incessantly, rocking forward and backward in chair, shifting weight from side to side).	5–60 days	3. Physician may change antipsychotic agent or give antiparkinsonian agent. Tolerance does not develop to akathisia, but akathisia disappears when neuroleptic is discontinued. Propranolol (Inderal), lorazepam (Ativan), or diazepam (Valium) may be used.
4. **Tardive dyskinesia:** ▶ **Facial:** Protruding and rolling tongue, blowing, smacking, licking, spastic facial distortion, smacking movements. ▶ **Limbs:** **Choreic:** rapid, purposeless and irregular movements **Athetoid:** slow, complex and serpentine movements ▶ **Trunk:** neck, shoulder, dramatic hip jerks and rocking, twisting pelvic thrusts.	6–24 mo to years	4. **No known treatment.** Discontinuing the drug does not always relieve symptoms. Possibly 20% or patients taking the drug for >2 years may develop tardive dyskinesia. Nurses and doctors should encourage patients to be screened for tardive dyskinesia at least every 3 months.

TABLE 22–10 DRUG INFORMATION: NURSING MEASURES FOR SIDE EFFECTS OF ANTIPSYCHOTIC MEDICATIONS *(Continued)*

SIDE EFFECTS	ONSET	NURSING MEASURES
	Cardiovascular Effects	
1. **Hypotension and postural hypotension**		1. Check blood pressure before giving; advise patient to dangle feet before getting out of bed to prevent dizziness and subsequent falls. A systolic pressure of 80 mm Hg when standing is indication to not give the current dose. This effect usually subsides when drug is stabilized in 1 to 2 weeks. Elastic bandages may prevent pooling. If condition is serious, physician orders volume expanders or pressure agents.
2. **Tachycardia**		2. Patients with existing cardiac problems should *always* be evaluated before the antipsychotic drugs are administered. Haloperidol is usually the preferred drug because of its low anticholinergic effects.
	Other Side Effects	
1. **Dermatologic changes:** hives, contact dermatitis, photosensitivity; these can reflect hypersensitivity to the drug		1. Notify physician; withdrawal of the drug may be indicated. Teach client to stay out of the sun and to use sunscreen, hat, and sunglasses.
2. **Photosensitivity:** extreme sensitivity to sun; patient is easily sunburned.		2. High with chlorpromazine (Thorazine). Advise patient to wear protective clothing and sunscreen when in the sun.
3. **Increased weight:** distressing side effect for many; increase in appetite is attributed to metabolic changes caused by the drug.		3. Nurse can work with client to monitor weight gain and to work with diets; if gain is severe, alternative drugs may be used.
4. **Endocrine changes:** moderate breast enlargement and galactorrhea in women; in both men and women, changes in sexual drive—usually loss of libido; amenorrhea seen occasionally in women.		4. Alert physician, who may change medication.
5. **Sedation:** may be a desired effect in early treatment but may become a liability to a person later in treatment or during maintenance therapy.		5. Physician may change regimen to a less sedative neuroleptic (fluphenazine [Prolixin], trifluoperazine [Stelazine]). Give full dose at bedtime. May relieve daytime sedation.
	Rare and Toxic Effects	
1. **Agranulocytosis:** symptoms include sore throat, fever, malaise, and mouth sore. It is a rare occurrence, but one the nurse should be aware of; any flulike symptoms should be carefully evaluated.	Usually occurs suddenly and becomes evident in the first 12 weeks	1. Notify medical staff STAT. Do not give medication. Physician may order blood work to determine presence of leukopenia or agranulocytosis. If test results are positive, the drug is discontinued, and reverse isolation may be initiated. Mortality is high if the drug is not ceased and if treatment is not initiated.
2. **Cholestatic jaundice:** Rare, reversible, and usually benign if caught in time; prodromal symptoms are fever, malaise, nausea, and abdominal pain; jaundice appears 1 week later.		2. Drug is discontinued; bed rest and high-protein, high-carbohydrate diet are given. Liver function tests should be performed every 6 months.

Continued on following page

TABLE 22–10 DRUG INFORMATION: NURSING MEASURES FOR SIDE EFFECTS OF ANTIPSYCHOTIC MEDICATIONS *(Continued)*

SIDE EFFECTS	ONSET	NURSING MEASURES
3. **Neuroleptic malignant syndrome:** Somewhat rare, potentially fatal. ▸ **Severe extrapyramidal:** e.g., severe muscle rigidity, oculogyric crisis, dysphasia, flexor-extensor posturing, cog wheeling. ▸ **Hyperthermia:** elevated temperature (≤107° F) ▸ **Autonomic dysfunction:** e.g., hypertension, tachycardia, diaphoresis, incontinence.	Can occur in the first week of drug therapy but often occurs later. Rapidly progresses over 2 to 3 days after initial manifestation	3. ▸ Stop neuroleptic. ▸ Transfer STAT to medical unit. ▸ Bromocriptine can relieve muscle rigidity and reduce fever. ▸ Dantrolene may reduce muscle spasms. ▸ Cool body to reduce fever. ▸ Maintain hydration with oral and IV fluids. ▸ Correct electrolyte imbalance. ▸ Arrhythmias should be treated. ▸ Small doses of heparin may decrease possibility of pulmonary emboli. ▸ Early detection increases client's chance of survival.

Data from Schatzberg, A. F., and Cole, J. O. (1991). *Manual of clinical psychopharmacology* (2nd ed.). Washington, DC: American Psychiatric Press; Maxmen, J. S., and Ward, N.G. (1995). *Psychotrophic drugs: Fast facts.* (2nd Ed.). New York: W. W. Norton; Berkow, R. et al. (Eds.) (1992). *Merck manual* (6th ed.). Rahway, NJ: Merck Research Laboratories; Guze, B., Richeimer, S., and Szuba, M. (1995). *The psychiatric drug handbook.* St. Louis: Mosby–Year Book.

IM, intramuscular; IV, intravenous; STAT, immediately.

used drugs include trihexyphenidyl (Artane), benztropine mesylate (Cogentin), diphenhydramine hydrochloride (Benadryl), and amantadine hydrochloride (Symmetrel). The first two in this list are antiparkinsonian drugs. Treatment with antiparkinsonian drugs is not completely benign, because the anticholinergic side effects of the antipsychotics may be intensified (e.g., urinary retention, constipation, failure of visual accommodation [blurred vision], cognitive impairment, and delirium) (Berkow et al. 1992).

Table 22–10 identifies common side effects and nursing and medical interventions for patients taking these antipsychotic medications. Box 22–1 identifies nursing measures for the administration of antipsychotic drugs.

Most clients develop tolerance to EPSs after a few months. Effective nursing and medical management is important during this time, to encourage compliance with the medications until the disturbing and frightening side effects have been properly managed. Table 22–11 identifies some of the more commonly used drugs for the treatment of EPS.

Perhaps the most troubling side effects for outpatients taking antipsychotics are weight gain, impotence, and tardive dyskinesia. Weight gain is most frequently a problem with women and may result in as much as a 100-pound gain in some clients. Discontinuation of the antipsychotic medication may be necessary, along with the use of an alternative drug. Impotence is occasionally reported (but frequently experienced) by men and may also necessitate switching to alternative drugs. Sexual dys-

BOX 22–1 DRUG INFORMATION: NURSING MEASURES FOR GIVING ANTIPSYCHOTIC AGENTS

FORMULATION	MEASURE
Oral	Dilute with milk, orange juice or semisolid food to reduce bitter taste. Check mouth; make sure medication is not held in cheek or under tongue.
Oral liquid	Protect oral liquid from light.
Intramuscular	▸ Do not hold drug in syringe for more than 15 minutes—may absorb plastic. ▸ Give slowly. ▸ Give in deltoid (absorbs more rapidly) or buttocks (upper outer quadrant). ▸ Tell patient injection may sting. ▸ Massage area slowly after injection. ▸ Alternate sites. ▸ Watch for orthostatic hypotension.
Decanoate	Long-acting intramuscular injection is oil based and requires a 20- or 21-gauge needle. ▸ Use a dry needle, at least 20 gauge, 1.5 inches long. ▸ Give deep intramuscularly with Z-track method. ▸ Do *not* massage.

TABLE 22–11 TREATMENT OF NEUROLEPTIC-INDUCED EXTRAPYRAMIDAL SIDE EFFECTS

DRUG	ORAL DOSE (MG)	INTRAMUSCULAR OR INTRAVENOUS DOSE (MG)	CHEMICAL GROUP
Amantadine hydrochloride (Symmetrel)	100 bid or tid	—	Dopaminergic agent
Benztropine mesylate* (Cogentin)	1–3 bid	1–2	ACA
Biperiden* (Akineton)	2 bid or qid	2	ACA
Trihexyphenidyl* (Artane)	2–5 tid	—	ACA
Diphenhydramine hydrochloride (Benadryl)	25–50 tid or qid	25–50	Antihistamine
Procyclidine hydrochloride (Kemadrin)	2.5–5 tid	—	ACA

From Maxmen, J. S., and Ward, N.G. (1995). *Psychotropic drugs: Fast facts* (2nd Ed.). New York: W. W. Norton.
*Antiparkinsonian drug.
ACA, anticholinergic agent (after 1 to 6 months of long-term maintenance antipsychotic therapy, most ACAs can be withdrawn); bid, twice a day; tid, three times a day; qid, four times a day.

functions are perhaps the most common reasons for male noncompliance.

Tardive dyskinesia, an EPS that usually appears after prolonged treatment, is more serious and not always reversible. Tardive dyskinesia consists of involuntary tonic muscular spasms that typically involve the tongue, fingers, toes, neck, trunk, or pelvis. This potentially serious EPS most frequently affects women, older clients, and up to 50% of people receiving long-term large-dose therapy. Tardive dyskinesia varies from mild to moderate and can be disfiguring or incapacitating. Early symptoms of tardive dyskinesia are fasciculations of the tongue or constant smacking of the lips. These early oral movements can develop into uncontrollable biting, chewing, sucking motions, an open mouth, and lateral movements of the jaw. In many cases, the early symptoms of tardive dyskinesia disappear when the antipsychotic medication is discontinued. In other cases, however, early symptoms are not reversible and may progress. No proven cure for advanced tardive dyskinesia exists.

The National Institute of Mental Health has developed a brief test for the detection of tardive dyskinesia. The test is referred to as the Abnormal Involuntary Movement Scale (Box 22–2), which is also included in Chapter 3. (A copy of the Abnormal Involuntary Movement Scaletest is free to those who write to the National Institute of Mental Health, Schizophrenic Disorders Section, Somatic Treatments Branch, Rockville, MD 20857.) The three areas of examination are facial and oral movements, extremity movements, and trunk movement.

Nurses need to know about some rare—but serious and potentially fatal—side effects of these drugs. Side effects include neuroleptic malignant syndrome, agranulocytosis, and liver involvement.

Neuroleptic malignant syndrome may occur in about 0.2% to 1% of clients who have taken antipsychotic agents (Caroff and Mann 1993). It is believed that the acute reduction in brain dopamine activity plays a role in the development of neuroleptic malignant syndrome. Neuroleptic malignant syndrome is fatal in about 10% of the cases. It usually occurs early in the course of treatment but has been reported in people after 20 years of treatment.

Neuroleptic malignant syndrome is characterized by decreased level of consciousness, greatly increased muscle tone, and autonomic dysfunction, including hyperpyrexia, labile hypertension, tachycardia, tachypnea, diaphoresis, and drooling. Treatment consists of early detection, discontinuation of the antipsychotic agent, management of fluid balance, reduction of temperature, and monitoring for complications. Dopamine antagonists or dantrolene (Dantrium) and even electroconvulsive therapy are used in some cases (see Table 22–10) (Caroff and Mann 1993).

Agranulocytosis is also a serious side effect and can be fatal. Liver involvement may occur. Nurses need to be aware of the prodromal signs and symptoms of these side effects and to teach them to their clients and clients' families.

Atypical Antipsychotics

Recent research into the neurobiological changes of schizophrenia has led to advances in the development of drugs that alleviate both the positive and the negative symptoms of schizophrenia. These newer "atypical" medications (Table 22–12) permit more than just control of the most alarming symptoms of this disease (e.g., hallucinations, delusions); they also allow for improvement in the quality of life for people with schizophrenia. The first of these newer drugs was clozapine, which caused dramatic changes in some clients resistant to the standard antipsychotics. It has as its major drawback a high incidence of agranulocytosis and seizures. Next came risperidone, which has also had a beneficial effect on the functioning of people with schizophrenia and could be used as a first-line drug without the hematological concerns of clozapine. One of the most recent, olanzapine, promises to set a new standard because of its low side-effect profile

BOX 22-2 ABNORMAL INVOLUNTARY MOVEMENT SCALE

DEPARTMENT OF HUMAN SERVICES
PUBLIC HEALTH SERVICE
Alcohol, Drug Abuse, and Mental Health Administration
NIMH Treatment Strategies in Schizophrenia Study

ABNORMAL INVOLUNTARY MOVEMENT SCALE (AIMS)

PATINET NUMBER	DATA GROUP	EVALUATION DATE
— — — —	aims	M M D D Y Y

PATIENT NAME

RATER NAME

RATER NUMBER — — —

EVALUATION TYPE (*Circle*)

1 Baseline	4 Start double-blind	7 Start open meds	10 Early termination
2 2-week minor	5 Major evaluation	8 During open meds	11 Study completion
3	6 Other	9 Stop open meds	

INSTRUCTIONS: Complete Examination Procedure (reverse side) before making ratings.
MOVEMENT RATINGS: Rate highest severity observed.

Code: 1 = None; 2 = Minimal, may be extreme normal; 3 = Mild; 4 = Moderate; 5 = Severe

		(Circle One)				
FACIAL AND ORAL MOVEMENTS:	**1. Muscles of facial expression** e.g., movements of forehead, eyebrows, periorbital area, cheeks; include frowning, blinking, smiling, grimacing	1	2	3	4	5
	2. Lips and perioral area e.g., puckering, pouting, smacking	1	2	3	4	5
	3. Jaw e.g., biting, clenching, chewing, mouth opening, lateral movement	1	2	3	4	5
	4. Tongue Rate only increase in movement both in and out of mouth, NOT inability to sustain movement	1	2	3	4	5
EXTREMITY MOVEMENTS:	**5. Upper** (*arms, wrists, hands, fingers*) Include choreic movements (i.e., rapid, objectively purposeless, irregular, spontaneous), athetoid movements (i.e., slow, irregular, complex, serpentine). Do NOT include tremor (i.e., repetitive, regular, rhythmic)	1	2	3	4	5
	6. Lower (*legs, knees, ankles, toes*) e.g., lateral knee movement, foot tapping, heel dropping, foot squirming, inversion and eversion of foot	1	2	3	4	5
TRUNK MOVEMENTS:	**7. Neck, shoulders, hips** e.g., rocking, twisting, squirming, pelvic gyrations	1	2	3	4	5

GLOBAL JUDGMENTS:	**8. Severity of abnormal movements**	None, minimal Minimal Mild Moderate Severe	1 2 3 4 5
	9. Incapacitation due to abnormal movements	None, minimal Minimal Mild Moderate Severe	1 2 3 4 5
	10. Patient's awareness of abnormal movements Rate only patient's report	No awareness Aware, no distress Aware, mild distress Aware, moderate distress Aware, severe distress	1 2 3 4 5
DENTAL STATUS:	**11. Current problem with teeth and/or dentures?**	No Yes	1 2
	12. Does patient usually wear dentures?	No Yes	1 2

BOX 22-2 ABNORMAL INVOLUNTARY MOVEMENT SCALE *(Continued)*

EXAMINATION PROCEDURE

Either before of after completing the Examination Procedure observe the patient unobrtusively, at rest (e.g., in waiting room).

The chair to be used in this examination should be a hard, firm one without arms.

1. Ask patient to remove shoes and socks.
2. Ask patient whether there is anything in his/her mouth (i.e., gum, candy, etc.) and if there is, to remove it.
3. Ask patient about the *current* condition of his/her teeth. Ask patient if he/she wears dentures. Do teeth or dentures bother the patient *now?*
4. Ask patient whether he/she notices any movements in mouth, face, hands, or feet. If yes, ask to describe and to what extent they *currently* bother patient or interfere with his/her activities.
5. Have patient sit in chair with hands on knees, legs slightly apart, and feet flat on floor. (Look at entire body movements while in this position.)
6. Ask patient to sit with hands hanging unsupported: if male, between legs; if female and wearing a dress, hanging over knees. (Observe hands and other body areas.)
7. Ask patient to open mouth. (Observe tongue at rest within mouth.) Do this twice.
8. Ask patient to protrude tongue. (Observe abnormalities of tongue movement.) Do this twice.
9. Ask patient to tap thumb, with each finger, as rapidly as possible for 10 to 15 seconds: separately with right hand, then with left hand. (Observe each facial and leg movement.)
10. Flex and extend patient's left and right arms (one at a time). (Note any rigidity.)
11. Ask patient to stand up. (Observe in profile. Observe all body areas again, hips included.)
12. Ask patient to extend both arms outstretched in front with palms down. (Observe trunk, legs, and mouth).
13. Have patient walk a few paces, turn, and walk back to chair. (Observer hands and gait.) Do this twice.

TABLE 22–12 DRUG INFORMATION: ATYPICAL ANTIPSYCHOTIC MEDICATION

DRUG	ACUTE (MG/DAY)	MAINTENANCE (MG/DAY)	TOXIC/SIDE EFFECTS	SPECIAL CONSIDERATIONS
Clozapine (Clozaril)	300–900	200–400 (start with low doses)	Agranulocytosis (0.8%–2% of patients) Seizures Hypersalivation Persistent tachycardia	Atypical antipsychotic, used when clients fail to respond to other neuroleptics. Can target the negative as well as the positive symptoms of schizophrenia. 1%–2% incidence of agranulocytosis. Weekly white blood cell counts are required. High incidence of dosage-related seizures Can cause sedation, hypotension, tachycardia, and severe drooling.
Risperidone (Risperdal)		4–6	Insomnia (26%) Agitation (22%) EPS (17%) Headache (17%) Rhinitis (10%) Hypotension Anxiety (12%) Weight gain	Low EPS profile. Generally low side effects. Targets both positive and negative symptoms. Start at 5 mg/day and gradually increase dose to minimize orthostatic hypotension in the elderly. Effective first-line antipsychotic.
Olanzapine (Zyprexa)	10–20	7.5–12.5–20	Agitation Insomnia (10.4%) Headache Nervousness (5.6%) Drowsiness Dizziness Akathisa (6.6%) Dry mouth (7.5%) Weight gain	Low side effect profile, especially for cardiac and hematological problems. Targets both positive and negative symptoms. Effective first-line antipsychotic. Long half-life allows once-a-day dosage. Interactions with SSRIs and other antidepressants may occur.
Sertindole* (Serlect)		12–20–24	Rhinitis Decreases ejaculatory volume in men (17%) but not associated with erectile disturbance or decreased libido. Orthostatic hypotension Tachycardia	Can cause a dose-related lengthening in the QT interval on ECG. ECG monitoring may be encouraged. Monitor for signs of dizziness or lightheadedness because of above ECG changes. Start with 4 mg/day and increase by 4 mg every 2–3 days to minimize orthostatic hypotension.

Data from Kaplan, H. I., and Sadock, B. J. (1995). *Synopsis of psychiatry* (6th ed.). Baltimore: Williams & Wilkins; Kane, J. M. (1995). Clinical psychopharmacology of schizophrenia. In G. O. Goddard (Ed.), *Treatment of psychiatric disorders* (2nd ed., Vol. 1, pp. 970–986). Washington, DC: American Psychiatric Press; Littrell, K. (1996). Olanzapine: An exciting new antipsychotic. *American Psychiatric Nurses' Association*, 8(4):4. Marder, S. R., Wirshing, W. C., and Ames, D. (1997). New antipsychotic drugs. In D. L. Dunner and J. F. Rosenbaum (Eds.), *Psychiatric Clinic of North America annual of drug therapy* (pp. 195–207). Philadelphia: W. B. Saunders. American Psychiatric Association (1997). Practice guidelines for the treatment of patients with schizophrenia. *American Journal of Psychiatry* (Suppl.) 154(4):21–23.
EPS, extrapyramidal side effects.
*Not yet FDA approved as of this printing.

and need for only once-a-day dosing. As this textbook goes to print, many other newer atypical antipsychotics are in development.

CLOZAPINE (CLOZARIL). In the early 1990s, clozapine was released in the United States for use in clients with treatment-resistant schizophrenia and intolerance of the side effects of the standard antipsychotics. Clozapine is credited with causing dramatic changes in some clients who had not responded to treatment with standard antipsychotics. One of the advantages of this drug is that both the negative (lack of motivation, anergia, and impaired judgment) and the positive symptoms of schizophrenia (hallucinations, delusions, and aggression) are greatly reduced. Another is that many of the side effects of the standard or traditional antipsychotics are absent and do not appear with clozapine. Because clozapine causes minimal or no dopamine blockade, there have been no reported cases of pseudoparkinsonism or dystonia and much less akathisia. Clozapine also seems unlikely to cause tardive dyskinesia.

However, notable disadvantages include a high incidence of agranulocytosis (0.8% to 2% in all clients in the United States). The need to monitor a client's white blood cell count weekly keeps the cost of this drug relatively high and out of reach for many clients. All clients taking this drug must be monitored by a client management system. The incidence of seizures is also high with use of this drug, 1% to 2% at low doses and 5% at higher doses (Preston and Johnson 1995). Many physicians use clozapine as the drug of last resort. Clozapine can also be sedating, can cause hypotension and tachycardia, and, in some clients, can cause severe drooling. Early research studies indicate that clozapine may play a substantial role in reintegrating clients into the community (Gordon and Milke 1995).

RISPERIDONE (RISPERDAL). This drug was introduced in 1993, is a serotonin and a dopamine blocking agent, and has proved to be an effective antipsychotic medication. Risperidone targets the negative and the positive symptoms of schizophrenia. Risperidone, like clozapine, is also free of many of the disturbing and disabling neurological side effects of the older, phenothiazine-like, antipsychotics. Risperidone, however, does not cause agranulocytosis and is being used as an effective first-line treatment in many facilities (Klausner and Brecher 1995). Risperidone has a low ESP profile and targets negative symptoms at lower doses. Studies reveal that both clozapine and risperidone may have an ameliorating effect on the symptoms of tardive dyskinesia. Risperidone appears to be well tolerated. Six mg/day appears to be the optimal dose for most clients. Doses of 10 mg/day are associated with significantly more EPSs. The most common adverse effects in clients receiving 10 mg/day or less are insomnia, agitation, EPSs, headache, anxiety, and rhinitis. Lower dosing and morning dosing can eliminate or reduce the incidence of insomnia and agitation. Doses should be titrated over 3 days, beginning with 1 mg twice a day and reaching 3 mg twice a day on the third day (Kane 1995).

OLANZAPINE (ZYPREXA). Olanzapine, which was introduced in 1996, represents a major advance in the pharmacological treatment of schizophrenia (Littrell 1996). Olanzapine has a high efficacy for both positive and negative symptoms of schizophrenia in the absence of hematological or cardiac problems. Olanzapine shows a relatively limited side-effect profile and is thought to be safer than currently used drugs. All drugs have side effects, but in clinical trials, olanzapine's side effects were milder than those of older medications, and far fewer people were forced to stop treatment as a result of adverse reactions. The most common side effects include drowsiness, dizziness, agitation, insomnia, headache, nervousness, and akathisia. Dry mouth and weight gain seem to be dose-related responses. Because of the long half-life of the drug (27 hours), olanzapine can be given just once a day. The recommended initial dose of olanzapine is 2.5 to 7.5 mg/day, and the effective dose ranges from 7.5 to 20 mg/day. (Marder et al 1997). Littrell (1996) stated that the combined positive features of olanzapine enable this drug to become the new "gold standard" in antipsychotic pharmacotherapy.

Other Atypical Antipsychotics

Other atypical antipsychotics are being introduced into widespread use, or will be soon. Drugs in clinical trials include sertindole (Serlect), quetiapine (Seroquel), and ziprasidone. Although schizophrenia is not curable, the newer, atypical antipsychotics make this disorder even more tractable and manageable (Marder et al. 1997). At present, there is more reason for optimism regarding clients with schizophrenia and their families than at any other time in medical history.

Adjuncts to Antipsychotic Drug Therapy

Other drugs are often used in the treatment of drug-resistant schizophrenia. For example, lithium can be useful for suppressing episodic violence in schizophrenia as well as for targeting many of the more disturbing symptoms when the agent is used along with a more traditional antipsychotic. Carbamazepine and valproic acid (Depakene) have also been found to alleviate symptoms in some drug-resistant clients who have schizophrenia when it is used along with a standard antipsychotic (see Chapter 21).

Benzodiazepines are also being studied as possible adjuncts in the treatment of selected clients with schizophrenia. For example, in one study, diazepam (Valium) was found to be useful in controlling psychotic symptoms in a small sample of people with paranoid schizophrenia. In several small studies, alprazolam (Xanax) has been found to be useful in controlling panic attacks and anxiety symptoms in schizophrenic clients taking antipsychotic drugs (see Chapter 17) (Schatzberg and Cole 1991).

When to Change an Antipsychotic Regimen

The following conditions suggest the need for a different antipsychotic agent (Nehart 1996):

- Clear lack of efficacy of the current drug regimen
- Need for supplemental medications (lithium, carbamazepine, valproate)
- Occurrence of intolerable or persistent side effects

Electroconvulsive Therapy

In several studies of first-admission schizophrenic clients, electroconvulsive therapy (ECT) was found to be as effective as antipsychotic medication during the acute phase (APA 1997). ECT may be used for severely catatonic clients. It is also indicated when antipsychotic drug therapy fails or is contraindicated. Electroconvulsive therapy may be helpful for people who do not respond satisfactorily to drugs and are too old to be discharged—for example, for a client who appears to be tormented by hallucinations or delusional fears, or who has rapid or dramatic onset of psychosis, or who presents an ongoing or acute risk to his or her life (refusing food or fluids, maintaining active suicidal intent) (Johns 1996). However, electroconvulsive therapy is mostly used for people with psychotic depression who are violent, suicidal, or participating in self-starvation.

Milieu Therapy (Basic Level)

Activities

Effective hospital care involves more than protection of the client from a confusing family, social, or vocational environment. Slately (1994) reported finding that a structured milieu contributes to greater improvement with schizophrenic clients in the acute phase than does an open unit where the clients have more freedom. The milieu should also provide healthy substitutes for erecting new identifications, resources for resolving conflicts, and opportunities for learning social and vocational skills.

Group work with schizophrenic clients is oriented toward providing support, an environment in which a client can develop social skills, and a format that allows friendships to begin (Black et al. 1988). Structured group therapy can target some of the negative symptoms of schizophrenia. For example, participation in activity groups, which is determined by the client's level of functioning, has been found to decrease withdrawal, promote motivation, modify unacceptable aggression, and increase social competence. People who respond to group therapy while hospitalized may benefit from group therapy on an outpatient basis, and group therapy would thus be an important part of the client's community milieu.

Group work with schizophrenic clients can result in increased self-concept scores. Such activities as drawing pictures, reading poetry, and listening to music can be used as a focus of conversation to reduce anxiety and promote socialization. Group functions, such as picnics, can result in growth in social concern for others and the ability to set limits on self and others. Nurses can use activity group therapy in many settings. Success at tasks and increased involvement with objects and individuals can lead to greater self-esteem in many settings.

In the hospital and outpatient settings, the nurse may participate with other members of the health care team in providing appropriate, structured, and useful activities for the clients. Recreational, occupational, art, and dance therapists are available on many psychiatric units as well as in structured community settings (see Chapter 8).

Safety

A client, especially on in the acute phase, may become physically violent, often in response to hallucinations or delusions. During this time, measures need to be taken to ensure the client's safety as well as the safety of others. After unsuccessful verbal de-escalation efforts, and if chemical restraints (antipsychotic medication) fail to lessen the person's aggression, measures such as physical restraints and isolation may be indicated. (see Chapters 12 and 21 for indications and general guidelines for management of a client in seclusion.)

Psychotherapy (Advanced Practice)

Medication maintenance has been shown to be the single most important factor in the prevention of relapse in a schizophrenic person. Drugs reduce most of the disturbing, disorganizing, and destructive aspects of the schizophrenic person's behavior (positive symptoms). The new antipsychotics do alter in part some of the negative symptoms, such as the underlying apathy, unresponsiveness, and lack of initiative. However, supportive psychotherapy, in addition to drug therapy, results in an even lower rate of relapse than does drug therapy alone. Zahniser and colleagues (1991) identified relationship problems, family concerns, depression, losses, and medication as the most common concerns of schizophrenic clients in therapy. Hilde Bruch (1980) cited a study that identified the elements that contribute to successful therapeutic outcomes with schizophrenic clients, even though the therapists' disciplines were diverse:

> The highest improvement rate was associated with "active participation," with the therapist showing initiative in a sympathetic inquiry, challenging the client's self-deprecatory attitude, and identifying realistic limits as to what is acceptable in the client's behavior.

Individual Therapy

For people with schizophrenia, the most useful therapeutic modality is supportive therapy. Supportive therapy over long periods has great value and helps people make adjustments to a more useful and satisfactory life. Individual therapy, ideally combined with group therapy, should be made available to the client on an outpatient basis as well as being part of inpatient treatment.

Group Therapy

Group therapy is particularly useful for clients who have had one or more psychotic episodes. It has been shown that groups can help the client develop

- Interpersonal skills.
- Resolution of family problems.
- Effective use of community supports.

Groups provide opportunities for socialization in safe settings, for expression of tensions, and for sharing problems.

The most useful types of groups for schizophrenic clients are those that help clients develop abilities to deal with such issues as solving day-to-day problems, sharing relevant experiences, learning to listen, asking questions, and keeping topics in focus. Groups available on a continuing outpatient basis allow individual growth in these areas.

Some day, hospitals and clinics may offer medication groups for clients. Medication groups can help clients

- Deal more effectively with troubling side effects.
- Alert the nurse to potential adverse side effects or toxic effects.
- Minimize isolation among clients receiving antipsychotics.
- Increase compliance.

Refer to Chapter 10 for more on group work with schizophrenic clients.

Family Therapy

Families with a schizophrenic member often endure considerable hardships while coping with the psychotic and residual symptoms of schizophrenia. Often, these families become isolated from their communities and relatives. To make matters worse, until recently, families were often blamed for causing or triggering episodes of schizophrenia in their schizophrenic member (Fenton and Cole 1995). The National Alliance for the Mentally Ill (NAMI) and the National Association for Research in Schizophrenia and Depression are actively involved in efforts to develop new and effective treatment strategies that involve families, making them partners in the treatment process (Fenton and Cole 1995). Families can play an important role in the course of the illness of their schizophrenic member. Family education and family therapy are known to diminish the negative effects of family life on schizophrenic clients. It is well established that when family therapy is added to pharmacological therapy, the relapse rate is reduced to about half. The results of eight studies in the United States and England found that family intervention has reduced the average relapse rate from 44% to 12% (McFarlane 1995).

Programs that provide support, education, coping skills training, and social network development are extremely effective. This approach is called *psychoeducational*, and it combines educational with behavioral approaches to family treatment. The psychoeducational approach assumes that families are not to be blamed for their schizophrenic member's illness but in fact are secondary victims of a biological illness (McFarlane 1995).

In family therapy sessions, the family can identify fears, faulty communications, and distortions. Improved problem-solving skills can be taught, and healthier alternatives to situations of conflict can be explored. Family guilt and anxiety can be lessened, which facilitates change.

In a recent study investigators concluded that families with schizophrenic members who have a high risk for relapse and who received psychoeducational treatment in multiple family groups did even better than those treated in single family groups. Over a 2-year follow-up, those treated in single family therapy had a 27% relapse, while those treated in multiple family therapy groups had only a 16% relapse (Gabbard and Callaway 1995). Both single and multiple family treatments are cost effective; multiple family groups are the more cost effective and the most advantageous to families and their schizophrenic member. Some factors that seem to be involved in improvement follow (Gabbard and Callaway 1995):

- Expands the client's and their relatives' social network
- Expands the problem-solving capacity available in groups
- Lowers the emotional overinvolvement of families
- Increases the overall positive tone that characterizes such groups

The family self-help movement has been an important development in the mental health field. Families of schizophrenic clients have formed local and national self-help and advocacy organizations.

Families with schizophrenic members have very real needs. They need to be part of the decision-making process, to have adequate and appropriate help in crises, and to have periodic respite from the hard work of coping with a schizophrenic member (Lamb et al. 1986). Families need help in

- Understanding the disease and the role of medications.
- Setting realistic goals.
- Developing problem-solving skills for handling tensions and misunderstandings within the family environment.

Whether this is in the form of family therapy, psychoeducational multiple family therapy, or educational counseling, the family unit needs to be included in the treatment plan and counseling made available if the schizophrenic member is to become stabilized.

Case Management (Basic Level)

Discharge planning is a vital part of managing schizophrenic clients. With the shifting of care for the seriously mentally ill from inpatient to community-based treatment centers, the need for transitional care is heightened. Case management by nurses and other health care professionals is one way that clients can be effectively monitored. Because of the limits to hospital stay length that have been established by third-party payers, clients are discharged to the community while they are still severely impaired and even frankly psychotic. Alternatives to hospitalization that work for many include partial hospitalization, halfway houses, and day treatment programs (Baldessarini 1996):

Partial hospitalization	Clients sleep at home and attend treatment sessions during the day or evening.
Halfway houses	Client live in the community with a group of other clients, sharing expenses and responsibilities. Clients are supervised by social workers or psychologists who are present in the house 24 hours a day, 7 days a week.
Day treatment programs	Clients live in halfway house or on their own, sometimes with home visits. Clients attend a structured program during the day. Program may consist of ▸ Group therapy ▸ Supervised activities ▸ Individual counseling ▸ Specialized training and rehabilitation

Nurses, physicians, and social workers should be aware of the community resources for clients who are to be discharged and their families. Some clients may feel more comfortable with self-help community groups, such as Recovery Inc. and Schizophrenics Anonymous. Information on community resources should be made available to clients and families alike. Examples include community mental health services, home health services, work support programs, day hospitals, social skills/supportive groups, family educational skills groups, and respite care. Clients, families, or siblings should be given telephone numbers and addresses of local support groups that are affiliated with the National Alliance for the Mentally Ill. (Information can be obtained at National Alliance for the Mentally Ill, 1901 North Fort Myers Drive, Suite 500, Arlington, VA 22209 (703) 525-7600. 1-800-950-NAMI can provide information regarding chapters nearest the reader.)

A study by Dowart and Hoover (1994) revealed that 74% of nonfederal inpatient mental health facilities provided no case management services. Effective follow-up and appropriate services are critical in minimizing future need for hospitalization and in offering some hope for people with schizophrenia and their families.

SCHIZOPHRENIA SUBTYPES

Figure 22–3 provides an overview of the subtypes of schizophrenia. The chart presents the different subtypes, and the data can be related with the case studies.

Paranoia

Any intense and strongly defended irrational suspicion can be regarded as **paranoia.** Paranoid ideas cannot be corrected by experiences and cannot be modified by facts or reality. *Projection* is the most common defense mechanism used by people who are paranoid. For example, when paranoid individuals feel self-critical, they experience others as being harshly critical toward them. When they feel anger, they experience others as being unjustly angry at them, as if to say "I'm not angry, you are!"

Paranoid states may occur in numerous mental or organic disorders. For example, a person experiencing a psychotic depression or manic episode may display paranoid thinking. Paranoid symptoms can be secondary to physical illness, organic brain disease, or drug intoxications.

Paranoid schizophrenia is one of the *primary* paranoid disorders (i.e., those in which the primary symptom is paranoid thinking). The others are paranoid delusional disorder and paranoid personality disorder. Chapter 19 addresses the paranoid personality disorder.

People with paranoid schizophrenia usually have a later age of onset (late twenties to thirties). Paranoid schizophrenia develops rapidly in individuals with good premorbid functioning and tends to be intermittent during the first 5 years of the illness. In some cases, paranoid schizophrenia is associated with a good outcome or with recovery (Fenton and McGlashan 1991). People with a paranoid disorder are usually frightened. Although not always consciously aware of their feelings, paranoid people have deep feelings of loneliness, despair, helplessness, and fear of abandonment. The paranoid facade is a defense against painful feelings. Useful nursing strategies are outlined in the following sections.

Counseling

Because persons who are paranoid are unable to trust the actions of those around them, they are usually guarded, tense, and reserved. Although clients may keep themselves aloof from interpersonal contacts, impairment in actual functioning may be minimal. To ensure interpersonal distance, they may adopt a superior, hostile, and sarcastic attitude. A common defense used by paranoid individuals to maintain self-esteem is to disparage others and dwell on the shortcomings of others. The client frequently misinterprets the messages of others or gives private meaning to the communications of others (**ideas of reference**). For example, a client might see his primary nurse talking to the physician and believe that they are planning to harm him in some manner. Minor oversights are often interpreted as personal rejection.

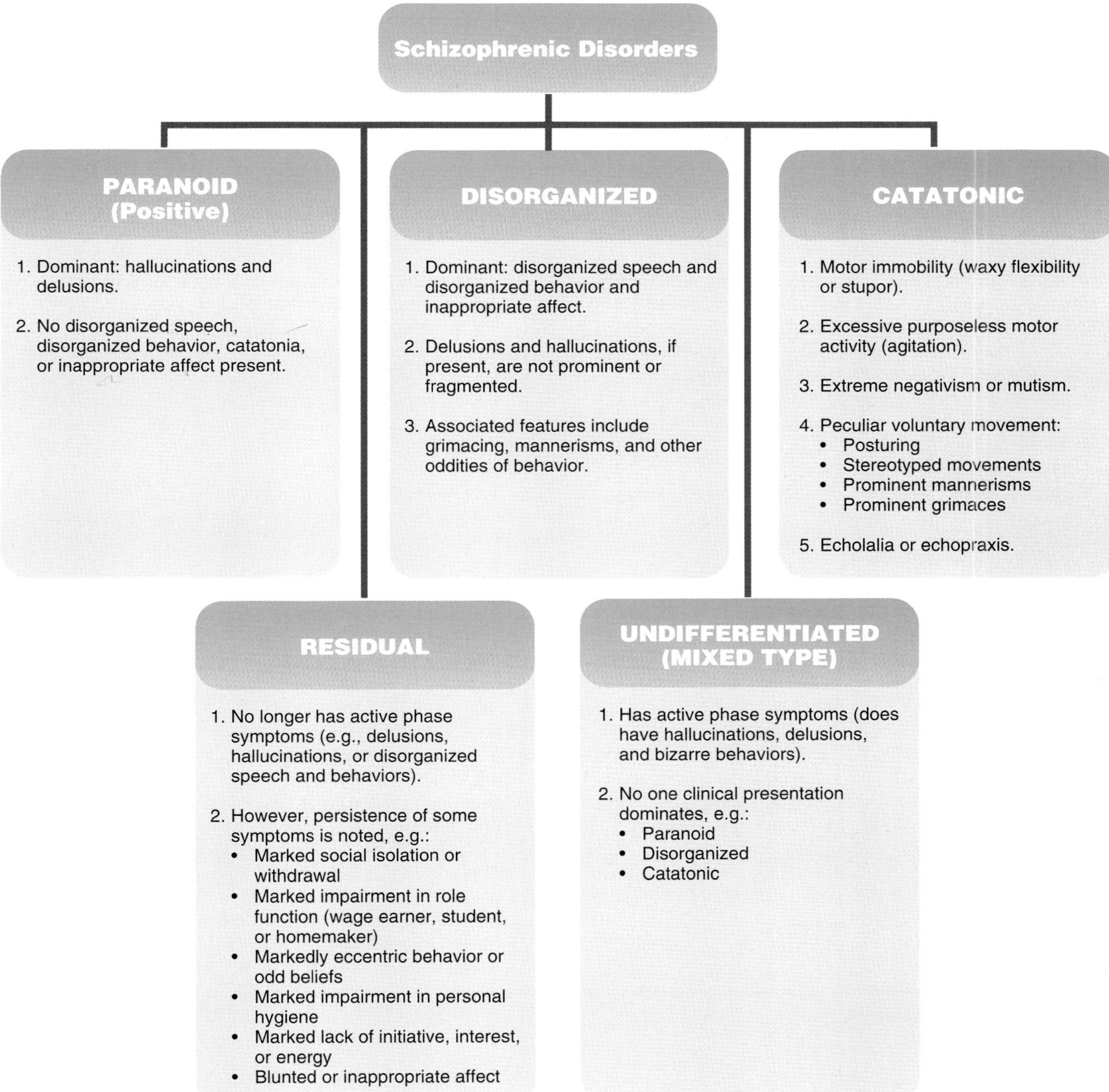

Figure 22–3 Diagnostic criteria for the subtypes of schizophrenia. (Adapted from American Psychiatric Association (1994). *Diagnostic and statistical manual of mental disorders*, 4th ed. Washington, DC: American Psychiatric Association. Reprinted with permission. Copyright 1994 American Psychiatric Association.)

During hospitalization, a paranoid client may make offensive yet accurate criticisms of staff and ward policies. It is important that staff not react to these criticisms with anxiety or rejection of the client. Staff conferences, peer group supervision, and clinical supervision are effective ways of looking behind the behaviors to the motivations of the client. This provides the opportunity to reduce the client's anxiety and increase staff effectiveness. Table 22–13 provides guidelines to communication approaches for a paranoid person.

Self-Care Needs

People with paranoid schizophrenic disorder usually have stronger ego resources than do individuals with other schizophrenic disorders, particularly with regard to occupational functioning and capacity for independent living. Grooming, dress, and self-care may not be a problem. In fact, in some cases, grooming may be meticulous. Nutrition, however, may pose a problem. A common distortion or delusion is that the food is poisoned. In this

TABLE 22–13 COUNSELING TECHNIQUES WITH A PARANOID CLIENT

INTERVENTION	RATIONALE
Communications	
Nursing Diagnosis: **Altered thought processes related to perceptual and cognitive distortions, as evidenced by suspicious thoughts and defensive behaviors**	
1. Honesty and consistency are imperative. If you say "I'll be back at 11 AM" or "I'll call your social worker this morning." *always* follow through with what you say you will do.	1. A person who is paranoid is quick to discern dishonesty. Honesty and consistency provide an atmosphere in which trust can grow.
2. Avoid a warm and gushing approach. A nonjudgmental, respectful, and consistent approach is most effective.	2. Warmth and gushing can be frightening to a person who needs emotional distance. Matter-of-fact consistency is not threatening.
3. Eliminate physical contact; do *not* touch the client. Ask the client's permission if touch is necessary.	3. Touch may be interpreted as a physical or sexual as sault.
4. Focus on maintaining ego boundaries, e.g., ▶ Do not get too physically close. ▶ Avoid touching the client. ▶ Limit the time of interaction.	4. Perceptions of having personal space invaded can increase the client's anxiety.
5. Evaluate the themes in hallucinations and delusions.	5. The themes are important to know (e.g., killing self or others) because protective action may have to be taken.
6. Do not argue with the content of hallucinations or delusions.	6. Arguing with hallucinations and delusions makes the person defend his or her beliefs more vigorously.
7. When speaking of the client's "voices," note that the client hears voices not experienced by you.	7. Increases trust while accepting and acknowledging the client's experience.
8. Resist getting caught up in content; rather, look for the feelings behind the delusions and hallucinations.	8. One cannot logically discuss illogical material, but one *can* discuss feelings, e.g., "I don't know about the FBI trying to harm you, but thinking that must be frightening."
9. Clarify and restate your role. Repeat with patience and understanding.	9. Prevent misinterpretations and minimizes misconstruing of the relationship.
10. Use simple and clear language when speaking to the client. Explain everything you are going to do before you do it.	10. Prevent misinterpretations and clarifies nurse's intent and actions.
11. Diffuse angry and hostile verbal attacks with a nondefensive stand. Explore with the client the origin of angry feelings.	11. The anger a paranoid client expresses is often displaced. When the staff become defensive, anger of both the client and the staff escalates. A nondefensive and nonjudgmental attitude provides an atmosphere in which feelings can be explored more easily.

FBI, Federal Bureau of Investigation.

case, special foods should be provided in enclosed containers to minimize the suspicion of tampering. If clients think that others will harm them when they are sleeping, they may be fearful of going to sleep. Therefore, adequate rest may become a problem that warrants nursing interventions.

Milieu Needs

A paranoid person may become physically aggressive in response to hallucinations or delusions. Hostile drives are projected onto the environment and then acted on. Homosexual urges may be projected onto the environment as well, and fear of sexual advances from others may stimulate aggression or homosexual panic.

An environment that provides the client with a sense of security and safety should minimize anxiety and environmental distortions. Activities that distract the client from ruminating on hallucinations and delusions can also help decrease anxiety. Table 22–14 provides strategies for meeting self-care and milieu needs for clients who are experiencing paranoia.

A case study of a client with paranoid schizophrenia follows. The case study follows the steps in the nursing process and integrates the material presented in this chapter.

TABLE 22–14 SELF-CARE AND MILIEU NEEDS FOR A PARANOID CLIENT

INTERVENTION	RATIONALE
Self-Care Needs	
Nursing Diagnosis: **Altered health maintenance related to fear of harm by others, as evidenced by refusal to eat or sleep**	
1. Provide the necessary toilet articles and facilities for the client to care for clothes.	1. Grooming and dress are rarely a problem.
2. If the client thinks food is poisoned, the nurse can provide foods in their own containers, e.g., milk cartons, hard-boiled eggs, or apples.	2. Delusions that food is poisoned are common with paranoid clients. Usually, these measures promote adequate nutrition. Tube feeding is instituted as a last resort.
3. If the client is unable to sleep, staying with the client for specific time periods can be helpful.	3. The client may feel too vulnerable to sleep. The nurse's presence often helps the client feel more secure, e.g., "I will stay with you 15 minutes," or "until you fall asleep."
4. Use of radio or tape player may decrease anxiety at bedtime.	4. Provides a focus at bedtime other than hallucinations.
Milieu Needs	
Nursing Diagnosis: **Risk for violence related to altered perceptions and cognitive distortion, as evidenced by increased agitation and hostile behaviors**	
1. Maintain low level of stimuli, e.g., avoid groups and provide quiet setting and subdued lighting.	1. Noisy environments may be perceived as threatening.
2. Observe client frequently, e.g., every 15 minutes.	2. Observing for increased agitation and increased motor behavior, and intervening in a timely manner, can help prevent a client from losing control. Frequent observation can help prevent a crisis that has potential to harm the client or others.
3. Provide verbal and physical limits to client's hostility, e.g., "We won't allow you to hit or hurt anyone here; if you can't control yourself, we will help you."	3. When anxiety is high, the client may feel out of control. Often, firm verbal limits are effective in calming the client. If not, a quiet room or medication may be necessary.
Nursing Diagnosis: **Diversional activity deficit related to panic level of anxiety**	
Assign solitary, noncompetitive activities that take some concentration (e.g., crossword puzzles, picture puzzles, photography, typing); when client feels less threatened, bridge and chess may be more appropriate, they require increased concentration.	When the client is extremely distrustful of others, solitary activities are best. Activities that demand concentration keep the client's attention on reality and minimize hallucinatory and delusional preoccupation.

CASE STUDY: WORKING WITH A PERSON WHO IS PARANOID

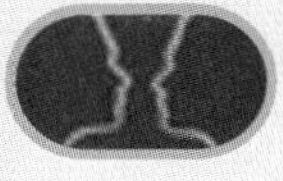

Tom is a 37-year-old man who is currently an inpatient at the Veterans Administration Hospital. He has been separated from his wife and four children for 6 years. His medical records state that because of his illness (which Tom describes as "hearing voices a lot"), he has been in and out of hospitals for 17 years. Tom is an ex-Marine who first "heard voices" at the age of 19, while he was stationed in Okinawa; he subsequently received a medical discharge.

The hospitalization was precipitated by an exacerbation of auditory hallucinations. "I thought people were following me. I hear voices, usually a woman's voice, and she's tormenting me. People say that it happens because I don't take my medications. The medications make me tired and I can't have sex." Tom also admits to using cocaine and marijuana. He is aware that marijuana and cocaine increase his paranoia and that taking drugs usually precedes hospitalization but says that "they make me feel good." Tom finished 11 years of school but did not graduate from high school. He says that he has no close friends. He was in prison for 5 years for manslaughter and told the nurse, "I was in prison because I did something bad." He was abusing alcohol and drugs at the time, and drug abuse has been related to each subsequent hospitalization.

Continued on following page

Case Study: Working With a Person Who is Paranoid

Ms. Lally is Tom's primary nurse. When Tom meets the nurse, he is dressed in pajamas and bathrobe. His hygiene is good and he is well nourished. He tells the nurse that he does not sleep much because "the voices get worse at night." Ms. Lally notes in Tom's medical record that he has had two episodes of suicidal ideation. During those times, the voices were telling him to jump "off rooftops" and "in front of trains."

During the first interview, Tom only occasionally makes eye contact and speaks in a low monotone. At times, he glances about the room as if distracted, mumbles to himself, and appears upset.

Nurse: Tom, my name is Ms. Lally. I will be your nurse while you're in the hospital. We will meet every day for 30 minutes at 10 AM. During that time, we can discuss areas of concern to you.

Tom: Well . . . don't believe what they say about me. I want to start a new. . . . Are you married?

Nurse: This time is for you to talk about *your* concerns.

Tom: Oh . . . *(Looks furtively around the room, then lowers his eyes.)* Someone is trying to kill me, I think . . .

Nurse: You appear to be focusing on something other than our conversation.

Tom: The voices tell me things . . . I can't say . . .

Nurse: I don't hear any voices except yours and mine. I am going to stay with you. Tell me what is happening and I will try to help you.

Tom: The voices tell me bad things.

Ms. Lally stays with Tom and encourages him to communicate with her. As Tom focuses more on the nurse, his anxiety appears to lessen. His thoughts become more connected, he is able to concentrate more on what the nurse is saying, and he mumbles less to himself.

ASSESSMENT

After the initial interview, Ms. Lally divides the data into objective and subjective components.

OBJECTIVE DATA

- Speaks in low monotone
- Poor eye contact
- Well nourished, adequate hygiene
- States that he has auditory hallucinations
- Has history of drug abuse—cocaine and marijuana
- Has no close friends
- Was first hospitalized at age 19 and has not worked since that time
- Has had suicidal impulses twice
- Imprisoned 5 years for violent acting out (manslaughter)
- Thoughts scattered when anxious

SUBJECTIVE DATA

- "Someone is trying to kill me . . . I think."
- "I don't take my medicine. It makes me tired and I can't have sex."
- "The voices get worse at night, and I can't sleep."
- Voices have told him to "jump off rooftops" and "in front of trains."

NURSING DIAGNOSIS

Ms. Lally formulates two nursing diagnoses on the basis of her assessment data.

1. **Altered thought processes** related to alteration in biochemical compounds, as evidenced by persecutory hallucinations and intense suspiciousness.
   - Voices have told him to "jump off rooftops" and "in front of trains."
   - "Someone is trying to kill me, I think."
   - Abuses cocaine and marijuana, although these increase paranoia, because "it makes me feel good."
2. **Noncompliance with medications** related to side effects of therapy, as evidenced by verbalization of noncompliance and persistence of symptoms.
   - Does not take prescribed medication because "it makes me tired and I can't have sex."
   - Chronic history of relapse of symptoms when client is out of hospital.

CASE STUDY: WORKING WITH A PERSON WHO IS PARANOID *(Continued)*

PLANNING

PLANNING OUTCOME CRITERIA

Ms. Lally decides that initial concentration should be placed on establishing a relationship in which Tom can feel safe with the nurse and comfortable enough to discuss his voices and the events that precipitate them. The nurse is aware that if Tom's anxiety level can be lowered and his suspicions can be diminished, he will be able to participate more comfortably in reality-based activities and will have an increased ability to solve problems. Because noncompliance with his medications seems to be a major factor in the persistence of Tom's disturbing symptoms, this becomes an important focus for discussion. Ms. Lally plans to evaluate the medication and side effects with the physician and to work with Tom on alternatives to increase his medical compliance.

NURSING DIAGNOSIS	OUTCOME CRITERIA	SHORT-TERM GOALS
1. **Altered thought processes** related to alteration in biochemical compounds, as evidenced by persecutory hallucinations and intense suspiciousness.	1. Tom will refrain from responding to his "voices" and suspicions, should they occur.	1a. By (date), Tom will state that he feels comfortable with the nurse. 1b. By (date), Tom will name two actions that precipitate voices and paranoia. 1c. By (date), Tom will name two actions he can take if the voices start to upset him.
2. **Noncompliance with medications** related to side effects of medication, as evidenced by verbalization of noncompliance and persistence of symptoms.	2. Tom will adhere to medication regimen.	2a. By (date), Tom will name actions he can take to offset the side effects of medication. 2b. Tom will attend weekly support group for people with schizoprenia.

NURSE'S FEELINGS AND SELF-ASSESSMENT

On the first day of admission, Tom assaults another male client, stating that the other client accused him of being a homosexual and touched him on the buttocks. After assessing the incident, the staff agrees that Tom's provocation came more from his own projections (Tom's sexual attraction to the other client) than from anything the other client did or said.

Tom's difficulty with impulse control frightens Ms. Lally. She has concerns regarding Tom's impulse control and the possibility of Tom's striking out at her, especially when Tom is hallucinating and highly delusional. Ms. Lally mentions her concerns to the nursing coordinator, who suggests that Ms. Lally meet with Tom in the day room until he demonstrates more control and less suspicion of others. After 5 days, Tom is less excitable, and the sessions are held in a room set aside for client interviews. Ms. Lally also speaks with a senior staff nurse regarding her fear. By talking to the senior nurse and understanding more clearly her own fear, Ms. Lally is able to identify interventions to help Tom regain a better sense of control.

INTERVENTION

Ms. Lally makes out an initial nursing care plan (Nursing Care Plan 22–1). An important part of her plan consists of conferring with the physician about the legitimate concerns Tom had regarding his medication. The concerns Tom has regarding not being able to sustain an erection are legitimate, and the physician states that he will put Tom on one of the newer atypical antipsychotics, olanzapine (Zyprexa), which has little known sexual inhibitors. Ms.

Continued on following page

CASE STUDY: WORKING WITH A PERSON WHO IS PARANOID *(Continued)*

Lally works with Tom on continuing his participation in the support group. During team conference, the social worker suggests that if Tom becomes able to maintain contact with a support group, he might be a good candidate for a group home in the future.

Antipsychotic medications seem to greatly lower Tom's suspiciousness and his hallucinatory symptoms. This enables Tom to discuss with the nurse more reality-based concerns and to be more amenable to attending the weekly support group. After their fourth meeting, Tom seems to view the group more favorably and even speaks of making a friend in the group.

EVALUATION

By discharge, Tom says he has a better understanding of his medications and what to do. He knows that marijuana and cocaine increase his symptoms, but he says that he sometimes got lonely and needed to "feel good." Tom continues with a supportive group and outpatient counseling. The reason he gives for deciding to attend outpatient therapy is that he feels that Ms. Lally had really cared about him, and that made him feel good. He reports sleeping much better and says that he has more energy during the day.

NURSING CARE PLAN 22–1 A PERSON WITH PARANOIA: TOM

NURSING DIAGNOSIS

Altered thought processes: related to alteration in biochemical compounds, as evidenced by persecutory hallucinations and intense suspiciousness

Supporting Data

- Voices have told him to "jump off rooftops" and "in front of trains."
- "Someone is trying to kill me, I think."
- Abuses cocaine and marijuana although paranoia increases: "It makes me feel good."

Outcome Criteria: Tom will state that he is able to function without interference from his "voices" by discharge.

SHORT-TERM GOAL	INTERVENTION	RATIONALE	EVALUATION
1. By (date), Tom will state that he feels comfortable with the nurse.	1a. Meet with Tom each day for 30 minutes.	1a. Short, consistent meetings help establish contact and decrease anxiety.	*GOAL MET* By the end of the first week, Tom says he looks forward to meeting with "my nurse."
	1b. Use clear, unambiguous statements.	1b. Minimizes potential for misconstruing of messages.	
	1c. Provide activities that need concentration and are noncompetitive.	1c. Increases time spent in reality-based activities and decreases preoccupation with delusional and hallucinatory experiences.	
2. By (date), Tom will name two actions that precipitate voices and paranoia.	2a. Investigate content of hallucinations with Tom.	2a. Identifies suicidal or aggressive themes.	*GOAL MET* Tom is able to identify that the voices are worse at nighttime. He also states that after smoking
	2b. Explore those time that voices are the most threatening and disturbing.	2b. Identifies events that increase anxiety.	

NURSING CARE PLAN 22–1 A PERSON WITH PARANOIA: TOM *(Continued)*

SHORT-TERM GOAL	INTERVENTION	RATIONALE	EVALUATION
			marijuana and taking cocaine, he always thought people were trying to kill him.
3. Tom will name two actions that he can take if the voices start to upset him by (date).	3. Explore with Tom possible actions that can minimize anxiety.	3. Offers alternatives while anxiety level is relatively low.	*GOAL MET* Tom has the telephone number of a physician he can call when hallucinations start to escalate.

NURSING DIAGNOSIS

Noncompliance with medications: related to side effects therapy, as evidenced by verbalization of noncompliance and persistence of symptoms

Supporting Data

- Does not take prescribed medication: "It makes me tired and I can't have sex."
- Chronic history or relapse symptoms when out of the hospital.

Outcome Criteria: Tom will adhere to medication regimen.

SHORT-TERM GOAL	INTERVENTION	RATIONALE	EVALUATION
1. By (date), Tom will name actions he can take to offset the side effects of medication.	1a. Evaluate medication response with physician in the hospital.	1a. Identifies drugs and dosages that have increased therapeutic value and decreased side effects.	*GOAL MET* Physician readjusts dose, with the large dose at bedtime to increase sleep and a small dose during the day to decrease fatigue. Tom states that he sleeps better at night but is still tired during the day.
	1b. Medication changed to olanzapine (Zyprexa)	1b. Olanzapine (Zyprexa) causes no known sexual difficulties.	
	1c. Educate Tom regarding side effects—how long they last and what actions can be taken.	1c. Can give increased sense of control over symptoms.	
2. Tom will attend weekly support group for people with schizophrenia by (date).	2. Encourage Tom to join support group for people with schizophrenia.	2. Mutual concerns and problems are discussed in an atmosphere of acceptance—concerns such as housing expenses, loneliness, and jobs. Group also provides peer support for drug therapy maintenance.	*GOAL MET* Week 1: Tom attends meeting. Week 2: Tom states that he has made a friend. He speaks in the group about "not feeling good" at times. Week 3: Tom says that he might go to group therapy after discharge from the hospital.

Catatonia

The essential feature of catatonia is abnormal motor behavior. Two extreme motor behaviors are seen in clients with catatonia: extreme motor agitation and extreme psychomotor retardation (with mutism, even stupor). Other behaviors identified with catatonia include posturing, waxy flexibility, stereotyped behavior, extreme negativism or automatic obedience, echolalia, and echopraxia. The onset of catatonia is usually abrupt and the prognosis favorable. With chemotherapy and improved individual management, severe catatonic symptoms are rarely seen today. Useful nursing strategies are discussed in the following sections.

Withdrawn Phase

COUNSELING TECHNIQUES. Clients in the withdrawn phase of catatonia can be so withdrawn that they appear comatose. They can be mute and may remain so for hours, days, or even weeks or months if they are not treated with antipsychotic medication. Although such clients may not appear to pay attention to events going on around them, the client is acutely aware of the environment and may remember events accurately at a later date. A withdrawn client has special needs, and the nurse can use the following guidelines. Developing skill and confidence in working with withdrawn clients takes practice (Table 22–15).

SELF-CARE NEEDS. When a client is extremely withdrawn, physical needs take priority. A client may need to be hand fed or tube fed for adequate nutritional status to be maintained. Normal control over bladder and bowel functions can be interrupted. Assessment of urinary or bowel retention must be made and acted on when found. Incontinence of urine and feces may cause skin breakdown and infection. Because physical movements may be minimal or absent, range-of-motion exercises need to be carried out to prevent muscular atrophy, calcium depletion, and contractures. Dressing and grooming usually need direct nursing interventions.

The client with catatonic symptoms may trigger staff resistance to nursing interventions because the client may refuse to participate in activities or cooperate voluntarily.

MILIEU NEEDS. During the withdrawn state, the catatonic person may be on a continuum from decreased

TABLE 22–15 COUNSELING TECHNIQUES FOR A WITHDRAWN CLIENT

INTERVENTION	RATIONALE
Communications Nursing Diagnosis: **Impaired verbal communication related to perceptual and cognitive distortions, as evidenced by severe withdrawal and anergia**	
1. Stay with the client and sit in silence for short intervals. Do not demand that the client reply. This is often the first step.	1. Meets the person at his or her own level. The client may be too anxious or confused to speak.
2. Initiate frequent, short, regular contacts with the withdrawn client.	2. Initially, short intervals are more tolerable for both the client and the nurse.
3. Visit the client regularly and be back when you say you will. Before you leave, be very specific as to when you will be back, e.g., "I will be back at 1 PM for 10 minutes." Always be on time and keep your word. If a delay is unavoidable, explain this to the client.	3. Disappointments cause by the nurse could interfere with the forming of a relationship.
4. When speaking to the client, use simple, short sentences.	4. The client's thoughts may be confused and his or her attention span short.
5. Make observations about happenings in the environment, e.g., "I see you brought your Bible with you this morning."	5. Focuses attention on common realities in the environment.
6. When the client begins to speak, keep topics neutral and simple.	6. Helps to minimize anxiety and frustration.
7. Clarify the client's use of the generalized "they."	7. Clients with loose ego boundaries have difficulty with differentiating others from self.
8. Meet hostility and rejection with a nonjudgmental and neutral response, e.g., "If you don't want to visit now, I'll be back at 1 PM to spend time with you."	8. Often, clients are verbally abusive to, or rejecting of, the nurse; this is rarely personal. When the client can experience acceptance and caring for how he or she is at that moment, feelings of self-worth may increase.
9. Always tell the client that you do not understand when you do not.	9. Clients may erroneously think that the nurse can know what they are thinking. By correcting this false belief, the nurse clarifies communications and delineates ego boundaries.

TABLE 22–16 SELF-CARE AND MILIEU NEEDS FOR A WITHDRAWN CLIENT

INTERVENTION	RATIONALE
Self-Care Needs	
Nursing Diagnosis: Altered health maintenance related to biochemical changes, as evidenced by apparent stupor	
1. Talk to the client who appears comatose while giving physical care and explain everything that you are doing. Talk as if the client fully understands. Address the client respectfully, e.g., "Mr. Jones, I am going to shave the other side of your face. The water may feel cold."	1. Even though clients may appear comatose, *they may be aware of everything that is going on.* Often, clients can remember verbatim the conversations of others around them during the time they were comatose.
2. Monitor intake.	2. Client may be too disorganized to eat or drink.
3. Monitor output.	3. Client may retain urine and feces or be incontinent of urine or feces.
4. Encourage involvement with hygiene and dressing at the client's own level. *Do not do for a client what he or she is able to do.*	4. Sometimes, giving short, simple reminders is sufficient for a disorganized client. At other times, the nurse may have to assist the client with grooming and dressing.
Milieu Needs	
Nursing Diagnosis: Impaired social interaction related to anxiety and inability to concentrate attention outward, as evidenced by poor attention span and withdrawal	
1. Increase participation with others at client's level of tolerance.	
a. **Stuporous to very withdrawn:** one-to-one simple activities with the nurse, e.g., talking, looking through a magazine, painting, working with clay.	a. Activities that require no verbal response and have no time limit or "right or wrong" are the least threatening.
b. **Less withdrawn:** simple, concrete activity with nurse and perhaps with one other client, e.g., card games, drawing, ping-pong.	b. Brings the client slowly into contact with others. This provides a greater opportunity for reality orientation and consensual validation.
c. Eventually, offer client group activities, e.g., ward meetings, occupational therapy, dance therapy, bingo games.	c. Increased participation with others can increase client's ability to validate reality and to experience satisfaction in reality-based activities.

spontaneous movements to complete stupor. *Waxy flexibility*, or the ability to hold distorted postures for extensive periods, is often seen. The term *waxy* refers to the holding of any posture that the staff may place the person in. For example, if someone raises the client's arms over his head, the client may maintain that position for hours or longer. This phenomenon is often used as a diagnostic sign. When less withdrawn, a client may demonstrate stereotyped behavior, echopraxia, echolalia, or automatic obedience.

Caution is advised because even after holding a single posture for long periods, the client may suddenly and without provocation have brief outbursts of gross motor activity in response to inner hallucinations, delusions, and change in neurotransmitters. Table 22–16 identifies intervention strategies for self-care needs and milieu needs for a catatonic client who is withdrawn or in a catatonic stupor. The following case study is for a client who is withdrawn.

CASE STUDY: WORKING WITH A PERSON WHO IS WITHDRAWN

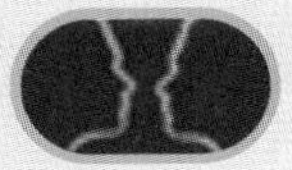

Mrs. Chou is a 25-year-old woman. She left China for the United States 6 months ago to join her husband. Before she came to the United States, she lived with her parents and worked in a button factory. In China, Mrs. Chou had been educated to speak and understand English. She had always been shy and looked to her parents and now to her husband for guidance and support. Shortly after she arrived in the United States, her mother developed pneumonia and died, and Mrs. Chou was not able to go back to China for the funeral. Mr. Chou states that his wife thought that if she had stayed in China, her mother would not have become ill. She told him recently that evil would come to their 1-year-old child because she was unable to take proper care of her mother. Three days before admission, Mrs. Chou became lethargic and spent most of the day staring into space and mumbling to herself. When Mr. Chou asked whom she was talking to, she would answer, "My mother." She has not

CASE STUDY: WORKING WITH A PERSON WHO IS WITHDRAWN *(Continued)*

eaten for 2 days; at the time of admission, Mrs. Chou sits motionless and mute and appears stuporous.

The physician notices that when he takes Mrs. Chou's pulse, her arm remains in midair until he replaces it by her side. Mr. Chou says that once his wife became extremely agitated and started to scream and cry while tearing the curtains and knocking over objects. Shortly afterward, she returned to a withdrawn, mute state. Mr. Chou is extremely distraught and confused, and he fears for the safety of their child. Mr. Nolan is assigned to Mrs. Chou as her primary nurse.

Mrs. Chou is sloppily dressed, and her hair and nails are dirty. She is pale, and her skin turgor is poor. She sits motionless and appears to be unaware of anything going on around her. Mr. Nolan introduces himself and explains what he will be doing beforehand—for example, that he will be taking her blood pressure and pulse and offering her fluids.

While taking her vital signs, he tells Mrs. Chou the date, the time, and where she is. When he is finished taking her vital signs, he offers Mrs. Chou some fluids. She is able to take sips from a straw when the straw is placed in her mouth. Mrs. Chou's intake and output are monitored, and she is placed in a four-bed room next to the nurses' station.

ASSESSMENT

Mr. Nolan assesses his data.

OBJECTIVE DATA

- Motionless and mute for 2 days
- Has not taken nourishment for 2 days
- Has had one episode of violent and destructive activity
- Eyes not focused, body limp
- Has had recent shock (mother's death)
- Skin turgor poor
- Poorly groomed
- Waxy flexibility

SUBJECTIVE DATA

Told husband "evil" would come to the baby because she did not take proper care of her mother

NURSING DIAGNOSIS

Mr. Nolan notes that Mrs. Chou is unable to take care of any basic needs (e.g., nutrition, hygiene, or proper toileting). He identifies **self-care deficit** as the primary initial priority.

PLANNING

PLANNING OUTCOME CRITERIA

Mr. Nolan formulates the following long-term and short-term goals:

NURSING DIAGNOSIS	OUTCOME CRITERIA	SHORT-TERM GOALS
1. **Self-care deficit** related to immobility, as evidenced by inability to feed, bathe, dress, or toilet herself.	1. Mrs. Chou will maintain nutritional intake and body weight.	1a. Mrs. Chou will take in 2000 ml of fluid each day. 1b. Mrs. Chou will eat three meals per day.
	2. Mrs. Chou will maintain normal bladder and bowel function.	2a. Mrs. Chou will void 1000 to 1500 ml per day. 2b. Mrs. Chou will have one bowel movement per day.
	3. Mrs. Chou will maintain present muscle tone and flexibility.	3a. Mrs. Chou will participate in passive range-of-motion exercises three times per day for 15 minutes.

NURSE'S FEELINGS AND SELF-ASSESSMENT

Mr. Nolan finds that initially, he becomes impatient with Mrs. Chou. He was used to carrying out nursing procedures quickly and efficiently. Mrs. Chou's morning care de-

CASE STUDY: WORKING WITH A PERSON WHO IS WITHDRAWN *(Continued)*

mands a great deal of time. For example, he finds himself being impatient with the long periods it takes to feed Mrs. Chou. He discusses his impatience with a colleague. During the discussion, it becomes apparent that it is actually Mrs. Chou's total dependency on him that makes him anxious. Mr. Nolan sees himself as highly organized and in control, often suppressing many of his own desires to be taken care of. "I guess her total dependency triggers some of my own unmet dependency needs." Once he is able to separate some of the personal concerns that have triggered his reaction, he is able to focus on Mrs. Chou's needs with more patience. He finds that the more he talks to Mrs. Chou as if she were able to understand everything he says, the easier it is for him to maintain a certain level of relatedness and interest.

INTERVENTION

Mr. Nolan assigns the psychiatric aide to bathe and dress Mrs. Chou in the mornings. He spends time with Mrs. Chou each morning and afternoon, doing range-of-motion exercises, offering her frequent sips of juice or milk, and talking to her (i.e., making observations about neutral happenings in the environment). Mr. Chou visits every day, and Mr. Nolan encourages him to talk to his wife about everyday occurrences in his life and about their future. He also cautions Mr. Chou that there is a possibility that Mrs. Chou could suddenly become agitated and aggressive, and that this is part of the disease.

With the aid of medication therapy and nursing management, Mrs. Chou begins to show signs of comprehension. By the end of the seventh day, Mrs. Chou is talking, feeding herself, and bathing herself. She appears to have developed a strong attachment to Mr. Nolan and tells her husband how kind he was to her while she was "away." She even remembers that Mr. Nolan brought in a Chinese music tape during the period when she was stuporous. The psychiatrists believe that Mrs. Chou's catatonic reaction was triggered by her mother's death, and strongly suggest counseling after discharge to facilitate the process of mourning.

EVALUATION

Catatonic episodes are generally acute and related to identifiable stressors, and the disorder has a favorable prognosis. Mrs. Chou responds rapidly to medication and Mr. Nolan's nursing intervention. After 3 weeks, Mrs. Chou is able to care for her activities of daily living with minimal supervision. Although much of Mrs. Chou's passivity is culturally determined, the psychiatrists suggest that Mrs. Chou develop more outlets for release of emotional tensions. Mrs. Chou agrees to counseling after discharge, and a referral is made to the mental health clinic in their area. Useful nursing strategies are provided in Table 22–17 for a client in the excited phase of catatonia.

Excited Phase

COUNSELING TECHNIQUES. During the excited, or acute, stage, the person talks or shouts continually, and verbalizations may be incoherent. Communication is clear and directed, and concern is for the client's and others' safety.

SELF-CARE NEEDS. A person who is constantly and intensely hyperactive can become completely exhausted and can even die if medical attention is not available. Most often, a standard antipsychotic agent is administered intramuscularly. The client may continue to be agitated, but within limits that are not potentially harmful. During this time of heightened physical activity, the client's body has an increased need for fluids, calories, and rest. During the hyperactive state, a client may be destructive and aggressive to others in response to hallucinations or delusions. Table 22–17 offers guidelines for meeting communication and self-care needs during the excited phase of catatonia. Many of these concerns and interventions are the same as for a bipolar client in a manic phase.

Disorganized Schizophrenia

The most regressed and socially impaired of all the schizophrenic disorders is the disorganized form. A person diagnosed with disorganized schizophrenia (formally hebephrenia) may have marked looseness of associations, grossly inappropriate affect, bizarre mannerisms, and incoherence of speech and may display extreme social with-

TABLE 22–17 NURSING MEASURES FOR A CLIENT WITH ACUTE, EXCITED CATATONIA

INTERVENTION	RATIONALE
Communications	
Nursing Diagnosis: **Ineffective coping related to panic level of anxiety, as evidenced by hyperactivity**	
1. Use firm, clear statements.	1. The client may be disorganized; needs clear statements. Firmness provides a sense of outside control.
2. Keep the client in quiet area.	2. Helps to decrease environmental stimuli and anxiety.
Self-Care Needs	
Nursing Diagnosis: **Altered health maintenance related to cognitive disturbances, as evidenced by inability to care for basic needs**	
1. Monitor weight and dietary intake.	1. The client may lose calories, fluids, and essential nutrients.
2. Offer high-calorie fluids and finger foods, e.g., milk, bananas, sandwiches, candy bars, hard-boiled eggs.	2. Foods that a client can carry with him or her when he or she is too active to sit during meals help replace and maintain adequate nutrition.
3. Provide rest periods.	3. Minimizes exhaustion and fatigue.
4. Supervise grooming and physical appearance.	4. The client may be too agitated to care for physical appearance.
Milieu Needs	
Nursing Diagnosis: **Risk for violence related to biochemical changes, as evidenced by agitation**	
1. Watch closely for signs of increased agitation.	1. The client may become increasingly agitated and may need a decrease in environmental stimuli or medication. Intervention should be made before anxiety escalates to panic levels, when intervention becomes traumatic for both the client and the staff.
2. Assess need for intervention if agitation increases (verbal, chemical, or seclusion or restraints).	2. Protect the client and others.
Nursing Diagnosis: **Diversional activity deficit related to cognitive disturbances, as evidenced by hyperactivity and poor concentration**	
Encourage simple physical activity using large muscle groups, e.g., pace with the client or play ping-pong, volleyball, when the client is no longer acute.	Gross motor activity that requires minimal concentration can reduce anxiety and tension.

drawal. Although delusions and hallucinations are present, they are fragmentary and not well organized. Behavior may be considered "odd," and giggling or grimacing in response to internal stimuli is common. Disorganized schizophrenia has an earlier age of onset (early to middle teens) and often develops insidiously. It is associated with poor premorbid functioning, a significant family history of psychopathological disorders, and a poor prognosis. Often, these clients are in state hospitals and can live in the community safely only in a structured and well-supervised setting. Unfortunately, these clients now make up a good portion of the homeless population. Other clients may live at home, and their families have significant needs for community support, respite care, and day hospital affiliations.

COMMUNICATION NEEDS. People with disorganized schizophrenia experience persistent and severe perceptual problems. Verbal responses may be marked by looseness of associations or incoherence. Clang associations or word salad may be present. **Blocking,** a sudden cessation in the train of thought, is frequently observed.

SELF-CARE NEEDS. Grooming is neglected. Hair may be dirty and matted, and clothes may be inappropriate and stained. The client has no awareness of social expectations. The client may be too disorganized to carry out simple activities of daily living.

Basic goals for nursing intervention include encouraging optimal level of functioning, preventing further regression, and offering alternatives for inappropriate behaviors whenever possible.

MILIEU NEEDS. Behavior is often described as bizarre. A client may twirl around the room or make strange gestures with the hands and face. Social behavior is often primitive or regressed. For example, a client may eat with the hands, pick the nose, or masturbate in public. Typical behaviors include posturing, grimacing or giggling, and mirror gazing. Table 22–18 provides communication strategies and interventions for self-care and milieu needs. A case study of a person with disorganized schizophrenia follows.

TABLE 22–18 NURSING MEASURES FOR A CLIENT WITH DISORGANIZED SCHIZOPHRENIA

INTERVENTION	RATIONALE
Communications	
Nursing Diagnosis: Ineffective coping related to perceptual and cognitive distortions, as evidenced by disorganized speech	
1. Speak in short, simple sentences	1. Thought patterns are disorganized. Simple phrases are best understood.
2. Constantly reinforce reality, e.g., call client by name, state the date, state your name.	2. Thinking if often autistic and confused. Stressing common environmental realities provides a tie with reality.
3. Initiate short, frequent contacts.	3. Helps establish a rapport and personal contact in a manner that is less threatening to client.
4. Allow client time to respond.	4. Because thought process of client is disorganized, time is needed for client to take messages in and compose a response.
Self-Care Needs	
Nursing Diagnosis: Altered health maintenance related to cognitive distortions, as evidenced by difficulty with activities of daily living	
1. Observe for signs and symptoms of physical illness, e.g., cold, thirst, pain.	1. Clients are often disorganized, out of touch with feelings, and unable to assess personal needs or ask for what they need.
2. Encourage appropriate dress and hygiene. Check for incontinence and provide fresh clothes when necessary. Use nonpunitive, matter-of-fact approach.	2. Client may be too disorganized to use toilet.
3. Help client with hygiene as needed, e.g., set up shaving, give step-by-step instructions; if unable to shave, help with shaving; help with putting on make-up, brushing hair, brushing teeth.	3. Can minimize anxiety and help client maintain self-esteem. Meets client at own level. When client is able to do partial care, even though slowly, this type of assistance encourages independent functioning.
4. Lay out clothes that are clean and appropriate. Give simple step-by-step instructions for dress, e.g., "Put in your left arm . . . now your right arm . . . pull sweater over your head."	4. Maintains optimal level of functioning and self-esteem.
5. Encourage appropriate social behaviors, e.g., have client eat with utensils and cover front with napkin. When discouraging unacceptable behavior, e.g., eating with hands, offer alternatives, e.g., large spoon with which to eat food.	5. Increases social interactions.
Milieu Needs	
Nursing Diagnosis: Diversional activity deficit related to inability to concentrate, as evidenced by purposeless activity and apathy	
1. Families need support in locating day hospitals, shelters, workshops, respite centers, and other community supports that can help them reduce family stress.	1. Provides socialization and structure for client and physical and emotional support for family.
2. Plan and initiate simple daily routine.	2. Consistent daily routine helps client maintain contact with reality with minimal anxiety.
3. Plan simple, concrete tasks that require minimal concentration and skill, e.g., drawing, walking with nurse, dancing, attending ward meeting, folding linen.	3. Tasks that match client's concentration and interest can promote socialization, increase contact with reality, provide exercise, and increase self-esteem.

CASE STUDY: WORKING WITH A PERSON WITH DISORGANIZED THINKING

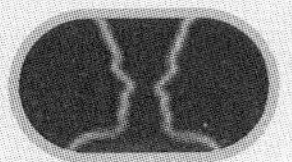

Martin Taylor, a 36-year-old white, unemployed man, has been referred to the mental health center. He is accompanied by his mother and sister. He had been hospitalized for 3 years in a state hospital with the diagnosis of chronic schizophrenia and was doing well at home until 2 months ago. His only employment was for 5 months as a janitor after high school graduation. Other significant family history includes a twin brother who died of a cerebral aneurysm in his teens.

Continued on following page

CASE STUDY: WORKING WITH A PERSON WITH DISORGANIZED THINKING *(Continued)*

Martin tells the nurse he has used every street drug available, including LSD and intravenous heroin. His mother states that as a teenager, before his substance abuse, he was an excellent athlete who received average grades. At the age of 17, he had his first psychotic break when taking a variety of street drugs. His behavior became markedly bizarre (e.g., eating cat food, swallowing a rubber-soled shoe that required an emergency laparotomy).

Ms. Lamb, a clinical nurse specialist, meets with Martin after speaking with his mother and sister. Martin is unshaven, and his appearance is disheveled. He is wearing a red headband in which he has placed popsicle sticks and scraps of paper. He chain smokes during the interview and frequently gets up and paces back and forth. He tells the nurse that he is Alice from *Alice in the underground* and that people from space hurt him with needles. His speech pattern is marked by associative looseness and occasional blocking. For example, he often stops in the middle of a phrase and giggles to himself. At one point, when he starts to giggle, Ms. Lamb asks him what he was thinking about. He stated "You interrupted me." At that point, he began to shake his head while repeating in a sing-song voice "Shake them tigers . . . shake them tigers . . . shake them tigers." He denies suicidal or homicidal ideation. Ms. Lamb notes that Martin has a great deal of difficulty accurately perceiving what is going on around him. He has markedly regressed social behaviors. For example, he eats with his hands and picks his nose in public. He has no apparent insight into his problems; he tells Ms. Lamb that his biggest problem is the people in space.

ASSESSMENT

OBJECTIVE DATA

- Associative looseness
- Giggles and mumbles to self
- Poorly and bizarrely dressed
- Low level of functioning
- History of bizarre behavior
- Restless, pacing, and chain smoking
- Regressed social behaviors
- Occasional blocking

SUBJECTIVE DATA

- "I am Alice in the underground."
- "People from space hurt me with needles."
- "You interrupted me," in response to being asked what he was thinking.
- Denies suicidal or homicidal impulses.
- "My biggest problems are the people from space."

NURSING DIAGNOSIS

Ms. Lamb identifies Martin's deterioration of functioning as a priority for intervention. Ms. Lamb's first diagnosis is **ineffective individual coping** related to confused thought processes and lack of motivation to respond, as evidenced by inability to meet basic needs:

- Regressed social behaviors.
- Poor and bizarre dress.
- Low level of functioning.
- Frequent looseness of association.

PLANNING

PLANNING OUTCOME CRITERIA

Ms. Lamb identifies Martin as a candidate for skills training and makes arrangements for him to live in a halfway house. She also encourages the family to participate in a multifamily psychoeducational group.

NURSING DIAGNOSIS	OUTCOME CRITERIA	SHORT-TERM GOALS
1. **Ineffective individual coping** related to confused thought processes and lack of motivation, as evidenced by inability to meet basic needs.	1. Martin will be able to perform three skills in daily living within 2 months.	1a. Martin will be able to bathe independently in 1 month. 1b. Martin will make his bed in 3 weeks. 1c. Martin will be able to make a sandwich with supervision in 5 weeks.

CASE STUDY: WORKING WITH A PERSON WITH DISORGANIZED THINKING *(Continued)*

NURSE'S FEELINGS AND SELF-ASSESSMENT

Working with a client who has limited potential for relating, poorly defined ego boundaries, and limited social skills and who demonstrates regressed bizarre behavior requires a great deal of skill, patience, and peer support. In the presence of delusions, bizarre behaviors, and regressed social skills, health care workers can experience helplessness, can feel overwhelmed, and can become anxious. Some anxiety may be caused by empathizing or acknowledging the client's deeply repressed feelings of inferiority, fear, and anger. At times, nurses may have similar repressed feelings that they have difficulty dealing with; these feelings may cause them to withdraw from the client in an attempt to minimize their awareness of uncomfortable feelings. Often, the more withdrawn and regressed the client is, the more taxing he or she is to health care workers.

INTERVENTION

Martin is placed in a group home, where skills training will be conducted. Because Martin has a chronic history of deterioration, concrete goals are set. A trial daily checklist for activities of daily living is devised and will be periodically reviewed. It includes such items as the following:

- Makes bed
- Brushes teeth
- Combs hair
- Shaves
- Showers
- Makes two sandwiches a week
- Wears clean clothing

EVALUATION

Martin gradually adapts to the group home, where skills training continues. The group home is helping Martin relearn self-care needs. After 3 months, Martin is able to carry out basic activities of daily living when constant reminders are given. He is able to bathe, shave, comb his hair, and dress more appropriately when given simple instructions and encouragement. The goal of making a sandwich or fixing a simple lunch has not yet been met; Martin starts to eat the food before the task of finishing the sandwich is completed. Martin and his family have been attending multiple-family psychoeducational group, and the stress on Martin and his family has been greatly reduced. Plans are for Martin to return home in the near future.

Undifferentiated Schizophrenia

In the undifferentiated type of schizophrenia, *active signs of the disorder* (positive or negative symptoms) are present, but the individual does not meet the criteria for paranoia, catatonia, or disorganized type (APA 1994). Undifferentiated schizophrenia has an early and insidious onset (early to middle teens), like that of disorganized schizophrenia. However, the premorbid state is less predictable, and the disability remains fairly stable, although persistent, over time (Fenton and McGlashan 1991).

Residual Type of Schizophrenia

In the residual type of schizophrenia, active phase symptoms are no longer present, but evidence of two or more residual symptoms persists. Residual symptoms include

- Lack of initiative, interests, or energy.
- Marked social withdrawal.
- Impairment in role function (wage earner, student, homemaker).
- Marked speech deficits (circumstantial, vague, and poverty of speech or content of speech).
- Odd beliefs, magical thinking, and unusual perceptual experiences.

Principles of care similar to those applying to withdrawn, paranoid, and disorganized schizophrenia apply to undifferentiated and residual schizophrenia, as dictated by the client's behavior.

EVALUATION

Evaluation is always an important step in the planning of care. Evaluation is especially important with people who have chronic psychotic disorders. Modifications may have to be made in the goals set for specific clients. All goals need to be realistic and obtainable. Often, the goals set for people with chronic disorders are too ambitious. A former short-term goal often becomes a long-term goal. Change is a process that occurs over time; with a person diagnosed with schizophrenia, the time period may be pronounced. Therefore, for preventing both client frustration and staff burnout, short-term goals should be realistic and obtainable.

Another advantage of regularly scheduled evaluations with chronically ill clients is that they allow the staff to consider new data and to reassess the client's problems. Is the client not progressing because a more important need is not being met? Is the staff using the client's strengths and interest to reach identified goals? Are more appropriate interventions available for this client to facilitate progress? If a newer antipsychotic agent is being tried, is there evidence of improvement or a lower level of functioning?

The active involvement of staff with the client's progress can help sustain interest and prevent feelings of helplessness and burnout. Input from the client can offer valuable data about why a certain desired behavior or situation has not occurred.

SUMMARY

Schizophrenia is a biologically based disease of the brain. Psychotic symptoms in schizophrenia are more pronounced and disruptive than are symptoms found in other disorders. The basic differences are in degree of severity, withdrawal, alteration in affect, impairment of intellect, and regression.

Neurochemical (catecholamines and serotonin), genetic, and neuroanatomical findings help explain the symptoms of schizophrenia. However, no one theory at present can account for all phenomena found in schizophrenic disorders.

During the nurse's work with schizophrenic clients, specific symptoms are evident. No one symptom is found in all cases. The positive and negative symptoms of schizophrenia are two of the major categories of symptoms. The *positive* symptoms are more florid (hallucinations, delusions, looseness of associations) and respond better to antipsychotic drug therapy. The *negative* symptoms of schizophrenia (poor social adjustment, lack of motivation, withdrawal) can be more debilitating and do not respond to antipsychotic (antipsychotic) therapy.

Some nursing diagnoses discussed include **sensory-perceptual alterations, altered thought process, impaired verbal communications, ineffective individual coping, risk for violence directed at self or others,** and **ineffective family coping: compromised or disabling.**

Planning outcomes involves setting short-term and long-term outcomes. An awareness of personal feelings and reactions to clients' feelings and behaviors is crucial.

Interventions for people with schizophrenia include special communication and counseling techniques, self-care strategies, and milieu intervention. Also necessary is an understanding of the properties, side effects, toxic effects, and doses of the traditional, atypical, and other medications used for schizophrenia.

Basic characteristics of paranoid, catatonic (withdrawn and excited), and disorganized schizophrenic are presented in this chapter. Specific nursing interventions are outlined in case studies.

REFERENCES

Addington, J., Addington, D., and Maticka-Tyndale, E. (1991). Cognitive functioning and positive and negative symptoms in schizophrenia. *Schizophrenia Research*, 5(2):123.

American Psychiatric Association (1994). *Diagnostic and statistical manual of mental disorders* (4th ed.). Washington, DC: American Psychiatric Association.

American Psychiatric Association (1997). *American Journal of Psychiatry* (Suppl). Practice guidelines for the treatment of patients with schizophrenia. 154(4):1.

Andreasen, N., and Munich, R. L. (1995). Introduction. In G. O. Goddard (Ed.), *Treatment of psychiatric disorders* (2nd ed., Vol. 1, pp. 944–946). Washington, DC: American Psychiatric Press.

Baldessarini, R. J. (1996). First episode psychosis: Effect of duration on hospital outcome. *Current Approaches to Psychosis*, 5(11):1, 4.

Berkow, R., et al. (Eds.) (1992). *Merck manual* (16th ed.). Rahway, NJ: Merck Research Laboratories.

Black, D. W., Yates, W. R., and Andreasen, N. C. (1988). Schizophrenia, schizophreniform disorders and delusional paranoid disorders. In J. A. Talbott, R. E. Hales and S. C. Yudofsky (Eds.), *Textbook of psychiatry*. Washington, DC: American Psychiatric Press.

Brekke, J. S., DeBonis, J. A., and Graham, J. W. (1994). The latent structure analysis of the positive and negative symptoms in schizophrenia. *Comprehensive Psychiatry*, 35(4):252.

Bruch, H. (1980). *Psychotherapy in schizophrenia: Historical considerations*. New York: Plenum.

Bugle, C., Andrew, S., Heath, J. (1992). Early detection of water intoxication. *Journal of Psychosocial Nursing*, 30(11):31.

Caroff, S. N., and Mann, S. C. (1993). Neuroleptic malignant syndrome. *Medical Clinics of North America*, 77(1):185.

Carpenter, W., and Buchanan, R. W. (1995). Schizophrenia: Introduction and overview. In H. I. Kaplan and B. J. Sadock (Eds.), *Comprehensive textbook of psychiatry* (6th ed., Vol. 1, pp. 889–902). Baltimore: Williams & Wilkins.

Dowart, R. A., and Hoover, C. W. (1994). A national study of transitional hospital services in mental health. *American Journal of Public Health*, 84(8):1229.

Duke, P. J. (1994). South Westminster schizophrenic survey: Alcohol use and its relationship to symptoms, tardive dyskinesia and illness onset. *British Journal of Psychiatry*, 164(5):630.

Fenton, W. S., and Cole, S. A. (1995). Psychosocial therapies of schizophrenia: Individual, group, and family. In G. O. Goddard (Ed.), *Treatment of psychiatric disorders* (2nd ed., Vol. 1, pp.988–1018). Washington, DC: American Psychiatric Press.

Fenton, W. S., and McGlashan, T. H. (1991). Natural history of schizophrenic subtypes: I. Longitudinal study of paranoid, hebephrenic, and undifferentiated schizophrenia. *Archives of General Psychiatry*, 48(11):969.

Gabbard, G. O., and Callaway, B. W. (1995). Multiple family groups reduce schizophrenia relapse. *The Menninger Letter*, 3(10):1.

Gordon, B. J., and Milke, D. J. (1995). Clozapine and recidivism. *Psychiatric Services*, 46(10):1079.

Grebb, J. A., and Cancro, R. (1989). Schizophrenia: Clinical features. In H. I. Kaplan, and B. J. Sadock (Eds.), *Comprehensive textbook of psychiatry* (Vol. I.). Baltimore: Williams & Wilkins.

Guze, B., Richeimer, S., and Szuba, M. (1995). *The psychiatric drug handbook*. St. Louis: Mosby–Year Book.

Johns, C. A. (1996). Managing the refractory patient. *Current Approaches to Psychosis*, 5(10):6.

Jones, R. M. (1994). Negative and depressive symptoms in schizophrenia. *Acta Psychiatrica Scandinavica*, 89(2):81.

Junginger, J. (1995). Common hallucinations and predictions of dangerousness. *Psychiatric Services*, 46(9):911.

Kahn, M. E. (1984). Psychotherapy with chronic schizophrenics: Alliance, transference and countertransference. *Journal of Psychosocial Nursing*, 22(7):20.

Kane, J. M. (1995). Clinical psychopharmacology of schizophrenia. In G. O. Goddard (Ed.), *Treatment of psychiatric disorders* (2nd ed., Vol. 1, pp. 970–986). Washington, DC: American Psychiatric Press.

Kaplan, H. I., and Sadock, B. J. (1995). *Synopsis of psychiatry* (6th ed.). Baltimore: Williams & Wilkins.

Klausner, M., and Brecher, M. (1995). Risperidone guidelines. *Psychiatric Services*, 46(9):950.

Kolb, L. C., and Brodie, H. K. H. (1982) *Modern clinical psychiatry* (10th ed.). Philadelphia: W. B. Saunders.
Lamb, R. H., et al. (1986). Families of schizophrenics: A movement in jeopardy. *Hospital and Community Psychiatry*, 37(4):353.
Levinson, D. F. (1991). Pharmacologic treatment of schizophrenia. *Clinical Therapy*, 13(3):326.
Lipton, A. A., and Cancro, R. (1995). Schizophrenia: Clinical features. In H. I. Kaplan and B. J. Sadock (Eds.), *Comprehensive textbook of psychiatry* (6th ed., Vol. 1, pp. 968–986). Baltimore: Williams & Wilkins.
Littrell, K. (1996). Olanzapine: An exciting new antipsychotic. *American Psychiatric Nurses' Association*, 8(4):4.
Marder, S. R., Wirshing, W. C., and Ames, D. (1997). New antipsychotics. In D. L. Dunner and J. F. Rosenbaum (eds.). *Psychiatric Clinics of North America annual of drug therapy*. Philadelphia: W. B. Saunders.
Maxmen, J. S., and Ward, N. G. (1995). *Psychotrophic drugs: Fast facts*. (2nd ed.). New York: W. W. Norton.
McFarlane, E. R. (1995). Families in the treatment of psychotic disorders. *The Harvard Mental Health Letter*, 12(4):4.
McGlashan, T. H., and Hoffman, R. E. (1995). Schizophrenia: Psychodynamic to neurodynamic theories. In H. I. Kaplan and B. J. Sadock (Eds.), *Comprehensive textbook of psychiatry* (6th ed., Vol. 1, pp 957–967). Baltimore: Williams & Wilkins.
Metzler, H. Y., Rabinowitz, J., Lee, M. A., et al. (1997). Age onset and gender of schizophrenic patients in relation to neuroleptic resistance. *American Journal of Psychiatry*, (154)4:475.
Menninger, W. W. (1984). Dealing with staff reactions to perceived lack of progress by chronic mental patients. *Hospital and Community Psychiatry*, 35(8):805.
Moller, M. D. (1989). *Understanding and communicating with an individual who is hallucinating* (video). Omaha, NE: NurScience.
Nehart, M. A. (1996). Neurobiology of schizophrenia. *Journal of the American Psychiatric Nurses Association*, 2(5):174.
Peralta-Martin, V., and Cuesta-Zorita, M. J. (1994). Validation of positive and negative symptom scale (PANSS) in a sample of Spanish schizophrenic patients. 22(4):171.
Preston, T., and Johnson, J. (1995). *Clinical psychopharmacology made ridiculously simple*. Miami: Med Master.
Roy, M. A., and DeVrient, X. (1994). Positive and negative symptoms in schizophrenia: A current review. *Canadian Journal of Psychiatry*, 39(7):407.
Schatzberg, A. F., and Cole, J. O. (1991). *Manual of clinical psychopharmacology* (2nd ed.). Washington, DC: American Psychiatric Press.
Schiller, L., and Bennett, A. (1994). *The quiet room*. New York: Warner Books.
Slately, A. E. (1994). *Handbook of psychiatric emergencies*. Norwalk, CT: Appleton & Lange.
Swonger, A., and Matejski, M. P. (1991). *Nursing pharmacology: An integrated approach to drug therapy and nursing practice* (2nd ed.). Philadelphia: J. B. Lippincott.
Talbott, J., Hales, R., and Yadofsky, S. C. (1994). *Textbook of psychiatry* (2nd ed.). Washington, DC: American Psychiatric Press.
Tollefson, G. (1995). *The neurobiology of schizophrenia*. U. S. Psychiatric and Mental Health Congress Conference and Exhibition, November 17, 1995.
Vidal, G. (1982). *The second American revolution and other essays (1976–1982)*. New York: Random House.
Willick, M. S. (1993). The deficit syndrome in schizophrenia: Psychoanalytic and neurobiological perspectives. *Journal of the American Psychoanalytic Association*, 41(4):1135.
Wright, P., et al. (1993). Genetics and the maternal immune response to viral infection. *American Journal of Medical Genetics*, 48(1):40.
Wyatt, R. J., Kirch, B. G., and Egan, M. F. (1995). Schizophrenia: Neurochemical, viral, and immunological studies. In H. I. Kaplan and B. J. Sadock (Eds.), *Comprehensive textbook of psychiatry* (6th ed., Vol. 1, pp. 927–941). Baltimore: Williams & Wilkins.
Yamamoto, B. K., and Meltzer, H. Y. (1995). Basic neuropharmacology of antipsychotic drugs. In G. O. Goddard (Ed.), *Treatment of psychiatric disorders* (2nd ed., Vol. 1, pp. 947–967). Washington, DC: American Psychiatric Press.
Zahniser, J. H., Courey, R. D., and Herghbarger, K. (1991). Individual psychotherapy with schizophrenic outpatients in the public mental health systems. *Hospital and Community Psychiatry*, 42(9):906.

Further Reading

Acker, C. (1993). Drug offers hope to schizophrenia. *Philadelphia Inquirer*, June 21, 1993.
Baldwin, L. J., et al. (1992). Decreased excessive water drinking by chronic mentally ill forensic patients. *Hospital and Community Psychiatry*, 43(5):507.
Dixon, et al. (1991). Drug abuse in schizophrenic patients: Clinical correlates and reasons for use. *The American Journal of Psychiatry*, 148(2):224.
Falloon, I. R. H. (1986). Family stress and schizophrenia: Theory and practice. *Psychiatric Clinics of North America*, 9(1):165.
Garza-Trevino, E. S., et al. (1990). Neurobiology of schizophrenic syndromes. *Hospital and Community Psychiatry*, 41(9):971.
Goldman, M. B. (1991). A rational approach to disorders of water balance in psychiatric patients. *Hospital and Community Psychiatry*, 42(5):488.
Javitt, D. C., and Zurkin, S. R. (1991). Recent advances in the phencyclidine model of schizophrenia. *American Journal of Psychiatry*, 148(10):1201.
Keefe, R. S. E., and Harvey, P. D. (1994). *Understanding schizophrenia: A guide to the new research on causes and treatment*. New York: Free Press.
Lehman, A. F. (1995). Schizophrenia: Psychosocial treatment. In H. I. Kaplan and B. J. Sadock (Eds.), *Comprehensive textbook of psychiatry* (6th ed., Vol. 1, pp. 998–1018). Baltimore: Williams & Wilkins.
MacKinnon, R. A., and Michels, R. (1971). *The psychiatric interview in clinical practice*. Philadelphia: W. B. Saunders.
Marder, S. R. (1995). Switching antipsychotic therapies. *Current Approaches to Psychosis*, 4(1):5.
Mueser, K. T., and Gingerich, S. (1994). *Coping with schizophrenia: A guide for families*. Oakland, CA: New Harbinger Publications.
Sandy, K. R., and Kay, S. R. (1991). The relationship of pineal calcification to cortical atrophy in schizophrenia. *International Journal of Neuroscience*, 57(3/4):179.
Schizophrenia: The present state of understanding (Part I) (1992). *Harvard Mental Health Letter*, 8(11):1.
Schizophrenia: The present state of understanding (Part II) (1992). *Harvard Mental Health Letter*, 8(12):1.
Schultz, S. C. (1995). Schizophrenia: Somatic treatment. In H. I. Kaplan and B. J. Sadock (Eds.), *Comprehensive textbook of psychiatry* (6th ed., Vol. 1, pp. 968–986). Baltimore: Williams & Wilkins.
Smoyak, S. A. (1994). Hildegard E. Peplau awarded honorary doctorate. *Journal of Psychosocial Nursing*, 32(11):45, 1994.
Wallace, C. J., and Liberman, R. P. (1995). Psychiatric rehabilitation. In G. O. Goddard (Ed.), *Treatment of psychiatric disorders* (2nd ed., Vol. 1, pp. 1020–1038). Washington, DC: American Psychiatric Press.

SELF-STUDY AND CRITICAL THINKING

Short answer

Write brief responses to the following.

1. Discuss the difference between a hallucination and a delusion and give examples.
2. Depersonalization and derealization are examples of ________________.
3. Give an example of

   A. Clang association ____________________________
   B. Neologism ____________________________

C. Word salad ______________________________

4. Formulate two possible short-term goals for a client with altered thought process.

A. ______________________________
B. ______________________________

True or false

Place T (true) or F (false) next to each statement. Correct the false statements.

5. __________ It is impossible to understand a person when his or her speech is characterized by looseness of association.

6. __________ Hallucinations, delusions, and neologisms are examples of positive symptoms.

7. __________ Ambivalence in relationships is found only in the mentally ill.

8. __________ A man hears the stock market is down and takes that as a sign that God will destroy the world. This is an example of an idea of reference.

Multiple choice

Circle all correct answers.

9. Circle possible outcomes of unresolved feelings by a nurse.

A. Denial
B. Withdrawal from client
C. Increase in nurse's self-esteem
D. Burnout

10. Circle all the possible outcomes of effective health teaching with client and family.

A. Increase compliance with medication
B. Increase problem-solving skills
C. Minimize misunderstanding of the schizophrenic member within the family or community group
D. Reduce the occurrence of schizophrenic symptoms caused by the ingestion of certain drugs (e.g., marijuana, amphetamines)
E. Help the family identify symptoms that may signal a possible relapse

11. Circle all the possible effects of antipsychotic medication.

A. Reduction in the intensity of hallucinations and delusions
B. Improvement in thought processes
C. Increase in affect and motivation
D. Decrease in the intensity of paranoid reactions
E. Increase in the ability to function socially

Place H (hallucinations), D (delusions), or HD (hallucinations and delusions) next to the appropriate intervention.

12. __________ Look for themes in the client's speech patterns.

13. __________ Tell the client that you do not hear the voices he or she hears.

14. __________ Point out reality and attempt to empathize with the client's experience

15. __________ Do not argue with the client over the validity of this thinking.

16. ________ Always validate reality.

17. ________ Clarify misinterpretations of the environment.

18. ________ Do not pretend to understand the client when you do not.

19. ________ Place the focus of difficulty in understanding on yourself (e.g., "I am having a difficult time understanding you.").

True or false

Place T (true) or F (false) next to each statement and correct those that are false.

20. ________ All the extrapyramidal side effects are reversible.

21. ________ Specific antipsychotics are often ordered because of their specific side effects.

22. ________ The only problem with antipsychotics is that tolerance develops.

23. ________ Tardive dyskinesia, weight gain, and impotence are among the most troubling side effects in outpatient management with the traditional antipsychotics.

24. ________ Fatal side effects from the antipsychotics, such as neuroleptic malignant syndrome, are rare.

25. ________ A person in a catatonic stupor is totally unaware of anything going on around him or her.

26. ________ Physical needs may take the highest priority when a person is in either extreme catatonic excitement or stupor.

27. ________ Only positive symptoms are targeted by antipsychotics.

The following can result from frequent team evaluation of the treatment plan for a chronic schizophrenic client.

28. ________ Reassessment of problems; important needs may have been missed.
29. ________ Re-evaluation of the client's strengths and identification of alternative interventions.
30. ________ Reassessment of goals can renew interest in the client.

A person with paranoid schizophrenia

31. ________ Often has better ego functions than a person with any other schizophrenic disorder.
32. ________ Uses sarcasm and hostility to maintain emotional distance and increase feelings of safety.
33. ________ Usually needs help with grooming and dress.

Multiple choice

Jerry, a 17-year-old youth, has a paranoid psychotic break after the death of his twin brother. He is sure everyone wants him dead and that his food is poisoned. He hears the voice of God demanding that he join his brother. He will not bathe or change his clothes because he believes that the warlocks could then take over his body.

34. Of the following possible nursing diagnoses, which has the highest priority?

A. Alteration in nutrition: less than body requirements
B. Alteration in health maintenance
C. Potential for self-harm
D. Alteration in thought processes

35. If Jerry thought his food was poisoned, the nurse should first

A. Discuss nutrition with Jerry.
B. Get an order for tube feedings.
C. Offer Jerry food in its own containers (e.g., milk, oranges).
D. Show him how irrational his thinking is.

36. When Jerry says, "You are wearing a red sweater. That means you are against me today," he is experiencing

A. Delusion.
B. Hallucination.
C. Idea of reference.
D. Fantasy.

37. When speaking to a person who is paranoid, you would consider all of the following *except*

A. Use simple, clear language.
B. Refrain from touching the client.
C. Be warm and enthusiastic.
D. Clarify and reiterate your role in a patient manner.

38. Which activity would you choose initially for a person who is paranoid?

A. Listening to music alone, going with the flow
B. Playing poker with two other people, to increase self-esteem
C. Playing team volleyball, to become more cooperative
D. Building model airplanes, to concentrate on a reality based activity.

39. Medication appropriate for a person in acute and extreme psychomotor agitation is

A. Lithium.
B. Chlorpromazine (Thorazine).
C. Chlordiazepoxide hydrochloride (Librium).
D. Trihexyphenidyl hydrochloride (Artane).

Critical thinking

40. Using Table 22–5, teach a group (study group, co-workers) about the acute and long-term needs of people with schizophrenia. Identify the basic focus and interventions for the different phases.

Case study

41. Jamie, a 29-year-old woman, is being discharged in 2 days from the hospital after her first psychotic break (paranoid schizophrenia). Jamie is recently divorced and has been working as a legal secretary, although her work had become erratic, and her suspicious behavior was calling attention to herself at work. Jamie will be discharged in her mother's care until she is able to resume working. Jamie's mother is overwhelmed and asks the nurse how she is going to cope. "Jamie has become so

distant, and she always takes things the wrong way. I can hardly say anything to her without her misconstruing everything. She is very mad at me because I called 911 and had her admitted after she told me she was going to get justice back in the world by blowing up evil forces that have been haunting her life, and then proceeded to try to run over her ex-husband, thinking he was the devil. She told me there is nothing wrong with her and I am concerned she won't take her medications once she is discharged. What am I to do?"

Answer the following questions relating to the above case study. It is best if you can discuss and analyze responses to these situations with your classmates.

A. What are some of the priority concerns that the nurse could address in the hospital setting before Jamie's discharge?
B. How would you explain to Jamie's mother some of the symptoms that Jamie is experiencing? What suggestions could you give her to handle some of her immediate concerns?
C. What issues could you bring up to the staff about Jamie's medical compliance? What would be some ways to deal with this issue? Keep in mind that Jamie has exhibited only positive symptoms of schizophrenia.
D. What are some of the community resources that the case manager could contact to help support this family and increase the chances of continuity of care? Identify some useful community referrals that would be supportive for Jamie and her mother. Name at least three and describe how they could be supportive to this family.
E. What do you think of Jamie's prognosis? Support your hypothesis with data on influences on the course of schizophrenia.

23

Cognitive Disorders

ELIZABETH M. VARCAROLIS

OUTLINE

KEY TERMS AND CONCEPTS

The key terms and concepts listed here also appear in bold where they are defined or discussed in this chapter.

cognitive disorder
delirium
dementia
amnestic disorder
illusions
hallucinations (tactile, visual)
hypervigilance
primary dementia

secondary dementia
Alzheimer's disease
pseudodementia
confabulation
perseveration
aphasia
apraxia
agnosia
mnemonic disturbance
agraphia
hyperorality
hypermetamorphosis

OBJECTIVES

After studying this chapter, the reader will be able to

1. Compare and contrast the clinical picture of delirium with the clinical picture of dementia.
2. Discuss three critical needs of a person with delirium and state them in terms of a nursing diagnosis.
3. Formulate three outcome criteria for a client with delirium.
4. Summarize the essential somatic and psychotherapeutic interventions for a client with delirium.
5. Describe three essential features of each of the four stages of Alzheimer's disease.
6. Demonstrate an example of the following phenomena assessed during the progression of Alzheimer's disease: (a) apraxia, (b) agnosia, (c) aphasia, (d) confabulation, and (e) hyperorality.
7. Formulate at least three nursing diagnoses suitable for a client with Alzheimer's disease and formulate two goals for each.
8. Identify at least three nursing interventions for a client with Alzheimer's disease in each of the following areas: (a) communication, (b) health teaching and maintenance, (c) milieu management, and (d) psychobiological interventions.
9. Role play the following with a classmate: teaching a family with a member who has Alzheimer's disease: (a) types of community resources, (b) actions the family can take in the home to make it safer for the client, and (c) teaching the family about the disease.

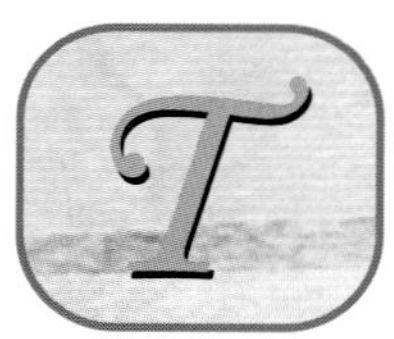

The *Diagnostic and statistical manual of mental disorders*, fourth edition (DSM-IV) (APA 1994) has replaced the former term *organic mental disorder* with **cognitive disorder.** The cognitive disorders include: delirium, dementia, and amnestic disorder and other cognitive disorders; mental disorders due to general medical conditions, and substance-related disorders.

Figure 23–1 identifies the three cognitive disorders and DSM-IV criteria for each. This chapter addresses the broad categories of delirium and dementia because these are by far the most common conditions that nurses encounter.

Delirium "is characterized by a disturbance of consciousness and a change in cognition such as impaired attention span and disturbances of consciousness, that develop over a short period" (APA 1994, p. 123). Delirium is always secondary to another condition, such as *general medical condition, substance induced* (drugs of abuse, a medication or toxin exposure), or delirium may have multiple causes. When the cause cannot be determined, delirium is coded as *delirium not otherwise specified* (NOS). By definition, delirium is a transient disorder, and if the underlying medical cause is corrected, complete recovery should occur (Goldberg 1995).

Delirium secondary to substance abuse is discussed in Chapter 25. This chapter will highlight delirium secondary to medical conditions as the example because delirium is one of the most commonly encountered mental disorders in medical practice. Delirium can affect up to half of all hospitalized and elderly medically ill people at some point (Goldberg 1995).

Dementia usually develops more slowly and is characterized by multiple cognitive deficits that include impairment in memory. In 80% to 95% of cases, dementias are irreversible (Goldberg 1995). The 5% to 20% of dementias that have a reversible component are *secondary* to other pathological processes (e.g., neoplasms, trauma, infections, and toxic disturbances). When the secondary, or underlying, causes are treated, the dementia often improves. However, most dementias, such as dementias of the Alzheimer type, involve a *primary* encephalopathy. Alzheimer's disease accounts for 70% of all dementias. Primary dementias have no known cause or cure; thus, they are progressive and irreversible.

Amnestic disorder is characterized by loss in both short-term memory (including the inability to learn in-

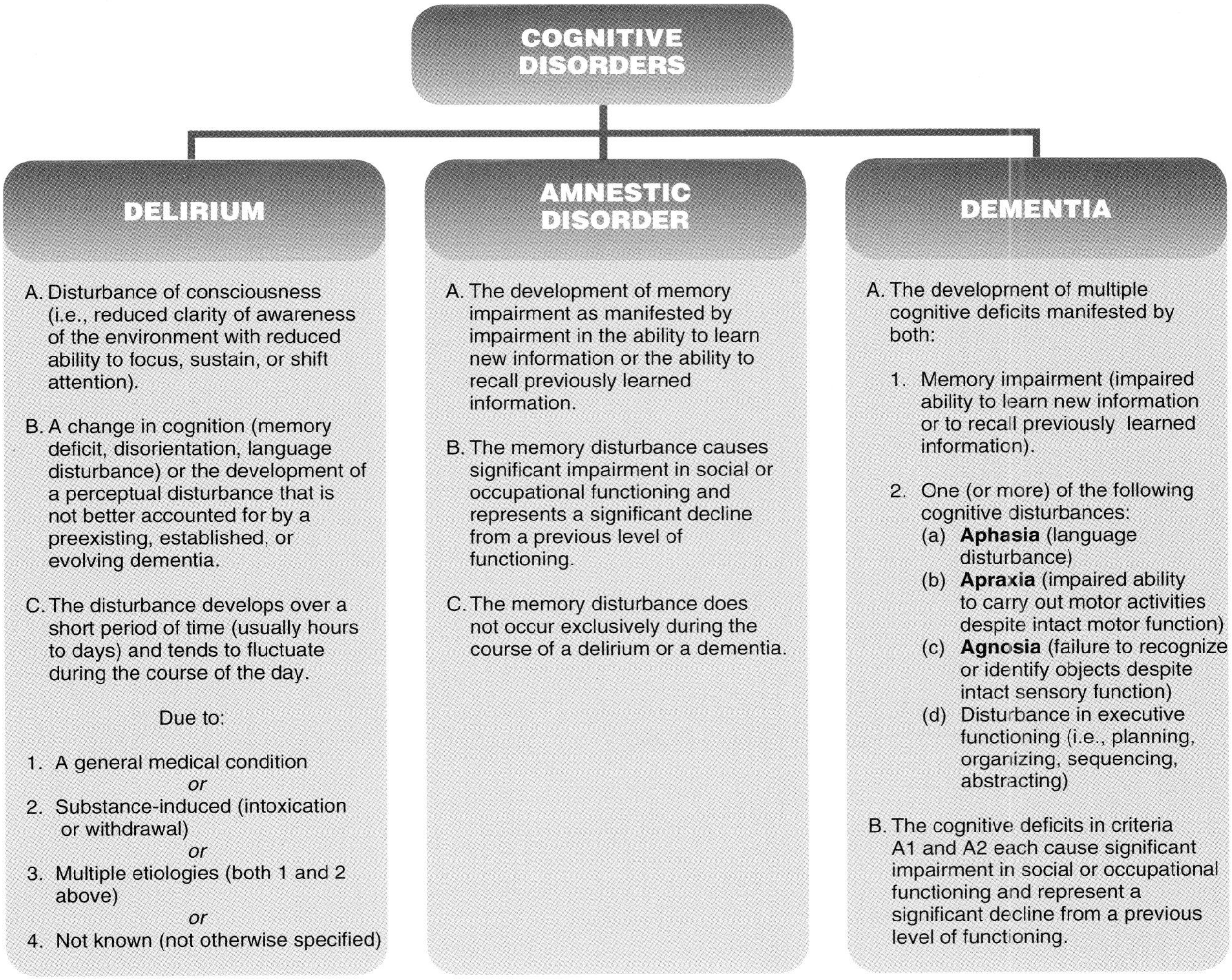

Figure 23–1 Diagnostic criteria for delirium, dementia, and amnestic disorder. (Adapted from American Psychiatric Association (1994). *Diagnostic and statistical manual of mental disorders (DSM-IV)*, 4th ed. Washington; DC: American Psychiatric Association. Reprinted with permission. Copyright 1994 American Psychiatric Association.)

formation) and long-term memory, sufficient to cause some impairment in the person's functioning (Goldberg 1995). This memory impairment exists in the absence of other significant cognitive impairments. These amnestic disorders are always *secondary* to underlying causes, such as *general medical condition, substance induced; persistent amnestic disorder;* and *amnestic disorder not otherwise specified.* Figure 23–2 shows the placement of the cognitive impairment disorders on the mental health continuum.

DELIRIUM

Nurses frequently encounter delirium on medical and surgical units in the general hospital setting. During certain phases of a hospital stay, confusion may be noted (e.g., after surgery or after the introduction of a new drug). The second or third hospital day may herald the onset of confusion for older people and difficulty adjusting to an unfamiliar environment.

Delirium occurs more frequently in elderly than in younger clients. Postoperative delirium, drugs, cerebrovascular disease, and congestive heart failure are some

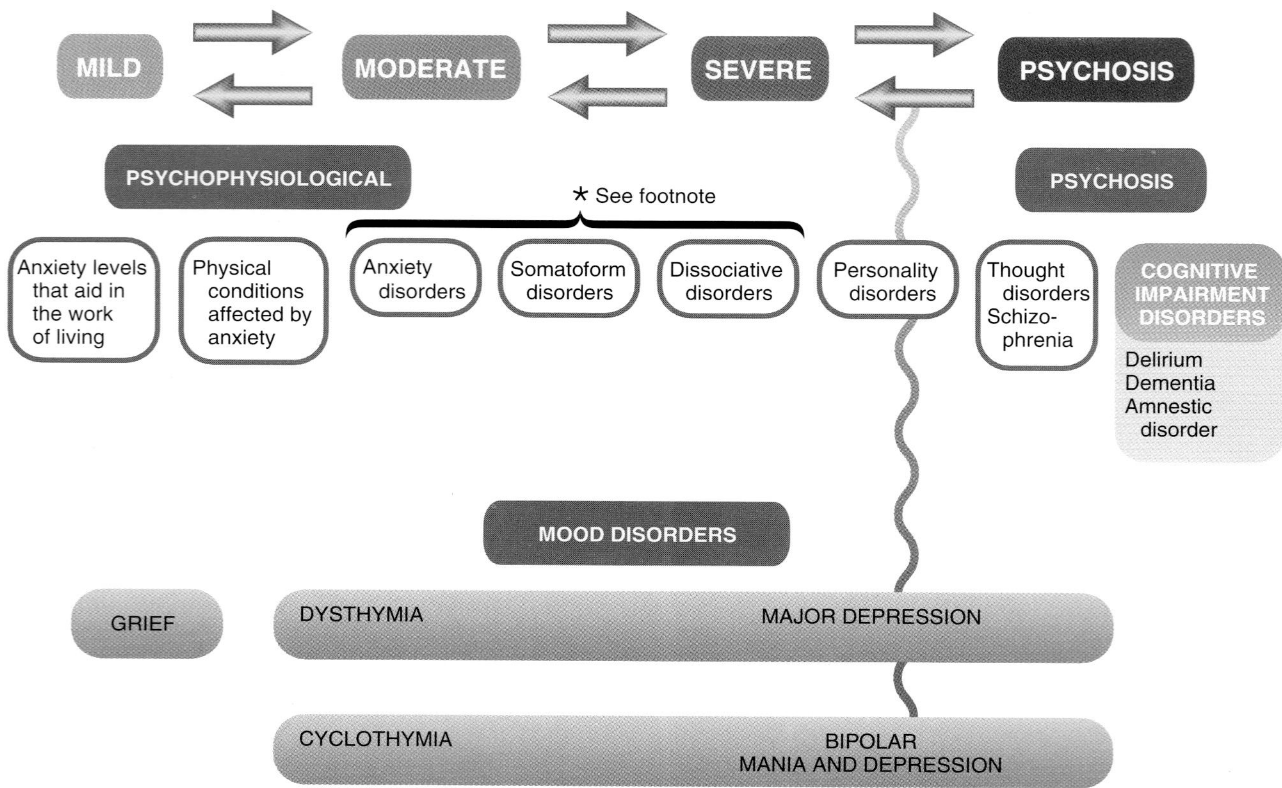

Figure 23–2 The mental health continuum for cognitive disorders.

of the most common causes. Delirium is also commonly seen in children with fever. Delirium is a common problem in terminally ill clients and, when recognized, is easily treated and may be reversible (de-Stoutz et al. 1995).

Symptoms of delirium can also be mistaken for depression. A delayed or missed diagnosis can have serious prognostic implications if delirium is not diagnosed in a timely manner (Nicholas and Lindsey 1995).

DSM-IV states that the essential feature of delirium is a *disturbance in consciousness* and that delirium is generally marked by cognitive difficulties. Thinking, memory, attention, and perception are typically disturbed. The clinical manifestations of delirium develop over a short period (hours to days) and tend to fluctuate during the course of the day.

Since delirious states fluctuate in intensity, nurses may note varying levels of consciousness and orientation during a short period. Delirium is characterized by progressive disorientation to time and place and can be classified as mild to severe. Mild delirium, which becomes more pronounced in the evening, is sometimes referred to as *sundowning*.

Because delirium increases psychological stress, supportive interventions that lower anxiety and reduce manifestations of the delirium can restore a sense of control (Foreman 1990). Clients with delirium may appear withdrawn, agitated, or psychotic. Also, underlying personality traits often become exaggerated; for example, a client may become more paranoid (Goldberg 1995), or a client may become disinhibited.

Delirium is always secondary to some physical disorder or drug toxicity. The priorities in medical care are to identify the cause and to make an appropriate medical or surgical intervention. If the underlying disorder is corrected and reversed, complete recovery is possible. If, however, the underlying disorder is not corrected and persists, sustained neuronal damage can lead to irreversible changes, such as dementia and even death.

Therefore, nursing concerns center on (1) assisting with proper health management to eradicate the underlying cause; (2) preventing physical harm due to confusion, aggression, or electrolyte and fluid imbalance; and (3) using supportive measures to relieve distress.

THEORY

Delirium can be caused by any number of pathophysiological conditions. Some of the most common causes of delirium include infections, postoperative states, metabolic abnormalities, hypoxic conditions, drug withdrawal states, and drug intoxications. Multiple drug use, or polypharmacy, is frequently implicated in delirium (Caine et al. 1995). Some drugs commonly responsible for delirium states are digitalis preparations and antihistamines, as well as medications used for treatment of hypertension, depression, and Parkinson's disease. Other likely offenders include anticholinergics, benzodiazepines, and analgesics, which induce central nervous system depression (Andresen 1992). Box 23–1 lists common causes of delirium.

BOX 23–1 COMMON CAUSES OF DELIRIUM

Postoperative states

Drug intoxications and withdrawals

- Alcohol, anxiolytics, opioids, and central nervous system stimulants (e.g., cocaine and crack cocaine)

Infections

- Systemic: pneumonia, typhoid fever, malaria, urinary tract infection, and septicemia
- Intracranial: meningitis and encephalitis

Metabolic disorders

- Hypoxia (pulmonary disease, heart disease, and anemia)
- Hypoglycemia
- Sodium potassium, calcium, magnesium, and acid-base imbalances
- Hepatic encephalopathy or uremic encephalopathy
- Thiamine (vitamin B_1) deficiency (Wernicke's encephalopathy)
- Endocrine disorders (e.g., thyroidism or parathyroidism)
- Hypothermia or hyperthermia
- Diabetic acidosis

Drugs

- Digitalis, steroids, lithium, levodopa, anticholinergics, benzodiazepines, central nervous system depressants, or tricyclic antidepressants
- Central anticholinergic syndrome due to use of multiple drugs with anticholinergic side effects

Neurological diseases

- Seizures
- Head trauma
- Hypertensive encephalopathy

Tumor

- Primarily cerebral

Psychosocial stressors

- Relocation or other sudden changes
- Sensory deprivation or overload
- Sleep deprivation
- Immobilization

ASSESSMENT

Problems in accurate assessment of delirium often arise. First, the degree of reversibility can be determined only retrospectively. Second, the relative acuity of the onset depends on how noxious the stimuli are. Third, delirium can occur simultaneously with, or be superimposed on, an irreversible mental syndrome (dementia), thereby further complicating accurate identification.

Generally, the nurse suspects the presence of delirium when a client *abruptly* develops a disturbance in consciousness that is manifested in reduced clarity of awareness of the environment. The person may have difficulty with orientation first to time, then to place, and last to person. For example, a man with delirium may think that the year is 1972 instead of the correct year, that the hospital is home, and that the nurse is his wife. Orientation to person is usually intact to the extent that the person is aware of the self's identity. The ability to focus, sustain, or shift attention is impaired. Questions need to be repeated because the individual's attention wanders, or the person might easily get off track and need to be refocused. Conversation is made more difficult because the person may be easily distracted by irrelevant stimuli (APA 1994).

Fluctuating levels of consciousness tend to be unpredictable. Disorientation and confusion are usually markedly worse at night and during the early morning. In fact, some clients may be confused or delirious only at night and may remain lucid during the day.

Some clinicians use standardized mental status examinations to screen or follow the progress of an individual with delirium or dementia. A commonly used test is the Mini-Mental State Examination (Table 23–1).

Nursing assessment should include assessment of (1) cognitive and perceptual disturbances, (2) physical needs, and (3) mood and behavior.

Cognitive and Perceptual Disturbances

It may be difficult to engage delirious persons in conversation because they are easily distracted and display marked attention deficits. *Memory* is often impaired. In mild delirium, memory deficits are noted on careful questioning. In more severe delirium, memory difficulties usually take the form of obvious difficulty in processing and remembering recent events. For example, the person might ask when a son is coming to visit, even though the son has left only an hour before.

Perceptual disturbances are also common. Perception is the processing of information about one's internal and

TABLE 23–1 THE MINI-MENTAL STATE EXAMINATION*

Maximum	Score	
		ORIENTATION
5	( )	What is the (year) (season) (date) (day) (month)?
5	( )	Where are we (state) (county) (town) (hospital) (floor)?
		REGISTRATION
3	( )	Name three objects, and ask patient to repeat them (e.g., glass, window, table). One point for each correct. Continue until patient learns them.
		ATTENTION AND CALCULATION
5	( )	Serial 7s. One point for each correct response. Stop after 5 answers (or as an alternative, spell "WORLD" backwards).
		RECALL
3	( )	Ask for the three objects from registration section. One point for each correct.
		LANGUAGE
2	( )	Point to a pencil and a watch. Ask the patient to name each. One point for each correct.
1	( )	Repeat: "No ifs, ands, or buts."
3	( )	Have patient follow a three-stage command. "(1) Take paper in your right hand, (2) fold it in half, and (3) put it on the floor." One point for each correct.
1	( )	Write the following in large letters: CLOSE YOUR EYES. Ask the patient to read and perform the task.
1	( )	Write a sentence. Score one point if sentence has a subject, object, and verb.
1	( )	Draw this design and have the patient copy it.
TOTAL SCORE 30	Pts. ____	

Assess level of consciousness

Alert Drowsy Stupor Coma

*Mini-mental State Examination. Points are assigned for correct answers. Scores of 20 points or less indicate dementia, delirium, schizophrenia, or affective disorders alone or in combination. Such scores are not found in normal elderly people or in those with neuroses or personality disorders.

Adapted from Folstein, M. F., Folstein, S. E., McHugh, P. R. (1975). Mini-mental state: A practical method for grading the cognitive state of patients for the clinician. *Journal of Psychiatric Research*, 12:189–198.

external environment. Various misinterpretations of reality may take the form of illusions or hallucinations.

Illusions are errors in perception of sensory stimuli. For example, a person may mistake folds in the bedclothes for white rats, or the cord of a window blind for a snake. The stimulus is a real object in the environment; however, it is misinterpreted and often becomes the object of the client's projected fear. Illusions, unlike delusions or hallucinations, can be explained and clarified for the individual.

Hallucinations are false sensory stimuli (see Chapter 22). Visual hallucinations are diagnostic of a more cognitive disorder. Tactile hallucinations may also be present. For example, delirious individuals may become terrified when they "see" giant spiders crawling over the bedclothes or "feel" bugs crawling on or under their bodies. Auditory hallucinations occur more often in other psychiatric disorders, such as schizophrenia and depression.

The delirious individual generally possesses an awareness that something is very wrong. For example, the delirious person may state "My thoughts are all jumbled." When perceptual disturbances are present, the emotional response is one of fear and anxiety. Verbal and psychomotor signs of agitation should be noted.

Physical Needs

Physical Safety

A person with delirium becomes disoriented and may try to "go home." Alternatively, a person may think that he or she *is* home and may jump out of a window trying to get away from "invaders." Wandering, pulling out intravenous lines and Foley catheters, and falling out of bed are common dangers that require nursing intervention.

An individual experiencing delirium has difficulty processing stimuli in the environment. Confusion magnifies the inability to recognize reality. The physical environment should be made as simple and as clear as possible. Elevating the head of the bed slightly can maximize orientation to place. Objects such as clocks and calendars can maximize orientation to time. Eyeglasses, hearing aids, and adequate lighting without glare can maximize the person's ability to interpret more accurately what is going on in the environment. Nagley (1986) recommended nurse-client interaction for periods of at least 5 to 10 minutes, when no other nursing actions are being carried out, to help decrease anxiety and increase awareness of reality.

Bacteriological Safety

Self-care deficits, injury, or hyperactivity or hypoactivity may lead to skin breakdown and may leave a person prone to infection. Often, this condition is compounded by poor nutrition, forced bed rest, and possible incontinence. These areas require nursing assessment and intervention.

Biophysical Safety

Autonomic signs, such as tachycardia, sweating, flushed face, dilated pupils, and elevated blood pressure, are often present. These changes must be monitored and documented carefully and may require immediate medical attention.

Changes in the sleep-wake cycle usually occur, and in some cases, a complete reversal of the night-day sleep-wake cycle can occur, as in the sundowner syndrome previously mentioned. The level of consciousness may range from lethargy to stupor or from semicoma to hypervigilance. The person with **hypervigilance** is extraordinarily alert and may have difficulty getting to sleep, or may be actively disoriented and agitated throughout the night.

It is also important that the nurse assess all medications because the nurse is in a position to recognize drug reactions or potential interactions before delirium actually occurs.

Moods and Physical Behaviors

The delirious individual's behavior and mood may change dramatically within a short period. Moods may swing back and forth from fear, anger, and anxiety to euphoria, depression, and apathy. These labile moods are often accompanied by physical behaviors associated with feeling states. A person may strike out from fear or anger or may cry, call for help, curse, moan, and tear off clothing one minute and become apathetic or laugh uncontrollably the next. In short, behavior and emotions are erratic and fluctuating. Lack of concentration and disorientation complicate interventions. The following vignette illustrates delirium.

◗ Mrs. Lew, 68 years of age, lives with her daughter, Jean, and son-in-law, Ted. Mrs. Lew takes care of the house, does the cooking and cleaning, and is active in church activities. She has a number of women friends and once a week goes to the movies or plays cards "with the girls." One day after work, her daughter Jean comes home to find her mother huddled in a darkened room, terrified. When asked what is wrong, Mrs. Lew states that the house is under siege and she has to hide in the dark: "Can't you hear them?" Outside, there is the sound of drilling and pounding by construction workers. Mrs. Lew is experiencing illusions. That night when Jean goes in to check on her mother, she discovers that her mother is gone. Jean finds her wandering in her nightclothes three blocks from the house.

◗ Jean becomes terribly alarmed, even though her husband insists that "it's normal for old people to become confused" and that they have just been fortunate up until now. Mrs. Lew is taken to the emergency department. On admission, she is oriented to person but not to time and place. She thinks it is 1941 and that she is back in London during the blitz. She keeps shouting "Get those men out of my house!" She "picks" at things in the air and is so restless, agitated, and incoherent that a mental examination is postponed.

◗ Physical examination of Mrs. Lew reveals bilateral rales in the lower lobes of the lungs, a high white blood cell count, a temperature of 101.3° F, and mild dehydration. A diagnosis of bilateral lower lobe pneumonia is made, and within 24 hours of treatment with intravenous fluids, antibiotics, and diligent nursing care, Mrs. Lew becomes oriented to time, place, and person, and the disturbance in her consciousness disappears.

◗ The nurse explains to the family that Mrs. Lew's temporary delirium had been secondary to the infectious process and that the symptoms of delirium often appear hours before the signs or symptoms of the underlying disorder.

NURSING DIAGNOSIS

Safety needs play a substantial role in nursing care. Clients often perceive the environment as distorted. Objects in the environment are often misperceived (illusions) or imagined (hallucinations), and people and objects may be misinterpreted as threatening or harmful. Clients often act on these misinterpretations. For example, if feeling threatened or thinking that common medical equipment is harmful, the client may pull off an oxygen mask, pull out an intravenous or nasogastric tube, or try to flee. In such a case, a person demonstrates a **risk for injury** related to confusion, as evidenced by sensory deficits or perceptual deficits.

Fever and dehydration may be present; thus, fluid and electrolyte balance may need to be managed. If the underlying cause of the client's delirium results in fever, decreased skin turgor, decreased urinary output or fluid intake, and dry skin or mucous membranes, then the nursing diagnosis of **fluid volume deficit** is appropriate. Fluid volume deficit may be related to fever, electrolyte imbalance, reduced intake, or infection.

Perceptions are disturbed during delirium. Hallucinations, distractibility, illusions, disorientation, agitation, restlessness, and misperception are often part of the clinical picture. When some of these symptoms are present, **acute confusion** would be an appropriate nursing diagnosis.

Because disruption in the sleep-wake cycle may be present, the client may be less responsive during the day and may become disruptively wakeful during the night. At no time, either during the day or the night, does the client experience a restful sleep; instead, he or she has a fragmented and fluctuating state of consciousness (McHugh and Folstein 1987). Therefore, **sleep-pattern disturbance** related to impaired cerebral oxygenation or disruption in consciousness is a likely diagnosis.

Because delirious people are usually dazed or drowsy, they can rarely sustain attention to any mental task. The client may be roused for a moment and coaxed to respond before slipping back to unresponsiveness. Memory is often impaired. Because sustaining communication with a delirious client is difficult, **impaired verbal communication** related to cerebral hypoxia or decreased cerebral blood flow, as evidenced by confusion or clouding of consciousness, may be diagnosed.

Other nursing concerns include **fear, self-care deficits,** and **impaired social interaction.** Fear is one of the most common of all nursing diagnoses, and may be related to illusions, delusions, or hallucinations, as evidenced by verbal and nonverbal expressions of fearfulness.

PLANNING

Planning Outcome Criteria

The client may present various needs; however, **risk for injury** is usually present. Appropriate outcome criteria might include the following:

- Client will remain safe and free from injury while in the hospital.
- During lucid periods, client will be oriented to time, place, and person with the aid of nursing interventions, such as clocks, calendars, and other orienting information.
- Client's tubes will remain in place (e.g., intravenous, nasogastric, catheter, or oxygen) while confused, with the aid of frequent orientation by nurse and medications, if necessary.
- Client will remain free from falls and injury while confused, with the aid of nursing safety measures.
- Client will respond to external controls if he or she becomes physically aggressive toward self, other clients, or staff.

Because **acute confusion** and **sensory-perceptual alterations** are usually evident, goals that enhance the client's ability to interpret reality are useful. For example:

- Client will be able to tell the nurse where he or she is by (date).
- Client will state that he or she understands that the nurse will provide support when the client is "hearing" or "seeing" frightening things.
- Client will correctly name environmental objects or sounds after experiencing an illusion, with aid of nursing interventions.
- Client will state hallucinations have decreased from (state number) to (state number) a day.

Maintaining fluid and electrolyte balance is crucial if the underlying disorder increases the person's metabolic rate and results in increased temperature and decreased circulating fluid volume. Outcome criteria for **fluid volume deficit** could include the following:

- Client will be well hydrated within 24 hours, as evidenced by normal skin turgor or appearance of mucous membranes, and specific gravity (urine) will be within normal limits.
- Client will take 8 ounces of protein fluid orally once every hour.
- Client's vital signs will become or will remain stable by (time).

Sleep-pattern disturbance can cause a problem not only for the delirious client but also for the other clients because it may lead to sleep deprivation and fatigue for all concerned. Creative nursing measures are often necessary. Possible outcome criteria and short-term goals follow:

- Client will sleep 4 to 6 hours per night within 3 days.
- Client will state that he or she is comfortable at night with aid of nursing measures (e.g., light, frequent orientation, or nurse's presence) within (time).
- Client will state accurately where he or she is and what is happening when he or she is awake at night.
- Client's self-reported anxiety level will decrease from (state level) to (state level) on a scale of 1 to 10 with aid of medication and nursing interventions.

Goals for improving the client's psychosocial status and reducing **fear** and **impaired social interaction** include the following:

- Client will recognize the presence of significant others.
- Verbal ("I am so afraid," "What's happening to me?") and nonverbal (e.g., staring, grimacing, or agitation) expressions of fear will measurably decrease.

Nurse's Feelings and Self-Assessment

In many cases, delirium is more easily associated with a medical disease. First, delirium is usually treated on a medical or surgical unit, and second, delirium usually responds to specific medical or surgical interventions, depending on the underlying cause. Frequently, this syndrome reverses within a few days or less when the underlying cause is identified and treated. Because the behaviors exhibited by the client can be directly attributed to temporary medical conditions, intense personal reactions are less likely to occur. In fact, intense conflicting emotions are less likely to occur in nurses working with a client with delirium than in nurses working with a client with dementia, which is discussed later in this chapter.

However, the nurse may find some behaviors associated with delirium especially challenging. Because delirium is predictably more severe and incapacitating during the night and early morning hours, night staff often find that a loud, frightened, agitated, and perhaps aggressive client can take up much of their time. Experienced nurses are aware that even though people with delirium may appear "out of it," they often respond to a calm and caring approach. Maximizing the person's contact with reality during the night can help reduce the anxiety and terror these clients often experience.

However, certain instances may cause staff to have strong negative feelings toward a client with delirium. Such incidents might include withdrawal. For example, nurses working with a client with alcohol withdrawal delirium might think that the client "did it to herself" or is "getting what he deserves." Often, nurses exhibit judgmental attitudes toward people experiencing withdrawal. Unfortunately, negative attitudes by staff serve only to increase the client's anxiety, intensifying feelings of terror, anger, and confusion and defensive behavior.

INTERVENTION

Medical management of delirium involves treating the underlying organic causes. If the underlying cause of delirium is not treated, permanent brain damage may ensue. Judicious use of antipsychotic or antianxiety agents may also be useful in controlling agitation and psychotic symptomatology.

Nursing care involves encouraging one or two significant others to stay with the delirious client to avoid the use of physical restraints (Sullivan et al. 1991). The nurse should promote adequate and accurate sensory input through the use of eyeglasses or hearing aids, if appropriate. Communication should occur face to face and should consist of simple, direct statements. Orientation may be aided by maintenance of familiar objects in the environment and by use of orienting devices, such as calendars and clocks. Although the use of reality orientation is extremely questionable in clients with chronic confusion, it may prove helpful during lucid periods in clients with acute confusional states, such as delirium.

The nurse should allow clients to care for themselves in areas of competency and should do only what is necessary for the client, while providing continual explanations when physical care is given. Safety may be aided by the use of night lighting and soothing music and by the involvement of significant others in supervising the client. As with any client exhibiting psychotic symptoms, a tolerant, calm, matter-of-fact approach by the nurse has proved to be the most helpful. Table 23–2 presents nursing guidelines for caring for a delirious client.

The following vignette highlights the fear and confusion a client may experience when admitted to an intensive care unit (ICU). What are some more useful interventions the nurse could have used in the case of Mr. Arnold (Table 23–2)?

A CLIENT WITH DELIRIUM

A 55-year-old married man, Mr. Arnold, is admitted to the ICU after having a three-vessel coronary artery bypass. Mr. Arnold's surgery has taken longer than usual and has necessitated his remaining on a cardiac pump for 3 hours. He arrives in the ICU without further complications. On awakening from the anesthesia, he hears the nurse exclaim "I need to get a gas." Another nurse answers in a loud voice "Can you take a large needle for the injection?" During this period, Mr. Arnold experiences the need to urinate and asks the nurse very calmly if he can go to the bathroom. Her reply is, "You don't need to go; you have a tube in." He again complains about his discomfort and assures the nurse that if she will let him go to the bathroom, he will be fine. The nurse informs Mr. Arnold that he cannot urinate and that he has to keep the "mask" on so that she can get the "gas" and check his "blood levels." On hearing this, Mr. Arnold begins to implore more loudly and states that he sees the bathroom sign. He assures the nurse that he will only take a minute. In reality, the sign is an exit sign.

To prove to him that a bathroom does not exist in the ICU and that the sign does not indicate a bathroom, the nurse takes off the restraints so that his head can be raised to see the sign. He abruptly breaks away from the nurse's grasp and runs toward the entrance to the ICU. He discovers a door, which is the entrance to the nurses' lounge, barricades himself in the room, and pulls out his chest tube, Foley catheter, and intravenous lines. Needless to say, he finds the bathroom that is connected to the lounge. Ten minutes later, the nurses and security personnel break through the barricade and escort Mr. Arnold back to bed.

When he becomes fully alert and oriented a day later, Mr. Arnold tells the nurses his perception of the previous events. Initially, he had thought he had been kidnapped and was being held against his will (the restraints had been tight). When the nurse yelled out about blood gas, he had thought she was going to kill him with noxious

TABLE 23–2 GUIDELINES FOR CARING FOR A DELIRIOUS CLIENT

INTERVENTION	RATIONALE
Nursing Diagnosis: Acute confusion related to transitory neurological dysfunction, as evidenced by fluctuating level of consciousness, perceptual disturbances (illusion or hallucination), and reduced awareness of environment	
1. Introduce self and call client by name at the beginning of each contact.	1. With short-term memory impairment, person is often confused and needs frequent orienting to time, place, and person.
2. Maintain face-to-face contact.	2. If client is easily distracted, he or she needs help to focus on one stimulus at a time.
3. Use short, simple, concrete phrases.	3. Client may not be able to process complex information.
4. Briefly explain everything you are going to do before doing it.	4. Explanation prevents misinterpretation of action.
5. Encourage family and friends (one at a time) to take a quiet, supportive role.	5. Familiar presence lowers anxiety and increases orientation.
6. Keep room well lit.	6. Lighting provides accurate environmental stimuli to maintain and increase orientation.
7. Keep head of bed elevated.	7. Helps provide important environmental cues.
8. Provide clocks and calendars.	8. These cues help orient client to time.
9. Encourage family members to bring in meaningful articles from home (e.g., pictures or figurines).	9. Familiar objects provide comfort and support and can aid orientation.
10. Encourage client to wear prescribed eyeglasses or hearing aid.	10. Helps increase accurate perceptions of visual auditory stimuli.
11. Make an effort to assign the same personnel on each shift to care for client.	11. Familiar faces minimize confusion and enhance nurse-client relationships.
12. When hallucinations are present, clarify reality, e.g., "I know you are frightened; I do not see spiders on your sheets. I'll sit with you a while."	12. Person feels understood and reassured while reality is validated.
13. When illusions are present, clarify reality, e.g., "This is a coat rack, not a man with a knife . . . see? You seem frightened. I'll stay with you for a while."	13. Misinterpreted objects or sounds can be clarified, once pointed out.
14. Inform client of progress during lucid intervals.	14. Consciousness fluctuates: client feels less anxious knowing where he or she is and who you are during lucid periods.
15. Ignore insults and name calling, and acknowledge how upset the person may be feeling. For example: **Client:** You incompetent jerk, get me a real nurse, someone who knows what they are doing. **Nurse:** You are very upset. What you are going through is very difficult. I'll stay with you.	15. Terror and fear are often projected onto environment. Arguing or becoming defensive only increases client's aggressive behaviors and defenses.
16. If client behavior becomes physically abusive, first, set limits on behavior, e.g., "Mr. Jones, you are not to hit me or anyone else. Tell me how you feel." or "Mr. Jones, if you have difficulty controlling your actions, we will help you gain control." Second, check orders for use of chemical or physical restraints (e.g., Posey belt).	16. Clear limits need to be set to protect client, staff, and others. Often, client can respond to verbal commands. Chemical and physical restraints are used as a last resort, if at all.

gas through his face mask (the reason he did not want to wear the face mask). All he could think about was escaping his tormentor and executioner. In this case, the nurse had not assessed the alteration in Mr. Arnold's mental status and allowed him to get out of bed. The medical jargon and loud voices had perpetuated his confusion and distortion of reality.

What could the nurses have done differently? What would you have done? What initial nursing actions would you have taken in order to assess his bladder?

For example, the nurses could have told Mr. Arnold where he was and that the nursing staff were caring for him; they could have better explained the function of his Foley catheter. Furthermore, the staff could have

TABLE 23–2 GUIDELINES FOR CARING FOR A DELIRIOUS CLIENT *(Continued)*

INTERVENTION	RATIONALE
Nursing Diagnosis: Risk for Injury related to neurological changes, as evidenced by unstable vital signs, potential for dehydration, skin breakdown, and sleep deprivation	
1. Check pulse periodically, e.g., every hour or every 4 hours, depending on underlying conditions.	1. Pulse is a good indicator of course of delirium.
2. Check temperature regularly.	2. Hyperthermia may occur.
3. Schedule medications and treatments so that they do not interfere with client's sleep or rest.	3. Fluctuating levels of consciousness prevent adequate rest.
4. Check for skin breakdown and apply appropriate interventions, e.g., turn every 2 hours, apply lotion to bony prominences, and ensure proper positioning.	4. Breakdown combined with dehydration can develop rapidly when client is on bed rest.
5. Monitor fluid intake and output and electrolyte levels.	5. Fluid and electrolyte imbalance cause or exacerbate delirium.
6. Check skin turgor and urine specific gravity. If client appears dehydrated, forcing fluids may be appropriate.	6. Forcing fluids replaces fluid volume.
7. If skin turgor and urine specific gravity are within limits, or if the client is overhydrated, fluids should *not* be forced.	7. Monitoring prevents fluid volume overload.

brought in family members to help calm and orient Mr. Arnold.

EVALUATION

Long-term outcome criteria for a delirious person include the following:

- The client will remain safe while in the hospital.
- The client will be oriented to time, place, and person by discharge.

However, the short-term outcomes or goals need constant assessment.

For example, are the client's vital signs within normal limits? Are all intravenous and nasogastric tubes, Foley catheters, and hyperalimentation lines intact? Are the client's skin turgor and urine specific gravity within normal limits? Is the client oriented to time and place? Has the client's anxiety level decreased from panic levels to severe or moderate levels? Frequent checking of the parameters of the short-term goals helps monitor successful treatment of the client's underlying medical condition, as well as the client's responses to nursing interventions, and helps prevent possible progression to more profound levels of illness or to irreversible neuronal changes.

DEMENTIA

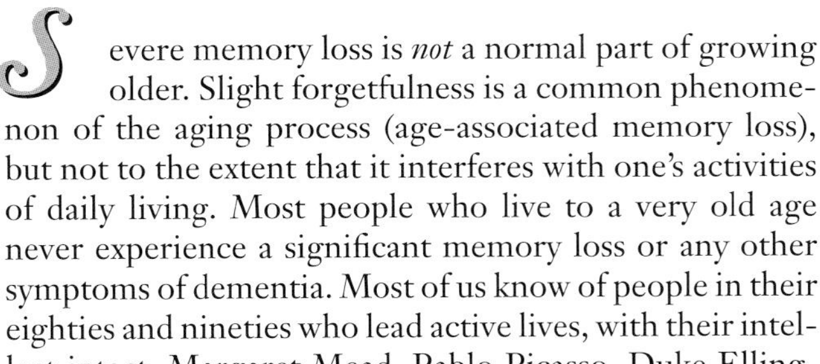

Severe memory loss is *not* a normal part of growing older. Slight forgetfulness is a common phenomenon of the aging process (age-associated memory loss), but not to the extent that it interferes with one's activities of daily living. Most people who live to a very old age never experience a significant memory loss or any other symptoms of dementia. Most of us know of people in their eighties and nineties who lead active lives, with their intellect intact. Margaret Mead, Pablo Picasso, Duke Ellington, Count Basie, Ansel Adams, Sonny Coles, and George Burns are all examples of people who were still active in their careers when they died; all were older than 75 years of age (Picasso was 91; George Burns was 100). The slow, mild cognitive changes associated with aging should not impede social or occupational functioning.

Dementia, on the other hand, is marked by progressive deterioration in intellectual functioning, memory, and ability to solve problems and learn new skills. Judgment and moral and ethical behaviors decline as personality is altered.

In dementia, progressive decline in activities of everyday life, the failure of memory and intellect, and the disorganization of the personality occur. A person's declining intellect often leads to emotional changes, lack of self-care, and finally, to hallucinations and delusions (i.e., psychotic symptoms brought on by neurological changes).

A person may have progressive dementia from various causes; dementia of the Alzheimer type (DAT), Pick's disease, Huntington's chorea, multi-infarct dementias, advanced alcoholism (such as in Korsakoff's syndrome), and Creutzfeldt-Jakob disease are a few examples.

Dementias can be classified as primary or secondary. **Primary dementia** is not reversible, is progressive, and is not secondary to any other disorder. For example, Alzheimer's disease accounts for about 70% of all dementias, and multi-infarct dementia accounts for about 20% of all dementias (Goldberg 1995). Both Alzheimer's and multi-infarct dementias are *primary*, progressive, and irreversible.

Secondary dementia occurs as a result of some other pathological process (e.g., metabolic, nutritional, or neurological). Acquired immunodeficiency syndrome (AIDS)–related dementia is an example of a secondary dementia that is increasingly seen in health care settings. The exact prevalence of AIDS-related dementia is not known, but it occurs in 20% to 40% of individuals with human immunodeficiency virus (HIV) infection and in up to 90% of clients dying of AIDS (Buzan and Dubovsky 1995). This phenomenon is now commonly referred to as HIV encephalopathy. Table 23–3 compares and contrasts Alzheimer dementia with AIDS-related dementia. Other secondary dementias can result from viral encephalitis, pernicious anemia, folic acid deficiency, and hypothyroidism.

Korsakoff's syndrome is an example of secondary dementia caused by thiamine (B_1) deficiency that may be associated with prolonged, heavy alcohol ingestion. Along with progressive mental deterioration, Korsakoff's syndrome is marked by peripheral neuropathy, cerebellar ataxia, confabulation, and myopathy (APA 1994).

Some secondary dementias are treatable. In about 5% to 20% of dementia cases, the symptoms of dementia can be reversed when the underlying cause is eliminated (Goldberg 1995). Box 23–2 lists the common causes of dementia. At times, it is necessary to distinguish delirium from dementia (Table 23–4).

TABLE 23–3 SELECTED CLINICAL SIGNS: HIV ENCEPHALOPATHY VERSUS DEMENTIA OF THE ALZHEIMER'S TYPE (DAT)

CLINICAL SIGN	HIV ENCEPHALOPATHY	DAT
Central nervous system changes	Subcortical	Cortical
Disease progression	More rapid	Slower
	Cognitive	
Aphasia (language)	Usually absent; may appear in later stages	Usually present
Agnosia (perception)	Usually absent; may appear in later stages	Usually present
Apraxia (intentional movements)	Usually absent; may appear in later stages	Usually present
Memory loss	Early state—"absentmindedness"	Recent events
	Later—severe loss	Recent and remote events
	Behavioral	
Depression	More frequent	Less frequent
Affect	Early stage—blunted	Present
Insight	Early stage—poor	Denial of losses
Socialness	Early stage—withdrawn	Present
Interest in social activities	Early stage—loss of interest	Present
	Motor/neurological	
Ataxia	Early signs; often present	Not usually present
Leg weakness	Early signs; often present	Not usually present
Progressive loss of balance, clumsiness	Early signs; often present	Not usually present
Nonspecific tremors or signs of peripheral	Early signs; often present	Not usually present
neuropathy	Early signs; often present	Not usually present

Adapted from Sabin, T. (1987). AIDS: The new "great imitator." *Geriatrics*, 35(5):467. Reproduced with permission. Copyright by Advanstar Communications, Inc.; Scharnhorst, S. (1992). AIDS dementia complex in the elderly. *Nurse Practitioner*, 17(8):41.
HIV, human immunodeficiency virus.

BOX 23–2 COMMON CAUSES OF DEMENTIA

PRIMARY DEMENTIAS

Alzheimer's disease (senile and presenile dementia)
Multi-infarct dementia
Pick's disease

SECONDARY DEMENTIAS

Infections

- Tuberculosis
- Tertiary neurosyphilis
- Fungal, bacterial, and viral infections of the brain (Creutzfeldt-Jacob disease)

Trauma; subdural hematoma, hypoxia
Toxic and metabolic disturbances

- Korsakoff's syndrome; Wernicke's encephalopathy (thiamine deficiency)
- Pernicious anemia (vitamin B_{12} deficiency)
- Folic acid deficiency
- Thyroid, parathyroid, or adrenal gland dysfunction
- Liver or kidney dysfunction
- Metal poisoning
- Carbon dioxide and some drugs

Neoplasms
Other neurological diseases

- Huntington's chorea
- Parkinson's disease
- Multiple sclerosis
- Cerebellar degenerations

Normal pressure hydrocephalus
AIDS-related dementia (HIV encephalopathy)

AIDS, acquired immunodeficiency syndrome; HIV, human immunodeficiency virus.

Because DAT (dementia of the Alzheimer type) accounts for 70% of all dementias and is the fourth most prevalent cause of death after heart disease, cancer, and stroke in the adult population (Powell and Courtice 1983), Alzheimer's disease is discussed here in detail as an example of dementia.

ALZHEIMER'S DISEASE

Alzheimer's disease attacks indiscriminately. Its victims are male and female, black and white, rich and poor, all with varying degrees of intelligence. Although the disease can strike at a younger age (early onset), most victims are 65 years of age or older (late onset). Alzheimer's is "a thief of minds, a destroyer of personalities, wrecker of family finances and filler of nursing homes" (American Association of Retired Persons 1986).

Yasmin Aga Khan (the daughter of the famous actress Rita Hayworth, who had Alzheimer's disease) once stated that to watch a once proud, beautiful, independent, dignified human being transformed into a dependent, mentally disabled person is terrifying. An estimated 4 million Americans have the disease; it occurs in up to 15% of the population over 65 years of age and 48% or more of the population over 85 years (Masterman et al. 1995).

A wide range of problems may masquerade as dementia and may be mistaken for Alzheimer's disease. For example, depression in the elderly is often misdiagnosed as dementia. It is important that nurses and other health care professionals be able to assess some of the important differences between depression and dementia. Table 23–5 outlines important differences between the two diseases.

Other disorders that often mimic dementia include drug toxicity, metabolic disorders, infections, and nutritional deficiencies. A disorder that mimics dementia is sometimes referred to as a **pseudodementia.** That is, although the symptoms may suggest dementia, a careful examination may reveal another diagnosis altogether. Newbern (1991) emphasized the critical nature of careful evaluation of tractable conditions and that histories of alcohol abuse and affective disorders must be considered. When a cognitive syndrome is suspected, clinical evaluation includes the following (Perry and Markowitz 1988):

1. Confirm the diagnosis
2. Search for underlying causes
3. Identify psychosocial stressors that may exacerbate related emotional and behavioral problems

The diagnosis of Alzheimer's disease includes ruling out all other pathophysiological conditions through the history and physical and laboratory tests, such as:

- Chest and skull x-ray studies.
- Electroencephalography.
- Electrocardiography.
- Urinalysis.
- Sequential multiple analyzer: 12-test serum profile.
- Thyroid function tests.
- Folate levels.
- Venereal Disease Research Laboratories (VDRL), HIV tests.
- Serum creatinine assay.
- Electrolyte assessment.
- Vitamin B_{12} levels.
- Vision and hearing evaluation.
- Neuroimaging (when diagnostic issues are not clear).

Computed tomography, positron-emission tomography, and other developing scanning technologies possess diagnostic capabilities because they reveal brain atrophy and rule out other conditions, such as neoplasms. Mental status questionnaires, such as that in Table 23–1, and various other tests to determine mental status deterioration and brain damage are important parts of the assessment.

In addition to a complete physical and neurological examination, the importance of a complete medical history and description of recent symptoms (including question-

TABLE 23–4 NURSING ASSESSMENT: DELIRIUM VERSUS DEMENTIA

DELIRIUM	DEMENTIA
Onset	
Acute impairment of orientation, memory, intellectual function, judgment, and affect.	Slow insidious deterioration in cognitive functioning.
Essential feature	
Disturbance in consciousness, fluctuating levels of consciousness, and cognitive impairment.	Progressive deterioration in memory, orientation, calculation, and judgment; symptoms do not fluctuate.
Cause	
The syndrome is secondary to many underlying disorders that cause temporary, diffuse disturbances of brain function.	The syndrome is either *primary* or *secondary* to other disease states or conditions.
Course	
The clinical course is usually brief (hour to days); prolonged delirium may lead to dementia.	Progresses over months or years; often reversible.
Speech	
May be slurred; reflects disorganized thinking.	Generally normal in early stages; progressive aphasia; confabulation.
Memory	
Short-term memory impaired.	Short-term, then long-term, memory destroyed.
Perception	
Visual or tactile hallucinations; illusions.	Hallucinations not prominent.
Mood	
Fear, anxiety, and irritability most prominent.	Mood labile; previous personality traits become accentuated, e.g., paranoid, depressed, withdrawn, and obsessive-compulsive.
EEG	
Pronounced diffuse slowing or fast cycles.	Normal or mildly slow.

EEG, electroencephalogram

TABLE 23–5 DEMENTIA VERSUS DEPRESSION

DEMENTIA	DEPRESSION
1. Recent memory is impaired. In early stages, client attempts to hide cognitive losses; is skillful at covering up.	1. Patient readily admits to memory loss; other cognitive disturbances may or may not be present.
2. Symptoms progress slowly and insidiously; difficult to pinpoint onset.	2. Symptoms are of relatively rapid onset.
3. Approximate or "near-miss" answers are typical; tries to answer.	3. "Don't know" answers are common; client does not try to recall or answer.
4. Client struggles to perform well but is frustrated.	4. Little effort to perform; is apathetic; seems helpless and pessimistic.
5. Affect is shallow or labile.	5. Depressive mood is pervasive.
6. Attention and concentration may be impaired.	6. Attention and concentration are usually intact.
7. Changes in personality, e.g., from cheerful and easygoing to angry and suspicious.	7. Personality remains stable.

ing significant others) cannot be overestimated (Souder 1992). Gray-Vickrey (1988) recommended a psychiatric history, a dietary evaluation, and a medication evaluation.

Studies have revealed that certain clinical diagnostic criteria can substantially improve the diagnostic accuracy in Alzheimer's disease. Four studies using the National Institute of Neurological and Communicative Disorders and Stroke and the Alzheimer's Disease and Related Disorders Association (NINCDS-ADRDA) guidelines found a 91% specificity for diagnosing Alzheimer's disease (Dewan and Gupta 1992).

As already mentioned, depression in the elderly is the disorder most often confused with dementia. Medical and nursing personnel should be cautioned, however, that dementia and depression *can* coexist in the same person. In fact, studies indicate that many people diagnosed with Alzheimer's dementia also meet DSM-IV criteria for a depressive disorder.

THEORY

Although the cause of Alzheimer's disease is not known, numerous hypotheses regarding its cause exist.

Genetic Model

Family members of people with DAT have a risk of acquiring the disease that is higher than that of the general population. Numerous twin studies have shown that, on average, a 40% concordance rate exists in monozygotic twins (Masterman et al. 1995). Studies have provided evidence that in some families with *early-onset* disease, there appears to be a defect on chromosome 21 and chromosome 14. Other studies have indicated that *late-onset* familial Alzheimer's disease may be linked to alterations on chromosome 19. This intriguing genetic link to Alzheimer's disease (DAT) is the apolipoprotein E4 allele in cases of late-onset familial DAT (Masterman et al. 1995).

Therefore, three chromosomes—14, 21, and 19—are all individually suspected of rendering individuals susceptible to DAT. These multiple potential genetic causes support the theory that DAT may not be a single disorder.

Toxic and Other External Agent Hypotheses

Aluminum exposure, low-calcium intake, organic solvents, malnutrition, smoking, thyroid disease, and head trauma have all been implicated as possible risk factors for Alzheimer's disease (Yi et al. 1994). Other causes under investigation include slow viral infection, autoimmune process, environmental factors, and decreased blood flow to the brain (Kaufman 1995).

Neurochemical Changes

Some studies have indicated that people with Alzheimer's dementia have drastically reduced levels of the enzyme acetyltransferase, which is needed to synthesize the neurotransmitter acetylcholine. Some theorists propose that the cognitive defects that occur in Alzheimer's disease, especially memory loss, are a direct result of the reduction in acetylcholine available to the brain.

Pathological Changes

ALZHEIMER'S TANGLES. Alzheimer's disease results in cerebral atrophy and in neuritic plaques and neurofibrillary tangles that are microscopic abnormalities in brain tissue. Beta-amyloid protein is the main component of neuritic plaques, one of the abnormal structures found in the brain of Alzheimer's clients. Beta-amyloid protein is now the subject of intense interest in Alzheimer's research (Alzheimer's Research 1994). A more detailed description follows:

1. *Neurofibrillary tangles* form mostly in the hippocampus, the part of the brain responsible for recent (short-term) memory as well as emotions. Therefore, memory and emotions are negatively affected.
2. *Senile plaques* are cores of degenerated neuron material that lie free of the cell bodies on the ground substances of the brain. The quantity of plaques has been correlated with the degree of mental deterioration.
3. *Granulovascular degeneration* is the filling of brain cells with fluid and granular material. Increased degeneration accounts for increased loss of mental function.

Brain atrophy is observable with wider cortical sulci and enlarged cerebral ventricles, as demonstrated by computed tomography or magnetic resonance imaging (APA 1994).

ASSESSMENT

Alzheimer's disease is commonly characterized by progressive deterioration of cognitive functioning. Initially, deterioration may be so subtle and insidious that others may not notice. In the early stages of the disease, the affected person may be able to compensate for loss of memory. Some people may have superior social graces and charm that give them the ability to hide severe deficits in memory, even from experienced health care professionals. This "hiding" is actually a form of *denial*, which is an unconscious protective defense against the terrifying reality of losing one's place in the world. Family members may also unconsciously deny that anything is wrong as a defense against the painful awareness of deterioration of a loved one. As time goes on, symptoms become more obvious, and other defensive maneuvers become evident. **Confabulation** (making up stories or answers to maintain self-esteem when the person does not remember) is noticed. For example, the nurse addresses a client who has remained in a hospital bed all weekend:

Nurse: Good morning, Ms. Jones. How was your weekend?

Client: Wonderful. I discussed politics with the President, and he took me out to dinner.
or I spent the weekend with my daughter and her family.

Confabulation is not the same as lying. When people are lying, they are aware of making up an answer; confabulation is an *unconscious* attempt to maintain self-esteem.

Perseveration (the repetition of phrases or behavior) is eventually seen and is often intensified under stress. The avoidance of answering questions is another mechanism by which the client is able to maintain self-esteem unconsciously in the face of severe memory deficits.

Therefore, (1) denial, (2) confabulation, (3) perseveration, and (4) avoidance of questions are four defensive behaviors the nurse might notice during assessment.

The following four signs of Alzheimer's disease have been described (Wolanin and Fraelich-Philips 1981):

1. **Aphasia** (loss of language ability), which progresses with the disease. Initially, the person has difficulty finding the correct word, then is reduced to a few words, and then is finally reduced to babbling or mutism.
2. **Apraxia** (loss of purposeful movement in the absence of motor or sensory impairment). The person is unable to perform once-familiar and purposeful tasks. For example, in apraxia of gait, the person loses the ability to walk. In apraxia of dressing, the person is unable to put clothes on properly (may put arms in trousers or put a jacket on upside down).
3. **Agnosia** (loss of sensory ability to recognize objects). For example, the person may lose the ability to recognize familiar sounds (auditory agnosia), such as the ring of the telephone, a car horn, or the doorbell. Loss of this ability extends to the inability to recognize familiar objects (visual or tactile agnosia), such as a glass, magazine, pencil, or toothbrush. Eventually, people are unable to recognize loved ones or even parts of their own bodies.
4. **Mnemonic disturbance** (loss of memory). Initially, the person has difficulty remembering recent events. Gradually, deterioration progresses to include both recent and remote memory.

The degeneration of neurons in the brain is the wasting away of working components in the brain. These cells contain memories, receive sights and sounds, and cause hormones to secrete, produce emotions, and command muscles into motion.

A person with Alzheimer's disease loses a personal history, a place in the world, and the ability to recognize the environment and, eventually, loved ones. Alzheimer's disease robs family and friends, husbands and wives, and sons and daughters of valuable human relatedness and companionship, resulting in a profound sense of grief. Alzheimer's disease robs society of productive and active participants. Because of these devastating effects, it challenges mental health professionals and social agencies, the medical and nursing professions, and researchers looking for possible solutions.

Alzheimer's disease has been classified according to the stages of the degenerative process. The number of stages ranges from three to seven, depending on the source. However, four stages, discussed subsequently, are commonly used to categorize the progressive deterioration seen in victims of Alzheimer's disease. Table 23–6 can be used as a guide to the next sections on the four stages of Alzheimer's.

Stage 1: Mild Alzheimer's Disease

The loss of intellectual ability is insidious. The person with mild Alzheimer's disease loses energy, drive, and initiative and has difficulty learning new things. Personality and social behavior remain intact, which often influences others to minimize and underestimate the loss of the individual's abilities. The individual may still continue to work, but the extent of the dementia becomes evident in a new or demanding situation. Depression may occur early in the disease but usually lessens as the disease progresses. Activities such as doing the marketing or managing finances are noticeably impaired during this phase.

▸ Mr. Collins, 56 years of age, is a lineman for a telephone company. He feels that he is getting old. He keeps forgetting things and writes notes to himself on scraps of paper. One day on the job, he forgets momentarily which wires to connect and connects all the wrong ones, causing mass confusion for a few hours. At home, Mr. Collins flies off the handle when his wife suggests they invite the new neighbors for dinner. It is hard for him to admit that anything new confuses him, and he often forgets names (aphasia) and sometimes loses the thread of conversations. Once, he even forgot his address when his car broke down on the highway. He is moody and depressed and becomes indignant when his wife finds 3 months' unpaid bills stashed in his sock drawer. Mrs. Collins is bewildered, upset, and fearful that something is terribly wrong.

The rate of progression varies from person to person. Some individuals with stage 1 Alzheimer's disease decline quickly and may be dead within 3 years. Others, although their condition worsens, may still function in the community with support. And still others may remain at this level for 3 years or more. The time of onset of symptoms to death averages 8 years but can range from 3 to 20 years.

TABLE 23-6 STAGES OF ALZHEIMER'S DISEASE

Stage	Characteristics
Stage 1 (Mild) *Forgetfulness*	Losses in short-term memory; loses things, forgets. Memory aids compensate; lists, routine, organization. Aware of the problem; concerns about lost abilities. Depression common, worsens symptoms. Not diagnosable at this time.
Stage 2 (Moderate) *Confusion*	Memory loss progressive; short-term memory impaired; interferes with all abilities. Withdrawn from social activities. Declines in instrumental activities of daily living (ADLs), e.g., money management, legal affairs, transportation, cooking, housekeeping. Denial common; fear of "losing their mind." Depression increasingly common; frightened because aware of deficits. Cover-up for memory loss through confabulation. Problems intensified when stressed, fatigued, out of own environment, ill. Commonly need day care or in-home assistance.
Stage 3 (Moderate-Severe) *Ambulatory Dementia*	ADL losses (in order): willingness and ability to bathe, grooming, choosing clothing, dressing, gait and mobility, toileting, communication, reading, and writing skills. Loss of reasoning ability, safety planning, and verbal communication. Frustration common; becomes more withdrawn and self-absorbed. Depression resolves as awareness of losses diminishes. Difficult communication; increasing loss of language skills. Evidence of reduced stress threshold; institutional care usually needed.
Stage 4 (Late) *End Stage*	Family recognition disappears; does not recognize self in mirror. Nonambulatory; little purposeful activity; often mute; may scream spontaneously. Forgets how to eat, swallow, chew; commonly loses weight; emaciation common. Problems associated with immobility; pneumonia, pressure ulcers, contractures. Incontinence common; seizures may develop. Most certainly institutionalized at this point. Return of primitive (infantile) reflexes.

From Hall, G. R. (1994). Caring for people with Alzheimer's disease using the conceptual model of progressively lowered stress threshold in the clinical setting. *Nursing Clinics of North America*, 29(1):129–141.

Stage 2: Moderate Alzheimer's Disease

Deterioration becomes evident during the moderate phase. Often, the person with moderate Alzheimer's disease cannot remember his or her address or the date. There are memory gaps in the person's history that may fluctuate from one moment to the next. Hygiene suffers, and the ability to dress appropriately is markedly affected. The person may put on clothes backward, button the buttons incorrectly, or not fasten zippers (apraxia). Often, the person has to be coaxed to bathe.

Mood becomes labile, and the individual may have bursts of paranoia, anger, jealousy, and apathy. Activities such as driving become hazardous; the person may suddenly speed up or slow down for no apparent reason or may go through stop signs. Care and supervision become a full-time job for family members. Denial mercifully takes over and protects people from the realization that they are losing control, not only of their mind but also of their life. Along with denial, people begin to withdraw from activities and others, since they often feel overwhelmed and frustrated when they try to do things that once were easy. The person may also have moments of becoming tearful and sad.

▶ For a short period, Mr. Collins is transferred to a less complicated work position after his inability to function is recognized. His wife drives him to work and picks him up. Mr. Collins often forgets what he is doing and stares blankly. He accuses the supervisor of spying on him. Sometimes, he disappears at lunch and is unable to find his way back to work. The transfer lasts only a few months, and Mr. Collins is forced to take an early retirement. At home, Mr. Collins sleeps in his clothes. He loses interest in reading and watching sports on television and often breaks into angry outbursts, seemingly over nothing. Often, he becomes extremely restless and irritable and wanders around the house aimlessly.

Stage 3: Moderate to Severe Alzheimer's Disease

At this stage, the person is often unable to identify familiar objects or people, even a spouse (severe agnosia). The person needs repeated instructions and directions for the simplest tasks (advanced apraxia): "Here is the face cloth, pick up the soap. Now, put water on the face cloth and rub the face cloth with soap. . . ." Often, the individual cannot remember where the toilet is and becomes incontinent. Total care is necessary at this point, and the burden on the family can be emotionally, financially, and physically devastating. The world becomes very frightening to the person with Alzheimer's disease because nothing makes sense any longer. Agitation, violence, paranoia, and delusions are commonly seen once the mechanisms of denial and withdrawal are no longer effective. Another problem that is frightening to family members and caregivers is wandering behavior. An estimated 70% of people with Alzheimer's disease may wander and are at risk for becoming lost (Alzheimer's Association 1993).

Institutionalization may be the most appropriate recourse at this time because the level of care is so demanding, and violent outbursts and incontinence may be crises that the family can no longer handle. Some criteria for placement in a nursing home follow:

- The person wanders.
- The person is a danger to self and others.
- The person is incontinent.
- The person's behavior affects the sleep of others.

▸ Mr. Collins is terrified. Memories come and then slip away. People come and go, but they are strangers. Someone is masquerading as his wife, and it is hard to tell what is reality and what is memory. Things never stay in the same place. Sometimes, people hide the bathroom where he cannot find it. He in turn has to hide things to keep them safe, but he forgets where he hides them. Buttons and belts are confusing, and he does not know what they are doing there, anyway. Sometimes, he tries to walk away from the terrifying feelings and the strangers. He tries to find something he has lost long ago . . . if he could only remember what it is.

Stage 4: Late Alzheimer's Disease

Williams (1986) described what is called a Klüver-Bucy–like syndrome in late Alzheimer's disease, which includes the following symptoms. **Agraphia** (inability to read or write), **hyperorality** (the need to taste, chew, and put everything in one's mouth), blunting of emotions, visual agnosia (loss of ability to recognize familiar objects), and **hypermetamorphosis** (touching everything in sight) are all associated with this syndrome.

At this stage, the ability to talk, and eventually the ability to walk, are lost. If death due to secondary causes (e.g., infection or choking) has not come, the end stage of Alzheimer's disease is characterized by stupor and coma.

▸ Mrs. Collins and the children keep Mr. Collins at home until his outbursts become frightening. Once, he is lost for 2 days after he somehow unlocks the front door. Mrs. Collins has her husband placed in a Veterans Administration (VA) hospital. When his wife comes to visit, Mr. Collins sometimes cries. He never talks and is always tied into his chair when she comes to visit. The staff explain to her that although Mr. Collins can still walk, he keeps getting into other people's beds and scaring them. They explain that perhaps he wants comfort and misses human touch. They encourage her visits, even though Mr. Collins does not seem to recognize her. He does respond to music. His wife brings a radio, and when she plays the country and western music he has always loved, Mr. Collins nods and claps his hands.

▸ Mrs. Collins is torn between guilt and love, anger and despair. She is confused and depressed. She is going through the painful process of mourning the loss of the man she has loved and shared a life with for 34 years.

▸ Three months after his admission to the VA hospital, and 8 years after the incident of the crossed wires at the telephone company, Mr. Collins chokes on some food, develops pneumonia, and dies.

NURSING DIAGNOSIS

Care for a client with dementia, especially with Alzheimer's disease, requires a great deal of patience, creativity, and maturity. The needs of such a client can be enormous for nursing staff and for families who care for their loved ones in the home. As the disease progresses, so do the needs of the client and the demands on the caregivers, staff, and family.

One of the most important areas of concern identified by both staff and families is the client's safety. Many people with Alzheimer's disease wander and may be lost for hours or days. Wandering, along with behaviors such as rummaging, may be perceived as purposeful to the person with Alzheimer's disease. Wandering may result from changes in the physical environment, fear caused by hallucinations or delusions, or lack of exercise (Alzheimer's Newsletter 1993.)

Seizures are common in the later stages of this disease. Injuries from falls and accidents can occur during any stage as confusion and disorientation progress. The potential for burns exists if the client is a smoker or is unattended at the stove. Prescription drugs can be taken incorrectly, or bottles of noxious fluids can be mistakenly ingested, resulting in a medical crisis. Therefore, **risk for injury** is always present.

Throughout the course of the disease, the nursing diagnosis problem statement may not change (e.g., risk for injury); however, the "related to" and "as evidenced by" components may, and these are the parameters from which meaningful and effective goals are formed. Risk for injury can be related to confusion, unsteady gait, faulty judgment, poisons, household hazards, and loss of short-term memory. **Risk for injury** can be evidenced by impaired mobility, sensory deficits, history of accidents, and lack of knowledge of safety precautions, all of which increase the risks of hospitalization (Hall 1991).

Communicating with the client who has Alzheimer's disease becomes progressively more difficult. Comprehension diminishes, and the person finds it difficult and then impossible to name objects (aphasia). Eventually, the person is unable to recognize objects (agnosia). Lowering the person's levels of fear and anxiety, providing a sense of safety, and emphasizing visual and verbal clues are helpful to clients with a diagnosis of **impaired verbal communication.** Impaired verbal communication may be related to many disorders, including aphasia and cerebral impairment. Supporting data include difficulty finding the correct word, and inappropriate speech or response.

Impaired environmental interpretation syndrome and **uncompensated memory loss** and **chronic confusion** inevitably occur. The person becomes more disoriented, memory diminishes, and attention span decreases, and the person is unable to maintain continuity in relationships, events, and the environment.

Delusions (usually paranoid) and illusions will complicate the individual's experience.

As time goes on, the person loses the ability to perform tasks that were once familiar and routine (apraxia). For example, the person's ability to dress diminishes. At first, supervision or simple directions may be sufficient; eventually, total assistance is needed. This progression applies to bathing, hygiene, grooming, feeding, and toileting—in fact, to all areas of daily living. Therefore, **self-care deficits** involving many functional abilities occur to varying degrees. Depending on the affected person's disability, goals and interventions are planned. The most effective and respectful goals are those that allow the client to carry out as much self-care as possible.

Functional incontinence is often evident, especially in the later stages, and it tremendously increases the individual's need for help with self-care activities.

It may be difficult to view the person with Alzheimer's disease as a once-competent, humorous, and caring person whose life included family and friends. Memory impairment robs people of their continuity and their place in life, along with cherished relationships and the joy of living. Unfortunately, in the early stages, the affected person often *is* aware of what is happening to him or her. The loss of one's sense of self causes terror, despair, and isolation. Therefore, **self-esteem disturbance, altered role performance,** and **personal identity disturbance** need to be addressed when care is planned. **Powerlessness, hopelessness,** and **grieving** are also important considerations.

Ineffective individual coping is evident in clients with Alzheimer's disease. In addition to being unable to function in one's occupational and personal life, longstanding personality traits may intensify and manifest in inappropriate behaviors. Common behaviors include hoarding, regression, and being overly demanding. Therefore, nurses and family members often intervene in behaviors that signal ineffective individual coping. Family caregivers may experience compromised or even disabling family coping.

Additional family issues may emerge. Perhaps some of the most crucial aspects of the client's care are support, education, and referrals for the family. The family loses an integral part of its unit. Family members lose the love, the function, the support, the companionship, and the warmth that this person had provided. **Caregiver role strain** is always present, and planning with the family and offering community support is an integral part of appropriate care. **Anticipatory grieving** is also an important phenomenon to assess for and may be an important target for intervention. Helping the family grieve can make the task ahead somewhat clearer and, at times, less painful.

PLANNING

Planning Outcome Criteria

For the nursing diagnosis **risk for injury,** many outcome criteria may be appropriate. Some follow:

- Client will remain safe in the hospital or at home.
- With the aid of an identification bracelet and neighborhood or hospital alert, client will be returned within 3 hours of wandering.
- Client will remain free of danger during seizures.
- With the aid of nursing interventions, client will remain burn free.
- With the aid of nursing guidance and environmental manipulation, client will not hurt himself or herself if a fall occurs.
- Client will ingest only correct doses of prescribed medications and appropriate food and fluids.
- Client will communicate needs.
- Client will answer yes or no appropriately to questions.
- Client will state needs in alternative modes when he or she is aphasic (e.g., will signal correct word on hearing it or will refer to picture or label).
- Client will wear prescribed glasses or hearing aid each day.

For a client with **self-care deficit,** possible outcomes and goals follow:

- Client will participate in self-care at optimal level.
- Client is able to follow step-by-step instructions for dressing, bathing, and grooming.
- Client will put on own clothes appropriately, with aid of fastening tape (Velcro) and nursing supervision.

- Client's skin will remain intact, despite incontinence or prolonged pressure.

Self-esteem disturbance should also be addressed. Often, nurses tend to treat older people or people with cognitive impairments as if they were children. Being treated like a child may very well foster childlike behaviors. Self-esteem is damaged, anxiety increases, and regressive behaviors are fostered. Some goals that might apply follow:

- Client will state both positive and negative comments about his or her personal level of functioning.
- Client will function at his or her highest level within the family.
- Client will state that he or she is aware that people care about him or her.
- Each day, client will participate in simple activities that bring enjoyment (e.g., singing with others, group exercises, or recounting past successes to others).

Impaired environmental interpretation syndrome, or **chronic confusion,** as evidenced by hallucinations, delusions, illusions, and severe memory impairment, may play a large role in the care provided by the nurse or families. Some nursing goals that might be appropriate follow:

- Client will acknowledge the reality, after it is pointed out, of an object or a sound that was misinterpreted (illusion).
- Client will state that he or she feels safe after experiencing delusions or illusions.
- Client will remain nonaggressive when experiencing paranoid ideation.

Ineffective individual coping, as evidenced by hoarding, regression, and demanding behaviors, can also be a challenge for both nurses and families. Goals include the following:

- Client will retain only hoarded items that do not include potentially dangerous materials, such as glass, metal, and food.
- Client will respond to suggestions by nurse to go to his or her room to masturbate when he or she masturbates in a public area.
- Number and intensity of client's demands on staff or family will decrease with the aid of nursing interventions.
- Client will discuss some aspects of his or her life that hold pleasant memories.

Families with a demented member are under tremendous stresses. The stress of caring for an ill family member, who in many ways has become a stranger, can trigger intense feelings of anger, guilt, hopelessness, despair, and grief within the family. If the family is caring for the ill member in the home, the combination of intense emotional conflicts and overwhelming demands to meet the ill family member's multiple physical needs can be tremendous. Therefore, **caregiver role strain** is almost always present. Divorces, separations, and other evidence of severe stress may result. Financial drains may leave the family bankrupt. Many supports are needed. Goals for caregiver role strain follow:

- Family members will have the opportunity to express "unacceptable" feelings in a supportive environment.
- Family members will have access to professional counseling.
- Family members will name two organizations within their geographical area that can offer support.
- Family members will participate in ill member's plan of care, with encouragement from staff.
- Family members will state that they have outside help that allows family members to take personal time for themselves (1 to 7 days) each week or month.
- Family members will have the names of three resources that can help with financial burdens and legal considerations.

In the moderate stages of the illness, nutritional intake may exceed bodily requirements. However, weight gain is not customary, perhaps because of agitation and wandering, which burn up additional calories. As the illness progresses into later stages, **altered nutrition: less than body requirements** typically ensues. According to Wilson (1990), problems range from clients' forgetting to eat to ingesting nonedible substances. Desired outcome criteria for **altered nutrition** include the following:

- The client will ingest adequate calories (at least 1200 to 1600 calories per day).
- The client will maintain an adequate fluid intake (at least 2400 to 3200 ml per day).

The incontinence of Alzheimer's disease may be classified under the nursing diagnosis of **functional incontinence,** i.e., no specific physiological problem exists other than that the person with Alzheimer's disease has lost the ability to negotiate the environment for adequate toileting. Outcomes include the following:

- Client will participate in a toileting program.
- As the disease progresses, however, a more realistic goal may be that the client will remain clean and dry.

Nurse's Feelings and Self-Assessment

Nurses working in any setting with cognitively impaired clients are aware of the tremendous responsibility placed on the caregivers. Severe confusion, psychotic states, and violent and aggressive behaviors can take their toll on staff and family (Burnside 1988). Taking care of clients who are unable to communicate and who have lost the ability to relate and respond to others is extremely difficult, especially for student nurses or nurses who do not understand dementia or Alzheimer's disease.

Nurses working in facilities for clients who are cognitively impaired (e.g., nursing homes and extended care facilities) need special education and skills. Education needs to include information about the process of the disease and effective interventions, as well as knowledge regarding antipsychotic drugs. Support and educational opportunities should be readily available, not just to nurses but also to nurse's aides, who are often directly responsible for administering basic care.

Burnout of staff can occur. Burnside (1988) identified three possible antidotes to burnout:

1. *Revise goals* so that they are realistic. Nurses sometimes set goals that are too high and unrealistic. Frustration and discouragement ensue when the goals cannot be met.
2. *Refrain from being swept into a hopeless stance.* Concentrate on finding satisfaction in small accomplishments (e.g., the client is comfortable, is participating in an activity, or is less delusional than previously). Indeed, for this person, such a situation may mark quite an accomplishment.
3. *Research* is a prime factor for eliminating staff burnout. Involving nurses in research can increase nurses' knowledge about caring for the demented client and can add a feeling of purpose to a demanding job that requires great patience and maturity.

INTERVENTION

The nurse's attitude of unconditional positive regard is the single most effective tool in caring for demented clients. It induces clients to cooperate with care, reduces catastrophic outbreaks, and increases family members' satisfaction with care.

More than 30% of individuals with dementia have a group of secondary behavioral disturbances, including depression, hallucinations and delusions, agitation, insomnia, and wandering (Corey-Bloom and Galasko 1995). Because these symptoms impair the person's ability to function, increase their need for supervision, and influence the need to institutionalize them, the control of these symptoms is a priority in managing Alzheimer's disease (Corey-Bloom and Galasko 1995):

> The basic principle underlying all care for the cognitively impaired is to facilitate the highest level of functioning a person is capable of in all areas (e.g., self-care and social and family relationships).

Intervention with family members is critical. The effects of losing a family member to dementia—that is, watching a person who has an important role within the family unit and who is loved and is a vital part of his or her family's history deteriorate—can be devastating. The interventions discussed subsequently are useful.

Counseling (Basic Level)

How nurses choose to communicate with these clients has a major impact on their maintenance of self-esteem and their ability to participate in care. For example:

"I see you are ready to brush your teeth. May I help you get the toothpaste?"	Offers assistance. Points out next step in care without highlighting memory loss.
"I know it isn't familiar but this is the room we have fixed up for you while you're staying with us."	Accesses client's long-term memories, which are retained longer. Acknowledges client's feelings.

Burnside (1988) suggested the following guidelines for implementing interventions or teaching a severely cognitively impaired person:

1. Provide only one visual clue (object) at a time.
2. Know that the client may lack understanding of the task assigned.
3. Remember that relevant information is remembered longer than irrelevant information.
4. Break tasks into very small steps.
5. Give only one instruction at a time.
6. Report, record, and document all data.

Table 23–7 gives special guidelines for nurses and family members to use to communicate with a cognitively impaired person.

Health Promotion and Health Maintenance (Basic Level)

Health teaching and support for families are vital components of care for individuals with dementia. Educating families who have a cognitively impaired member is one of the most important areas for nurses. Families who are caring for a member in the home need to know about strategies for communicating and for structuring self-care activities (Table 23–8).

Most important, families need to know where to get help. Help includes professional counseling and education regarding the process and the progression of the disease. Families especially need to know about, and be referred to, community-based groups that can help shoulder this tremendous burden (e.g., day care centers, senior citizen groups, organizations providing home visits and respite care, and family support groups). A list with definitions of some of the types of services available in the client's community should be provided to the family, as well as the names and telephone numbers of these services.

A recent addition to resources that can provide caregivers of persons with Alzheimer's disease with information, communication, and decision-support functions is Computer Link, a computer bulletin board (Brennan et al. 1995).

TABLE 23–7 COMMUNICATION WITH A COGNITIVELY IMPAIRED PERSON

INTERVENTION	RATIONALE
Nursing Diagnosis: Impaired communication related to neurological changes, as evidenced by impairment in memory and judgment and difficulty defining words and concepts	
1. Always identify yourself and call the person by name at each meeting.	1. Client's short term memory is impaired—requires frequent orientation to time and environment.
2. Speak slowly.	2. Gives client time to process information.
3. Use short, simple words and phrases.	3. Client may not be able to understand complex statements or abstract ideas.
4. Maintain face-to-face contact.	4. Maximizes verbal and nonverbal clues.
5. Be near client when talking, one or two arm-lengths away.	5. This distance can help client focus on speaker as well as maintain personal space.
6. Focus on one piece of information at a time.	6. Attention span of client is poor and easily distracted—helps client focus. Too much data can be overwhelming and can increase anxiety.
7. Talk with client about familiar and meaningful things.	7. Allows self-expression and reinforces reality.
8. Encourage reminiscing about happy times in life.	8. Remembering accomplishments and shared joys helps distract client from deficit and gives meaning to existence.
9. When client is delusional, acknowledge client's feelings and reinforce reality. Do not argue or refute delusions.	9. Acknowledging feelings helps client feel understood. Pointing out realities may help client focus on realities. Arguing can enhance adherence to false beliefs.
10. If a client gets into an argument with another client, stop the argument and get them out of each other's way. After a short while (5 minutes), explain to each client matter-of-factly why you had to intervene.	10. Prevents escalation to physical acting out. Shows respect for client's right to know. Explaining in an adult manner helps maintain self-esteem.
11. When client becomes verbally aggressive, acknowledge client's feelings and shift topic to more familiar ground, e.g., "I know this is upsetting for you, since you always cared for others . . Tell me about your children."	11. Confusion and disorientation easily increase anxiety. Acknowledging feelings makes client feel more understood and less alone. Topics client has mastery in can remind him or her of areas of competent functioning and can increase self-esteem.
12. Have client wear prescription eyeglasses or hearing aid.	12. Increases environmental awareness, orientation, and comprehension, which in turn increases awareness of personal needs and the presence of others.
13. Keep client's room well lit.	13. Maximizes environmental clues.
14. Have clocks, calendars, and personal items (e.g., family pictures or Bible) in clear view of client while he or she is in bed.	14. Assists in maintaining personal identity.
15. Reinforce client's pictures, nonverbal gestures, Xs on calendars, and other methods used to anchor client in reality.	15. When aphasia starts to hinder communication, alternate methods of communication need to be instituted.

Scott and colleagues (1986) confirmed in their research that family support was positively associated with the caregiver's coping effectiveness. Each stage of Alzheimer's disease involves new and different stresses, which can be diminished by professional assistance.

The Alzheimer's Association is a national umbrella agency that provides various forms of assistance to persons with the disease and their families. The Alzheimer's Association has launched Safe Return, the first nationwide program to help locate and return missing people with Alzheimer's disease and other memory impairments. Information regarding housekeeping, home health aides, and companions should also be available. Such outside resources can help prevent the total emotional and physical fatigue of family members. Family members can call (800) 272-3900 to locate the Alzheimer's Association nearest them. Types of resources that might be available in some communities are found in Table 23–9.

Family members often feel guilty that they did not do or are not doing enough. They may feel frustrated and angry, and they may blame staff, nurses, and doctors. The use of projection helps protect family members from their own feelings of helplessness and hopelessness. It is *vital* that the health care providers understand this phenomenon to minimize defensive responses. Consultation with family members and education about the disease are of enormous benefit.

Family members need to know where and how to place the ill member when this becomes necessary. Even-

TABLE 23–8 STRUCTURING SELF-CARE ACTIVITIES FOR A COGNITIVELY IMPAIRED PERSON

INTERVENTION	RATIONALE
Nursing Diagnosis: Self-care deficit related to cognitive impairment, as evidenced by deficit in	
Dressing and Bathing	
1. Always have client perform all tasks that he or she is capable of.	1. Maintains client's self-esteem and uses muscle groups; impedes staff burnout; minimizes further regression.
2. Always have client wear own clothes, even if in the hospital.	2. Helps maintain client's identity and dignity.
3. Use clothing with elastic, and substitute fastening tape (Velcro) for buttons and zippers.	3. Minimizes client's confusion and eases independence of functioning.
4. Label clothing items with client's name and name of item.	4. Helps identify client if he or she wanders and gives client additional clues when aphasia or agnosia occurs.
5. Give step-by-step instructions whenever necessary, e.g., "Take this blouse . . . put in one arm . . . now the next arm . . . pull it together in the front . . . now . . ."	5. Client can focus on small pieces of information more easily; allows client to perform at optimal level.
6. Make sure that water in faucets is not too hot.	6. Judgment is lacking in client; is unaware of many safety hazards.
7. If client is resistant to doing self-care, come back later and ask again.	7. Moods may be labile, and client may forget but often complies after short interval.
Nutrition	
1. Monitor food and fluid intake.	1. Client may have anorexia or be too confused to eat.
2. Offer finger food that client can walk around with.	2. Increases input throughout the day; client may eat only small amounts at meals.
3. Weigh client regularly (once a week).	3. Monitors fluid and nutritional status.
4. During period of hyperorality, watch that client does not eat nonfood items (e.g., ceramic fruit or food-shaped soaps).	4. Client puts everything into mouth; may be unable to differentiate inedible objects made in the shape and color of food.
Bowel and Bladder Function	
1. Begin bowel and bladder program early; start with bladder control.	1. Same time of day for bowel movements and toileting—in early morning, after meals and snacks, and before bedtime—can help prevent incontinence.
2. Evaluate use of disposable diapers.	2. Prevents embarrassment.
3. Label bathroom door as well as doors to other rooms.	3. Additional environmental clues can maximize independent toileting.
Sleep	
1. Since client may become awake, be frightened, or cry out at night, keep area well lit.	1. Reinforces orientation, minimizes possible illusions.
2. Maintain a calm atmosphere during the day.	2. Encourages a calming night's sleep.
3. Nonbarbiturates may be ordered (e.g., chloral hydrate)	3. Barbiturates can have a paradoxical reaction, causing agitation.
4. If medications are indicated, neuroleptics with sedative properties may be the most helpful (e.g., haloperidol [Haldol]).	4. Helps clear thinking and sedates.
5. Avoid the use of restraints.	5. Can cause client to become more terrified and fight against restraints until exhausted to a dangerous degree.

tually, the ill person's labile and aggressive behavior, incontinence, wandering, unsafe habits, or disruptive nocturnal activity can no longer be appropriately dealt with in the home. Families need information, support, and legal and financial guidance at this time. When the nurse is unable to provide the relevant information, proper referrals by the social worker are needed. Information regarding advance directives, durable power of attorney, guardianship, and conservatorship should be included in the communication with the family (Weiler and Buckwalter 1988).

Milieu Management (Basic Level)

According to Ninos and Makohon (1985), assisting clients to cope with their environment is the basis for therapy, particularly nursing therapy. Thus, nurses must identify and modify, where possible, specific functional disturbances and must assist clients and families in compensating for such disturbances.

A therapeutic environment can be divided into (1) safety considerations and (2) activities that increase socialization and minimize loneliness. Table 23–10 gives

TABLE 23-9 DEFINITIONS OF CARE SERVICES FOR PERSONS WITH DEMENTIA

Adult day care: a program of medical and social services, including socialization, activities, and supervision, provided in an outpatient setting.

Case management: client assessment, identification and coordination of community resources, and follow-up monitoring of client adjustment and service provision.

Chore services: household repairs, yard work, errands.

Congregate meals: meals provided in a group setting for people who may benefit both from the nutritionally sound meal and from social, educational, and recreational services provided at the setting.

Home-delivered meals: meals delivered to the home for individuals who are unable to shop or cook for themselves.

Home health aide services: assistance with health-related tasks, such as medications, exercises, and personal care.

Homemaker services: household services, e.g., cooking, laundry, cleaning, and shopping, and escort service to accompany patients to medical appointments and elsewhere.

Hospice services: medical, nursing, and social services to provide support and alleviate suffering for dying persons and their families.

Information and referral: provision of written or verbal information about community agencies, services, and funding sources.

Legal services: assistance with legal matters, e.g., advance directives, guardianship, power of attorney, and transfer of assets.

Mental health services: psychosocial assessment and individual and group counseling to address psychological and emotional problems of patients and families.

Occupational therapy: treatment to improve functional abilities; provided by an occupational therapist.

Paid companion/sitter: an individual who comes to the home to provide supervision, personal care, and socialization during the absence of the primary caregiver.

Personal care: assistance with basic self-care activities, e.g., bathing, dressing, getting out of bed, eating, and using the bathroom.

Personal emergency response systems: telephone-based systems to alert others that an individual who is alone is experiencing an emergency and needs assistance.

Physical therapy: rehabilitative treatment provided by a physical therapist.

Physician services: diagnosis and ongoing medical care, including prescribing medications and treating intercurrent illness.

Protective services: social and law enforcement services to prevent, eliminate, or remedy the effects of physical and emotional abuse or neglect.

Recreational services: short-term, inpatient or outpatient services intended to provide temporary relief for the caregiver.

Skilled nursing: medically oriented care provided by a licensed nurse, including monitoring acute and unstable medical conditions; assessing care needs; supervising medications, tube and intravenous feeding, and personal care services; and treating pressure ulcers and other conditions.

Supervision: monitoring an individual's whereabouts to ensure his or her safety.

Telephone reassurance: regular telephone calls to individuals who are isolated and often homebound.

Transportation: transporting people to medical appointments, community facilities, and elsewhere.

Adapted from Mace, N. L., and Rabins, P. B. (1981). *The 36 hour day* (p. 180). Baltimore: Johns Hopkins University Press.

some guidelines for providing a therapeutic milieu that can be helpful to family members.

Minimizing fatigue can greatly help the eruption of dysfunctional or catastrophic episodes. Fatigue is probably one of the most common factors in producing such episodes (Hall 1994). Early in the disease, clients are able to prevent fatigue by taking breaks and resting quietly twice daily. As the disease progresses, clients may nap for one or more rest periods (Hall 1994). To reduce disorientation to time, clients should nap in daytime clothing on top of the bed covers to distinguish daytime naps from nighttime sleep.

Psychobiological Interventions (Basic Level)

Cognitive Impairment

Tacrine (THA, Cognex) was the first cholinesterase inhibitor to be approved by the US Food and Drug Administration (FDA) for the treatment of mild to moderate symptoms of Alzheimer's disease. It has shown to improve functioning and slow the progress of the disease, particularly in the area of cognition and memory in about 20% to 50% of clients with Alzheimer's disease. Unfortunately, tacrine is associated with a high frequency of side effects, including elevated liver transaminase levels, gastrointestinal effects, and liver toxicity (Eagger and Harvey 1995). Weekly blood tests are necessary to monitor liver functions. The delay in the progression of Alzheimer's disease by long-term tacrine treatment was supported in a study by Minthon and associates (1995). Donepezil (Aricept), approved by the FDA in December 1996, also appears to slow down deterioration in cognitive functions but without the potentially serious liver toxicity attributed to tacrine. In client studies with donepezil, some individuals with Alzheimer's disease did experience diarrhea and nausea. Both tacrine and donepezil have been shown to slow down cognitive deterioration by about 2 months.

The results of studies on drug substances that are already on the market are showing promising results in

TABLE 23–10 MAINTAINING A THERAPEUTIC MILIEU FOR A COGNITIVELY IMPAIRED PERSON

INTERVENTION	RATIONALE
Safe Environment	
Nursing Diagnosis: Risk for injury related to cognitive impairment	
If client lives with family:	
1. Gradually restrict use of the car.	1. As judgment becomes impaired, client may be dangerous to self and others.
2. Remove throw rugs and other objects in person's path.	2. Minimizes tripping and falling.
If client is in hospital or living with family:	
3. Minimize sensory stimulation.	3. Decreases sensory overload, which can increase anxiety and confusion.
4. If client becomes verbally upset, listen briefly, give support, then change the topic.	4. Goal is to prevent escalation of anger. When attention span is short, client can be distracted to more productive topics and activities.
5. Label all rooms and drawers. Label often-used objects (e.g., hairbrushes and toothbrushes).	5. May keep client from wandering into other client's rooms. Increases environmental clues to familiar objects.
6. Install safety bars in bathroom.	6. Prevents falls.
7. Supervise client when he or she smokes.	7. Danger of burns is always present.
8. If client has history of seizures, keep padded tongue blades at bedside. Educate family and observe.	8. Seizure activity is common in advanced Alzheimer's disease.
If client wanders:	
9. If client wanders during the night, put mattress on the floor.	9. Prevents falls when client is confused.
10. Have client wear Medic-Alert bracelet that cannot be removed (with name, address, and telephone number). Provide police department with recent pictures.	10. Client can easily be identified by police, neighbors, or hospital personnel.
11. Alert local police and neighbors about wanderer.	11. May reduce time necessary to return client to home or hospital.
12. If client is in hospital, have him or her wear brightly colored vest with name, unit, and phone number printed on back.	12. Makes client easily identifiable.
13. Put complex locks on door.	13. Reduces opportunity to wander.
14. Place logs at top of door.	14. In moderate and late DAT, ability to look up and reach upward is lost.
15. Encourage physical activity during the day.	15. Physical activity may decrease wandering at night.
16. Explore the feasibility of installing sensor devices.	16. Provides warning if client wanders.
Activities	
Nursing Diagnosis: Impaired social interaction related to cognitive impairment	
1. Provide picture magazines and children's books when client's reading ability diminishes.	1. Allows continuation of usual activities that the client can still enjoy; provides focus.
2. Provide simple activities that allow exercise of large muscles.	2. Exercise groups, dance groups, and walking provide socialization as well as increased circulation and maintenance of muscle tone.
3. Encourage group activities that are familiar and simple to perform.	3. Such activities as group singing, dancing, reminiscing, and working with clay and paint all help to increase socialization and minimize feelings of alienation.

DAT, dementia of the Alzheimer's type.

delaying the deterioration of clients with Alzheimer's disease. For example, selegiline (Eldepryl) and alpha tocopherol (vitamin E) have both been seen to delay progression of some aspects of the disease (loss of daily activities including bathing, dressing, and handling money) (NIH 1997). Observational studies indicate that estrogen or anti-inflammatory agents may also have some positive benefits on Alzheimer's disease (NIH 1997). Other cholinesterase inhibitors are being developed in other countries and are being studied in clinical trials.

Other medications are often useful in managing behavioral symptoms of individuals with dementia, but these need to be used with caution (Goldberg 1995).

PSYCHOTIC SYMPTOMS (DELUSIONS AND HALLUCINATIONS)	COMMENTS AND CAUTIONS
Antipsychotics	Can produce akathisia, with increased restlessness and agitation. Clients can become more incapacitated by the parkinsonian and anticholinergic side effects.

AFFECTIVE SYMPTOMS (DEPRESSION)	
Antidepressants	Agents with high anticholinergic activity should be avoided. The selective serotonin reuptake inhibitors appear to be well tolerated and effective in geriatric clients.

ANXIETY	COMMENTS AND CAUTIONS
Buspirone (Buspar)	Does *not* produce psychomotor impairment, drowsiness, or cognitive impairment, as do the benzodiazepines. It has no serious side effects for the elderly and should be considered.
Benzodiazepines	Have side effects mentioned above; shorter-acting agents should be used at doses as low as possible.

Agitated Behaviors

Numerous drugs have been used to treat agitated behaviors, but the drug group, and the medication within that group, should be used with careful assessment of the other behaviors and characteristics of the demented individual in mind.

Antipsychotics	When the behavior is a consequence of underlying psychotic process only.
Buspirone	Can decrease episodic agitation in dementia clients (5 mg TID).
Trazodone	Appears to decrease aggressive behavior in agitated demented clients over 3–4 weeks.
Benzodiazepines	May nonspecifically sedate agitated clients, however, over sedation impairs function and can increase cognitive ability and psychomotor impairment.

EVALUATION

Outcome criteria set for clients with cognitive impairment need to be measurable, be within their capabilities, and be evaluated frequently. As the person's condition continues to deteriorate, outcomes (goals) need to be altered to reflect the person's diminished functioning. Frequent evaluation and reformulation of outcome criteria and short-term goals also help diminish staff and family frustration, as well as minimize the client's anxiety by ensuring that tasks are not more complicated than the person can accomplish. The overall goals in treatment are to promote the client's optimal level of functioning and to retard further regression, whenever possible. Working closely with the family and providing them with the names of available resources and support may help increase the quality of life for both the family and the client.

CASE STUDY: WORKING WITH A PERSON WHO IS COGNITIVELY IMPAIRED

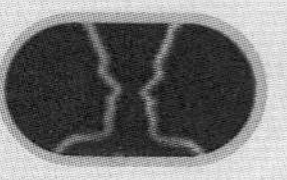

During the past 4 years, Mr. Ludwik has demonstrated rapidly progressive memory impairment, disorientation, and deterioration in his ability to function, related to Alzheimer's disease. He is a 67-year-old man who retired at age 62 to spend some of his remaining "youth" with his wife and to travel, garden, visit family, and finally experience the plans they made over the past 40 years. He was diagnosed with Alzheimer's disease at age 63.

Mr. Ludwik has been taken care of at home by his wife and daughter, Daisy. Daisy is divorced and has come home to live with her two young daughters.

The family members find themselves progressively closer to physical and mental exhaustion. Mr. Ludwik has become increasingly incontinent when he cannot find the bathroom. He wanders away from home constantly, despite close supervision. The police and neighbors bring him back home an average of four times a week. Once, he was lost for 5 days, after he

CASE STUDY: WORKING WITH A PERSON WHO IS COGNITIVELY IMPAIRED *(Continued)*

had somehow boarded a bus for Pittsburgh, 100 miles from home. He was robbed and beaten before being found by the police and returned home.

He frequently wanders into his granddaughters' rooms at night while they are sleeping and tries to get into bed with them. Too young to understand that their grandfather is lonely and confused, they fear that he is going to hurt them. Four times in the past 2 weeks, he has fallen while getting out of bed at night, thinking he is in a sleeping bag camping out in the mountains.

After a conflicting and painful 2 months, the family places him in a special hospital for people with Alzheimer's disease.

Mrs. Ludwik tells the admitting nurse, Mr. Jackson, that her husband wanders almost all the time. He has difficulty finding the right words for things (aphasia) and becomes frustrated and angry when that happens. Sometimes, he does not seem to recognize the family (agnosia). Once, he thought that Daisy was a thief breaking into the house and attacked her with a broom handle. This story causes Daisy to break down into heavy sobs: "What's happened to my father? He was so kind and gentle. Oh God . . . I have lost my father."

Mrs. Ludwik tells Mr. Jackson that her husband can sometimes participate in dressing himself; at other times, when he appears confused over what goes where, he needs total assistance. At this point, Mrs. Ludwik begins to cry uncontrollably, saying "I can't bear to part with him . . . but I can't do it any more. I feel as if I've betrayed him."

Mr. Jackson then focuses his attention on Mrs. Ludwik and her experience. He states, "This a difficult decision for you." He says that he supports their decision to move Mr. Ludwik to the Alzheimer's unit. However, he is also aware that families usually have conflicting and intense emotional reactions of guilt, depression, loss, anger, and other painful feelings. Mr. Jackson suggests that Mrs. Ludwik talk to other families with a cognitively impaired member. "It might help you to know that you are not alone, and having contact with others to share your grief can be healing." One of the groups he suggests is the Alzheimer's Disease and Related Disorders Association (ADRDA), or simply Alzheimer's Association, a well-known self-help group.

ASSESSMENT

Because, indeed, the family is just as much the client as the family member with Alzheimer's disease, Mr. Jackson tries to take the most pressing immediate needs into consideration. He obtains the following data on initial assessment:

OBJECTIVE DATA

- Wanders away from home about four times a week
- Was lost for 5 days and was robbed and beaten
- Often incontinent when he cannot find the bathroom
- Has difficulty finding words
- Has difficulty identifying members of the family at times
- Has difficulty dressing himself at times
- Falls out of bed at night
- Has memory impairment
- Is disoriented much of the time
- Gets into bed with granddaughters at night when wandering
- Family undergoing intense feelings of loss and guilt

SUBJECTIVE DATA

- "I can't bear to part with him."
- "I feel I've betrayed him."
- "I've lost my father."

NURSING DIAGNOSIS

Mr. Jackson evaluates the data. Indeed, many potential nursing diagnoses and several client needs are identified that require intervention by the nursing staff. Mr. Jackson chooses four initially; the first one deals with client safety, two address maintaining an optimal level of functioning and preventing further regression, and the fourth deals with the very real and immediate needs of a family in crisis. Therefore, Mr. Jackson makes the following diagnoses:

1. **Risk for injury** related to confusion, as evidenced by wandering
   - Wanders away from home about four times a week
   - Wanders despite supervision
   - Falls out of bed at night
   - Gets into other people's beds

Continued on following page

CASE STUDY: WORKING WITH A PERSON WHO IS COGNITIVELY IMPAIRED *(Continued)*

- Wanders at night

2. **Functional incontinence** related to disturbed cognition, as evidenced by inability to find the toilet
   - Incontinent when he cannot find the bathroom
3. **Self-care deficit** (self-dressing deficits) related to impaired cognitive functioning, as evidenced by impaired ability to put on and take off clothing
   - Sometimes is able to dress with help of wife
   - At other times is too confused to dress self at all
4. **Anticipatory family grieving** related to loss and deterioration of family member
   - "I can't bear to part with him."
   - "I feel I've betrayed him."
   - "I've lost my father."
   - Family undergoing intense feelings of loss and guilt

PLANNING

PLANNING OUTCOME CRITERIA

Although Mr. Ludwik has many unmet needs that require nursing interventions, Mr. Jackson decides to focus on the four initial nursing diagnoses. As other problems arise, they will be addressed.

NURSING DIAGNOSIS	LONG-TERM OUTCOME	SHORT-TERM GOALS
1. **Risk for injury** related to confusion, as evidenced by wandering.	1. Client will remain safe in nursing home.	1a. Client will remain in bed injury free. 1b. Client will wander only in protected area. 1c. Client will be returned within 2 hours if he leaves the unit.
2. **Functional incontinence** related to disturbed cognition, as evidenced by inability to find the toilet.	2. Client will experience less incontinence (fewer episodes) by fourth week of hospitalization.	2a. Client will participate in toilet training. 2b. Client will find the toilet most of the time.
3. **Self-care deficit** (self-dressing) related to impaired cognitive functioning, as evidenced by impaired ability to put on and take off clothes.	3. Client will participate in dressing himself most of the time.	3a. Client will follow step-by-step instructions for dressing most of the time. 3b. Client will dress in own clothes with aid of fastening tape.
4. **Anticipatory family grieving** related to loss and deterioration of family member.	4. All family members will state, in 3 months' time, that they feel more supported and able to talk about their grieving.	4a. Family members will state that they have opportunity to express "unacceptable" feelings in supportive environment. 4b. Family members will state that they have found support from others who have a family member with Alzheimer's disease.

CASE STUDY: WORKING WITH A PERSON WHO IS COGNITIVELY IMPAIRED *(Continued)*

NURSE'S FEELINGS AND SELF-ASSESSMENT

Mr. Jackson has worked on this particular unit for 4 years. It is a unit especially designed for cognitively impaired individuals, which makes nursing care easier than on a regular unit. However, Mr. Jackson would be the first to admit that he has come a long way during the time he has worked on the unit.

Four years ago, he found himself getting constantly frustrated and angry. He had entered this special unit enthusiastically and had worked hard setting goals and trying to implement them. However, he thought no one, especially the clients, cared about what he was doing for them. When the nursing coordinator asked him what made him come to that conclusion, he burst out "Nothing I do seems to make any difference . . . no one listens to me."

Mr. Jackson had a lot to learn about Alzheimer's disease, and he found that the more he learned, the more he understood about why change took so long or, in some cases, could not take place. He, like everyone before him, learned to become more realistic in formulating goals, thereby lessening his frustration.

From his co-workers, he also learned many nursing care strategies that increased competent care and decreased frustration. For example, he learned that he could distract certain clients from inappropriate behaviors (e.g., arguing with others or taking things out of other people's rooms) by engaging them in another, enjoyable activity, such as talking about something they were interested in. This reduced Mr. Jackson's initial response of scolding the client, which had usually resulted in escalating the client's anxiety, confusion, and sometimes aggression, and left Mr. Jackson annoyed and upset.

As time progressed, Mr. Jackson found that he was well suited to this kind of nursing. He has an enthusiastic manner, and his patience, wit, and genuine liking of his clients make him an ideal role model for staff new to the unit. He does a lot of teaching on the unit, both formal and informal. He is compiling a workbook for caregivers of the cognitively impaired.

INTERVENTION

Mr. Jackson gives Mrs. Ludwik the names of two organizations in her community that work with families of a cognitively impaired member. He emphasizes that the Alzheimer's Association support group consists of other family members who are going through similar circumstances.

He gives Mrs. Ludwik the name of the social worker and the nurse clinician assigned to the unit, who could give the family information on the disease, answer questions, and provide support and further referrals. Mr. Jackson asks Mrs. Ludwik to let him know after 1 week how things are going, and he says that further plans could be made at that time.

Wandering is a common phenomenon, especially in men with Alzheimer's disease. However, because night wandering may be indicative of cardiac decompensation, Mr. Jackson alerts the medical staff. Mr. Ludwik's mattress is placed on the floor to prevent falls, and there is a large area on the unit where he can wander safely. A bright orange vest is made for Mr. Ludwik with his name, unit, and phone number taped on the back, in case he does wander off the unit. A Medic-Alert bracelet is also made up for him, containing the same information. He is encouraged to participate in activities that encourage the exercise of large muscle groups (e.g., exercise and dance groups). He seems to wander less at night if he has been involved in physical exercise during the day. On the nights that he does wander out of his room, the staff allow him to wander in the safe area. He is offered snacks, and the room is kept well lit. Sometimes, Mr. Ludwik curls up on the couch and falls asleep.

On the unit, Mr. Jackson and the staff begin toilet training Mr. Ludwik (i.e., they take him to the toilet early in the morning, after each meal and snack, and in the evening). On this unit, all the rooms, including the bathrooms, are clearly labeled in large, colorful letters; clocks are placed

Continued on following page

CASE STUDY: WORKING WITH A PERSON WHO IS COGNITIVELY IMPAIRED *(Continued)*

in every room in clear view, and each room has a large calendar with Xs marking off the days.

Mr. Jackson finds that on most mornings, Mr. Ludwik is able to follow simple step-by-step instructions for dressing, but that he is much better at this after breakfast than in the early-morning hours. Therefore, a schedule is set up that includes toileting, breakfast, toileting, and then dressing. When Mr. Ludwik becomes irritable and refuses to dress, Mr. Jackson involves Mr. Ludwik in another activity and, after 15 or 20 minutes, suggests dressing. This seems to work most of the time. Mr. Ludwik always wears his own clothes, unaltered except for the fastening tape that replaces the original buttons and zippers. This seems to lessen Mr. Ludwik's frustration during dressing.

Mr. Ludwik's love for gardening is sublimated into activities such as finger painting and clay modeling. The activity therapist finds that Mr. Ludwik is most content during these times. Nursing Care Plan 23–1 provides more details on Mr. Ludwik's treatment.

EVALUATION

At the end of 4 weeks, Mr. Ludwik is still free from injuries. Placing his mattress on the floor has solved one potential problem. Mr. Ludwik continues to wander at night, but more often, he naps on the couch after having a snack. He does wander off the unit once, when visitors are coming in, but is returned to the unit by the security guard as Mr. Ludwik prepares to leave the hospital. The familiar orange vest was spotted immediately.

When Mr. Ludwik first came to the unit he had been very disoriented. However, getting used to certain staff members and set routines helped to overcome his disorientation. With the aid of the tape fasteners and constant, short reminders, Mr. Ludwik dresses himself with minimal assistance.

Urinary incontinence shows great improvement over the 4-week period. Although Mr. Ludwik is still incontinent, the episodes now occur only 4 times a week. He is amenable to the toileting schedule and usually complies without problems.

The family begins short-term counseling together. Counseling sessions not only give Mrs. Ludwik and Daisy an opportunity to express pent-up feelings and receive guidance, but also give Mr. Ludwik's granddaughters time to express their own fears and confusion.

Mrs. Ludwik has been to two meetings of an Alzheimer's support group, at which she finds great relief. She says that she has felt isolated for so long. Her daughter Daisy is planning to go with her to the next meeting.

NURSING CARE PLAN 23–1 A PERSON WITH COGNITIVE IMPAIRMENT*

NURSING DIAGNOSIS

Risk for Injury: related to altered cerebral functioning, as evidenced by wandering

Supporting Data

- Wanders despite supervision
- Falls out of bed
- Gets into other people's beds

Outcome Criteria: Client will remain safe

NURSING CARE PLAN 23–1 A PERSON WITH COGNITIVE IMPAIRMENT *(Continued)*

SHORT-TERM GOAL	INTERVENTION	RATIONALE	EVALUATION
1. Client will not fall out of bed at any time.	1a. Spend time with client on admission.	1a. Lowers anxiety, provides orientation to time and place. Client's confusion is increased by change.	*GOAL MET*
	1b. Label client's room in big, colorful letters.	1b. Offers clues in new surroundings.	
	1c. Remove mattress from bed and place on floor.	1c. Prevents falling out of bed.	Mattress on floor prevents falls out of bed.
	1d. Keep room well lit at all times.	1d. Provides important environmental clues; helps lower possibility of illusions.	
	1e. Show client clock and calendar in room.	1e. Fosters orientation to time.	
	1f. Keep window shade up.	1f. Allows day-night variations.	
2. Client will wander only in protected area.	2a. At night, take client to large, protected, well-lit room.	2a. Client is able to wander safely in protected environment.	*GOAL MET* Client continues to wander at night; with supervision, keeps out of other clients' rooms most of the time.
	2b. Alert physician to check client for cardiac decompensation.	2b. Possible underlying cause of nocturnal wakefulness and wandering.	
	2c. Offer snacks when client is up—milk, decaffeinated tea, sandwich.	2c. Helps replace fluid and caloric expenditure.	By fourth week, client starts to nap on couch in large room after snacks during the night.
	2d. Allow soft music on radio.	2d. Helps induce relaxation.	
	2e. Spend short, frequent intervals with client.	2e. Decreases client's feelings of isolation and increases orientation.	
	2f. Take client to bathroom after snacks.	2f. Helps prevent incontinence.	
	2g. During day, offer activities that include use of large muscle groups.	2g. For some clients, helps decrease wandering.	
3. Client will be returned within 2 hours if he leaves the unit.	3a. Order Medic-Alert bracelet for client (with name, unit or hospital, phone number).	3a. If client gets out of hospital, he can be identified.	*GOAL MET* By fourth week, client wanders off unit only once; is found in lobby and returned by security guard within 45 minutes.
	3b. Place brightly colored vest on client with name, unit, and phone number taped on back.	3b. If client wanders in hospital, he can be identified and returned.	

Continued on following page

NURSING CARE PLAN 23–1 A PERSON WITH COGNITIVE IMPAIRMENT *(Continued)*

SHORT-TERM GOAL	INTERVENTION	RATIONALE	EVALUATION
	3c. Check client's whereabouts periodically during the day and especially at night.	3c. Helps monitor client's activities.	

NURSING DIAGNOSIS

Functional Incontinence: related to a cerebral impairment when client cannot find the toilet

Supporting Data

- Increasingly incontinent when client cannot find the bathroom

Outcome Criteria: Client will experience a decrease in incontinence by fourth week of hospitalization.

SHORT-TERM GOAL	INTERVENTION	RATIONALE	EVALUATION
1. Client will participate in toilet training.	1a. Start toilet training in early morning, after meals and snacks, and before bed.	1a. Reduces risk of incontinence.	*GOAL MET* For first 2 weeks, client is very confused in new environment.
	1b. Simplify steps involved in task; present steps one at a time (e.g., "Unbuckle pants, sit down. . .")	1b. Cueing and task segmentation increase likelihood of desired behavior.	Client gradually adjusts to toileting.
2. Client will find toilet and be less incontinent by the fourth week.	2a. Frequently identify large sign (or picture) on bathroom.	2a. Frequent orientation to place is helpful to client.	*GOAL MET* By fourth week, incontinent episodes decrease from three times a day (rate in first week) to four times a week.
	2b. Simplify clothing. Sweat pants or jogging suits are ideal. Replace any buttons and zippers with fastening tape (Velcro).	2b. Modified clothing improves ease of toileting and reduces delay.	
	2c. Evaluate use of incontinence pad.	2c. Can provide dignity and help maintain self-esteem.	

NURSING DIAGNOSIS

Self-Care Deficit: (self-dressing deficit) related to diminished cognitive functioning, as evidenced by impaired ability to put on and take off clothing

Supporting Data

- Sometimes is able to dress with wife's help
- At other times is too confused to dress self at all

Outcome Criteria: Client will be less incontinent by fourth week of hospitalization

SHORT-TERM GOAL	INTERVENTION	RATIONALE	EVALUATION
1. Client will follow step-by-step instructions for dressing.	1a. Refrain from rotating staff.	1a. Minimizes confusion and disorientation.	*GOAL MET* By fourth week, client is able to follow instructions for dressing most of the time.
	1b. Always provide client's own clothes.	1b. Maintains client's identity and sense of dignity.	

NURSING CARE PLAN 23–1 A PERSON WITH COGNITIVE IMPAIRMENT *(Continued)*

SHORT-TERM GOAL	INTERVENTION	RATIONALE	EVALUATION
	1c. Divide tasks into very small steps.	1c. Client can understand one simple comment at a time.	
	1d. Do not hurry client.	1d. Hurrying client can cause increased anxiety, agitation, and disorientation.	
	1e. Calmly give instructions: "Put one leg in trousers . . . now the next leg. . ."	1e. Support and encouragement help lower anxiety and maximize ability to follow instructions.	
2. Client will dress in own clothes with aid of fastening tape.	2a. Have family replace buttons and zippers with fastening tape.	2a. Fastening shirts and pants is easier.	*GOAL MET* Client is able to use fastening tape much of the time to dress self, with close supervision.
	2b. Have client wear pants with elastic in waist.	2b. Lessens need for fastening.	
	2c. Work with client on how to use fastening tape.	2c. Client responds to frequent orientation and step-by-step instruction.	
	2d. When client refuses or is too agitated to follow instructions, come back later.	2d. Client's moods are often labile; forgets easily. Can be redirected later (15 to 20 minutes).	

NURSING DIAGNOSIS

Anticipatory Family Grieving: related to deterioration of client's mental status

Supporting Data

- "I've lost my father."
- "I can't bear to part with him."
- "I feel like I've betrayed him."

Outcome Criteria: All family members will state that they feel more supported and able to talk about their grieving in 3 months' time.

SHORT-TERM GOAL	INTERVENTION	RATIONALE	EVALUATION
1. Family members will state that they have opportunity to express "unacceptable" feelings in supportive environment.	1a. Make arrangements for family to meet with counselor (e.g., nurse clinician, social worker, psychologist).	1a. Family is in crisis: family needs to identify feelings and define some plan to regain sense of control and facilitate grief work.	*GOAL MET* By the end of the third week, family starts attending short-term family counseling sessions.
	1b. Encourage spouse's input.	1b. Helps maintain spouse's involvement and may help reduce feelings of guilt.	

Continued on following page

NURSING CARE PLAN 23–1 A PERSON WITH COGNITIVE IMPAIRMENT *(Continued)*

SHORT-TERM GOAL	INTERVENTION	RATIONALE	EVALUATION
	1c. Encourage family members to stay with client and arrange outings (e.g., home visits for holidays, picnics, and weekends).	1c. Increases client's personal identity and aids family members in gradually "letting go."	
	1d. Encourage family members to express feelings; encourage ongoing sessions with counselor.	1d. Family members need to have a place where they can get support and understanding.	
2. Family will state that they have found support from others who have a family member with Alzheimer's disease.	2a. Offer family written names and phone numbers of available support groups in their vicinity.*	2a. The more support a family has, the better they are able to cope with a complex and painful situation.	*GOAL MET* Mrs. Ludwik attends two meetings of an Alzheimer's support group and finds it enormously supportive. The daughter plans to attend the next meeting.
	2b. Follow up periodically.	2b. Continues to assess needs and encourage family members to obtain support.	

* A family caring for a client in the home would benefit from, along with the above, (1) companions, (2) other volunteers, (3) home health aides, (4) visiting nurses, (5) day care centers, (6) senior citizen groups, (7) respite care, and (8) financial and legal counseling. Caring for a cognitively impaired family member can quickly lead to physical and emotional exhaustion and can throw the family into crisis.

SUMMARY

Cognitive disorder is the term that refers to disorders marked by disturbances in orientation, memory, intellect, judgment, and affect resulting from changes in the brain. Delirium and dementia were discussed in this chapter because they are the cognitive disorders most widely seen by health care workers.

Delirium is marked by acute onset, disturbance in consciousness, and symptoms of disorientation and confusion that fluctuate by the minute, hour, or time of day. Delirium is always secondary to an underlying condition; therefore, it is temporary, transient, and may last from hours to days once the underlying cause is treated. If the cause is not treated, permanent damage to the neurons could result in dementia or death.

Nursing diagnoses for delirium were suggested, including **risk for injury, fluid volume deficit, acute confusion, sleep-pattern disturbance, impaired verbal communication, fear, self-care deficits,** and **impaired social interaction.** Goals for each of these nursing diagnoses were identified.

The clinical picture of delirium in an intensive care unit was described, and medical and nursing interventions were delineated.

Dementia usually has a more insidious onset than delirium. Global deterioration of cognitive functioning (e.g., memory, judgment, ability to think abstractly, and orientation) is often progressive and irreversible, depending on the underlying cause. If dementia is primary (e.g., Alzheimer's disease, multi-infarct dementia, or Pick's disease), the course is irreversible. However, if the underlying cause is treatable, then the progression of the dementia may be halted or reversed.

Alzheimer's disease accounts for up to 70% of all cases of dementia, and multi-infarct disease accounts for about 20%; however, these percentages may change with the rising incidence of AIDS-related dementia (HIV encephalopathy).

Various theories exist about the cause of Alzheimer's disease; none of these is conclusive, although the genetic theory identifies familial tendencies. In this chapter signs and symptoms were noted during the progression of the disease through four stages: stage 1 (mild), stage 2 (moderate), stage 3 (moderate to severe), and stage 4 (late). The phenomena of confabulation, perseveration, aphasia, apraxia, agnosia, and hyperorality were explained.

No known cause or cure exists for Alzheimer's disease, although the drugs tacrine (Cognex) and donepezil (Aricept) offer some hope for slowing down the progression of the disease. Much research is still needed for unraveling the mysteries of this devastating illness. Duffy and colleagues (1989) described a nursing research agenda that included better care and management of clients with Alzheimer's disease and an emphasis on research-based practice.

People with Alzheimer's disease have many unmet needs and present many management challenges to their families, as well as health care workers, once clients with the disease are institutionalized. There is often **risk for injury, impaired verbal communication, self-care deficit, self-esteem disturbance, impaired environmental interpretation syndrome, chronic confusion, ineffective individual coping,** and always, **caregiver role strain.** Functional incontinence and nutritional deficits were also discussed in this chapter.

Specific nursing interventions for cognitively impaired individuals can enhance the optimal functioning of the client, especially in the areas of communication, activities of daily living, health teaching of families, and therapeutic environment.

REFERENCES

Alzheimer's Association Newsletter 13(2):4, 1993.
Alzheimer's Disease (Part I). (1992). *The Harvard Mental Health Letter*, 9(3):1.
Alzheimer's in the skin (1993). *Discover*, 12:26.
American Association of Retired Persons (AARP) (1986). *Coping and caring: Living with Alzheimer's disease*. Washington, DC: American Association of Retired Persons.
American Psychiatric Association (1987). *Diagnostic and statistical manual of mental disorders* (3rd ed., Revised). Washington, DC: American Psychiatric Association.
American Psychiatric Association (1994). *Diagnostic and statistical manual of mental disorders* (4th ed.). Washington, DC: American Psychiatric Association.
Andresen, G. (1992). How to assess the older mind. *RN*, 55(7):34.
Brennan, P. F., et al. (1995). The effects of a special computer network on caregivers of persons with Alzheimer's disease. *Nursing Research*, 44(3):155.
Burnside, I. (1988). *Nursing and the aged* (3rd ed.). New York: McGraw-Hill.
Buzan, R. D., and Dubovsky, S. L. (1995). Dementia due to other general medical conditions and dementia due to multiple etiologies. In G. O. Gabbard (Ed.), *Treatments of psychiatric disorders* (Vol. 1, pp. 535–554). Washington, DC: American Psychiatric Press.
Caine, E. D., et al. (1995). Delirium, dementia, and amnestic and other cognitive disorders and mental disorders due to a general medical condition. In H. I. Kaplan and B. J. Saddock (Eds.), *Comprehensive textbook of psychiatry* (6th ed., Vol. 1, pp. 705–754). Baltimore: Williams & Wilkins.
Corey-Bloom, J., and Galasko, D. (1995). Adjunctive therapy in patients with Alzheimer's disease: A practical approach. *Drugs and Aging*, 7(2):79.
de-Stoutz, N. D., et al. (1995). Reversible delirium in terminally ill patients. *Journal of Pain and Symptom Management*, 10(3):249.
Dewan, M. J., and Gupta, S. (1992). Toward a definite diagnosis of Alzheimer's disease. *Comprehensive Psychiatry*, 33(4):282.
Duffy, L. M., et al. (1989). A research agenda in care for patients with Alzheimer's disease. *Journal of Nursing Scholarship*, 21(4):254.
Eagger, S. A., and Harvey, R. J. (1995). Clinical heterogeneity: Responders to cholinergic therapy. *Alzheimer's Disease and Associated Disorders*, 9(2):37.
Foreman, M. D. (1990). Complexities of acute confusion. *Geriatric Nursing*, 11:136.
Goldberg, R. J. (1995). *Practical guide to the care of the psychiatric patient*. St. Louis: Mosby–Year Book.
Gray-Vickrey, P. (1988). Evaluating Alzheimer's patients. *Nursing 88*, 18:34.
Hall, G. R. (1991). This hospital patient has Alzheimer's. *American Journal of Nursing*, 91(10):44–50.
Hall, G. R. (1994). Caring for people with Alzheimer's disease using the conceptual model of progressively lowered stress threshold in the clinical setting. *Nursing Clinics of North America*, 29(1):129.
Kaufman, D. M. (1995). *Clinical neurology for psychiatrists* (4th ed.). Philadelphia: W. B. Saunders.
Mace, N. L., and Rabins, P. B. (1981). *The 36 hour day*. Baltimore: Johns Hopkins University Press.
Masterman, D. L., et al. (1995). Alzheimer's disease. In G. O. Gabbard (Ed.), *Treatments of psychiatric disorders* (Vol. 1, pp. 535–554). Washington, DC: American Psychiatric Press.
McHugh, P. R., and Folstein, M. F. (1987). Organic mental disorders. In R. Michels and J. O. Cavenar (Eds.), *Psychiatry* (Vol. I). Philadelphia: J. B. Lippincott.
Minthon, L., et al. (1995). Long-term effects of tacrine on regional cerebral flow changes in Alzheimer's disease. *Dementia*, 6(5):245.
Nagley, S. J. (1986). Predicting and preventing confusion in your patients. *Journal of Gerontological Nursing*, 12(3):27.
National Institutes of Health (1997). New drug therapies delay effects of Alzheimer's disease. Washington, DC: NIH Press Release, April 23, 1997.
Newbern, V. B. (1991). Is it really Alzheimer's? *American Journal of Nursing*, 2:51.
Nicholas, L. M., and Lindsey, B. A. (1995). Delirium presenting with symptoms of depression. *Psychosomatics*, 36(5):471.
Ninos, M., and Makohon, R. (1985). Functional assessment of the patient. *Geriatric Nursing*, 6:139.
Parnetti, L. (1995). Clinical pharmacokinetics of drugs for Alzheimer's disease. *Clinical Pharmacokinetics*, 29(2):110.
Perry, S. W., and Markowitz, J. (1988). Organic mental disorders. In J. A. Talbott, R. E. Hales and S. C. Yudofsky (Eds.), *Textbook of psychiatry*. Washington, DC: American Psychiatric Press.
Powell, L. S., and Courtice, K. (1983). *Alzheimer's disease: A guide for families*. Reading, MA: Addison-Wesley.
Reisberg, B. (1984). Stages of cognitive decline. *American Journal of Nursing*, 84:225.
Scott, J. P., Roberto, K. A., Hutton, J. T. (1986). Families of Alzheimer's victims: Family support to the caregivers. *Journal of American Geriatrics Society*, 34:348.
Souder, E. (1992). Diagnosing dementia: Current clinical concepts. *Journal of Gerontological Nursing*, 18(2):5.
Sullivan, E. M., Wanich, C. K., and Kurlowicz, L. H. (1991). Elder care. *AORN Journal*, 53(3):820.
Tacrine update. (1993). *Alzheimer's Research Review*, Summer.
Weiler, K., and Buckwalter, K. C. (1988). Care of the demented client. *Journal of Gerontological Nursing*, 14(7):26.
Williams, L. (1986). Alzheimer's: The need for caring. *Journal of Gerontological Nursing*, 12(2):21.
Wilson, H. S. (1990). Easing life for the Alzheimer's patient. *RN*, 53(12):24.
Wolanin, M. O, and Fraelich-Philips, L. R. (1981). *Confusion, prevention and cure*. St. Louis: C. V. Mosby.
Yi, E. S., et al. (1994). Alzheimer's disease and nursing: New scientific and clinical insights. *Nursing Clinics of North America*, 29(1):85.

Further Reading

Alexopoulas, G. S., and Abrams, R. C. (1991). Depression in Alzheimer's disease. *Psychiatric Clinics of North America*, 14(2):327.
Breitner, J. C., and Welsh, K. A. (1995). Genes and recent developments in the epidemiology of Alzheimer's disease and related dementia. *Epidemiology Review*, 17(1):39.
Foreman, M. D. (1986). Acute confusional states in hospitalized elderly: A research dilemma. *Nursing Research*, 35(1):34.
Li, G., Silverman, J. M., Mohs, K. C. (1991). Clinical genetic studies of Alzheimer's disease. *Psychiatric Clinics of North America*, 14(2):267.
Mass, M. L., and Buckwalter, K. C. (1988). A special Alzheimer's unit: Phase 1 of baseline data. *Applied Nursing Research*, 1(1):41.
Morency, C. R. (1990). Clinical updates. *Journal of Professional Nursing*, 6(6):356.
Neimoller, J. (1990). Change of pace for Alzheimer's patients. *Geriatric Nursing*, 4:86.
Roper, J. M., Shapira, J., Change, B. L. (1991). Agitation in the demented patient: A framework for management. *Journal of Gerontological Nursing*, 17(3):17.

SELF-STUDY AND CRITICAL THINKING

Matching questions

Write DEL (delirium) or DEM (dementia) to categorize each of the following symptoms:

1. ________ Disorder has acute onset.
2. ________ Eventually, both short-term and long-term memory are affected.
3. ________ No or slow changes are seen on electroencephalogram.
4. ________ Fluctuating levels of consciousness exist.
5. ________ Aphasia and agnosia are commonly observed.
6. ________ Disorientation is most severe at night; client may be oriented during the day.
7. ________ Confabulation or perseveration is commonly observed.
8. ________ Visual tactile hallucinations are most common in this syndrome.

Match the terms in the right column with the definitions in the left column.

9. ________ The inability to name objects
10. ________ Difficulty finding the right word—can deteriorate to muteness
11. ________ Unable to perform once-familiar and simple tasks
12. ________ The need to taste, chew, and put everything in one's mouth
13. ________ Repeating the same word or behavior over and over again

A. Hypermetamorphosis
B. Perseveration
C. Hyperorality
D. Apraxia
E. Mnemonic disturbance
F. Agnosia
G. Aphasia
H. Confabulation

Short answer

Mark Peters, 51 years old and a Vietnam veteran, has just been admitted and diagnosed with acute bacterial endocarditis. His temperature is 103° F, his skin turgor is poor, and his urine is dark amber and scanty. He is agitated and screams in terror when he hears the bleeps from the electrocardiographic monitor. He thinks that he has been captured in Vietnam and that the bleeps are coming from a time bomb, and he is desperate to flee. He thinks it is 1971 and that you are the enemy.

14. Formulate two nursing diagnoses and identify at least one short-term goal for each diagnosis.

    Nursing diagnosis: ________________________
    related to ________________________
    as evidenced by ________________________
    Short-term goal: ________________________

Nursing diagnosis: ____________________
related to ____________________
as evidenced by ____________________
Short-term goal: ____________________

15. Describe the deterioration of a client who is going through the four stages of Alzheimer's disease and identify essential features during each stage.

 A. Stage 1 (mild)

 ____
 ____

 B. Stage 2 (moderate)

 ____
 ____

 C. Stage 3 (moderate to severe)

 ____
 ____

 D. Stage 4 (late)

 ____
 ____

Critical thinking

Mrs. Kendel is a 52-year-old woman who has progressive Alzheimer's disease. She lives with her husband, who has been trying to care for her in their home. Mrs. Kendel often wears evening gowns in the morning, puts her blouse on backward, and sometimes puts her bra on backward outside her blouse.

She often forgets where things are. She makes an effort to cook but often confuses frying pans and pots and sometimes has trouble turning on the stove.

Once in a while, she cannot find the bathroom in time, often mistaking it for a broom closet. She becomes frightened of noises and is terrified when the telephone or doorbell rings.

At other times, she cries because she is aware that she is losing her sense of her place in the world. She and her husband have always been close, loving companions, and he wants to keep her at home as long as possible.

16. Help Mr. Kendel by writing out a list of suggestions that he can try at home that might help facilitate (a) communication, (b) activities of daily living, and (c) therapeutic environment.
17. Identify at least seven interventions that are appropriate to this situation for each of the areas cited above.
18. Identify possible types of resources available for maintaining Mrs. Kendel in her home for as long as possible. Identify the name of one self-help group that you would urge Mr. Kendel to join.
19. Share with your clinical group the name and function of at least three community agencies in your area that could be an appropriate referral for a family in your neighborhood with a member with dementia. (For one, you can call the Alzheimer's Association [800-272-3900] to find a local chapter that might help you with this information; another resource is the Alzheimer's Disease Education and Referral [ADEAR] Center [800-438-4380], website: http://www.alzheimers.org/adear.)

UNIT SIX

People Who Employ Self-Destructive Behaviors

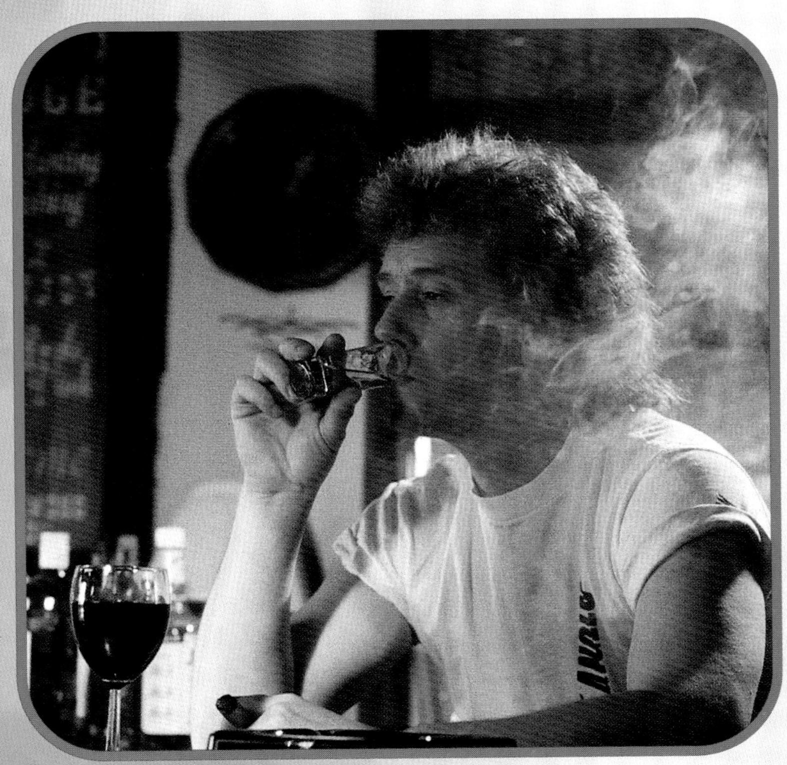

. . . man will occasionally stumble over the truth, but usually manages to pick himself up, walk over or around it, and carry on.

WINSTON S. CHURCHILL

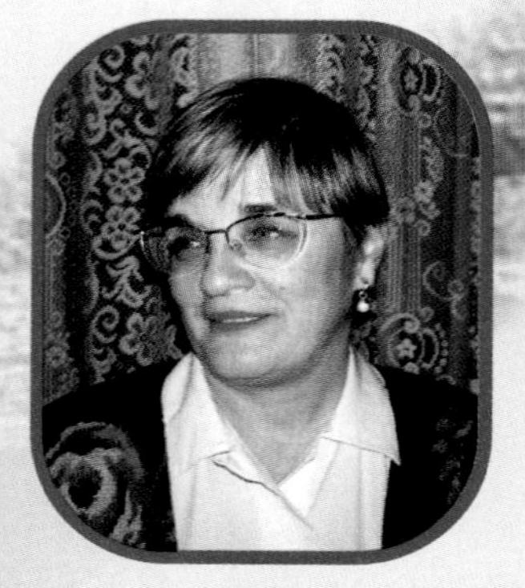

A Nurse Speaks

Sharon Shisler

Facilitating a weekly support group of women with HIV for the past 4 years has shown me how group work can help women. This group helps them deal with their fears, increases their knowledge, and empowers them to voice their concerns and to obtain responses and action from others.

When I was asked to begin a support group for women with HIV, I blithely responded "Well, of course." I had been providing emotional support to patients with HIV/AIDS, their lovers, and their family members for at least 3 years. It was not until I began to prepare for the first evening session that I began to feel anxious. The previous attempts to organize a women's group never got off the ground, and women with HIV were still relatively rare back in the early 90s.

I was terrified; I was fearful of being "pulled down by their depression." I feared that no one would show up. I wondered if I would have the skills to handle their problems. The group started with two members who are still very active in the group. A total of 14 different women have attended over the years. A core of five women currently attend on a regular basis.

The group meets in a community space similar to a living room. The women range in age from the twenties to the fifties. The group combines medically recommended treatments with alternative therapies. The group starts out with Tái Chi exercises, taught by one of the members. The participants also practice breathing exercises, affirmations, relaxation skills, and visualizations.

Members share their worries and their accomplishments. They have developed a special kind of quiet listening and "having been there" when recently diagnosed women attend their first group meeting and tell their story. This special quality is not something learned in psychiatric nursing 101. They just have it.

The women's group is a microcosm of women in our society. They are in the highest to the lowest socioeconomic classes, from being independently wealthy to being homeless during some periods of their life. They are single, married, and widowed. Some have children; some are hoping to have children. Some are in relationships; some are hoping to have relationships. Some get along with their families and some don't.

These women are also very different from other women by virtue of their infection. They have been diagnosed with their infection from 6 months to 12 years before. They have acquired HIV by most of the familiar methods of infection: one woman had sexual relations with a man who had hemophilia and AIDS, another woman with her secretly bisexual husband, and another woman with an infected intravenous (IV) drug abuser who is now in jail for violence. One woman was infected from a transfusion with infected blood, while another woman was a former IV drug abuser. In fact, the method of infection is for many of these women the pivotal point around which they feel stigmatized and avoided. A subtle web of rejection related to the assumed mode of infection has been felt by every woman from many of their friends, families, and health professionals.

Many of the women tell stories of health providers responding to them as if they were an illness, not a person with an illness. DeDe (her pen name) tells a story about confronting a dentist who failed to provide proper pain relief during dental work because he assumed that she had become infected from IV drug abuse and didn't want to get her "rehooked" by giving her pain medication. DeDe corrected his misperception, admittedly a bit late, by informing him that she had acquired her infection by having sex with an infected man who had hemophilia.

HIV/AIDS is often on their minds and part of their everyday activities and decisions. Where will I be when I need to take my medications? How can I pay for all this treatment? Can I get the services I need? If I become vocal on a local or national level, how will this affect my family and children? No member of the group has died, but each member has experienced many losses of friends from HIV-related infections. An often-heard remark is that they will die of other causes, such as an automobile accident. In fact, one of the women suffered from a heart attack and another had a mastectomy for breast cancer.

Paradoxically, they lead relatively normal lives despite having a chronic illness. They are women you see in your grocery stores, in the post office, and in every walk of life. You would not know that they are infected.

Many of these women had not found their voice until they joined the group. Their voice seems to be related to two factors: (1) their level of comfort with disclosure, that is, to tell or not, to whom, when, and how; and (2) their ability to deal productively with the stigma and shame associated with HIV.

Disclosure is a big issue for each woman. Each told her circle of friends and family in different ways with various responses. Ellen told many of her significant others all at once, only to later regret her impulsive decision. Gertrude told a select few and was surprised on the one hand at the increased strength of a friendship with a previously casual friend and on the other by the precipitous loss of a long-term friend.

Rebecca is a mother of 6-year-old twins, an infected girl and a noninfected boy. In preparation for leading a group of parents who have children with HIV on the topic of disclosure, the two of us spent hours reading books, reviewing brochures and lecture notes, and discussing the ramifications of telling or not telling your child. Shortly after the parents' meeting, Rebecca felt comfortable to tell her twins about the sister of the pair being infected. She found her voice. She became active on a national and international level. She started writing articles, assisting with all day workshops, and going to international conferences, first as a participant and later as a presenter. She is the current editor of a handbook the group is developing for assisting newly diagnosed women with simple and accurate information.

Women in the group find their voice by knowing their medical information, knowing themselves and their bodies, and knowing the ways that others need to treat them regarding their illness, their questions, and their concerns. They generate a wealth of up-to-date information about medications, protocols, alternative treatments, financial resources, legal options, and names of sensitive and insensitive health professionals. The initial din resulting from the exchange of information is enough to make one at risk for hearing loss. Literature flies about; books are exchanged. Genuine and well-founded support for dealing with side effects of medications is gratefully received.

Every one of these women has increased her voice in advancing the awareness and knowledge of people with whom they come into contact. DeDe writes a monthly column about personal issues in an AIDS newsletter. Moira is great at connecting other women with needed resources. Gertrude volunteers to do the paper work for one of the drug protocols. Rebecca is the fund raiser, writing personal letters to secure funding for children infected with the virus. Many of the women have spoken with groups of teenagers and on national television programs. The group has been active in informing legislators of the lack of research including women and gaps in services for women. The group has been involved in advocating for pediatric doses and medication formulations more receptive to children. During 1 year of correspondence, our group received three letters from President Clinton. A group of women spoke about their experiences on a local radio program, hoping to lower the shame and stigma of having AIDS. Sylvia helps with printing and is now chair of the group's public relations and recruitment. Our group has joined with other women's groups to share information and support action in Washington. Fatigue and conflicting demands of family and work have regretfully prevented us from being able to attend group demonstrations in Washington and meeting with legislators.

The other issue, fear woven with shame, is highlighted by Sylvia's story. She suspected that she was infected for almost 5 years before being tested. It was not until after she successfully survived AFF (Accelerated Free Fall) that she felt competent and strong enough to be tested. In AFF an individual, who has had hours of training and practice, falls from a plane flying about 10,000 feet. The individual has an instructor at each side and opens her parachute at the end of the fall.

Although AIDS and HIV were always woven into the discussion, these brave and caring women taught and inspired me much more than I ever imagined on that first night. Ted Menten in *Gentle Closing: How to Say Goodbye to Someone You Love* states "People who know they are going to die spend their remaining time either (a) being alive or (b) staying alive. Those being alive enjoy the time they have left, while those staying alive desperately seek a cure." My being with these women has shown me how they walk the tightrope between the two ends of this dichotomy. Their walk depends upon many factors, some of which are the length of infection, their own way of handling stress, and their current level of stress.

I came to the group with many preconceived notions about how I was going to help them. I leave the group after 1½ to 2 hours in the evening, not tired, but rejuvenated and tingling with energy. But most of all, I leave with hope: hope for them; hope for their families; hope for the future. HIV is not a death sentence; it is a wake-up call to live every moment of one's life to the fullest, learning everything one can about the infection and about ways of treating and coping with the virus.

These women are more than surviving with HIV/AIDS, they are thriving. Through their well-educated and empowered voices, they are making a difference with themselves, their families, their friends, their communities, and me.

REFERENCE

Menten, T. (1991). *Gentle Closings: How to Say Goodbye to Someone You Love.* Philadelphia: Running Press.

24

People Who Contemplate Suicide

ELIZABETH M. VARCAROLIS

OUTLINE

KEY TERMS AND CONCEPTS

The key terms and concepts listed here also appear in bold where they are defined or discussed in this chapter.

suicide
completed suicide
suicide attempt
suicidal ideation
SAD PERSONS scale
primary intervention
secondary intervention
tertiary intervention/postvention
no-suicide contract

OBJECTIVES

After studying this chapter, the reader will be able to

1. Describe the profile of suicide in the United States, including clues, professions at risk, most common psychopathology, populations at risk, and when people may commit suicide.
2. Identify common precipitating events.
3. Role-play two verbal and two nonverbal clues that might signal suicidal ideation.
4. Using the SAD PERSONS scale, explain the ten risk factors to consider when assessing for suicide.
5. Describe three expected reactions a nurse may have when beginning work with suicidal clients.
6. Give examples of primary, secondary, and tertiary (postvention) interventions.
7. Distinguish among the interventions that a nurse may carry out (a) in the community, (b) in the hospital, and (c) on a telephone hotline.
8. Formulate a "no-suicide contract."
9. Develop a care plan including two nursing diagnoses and four goals for a suicidal client.

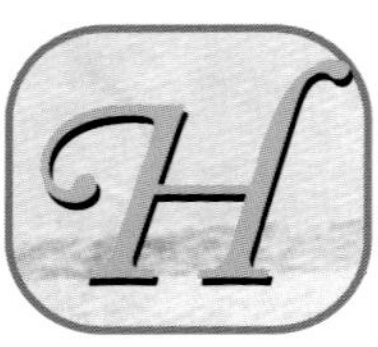

Humans are the only creatures that are aware of their own mortality. They are able to contemplate the past as well as the future, to consider their personal end, and to be cognizant of their own death (Mowshowitz 1984).

Whether to live or die is a universal question that has been debated for centuries. Whether a person has the right to suicide is an intensely complex moral, ethical, religious, and legal issue.

The U.S. government grants people the right to "life, liberty, and the pursuit of happiness." Health care professionals, however, are in frequent contact with people who are following more self-destructive pursuits. Compulsive use of drugs and alcohol, hyperobesity, gambling, self-harmful sexual behaviors, medical noncompliance, and high-risk life styles are examples of covert, self-destructive behaviors. People who engage in self-destructive behavior often take part in hastening their own death. This participation in one's own death may be on a covert, or unconscious, level. Hoff (1995) refers to this group as chronically self-destructive.

Suicide is the ultimate act of self-destruction. In most cases of suicide, crisis precedes the attempt. Suicidal risk should always be assessed in any crisis situation. Suicidal thoughts, threats, or attempts are signals of a person or family in crisis.

The act of purposeful self-destruction represented by taking one's own life arouses intense and complex emotions in others. Suicide, which is the act of opting for nonexistence, is an option that some members of our society are choosing at increasing and alarming rates.

In the United States, suicide is the ninth leading cause of death; among adolescents, it is the third cause of death; and among white adolescents, it is the second cause of death (Roy 1995a). These figures do not take into account the many suicides disguised as accidents. However, the group that has the highest suicide rate of any other is the elderly, who account for 25% of suicides, although they make up only 10% of the population (Roy 1995a).

Among youths who commit suicide, drug use and antisocial personality disorder are found more often in those under 30 years of age. Depression, alcoholism, and illness stressors are found more often among suicide victims over 30 (Roy 1995a). However, more important than the degree of depression, *hopelessness about the future* has been highly correlated with the seriousness of suicidal intent (Hendrin 1992). Box 24–1 provides U.S. statistics on suicide.

Although the suicide rate among whites is about twice that in nonwhites, the rate among black women has increased 80% since the mid-1970s (Berkow and Fletcher 1992). The suicide rate among ghetto youths and certain Native Americans exceeds the national rate, and in some tribes it is five times the national average (Berkow and Fletcher 1992).

The following summary of statistical findings provides a profile of suicide in America:

- About 75% to 80% of people who go on to commit suicide give clues and warnings and often seek help. An estimated 75% of all suicide victims seek help within the 4 months before they take their lives.
- Of those who commit suicide, 65% to 70% have made previous attempts. A person who has attempted suicide in the past is at great risk for successful suicide. The risk is highest in the first 2 years after a suicide attempt, *especially in the first 3 months.*
- The incidence of suicide is higher in urban areas than in rural areas. It is also higher for those who are socially mobile or who are migrants. It is likewise higher in stu-

BOX 24–1 SUMMARY OF SUICIDE STATISTICS

- Suicide is the ninth leading cause of death in the United States.
- Suicide is the *third* cause of death among young people 15–24 years of age.
- The highest suicide rate is for persons over 65 years.
- It is estimated that there are about ten attempted suicides to one completion.
- 72% of all suicides are committed by white males.
- The male-to-female gender ration is 4:1.
- Suicide by firearms is the most common method (60% of all suicides).
- Nearly 80% of all firearm suicides are committed by white men.
- Professional persons including lawyers, dentists, military men, and physicians, have higher than average suicide rates.
- Suicide is less frequent among practicing members of most religious groups.

Data from National Institute of Mental Health (1995); *Merck manual* 1992.

dents, the elderly, gifted individuals, immigrants, and Alaskan and Canadian Native Americans.

- The incidence of suicide also appears to be higher in certain occupations. Doctors, dentists, lawyers, police officers, and air-traffic controllers have higher suicide rates than in the general population. People who are physically ill are also at higher risk than the general population. The suicide rate is higher for single people than for married people and is higher for divorced males than for divorced females. See Table 24–1 for myths and facts about suicide.
- A significantly greater number of suicide attempters stated that they did not participate in religious activities, according to one study.

Monday is the most frequent day for suicide, morning the most frequent time, and April the most frequent month.

People who have problems with impulse control (e.g., those who use drugs, alcohol, violence), are depressed, are psychotic, or have a family member who committed suicide are at greater risk than the general public. Up to 75% of clinically depressed people have suicidal ideation or intent (Mullis and Byers 1988).

The "right to die" issue is presently controversial. The dilemma is most debated in cases of terminal illness, severe debilitation, intractable pain, and progressive illnesses such as multiple sclerosis. Does someone with a terminal disease who is in severe pain have a moral and ethical right to take his or her own life? Can rational suicide in such cases be legally and ethically sanctioned? The question of whether intentionally ending one's life can ever be rational or praiseworthy, and if so under what circumstances, continues to be hotly debated in classrooms, courtrooms, medical and ethical journals, and popular news media. In November 1995, Oregon became one of the first jurisdictions outside the Netherlands to allow physician-assisted suicide. The passage of the Death with Dignity Act allows terminally ill patients to receive a fatal prescription from a doctor after they meet several criteria (Mullens 1995). The issues of the right to die with dignity and respect for the wishes of a person to die in the face of unbearable suffering or progressive disability are presently challenging the health professions, both in the United States and abroad.

Transient thoughts of death and dying are a universal phenomenon. Almost everyone will experience momentary self-destructive thoughts. Obsessive preoccupation with thoughts of suicide, however, is pathological.

The Center for Study of Suicide Prevention of the United States Public Health Service has classified suicidal behavior into three categories, according to intent:

1. **Completed suicide** includes all willful, self-inflicted, life-threatening acts leading to death.
2. **Suicide attempt** includes all willful, self-inflicted, life-threatening attempts that have not led to death.
3. **Suicidal ideation** means that the person is thinking about harming himself or herself.

THEORY

Because the subject of suicide arouses strong feelings and reactions in all persons, it is wise to examine personal thoughts and ethical beliefs regarding another person's attempt at suicide.

Theoretical considerations and research findings can clarify or modify one's understanding of the phenomena surrounding overt self-destructive behavior.

Much information has been gathered on suicide from clinical observations, studies, and research. However, no single theory can account for all the data available. Two theoretical models presented here are (1) sociological theories and (2) a more recent area of study, biochemical-genetic theories.

Sociological Theories

Suicidal crisis involves the unique characteristic of rejecting society, as well as rejecting oneself. The threat of death carries enormous impact for all concerned. No other kind of death leaves family and friends with such long-lasting feelings of shame, guilt, puzzlement, and distress (Van Dongen 1988).

Sociological theory refers to the social and cultural context in which a person lives. "Suicide or dying behaviors do not exist in a vacuum, but are an integral part of the life style of the individual" (Schneidman 1963). Cir-

TABLE 24–1 MYTHS VERSUS FACTS: SUICIDE

MYTH	FACT
1. Only people who are mentally ill commit suicide.	1. Suicide can be a decision made by a sane individual. Although many people may be in emotional turmoil or depressed at the time, it is not the same as being crazy.
2. Suicidal persons are fully intent on dying.	2. Most persons who contemplate suicide are highly ambivalent about dying. They don't want death; they want the pain to stop.
3. If a nurse suspects that a person is thinking about suicide, the nurse should not bring up the subject lest the person kill himself or herself.	3. Open dialogue is most often a relief fot the suicidal person. Talking can decrease the risk of suicide.
4. Suicide is an impulsive act.	4. The act may be impulsive, but most often suicide has been carefully thought out.
5. The chance of suicide lessens as depression lessens.	5. When depression is lifting, there is more energy to carry out a previously pondered suicide plan.
6. Suicide can be an inherited trait.	6. Alcoholism and depression most likely are genetic, and having a relative who has committed suicide is a risk factor; however, there are as yet no genetic markers for suicide.
7. Most suicidal persons give no warning.	7. Most people who attempt or commit suicide give definite clues and warnings.
8. All nonwhites have a lower suicide rate than whites.	8. This is true with the exception of young black males.
9. Professionals such as lawyers, doctors, dentists, police officers, and air-traffic controllers have a low suicide rate.	9. All have higher suicide rates than people in the general population.
10. People with definite psychopathology have the greatest chance of killing themselves.	10. People with depression and alcoholism are at greatest risks for suicide among people with psychopathology, although psychosis is also a risk factor.
11. Only people with grave problems, mental illness, or physical illness think about suicide.	11. At one time or another, almost everyone contemplates suicide.
12. People who just want attention use suicidal threats as manipulation.	12. Even if a suicide threat is manipulative, the person may actually go on to commit suicide. **All threats should be taken seriously.**
13. Young people who have antisocial and borderline personality disorders never attempt suicide.	13. Both have higher suicide rates that the general population.
14. People who go from "rags to riches" are better protected against suicide than those who go from fortune to poverty.	14. Persons with a sudden change in fortune (success, riches, acclaim) are also at risk for suicide. Actually, rates tend to be the highest among both the lowest and highest socioeconomic classes.
15. When gay, lesbian, and bisexual people recognize the "sinfulness" of their lives, most of them kill themselves.	15. Although a significant number of this group commit suicide or make suicide attempts, they do so most often because of the prejudice, hatred, and sometimes violence they have endured from mainstream society.

Data from Harvard Medical School 1986; Roy 1995; Hoff 1994.

cumstances in a person's cultural and social environment may correlate with a person's opting for death over life. Durkheim is the pioneer of sociological research in the study of suicide. The principal types of suicide found in his studies are as follows:

1. *Egotistic suicide* occurs when a person lacks purpose in life and feels insufficiently integrated into society.
2. *Anomic suicide* occurs when a person feels isolated from others through changes in social status or social norms.
3. *Altruistic suicide* occurs as a response to societal demands, for example, as in the deaths of Buddhist monks and of nuns who set themselves on fire to protest the Vietnam War.

One extension of Durkheim's theory proposes that the more integrated individuals are in a given society, the lower is the risk of suicide. For example, the more meaningful the occupational roles and the higher the status of integration, the lower is the suicidal risk (Adam 1985).

Biochemical-Genetic Theories

It is difficult to distinguish biochemical or genetic predispositions to suicide from predispositions to depression or alcoholism. Both of these disorders run in families and most likely have a genetic component. However, low levels of the neurotransmitter serotonin (5-HT) are thought to play a part in the decision to commit suicide. Low serotonin levels are related to depressed moods. In a study of people hospitalized for suicide attempts, those with low serotonin levels were more likely to commit suicide than those with normal levels (Roy 1995a). A study by Pandey and colleagues (1995) observed a higher number of serotonin-2 receptors (5-HT-2) in both the brain and platelets of suicidal patients. Therefore, it is possible that 5-HT-2 receptors may represent biological markers for identifying suicide-prone patients.

From a genetic point of view, a study of groups of twins in which one twin had committed suicide found a significant concordance rate for the monozygotic twins (those that shared the same genetic make-up) as compared with dizygotic twins (those with separate genetic material) (Roy et al. 1995).

ASSESSMENT

Nurses in all areas of work are in contact with people who have a high potential for suicidal behaviors. Patients on the general medical-surgical units often suffer losses in health or losses of function. Many people are hospitalized for alcohol-related medical problems or have alcoholism as a secondary diagnosis. These two groups make up about one half of all completed suicides.

On maternity wards, women are often undergoing situational crises that may be related to an unwanted newborn or loss of a newborn. On gynecological or surgical units, removal of a breast or uterus can be experienced as traumatic mutilation, resulting in alteration in self-concept and personal identity. In specialized areas, such as burn units and intensive care units, nurses are continually dealing with people in physical and emotional crises.

Nurses working with women who are battered or people with a history of child abuse sshould know that this population is also at high risk for suicide. Appropriate interventions through referral for a psychiatric consultation or for counseling can prevent a suicide attempt or the actual act of suicide in many high-risk clients.

Three areas of assessment will be discussed: (a) verbal and nonverbal suicidal clues, (b) the lethality of the suicide plan, and (c) high-risk factors.

Verbal and Nonverbal Clues

Almost all people considering suicide send out clues, especially to people they think of as supportive. Nurses often fit this category. Clues may be verbal, behavioral, somatic, or emotional.

VERBAL CLUES	EXAMPLES
Overt statements	"I can't take it anymore." "Life isn't worth living anymore." "I wish I were dead." "Everyone would be better off if I died."
Covert statements	"It's OK now, soon everything will be fine." "Things will never work out." "I won't be a problem much longer." "Nothing feels good to me anymore, and probably never will." "How can I give my body to medical science?"

The nurse should always make overt what is covert. Most often it is a relief for people contemplating suicide to finally talk to someone about their despair and loneliness. Asking someone if he or she is thinking of suicide does *not* "give a person ideas." Self-destructive ideas are a personal decision. Making covert indications of suicide overt *does* make possible a decrease in isolation and can increase problem-solving alternatives for living. Pallikkathayil and McBride (1986) found that suicide attempters were extremely receptive to talking about their suicide crisis, even those who regretted the failure of their attempt. Often these people expressed gratitude for the opportunity to talk to someone. Specific questions to ask include the following (Stevenson 1988):

- Are you experiencing thoughts of suicide?
- Have you ever had thoughts of suicide in the past?
- Have you ever attempted suicide?
- Do you have a plan for committing suicide?
- If so, what is your plan for suicide?

The following dialogue illustrates how the nurse can make covert messages overt:

Nurse: You haven't eaten or slept well for the past few days, Mary.
Mary: No, I feel pretty low lately.
Nurse: How low are you feeling?
Mary: Oh, I don't know. Nothing seems to matter to me anymore. It's all so meaningless. . .
Nurse What is meaningless, Mary?
Mary: Life . . . the whole thing . . . nothingness. Life is a bad joke.
Nurse: Are you saying that you don't think life is worth living?
Mary: Well . . . yes. It's all so hopeless anyway.
Nurse: Are you thinking of killing yourself, Mary?
Mary: Oh, I don't know. Well, sometimes I think about it. I probably would never go through with it.
Nurse: Let's talk more about what you are thinking and feeling. Since this is important, Mary, I will need to share your thoughts with other members of the staff.

Be alert for behavioral clues, somatic clues, and emotional clues.

BEHAVIORAL CLUES	EXAMPLES
Sudden behavioral changes may be noted, especially when depression is lifting and when the person has more energy available to carry out a plan.	Signs include giving away prized personal possessions, writing farewell notes, making out a will, and putting personal affairs in order.

SOMATIC CLUES	EXAMPLES
Physiological complaints can mask psychological pain and internalized stress.	Symptoms associated with chronic stress include headaches, muscle aches, difficulty sleeping, irregular bowel habits, unusual appetitie, and weight loss.

EMOTIONAL CLUES	EXAMPLES
Various emotions can signal possible suicidal ideation.	Symptoms include social withdrawal, feelings of hopelessness and helplessness, confusion, irritability, and complaints of exhaustion.

Lethality of Suicide Plan

The evaluation of a suicide plan is extremely important in determining the degree of suicidal risk. There are three main elements to be considered when evaluating the lethality of a suicide plan: (1) specificity of details, (2) lethality of the proposed method, and (3) availability of means (Farberow 1967). People who have definite plans for the time, place, and means are at high risk. Someone who is considering suicide but has not thought about when, where, or how is at a lower risk.

The lethality of method also indicates the level of risk, such as how quickly the person would die by that method, thereby lessening the probability of intervention. Higher-risk methods, also referred to as "hard" methods, include

- Using a gun.
- Jumping off a high place.
- Hanging.
- Carbon monoxide poisoning.
- Staging a car crash.

Example of lower-risk methods, also referred to as "soft" methods, include

- Slashing one's wrists.
- Inhaling house gas.
- Ingesting pills.

One study of persons who had attempted suicide showed that those who used hard methods displayed more social disintegration, were more often psychiatrically ill, and had more negative self-esteem (Schmitt and Mundt 1991).

When the means are available, the situation is more serious. For example, a man who has access to a high building and states that he will jump from it, or a woman who has a gun and says that she will shoot herself, is a serious risk. When people are psychotic, they are at high risk regardless of the specificity of details, lethality of method, and availability of means, because impulse control, judgment, and thinking are all grossly impaired. A psychotic person is particularly vulnerable if experiencing command hallucinations.

High-Risk Factors

Data gathered from numerous studies have identified risk factors. The act of suicide may be precipitated by many internal, external, and coexisting conditions and events. Studies in the literature find that social isolation and severe life events often precede a suicide attempt.

Social Isolation

Suicidal individuals frequently have difficulty forming and maintaining relationships. Usually there is a high rate of divorce, separation, or single marital status (Roy 1995b). Norman Cousins maintains that all human history is an endeavor to shatter loneliness. He tells the story of a woman who had committed suicide. She had written in her diary every day during the week before her death, "Nobody called today, nobody called today, nobody called today" (Mowshowitz 1984).

Severe Life Events

Severe life events often precede a suicide attempt. Paykel and colleagues (1975) found that people who attempted suicide were four times as likely to suffer severe life events (e.g., divorce, death, sickness, blows to self-esteem, legal problems, interpersonal discord) in the 6 months before their attempts as people in the general population. Having serious arguments with a spouse, having a new person in the home (baby, elderly parent), and having to appear in court were more frequent occurrences for persons who attempted suicide than for nonsuicidal persons (Hoff 1995). A study by Parker (1988) found that adolescents attempting suicide experienced more life changes than other adolescents and had a history of emotional illness in the family.

Disadvantageous childhood and family circumstances can lend increased risk and vulnerability to adolescent suicidal behaviors (Fergusson and Lynsky 1995). Low

BOX 24–2 NURSING ASSESSMENT: SAD PERSONS SCALE

S	Sex	Men kill themselves three times more often than women, although women make attempts three time more often than men.
A	Age	High-risk goups: 19 years or younger; 45 years or older, especially the elderly of 65 years or over.
D	Depression	Studies report that 35%–79% of those who attempt suicide manifested a depressive syndrome.
P	Previous attempts	Of those who commit suicide, 65% to 70% have made previous attempts.
E	ETOH	ETOH (alcohol) is associated with up to 65% of successful suicides. Estimates are that 15% of alcoholics commit suicide. Heavy drug use is considered to be in this group and is given the same weight as alcohol.
R	Rational thinking loss	People with functional or organic psychoses are more apt to commit suicide than those in the general population.
S	Social supports lacking	A suicidal person often lacks significant others (friends, relatives), meaningful employment, and religious supports. All three of these areas need to be assessed.
O	Organized plan	The presence of a specific plan for suicide (date, place, means) signifies a person at high risk.
N	No spouse	Repeated studies indicate that persons who are widowed, separated, divorced, or single are at greater risk than those who are married.
S	Sickness	Chronic, debilitating, and severe illness is a risk factor.

Data from Patterson W., et al. (1983). Evaluation of suicidal patients: The SAD PERSONS scale. *Psychosomatics,* 24(4):343; Adam 1989; *Merck manual* 1992; Mueller and Leon 1996.

self-esteem is closely related to feelings of depression and hopelessness and suicidal tendencies. Assessment of adolescents should include an evaluation of self-esteem, and therapies should include the targeting of self-esteem deficits (Overholser et al. 1995).

An important, previously unrecognized risk factor in jail suicide is the charge of manslaughter or murder, as revealed by a study by Durand and associates (1995).

A panel from the National Institute of Mental Health (1995) came to the following conclusions:

- The strongest risk factors for youths are alcohol or other drug use disorders and aggressive or disruptive behaviors.
- The strongest risk factors for adults are depression, alcohol abuse, cocaine use, and separation or divorce.
- Most elderly suicides have visited their primary care physician in the month before their suicide. Recognition and treatment of depression in the medical setting is a promising way to prevent suicide in the elderly.

Many tools can be used to aid a health care worker in assessing suicidal potential. Patterson and co-workers (1983) devised an assessment aid using a brief acronym (**SAD PERSONS scale**) to evaluate ten major risk factors for suicide potential (Box 24–2). The SAD PERSONS assessment is a simple, clear-cut, and practical guide for gauging suicide potential. Ten categories are described in the assessment tool, and the person being evaluated is assigned one point for each applicable category. The person's total points are compared with a scale, which assists health care workers in determining whether hospital admission is necessary. The decision to admit someone to a hospital unit depends on many variables, such as whether the person (1) lives alone, (2) has access to a high-risk weapon, or (3) has attempted suicide previously. The following scale serves as a general guideline:

POINTS	GUIDELINES FOR INTERVENTION
0–2	Treat at home with follow-up care
3–4	Closely follow up and consider possible hospitalization
5–6	Strongly consider hospitalization
7–10	Hospitalize

NURSING DIAGNOSIS

The nursing diagnoses for a person who is suicidal may address many areas. However, the nursing diagnosis with the highest priority is **risk for violence—self-directed,** which may be evidenced by various emotional states. Feelings of hopelessness, anger, poor impulse control, frustration, abandonment, and rejection are common among people who are suicidal. Suicide is often related to a loss. The loss of a significant person can leave a person feeling isolated, panicky, and confused. Loss of job, status, and money, when combined with sickness, can be overwhelming. Risk for self-harm can also be related to crises in adolescents, adults, and the elderly. Identity crisis in adolescents and isolation and loss of spouse in the elderly are situations signaling individuals in trouble.

Ineffective individual coping is also usually present. For example, a person who is clinically depressed, relies heavily on drugs and alcohol, is facing situational or maturational crises, or has chronic mental or physical problems may have impaired problem-solving and coping skills. Therefore, ineffective individual coping may be evidenced by the inability to meet role expectations or to meet basic needs related to heavy use of alcohol or drugs, inadequate psychological resources, or unsatisfactory support systems.

Ineffective family coping is often present. Children or teenagers may be unable to get the guidance, support, and love they need from home. Withdrawal of support by other family members can leave a child feeling abandoned, overwhelmed, and confused. This withdrawal of love and support may be related to the parent's own problems with alcohol or drugs, mental disorders, or perceived desertion through divorce or separation. When there are intense feelings of hostility and intolerance between parents, children often get left out or are manipulated and pitted against either or both parents. Therefore, examples of ineffective family coping may be evidenced by behavior problems in children, break-up of the family unit, chaotic family communication, or highly ambivalent family relationships.

Suicide is an attempt to end an intolerable life situation or state of mind that people feel helpless or powerless to change. Therefore, feelings of hopelessness and powerlessness are often described by people who contemplate suicide.

Hopelessness (the belief that nothing can help change an intolerable situation or experience), plays a major role in most suicides. Hopelessness can be related to a multitude of physical conditions (e.g., acquired immunodeficiency syndrome, cancer) and situations (e.g., financial difficulties, alterations in significant relationships). It can be evidenced by verbal statements and cognitive difficulties (e.g., decreased judgment, decreased problem solving). Hopelessness is particularly prevalent in depressed individuals.

Powerlessness (thinking one has no control over events) may be related to a life style of helplessness or a current situation that the person perceives as untenable and unalterable. An interpersonal interaction may also be regarded as unalterably painful or psychologically traumatic. The person may be left feeling powerless or isolated.

People who think of ending their lives often do not feel very good about themselves. Feelings of worthlessness and expressions of shame or guilt are common among some. Therefore, the diagnoses **disturbance in self-esteem, chronic low self-esteem,** and **spiritual distress** all need serious consideration.

PLANNING

Planning Outcome Criteria

Outcome criteria/goals are set for each nursing diagnosis. The nurse works with the client to set goals that are consistent with the suicidal person's perceptions and ability to carry out the goals. If a person is thought to be actively suicidal, hospitalization may be appropriate.

For the nursing diagnosis **risk for violence—self-inflicted,** the following goals may apply:

OUTCOME CRITERIA

- Client will state by (date) that he or she wants to live.
- By (date), client will name two people he or she can call if thoughts of suicide recur.
- Client will name one acceptable alternative to his or her situation by (date).

SHORT-TERM GOALS

- Client will remain safe while in the hospital.
- Client will make a no-suicide contract with the nurse covering the next 24 hours.
- Client will talk about painful feelings (guilt, anger, loneliness) by (date).

Ineffective Individual Coping. When people are depressed or suicidal, they are often unable to see choices or make decisions that could change their situation. This phenomenon is referred to as *tunnel vision.* Clarifying hazards for the client and facilitating the expression of negative feelings are basic interventions. When clients are able to explore alternatives to their situation, changes in thinking and behavior are possible. When alternatives to suicide are acceptable, feelings of hopelessness diminish.

Therefore, outcome criteria for **ineffective individual coping,** as evidenced by faulty problem solving, could include the following:

OUTCOME CRITERIA

- Client will describe two new coping mechanisms used successfully in a stressful situation.
- Client will state one decision that he or she has made that will improve the situation.
- Client will name signs and symptoms that indicate that he or she is starting to feel overwhelmed.
- Client will name two persons to whom he or she can talk if suicidal thoughts recur in the future.

SHORT-TERM GOALS

- Client will discuss with the nurse situations that trigger suicidal thoughts, and feelings about these situations, by (date).
- Client will identify three past coping mechanisms, and state which were useful and which were not by (date).
- Client will name two effective ways to handle difficult situations in the future by (date).
- Client will state that he or she feels comfortable with one new technique after three sessions of role playing.

Ineffective Family Coping. Often a suicidal person is living within a family unit (with spouse, children, parent(s), or other significant others). The hopelessness, desperation, irritability, and withdrawal of the suicidal person profoundly affect other members of the family. Feelings of anxiety, denial, guilt, anger, frustration, and hopelessness arise in those close to a suicidal person. In many cases the suicidal behavior is a reaction to dysfunctional family behavior. If the motive is to instill guilt in a significant person to control and extract revenge, the whole family unit may be in crisis. Therefore, the whole family needs support and counseling.

For a diagnosis of **ineffective family coping** related to ineffective patterns of communication, the following outcome criteria may be included:

OUTCOME CRITERIA

- Each family member will state that he or she feels less guilty, angry, or manipulated now (using a scale from 1 to 10) than before working with the nurse.
- Each family member will describe how he or she has been better able to communicate with the suicidal member.
- Each family member will state that he or she feels supported (by nurse, counselor, or therapist) and less confused and angry.
- Each family member will state that the communication among all members of the family has improved.

SHORT-TERM GOALS

- Each family member will describe two feelings toward the suicidal member by (date).
- Each family member will state what he or she thinks the problem is by (date).
- Each family member will state three referral sources available for individual or family counseling, support, and guidance during the crises.

Disturbance in Self-Esteem, Chronic Low Self-Esteem, and Spiritual Distress. Although the motives for suicide may vary and the number of precipitating events may be infinite, all persons with suicidal ideation suffer similar feelings. Intense feelings of deprivation of affection, lack of hope for the future, and profound feelings of worthlessness and having nowhere to turn or no one (or no power) to trust in are common.

The diagnosis of **disturbance in self-esteem, chronic low self-esteem,** or **spiritual distress** related to feelings of worthlessness may have the following associated outcomes:

LONG-TERM OUTCOMES

- Client will name three personal strengths.
- Client will participate in two activities that he or she enjoys and does well.
- Client will state that he or she feels more comfortable around people.
- Client will name one project he or she has completed and feels proud of.
- Client will report feeling better about self.
- Client will state that belief in "a higher power" is a renewed source of strength.

SHORT-TERM GOALS

- Client will state that he or she will continue meeting with the nurse/counselor on a regular basis by (date).
- Client will talk about painful feelings with the nurse/counselor by (date).
- Client will begin to look at personal strengths as well as weaknesses by (date).
- Client will participate in his or her treatment plan by (date).
- Client will participate in religious activities that had previously been a source of strength by (date).

Nurse's Feelings and Self-Assessment

People who are suicidal present affect and behavior that are difficult for nurses to deal with effectively. *All* health care professionals who work with suicidal people need supervision and guidance by a more experienced health care professional. Most people who are suicidal experience extreme hopelessness and helplessness, are withdrawn and keenly sensitive to rejection, are ambivalent, and may be hostile and angry. Affects such as these can stir up strong negative reactions in others. Birtchnell (1983) identified in the literature numerous reactions that often arise in health care workers when working with a client who is suicidal. If these and other intense emotional responses are not made known and discussed with a more experienced practitioner, effective intervention will be limited, especially if these feelings are perceived by the suicidal client.

When these feelings are *not* identified, discussed, and resolved, the least that may happen is that the nurse will feel incompetent, experience low self-esteem, and become angry at the client for arousing these feelings. The worst that may happen is escalation or perpetuation of the client's painful feelings. Clients may interpret the nurse's anxiety, irritation, and avoidance as validation for their own feelings of poor self-regard and self-hate. When feelings of hopelessness and poor self-esteem escalate, so does the potential for suicide.

The universal reactions of anxiety, irritation, avoidance, and denial in any health care worker caring for a suicidal person are discussed below.

ANXIETY. Anxiety may have numerous sources. However, it is important to recognize that two common sources of anxiety are activated when a nurse is working with a suicidal client. First, Birtchnell (1983) states that there are suicidal inclinations in all of us. A suicidal patient has the capacity to arouse these latent emotions and perhaps bring them out more strongly. Second, suicidal behavior or ideations on the part of the client may be interpreted by concerned health care personnel as personal rejection. Both sources of anxiety are usually working at an unconscious level. Nurses must become aware of their own anxiety and attempt to identify the source, or the unmet need or expectation. Personal anxiety can then be reduced and not transferred to the client.

IRRITATION. People who make repeated suicide attempts are often accused by family as well as health care workers of just "trying to get attention" or "looking for sympathy." It is common to hear of friends or family members out of frustration telling a suicidal person to "go ahead and get it over with." Such remarks by family and health providers strip the suicidal person of all hope and act as an encouragement to kill himself or herself. No matter how trivial the suicidal attempt may appear, it is a genuine communication that the person is despairing and is unable to find a way out of a desperate situation or state of mind.

AVOIDANCE. People who are suicidal and people who are psychotic are frequently kept at a distance and "handled with kid gloves" by both medical and nursing personnel (Birtchnell 1983). Nurses and physicians may get caught up into taking responsibility for the actions of the suicidal person (rescue fantasy). Then, when things do not go the way the nurse or physician would like them to go, helplessness sets in. Staff then avoid situations or people that stimulate feelings of helplessness and incompetence. When the need to feel in control and responsible for other people's decisions is lessened through experience and supervision, the nurse is better able to refocus energies back to the client.

DENIAL. Denying or minimizing suicidal ideation or gestures is a defense against experiencing the feelings aroused by a suicidal person. Denial can be seen in such statements as "I can't understand why anyone would want to take his own life." Often, family members and health care professionals are unable to acknowledge suicidal tendencies in someone close to them. Denial also occurs when identification with a suicidal person is strong, such as when a colleague commits suicide or a respected figurehead sends forth covert suicidal messages.

PERSONAL STAGES HEALTH CARE WORKERS PASS THROUGH. Hammel-Bissell (1985) documents the "rites of passage" that psychiatric nurses must go through in order to work effectively with a suicidal person. Four stages are presented, each progressing to the next as the nurse works through expected feelings and reactions.

1. Stage 1: *naïveté*, in which feelings of shock and denial are prominent.
2. Stage 2: *recognition*, which involves feelings of anxiety, fear, helplessness, and confusion.
3. Stage 3: *responsibility*, which brings with it a cycle of feeling responsible, guilty, and then angry. This is a very conflicting time for people working with suicidal persons. It is crucial that during this time the nurse is helped by supervision and peer support. Nurses need to vent these feelings and benefit from the experience of others who have gone beyond this stage. Otherwise, they may suffer burnout, may distance themselves from colleagues and clients, or may leave the work situation altogether.
4. Stage 4: *individual choice*, which stems from awareness gained through supervision, continuing education, and/or personal therapy. This is the stage when the nurse comes to the realization that the client is the only one in charge of his or her life. This frees the nurse to do whatever is humanly possible to help the client, while realizing that one person cannot ultimately control the decisions of another.

IMPLEMENTATION

Suicide intervention can be divided into three distinct areas: primary, secondary, and tertiary.

Primary intervention includes activities that provide support, information, and education in situations that could otherwise become more serious and even lethal. Primary intervention can be practiced in schools, home, hospitals, and industrial settings.

Secondary intervention is treatment of the actual suicidal crisis. It is practiced in clinics, in hospitals, and on telephone hotlines. Most people who are suicidal do not necessarily want to die; they just do not know how to go on living in an intolerable situation or state of mind. The client's ambivalence is one of the most important tools a nurse has when working with a suicidal person.

Tertiary intervention/postvention can refer to (1) interventions with family and friends of a person who has committed suicide or (2) interventions with a person who has recently attempted suicide. Tertiary intervention for the latter is geared toward minimizing the traumatic after-effects of the suicide attempt.

Counseling (Basic Level)

Counseling skills used by the nurse working with a client who is suicidal are practiced (1) in the community, (2) in hospitals, and (3) on telephone hotlines. The key element is the establishment of a workable relationship. There is general agreement by workers in this field on the importance of warmth, sensitivity, interest, concern, and consistency on the part of the helping person. Studies indicate that any treatment modality can be effective as long as it (1) includes the establishment of a personal relationship with the suicidal person, (2) encourages more realistic problem-solving behavior, and (3) reaffirms hope (Evans 1983).

Material from the McKinley Health Center (1996) states that most suicides can be prevented by sensitive response to the person in crisis. You should

- *Remain calm.* In most instances, there is no rush. Sit and listen—really listen—to what the person is saying. Give understanding and active emotional support for his or her feelings.
- *Deal directly with the topic of suicide.* Most individuals have mixed feelings about death and dying and are open to help. Don't be afraid to ask or talk directly about suicide.
- *Encourage problem solving and positive actions.* Remember that the person involved in emotional crisis is not thinking clearly; encourage him or her to refrain from making any serious, irreversible decisions while in a crisis. Talk about the positive alternatives that may establish hope for the future.
- *Get assistance.* Although you want to help, do not take full responsibility by trying to be the sole counsel. Seek out resources that can lend qualified help, even if it means breaking a confidence. Let the troubled person know you are concerned—so concerned that you are willing to arrange help beyond that which you can offer.

The University of California at Los Angeles (UCLA) suicide prevention experts have summarized the information to be conveyed to the person in crisis as follows:

1. The crisis is temporary.
2. Unbearable pain can be survived.
3. Help is available.
4. You are not alone.

There is no place for hostility, sarcasm, or power struggles in the treatment of a suicidal person. These responses only enhance poor self-esteem and feelings of hopelessness. Efforts should be geared toward maintaining or raising the suicidal person's self-esteem and self-respect. Cassem (1980) states that "self-esteem or self-respect is the most basic psychic condition to be guarded if life is to continue."

Community

Usually, people in suicidal crisis are seen in emergency rooms and referred to an outpatient clinic. Indeed, if after initial assessment the person is thought to be at low risk and not in need of hospitalization, referral to a clinic for crisis counseling is always indicated. Hoff (1995) names six techniques that are useful in an outpatient community setting:

TECHNIQUE	ACTION
1. Relieve isolation	1. Arrange for the person to stay with family or friends. If no one is available and the person is highly suicidal, hospitlization must be considered.
2. Remove all weapons.	2. Weapons and pills are removed by friends, relatives, or the nurse.
3. Encourage alternative expression of anger.	3. Have the person talk freely about feelings, unmet expectations, and disappointments. Plan with the person alternative ways of handling frustration and anger.
4. Avoid final decision for suicide during crisis.	4. Assure the person that the suicidal crisis is a temporary state. Encourage the person to avoid a decision until alternatives can be considered during a noncrisis state (see subsequent discussion of no-suicide contract).
5. Re-establish social ties.	5. Contact family members. Arrange for family crisis counseling. Activates links to self-help groups: e.g., Widow-To-Widow, Parents Without Partners, and Al-a-Teen.
6. Relieve extreme anxiety and sleep loss.	6. After thorough assess ment, a tranquilizer may be prescribed to induce sleep and lower anxiety. **Note: only a 1- to 3-day supply should be given, and only with a return appointment for crisis counseling.**

All persons receiving crisis counseling for suicidal ideations or actual suicide attempts should be given the opportunity for follow-up counseling or psychotherapy after the immediate crisis is over. A **no-suicide contract** between a counselor and a suicidal client has been used successfully in numerous settings, such as individual therapy, family therapy, group work, and behavioral therapy. The contract is outlined in clear and simple language. The purpose of the no-suicide contract is to give the counselor time to explore alternatives with the client. When the time of the contract is up, the contract is renegotiated. Examples of entries in a no-suicide contract include the following:

- "I will talk to my counselor if I have thoughts of harming myself."

- "I will wait until next week when I see my counselor before I take any action to harm myself."
- "I will go to the hospital emergency room if I start to have suicidal impulses."
- "I won't kill myself, either on purpose or accidentally, for any reason."

A 1-page written contract is signed by the client. Some counselors insert a clause stating that the person will report the importance of the contract to someone (e.g., counselor, friend, wife) at least once daily. If the client is in the hospital, he or she will talk to the nurse.

Crisis counseling is imperative for a person who is suicidal. Such a person may be in an acute crisis situation or may be chronically suicidal. A person who is chronically suicidal usually has the following clinical history (Hatton et al. 1977):

1. Has eliminated all resources—is isolated and withdrawn from significant others.
2. Abuses alcohol, drugs, or both.
3. Has recurrent depression.
4. Has made several previous suicide threats or attempts over a period of several years.
5. Has made numerous bids for help, with little or no relief.
6. Presents with instability in job performance, interpersonal relationships, or both.

Crisis counseling can be effective for the chronically suicidal person; however, it cannot alter personality patterns. More research and clinical study are needed in the areas of formulating a treatment plan and intervening successfully with such persons.

Hospital

How and when to use hospitalization is somewhat controversial. *Danger to self or others* is a general guideline. Legalities are often an important consideration. Either too much or too little restraint may be grounds for liability. Too much restraint may be grounds for abridgment of civil rights; too little restraint may be grounds for malpractice. Generally, if the primary counselor (e.g., nurse, social worker, psychologist) determines that the person is highly suicidal, has no immediate supports, and is exhausted and unable to carry out an alternative to suicide, hospitalization is indicated (Hatton et al. 1977). However, some people are more responsive to treatment when they are not under constant observation.

Even when the decision for hospitalization is made, there are no hospitals that are 100% "suicide proof." Every hospital should have a suicide protocol that attempts to ensure the suicidal client's safety. *Students are advised to become familiar with the suicide protocol in the hospital or community setting they are affiliated with.* Box 24–3 lists guidelines for minimizing suicidal behavior on a psychiatric unit.

Box 24–3 GUIDELINES FOR MINIMIZING SUICIDAL BEHAVIOR ON A PSYCHIATRIC UNIT

THE CLIENT

1. Suicide **precaution**, include one-on-one monitoring, having client in view at all times (one arm's length distance between staff member and client).
   a. Includes during toileting
   b. Includes during the night
2. Suicide **observation** includes a 15-minute visual check of suicidal client.
3. For each of the above, behavior, mood, and verbatim statements are recorded in the chart every 15 minutes.

THE ENVIRONMENT

1. Use plastic utensils.
2. Do not allow clients to spend too much time alone in their rooms. Do not assign to a private room.
3. Jump-proof and hang proof the bathrooms by installing break-away shower rods and recessed shower nozzels.
4. Keep electrical cords to a minimal length.
5. Install unbreakable glass in windows. Install tamper-proof screens or partitions too small to pass through. Keep all windows locked.
6. Lock all utility rooms, kitchens, adjacent stairwells, and offices. All nonclinical staff (e.g., housekeepers, maintenance workers) should receive instructions to keep doors locked.
7. Take all potentially harmful gifts (e.g., flowers in glass vases) from visitors before allowing them to see clients.
8. Go through client's belongings with client and remove all potentially harmful objects (e.g., belts, shoelaces, metal nail files, tweezers, matches, razors).
9. Ensure that visitors do not leave potentially harmful objects in client's room (e.g., matches, nail files).
10. Search clients for harmful objects (e.g., drugs, sharp objects, cords) on return from pass.

Data from Schultz, B. M. (1982). *Legal liability in psychotherapy.* San Francisco: Jossey-Bass.

Suicide precautions are meant to provide the client with a sense of security. If the client loses control and makes a suicidal attempt, the staff will step in and assume control. Built into the suicide protocol are frequent interactions between staff and the suicidal client, for example, once every 30 minutes or three times a day for 15 minutes. (See "Milieu Therapy" for structuring a therapeutic environment while the suicidal person is in the hospital.)

When suicidal adolescents are admitted to a psychiatric unit, further restrictions may be imposed. Phone calls and visitation rights are often limited to the family only; friends, schoolmates, and girlfriends and boyfriends are restricted. This is done to reduce the incidence of *secondary gains* and maintain personal dignity. (Secondary gains are discussed and defined in Chapter 18.) It is best to minimize positive reinforcement of suicide as a means of receiving attention and sympathy and of temporarily relieving feelings of isolation. Better problem-solving techniques and more satisfying ways of achieving attention, affection, and a sense of belonging are explored with the adolescent client.

Telephone Hotlines

A counselor on a telephone hotline is often a lay person or volunteer who has had special training. At other times, friends, neighbors, relatives, police officers, nurses, and the clergy find themselves at the other end of a telephone cry for help. Almost all persons who are suicidal are ambivalent.

Ambivalence is one of the best tools a nurse has when working with a suicidal individual. Talking with a helping person can help increase the suicidal person's likelihood of staying alive and can provide time to evaluate alternative actions. Essentially, the helping person attempts to establish rapport, identify the problem, assess the lethality of the situation, determine appropriate resources, and establish a plan with the caller.

Establish Rapport

Keeping the person on the line as long as possible is the most important thing. As long as the person keeps talking, he or she is not acting out suicidal threats. It is often helpful to acknowledge the person's distress. Although you do not know how people feel, you can tell them that you understand they are in distress and are extremely unhappy. This lets them know that

- You take their concerns seriously.
- There is no need to complete the suicidal act to make it clear that they are in distress.
- Other alternatives are available.

For example (Neville and Barnes 1985), "The fact that you are considering suicide makes it clear that you are feeling overwhelmed and need some assistance, but there is no need for you to hurt yourself without first talking about what can be done to help you."

Establishing rapport may also be contingent on allowing ventilation of the caller's feelings. The helping person often has to accept angry or manipulative communication. The goal is to keep the caller talking and provide a psychological lifeline.

Reinforcing the caller's positive responses is also useful. Any positive responses, thoughts, and actions that the person communicates need to be met with a validation that these were positive and in the person's best interests. For example, if the caller says that he or she was thinking about suicide but decided to call first, this should be reinforced as a positive move (Neville and Barnes 1985): "Your calling me at this time was a very positive move; I am glad you decided to call now."

Identify the Problem

The problem needs to be clearly identified. As with all crisis situations, the problem-solving approach is used. Reflection and restating are often *not* useful in crisis situations (see Chapter 14 for interventions in crisis). The use of problem-solving approaches is helpful. Problem-solving statements help define the problem and explore avenues of action. For example:

- To whom have you talked about your parent's divorce?
- How do you think the divorce will change your relationship with your parents?
- Have you told them/him/her?
- Do you think that they no longer love you?

Assess the Lethality of the Situation

1. If the caller is threatening suicide, evaluate the lethality of the plan.
2. If the caller has already taken pills, determine what kind and how many, whether he or she has been drinking, and other relevant medical information.
3. Determine whether there is someone nearby—neighbor, bystander, housekeeper, or manager. If the answer is yes, tell the caller that you want to speak to that person right now.
4. If not, try to get the caller's address and explain that you want to get help for him or her.
5. If the caller does not want to give you the address, instruct him or her on first aid:
   - Taking pills—induce vomiting.
   - Bleeding—apply pressure with bandage.
   - Inhalation poisoning—get fresh air, loosen tight clothing.
6. Pass a note to a staff member to attempt to have the call traced. Notify the telephone operator and then the police.

Evaluate Positive Coping and Encourage Alternatives

Has the caller felt this way in the past? What did he or she do then? What works best? What could the caller do differently in this situation? What does the caller think would help change his or her situation? Give referrals to appropriate places in the community that may help alter the situation.

Negotiate a No-Suicide Plan

As stated, a clearly worded contract with the caller may give the helping person time to work with the caller on more alternatives. Ideally, the aim is to get the caller into crisis counseling. If that is not possible, a relationship can be attempted over the phone. The wording in the contract should be clear and not conditional. Words such as "try" and "unless" are *not* used.

NOT USEFUL	MORE USEFUL
"I will *try* not to kill myself."	"When I have thoughts of killing myself, I will go see my counselor."
"I will not kill myself *unless* my wife leaves me."	"If my wife does leave me, I will call my counselor right away."
"I will not kill myself *until* I call you."	"When I have thoughts of killing myself, I will talk to you."

Densmore (1997) cautions against using the words *should* or *would* when writing a no-suicide contract. These terms may seem critical and authoritarian to some clients and be experienced as infantilizing. Densmore further states that training and experience are still the most important variables in soliciting a no-suicide contract.

It is necessary that the person staffing the telephone hotline have numerous community resources available for referral. Besides the names and addresses of the resource, telephone numbers and names of contact persons should also be given whenever possible. Dependence is placed on the caller to contact resources for more long-term assistance.

It is important that callers be made aware that they do have control over their own decisions and that they believe someone cares about the situation and is available.

Research on the ability of telephone counseling to reduce suicide rates and effect behavioral change is sparse. However, one study evaluating the effectiveness of telephone contact with a group of elderly people living alone suggests that it was useful in minimizing the suicide rate of this population (DeLeo et al. 1995).

Health Teaching (Basic Level)

Primary intervention in the form of health teaching is an important way to lessen suicidal attempts. The goal is to reach people before they become so overwhelmed that suicide appears to be a rational alternative. Primary intervention relates to the principles of good mental health. The following programs provide support, information, and education:

- Programs on emotional health in junior and senior high schools
- Drug and alcohol courses that allow "rap sessions" in grade schools and junior and senior high schools
- Special programs in industry for the drug and alcohol abuser
- Seminars for all health care providers on assessment and intervention in suicide, especially for those working in schools, industry, and well-baby clinics
- Seminars and group activities for the elderly that focus on (1) physical concerns such as reactions to medications and physical changes and (2) emotional concerns such as how to cope with loneliness, separations from family, and loss of friends through death

Milieu Therapy (Basic Level)

Hospitalization is sometimes the most therapeutic environment during the acute suicidal phase. Placing a highly suicidal person in a controlled hospital environment can provide structure and control and can give the person time to evaluate his or her situation with professional staff. During hospitalization, the client's suicidal risk and the level of suicidal precaution needed are continually assessed. Table 24–2 lists guidelines for suicide precautions. Repeated monitoring of a person's suicidal intent and extent of hopelessness is ongoing. The decision to discontinue suicide precautions is ideally based on clinical observations of nursing staff, physicians, and social workers, as well as on input from the client. Therefore, the decision to continue or discontinue suicide precautions should be based on subjective data and objective clinical observations.

After the acute phase, more long-term goals can be put into place. Because social isolation and withdrawal are often present, active encouragement and advice about contacting significant persons and loved ones needs to be given. Renewal of friendships and important relationships can help foster self-esteem. When the crisis pertains to a significant other (e.g., spouse, parent, child), therapies such as family, couple, or group counseling may be indicated.

Community agencies may be useful in helping a person renew or initiate activities related to work, special interests, hobbies, sports, and other activities that can help enhance self-esteem.

Psychobiological Interventions (Basic Level)

In cases in which extreme anxiety and lack of sleep last for several days, the risk of suicide can increase. An anxiolytic will usually take care of both the anxiety and the sleeping problem. If medication is given, the supply should be *for 1 to 3 days only*, with a return appointment scheduled for re-evaluation. Anxiolytics, however, should never be given to a highly suicidal individual. Generally, a lethal dose for anxiolytics is ten times the normal dose. When a drug is combined with alcohol, only half that amount can cause death (Hoff 1995).

When a coexisting psychiatric condition is present in a person who is suicidal, somatic intervention is dictated according to the psychopathology. For example, a person who is suicidal and also has the diagnosis of schizophrenia may need increased antipsychotic medication. Similar

TABLE 24–2 SUMMARY OF LEVELS OF SUICIDE PRECAUTIONS

POPULATION	EXAMPLES OF CLIENT SYMPTOMS	NURSING CARE
	Level I	
Clients who have suicidal ideations and who, after assessment by staff, are assessed to be in minimal danger of actively attempting suicide.	1. The client with vague suicidal ideation but without plan 2. The client who is willing to make a no-suicide contract 3. The client with insight into existing problems	1. Check client's whereabouts every 15–30 minutes. 2. Maintain frequent verbal contact while client is awake. 3. Chart client's whereabouts, mood, verbatim statements, and behavior every 15–30 minutes. 4. *
	Level II	
Clients with suicidal ideations and who, after assessment by unit staff, present clinical symptoms that indicate a suicide potential higher than level I.	1. The client with a concrete suicide plan 2. The client who is ambivalent about making a no-suicide contract 3. The client with minimal insight into existing problems 4. The client with limited impulse control	1. Conduct close observation* (i.e., within visual range of staff) while client is awake. Accompany to bathroom. Place client in multiple-client room. Check client every 15–30 minutes while client is awake. 2. Chart client's whereabouts, mood, verbatim statements, behavior every 15–30 minutes. 3. Ensure that meal trays contain no glass, metal silverware, or other sharps. 4. *
	Level III	
Clients with suicidal ideations or delusions of self-mutilation who, according to assessment by unit staff, present clinical symptoms that suggest a clear intent to follow through with the plan or delusion.	1. The client who is currently verbalizing a clear intent to harm self 2. The client who is unwilling to make a no-suicide contract 3. The client who presents with no insight into existing problems 4. The client with poor impulse control 5. The client who has already attempted suicide in the recent past by a particularly lethal method (e.g., hanging, gun, carbon monoxide poisoning)	1. Conduct one-to-one nursing observation and interaction 24 hours a day (never out of staff's sight). 2. Maintain arm's length at all times. 3. Chart client's whereabouts, mood, verbatim statements, and behavior every 15–30 minutes. 4. Ensure that meal trays contain no glass or metal silverware. 5. *

*The nurse and physician explain to the client what the nurse will be doing and why. Both nurse and physician document this in the chart.
Data adapted from: Busteen, E. L., and Johnstone, C. (1983). The development of suicide precautions for an inpatient unit. *Journal of Psychosocial Nursing and Mental Health Services, 21* (5): 18.

considerations are made for people who are clinically depressed as well as suicidal. Electroconvulsive therapy can save the life of a seriously depressed and highly suicidal person. See Chapter 20 for further information regarding electroconvulsive therapy. It can take 1 to 3 weeks of antidepressant therapy before the person experiences an elevation of mood. Electroconvulsive therapy can have more immediate effects.

Psychotherapy (Advanced Practice)

Suicidal Person

Initial intervention for a suicidal person consists of crisis intervention. However, all persons should be offered the opportunity for further therapy after the crisis is over. A nurse educated at the master's level may work with suicidal clients in several modalities. Suitable therapies have been mentioned. Couple, individual, family, and group counseling are all useful. This is especially true if a person is chronically suicidal or has coexisting psychopathology, such as depression, borderline symptoms, and schizophrenic disorders.

Family

A variety of family interventions have been applied to the treatment of families with a suicidal member. Carlson and Asarnow (1995) report a cognitive-behavioral model that is a six-session family treatment for adolescent suicide attempters and their families. This approach employs six intervention strategies:

1. Exercises designed to establish a positive family atmosphere
2. Exercises designed to help family members recognize and label their feelings

3. Exercises designed to teach a basic approach to problem solving
4. Use of role playing, scripts, and interactions with feedback to try out new ways of relating
5. Negotiating skills with practice
6. Practicing enjoying pleasant activities and sharing positive feelings

Survivors of Completed Suicide: Postvention

Intervention for family and friends ("survivors") of a person who has committed suicide should be initiated within 24 to 72 hours after the death. Natural feelings of denial and avoidance predominate during the first 24 hours (Thompson 1996). Mourning the death of a loved one who has committed suicide is painful at all times. The family of a person who has committed suicide is often faced with the process of mourning without the normal informal social supports usually provided. Unfortunately, neighbors, acquaintances, and even family friends are often confused and may blame the family for the death. Families of members who have committed suicide are often stigmatized and cut off and isolated from the usual supports during the time of mourning. Survivors often feel that they are "going crazy." They need to be told that these feelings are normal. Survivors need to find outlets for the undercurrent of anger against the deceased, who is responsible for the trauma, confusion, and pain inflicted on them. Unfortunately, few friends or family members of a person who has committed suicide seek out counseling. Pronounced feelings of anger and guilt are common reactions.

Thompson (1996) states that persons exposed to traumatic events such as suicide or sudden loss often manifest the following posttraumatic stress reactions: irritability, sleep disturbance, anxiety, startle reaction, nausea, headache, difficulty concentrating, confusion, fear, guilt, withdrawal, anger, and reactive depression. The particular pattern of the emotional reaction and type of response will differ with each survivor depending on the relationship of the deceased, circumstances surrounding the death, and coping mechanisms of the survivors. The ultimate contribution of suicide or sudden loss intervention in survivor groups is to create an appropriate and meaningful opportunity to respond to suicide or sudden death. (Refer to Chapter 17 for posttraumatic stress reaction.)

To reduce the trauma associated with the sudden loss, posttraumatic loss debriefing can help initiate an adaptive grief process and prevent self-defeating behaviors. Stages of posttraumatic loss debriefing are as follows (Thompson 1996):

1. *Introductory stage.* Introduce survivors to the debriefing process.
2. *Fact stage.* Information is gathered to "recreate the event" from what is known about it.
3. *Life review stage.* The opportunity to share "remember when . . ." stories lessens tension and anxiety within the survivor group.
4. *Feeling stage.* Feelings are identified and integrated into the process.
5. *Reaction stage.* Explore the physical and cognitive stress reactions to the traumatic event.
6. *Learning stage.* Assist survivors in learning new coping skills to deal with their grief reactions.
7. *Closure stage.* Wrap up loose ends, answer outstanding questions, provide final assurances, and create a plan of action that is life centered.

Self-help groups have been found to be extremely beneficial for survivors of a suicidal family member or friend. Many people join self-help groups even if the suicide took place 25 to 30 years before.

Self-help groups for the survivors of a family member or friend who committed suicide are similar to all other self-help groups. Essentially, these groups for family survivors are run by people who have lost someone through suicide. When a professional is involved, it is in the role of facilitator, consultant, or educator—not that of leader. Ideally, lay leaders should have some professional training in group processes and awareness of the limitations of the group experience. Professional therapists (e.g., nurses, social workers, psychiatrists, psychologists) should be used as a source of referral and should be available for consulting. Referral for individual and family therapy is advised once individual and family problems have been identified.

Counselors and Nursing Staff: Postvention

Staff and therapists who have been working with a client who successfully commits suicide also need support. Staff should have the opportunity to make adequate emotional expression of feelings of self-blame, guilt, and anger. If one of the staff has been closely involved over a long period with the client who has committed suicide, the staff member will also pass through a period of grief. Suicide can be a real possibility for a therapist involved in direct client care. Feelings of anger and guilt, loss of self-esteem, and intrusive thoughts about the suicide are common. Symptoms similar to those of posttraumatic stress disorder were experienced by a significant percentage of psychiatrists who had a client who committed suicide (Chemtob et al. 1988). Peer support and supervision help work through the loss.

A thorough psychological postmortem assessment should be carried out among staff. This can be a traumatic time for staff and group support, and processing the event can be healing. The suicidal event is reviewed to identify overlooked clues, faulty judgments, or changes in protocols that could be useful when evaluating future clients. Discussion during the postmortem should center on piecing together the pressures that led up to the client's taking his or her life.

CASE STUDY: Working With a Person Who is Suicidal

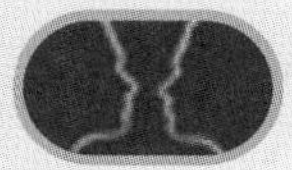

Thomas Martin, a 46-year-old social worker, was brought to the hospital for evaluation after an attempted suicide. When he did not show up for work, his co-worker called to check on him. His landlady stated that his car was still in the driveway and that she would check his room. She found Mr. Martin lying on the bed, beside him an empty bottle of sleeping pills. A strong smell of liquor filled the room and a nearly empty bottle of scotch was on a table by the bed. An ambulance took Mr. Martin to the emergency department, where his stomach was lavaged. He stayed in the emergency room (ER) for 16 hours until he was no longer groggy. He was then seen by a psychiatric nurse, Mrs. Ruiz, for evaluation.

He told Mrs. Ruiz that he had been separated from his wife for 2 years but had seen his 8-year-old son every week during that time. Three days before his suicide attempt, his wife sent him a letter stating that she wanted to remarry and move to Oklahoma with her son and new husband.

ASSESSMENT

Mr. Martin's manner was hostile and sarcastic. He told the nurse that it did not matter what anyone did, he would "do it again," and that next time he would succeed. He sat sneering at the nurse, saying "I never liked nurses anyway."

Nurse: What is it about nurses that you don't like?

Mr. M: *(mimicking the nurse's tone)* What is it about nurses that you don't like—what drivel. Don't try that therapeutic garbage on me. I don't need help from you or anyone else.
(Silence)
You're all castrating bitches . . . all women are. I hate all women.

Nurse: Tell me about one woman who has hurt you.

Mr. M: *(angrily)* . . . Stop prying into my business with your little therapeutic diddies.
(Silence)
Well . . . my wife . . . she . . . she . . . oh God . . . *At this point Mr. Martin starts sighing deeply, then bursts into tears.*

Nurse: *Waits a few minutes.* This situation with your wife and son moving away has upset you deeply.

Mr. M: I don't want to live if I can't see my son. He is all I have left. He is the only thing that ever mattered to me.

Nurse: You have no friends or family?

Mr. M: All my family died when I was a kid. As for friends . . . I don't need other people. Anyway, people don't seem to like me much. Look, don't spend time worrying about me. I've got a few more tricks up my sleeve.

Nurse: Do you mean that you will try to kill yourself again?

Mr. M: What could it possibly mean to you?

Nurse: I *am* concerned about you, Mr. Martin.

Mr. M: Well . . . isn't that the nursie thing to say. . . . Such great understanding.

Nurse: I do understand that you are very troubled right now and have no one to go to.

Mrs. Ruiz organized her data into objective and subjective components.

OBJECTIVE DATA

1. Male, age 46, no support systems
2. Impending loss of significant relationship with son
3. Possible drinking problem, need more data
4. Suicide attempt
5. Holds responsible job
6. Estranged wife and son moving away from area
7. Appears articulate and bright

SUBJECTIVE DATA

1. "I don't want to live if I can't see my son."
2. "I've got a few more tricks up my sleeve."
3. "He (son) is the only thing that ever mattered to me."
4. "All my family died when I was a kid."
5. "I don't need other people."
6. "People don't seem to like me much."

Continued on following page

NURSING DIAGNOSIS

Mrs. Ruiz analyzed her data and set up her nursing diagnoses in order of priority.

Risk for violence—self-directed related to suicidal behavior and belief that he has no reason to live

- Suicide attempt
- "I don't want to live if I can't see my son."
- "He is the only thing that ever mattered to me."
- "I've got a few more tricks up my sleeve."
- Is holding a responsible job

Impaired social interaction related to inability to engage in satisfying relationships

- "He (son) is all I have left."
- "All my family died when I was a kid."
- "I don't need other people."
- "People don't seem to like me much."

Mrs. Ruiz discussed the case with the admitting resident. Because Mr. Martin stated that he wanted to kill himself, had no family or friends that could stay with him, and had access to drugs, the decision was made to hospitalize him for further evaluation. Ordinarily, Mrs. Ruiz would follow him in clinic after discharge. In this case, Mrs. Ruiz told the physician that she thought it best for a male psychiatric nurse to work with Mr. Martin after discharge. Mrs. Ruiz explained that she thought Mr. Martin would have a strong negative transference with a female nurse, and at this time working with him on alternatives in his life was the main goal. After the immediate crisis was over, working on his interpersonal relationships would take priority.

PLANNING

Mr. Martin was kept in the hospital for 3 days. During that time he was placed on suicide precautions, as outlined in Table 24–2. He was discharged to the community outpatient division of the hospital after the staff thought that he was no longer a suicidal risk. When asked if he wanted a male nurse instead of a female nurse, he stated, "No . . . I'll talk to the little nursie . . . she's got a thing for me."

PLANNING OUTCOME CRITERIA

The nurse met with Mr. Martin, and both worked out the following goals.

Nursing Diagnosis	Long-Term Outcome	Short-Term Goals
1. **Risk for violence—self-directed** related to loss of a son	1. Mr. Martin will state that he wants to live.	1a. Mr. Martin will make a no-suicide contract with the nurse by the end of the first session. 1b. Mr. Martin will talk about painful feelings by (date). 1c. Mr. Martin will look at alternative ways he can keep in touch with his son by (date).
2. **Impaired social interaction** related to social isolation	2. Mr. Martin will state that he feels less isolated and is participating in at least one activity involving other people.	2a. Mr. Martin will discuss feelings of isolation and loneliness by (date). 2b. Mr. Martin will identify three positive aspects of self and job by (date). 2c. Mr. Martin will state that he enjoys one new weekly activity by (date).

NURSE'S FEELINGS AND SELF-ASSESSMENT

Mrs. Ruiz knew that working with Mr. Martin was going to evoke high anxiety. In talking to her clinical supervisor, it became apparent that the idea of sending Mr. Martin to a male nurse therapist, while logical on the surface, was motivated by Mrs. Ruiz's own anxiety. She was trying to avoid Mr. Martin. "I guess I did try to shove him off. His sarcasm and belittling made me feel put down and angry."

Reviewing that first session with the supervisor clarified a number of important dynamics. First, it became evident that Mr. Martin was experiencing low self-esteem as a result of the impending loss of his son's companionship. Mr. Martin's rage at the loss and his inability to change the situation resulted in intense feelings of helplessness. Second, it appeared from the data that Mr. Martin was extremely isolated. It also seemed that most of this isolation was self-imposed. His sarcasm and belittling remarks appeared to be devices to (1) push people away, (2) temporarily lift sagging self-esteem through "one-upmanship," and (3) divert attention from his own fears. The supervisor and Mrs. Ruiz saw the need to relieve Mr. Martin's isolation without increasing his anxiety to severe levels.

It was important for Mr. Martin to talk about some of his feelings. Identifying and expressing pent-up feelings could have a number of benefits. First, it could minimize feelings of isolation. Second, it could reduce the need to act them out through self-destructive channels. Third, once identified, these feelings could be more positively discharged and worked through.

INTERVENTION

At first, Mr. Martin was sarcastic, belittling, flirtatious, and hostile. Mrs. Ruiz kept her responses neutral and continued to focus her concern on Mr. Martin's situations and on working with alternatives. She gave him frequent opportunities to talk about his feelings. Initially, Mr. Martin would ridicule the nurse and belittle the idea: "Oh . . . you want to know about my precious painful feelings." Gradually, the testing-out behavior began to diminish. Slowly, and with some reluctance, Mr. Martin began talking about his feelings of loneliness and despair and sense of being a failure as a husband and father. He talked about the pain of his separation from his wife and his feelings of being a failure to his son.

The nurse continued to be neutral, not getting involved with power struggles or becoming defensive. Mrs. Ruiz began to see more clearly how these sarcastic and belittling behaviors helped Mr. Martin to defend against painful feelings of failure and low self-esteem. Refer to Nursing Care Plan 24–1 below for specific interventions used with Mr. Martin.

EVALUATION

After 2 months, Mr. Martin stated that although he missed his son desperately, he no longer thought of suicide. He did not want to leave his son that legacy. He was planning his next vacation in Oklahoma, camping with his son for 2 weeks. His interpersonal relationships were still strained. He was beginning to look at situations that gave rise to his sarcasm and belittling and to relate his actions to feelings that had been unconscious. His sarcasm toward and belittling of Mrs. Ruiz had diminished a great deal, although he still resorted to them when he felt threatened. He spent more time examining his life, his feelings, and where he wanted to go, and less on defensive behaviors. Although by this time the crisis was over, Mr. Martin continued counseling with Mrs. Ruiz. He was able to say that at times he felt more comfortable with his co-workers, although he still did not feel at home with others. He had resumed weekly bowling. He said he was surprised to find that he enjoyed it. He had even started talking to a "fellow there who is also divorced and got a rough deal. He's not a bad guy."

NURSING CARE PLAN 24–1 A SUICIDAL CLIENT AFTER DISCHARGE: MR. MARTIN

NURSING DIAGNOSIS

Risk for violence—self-directed: related to loss of son

Supporting Data

- Suicide attempt
- "I don't want to live if I can't see my son."
- "I've fot a few more tricks up my sleeve."
- Impending loss of son

Outcome Criteria: Mr. Martin will state that he wants to live.

SHORT TERM GOAL	INTERVENTION	RATIONALE	EVALUATION
1. Mr. Martin will make a no-suicide contract with nurse by end of first session.	1a. Assess suicide status.	1a. Ongoing periodic check of suicidal status. Higher rate of suicide for those who have attempted suicide.	*GOAL MET* Mr. Martin signed contract: "I will talk to the nurse if I think about killing myself. If she isn't available, I will call the crisis hotline." (first session).
	1b. Even if Mr. Martin denies suicide, make a no-suicide contract.	1b. Demonstrates concern and offers alternatives if suicidal thoughts return.	
2. Mr. Martin will talk about painful feelings by (date).	2a. Remain neutral in face of hostility and put-downs.	2a. Diminishes power struggles and discourages continuing acting out behaviors.	*GOAL MET* During first to third week, hostile and sarcastic communication was constant. By fourth week, Mr. Martin stated, "You really want to know." Mr. Martin talked of feeling like a failure as a husband and father.
	2b. Refocus attention back to Mr. Martin.	2b. Arguments and power struggles keep attention focused away from important issues.	
	2c. Give frequent opportunitites for discussion of feelings through verbal invitation and stated concern.	2c. Aggressive, hostile communications are cover for painful feelings. When client can express feelings in words, there is less need to act them out.	
3. Mr. Martin will look at alternative ways he can keep in touch with his son by (date).	3. Alternative solutions can be problem-solved once feelings and problems are identified.	3. Acceptable alternatives increase a future orientation and decrease hopelessness. Client can experience feelings of control over situation.	*GOAL MET* By fifth week, Mr. Martin talked about taking son on a camping trip during summer recess.

NURSING DIAGNOSIS

Impaired social interaction: related to social isolation

Supporting Data

- "He (son) is all I have left."
- "All my family died when I was a kid."
- "I don't need other people."
- "People don't seem to like me much."

NURSING CARE PLAN 24–1 A SUICIDAL CLIENT AFTER DISCHARGE: MR. MARTIN *(Continued)*

Outcome Criteria: Mr. Martin will state that he feels less isolated and less frightened of people by (date).

SHORT TERM GOAL	INTERVENTION	RATIONALE	EVALUATION
1a. Assess suicide 1. Mr. Martin will discuss feelings of isolation and loneliness by (date).	1. Provide opportunities for Mr. Martin to express feelings and thoughts regarding his self-imposed isolation.	1. Before change can take place, clarification of personal feelings and thoughts is necessary.	*GOAL MET* By fourth week, Mr. Martin spoke of feeling alone—son is only contact to life.
2. Mr. Martin will identify three positive aspects of self and job by (date).	2a. Validate Mr. Martin's strengths.	2. Positive as well as negative feedback aid in more realistic perception of self.	By fifth week, Mr. Martin stated that he thinks he is a good worker and is respected (if not liked) by his peers.
	2b. Encourage self-evaluation of positive as well as negative aspects of Mr. Martins's life.	2b. Client can begin to see himself more clearly, with increase in self-esteem.	
3. Mr. Martin will state that he enjoys one new weekly activity with at least one other person by (date).	3a. Review previous activities that Mr. Martin enjoyed before his marriage ended.	3a. Change focus from negative present to positive aspects of his past. Can help increase hope and self-esteem.	*GOAL MET* By seventh week, Mr. Martin stated that he started bowling again and was surprised that he had a good time.
	3b. Have Mr. Martin choose an activity that he is willing to participate in.	3b. Participating in own problem solving and decision making offers a sense of control and an increase in self-esteem.	

EVALUATION

Evaluation of a suicidal client is an ongoing part of the assessment. The nurse must be constantly alert to changes in the suicidal person's mood, thinking, and behavior. As mentioned, sudden behavioral changes can signal suicidal intent, especially when the client's depression is lifting and more energy is available to carry out a preconceived plan. A person with a diagnosis of schizophrenia is also at risk when recovering from a psychotic episode. Anniversaries of losses and holiday seasons are particularly difficult times for some people.

Evaluation includes identifying the presence or absence of any clues or thoughts of suicide. The nurse also looks for indications that people are communicating thoughts and feelings more readily and that their social network is widening. For example, if people are able to talk about their feelings and engage in problem solving with the nurse, this is a positive sign. Are the clients increasing their social activities and expanding their interests? Do they state that they have more or fewer suicidal thoughts? Essentially, the nurse evaluates the goals and establishes new ones as different situations arise. Outcome criteria for a client who is in a crisis situation may differ from those for one who is chronically suicidal.

SUMMARY

Suicide is the willful act of ending one's life. People can also hasten their death by covert self-destructive behaviors, such as alcoholism, medical noncompliance, hyperobesity, and anorexia nervosa. Death from such causes is a result of chronic self-destructive behavior.

Suicidal behavior can be classified into three categories: (1) completed, (2) attempted, and (3) ideation. Statistics surrounding suicide provide a profile that can be useful when assessing a person's suicidal intention. Many complex factors contribute to a person's decision to commit suicide, including psychodynamic, sociological, and biochemical theories.

It is critical for the nurse to assess the client's suicidal intent. The nurse assesses verbal and nonverbal clues, the lethality of the suicide plan, and high-risk factors. Nursing diagnoses may include a number of problem areas; however, **violence—self-directed** is the most crucial initially. When planning care, the nurse plans specific goals. Personal reactions to suicide and the suicidal client need to be dealt with. Common and expected reactions have been discussed, and supervision with a more experienced health care professional emphasized.

Intervention in suicide can be on a primary, secondary, or tertiary level. Secondary interventions take place in the ER, hospital unit, and community settings and on suicide hot-lines. Evaluation is ongoing, especially with a person who has a potential for suicide, because the incidence is often higher when depression is lifting or when a person is recovering from a psychotic episode. Goals are evaluated and reset, according to changes in the assessment and progress by the client toward mutually agreed upon goals. The case study highlighted nurses' work with a suicidal client.

REFERENCES

Adam, K. S. (1985). Attempted suicide. *Psychiatric Clinics of North America*, 8(2):183.

Berkow, R., and Fletcher, A. J. (Eds.)(1992). *Merck manual of diagnosis and therapy.* Rahway, NJ: Merck Research Laboratories.

Birtchnell, J. (1983). Psychotherapeutic considerations in the management of the suicidal patient. *American Journal of Psychotherapy*, 37(1):24.

Busteen, E. L, and Johnstone, C. (1983). The development of suicide precautions for an inpatient psychiatric unit. *Journal of Psychosocial Nursing and Mental Health Services*, 21(5):15.

Carlson, G. A., and Asarnow, J. R. (1995). Mood disorders and suicidal behavior. In G. O. Gabbard (Ed.), *Treatments of psychiatric disorders* (Vol. I, pp. 253–285). Washington, DC: American Psychiatric Press.

Cassem, N. H. (1980). Treating the person confronting death. In A. M. Nicholi (Ed.), *The Harvard guide to modern psychiatry.* Cambridge, MA: Belknap Press of Harvard University Press.

Chemtob, C. M., et al. (1988). Patients' suicide: Frequency and impact on psychiatrists. *American Journal of Psychiatry*, 145(2):224.

DeLeo, D., Carollo, G., and Dello-Buono, M. (1995). Lower suicide rates associated with a Tele-Help/Tele-Check service for the elderly at home. *American Journal of Psychiatry*, 152(4):632.

Densmore, W. E. (1997). Take caution with "no-suicide contract" (letter). *Journal of Psychosocial Nursing*, 35(5):11.

Durand, C. J., et al. (1995). A quarter century of suicide in a major urban jail: Implications for community psychiatry. *American Journal of Psychiatry*, 152(7):1077–1080.

Evans, D. L. (1983). Explaining suicide among the young: An analytic review of the literature. *Journal of Psychosocial Nursing and Mental Health Services*, 21(5):9.

Farberow, N. L. (1967). Crisis, disaster and suicide: Theory and therapy. In E. S. Schneidman (Ed.), *Essays in self-destruction.* New York: Jason Aronson.

Fergusson, D. M., and Lynsky, M. T. (1995). Childhood circumstances, adolescent adjustment, and suicide attempts in a New Zealand birth cohort. *Journal of American Academy of Child and Adolescent Psychiatry, 34(5):612.*

Hammel-Bissell, B. P. (1985). Suicidal casework: Assessing nurses' reactions. *Journal of Psychosocial Nursing and Mental Health Services*, 23(10):20.

Harvard Medical School Mental Health Letter (1986). *Suicide— Part II.* 2:1.

Hatton, C. L., et al. (1977). Theoretical framework. In C. L. Hatton (Ed.), *Suicide: Assessment and intervention.* New York: Appleton-Century Crofts.

Hendrin, H. (1992). Suicidality and the young. *American Journal of Psychiatry*, 149(6):850.

Hoff, L. A. (1995). *People in crisis: Understanding and helping* (4th ed.). San Francisco: Jossey-Bass.

Hornblow, A. R. (1986). The evolution and effectiveness of telephone counseling services. *Hospital and Community Psychiatry*, 37(7):731.

McKinley Health Center (1996). University of Illinois, Champaign Urbana. On-line Psychological Services, 1996.

Mowshowitz, I. (1984). The special role of the pastoral counselor. In *The will to live vs. the will to die.* New York: Human Sciences Press.

Mueller, T. I., and Leon, A. C. (1996). Recovery, chronicity, and levels of psychopathology in major depression. *Psychiatric Clinics of North America*, (19) 1:85.

Mullens, A. (1995). The Oregon vote may mark watershed for right-to-die debate in Canada, U.S. *Canadian Medical Association Journal*, 152(1):91.

Mullis, M. R, and Byers, P. H. (1988). Social support. *Journal of Psychosocial Nursing*, 25(4):16.

Neville, D., and Barnes, S. (1985). The suicidal phone call. *Journal of Psychosocial Nursing*, 23(8):14.

Overholser, J. C., et al. (1995). Self-esteem deficits and suicidal tendencies among adolescents. *Journal of American Academic Child Adolescent Psychiatry*, 34(7):919.

Pallikkathayil, L., and McBride, A. B. (1986). Suicide attempts. *Journal of Psychosocial Nursing*, 24(8):13.

Pandey, G. N., et al. (1995). Platelet serotonin-2A receptors: A potential biological marker for suicidal behavior. *American Journal of Psychiatry*, 152(6):850.

Parker, S. D. (1988). Accidents or suicide: Do life change events lead to adolescent suicide? *Journal of Psychosocial Nursing*, 26(6):15.

Patterson, W., et al. (1983). Evaluation of suicidal patients: The SAD PERSONS scale. *Psychosomatics*, 24(4):343.

Paykel, E. S., et al. (1975). Suicide attempts and recent life events. *Archives of General Psychiatry*, 33:327.

Roy, A. (1995a). Psychiatric emergencies. In H. I. Kaplan and B. J. Sadock (Eds.), *Comprehensive textbook of psychiatry VI.* Baltimore: Williams & Wilkins.

Roy, A. (1995b). Suicide. In H. I. Kaplan and B. J. Sadock (Eds.), *Comprehensive textbook of psychiatry VI.* Baltimore: Williams & Wilkins.

Roy, A., et al. (1995). Attempted suicide among living co-twins of twin suicide victims. *American Journal of Psychiatry*, 152(7):1075.

Schmitt, W., and Mundt, C. (1991). Differential typology among patients with hard and soft suicide methods. *Nervenarzt*, 62(7):440.

Schneidman, E. S. (1963). Orientation towards death: A vital aspect of the study of lives. In R. W. White (Ed.), *The study of lives.* New York: Atherton Press.

Stevenson J. M. (1988). Suicide. In J. A. Talbott, R. E. Hale and S. C. Yudofsky (Eds.), *Textbook of psychiatry.* Washington, DC: American Psychiatric Press.

Thompson, R. (1996). Post-traumatic loss debriefing: Providing immediate support for survivors of suicide or sudden loss. Ann Arbor, MI: ERIC Clearinghouse on Counseling and Personnel Services.

Van Dongen, C. J. (1988). The legacy of suicide. *Journal of Psychosocial Nursing*, 26(1):9.

Yang, B., and Lester, D. (1995). Social stress and suicide: Replicating an Asian study with American data. *Psychological Reports*, 76(2):553.

SELF-STUDY AND CRITICAL THINKING

True or false

Place T (true) or F (false) next to each statement. Correct all false statements.

1. ________ Attempted suicide is associated with depression and alcoholism.
2. ________ People with antisocial disorders have a low suicide rate.

3. __________ Once a person is over the suicide crisis, he or she most likely will not attempt suicide in the future.

4. __________ Nonwhites in a low socioeconomic status have the highest rates for suicide.

5. __________ If the nurse thinks that a client may be thinking of suicide, the nurse should not bring up the subject, lest the person get ideas.

6. __________ The suicide rate is higher among gifted individuals, immigrants, police officers, doctors, and the elderly than in the general population.

7. __________ A person who has had a family member commit suicide, is divorced, or has suffered multiple losses is a risk for possible suicide.

Multiple choice

Choose the most appropriate response in each case.

8. Choose the type of suicide that is included in Durkheim's theory:

   A. Murder in 180th degree
   B. Low serotonin levels
   C. Anomic
   D. Alcohol abuse or depression

9. The statement by a suicidal person "How can I go about giving my body to medical science?" is an example of

   A. An overstatement.
   B. A behavioral clue.
   C. An emotional clue.
   D. A covert statement.

10. The best response to a client who states "Things will never work out, but I have an answer now" is

    A. Things have a way of working out in time.
    B. I feel the same sometimes.
    C. I knew you would find a better solution.
    D. What things . . . What kind of answer have you found?

11. Charles Brown, age 52, lost his wife in a car accident 4 months ago. Since that time, he has been severely depressed and has taken to drinking to "numb the pain." Using the SAD PERSONS assessment scale, how many points does Mr. Brown have?

    A. Three
    B. Four
    C. Five
    D. Six

12. Which of the following is the best way to phrase a no-suicide contract?

    A. "I will call my therapist before I harm myself."
    B. "I will not kill myself unless my husband leaves me."
    C. "When I have thoughts of killing myself, I will talk to my counselor."
    D. "I will not try to kill myself until next week."

Completion

Next to the intervention, put a P for primary intervention, an S for secondary intervention, or a T for tertiary intervention.

13. ________ Work with the family of a recent suicide victim.
14. ________ Relieve isolation, remove all weapons, and encourage alternative expressions of anger.
15. ________ Place the suicidal person on suicide precautions when he or she is first admitted to the hospital.
16. ________ Work with a teenager who has recently attempted suicide.
17. ________ Provide seminars for the elderly that focus on physical and emotional concerns.
18. ________ Keep the person on the telephone, find out if the person has ingested any drugs, assess the lethality of the plan, and work on alternatives.

Formulate two short-term goals for the following nursing diagnoses:

19. *High risk for violence—self-directed* related to loss of a loved one

    1. ______________________________

    2. ______________________________

20. *Ineffective family coping* related to lack of sleep and inability to concentrate

    1. ______________________________

    2. ______________________________

Critical thinking

21. Identify three common and expected emotional reactions that a nurse might have when initially working with people who are suicidal. How do you think you might react? What actions could you take to process the event and obtain support?
22. How would you respond to a staff person who expresses guilt over the completed suicide of a client on your unit?
23. How would you respond to a person who expresses the view that not only should physician-assisted suicide be legal for the terminally ill, but any person who decides life isn't worth living has the right to act on this decision?
24. How would you respond to a person expressing suicidal thoughts who believes that the act of suicide is a sin? How would you respond to family members who believe that their relative who died by suicide committed a sin?
25. Compare the suicide protocol at your hospital unit/community center with the one in the text. What are the commonalities? Are there any steps you anticipate having difficulty carrying out? What suggestions do your peers/clinical group have regarding these difficulties that you could implement?

25

People Who Depend Upon Substances of Abuse

KATHLEEN SMITH-DIJULIO

OUTLINE

KEY TERMS AND CONCEPTS

The key terms and concepts listed here also appear in bold where they are defined or discussed in this chapter.

addiction
tolerance
withdrawal
polydrug abuse
CAGE questionnaire
toxicological screening
blood alcohol level
crack
Cannabis sativa
tetrahydrocannabinol (THC)
LSD
mescaline
psilocybin
psychedelic
synesthesia
PCP
flashbacks
naloxone (Narcan)
synergistic effect
antagonistic effect
predictable defensive style
comorbid dual diagnosis
Alcoholics Anonymous
enabling
intervention
Al-Anon
Al-a-Teen
Narc-Anon
Adult Children of Alcoholics
co-dependence
therapeutic communities
Wernicke's syndrome
hypomagnesemia
naltrexone (Trexan, ReVia)
disulfiram (Antabuse)
methadone (Dolophine)
LAAM (L-alpha acetylmethadol)
clonidine
HALT
skills training
assertiveness training
relaxation training
relapse prevention
lapse
relapse
aversive conditioning

OBJECTIVES

After studying this chapter, the reader will be able to

1. Compare and contrast the terms *substance abuse* and *substance dependence,* as defined by the *Diagnostic and statistical manual of mental disorders,* fourth edition (DSM-IV).
2. Explain the difference between tolerance and withdrawal, and give a clinical definition of each.
3. Discuss four components of the assessment process to be used with a person who is chemically dependent.
4. Describe the difference between the relationship of blood alcohol levels and behavior in an alcoholic person and that in a nondrinker.
5. Distinguish between the symptoms seen in alcohol withdrawal and those of alcohol delirium.
6. Discuss five physical and five psychological signs of sedative-hypnotic intoxication.
7. Compare and contrast the signs of intoxication, overdose, and withdrawal symptoms from cocaine and amphetamine use.
8. Distinguish between the symptoms of narcotic intoxication and those of narcotic withdrawal.
9. Discuss what is meant by *synesthesia* and give two examples.
10. Define *flashback* and give an example.
11. Identify physiological risk factors associated with inhalant use.
12. Discuss treatment for a person who is withdrawing from a central nervous system depressant.
13. Discuss the synergistic and antagonistic effects of drugs in polydrug abusers and give an example of each.
14. Formulate six nursing diagnoses that might apply to substance-abusing clients, including related causal factors.
15. Develop three short-term goals that might be useful steps in achieving long-term sobriety.
16. Analyze the pros and cons of the following treatments for narcotic addictions: (a) methadone or L-alpha acetylmethadol (LAAM),

(b) maintenance, (c) therapeutic communities, and (d) self-help, abstinence-oriented model.
17. Apply four principles of psychotherapeutic intervention to be used with a substance-abusing client.
18. Discuss two issues that a therapist should address when treating clients who abuse substances.
19. Recognize the phenomenon of relapse as it effects substance abusers during different phases of treatment.
20. Discuss three therapeutic modalities used with substance abusers.
21. Role play some of the reactions a nurse might have when working with a chemically impaired nurse.
22. Explain six ways that you as a nurse can help a chemically impaired colleague.
23. Evaluate four indications that a person is successfully recovering from substance abuse.

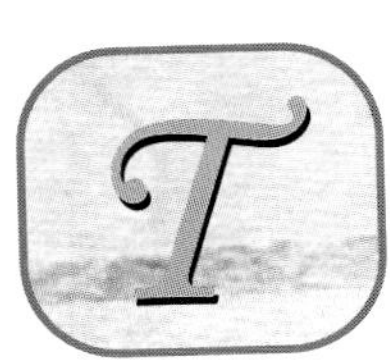

he United States is a drug-oriented society. People use a host of drugs for various purposes: to restore health, to reduce pain, to reduce anxiety, to increase energy, to create a feeling of euphoria, to induce sleep, and to enhance alertness. Many substances are available to alter mood or state of consciousness, and people take drugs for reasons other than medical need. Drugs may relieve stress or tension or may provide a temporary escape from difficulties. Peer pressure and advertising are strong factors in the use of drugs by young people. In many parts of our society, the use of drugs has become a rite of passage. Sometimes, drug use is part of the thrill of taking a risk.

Alcohol is the most widely used, and misused, drug in America. The impact of excessive alcohol use on human health and well-being is substantial, and no one is immune from the gamut of medical, social, emotional, familial, legal, and economic problems that uncontrolled alcohol use creates.

Two thirds of the nation's adults consume alcohol regularly. One in 10 of these has problems associated with alcohol use. It has been estimated that one third of hospital admissions are alcohol related. Alcohol-related traffic accidents continue to be a major problem in our society. Alcohol contributes significantly to the incidence and severity of problems in the home and the workplace. Other drugs contributing to these problems are other central nervous system (CNS) depressants, amphetamines, cocaine and crack, narcotics (especially heroin), marijuana, hallucinogens including lysergic acid diethylamide (LSD) and phencyclidine piperidine (PCP), and inhalants.

Because of the broad social impact of alcohol and drug use, it is critical that nurses learn to recognize the indicators of a developing problem. Substance abuse problems in most persons are progressive; therefore, early detection is critical for a positive prognosis. No arena of nursing practice can ignore problems caused by substance abuse. People with these problems are seen in clinics, inpatient hospital units, schools, and the workplace. Substance abuse contributes to emotional problems in the aged. Substance abuse in adolescents is increasing rapidly and is becoming more severe. Substance abuse in women is also increasing. Alcohol use during pregnancy can result in negative consequences for the fetus (i.e., fetal alcohol syndrome). Health care providers themselves are another population with a high proportion of substance abuse. The subject of impaired health care workers is addressed later in this chapter.

This chapter provides fundamental knowledge about substance abuse and focuses on the role of the nurse in assessment, care planning, intervention, and evaluation. Substance abuse can be conceptualized as an automatic behavior occurring in response to stress that becomes progressively more self-destructive over time. It occurs on a continuum, as illustrated in Figure 25–1.

THEORY

Addiction incorporates the concepts of (1) loss of control of substance ingestion, (2) substance use despite associated problems, and (3) tendency to relapse. The reason one person becomes addicted and another does not seems to depend on physical, developmental, psychosocial, and environmental factors as well as on genetic predisposition. The difficulty in determining cause and effect is that the diagnosis of addiction generally occurs many years after the onset of use. Various factors are involved over the course of those years. Biological, psychological, and sociocultural theories are briefly examined here.

Biological Theories

Interest in biological theories was augmented by the observation that substance problems seemed to run in families. If a person's ancestors had such problems, the likelihood seemed to be increased that the person would, too. Alcoholism is more likely to occur in children of alcoholic parents than in children of nonalcoholic parents. Sons of alcoholic parents are more likely to become alcoholics than are daughters.

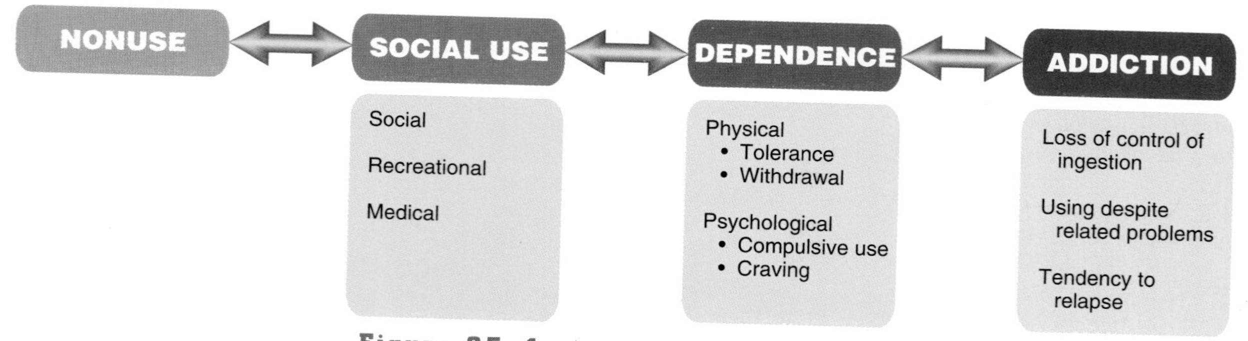

Figure 25–1 A continuum of substance use.

Current research describes two biological (genetic) pathways to substance abuse and dependency. The first is a direct effect from an alcohol-abusing or alcohol-dependent biological parent. The second starts with antisocial biological parents and leads to sons a significant proportion of whom are aggressive in adolescence, with the end result of both an antisocial personality diagnosis and drug abuse or dependence (Cadoret et al. 1995).

It has been demonstrated more recently that alcohol and drug use has specific effects on selected neurotransmitter systems. Neurotransmitters are chemicals in the brain that transmit impulses from one cell to another. Certain drugs interfere with the work of neurotransmitters. Alcohol and other CNS depressants act on gamma-aminobutyric acid (Bohn 1993). This finding helps explain the addictive and cross-tolerance effects that occur when the use of alcohol is combined with barbiturates and benzodiazepines. Cocaine dependence is primarily associated with a deficiency in the neurotransmitters dopamine and norepinephrine (Thomas 1993). It is hoped that correcting this deficiency can reduce an individual's craving for cocaine.

Psychological Theories

Although no known addictive personality type exists, associated psychodynamic factors exist, including

1. An intolerance for frustration and pain. This intolerance is exhibited in response to both psychological and physical pain. The myths that happiness should be an enduring state and that anxiety, depression, and loneliness are unnatural and should be avoided at all costs have contributed to the American "pill-popping" phenomenon.
2. Lack of success in life.
3. Lack of affectionate and meaningful relationships.
4. Low self-esteem; lack of self-regard. Substance abusers often feel worthless, hopeless, and helpless about themselves and the possibility of their lives ever being any different.
5. Risk-taking propensity.

According to psychological theories, a person uses substances to feel better. The habit of using a substance in response to psychological needs then becomes reinforced, and over time, the behavior develops into an addiction.

Sociocultural Theories

Sociocultural theories attempt to explain differences in the incidence of substance use in various groups. Social and cultural norms influence when, what, and how a person uses substances. For example, Italians and Jews are thought to have lower alcoholism rates because of cultural norms about when and how much to drink. Drinking occurs in the context of meals and serves specific social and religious purposes. Drunkenness is frowned on. The French, in contrast, are said to have high alcoholism rates because it is socially acceptable to drink anywhere and any time, and drunkenness is tolerated.

Another theory correlates substance use with the degree of socioeconomic stress people experience. Being a "drug addict" can give a person a place in a subculture where he or she can be accepted. This is most true in economically deprived and unstable environments, where drugs may be taken to provide a person with a sense of belonging and identity. The dominance of the drug subculture in highly stressed communities can make it almost impossible *not* to develop a problem.

Women in general have lower rates of substance use because of the cultural mores that have prohibited women from heavy use in public. Addicted women are viewed much more negatively than addicted men in many cultural groups.

In summary, there is no single cause of substance abuse. Multiple factors contribute to substance use, abuse, and addiction in any individual. For example, a child of an alcoholic may have a biochemical deficiency predisposing to alcoholism and may grow up with low self-esteem in a society that has no rituals governing alcohol use. Because of complex biological, psychological, and sociocultural factors, this person is at risk for developing alcoholism.

SUBSTANCE ABUSE vs. DEPENDENCE

SUBSTANCE ABUSE	SUBSTANCE DEPENDENCE
Maladaptive pattern of substance use leading to clinically significant impairment or distress, manifested by one or more of the following within a 12-month period:	Maladaptive pattern of substance use leading to clinically significant impairment or distress, manifested by three or more of the following within a 12-month period:
1. Inability to fulfill major role obligations at work, school, and home.	1. Presence of tolerance to the drug or
2. Recurrent legal or interpersonal problems.	2. Presence of withdrawal syndrome.
3. Continued use despite recurrent social and interpersonal problems.	3. Substance is taken in larger amounts/for longer period than intended.
4. Participation in physically hazardous situations while impaired (driving a car, operating a machine, exacerbation of symptoms, e.g., ulcers).	4. Reduction or absence of important social, occupational, or recreational activities.
	5. Unsuccessful or persistent desire to cut down or control use.
	6. Increased time spent in getting, taking, and recovering from the substance. May withdraw from family or friends.

Figure 25–2 DSM-IV criteria for substance abuse and dependence. (Adapted from American Psychiatric Association (1994). *Diagnostic and statistical manual of mental disorders (DSM-IV)* (4th ed.) (pp. 181–183). Washington DC: American Psychiatric Association. Reprinted with permission. Copyright 1994 American Psychiatric Association.)

Definitions

The diagnostic scheme in the *Diagnostic and statistical manual of mental disorders*, fourth edition (DSM-IV) (APA 1994) focuses on the behavioral aspects and the pathological patterns of use, emphasizing the physical symptoms of tolerance and withdrawal. An overview of DSM-IV diagnostic criteria for substance abuse and dependence is shown in Figure 25–2.

The concept of substance dependence includes the concepts of tolerance and withdrawal. **Tolerance** is a need for higher and higher doses to achieve the desired effect. **Withdrawal** occurs after a long period of continued use, so that stopping or reducing use results in specific physical and psychological signs and symptoms. Since alcohol is still the most common drug of abuse in the United States and poses the greatest withdrawal danger, DSM-IV diagnostic criteria for alcohol intoxication, withdrawal, and delirium are highlighted in Figure 25–3. Information on signs and symptoms of intoxication and withdrawal for other substances of abuse are identified later in this chapter.

ASSESSMENT

An objective assessment strategy allows nurses to obtain concrete data that are useful in diagnosis, planning, referral, and treatment. Most of the information needed for a complete and accurate health assessment is obtained by means of the nursing history. A thorough nursing history is designed to elicit information about the various physical and psychosocial problems that can occur in substance-dependent people. Multicultural and racial issues are important in interpreting symptoms, making diagnoses, providing clinical care, and designing prevention strategies.

Assessment is becoming more complex because of the increase in the simultaneous use of many substances (**polydrug abuse**). An additional assessment challenge is the deteriorated physical condition of people infected with the human immunodeficiency virus (HIV). During the assessment process, questions may arise as to whether the client has a specific CNS disease, such as dementia, encephalopathy, and acquired immunodeficiency syndrome (AIDS)–associated opportunistic infection that affects the brain, or a situational depression or the effects of substance abuse.

The following guidelines are helpful in the history-taking process:

1. *Begin by asking the client about the use of prescribed drugs.* The client is usually honest about these because they are ordered by a physician and are thus perceived to be needed. From the answer to this question, an impression can be gained about the person's drug orientation. Some people express their practice of using medications only when they are absolutely required (e.g., antibiotics for specific infections). Others state

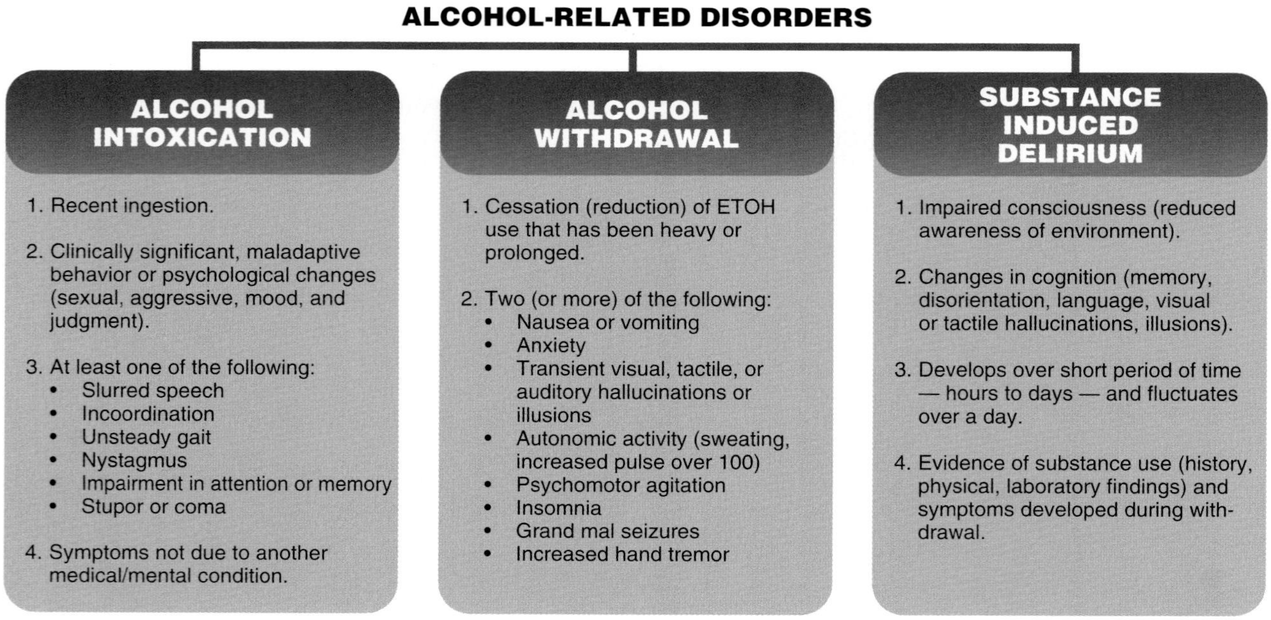

ALCOHOL-RELATED DISORDERS

ALCOHOL INTOXICATION

1. Recent ingestion.
2. Clinically significant, maladaptive behavior or psychological changes (sexual, aggressive, mood, and judgment).
3. At least one of the following:
   - Slurred speech
   - Incoordination
   - Unsteady gait
   - Nystagmus
   - Impairment in attention or memory
   - Stupor or coma
4. Symptoms not due to another medical/mental condition.

ALCOHOL WITHDRAWAL

1. Cessation (reduction) of ETOH use that has been heavy or prolonged.
2. Two (or more) of the following:
   - Nausea or vomiting
   - Anxiety
   - Transient visual, tactile, or auditory hallucinations or illusions
   - Autonomic activity (sweating, increased pulse over 100)
   - Psychomotor agitation
   - Insomnia
   - Grand mal seizures
   - Increased hand tremor

SUBSTANCE INDUCED DELIRIUM

1. Impaired consciousness (reduced awareness of environment).
2. Changes in cognition (memory, disorientation, language, visual or tactile hallucinations, illusions).
3. Develops over short period of time — hours to days — and fluctuates over a day.
4. Evidence of substance use (history, physical, laboratory findings) and symptoms developed during withdrawal.

Figure 25–3 DSM-IV criteria for alcohol-related disorders. ETOH, ethyl alcohol. (Adapted from American Psychiatric Association (1994). *Diagnostic and statistical manual of mental disorders (DSM-IV)* (4th ed.) (pp. 131–132, 197–199). Washington DC: American Psychiatric Association. Reprinted with permission. Copyright 1994 American Psychiatric Association.)

that they cannot get the correct prescriptions from any of the doctors they see. "Doctor shopping" and repeated client requests for medications, especially psychotropic medications, are indicators of a possible drug problem. These responses should be kept in mind when other questions are asked.

2. *Next, question the person about over-the-counter-drugs.* Many do not consider these substances to be drugs, because they are so readily available and advertised. These questions provide an opportunity for client education about drug effects.
3. *Finally, ask the person about commonly used social drugs.* The client may be puzzled or bewildered about this category. An explanation that caffeine and nicotine are drugs, followed by an assessment of their use by the client, sets the stage for taking a history of alcohol and then other drug use. The nurse should emphasize the fact that alcohol is a commonly used drug and should elicit the role that alcohol plays in the everyday functioning of the client. Then, the nurse should ask about the use of other substances, in descending order of commonality (e.g., marijuana, cocaine, heroin). The nurse should ask about all drugs taken, the amount, the length of use, the route, and the drug preference. It is important to determine how the drugs were used—that is, whether they were taken intravenously, intramuscularly, intradermally ("skin-popped"), or intranasally ("sniffed" or "snorted"); smoked; or taken by mouth. Many adverse physiologic drug effects are associated with the route of administration (Table 25–1). Asking about the extent and the duration of problems associated with substance use can also assist in determining the degree of severity of the dependence. Asking about family history of alcohol or drug problems allows further evaluation of a client's risk for problems with dependence.

The nurse should ask questions in a matter-of-fact, nonjudgmental fashion:

- What drug(s) did you take before coming to the emergency room (hospital, clinic)?
- How did you take the drug(s) (e.g., intravenously, intramuscularly, orally, subcutaneously, smoking, intranasally)?
- How much did you take? (When asking about alcohol, the nurse should ask about beer, wine, and liquor individually. The more questions the nurse asks, the more information she or he is likely to obtain.) (see Fig. 25–4 for alcohol equivalents.)
- When was (were) the last dose(s) taken?
- How long have you been using the substance(s)? When did you start this episode of use?
- How often and how much do you usually use?
- What kinds of problems has substance use caused for you? With your family? Friends? Job? Health? Finances? The law?

It is useful to incorporate the **CAGE questionnaire** as part of the assessment protocol. These questionnaires consist of four questions that focus on the main ideas of *cutting* down consumption, *annoyance* about criticism of use, *guilty* feelings associated with use, and *eye-openers*, or *early morning use*. The title of the questionnaire was derived by extracting the first letters of the four main ideas,

TABLE 25–1 DRUG INFORMATION: PHYSICAL COMPLICATIONS RELATED TO DRUG ABUSE

DRUG	PHYSICAL COMPLICATIONS
	Route: Intravenous*
Narcotics (e.g., heroin) Phencyclidine piperidine (PCP) Cocaine/crack	Acquired immunodeficiency syndrome Hepatitis Bacterial endocarditis Renal failure Cardiac arrest Coma Seizures Respiratory arrest Dermatitis Pulmonary emboli Tetanus Abscesses—osteomyelitis Septicemia
	Route: Intravenous, Intranasal, Smoking
Cocaine	Perforation of nasal septum (when taken intranasally) Respiratory paralysis Cardiovascular collapse Hyperpyrexia
	Route: Ingestion
Caffeine	Gastroesophogeal reflux Peptic ulcer Increased intraocular pressure in unregulated glaucoma Tachycardia Increased plasma glucose and lipid levels
	Route: Smoking, Ingestion
Marijuana	Impaired lung structure Chromosomal mutation—increased incidence of birth defects Micronucleic white blood cells—increased risk of disease due to decreased resistance to infection Possible long-term effects on short-term memory
	Route: Smoking, Chewing
Nicotine	*Heavy chronic use associated with* Emphysema Cancer of the larynx and esophagus Lung cancer Peripheral vascular diseases Cancer of the mouth Cardiovascular disease Hypertension
	Route: Intravenous,* Smoking
Heroin	Constipation Dermatitis Malnutrition Hypoglycemia Dental caries Amenorrhea
	Route: Ingestion*
Phencyclidine piperidine (PCP)	Respiratory arrest
	Route: Sniffing, Snorting, Bagging (Fumes Inhaled from a Plastic Bag), Huffing (Inhalant-soaked Rag in the Mouth)
Inhalants	Respiratory arrest Tachycardia Arrhythmias Nervous system damage

*__Note:__ The complications listed can result from any drug taken intravenously.

The amount of alcohol in one drink approximates the quantity of alcohol that can be metabolized by the body in 1 hour.

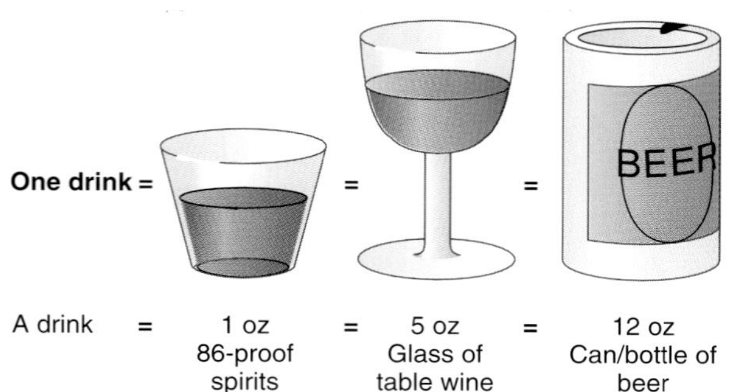

Figure 25–4 Alcohol equivalents.

formulating the acronym CAGE. The specific questions follow (Brown 1992; Ewing 1984; Mayfield et al. 1974):

1. Have you ever felt you should *cut down* on your drinking/(specific drug) use?
2. Have people *annoyed* you by criticizing your drinking/(specific drug) use?
3. Have you ever felt bad or *guilty* about your drinking/(specific drug) use?
4. Have you ever had a drink/used (specific drug) first thing in the morning to steady your nerves, get rid of a hangover *(eye-opener)*, or get the day started?

Two or three "yes" answers to these questions strongly suggest substance dependence, especially physical dependence in terms of the inability to cut down and the need for an eye-opener. The nurse should also ask how much is used on a given occasion and what happens when substance use is curtailed. A useful measure for assessing alcohol use in the past year is the Alcohol Use Disorder Identification Test (AUDIT) (USDHHS 1993).

How a person responds to interview questions is significant for assessment purposes. Most people give thoughtful, matter-of-fact responses that suggest no alcohol/drug problem. Some express concern and ask for information and referral. It may have been the first time anyone has asked about their substance use. Others say that they abstain. The reasons for abstinence are important. Do they abstain for religious or health reasons? Are they acknowledged addicts in recovery? Are they trying to prove to someone else that they can be abstinent? For example: "My husband thinks I drink too much, so I'm going to show him. I'm not going to have a drop for 2 weeks. I can take it or leave it." Such a response indicates possible problems, and further assessment is required. Other responses that serve as red-flag indicators of the need for further assessment are rationalizations: "You'd smoke dope, too, if . . . "; automatic responses, as if predicted; or slow, prolonged responses, as if the person is being careful about what to say. Last are the practicing addicts who admit they have a problem but project an air of hopelessness about ever achieving sobriety.

If the person is not able to provide a drug history, the nurse should assess for indications of substance abuse, such as dilated or constricted pupils, abnormal vital signs, needle marks, tremors, alcohol on the breath, and history from family and friends. The clothing is checked for drug paraphernalia, such as used syringes, crack vials, and evidence of white powder, razor blades, bent spoons, and pipes.

A urine **toxicology screening** and/or **blood alcohol level** (BAL) can also be useful for assessment purposes.

Level of Intoxication and Physiological Changes

Often, attitude and expectations, or mental "set," and environment combine with pharmacological effects to produce intoxication. Alcohol, however is the only drug for which objective measures of intoxication exist. The relationship between BAL and behavior in a *nontolerant individual* is shown in Table 25–2. Knowledge of the BAL assists the nurse in determining the level of intoxication, the level of tolerance, and whether the person accurately reported recent drinking during the nursing history. These factors are also assessed by means of behavioral cues.

TABLE 25–2 RELATIONSHIP BETWEEN BLOOD ALCOHOL LEVELS AND BEHAVIOR IN A NONTOLERANT DRINKER

BLOOD ALCOHOL LEVELS	BLOOD ALCOHOL ACCUMULATION*	BEHAVIOR
0.05 mg%	1–2 drinks	Changes in mood and behavior; judgment is impaired
0.10 mg%	5–6 drinks	Voluntary motor action becomes clumsy; **legal level of intoxication in most states**
0.20 mg%	10–12 drinks	Function of entire motor area of the brain is depressed, causing staggering and ataxia; emotional lability is present
0.30 mg%	15–18 drinks	Confusion; stupor
0.40 mg%	20–24 drinks	Coma
0.50 mg%	25–30 drinks	Death due to respiratory depression

As tolerance develops, a discrepancy exists between BAL and expected behavior. A person with tolerance to alcohol may have a high BAL but minimal signs of impairment, as indicated in the following example.

◗ Clarence presents in the emergency department with a BAL of 0.51 mg%. He is stuporous and ataxic and has slurred speech. The fact that he is still alive indicates a high tolerance for alcohol. A nursing history conducted as the client sobers up revealed an extensive drinking history. When the blood alcohol is this high, assessing for withdrawal symptoms is important.

A list of the physiological effects of alcohol use is presented in Box 25–1. The nursing history, physical examination, and laboratory tests are methods used to gather data about drug-related physical problems. The extent of impairment depends on individual susceptibility as well as on amount of drug used and route of administration (see Table 25–1).

Each class of drugs has its own physiological signs and symptoms of intoxication, which are summarized in Tables 25–3 to 25–8.

Central Nervous System Depressants

This class of drugs includes alcohol, benzodiazepines, and barbiturates. Symptoms of intoxication, overdose, and withdrawal, along with possible treatments, are presented in Table 25–3.

Central Nervous System Stimulants

Table 25–4 outlines the physical and psychological effects of intoxication from abuse of amphetamines and other psychostimulants, possible life-threatening results of overdose, and emergency measures for both overdose and withdrawal.

All stimulants accelerate the normal functioning of the body and affect the CNS. Common signs of stimulant abuse include dilation of the pupils, dryness of the oronasal cavity, and excessive motor activity.

When a person who has ingested a stimulant experiences chest pain, has an irregular pulse, or has a history of heart trouble, the person should be taken to an emergency department immediately.

COCAINE AND CRACK. Cocaine is a naturally occurring stimulant extracted from the leaf of the coca bush. **Crack** is a cheap, widely available alkalinized form of cocaine. When crack is smoked, it takes effect in 4 to 6 seconds. Dependence on crack develops rapidly. A popular rock star recovering from crack addiction stated "If you are on crack, you have three choices: you can get off, you can go crazy, or you can die." The fleeting high obtained from crack (lasting 5 to 7 minutes) is followed by a period

BOX 25–1 PHYSIOLOGICAL EFFECTS RELATED TO ALCOHOL USE

Metabolic
Hypoglycemia
Hyperlipidemia
Hyperuricemia

Gastrointestinal System
Increased incidence of cancer of the oral mucosa
Increased acid production
Nausea and vomiting; diarrhea
Esophagitis and varices
Malabsorption of nutrients, especially folic acid, vitamin B_1 (thiamine), and vitamin B_{12}
Ulcer—gastric and duodenal
Gastritis, enteritis, colitis, hemorrhoids
Fatty liver, alcoholic hepatitis, cirrhosis
Pancreatitis

Neurological System
Sleep disturbance
Peripheral neuropathies
Brain syndromes
Wernicke-Korsakoff syndrome
Cerebellar degeneration

Cardiovascular System
Hypertension, tachycardia due to withdrawal
Decreased mechanical performance of the heart
Cardiomyopathy, after 10 or more years

Respiratory System
Impaired diffusion
Increased incidence of lung infections (e.g., bronchitis, pneumonias)
Smoking effects (e.g., chronic obstructive pulmonary disease)

Genitourinary System
Increased urinary excretion of potassium and magnesium leads to hypomagnesemia and hypokalemia
Hypogonadism, hypoandrogenization, hyperestrogenization in men
Diminished sexual performance
Impotency in men
Decreased menstruation, leading to infertility

Musculoskeletal System
Myopathies
Skin Infections
Lesions, burns, scars

Hematological System
Anemias
Impaired phagocytosis, which reduces body's response to invasion by bacteria
Leukopenia, which can affect the body's immune system
Hematomas

TABLE 25–3 DRUG INFORMATION: DEPRESSANTS*

		OVERDOSE		WITHDRAWAL	
DRUG	**INTOXICATION**	**Effects**	**Possible Treatments**	**Effects**	**Possible Treatments**
Barbiturates Amobarbital (Amytal) Pentobarbital (Nembutal) Secobarbital (Seconal) **Benzodiazepines** Diazepam (Valium) Chlordiazepoxide (Librium) Lorazepam (Ativan) Oxazepam (Serax) Alprazolam (Xanax) **Chloral hydrate** **Glutethimide** (Doriden) **Meprobamate** (Equanil, Miltown) **Alcohol**	*Physical:* Slurred speech Incoordination Unsteady gait Drowsiness Decreased blood pressure *Psychological/ perceptual:* Disinhibition of sexual or aggressive drives Impaired judgment Impaired social or occupational function Impaired attention or memory Irritability	Cardiovascular or respiratory depression or arrest (mostly with barbiturates) Coma Shock Convulsions Death	*If awake:* Keep awake Induce vomiting Give activated charcoal to aid absorption of drug Every 15 minutes check vital signs (VS) *Coma:* Clear airway—endotracheal tube Intravenous (IV) fluids Gastric lavage with activated charcoal Frequent VS checks for shock and cardiac arrest after client is stable Seizure precautions Possible hemodialysis or peritoneal dialysis Flumazenil (Romazicon) IV	*Cessation of prolonged/ heavy use:* Nausea/vomiting Tachycardia Diaphoresis Anxiety or irritability Tremors in hands, fingers, eyelids Marked insomnia Grand mal seizures *After 5–15 years of heavy use:* Delirium	Carefully titrated detoxification with similar drug **NOTE: Abrupt withdrawal can lead to death.**

Data from American Psychiatric Association (1994). *Diagnostic and statistical manual of mental disorders* (4th ed.). Washington, DC: American Psychiatric Association; Bohn, M. J. (1993). Alcoholism. *Psychiatric Clinics of North America*, 16(4):679.

***DEFINITION: Known as minor tranquilizers, sedatives, hypnotics, and antianxiety agents, these drugs reduce pathological anxiety, tension, and agitation without therapeutic effects on disturbed cognitive or perceptual processes. High potential for dependency; all act differently in the body but produce symptoms of intoxication and withdrawal similar to those of alcohol.**

of deep depression that reinforces addictive behavior patterns and guarantees continued use of the drug.

Cocaine has been classified by the federal government as a schedule II substance—a drug officially considered to have "high abuse potential with some recognized medical use." Cocaine is consumed in three ways: sniffed intranasally, smoked as freebase or crack, or injected. Various medical problems may develop, depending on the route used. People who sniff cocaine have problems that relate to deterioration of the nasal passages: sores, hoarseness, and throat infections. Those who smoke the drug can have lung damage, upper gastrointestinal tract problems, and throat damage from the harsh smoke. Intravenous users may experience endocarditis, heart attacks, angina, and needle-related diseases, such as hepatitis and HIV.

Cocaine exerts two main effects on the body—anesthetic and stimulant. As an anesthetic, it blocks the conduction of electrical impulses within the nerve cells that are involved in sensory transmissions, primarily pain. It also acts as a stimulant for both sexual arousal and violent behavior.

The body's peak reaction to cocaine occurs about 5 minutes after it is taken and declines steadily over the following 2 to 5 hours. After the initial euphoria, however, most of cocaine's effects take place between 20 to 40 minutes after use.

Some common effects of cocaine use are euphoria, talkativeness, contentment, alertness, reduced need for sleep, heightened self-awareness, altered sexual feelings, humor, physical neglect, perceptual changes, and compulsive behavior.

Table 25–4 Drug Information: Stimulants

Drug	Intoxication	Overdose: Effects	Overdose: Possible Treatments	Withdrawal: Effects	Withdrawal: Possible Treatments
Amphetamines (Long acting) Dextroamphetamine (Dexedrine) Methamphetamine (Methadrine) Ice (synthesized for street use)	*Physical:* Tachycardia Dilated pupils Elevated blood pressure Nausea and vomiting Twitching *Psychological/ perceptual:* Assaultive Grandiose Impaired judgment Impaired social and occupational functioning Euphoria Increased energy *Severe effects:* Resembles paranoid schizophrenia Paranoia with delusions Psychosis Visual, auditory, and tactile hallucinations Severe to panic levels of anxiety Potential for violence **NOTE: Paranoia and ideas of reference may persist for months afterward.**	Respiratory distress Ataxia Hyperpyrexia Convulsions Coma Death associated with hyperpyrexia, convulsions, cardiovascular shock	*Supportive measures:* Acidify urine (ammonium chloride) Phenothiazines to treat psychotic reactions *Medical and nursing management for* Hyperpyrexia Convulsions Respiratory distress Cardiovascular shock	Depression Agitation Apathy Sleepiness Disorientation Fatigue Lethargy	Antidepressants for depression
Cocaine/crack (Short acting) **NOTE:** *High obtained:* Snorted—3 min Injected—30 sec Smoked—4–6 sec (crack) *Average high lasts* Cocaine—15–30 min Crack—5–7 min	*Physical:* Tachycardia Dilated pupils Elevated blood pressure Insomnia Anorexia *Psychological/ perceptual:* Elation Grandiosity Resistance to fatigue Impaired judgment Paranoid thinking Disturbed concentration Psychosis Violent temper outbursts	Seizures Cardiac arrest Respiratory depression/ arrest Convulsions Hyperpyrexia Death	*Medical and nursing life-saving measure for* Convulsions (prescribe diazepam) Hyperpyrexia (use hypothermia mattress) Respiratory depression/ cardiac arrest	Fatigue Depression Apathy Anxiety Chronic users often abuse or are dependent on a narcotic, alcohol, or an anxiolytic to lessen the withdrawal symptoms of cocaine/crack Craving	*Detoxification:* Experimental at present: 1. Amino acids (tyrosine and tryptophan) 2. Dopamine agonist 3. Antidepressants (desipramine)

Continued

TABLE 25–4 DRUG INFORMATION: STIMULANTS *(Continued)*

Drug	Intoxication	Overdose: Effects	Overdose: Possible Treatments	Withdrawal: Effects	Withdrawal: Possible Treatments
	Severe effects (Chronic use): **Formication** (tactile hallucinations involving animals or bugs); "cocaine bugs" refer to the sensation some chronic users experience of bugs crawling under their skin *Chronic user complaints:* ▸ Chronic insomnia ▸ Chronic fatigue ▸ Severe headaches ▸ Nasal problems ▸ Poor/decreased sexual performance ▸ Potential toxic cardiovascular effects				
Nicotine	None known: however, dependence caused by at least several weeks of smoking 10 cigarettes (0.5 mg nicotine each) per day			Cravings—"nicotine fits" Anxiety Restlessness Difficulty concentrating Disruption in sleep patterns Excessive eating Irritability Constipation Headaches Gastrointestinal disturbances	None known
Caffeine	*Physical:* Restlessness Excitement Insomnia Flushed face Diuresis Gastrointestinal complaints Cardiac arrhythmias Psychomotor agitation Periods of inexhaustibility Nervousness Rambling flow of thought			Headache Fatigued feeling Irritability	

Data from American Psychiatric Association (1994). *Diagnostic and statistical manual of mental disorders* (4th ed.). Washington, DC: American Psychiatric Association; O'Connor, P. G., Samet, J. H., and Stein, M. D. (1994). Management of hospitalized intravenous drug users: Role of the internist. *American Journal of Medicine*, 96:551; Bell (1992).

Cocaine produces an imbalance of neurotransmitters (dopamine and norepinephrine) that may be responsible for many of the physical withdrawal symptoms reported by heavy chronic cocaine users: depression, paranoia, lethargy, anxiety, insomnia, nausea and vomiting, and sweating and chills—all signs of the body struggling to regain its normal chemical balance.

NICOTINE AND CAFFEINE. Nicotine can act as a stimulant, depressant, or tranquilizer. Most people ingest caffeine by way of coffee, tea, or cola drinks. People ingest coffee as a drug: "I've got to have two cups in the morning to function"; for social reasons: "Let's get together for coffee"; or as a reward: "After I finish this job, I'm going to take a coffee break." Restlessness, excitement, cardiac arrhythmias, and nervousness are some of the signs of caffeine intoxication. Nicotine can also be chewed (smokeless tobacco), which adds cancer of the mouth to the list of dangers; cancer of the lungs is highly correlated with smoking tobacco (see Table 25–4).

Opiates

This class of drug includes opium, morphine, heroin, codeine, fentanyl and its analogs, methadone, and meperidine. Table 25–5 lists signs and symptoms of intoxication, overdose, withdrawal, and possible treatments.

Fentanyl analogs can be made to look like heroin, so that users do not know the difference when buying the drug. They are extremely dangerous because most illegal manufacturers are unable to control the strength of the substance they synthesize. (Fentanyl itself is 80 to 100 times as potent as morphine.) The only way to test potency is to try it, which often results in overdose and death. Fentanyl has caused severe damage to the brain and has left people in catatonic-like frozen states and with parkinson-like symptoms (Bell 1992). Also, because of the small amount of analog needed in comparison with heroin, the drug is often diluted with many toxic substances, such as talcum powder, corn starch, and flour. These substances can cause local and systemic complications when they are injected into the body. Fentanyl and its analogs are not detected through routine drug analysis, because only small amounts are present and 80% of it is excreted within 24 hours (Bell 1992).

Marijuana *(Cannabis sativa)*

Cannabis sativa is an Indian hemp plant. **Tetrahydrocannabinol (THC)** is the active ingredient found in the resin secreted from the flowering tops and leaves of the cannabis plant. THC has mixed depressant and hallucinogenic properties. Marijuana, the leaves of the cannabis plant, is generally smoked ("joint," "reefer,"

TABLE 25–5 DRUG INFORMATION: OPIATES*

		Overdose		Withdrawal	
Drug	**Intoxication**	**Effects**	**Possible Treatments**	**Effects**	**Possible Treatments/ Comments**
Narcotics Opium (paragenic) Heroine Meperidine (Demerol) Morphine Codeine Methadone (Dolophine) Hydromorphone (Dilaudid) Fentanyl (Sublimaze) Fentanyl analogs	*Physical:* Pupils constricted Decreased respiration Drowsiness Decreased blood pressure Slurred speech Psychomotor retardation *Psychological/ perceptual:* Euphoria Dysphoria Impairment of attention/ memory Impaired judgment	*Pupils may be dilated due to anoxia* Respiratory depression/ arrest Coma Shock Convulsions Death	Narcotic antagonist-e.g., naloxone (Narcan) quickly reverses central nervous system depression	Yawning Anorexia Insomnia Irritability Runny nose (rhinorrhea) Panic Diaphoresis Cramps Nausea Bone pain Chills Dilated pupils Fever Piloerection Lacrimation Diarrhea	Supportive measures *Short-acting drugs, e.g., heroin, morphine:* Peak 48–72 hours Course 7–10 days *Long-acting drugs, e.g., methadone* Peak 3–8 days Course several weeks

Data from American Psychiatric Association (1994). *Diagnostic and statistical manual of mental disorders* (4th ed.). Washington, DC: American Psychiatric Association; O'Connor, P. G., Samet, J. H., and Stein, M. D. (1994). Management of hospitalized intravenous drug users: Role of the internist. *American Journal of Medicine*, 96:551; Bell (1992).

***DEFINITION:** **An opiate derivative or synthetic that affects the central nervous system and the autonomic nervous system. Medically used primarily as an analgesic (pain killer). Consistent use causes tolerance and distressing withdrawal symptoms.**

"roach"), but it can be ingested. It is the most widely used illicit drug in the United States. Desired effects include detachment, relaxation, and others listed in Table 25–6. Overdose and withdrawal (other than craving) rarely occur. Medical indications exist for the use of THC (e.g., control of chemotherapy-induced nausea, reduced intraocular pressure in glaucoma, and appetite stimulation in AIDS wasting syndrome).

Hallucinogens

Hallucinogens can be defined loosely as drugs that alter one's mental state in a short period (National Institute on Drug Abuse [NIDA(a)] 1994).

LSD AND LSD-LIKE DRUGS. LSD (acid), **mescaline** (peyote), and **psilocybin** (magic mushroom) are hallucinogens. Mescaline and the mushroom *Psilocybe mexicana* (from which psilocybin is isolated) have been used for centuries in religious rites by Native Americans living in the southwestern United States and northern Mexico. A term popular in the 1960s for the hallucinogens was **psychedelic,** which in Greek means "for the soul to be manifest," emphasizing the subjective experience of expansion of consciousness reported by some users. The hallucinogenic experience produced by LSD is called a "trip." A good trip is characterized by a marked slowing of time, lightheadedness, perception of images in intense colors, and visions in sound (synesthesia). **Synesthesia** is the subjective experience of a sensation through a different sense than the one being stimulated (e.g., hearing colors, seeing music). People report experiencing spiritual ecstasy or being united with humankind. During a bad trip, a person may experience severe anxiety, paranoia, and terror compounded by distortions in time and distance. The terrorized person may become violent, unpredictably suicidal, or dangerously grandiose (e.g., thinking that he or she can fly). The trip ends when the effects of the drug wear off (8 to 12 hours for LSD). The best treatment for a person experiencing a bad trip is reassurance, companionship, and protection. Occasionally, an anxiolytic (diazepam [Valium] or chloral hydrate) is indicated.

PHENCYCLIDINE PIPERIDINE. PCP is also known as angel dust, horse tranquilizer, or peace pill.

TABLE 25–6 DRUG INFORMATION: CANNABIS SATIVA (MARIJUANA, HASHISH)

		OVERDOSE		WITHDRAWAL	
DRUG	INTOXICATION	Effects	Possible Treatments	Effects	Comments
Cannabis sativa (marijuana, hashish)	*Physical:* Tachycardia Conjunctival injection Increased appetite Impaired motor ability Talkativeness *Psychological/ perceptual:* Euphoria Intensification of perceptions Apathy Excessive anxiety/paranoia Impaired judgment Slowed perception of time Inappropriate hilarity Impaired memory Heightened sensitivity to external stimuli	Fatigue Paranoia Psychosis—rarely seen Anxiety/panic reactions			*Duration of effects:* Smoking 2–4 hr Ingestion: 5–12 hr **NOTE:** Cannabis dependence is associated with such psychological symptoms as ▸ **Lethargy** ▸ **Anhedonia (inability to enjoy life)** ▸ **Difficulty concentrating** ▸ **Memory problems**

Data from American Psychiatric Association (1994). *Diagnostic and statistical manual of mental disorders* (4th ed.). Washington, DC: American Psychiatric Association; Thomas, H. (1993). Psychiatric symptoms in cannabis users. *British Journal of Psychiatry*, 163:141; Bell (1992).

The route of administration plays a significant role in the severity of PCP intoxication. The onset of symptoms from oral ingestion occurs about 1 hour later. When taken intravenously, sniffed, or smoked, the onset of symptoms may occur within 5 minutes (APA 1994). The signs and symptoms of PCP intoxication range from acute anxiety to acute psychosis. The cardinal signs include a "blank stare," ataxia, muscle rigidity, vertical and horizontal nystagmus, tendency toward violence, and generalized anesthesia that lessens the sensations of touch and pain, making staff interventions difficult. *High doses* may lead to hyperthermia, agitated and repetitive movements, chronic jerking of the extremities, hypertension, and kidney failure. Persons with PCP intoxication may become stuporous with their eyes open, may be comatose, or may experience status epilepticus or respiratory arrest (Table 25–7).

Flashbacks are a common effect of hallucinogenic drugs. Flashbacks are the transitory recurrence of psychotomimetic drug experiences when a person is drug free. Such experiences as visual distortions, time expansion, loss of ego boundaries, and intense emotions are reported. Flashbacks are often mild and perhaps pleasant, but at other times, individuals experience repeated recurrences of frightening images or thoughts. Flashbacks are more likely to occur when a person is fatigued or has smoked marijuana in addition to ingesting a hallucinogenic drug.

Inhalants

About 17% of adolescents in the United States say that they have sniffed inhalants—usually volatile solvents, such as spray paint, glue, cigarette lighter fluid, and propellant gases used in aerosols—at least once in their lives (NIDA 1993). In children younger than 18 years, the level of inhalant use is comparable to that of stimulants and is exceeded only by the use of marijuana, alcohol, and cigarettes (NIDA 1994c). Types of inhalants, signs of intoxication, and side effects are given in Table 25–8. No one knows how many young people die each year from inhalant abuse, in part because medical examiners often attribute deaths from inhalant abuse to suffocation, suicide, or accident (NIDA 1994c). Inhalant use may be an early marker of substance abuse and should be the focus of increased prevention and early diagnosis and treatment (Hansen and Rose 1995).

Effects of Polydrug Abuse

The pathological use of more than one drug over a period of time is termed polydrug abuse. This phenomenon is seen in young, adult, and elderly clients. Polydrug abuse poses hazards to both the individual taking the drugs and the health care worker involved in treating a person who is intoxicated or in withdrawal. Polydrug abuse can have synergistic effects and antagonistic effects.

SYNERGISTIC EFFECT. Some drugs when taken together intensify or prolong the effect of either or both of the drugs (**synergistic effect**). For example, combinations of alcohol plus a benzodiazepine, alcohol plus an opiate, and alcohol plus a barbiturate all produce a synergistic effect. All these drugs are CNS depressants. Two of these drugs taken together result in far greater CNS depression than the sum of the effects of each drug added together. Many unintentional deaths have resulted from lethal combinations of drugs.

ANTAGONISTIC EFFECT. Many people may take a combination of drugs to weaken or inhibit the effect of another drug. For example, cocaine is often mixed with heroin (speedball). The heroin (CNS depressant) is meant to soften the intense letdown of cocaine (CNS stimulant) withdrawal. **Naloxone (Narcan),** an opiate antagonist, is often given to people who have overdosed on an opiate (usually heroin) to reverse respiratory and CNS depression (**antagonistic effect**). Since the duration of naloxone action may be less than that of the narcotic that was taken, further monitoring and possible additional doses of naloxone may be needed.

Severity of Withdrawal

Alcohol and other CNS depressant withdrawal reactions are associated with severe morbidity and mortality, unlike withdrawal from other drugs (see Tables 25–3 to 25–8.) The syndrome for alcohol withdrawal is the same for this entire class of CNS depressant drugs. Alcohol is used here as the prototype. The time intervals are delayed when other CNS depressants are the main drugs of choice or are used in combination with alcohol. In addition, as clients age, their symptoms of withdrawal continue for longer periods and appear to be more severe than in younger clients (Mudd et al. 1994).

Alcohol withdrawal reactions range from mild to severe, depending on the length of the drinking period and the amount of alcohol consumed. The most important assessment questions for planning care include (Wilson 1994)

- When did you last have a drink?
- What did you drink (beer, wine, hard liquor)?
- How much do you usually drink?
- How long have you been drinking?

Multiple drug and alcohol dependencies can result in simultaneous withdrawal syndromes that present a bizarre clinical picture and may pose problems for safe withdrawal. Family and friends may help provide important information that can assist in care planning. DSM-IV (APA 1994) identifies two alcohol withdrawal syndromes: (1) alcohol withdrawal and (2) the more severe alcohol withdrawal delirium (see Fig. 25–3).

TABLE 25–7 DRUG INFORMATION: HALLUCINOGENS*

		Overdose		Withdrawal	
Drug	Intoxication	Effects	Possible Treatments	Effects	Possible Treatments/ Comments
Hallucinogens Lysergic acid diethylamide (LSD) Mescaline (peyote) Psilocybin	*Physical:* Pupils dilated Tachycardia Diaphoresis Palpitations Tremors Incoordination Elevated temperature, pulse, respiration *Psychological/ perceptual:* Fear of going crazy Paranoid ideas Marked anxiety/ depression *Synesthesia,* e.g., colors are heard; sounds are seen Depersonalization Hallucinations occur although sensorium is clear Grandiosity, e.g., thinking one can fly	Psychosis Brain damage Death	Keep client in room with low stimuli—minimal light, sound, activity Have one person stay with client—reassure client, "talk down client" Speak slowly and clearly in low voice. Give diazepam or chloral hydrate for extreme anxiety/tension **NOTE: PCP and LSD-like drugs have different treatments.**	None known	**NOTE: Tolerance develops quickly.**
Phencyclidine piperidine (PCP)	*Physical:* Vertical or horizontal nystagmus Increased blood pressure, pulse, and temperature Ataxia Muscle rigidity Seizures Blank stare Chronic jerking Agitated, repetitive movements *Psychological/ perceptual* Maladaptive behavior changes	Psychosis Possible hypertensive crisis/ cardiovascular accident Respiratory arrest Hyperthermia Seizures	*If alert:* *Caution:* Gastric lavage can lead to laryngeal spasms or aspiration Acidify urine (cranberry juice, ascorbic acid); in acute stage, ammonium chloride acidifies urine to help excrete drug from body—may continue for 10–14 days Room with minimal stimuli **Do *not* attempt to talk down!** Speak slowly, clearly, and in low voice	*Tolerance and withdrawal reactions have been reported:* Lethargy Craving Depression **NOTE:** Takes 24–48 hr to recover from a high Drug stays in urine for a week or more Long-term effects of chronic PCP abuse may include ▶ Dulled thinking ▶ Lethargy ▶ Loss of memory and impulse control ▶ Depression	

TABLE 25-7 DRUG INFORMATION: HALLUCINOGENS* *(Continued)*

		Overdose		Withdrawal	
Drug	**Intoxication**	**Effects**	**Possible Treatments**	**Effects**	**Possible Treatments/ Comments**
	Belligerence, assaultiveness, impulsiveness, Impaired judgment, social and occupational functioning		Diazepam may be used for agitation Haloperidol may be used for severe behavioral disturbance (*not* a phenothiazine)		
	Severe effects: Hallucinations, paranoia Bizarre behaviors, e.g., barking like a dog, grimacing, repetitive chanting speech Regressive behavior Violent bizarre behavior Very labile behaviors		*Medical intervention for* Hyperthermia High blood pressure Respiratory distress Hypertension		

Data from American Psychiatric Association (1994). *Diagnostic and statistical manual of mental disorders* (4th ed.). Washington, DC: American Psychiatric Association; Bell (1992).

***DEFINITION: Produce *abnormal mental phenomena* in the cognitive and perceptual spheres. For example, distortion in space and time, hallucinations, delusions (paranoid or grandiose), and synesthesia may occur.**

Alcohol Withdrawal

The early signs of withdrawal develop within a few hours after cessation or reduction of alcohol (ethanol) intake; they peak after 24 to 48 hours and then rapidly and dramatically disappear, unless the withdrawal progresses to alcohol withdrawal delirium.

Early signs of withdrawal include anxiety, anorexia, insomnia, and tremor. The person may appear hyperalert, manifest jerky movements and irritability, startle easily, and experience subjective distress often described as "shaking inside." The person may also report transient, poorly formed hallucinations, illusions, or vivid nightmares. Nausea and vomiting may also occur.

People experiencing withdrawal are often terrified, confused, and anxious. A kind, warm, and supportive manner on the part of the nurse can allay anxiety and provide a sense of security. Consistent and frequent orientation to time and place may be necessary. Encouraging the family (one at a time) or close friends to stay with the client in quiet surroundings can also help increase orientation and minimize confusion and anxiety. *Illusions* are usually terrifying for the client. Illusions are misinterpretations of objects in the environment, usually of a threatening nature. For example, a person may think that spots on the wallpaper are blood-leaching ants. However, illusions can be clarified; this reduces the client's terror: "See, they are not ants, they are just part of the wallpaper pattern."

Panic may occur when an alcoholic craves a drink and realizes that no bottle is handy. If a person experiencing withdrawal is argumentative, hostile, or demanding, it is often because of this deep-seated anxiety as well as feelings of guilt and shame. The nurse can help the client overcome these feelings, making relief and hope possible by demonstrating an accepting attitude and showing strong support for efforts at recovery (Wilson 1994).

Pulse and blood pressure are usually elevated. Grand mal seizures may also develop; these usually appear 7 to 48 hours after cessation of ethanol intake, particularly in people with a history of seizures.

A client in alcohol withdrawal should be monitored to prevent progression into alcohol withdrawal delirium. Careful assessment followed by appropriate medical and nursing interventions can prevent the more serious withdrawal reaction of delirium.

TABLE 25–8 DRUG INFORMATION: INHALANTS

DRUG	INTOXICATION	SIDE EFFECT/OVERDOSE	TREATMENT
Volatile solvents: (gases or liquids that vaporize at room temperature) ▶ Butane ▶ Gasoline ▶ Spray paint ▶ Paint thinner ▶ Paint and wax removers ▶ Odorants ▶ Air fresheners ▶ Cigarette lighter fuels ▶ Analgesic sprays ▶ Propellant gases used in aerosols, e.g., whipped cream dispensers, hair spray ▶ Airplane glue ▶ Rubber cement ▶ Nail polish remover ▶ Dry cleaning fluid ▶ Spot remover ▶ Typing correction fluid or thinner	Excitation followed by drowsiness, disinhibition, staggering, lightheadedness, and agitation	Damage to the nervous system Death	Support affected systems
Nitrates ▶ Room odorizers (less common because products containing butyl and propyl were banned in 1991).	Enhance sexual pleasure		
Anesthetics ▶ Gas—especially nitrous oxide ▶ Liquid ▶ Local	Giggling, laughter	Peripheral nerve damage, death	

Data from National Institute on Drug Abuse Research Report Series (1994c). Inhalant abuse (NIH Publication No. 94-3818). Washington, DC: US Department of Health and Human Services.

Alcohol Withdrawal Delirium

Alcohol withdrawal delirium is considered a medical emergency and has up to a 20% mortality rate if it is left untreated. Death is usually due to myocardial infarction, fat emboli, peripheral vascular collapse, hyperthermia, or aspiration pneumonia. The state of delirium usually peaks 2 to 3 days (48 to 72 hours) after cessation or reduction of intake (can occur later) and lasts 2 to 3 days.

Along with anxiety, insomnia, anorexia, and delirium, additional features include

1. Autonomic hyperactivity (e.g., tachycardia, diaphoresis, elevated blood pressure).
2. Severe disturbance in sensorium (e.g., disorientation, clouding of consciousness).
3. Perceptual disturbances (e.g., visual or tactile hallucinations).
4. Fluctuating levels of consciousness (e.g., ranging from hyperexcitability to lethargy).
5. Delusions (paranoid), agitated behaviors, and fever (100° to 103°F).

Box 25–2 presents a vignette of a person going through alcohol withdrawal delirium.

Possible Traumatic Injuries

People may present for treatment after a fight or accident, with head injuries as well as the noticeable odor of alcohol on their breath or suspicion of other drug use. Intoxication can greatly interfere with an accurate physical and neurological assessment. Intracranial hematomas, subdural hematomas, and other conditions can go unnoticed if symptoms of acute alcohol intoxication and withdrawal are not distinguished from the symptoms of a brain injury. Therefore, neurological signs (pupil size, equality, and reaction to light) should be assessed, especially with comatose clients suspected of having traumatic injuries.

Levels of Anxiety and Coping Styles

Substance-abusing people are threatened on many levels in their interactions with nurses. First, they are concerned about being rejected. They are acutely aware that not all nurses are equally willing to care for addicted people, and in fact, many clients may have experienced instances of rejection in past encounters with nursing personnel. Therefore, vulnerability is increased each time that they must interact with the health care system.

BOX 25–2 CLINICAL VIGNETTE: A CLIENT WITH ALCOHOL WITHDRAWAL DELIRIUM

After her divorce, Mary started having a few drinks after coming home from work. She initially found that these drinks helped her relax and "put me in a good mood." Over time, Mary found that two drinks no longer did the trick and that she required three and then four drinks to achieve the relaxed feeling and mild euphoria she sought. Mary's body was building up a tolerance for the drug, and it took larger and larger doses to get the desired effect. The body is able to adjust to gradually increased doses of certain drugs over time and begins to require a certain level of the drug to function "normally." After 10 years, Mary was having a couple of drinks at lunch, before dinner, and during the evening. However, on first glance, the effects of alcohol did not show. Mary was able to appear normal with a high blood alcohol level. Mary eventually developed the habit of taking a drink every morning to settle the "shakes" and prevent tremulousness. She drank in the morning not to feel good but to prevent feeling bad.

In the spring of 1998, after suffering an acute attack of pancreatitis, Mary was hospitalized; she was given intravenous fluids and had a nasogastric tube in place. After 3 days, Mary became extremely agitated. She screamed that she was being held hostage by Iranian terrorists. She mistook her water carafe for a time bomb *(illusion)*. She became terrified at night, believing that she saw giant ants on the walls.

Mary's blood pressure increased from 120/70 mm Hg on admission to 150/100 mm Hg. Her pulse increased from 88 to 140. She thought it was the winter of 1985, about the time of her divorce.

After alcohol withdrawal delirium was diagnosed, Mary was given 100 mg of chlordiazepoxide hydrochloride (Librium) intravenously and then orally every 4 hours. Her pulse and blood pressure were monitored every hour. She was given 100 mg of thiamine intramuscularly, prophylactically against encephalopathy, as well as magnesium sulfate. Mary had normal skin turgor, and her urine specific gravity was within normal limits; therefore, fluids were not forced.

Her terror at seeing large ants was reduced by the nurse's presence and assurances that the nurse did not see the ants. Once the nurse showed her the carafe and poured some of the water into a glass, Mary understood that it was not a bomb.

Mary's agitation and aggressiveness became worse at night, and a friend stayed with her, talking in a calm manner and orienting her to her surroundings. When the nurses came to give medication and check vital signs and urinary output, they carefully explained everything they were going to do beforehand to allay misinterpretation of their actions by Mary.

Mary was placed in a private, well-lit room. A minimal amount of environmental stimuli were allowed (e.g., no radios or television, one visitor at a time). A clock was placed in clear view. The head of her bed was kept elevated to increase environmental orientation, and her bed faced the window to provide further orientation to time of day.

Three days later, Mary was fully oriented although still taking chlordiazepoxide. The episode had frightened her. She agreed to go to an Alcoholics Anonymous meeting and learn about other available avenues to sobriety.

Second, substance abusers may be anxious about recovering because to do so they must give up the substance they think they need to survive. Third, addicts are concerned about failing at recovering. Addiction is a chronic relapsing condition. In fact, relapse is one of the criteria for diagnosing addiction. Most addicts have tried recovery at least once before and have relapsed. As a result, many become discouraged about their chances of ever succeeding.

The aforementioned concerns can threaten the addict's sense of security and sense of self; thus, anxiety levels are increased. To protect against overwhelming anxiety, the addict establishes a **predictable defensive style.** The elements include defense mechanisms (denial, projection, rationalization), as well as characteristic thought processes (all-or-none thinking, selective attention) and behaviors (conflict minimization and avoidance, passivity, and manipulation). The addict is not able to give up these maladaptive coping styles until more positive and functional skills are learned.

Anxiety can also occur as a direct effect of the substance used. DSM-IV diagnostic criteria for substance-induced anxiety disorder are presented in Figure 25–5.

Psychological Changes

Certain psychological characteristics are associated with substance abuse, including denial, depression, anxiety, dependency, hopelessness, low self-esteem, and various psychiatric disorders. It is often difficult to determine which came first, psychological changes or substance abuse. Some people self-medicate to cope with psychiatric symptoms. For these people, symptoms of psychological difficulty remain, even after months of sobriety. Psychological changes that occurred as a result of drinking resolve quickly with sobriety.

Psychiatric disorders that may be seen concurrently in addicts include acute and chronic cognitive impairment disorders, attention deficit disorder, schizophrenia, borderline personality disorder, antisocial personality disorder, anxiety disorders, and disorders of mood (Fig. 25–5).

Suicidal ideation is always assessed, especially in cases of toxicity or coma. If the client appears to be suicidal,

PSYCHIATRIC DIAGNOSIS SECONDARY TO SUBSTANCE USE

SUBSTANCE-INDUCED ANXIETY DISORDER

A. Prominent anxiety, panic attacks, or obsessions or compulsions predominate the clinical picture.

SUBSTANCE-INDUCED MOOD DISORDER

A. A prominent and persistent disturbance in mood predominates in the clinical picture and is characterized by either (or both) of the following:

(1) Depressed mood or markedly diminished interest or pleasure in all, or almost all, activities
or
(2) Elevated, expansive, or irritable mood.

SUBSTANCE-INDUCED DISORDER

B. Evidence from the history, physical examination, or laboratory findings of either (1) or (2):

(1) The symptoms in criterion A developed during, or within 1 month of, substance intoxication or withdrawal.

(2) Medication use is etiologically related to the disturbance.

C. The disturbance is not better accounted for by an anxiety disorder/mood disorder that is not substance induced. Evidence that the symptoms are better accounted for by an anxiety disorder/mood disorder that is not substance induced might include the following: the symptoms precede the onset of the substance use (or medication use); the symptoms persist for a substantial period of time (e.g., about 1 month) after the cessation of acute withdrawal or severe intoxication or are substantially in excess of what would be expected given the type or amount of the substance used or duration of use; or there is other evidence suggesting the existence of an independent non–substance-induced anxiety disorder (e.g., a history of recurrent non–substance-related episodes)/mood disorder (e.g., a history of recurrent major depressive episodes).

D. The disturbance does not occur exclusively during the course of delirium.

E. The disturbance causes clinically significant distress or impairment in social, occupational, or other important areas of functioning.

Figure 25–5 DSM-IV criteria for substance-induced anxiety disorder and substance-induced mood disorder. (Adapted from American Psychiatric Association (1994). *Diagnostic and statistical manual of mental disorders (DSM-IV)* (4th ed.) (pp. 374–375, 439). Washington DC: American Psychiatric Association. Reprinted with permission. Copyright 1994 American Psychiatric Association.)

the nurse should determine whether previous suicide attempts have occurred. Information regarding suicide history of family members is also elicited (see Chapter 24 for assessment of suicidal potential).

Close attention to mental status often provides clues to these disorders. If addiction is present along with a well-defined psychiatric disorder, treatment consists of viewing both co-existing disorders as primary **(comorbid dual diagnosis)** and treating each separately. A well-monitored detoxification period allows for observation of mental symptoms. Skilled psychiatric nursing care is required when a detoxifying client begins to exhibit the symptoms of major psychiatric problems that must be treated as well.

Assessment strategies include data collection pertaining to both substance dependence and psychiatric impairment. Problem areas in assessment that are of particular relevance in a population with comorbidity include the masking of withdrawal by the subtle symptoms of psychiatric impairment (e.g., irritability, depression, restlessness). A further complication is the difficulty in differentiating normal aspects of the substance abuse recovery process from psychiatric impairment, such as major depression (Riley 1994). Ziedonis and colleagues (1994) found that the rate of psychiatric **comorbidity** (dual diagnosis) among cocaine addicts varied by race and gender.

Tolerance and progression of substance use and abuse also may be difficult to assess. Individuals with comorbid illnesses often follow a pattern of sporadic abuse with bingeing. These individuals are often poor historians and may have impaired capacities for honesty, recall, and insight.

Individuals with previously established psychiatric impairment may be experiencing substance abuse or dependence if they exhibit increasing frequency of symptoms, exacerbation without obvious reason, chronic noncompliance with treatment regimens, and self-medication or use of a substance in response to symptomatology secondary to psychiatric impairment or social stressors (Riley 1994). Substance abuse can go undetected in those who are depressed, suicidal, or anxious unless a thorough history is taken. Similarly, the understanding and treatment of substance-dependent people is enhanced by inquiries about symptoms of depression and anxiety (Madden 1993).

Compared with people who have a mental health disorder or a substance-abuse problem alone, clients with comorbid or coexisting diagnoses often experience more severe and chronic medical, social, and emotional problems. Because they have two or more disorders, they are vulnerable to both substance relapse and worsening of the psychiatric disorder. Further, substance relapse often leads to psychiatric decompensation, and worsening of psychiatric problems often leads to substance relapse. Thus, relapse prevention must be specially designed for clients with dual and comorbid disorders. Relapse prevention is discussed later in this chapter. Compared with clients who have a single disorder, clients with dual disorders often require longer treatment, have more crises, and progress more gradually into treatment (Ries 1994). Common examples of dual disorders include the combinations of major depression with cocaine addiction, alcohol addiction with panic disorder, alcoholism and polydrug addiction with schizophrenia, and borderline personality disorders with episodic polydrug abuse (Ries 1994).

Social Changes and Available Support Systems

Deterioration in a person's social status and social relationships often occurs as a result of addiction. Job demotion or loss of job, with resultant reduced or nonexistent income, may occur. Meeting basic needs for food, shelter, and clothing is thereby hampered. Marriages and other close relationships deteriorate and fail, and the person is often left alone and isolated. The lack of interpersonal and social supports is a complicating factor in treatment planning for the addict.

NURSING DIAGNOSIS

Appropriate nursing diagnoses depend on an accurate assessment. Whereas DSM-IV criteria emphasize patterns of use and physical symptoms, nursing diagnoses identify how dependence on substances of abuse interferes with a person's ability to meet the activities and demands of daily living.

Nursing diagnoses for clients with psychoactive substance use disorders are many and varied as a result of the large range of physical and psychological effects of drug abuse or dependence on the user and his or her family. Potential nursing diagnoses for people with substance use disorders are as follows (see also Table 25–9):

- **Anxiety**
- **Ineffective individual coping**
- **Altered health maintenance**
- **Risk for injury**
- **Altered cardiac output**
- **Impaired communication**
- **Fear**
- **Ineffective denial**
- **Defensive coping**
- **Sensory-perception alterations**
- **Hopelessness**
- **Risk for infection**
- **Altered parenting**
- **Ineffective breathing pattern**
- **Risk for self-harm**
- **Sexual dysfunction**
- **Sleep-pattern disturbance**
- **Impaired social interaction**
- **Altered thought processes**
- **Risk for violence: self-directed or directed at others**
- **Altered family process**
- **Self-care deficit**
- **Personal identity disturbance**
- **Risk for trauma**
- **Diversional activity deficit**
- **Altered nutrition: less than body requirements**
- **Powerlessness**
- **Self-esteem disturbance**
- **Spiritual distress**
- **Impaired skin integrity**

PLANNING

On completion of the assessment process, identified problems are assigned priorities, and a plan of care is developed. A plan of care is a guide to action for improvement or recovery from addiction. Planning care is guided by identification of long-term outcomes and awareness of common personal reactions.

Planning Outcome Criteria

Planning care requires attention to the client's social status, income, ethnic background, sex, age, substance use history, and current condition. It is safest to propose abstinence as a treatment goal for all addicts. Abstinence is strongly related to good work adjustments, positive health status, comfortable interpersonal relationships, and general social stability. Treatment must also address the client's major psychological and social problems as well as the substance-using behavior. Involvement of ap-

TABLE 25–9 NURSING DIAGNOSES: SUBSTANCE ABUSERS

NURSING DIAGNOSIS	RELATED PHENOMENA AND RATIONALE
Activity intolerance	Malnutrition. Peripheral neuropathies. Bacterial endocarditis.
Ineffective airway clearance	Pneumonias.
Anxiety	Drug withdrawal. Abstinence.
Diarrhea	Inflammation, irritation of the bowel due to ingestion. Black, tarry stools from gastrointestinal bleeding.
Ineffective breathing pattern	Alcohol or drug overdose.
Decreased cardiac output	Alcoholic cardiomyopathy.
Ineffective family coping: disabling	Social patterns often become dysfunctional.
Ineffective individual coping	A drug-dependent person has come to see substances as the solution to every problem; excessive drug taking is maladaptive, and problem-solving abilities are impaired. • Loses most or all significant others. • Not able to perform on the job. • Usually does not meet basic needs. • Risk of suicide increases. • Denial becomes a major barrier to overcome in effecting change. • Illness rates increase owing to effects of life style as well as drugs. • Accident rate increases owing to intoxication.
Risk for fluid volume deficit	Secondary to protracted vomiting or diarrhea.
Altered health maintenance	Substance abuse impairs health status; when intoxicated, the person is not concerned with being healthy and often does not take responsibility for basic care.
Risk for injury	Use of substances impairs judgment and increases risk-taking behavior; accidents and injury often result; with alcohol dependence, the blood profile becomes abnormal—liver function test results are elevated, and hemoglobin and hematocrit values are decreased.
Knowledge deficit	Learning needs about alcohol/drug effects. Learning needs about withdrawal process.
Noncompliance	Resumption of alcohol/drug-taking behavior after treatment.
Altered nutrition: less than body requirements	Nutritional deficits are frequent because an intoxicated person is not interested in food; money is spent on the substance of choice. Nutrient absorption is impaired.
Altered oral mucous membrane	Combined with the effects of smoking, leads to an increased incidence of carcinoma of the oropharynx.
Altered parenting: actual or risk for	Adults focused exclusively on their own needs to manage drug dependence do not pay attention to the needs of their children. Ineffective role modeling. Emotional neglect. Increased incidence of physical, sexual abuse.
Powerlessness	Central feelings in substance dependent people.
Self-esteem disturbance **Chronic low self-esteem**	Evidenced by the self-destructive nature of substance dependence and by nonparticipation in treatment. Not taking responsibility for self.
Sensory-perceptual alteration: auditory-visual	Audiovisual hallucinations due to withdrawal.
Sexual dysfunction	Substance abuse and dependence interfere with sexual arousal and performance: • Impotence in men. • Decreased vaginal lubrication in women.
Sleep-pattern disturbance	Central nervous system depressants interfere with rapid eye movement and stage IV (deep) sleep.
Altered thought processes	Judgment impaired; memory deficits with Wernicke-Korsakoff syndrome; when intoxicated, the alcohol- or drug-dependent person is less able to grasp ideas, reason, solve problems, calculate, attend to task.
Risk for violence or self-harm	Increased risk of suicide; increased incidence of child abuse and domestic violence, including battered woman syndrome.
Spiritual distress	Because feelings of hopelessness and helplessness are common and social relationships are often impaired, people often feel abandoned and alienated from others and from a higher power.

propriate family members is now considered essential by most treatment providers.

Goals for treatment need to be developed with the client and must reflect the client's goals and expectations for the future. Both short-term and long-term outcomes must be established.

Long-term outcome criteria are usually more comprehensive and tend to be viewed as the end product of a hard struggle—for example, sobriety. Short-term goals are the intermediate steps toward the long-term goal and often include target dates. For example, for the nursing diagnosis **ineffective individual coping** related to biochemical changes caused by alcohol and/or drug ingestion, the goals would be as follows:

LONG-TERM OUTCOME

- Client will maintain sobriety or drug-free status.

SHORT-TERM GOALS

- Client will attend a self-help group (e.g., **Alcoholics Anonymous** [AA]) every night for 1 month (by date).
- Client will be actively involved with his or her sponsor within 2 weeks.
- Client will participate in treatment center aftercare (group and individual or family counseling) (by date).
- Client will name two people to call when experiencing an urge to drink or use substance at end of week.
- Client will participate in relapse prevention training (identifying the individual's high-risk situations for drinking).
- Client will name two "problem areas" that he or she wants to work on at the beginning of each session.

Another important area for initial intervention is self-esteem. Therefore, for the nursing diagnosis self-esteem disturbance or **chronic low self-esteem,** the goals might be as follows.

LONG-TERM OUTCOMES

- Client will state that he or she feels good about self and about potential for the future.
- Client will demonstrate responsibility in implementing personal treatment goals.
- Client will demonstrate responsibility in implementing personal life goals.

SHORT-TERM GOALS

- Client will state that the self-help group (e.g., AA) is assisting self to "live one day at a time" (by date).
- Client will participate in social skills training (by date).
- Client will role play assertive communication skills to get needs met and maintain self-esteem (by date).
- Client will demonstrate one new skill learned each week.
- Client will discuss negative aspects of his or her life while keeping the focus on ways to effect positive change (by date).
- Client will identify three positive characteristics of self (by date).
- Client will state that he or she is more comfortable accepting positive feedback from others regarding personal strengths and positive qualities (by date).

Nurse's Feelings and Self-Assessment

Although nurses may identify with, and have empathy for, clients addicted to caffeine or tobacco, their responses to clients who abuse substances may not be so empathetic. A client who has overdosed on heroin, LSD, or cocaine may be viewed with disapproval, intolerance, and condemnation or may be considered morally weak. Also, manipulative behaviors often seen in these clients may lead nurses to feel angry and exploited. A nurse might want to help but may perceive the client who abuses drugs to be willful, uncooperative, and unworkable.

In some areas of the United States, the recreational use of cocaine, marijuana, and amphetamine is so common that the nurse may view this occurrence of intoxication or overdose as "normal" and may not have much emotional reaction. This attitude is as detrimental as strong emotional disapproval because the nurse may underestimate the importance of supportive measures and client education and the need for follow-up psychotherapeutic intervention.

Perhaps the most detrimental attitude in nurses and other health care workers is that of **enabling.** Enabling is supporting, or denying the seriousness of, the client's physical or psychological substance dependence. Behaviors that signal enabling by the nurse include

1. Encouraging denial by agreeing that the client only drinks or takes drugs "socially" or when he or she is a little nervous.
2. Ignoring cues to possible dependency—steers away from drugs to topics that are more comfortable for the nurse (e.g., anxiety or depression).
3. Demonstrating sympathy for the client's reasons (e.g., work, family, or financial problems) for abusing drugs rather than pointing out that these difficulties are often the result of—not the cause of—substance abuse.
4. Preaching that the problem can be overcome by will power, thus minimizing the fact that the person is physically or psychologically chemically dependent and has lost control over the use of the drug.

To come to a true personal understanding means that one must examine one's own attitudes, feelings, and beliefs about addicts and addiction. It often means that one must examine one's own substance use and that of others, and this is not always pleasant work.

A history of substance abuse in a nurse's own family can overshadow the nurse's interactions with addicts. The negative or positive experiences a nurse has had with addicted family members can influence interpersonal interactions with present or future clients.

Therefore, it is important that nurses attend to personal feelings that arise when they work with addicts. All health care professionals require supervision if they are not experienced in this area. Nurses who do not attend to, and work through, expected negative feelings that arise during treatment have power struggles with the clients, and the therapeutic process is generally ineffective. Each nurse must be free from the unconscious projection of negative feelings and of expectations and damaging stereotypes on clients. A therapeutic alliance is born, despite differences, when the client feels genuine empathy from the nurse (Wallace 1993).

INTERVENTION

Nurses interact with substance abusers in all areas of nursing practice. General approaches to interventions that apply to all contexts of care are described here.

The aim of treatment is self-responsibility, not compliance. A major challenge is predicting treatment outcome and improving treatment effectiveness by matching subtypes of clients to specific types of treatment. Although addicts share some characteristics and dynamics, significant differences exist within the addict population in regard to physiological, psychological, and sociocultural processes. These differences influence the recovery process, either positively or negatively.

Often, the choice of inpatient or outpatient care depends on cost and whether insurance coverage is available. Outpatient programs work best for employed substance abusers who have an involved social support system. People who have no support and structure in their day often do better in inpatient programs when and where available.

In addition, neuropsychological deficits have been associated with long-term alcohol abuse. Impairment has been found in abstract reasoning ability, ability to use feedback in learning new concepts, attention and concentration spans, cognitive flexibility, and subtle memory functions. These deficits undoubtedly have an impact on the process of alcoholism treatment.

At all levels of practice, the nurse can play an important role in the intervention process by recognizing the signs of substance abuse in both the client and the family and by knowing available resources to help with the problem. Nursing interventions and rationales are presented in Table 25–10. Specific interventions are discussed throughout the rest of the chapter.

Counseling (Basic Level)

Counseling involves working with behaviors that almost all substance abusers have in common, including dysfunctional anger, manipulation, impulsiveness, and grandiosity. Working with clients who frequently display these behaviors can be challenging and frustrating. However, supervision, peer support, and team cooperation lessen anxiety and feelings of helplessness in the staff and increase the client's opportunity to learn more adaptive coping styles. Table 25–11 identifies important interventions for nurses working with people who are recovering from substance abuse.

The nurse's ability to develop a warm, accepting relationship with an addicted client can assist the client in feeling safe enough to start looking at problems with some degree of openness and honesty. If the nurse lacks acceptance and empathy, knowledge and skill are not useful. Issues can become infinitely more complex if the client is a health care worker.

If the nurse has not worked through strong negative feelings related to the use of substances, the nurse should refer the client to another staff who has dealt with these issues and can begin promoting recovery. The client-counselor relationship is often considered to be more important than the type of treatment pursued. The follow-

TABLE 25–10 NURSING INTERVENTIONS AND RATIONALES: PEOPLE AFFECTED BY SUBSTANCE ABUSE

NURSING INTERVENTION	RATIONALE
1. Offering support/kindness.	1. Promotes ability to engage in treatment; minimizes anxiety.
2. Reinforcing disease concept of addiction.	2. Decreases guilt associated with behavior.
3. Communicating effectively.	3. Establishes trust; role modeling.
4. Setting limits.	4. Promotes ability to engage in treatment.
5. Maintaining consistency.	5. Fosters an objective and nonjudgmental milieu.
6. Providing information and education.	6. Client has learning needs related to ▸ Substance abuse as a chronic disease. ▸ The development of alternative coping skills to deal with stressful or problematic feelings or situations. ▸ Nutrition, hygiene, infection control.
7. Encouraging family therapy.	7. Promotes sharing of feelings and identification of destructive patterns that exist within the family system.

TABLE 25–11 NURSING INTERVENTIONS AND RATIONALES: PEOPLE RECOVERING FROM SUBSTANCE ABUSE

INTERVENTION	RATIONALE
1. Communicate empathy, focus on feelings. Avoid comments that seem judgmental.	1. Establish a therapeutic alliance based on understanding in an atmosphere of openness and support.
2. Evaluate extent of substance use (using a nursing history and standardized test), levels of anxiety, and coping styles as well as support systems.	2. Ascertain strengths and weaknesses, coping skills, available resources, and potential withdrawal reactions.
3. Continually assess ▶ Presence of predictable defense style. ▶ Psychophysiological responses.	3. Data collected in initial interview are not complete; assessment is ongoing.
4. Assess for relapse.	4. Substance abuse is a chronic condition; relapse should be addressed.
5. Refer to local resources—always include self-help groups.	5. Behavior change is long term; support, encouragement, and suggestions are needed throughout.
6. Refer to other community agencies as needed.	6. Assistance may be needed in other areas of life functioning (e.g., vocational rehabilitation, socialization, treatment of associated psychiatric disorders).

ing vignette illustrates the effective intervention that can occur when the nurse displays a nonthreatening style.

▶ Elyse, a 34-year-old recently divorced nurse, is brought into the hospital emergency department by two friends who had gone to her apartment after a frantic call from her. When she didn't answer the door, they had the superintendent let them in. They state that they found Elyse lying on the couch with a half-empty bottle of vodka as well as an empty bottle of diazepam pills that had recently been prescribed. When her friends tried to talk to Elyse, she responded with slurred speech. When she attempted to walk, her gait was unsteady. The friends report that when they questioned Elyse about her condition, she became extremely irritable. They say that as they sat with Elyse, they became increasingly alarmed and telephoned her physician, who encouraged them to take her to the hospital. The following initial interview takes place there after she is treated and determined to be stable.

DIALOGUE	THERAPEUTIC TOOL/COMMENT
Nurse: Elyse, I get the impression that life must have been getting very difficult for you lately.	Validating and empathizing.
Elyse: *(Silence)* . . . I don't think you would understand.	
Nurse: I guess sometimes it feels as if no one understands, but I would like to try.	Reflecting/empathizing
Elyse: At times . . . I feel I can't go on any more . . . so many losses.	
Nurse: Loss is difficult. Elyse, tell me about your losses.	Encouraging the client to share her painful feelings.
Elyse: My brother's sudden death . . . We were so close . . . I depended on him so much.	
Nurse: It must have been difficult for you to lose him so suddenly.	Empathizing.
Elyse: *(Silence)* . . . No one knows . . . then Harry, he left . . . *(Elyse starts to cry)*	
Nurse: Tell me what you are feeling right now.	Encouraging the expression of feelings while feelings are close to the surface.
Elyse: I don't know . . . angry maybe . . . why does everyone leave me? . . . Oh, I hate them . . . Oh, I wish I had a Valium now . . .	
Nurse: And what does the Valium do to help you?	Beginning to explore the drug dependence in a gently nonthreatening manner.

▶ Elyse becomes less defensive as time goes on and seems to relate best to the nurse. The nurse tells Elyse about a Narcotics Anonymous group that is made up of chemically impaired people from the health care professions. She states that substance-abuse disorders among nurses and doctors are a widespread, recognized problem. Elyse still has a tendency to minimize her drug dependence, but she is willing to work on her feelings about her divorce and her brother's death. She agrees to group and individual therapy on an outpatient basis.

Principles for counseling interventions include the following:

1. Expect abstinence/sobriety. The distortions, memory loss, and confusion that occur as a result of drug intoxication make communication and intervention ineffective when the person is intoxicated.
2. Individualize goals and interventions.
3. Set limits on behavior and on conditions under which treatment will continue.
4. Support and redirect defenses rather than attempting to remove them.
5. Recognize that the process of recovery is carried out in stages.
6. Look for therapeutic leverage. Make abstinence and sobriety worthwhile for the substance abuser (e.g., keeping one's job, family, friends).

The following vignette demonstrates the use of therapeutic leverage in addressing the role of drug use in the client's life. It is presented as a dialogue between a nurse and a 17-year-old young man. His parents are divorced, and his father abuses him when drinking. He was picked up three times during the preceding 7 months for possession of cocaine.

DIALOGUE	THERAPEUTIC TOOL/COMMENT
Nurse: I understand you entered the treatment program yesterday afternoon following your court appearance.	Placing the event in time and sequence, validating the precipitating event.
Frank: Yeah—it was my Dad's idea.	
Nurse: Well, what do you think of the idea?	Encouraging evaluation (actions first, thoughts, then feelings).
Frank: I don't like it. I don't need this place. I'm not a junkie—I just use cocaine, that's all. I can handle it.	
Nurse: From what I've heard, your involvement with cocaine has gotten you into trouble.	Pointing out realities.
Frank: Yeah, well, I guess I can't deny that . . . but I still don't think I need this place.	
Nurse: Are you saying that you don't think you need a treatment program?	Validating the client's perception.
Frank: Well, I don't know, I guess maybe I am messed up a bit.	
Nurse: "Messed up."	Restating
Frank: Yeah.	
Nurse: What is one thing about you that's messed up?	Encouraging client to be specific rather than global.
Frank: *(Silence)* I guess I feel like I don't belong anywhere.	
Nurse: Talk more about that.	

A useful tool for helping the resistant addict develop a willingness to engage in treatment is known as the **intervention.** The concept behind the intervention is that addiction is a progressive illness and rarely goes into remission without outside help. The strategies for the intervention are outlined in Box 25–3.

Counseling and support should be encouraged for all families with a drug-dependent member. **Al-Anon** and **Al-a-Teen** are self-help groups that offer support and guidance for adults and teenagers, respectively, in families with a chemically dependent member.

BOX 25–3 STEPS IN THE INTERVENTION

1. All the people concerned about, and affected by, the person's drinking are gathered together to present their case. The intervention must be rehearsed before it is actually carried out, usually with the support and guidance of a counselor.
2. Specific evidence related to the drinking is presented by each person, and it is written down so that each person does not have to rely on memory in a tense situation.
3. Timing must be right:
   - There must be current evidence available.
   - It must take place after a crisis is precipitated by alcohol use and *not* when the person is intoxicated or in severe withdrawal.
4. The intervention requires privacy. It is held in a place where no interruptions can occur.
5. Anticipate the use of defenses. Do not react to them.
6. Demonstrate genuine, but firm, concern.
7. Understand alcoholism as a disease.
8. Present treatment alternatives.
9. Prepare responses to possible outcomes. The goal is to get the affected person treatment. If the alcoholic person agrees to get treatment, then he or she is taken immediately to a detoxification unit, where arrangements have been previously made. If the person refuses, then family members state that his or her decision must force them to make decisions of their own because they are no longer willing to live with the alcoholic person's behavior.

Adapted from Johnson, V. E. (1986). *Intervention: How to help someone who doesn't want help.* Minneapolis: Johnson Institute.

Self-Care Activities (Basic Level)

Twelve-Step Programs

The most effective treatment modalities for all addictions have been the 12-step programs. AA is the prototype of all 12-step programs that were subsequently developed for any number and types of addictions. Three basic concepts are fundamental to all 12-step programs:

1. Individuals with addictive disorders are powerless over their addiction, and their lives are unmanageable.
2. Although individuals with addictive disorders are not responsible for their disease, they are responsible for their recovery.
3. Individuals can no longer blame people, places, and things for their addiction; they must face their problems and their feelings.

The 12 steps are considered the core of treatment (Box 25–4). Using the 12 steps is often referred to as "working the steps." They are designed to help a person refrain from addictive behaviors as well as to foster individual change and growth. They offer the behavioral, cognitive, and dynamic structure needed in recovery. In addition to AA, other 12-step programs include Pills Anonymous, Narcotics Anonymous, Cocaine Anonymous, and Valium Anonymous.

Self-help groups help family members deal with many common issues. Al-Anon and **Narc-Anon** are support groups for spouses and friends of alcoholics or addicts. Al-Anon, like AA, Al-a-Teen, and Adult Children of Alcoholics (discussed later), works through a combination of educational and operational principles centered around acceptance of the disease model of addiction. This acceptance can remove the burdens of guilt, hostility, and shame from family members. Al-Anon also offers pragmatic methods for avoiding enabling behaviors.

Al-a-Teen is a nationwide network for children older than 10 years of age who have alcoholic parents. It is structured under the guidance of members of Al-Anon. It offers the teenager the chance to share feelings and discuss problems with other teenagers who are having similar experiences; this process can be tremendously therapeutic. The group is open to children who have parents who use other substances as well.

Adult Children of Alcoholics (ACoA) groups offer support for those who experience difficulties and problems in their adult life as a result of having an alcoholic parent or parents. Adult children of alcoholics were often deprived of a nurturing parent in their formative years.

Self-help groups, like AA and the others described, offer camaraderie and a chance to talk about feelings in a comfortable, accepting, caring environment. A concept supported by these groups is the concept of the **co-dependent** or enabler; not buttressed by any research data, this concept describes a person who was often called addicted or sick and is said to benefit from "treatment."

Co-dependence as a Phenomenon

Co-dependence is a cluster of behaviors once thought to exist only in alcohol addiction. Since the mid-1980s, many disciplines have identified co-dependent behaviors that exist separately from addictions (Bradshaw 1988; Whitefield 1988). Some theorists believe that co-dependence behavior grows out of dysfunctional structures—whether one's family, one's profession, or one's society. In nursing, we see co-dependence surfacing in the form of addictions, eating disorders, unhappy primary relationships, burnout, and physical and mental illness.

BOX 25–4 THE TWELVE STEPS OF ALCOHOLICS ANONYMOUS

1. We admitted we were powerless over alcohol—that our lives had become unmanageable.
2. Came to believe that a power greater than ourselves could restore us to sanity.
3. Made a decision to turn our will and our lives over to the care of God **as we understood Him.**
4. Made a searching and fearless moral inventory of ourselves.
5. Admitted to God, to ourselves, and to another human being the exact nature of our wrongs.
6. Were entirely ready to have God remove all these defects of character.
7. Humbly asked Him to remove our shortcomings.
8. Made a list of all persons we had harmed, and became willing to make amends to them all.
9. Made direct amends to such people whenever possible, except when to do so would injure them or others.
10. Continued to take personal inventory, and when we were wrong, promptly admitted it.
11. Sought through prayer and meditation to improve our conscious contact with God, **as we understood Him,** praying only for knowledge of His will for us and the power to carry that out.
12. Having had a spiritual awakening as the result of these steps, we tried to carry His message to alcoholics, and to practice these principles in all our affairs.

People who are co-dependent usually have a constellation of dysfunctional thoughts, feelings, behaviors, and attitudes that effectively prevent them from living full and satisfying lives. Symptomatic of co-dependence is valuing oneself by what one does, what one looks like, and what one has, rather than by who one is. Refer to Box 25–5.

Living with a substance abusing or alcoholic individual is a source of stress and requires family system adjustments. Certain behaviors usually arise when a person attempts to cope with stressful situations. Often, these behaviors are designed to control the situation in an attempt to eliminate the source of the stress. In the case of alcoholism, whether these behaviors are any different from those present in response to other chronic conditions has yet to be demonstrated. In fact, the behaviors attributed to the co-dependent person are found in a large proportion of the general population; they are, in fact, skills at which women excel, namely, relationship building and maintenance.

The contemporary co-dependence literature and the recovery groups that draw on it characterize relationship dilemmas as pathological and vastly oversimplify problems of human dependency and interdependency. This has particular appeal now, with social roles being in flux and women feeling especially burdened by the combination of traditional caretaking responsibilities and roles introduced by their entry into the workforce. New forms of healthy interdependence between people have not been sufficiently realized as the old social contracts have been unraveling. Characterizing these symptoms of individual and social transition as pathological is not helpful to anyone, especially the minority group that already serves as the lightning rod for all sorts of psychological pathology, women. Recent studies seem to support the view that the overresponsible behavior of alcoholic spouses reflects their stressful circumstances more than their disturbed personalities. Table 25–12 offers some guidelines for a person in a co-dependent relationship.

Co-dependence is overresponsible behavior—doing for others what they could just as well do for themselves. Talking in terms of extremes of overresponsibility or underresponsibility points to a need for behavioral change rather than the need for recovery from a "disease."

BOX 25–5 OVERRESPONSIBLE (CO-DEPENDENT) BEHAVIORS

Co-dependent individuals find themselves

1. Attempting to control someone else's drug use.
2. Spending inordinate time thinking about the addicted person.
3. Finding excuses for the person's substance abuse.
4. Covering up the person's drinking/drugging or lying.
5. Feeling responsible for the person's drug use.
6. Feeling guilty for the addicted person's behavior.
7. Avoiding family and social events because of concerns or shame about the addicted member's behavior.
8. Making threats regarding the consequences of the alcoholic's/drug abuser's behavior and failing to follow through.
9. Eliciting promises for change.
10. Feeling like they are "walking on eggshells" on a routine basis to avoid causing problems, especially alcohol or drug use.
11. Allowing moods to be influenced by those of the addicted person.
12. Searching for, hiding, and destroying the abuser's source of supply, e.g., alcohol.
13. Assuming the alcoholic's/substance abuser's duties and responsibilities.
14. Feeling forced to increase control over the family's finances.
15. Often bailing the addicted person out of financial or legal problems.

Milieu Therapy (Basic Level)

It was formerly thought that addicted individuals could not be helped until they were ready for help. This is only partly true. It is true that most addicted people do not come readily for treatment. The motivation of an addicted client, like that of anyone else who is facing changes in life style, is mixed. Whatever motivation is there can be encouraged. It is part of the nurse's job to help clients become receptive to the possibility of change. This can occur in the context of the therapeutic environment.

Substance abusers often seem indifferent to the destruction they bring on themselves and their families. They also show marked dependency, and they may depend on others (most often loved ones) to solve their problems. This characteristic can give the family and friends an effective means of motivating the substance-abusing person toward treatment. When family and friends refuse to solve the person's problems, the individual is forced to face the consequences of his or her behavior. Al-Anon teaches family members the "three Cs" concept. Family members did not *cause* the disease, they cannot *control* it, nor can they *cure* it. They learn that they are not responsible for this disease or for the person who has it.

A significant relationship has been noted between a client's feelings of "belongingness" and treatment outcome. The more the client feels socially involved with peers, the better the chance for successful treatment outcome, continuation of treatment, and lower relapse rates. Nurses should evaluate the feelings of belongingness periodically by questioning clients about how they perceive themselves within their peer group. A client may be immersed in social events but perceive himself or herself as

TABLE 25–12 STRATEGIES FOR CO-DEPENDENT RELATIONSHIPS

STRATEGY	RATIONALE
I will not allow myself to	
1. **Argue** when my partner has been drinking/using or is angry, upset, or strung out because	1a. When I argue, it causes me to become defensive and justify myself. 1b. Arguments when we are upset accomplish nothing. 1c. Arguments cause me to become sad or mad. 1d. During arguments, we say things we regret.
2. **Be put down** and be abused verbally, because	2a. I am human and entitled to make mistakes. 2b. Putdowns cause me to become defensive. I do not need to defend myself. I am a responsible, caring, and loving individual. 2c. I cannot use putdowns. They do not give me any information about myself or about anything else. However, I can use support and guidance if this is a reciprocal process and my support and guidance are listened to. 2d. Putdowns cause me to become sad, to become mad, and to lose control of myself, and I do not like myself when I lose control, even when my partner provokes it.
3. **Accept more** than my share of responsibility, because	3a. Eventually, I would become resentful and angry. 3b. I would then feel used and abused. 3c. It would increase the stress I am feeling. 3d. I already have more responsibility than I can handle. 3e. If I accept more than my share of responsibility, I would not have energy and time left for myself first and others second.
4. **Hold in** my emotions, because	4a. I could become physically sick. 4b. I am entitled to express my feelings provided I do not put anybody else down. 4c. If I hold in my feelings, they could build up to the point of a blow-up. 4d. Expressing my feelings lets other people know that my feelings are important, because they are my feelings and I am important. 4e. Feelings are to be shared with those I love and who love me. If people do not care about my feelings, maybe they do not care about me. 4f. Sharing my feelings with those I love will give them a chance to share their feelings with me. 4g. Sharing my feelings will help people I love learn to know me better and appreciate me for what I am—an important person.
5. **Let anybody keep me from doing the things I enjoy doing,** because	5a. I deserve some enjoyment out of life. 5b. My family is part of my life. I enjoy being with them and I should be able to spend time with them without feeling guilty. 5c. It makes me happy and content to do things I enjoy, including doing absolutely nothing! I am important even when I am doing nothing.

From L'Abate, L. and Norreson, M. (1992). Treating codependency. In L. L'Abate, J. Farrar, and D. Serrilella (Eds.), *Handbook of differential treatments for addictions* (p. 296). Boston: Allyn & Bacon.

isolated. Clients with an isolated perception have a much greater chance of shorter lengths of stay in treatment programs and a higher rate of relapse. Mynatt (1996) stressed the vulnerability of teenagers and women in our society and offered holistic prevention and intervention strategies as outlined in Box 25–6.

Residential Therapeutic Communities

Many residential **therapeutic communities** expect the addict to remain for 12 to 18 months. It is difficult to say how these programs will be affected (i.e., by cutbacks on finances and emphasis on shorter-term care) by the changes in the health care system. The goal of treatment is to effect a change in life style, including abstinence from drugs. Other anticipated outcomes are development of social skills and elimination of antisocial behavior. Follow-up studies suggest that clients who stay 90 days or longer exhibit a significant decrease in illicit drug use and recorded arrests and an increase in legitimate employment. The residential therapeutic community is considered to be best suited for individuals who have a long history of antisocial behavior. Synanon, Phoenix House, and Odyssey House are three of the more familiar names among the 300-plus therapeutic communities in the United States.

Intensive Outpatient Programs

Most treatment for substance-abusing clients takes place in the community. With managed care, many people who would previously have been treated in the hospital

BOX 25–6 HOLISTIC PREVENTION AND INTERVENTION RECOMMENDATIONS

- Prevention and intervention strategies in vulnerable teens and recovering women should be used to increase self-esteem, assertiveness, coping mechanisms, problem solving, and other life skills, and to decrease depression, loneliness, and anxiety, with the goal of increasing resiliency to substance abuse disorders.
- Group strategies for women and teens would provide the social support and means to accomplish these changes.
- Fostering interest in a career in children and teenagers should increase self-esteem and increase the resiliency to the use of alcohol or drugs.
- Fostering the ability to maintain one's practice as a nurse should maintain the nurse's self-esteem and decrease the risk of relapse to alcohol or drugs as a maladaptive coping mechanism.
- Every nurse admitted to a treatment or monitoring recovery program should be assessed for the effects of previous or current victimization and the appropriate referral made.
- Every health care provider and employer should be aware of the risks and symptoms of relapse and the effects of unresolved familial issues of victimization on relapse.
- Further research aimed at women's needs must test the strength of the risk factors, develop treatment strategies, and test the efficacy of treatment.

From Mynatt, S. (1996). A model of contributing risk factors to chemical dependency in nurses. *Journal of Psychosocial Nursing,* 34(7):21.

setting will now be treated in intensive outpatient programs. Clinical Pathway 25–1 is an example of the steps addicted people follow in an intensive outpatient program until they "graduate" to the aftercare phase of the program.

Intensive outpatient treatment programs are becoming more popular because they are viewed as flexible, diverse, cost-effective, and responsive to the specific individual needs of a person.

Outpatient Drug-Free Programs and Employee Assistance Programs

Outpatient drug-free programs have the same goals as the therapeutic communities but aim to achieve these goals in an outpatient setting, thus allowing individuals to continue employment and family life. Outpatient drug-free programs are better geared to the polydrug abusing or alcoholic client rather than to the client who is heavily addicted to heroin. These centers may offer vocational education and placement, counseling, and individual or group psychotherapy. Employee assistance programs have been developed to provide the delivery of mental health services in occupational settings. Many hospitals and corporations offer their employees counseling and support as an alternative to being terminated when the employee's work performance is negatively affected by their impairment. Employee assistance programs offer employee counseling, information, and referral services.

Psychobiological Interventions (Basic Level)

The predominant somatic therapies are for detoxification (management of withdrawal) or for attempts to alter drug use (e.g., disulfiram [Antabuse], methadone, and naltrexone).

Alcohol Withdrawal

Not all people who stop drinking require management of withdrawal. This decision depends on the length of time and the amount the client has been drinking, the prior history of withdrawal complications, and the overall health status. Medication should not be given until the symptoms of withdrawal are seen. Early withdrawal symptoms are tremors, diaphoresis, rapid pulse (> 100), elevated blood pressure (> 150/90 mm Hg), and occasional transient tactile or visual hallucinations. Grand mal seizures can occur and are self-limited. The withdrawal process, not the seizure, needs to be treated. Drugs that are useful in treating alcohol withdrawal delirium are listed in Table 25–13.

Cross-dependent sedatives (chemical equivalents) are temporarily useful for reducing symptoms. Cross-dependent sedatives work by controlling the overactivity of the sympathetic nervous system. Chemical equivalents to alcohol that are used for this purpose include the benzodiazepines, such as diazepam and chlordiazepoxide hydrochloride (Librium) (Bird and Makela 1994). In uncomplicated withdrawal, 25 to 50 mg of chlordiazepoxide hydrochloride may be given every 2 to 4 hours. However, once alcohol withdrawal delirium appears, doses of 50 to 100 mg are given. Ten to 20 times the normal doses of these drugs may be needed because cross-tolerance from the drug of dependence often develops. Danger of an inadvertent overdose is always possible, and close nursing and medical observation is needed, especially during the first 24 hours.

The pulse and blood pressure should be checked hourly for the first 8 to 12 hours after admission, at least every 4 hours during the first 48 hours, and then 4 times a day thereafter. The pulse is a good indication of progress through withdrawal. Elevated pulse may indi-

CLINICAL PATHWAY 25–1 Substance Abuse-Intensive Outpatient Program

	1ST 4 WEEKS	NEXT 6 WEEKS	NEXT 2 WEEKS
Assessment	Evaluation (CAC) H & P (MDs)	Initial treatment plan completed Diagnostic summary completed First treatment plan review completed.	Continue ongoing monitoring of abstinence. Conduct second treatment plan review.
Diagnostic studies	Routine lab tests* Complete or partial physical exam	Review lab results	Repeat follow-up labs and work-up as needed
Medications	Written orders	Medication monitoring, PRN Routine lab and medication levels*	
Treatment activity	Individual counseling, psycho-educational groups, random drug screens—monitoring of results; random alcohol saliva tests—monitoring of results; attendance at AA/NA meetings.	→	→
Teaching	Disease concept of alcoholism/addiction explained. Family education sessions begin; Rules and regulations explained	Education on feelings, 12 steps, relapse prevention, post–acute withdrawal symptoms, anger management, spirituality of recovery	→
Discharge planning	Initial assessment of discharge needs.	Discharge status reviewed	Revise discharge needs. Transfer patient to aftercare phase.
Consults	Psychiatric evaluations. Subspecialists or legal authorities*	→	→
Patient outcomes	Verbalizes understanding of concept Attends 12-step Anonymous meetings 3 times per week Abstains from all mood-altering substances	Verbalizes feeling states Verbalizes relapse triggers → → Develops strategies to avoid relapse Prepares 1st step: relapse prevention	Presents 1st step Receives peer evaluation Gives life story Gives peer goals to complete Presents completed peer goals to peers Graduates to aftercare phase of program

Modified from Mary T. Pfister, RN, MHA. Mountainside Hospital, Glen Ridge/Montclair, NJ.
*As indicated.
CAC, community alcohol center; H & P, history and physical; PRN, as needed; AA, Alcoholics Anonymous; NA, Narcotics Anonymous; MDs, physicians.

cate impending alcohol withdrawal delirium, signaling the need for more rigorous sedation.

Thiamine (vitamin B_1) deficiency is often present, owing to poor dietary intake and malabsorption. Thiamine replacement is given in order to prevent **Wernicke's syndrome** (encephalopathy). Wernicke's syndrome is characterized by nystagmus, ptosis, ataxia, confusion, coma, and possible death.

Hypomagnesemia is another condition found in people with long-term drinking problems. Magnesium sulfate may be given to increase the body's response to thiamine and to raise the seizure threshold.

Anticonvulsants may or may not be used. Diazepam or phenobarbital may be used on a short-term basis to control seizures and prevent status epilepticus. Phenytoin (Dilantin) is less frequently used because seizures usually occur within the first 48 hours of withdrawal and an effective blood level of phenytoin takes days to reach; because alcohol withdrawal seizures *do not represent a primary seizure disorder*, a person without such a disorder should not be routinely given phenytoin.

Fluid and electrolyte replacements may be necessary, especially if the client is vomiting, has diarrhea, and is experiencing diaphoresis. In these cases, the client may be dehydrated and may need proper fluid and electrolyte replacement (e.g., potassium). However, caution is warranted. Diuresis occurs when BALs *rise*, but fluid retention may occur as BALs fall; therefore, a person in withdrawal may be *overhydrated*. Rigorous fluid therapy could cause serious complications, such as congestive heart failure.

Alcohol Treatment

NALTREXONE (TREXAN, REVIA). Naltrexone (an agent used for narcotic addiction) is also being used with success for some people in the treatment of alcoholism under the trade name ReVia. Naltrexone is proving to be a safe and useful adjunct in the treatment of alcoholism, especially for people with high levels of craving and somatic symptoms. A study by Volpkalli and associ-

TABLE 25–13 DRUG INFORMATION: TREATMENT OF ALCOHOL WITHDRAWAL DELIRIUM

DRUG	DOSE	PURPOSE
Sedatives Benzodiazepines Chlordiazepoxide (Librium) drug of choice	25–100 mg PO every 4 hours (for 5–7 days) in tapering doses	Chlordiazepoxide and diazepam provide *safe* withdrawal and have *anticonvulsant* effects.
Diazepam (Valium)	5–10 mg PO every 2–4 hours in tapering doses	
Phenobarbital/pentobarbital	100 mg PO in tapering doses	Control withdrawal. Caution: can depress respiration.
Thiamine (vitamin B_1) Given intramuscularly or intravenously before glucose loading	100 mg PO QD	Prevent Wernicke's encephalopathy.
Magnesium sulfate (especially if history of seizures)	1 g IM every 6 hours for 2 days	Increases effectiveness of vitamin B_1. Helps reduce status postwithdrawal seizures.
Anticonvulsant Phenobarbital Benzodiazepines Phenytoin (Dilantin)		For seizure control.
Folic Acid	1 mg PO QID	Most effective in short time. Takes days to reach therapeutic level.
Multivitamins	1 daily	Malabsorption due to heavy long-term alcohol abuse causes deficiencies in many vitamins.

PO, orally; QID, four times a day.

ates (1995) found that naltrexone-treated subjects had a greater decrease in alcohol craving, number of drinking days, and alcohol relapse rates than placebo-treated subjects.

DISULFIRAM (ANTABUSE). Disulfiram is used on motivated clients who have shown the ability to stay sober. Disulfiram works on the classical conditioning principle of inhibiting *impulsive* drinking because the client tries to avoid the unpleasant physical effects from the alcohol-disulfiram reaction. These effects consist of facial flushing, sweating, throbbing headache, neck pain, tachycardia, respiratory distress, a potentially serious decrease in blood pressure, and nausea and vomiting. The adverse reaction usually begins within minutes to a half hour after drinking and may last 30 to 120 minutes. These symptoms are usually followed by drowsiness and are gone after the person naps.

Disulfiram must be taken daily. The action of the drug can last from 5 days to 2 weeks after the last dose. It is most effectively used early in the recovery process while the individual is making the major life changes associated with long-term recovery from alcoholism. Disulfiram should always be prescribed with the full knowledge and consent of the client. The client needs to be told about the side effects and must be well aware that any substances that contain alcohol can trigger an adverse reaction. Three primary sources of "hidden" alcohol exist—food, medicines, and preparations that are applied to the skin. People also need to be careful to avoid inhaling fumes from substances that might contain alcohol, such as paints, wood stains, and "stripping" compounds. Unfortunately, voluntary compliance with the disulfiram regimen is often poor.

Opioid Treatment

METHADONE (DOLOPHINE). Methadone is a synthetic opiate that at certain doses (usually 40 mg) blocks the craving for, and effects of, heroin. It has to be taken every day, is highly addicting, and when stopped produces withdrawal. To be effective, the client must take a dose that will prevent withdrawal symptoms, block drug craving, and block any effects of illicit use of short-acting narcotics through the development of tolerance and cross-tolerance (NIDA 1994b).

A methadone maintenance program is not considered to be an effective treatment in itself. At times, it keeps the client out of the illegal drug subculture, but, to be successful, programs must include counseling and job training. Methadone maintenance reduces heroin addicts' risk of infection with HIV by reducing the occurrence of drug injection (Caplehorn and Ross 1995).

Methadone is the only medication currently approved for the treatment of the pregnant opioid addict. The clinical studies available demonstrate that methadone maintenance at the appropriate dose, when combined with prenatal care and a comprehensive program of support, can significantly improve fetal and neonatal outcome (Jarvis and Schnoll 1994).

Although abstinence from drug use during pregnancy is the ideal goal, it is not attainable for most addicted women. They may repeatedly withdraw and then use the substance again, which results in a continuing variation of blood levels of opiates and other drugs; this phenomenon appears to have severe consequences for fetal development. Methadone maintenance prevents this cycling and reduces the risk of other medical consequences of street drug use (e.g., HIV infection, hepatitis, sexually transmitted diseases) (Jarvis and Schnoll 1994).

L-ALPHA ACETYLMETHADOL. As an alternative to methadone, **LAAM** is effective for up to 3 days (72 to 96 hours), so clients need to come to an outpatient service for their dose only three times a week. This regimen makes it easier for clients to keep jobs and gives them more freedom than is available with methadone maintenance. LAAM is also an addictive narcotic: its therapeutic effects and side effects are the same as those of morphine.

NALTREXONE (TREXAN, REVIA). Naltrexone is a relatively pure antagonist that blocks the euphoric effects of opioids. It has low toxicity with few side effects. A single dose provides an effective opiate blockade for up to 72 hours. Taking naltrexone three times a week is sufficient to maintain a fairly high level of opiate blockade. For many clients, long-term use results in gradual extinction of drug-seeking behaviors. Naltrexone does not produce dependence. As previously mentioned, it has also been approved for the treatment of alcoholism because it decreases the pleasant, reinforcing effects of alcohol (Swift 1995).

Clonidine, which was initially marketed for high blood pressure, is also an effective somatic treatment for some chemically dependent individuals when combined with naltrexone. Clonidine is a nonopioid suppresser of opioid withdrawal symptoms. It is also nonaddicting.

Nicotine Addictions

Transdermal nicotine doubles long-term abstinence rates. It is preferred over nicotine gum because of its improved compliance, steadier blood levels, little long-term dependence, and less complicated instructions (Hughes et al. 1994).

Health Promotion and Health Maintenance (Basic Level)

Health maintenance for people who are abusing drugs and plan to continue to use them includes the following information. The nurse could say something like, "I would rather you seek treatment and not use drugs, but since you are choosing this behavior, here are some ways to minimize your risk." The nurse's counseling includes

1. Instruction on how to administer the drug under antiseptic conditions if the intravenous route is being used (reduces risk for HIV and hepatitis).
2. Education as to the properties, side effects, and long-term physical or emotional effects of the drug.
3. Referral information about community-based clinics, telephone numbers for hotlines, self-help groups, and halfway houses for possible future use.
4. Nutritional information. Many people who use drugs have malnutrition, either because of their life style or because of the properties of the drugs themselves.

Primary prevention through health teaching can have an important impact on how youngsters and adolescents choose to solve problems and relate interpersonally. Primary prevention programs aimed at youth must emphasize a "decision about substance use" theme and must educate youngsters about the effect of substances on mental and physical processes as well as mood. Peer teaching is often most effective, especially in adolescents. Teaching about alcohol's effects on unborn babies should occur in the preteen and teenage years as well as in gynecologists' offices and obstetrics clinics.

Many communities have youth organizations, such as scouting, 4-H clubs, school clubs, and organized church activities for youth. It has been found that the young people who participate in these groups are at a lower risk for substance abuse. Activities such as these help develop self-confidence and self-esteem in young people. Neighborhood recreational and occupational opportunities are an important investment not only for youth but also for communities as a whole. More such programs are sorely needed.

Part-time job placement can be an important alternative to substance abuse. Earning money on one's own can increase feelings of self-worth and confidence.

Primary prevention of HIV infection in the drug population is facilitated by needle exchange programs, in which addicts return their used needles for sterile ones. One of three people with AIDS in the United States is an intravenous drug user or the sexual partner of an intravenous drug user. Reducing needle sharing reduces the spread of HIV.

Case Management (Basic Level)

The prevailing care delivery model for dually diagnosed clients or those with comorbid illnesses is multidisciplinary case management. Practitioners are cross-trained in both substance dependency and psychiatry and thus can provide more comprehensive services. The case manager coordinates the services provided. Advanced practice psychiatric mental health nursing, with its holistic approach, is in a prime position to demonstrate the delivery of integrative care to the psychiatrically impaired and substance-abusing population (Riley 1994). Intensive case management has been shown to be as effective as behavioral skills training and more effective than 12-step programs in treating dually diagnosed clients (Jerrell and Ridgely 1995).

Psychotherapy (Advanced Practice)

Nurses with advanced training may be involved in psychotherapy with substance-using clients. Psychotherapy assists clients in identifying and using alternative coping mechanisms to reduce reliance on substances. Eventually, psychotherapy can assist recovering addicts to become increasingly comfortable with sobriety.

Psychotherapy with substance-using clients takes many forms. It can be individual, group, or family therapy; directive or nondirective therapy; goal-centered or insight-oriented therapy. Whatever type is used, clients need to be informed of what they can and cannot expect from the therapy and, likewise, what is expected from them.

Clients may ask nurses-therapists about their own habits of substance use. It is best to deal with this issue by exploring clients' underlying concerns about whether the nurse can understand and help them.

Confidentiality must be maintained throughout therapy except when this conflicts with events that require mandatory reporting (e.g., child abuse).

Many critical issues arise during the first 6 months of sobriety. These include the following:

1. Physical changes take place as the body adapts to functioning without substances.
2. Numerous signals occur in the client's internal and external world that previously were cues to drinking and drug use. Different responses to these cues need to be learned.
3. Emotional responses (feelings that were formerly diluted with substances) are now experienced full strength. Because they are so unfamiliar, they can produce anxiety.
4. Responses of family and co-workers to the client's new behavior must be addressed. Sobriety disrupts a system, and everyone in that system needs to adjust to the change.
5. New coping skills must be developed to prevent relapse and ensure prolonged sobriety. AA makes use of the acronym **HALT:** "Don't get too Hungry, Angry, Lonely, or Tired." When alcoholics experience these feelings, they are to "halt" and implement alternative coping strategies.

Psychotherapy during this early stage of treatment needs to be directive, open and honest, and friendly and caring. Slogans from AA can be helpful in providing initial as well as ongoing motivation for adjusting to life without alcohol. Some examples are "One day at a time," "Easy does it," and "Utilize, don't analyze." These phrases can provide a focus for clients who are new to recovery. The therapeutic process involves teaching the client to identify the physical and emotional changes that are occurring in the here and now. The nurse therapist can then assist in the problem-solving process.

Recovery programs that are successful in producing abstinence, such as AA and Narc-Anon, owe some of their success to the intuitive recognition of the fact that in the early stages of recovery, the addict protects his or her self-esteem by attempting to minimize the anxiety associated with change and growth. Often, the best time for a recovering alcoholic to engage in insight psychotherapy is after 2 to 5 years of sobriety—once defenses have been loosened.

Psychotherapy must be geared toward the individual's phase in the recovery process. A particular therapeutic intervention for an addict who has recently used the substance or substances may be entirely inappropriate for a client who has managed to achieve several years of sobriety, and vice versa. Besides individual therapy, other specific psychotherapeutic techniques used with addicts include behavior therapy and group, family, and marital therapy.

Individual Therapy

Individual psychotherapy may be a significant and sometimes essential contribution to the recovery process. Control mastery therapy helps to provide addicted and recovering clients with a therapeutic relationship in which they may work to challenge their belief system about the role of substances in their lives. This is a valuable treatment method for helping clients enter and remain in a successful and abstinent recovery (O'Connor and Weiss 1993).

Relapse Prevention

Relapses are common during a person's recovery. Behavioral techniques have been formed that are extremely successful in helping people maintain sobriety or abstinence. Various behavioral techniques are used for situations that the client may face during recovery. Included are **skills training** (for situations requiring refusal of substances), **assertiveness training, relaxation training,** and **relapse prevention** training, which focuses on interrupting signals to drink. The last approach realistically recognizes that addiction is a chronic condition marked by relapses. The possibility of a **lapse** (a single incident of substance use after treatment or abstinence) should be discussed, therefore, and options for preventing escalation into a full-blown **relapse** (continuing drug use) should be explored. The goal is to help the person learn from those situations so that periods of sobriety can be lengthened over time and so that lapses and relapses are not viewed as total failure.

◗ Bill, a 20-year-old single man, is brought to the emergency department in a coma. He is accompanied by his mother, with whom Bill lives in a small apartment. Bill had been in his room at home. When his mother was not able to arouse him, she dialed 911 for an ambulance. A syringe and some white powder were found next to Bill.

◗ Bill's breathing is labored, and his pupils are constricted. Vital signs are taken; his blood pressure is 60/40 mm Hg, and his pulse is 132. Bill's situation is determined to be life threatening.

◗ Bill's mother is extremely distressed, but she is able to report to the staff that Bill has a substance-abuse problem and had been taking heroin for 6 months before entering a methadone maintenance program.

◗ It is determined at this point to administer a narcotic antagonist, and naloxone (Narcan) is given intramuscularly. After this, Bill's breathing improves, and he responds to verbal stimuli.

◗ Bill's mother later tells staff that Bill has been in the methadone maintenance program for the past year but has not attended the program or received his methadone for the past week. At their urging, she calls the program, which arranges to send an outreach worker, Mr. Rodriguez, to talk to her and Bill. Bill makes an appointment with Mr. Rodriguez for the following Monday.

◗ Mr. Rodriguez knows that Bill's future ultimately rests with Bill. On Monday, Mr. Rodriguez talks to Bill regarding his perceptions of his situation, where Bill wants to go, and what Bill thinks he needs to get there.

DIALOGUE	THERAPEUTIC TOOL/ COMMENT
Mr. Rodriguez: I was in the emergency room Friday afternoon when you were brought in by ambulance.	Placing the event in time and sequence, validating the precipitating event.
Bill: Were you? I guess a lot of people thought it was over for me.	
Mr. Rodriguez: It certainly looked quite serious.	Emphasizing the reality—prevents minimizing situation.
Bill: Yeah. I should never have left the program. I was doing better, and I just didn't think I needed it anymore.	
Mr. Rodriguez: You said you were doing well.	Reflecting.
Bill: Yeah. I had a job, and I was beginning to save some money. Wow! I can't believe I blew this whole thing.	
Mr. Rodriguez: I don't know that you really did. Your counselor for the program phoned your doctor this morning to find out how you were doing.	Pointing out reality.
Bill: Do you think they will take me back?	
Mr. Rodriguez: Why don't we talk some more, and after we finish, I'll speak with the other staff about your situation. If you would like to get back into the program, you can call your counselor and we'll support your decision.	Gathering information.

◗ After reviewing Bill's history, the health care team decides that the self-help, abstinence-oriented recovery treatment might be the most helpful program. Bill has not been taking drugs a long time, he has a job, and he appears motivated. Naltrexone (Trexan) will be given in conjunction with relapse prevention training and regular attendance at Narcotics Anonymous meetings.

Relapse prevention strategies focus on training clients to anticipate and cope with the possibility of relapse and on helping clients modify their lives to reduce their exposure to high-risk situations (drug cravings and social pressures to use drugs) and strengthen their overall coping abilities. Relapse prevention should be integrated into all treatment approaches. The major tenets of relapse prevention (NIDA 1994b) are as follows:

- Abstinence, not controlled use, must be the ultimate goal.
- Clients should be helped to recognize that one or more temporary lapses are likely to occur. This recognition must be instilled in a way that does not appear to give permission for occasional drug use.
- Clients should be taught skills for anticipating, avoiding, and coping with their personal high-risk situations.
- Clients should be taught constructive responses to cope with lapses when they do occur.
- Any positive expectations that clients have about drug use should be countered with reminders about the lows that follow the highs and about the long-term negative consequences of substance abuse.

General strategies for relapse prevention are cognitive and behavioral: recognizing and learning how to avoid or cope with threats to recovery; changing life style; learning how to participate fully in society without drugs; and securing help from other people, or social support (DeJong 1994; NIDA 1994b).

Group Therapy

Group therapy has been helpful for many people recovering from addiction. The advantages of group therapy are the following:

- Social isolation is decreased.
- Newly recovering addicts have models in people with longer histories of sobriety.
- Addicts are encouraged to seek support and encouragement from a variety of people.
- The therapist can observe the interpersonal behavior of the clients without always being directly involved.

Groups can be closed or open, homogeneous or mixed, education oriented or therapy oriented. Clients should be screened for admission to the group, and the therapist should maintain good record keeping throughout. Ground rules must be developed that include commitments to the following points:

- Minimal stay in the group
- Expectations of regular attendance or advance notice of absences
- Advance notice to the group if the client is considering leaving
- Abstinence and willingness to talk about fears of drinking or actual lapses should they occur
- Communication about other difficult issues in the client's life
- Communication about group dynamics
- Confidentiality

Goals for therapy include

- Maintaining sobriety.
- Developing motivation to continue to grow and change.
- Recognizing and identifying behavior patterns that led to drinking.
- Learning new ways to handle old problems.
- Developing an emergency plan for high-risk situations that might lead to relapse.
- Recognizing and identifying feelings (especially guilt, anger, depression, fear).
- Learning to enjoy life without psychoactive substances.

Family Therapy

Family therapy for substance abusers is based on the premise that the addiction is a "family illness" because all members are affected. Family members of substance abusers lack trust in each other, lack nurturing closeness, and inadequately solve problems. Children become used to extra and inappropriate responsibilities. Parental role models are distorted. In fact, family equilibrium is established around the substance use. Therefore, removal of the "using" behavior becomes a threat.

As with any form of therapy, abstinence must be a goal. The family must begin to learn healthy ways to solve problems. Children of substance users are at high risk for developing their own addiction. This risk should be discussed openly at family therapy sessions. The basic purpose of intervention is to assist the family to change their ineffective communication and response patterns (Alexander and Gwyther 1995). Instilling hope in the family's future is one of the nurse's greatest responsibilities.

When the addict is in inpatient treatment, the family frequently has the opportunity to learn about the physiology of substance abuse, family dynamics, communication, and recovery. Structured family therapy may begin during this time of hospitalization. Past behavior, anger, and alcohol use—and the family's role in these—are brought up and dealt with. Plans are made to change behavior as sobriety becomes a part of daily life. The carrying out of these plans must be rehearsed and practiced.

After inpatient treatment of the addicted client, family members are usually concerned about the client's return to substance use. Members frequently "walk on eggshells," not talking about substance use or other problems, in an attempt to prevent a relapse. Ongoing therapy helps family members change roles as the need for control is lessened. (Spouses frequently are reluctant to give up the position of power they had when their spouse was intoxicated.) Responsibility needs to be renegotiated. Children's roles and changes in behaviors also need to be examined.

Marital Therapy

For the married couple, issues about time spent at home and about sex are prominent. The substance abusing client may not have much libido as she or he begins to recover. Sex is not a paramount urge. Having felt deprived in many areas, the spouse may want gratification of unmet needs soon after recovery begins. Couples need further education in the recovery process as they deal with major changes in how they function. For example, the wife may not understand the anger of the recovering husband. She may balk at his attendance at 12-step meetings or his kindness to people he meets there. She may feel rejected and not needed. These issues predominate in the early months of recovery.

Behavioral marital therapy helps substance abusers stay in treatment and helps couples better maintain their marital satisfaction after treatment.

The Chemically Impaired Nurse

Substance dependency in nurses is a serious problem for both the nurse and those under the nurse's care. Nurses have a 50% higher rate of chemical dependency than the general population. Among practicing nurses, estimates of nurses who are chemically dependent range from 10% to 20%. Helping the chemically impaired nurse is difficult but not impossible. The choices for actions are varied, and **the only choice that is clearly wrong is to do nothing.** Nurses who have worked with other nurses who are chemically impaired state that most want to be helped, not protected.

Descriptive studies of nurses recovering from dependency suggest the following profile: the nurse has a family history of substance abuse, depression, and sexual abuse; is academically and professionally successful; is often divorced; has received professional treatment for substance abuse; and regularly attends recovery self-help groups. A study by Mynatt (1996) found that most nurses (55%) began using drugs in their preteens and teens and 85% of chemically dependent nurses had begun by the age of 30. Mynatt (1996) proposed a triad of chaotic family of origin, victimization, and low self-esteem.

A demanding professional life has an impact on nurses who have experienced stressful family relationships in which alcohol or drug use was problematic. Nurses from such backgrounds frequently strive to be "supernurses" and deal with doubts about their feelings of inadequacy by overachieving or overfunctioning. Drug or alcohol use can become a facilitator for overfunctioning. Substance abuse can temporarily help the nurse feel adequate. However, in order to continue the overfunctioning behavior and sustain the temporary feelings of adequacy, the use and abuse of the drug need to continue.

Some early indicators of a substance-abuse problem that can alert peers (nurses) and nurse-managers who are sensitive to job performance problems include

- Changing a life style to focus on activities that encourage substance use.
- Showing inconsistency between statements and actions.
- Displaying increasing irritability.
- Projecting blame on others.
- Isolating oneself from social contacts.
- Showing deteriorating physical appearance.
- Having frequent episodes of vaguely described illness.
- Having frequent tardiness and absenteeism.
- Manipulating possession of the narcotic keys for a particular shift.
- Having deepening depression.

Often, the impaired nurse volunteers to work additional shifts to be nearer to the source of the drug. The nurse may leave the unit frequently or spend a lot of time in the bathroom. When the impaired nurse is on duty, more clients may complain that their pain is unrelieved by their narcotic analgesic or that they are unable to sleep, despite getting sedative medications. Increases in inaccurate drug counts and vial breakage may occur.

Direct confrontation results in hostility and denial. A nurse who demonstrates behaviors consistent with drug abuse or dependence should be reported immediately to a supervisor. This measure can prevent harm to clients under the nurse's care and can save a colleague's professional career or life. By dealing with the problem early on, the nurse may help stop the process of addiction before more devastating and permanent consequences affect the nurse's life. However, the peer's and supervisor's major concern must be with job performance. Clear and accurate documentation is vital, and referral to a drug and alcohol treatment program should always be an option. When a report is sent to the state board of nursing, it needs to contain factual documentation of specific dates, events, and consequences.

There are some things that one should not do, under any circumstances, when dealing with an alcohol-addicted or a drug-addicted nurse:

1. *Don't* lecture, moralize, scold, blame, threaten, or argue with the person about the problem. Document the behavior. The nurse's supervisor can use it to counsel the nurse about job performance.
2. *Don't* lose your temper.
3. *Don't* "enable" the problem to continue by covering up the consequences, trying to protect the person, making excuses, or doing the addicted nurse's job.
4. *Don't* give the person an easier work schedule.
5. *Don't* have a holier-than-thou attitude.
6. *Don't* be too sympathetic. You are not a counselor or a big sister or brother.
7. *Don't* accept what you know is a lie. When you know the person is lying, say so. Accepting lies only encourages more lying, and you will lose the person's respect at the same time.
8. *Don't* accept promises to "do better," and don't keep switching agreements. When you say that a job is in jeopardy (suspension or termination) if the person's performance does not improve, you must follow through.
9. *Don't* accept the responsibility of letting someone work on your unit or team if he or she is impaired by alcohol or drugs. Judgment is the first casualty of alcohol or drug use.
10. *Don't* put off facing the problem, hoping it will get better with time. It will not.

Programs for chemically dependent nurses have been developed in some states in response to a policy statement issued by the American Nurses' Association. Some state boards of nursing allow impaired nurses to avoid disciplinary action if they seek treatment. Other states may refuse to grant or restore the impaired nurse's license. Some state boards of nursing administer the treatment program themselves. The aim of these programs is to protect clients and to keep the nurse in active practice (perhaps with limitations) or to return the nurse to practice after suspension and professional help. Mynatt (1996) advocated a holistic approach to prevention and intervention in order to deal with the complex issues in the workplace and in the lives of impaired nurses. Box

25–6 recommends critical areas for prevention and intervention. Mynatt stressed that nurses who have completed treatment for chemical dependency should receive long-term continuing care since relapse rates are often high. Relapse occurs in 60% to 75% of clients within 90 days of completion of a treatment program and in 80% to 90% within 1 year of treatment (Mynatt 1996) (see Box 25–6).

Both the medical and nursing professions are formally recognizing this problem, and there is an increased commitment to the rehabilitation of chemically impaired health care professionals, in the form of self-help peer-support groups, hotlines, crisis information, and treatment referral.

EVALUATION

Treatment outcome is judged by increased lengths of time in abstinence, decreased symptomatic denial, acceptable occupational functioning, improved family relationships, and, ultimately, ability to relate normally and comfortably with other human beings.

The ability to use existing supports and skills learned in treatment is important for ongoing recovery. For example, recovery is actively viable if, in response to cues to use the substance, the client calls his or her sponsor or other recovering persons; increases attendance at 12-step meetings, aftercare, or other group meetings; or writes feelings in a log and considers alternative action.

Other factors, such as environmental stressors, coping responses, and social resources, may have as much influence on the recovery process as the client's treatment experiences and initial symptoms. Addicted clients recover not so much because nurses treat them as because they treat themselves. Four factors that are closely associated with remission from substance abuse are

1. Finding a substitute dependency, such as a compulsive hobby, to replace the drug.
2. Experiencing a consistent aversive event related to using the drug of choice (**aversive conditioning**), such as that occurring with disulfiram or an obvious adverse health effect (abscesses from "skin popping").
3. Discovering a fresh source of hope and self-esteem.
4. Obtaining new social supports, such as new friends and a new job.

Awareness and clinical assessment of extra-treatment factors make the evaluation process more meaningful, in that the nurse can more adequately understand posttreatment functioning and the process of recovery and relapse. Continuous monitoring and evaluation lead to a better chance for prolonged recovery.

CASE STUDY: WORKING WITH A PERSON DEPENDENT ON ALCOHOL

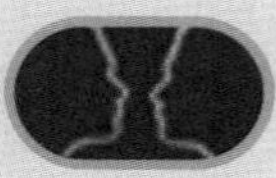

Mr. Young, aged 49 years, and his wife arrive in the emergency department one evening, fearful that he has had a stroke. His right hand is limp and he is unable to hyperextend his right wrist. Sensation to the fingertips in his right hand is impaired.

Mr. Young looks much older than his stated age; in fact, he looks to be about 65. His complexion is ruddy and flushed. History taking is difficult. Mr. Young answers only what is asked of him, volunteering no additional information. He states that he took a nap that afternoon and that when he awakened, he noticed the problems with his right arm.

Mr. Young reveals that he has been unemployed for 4 years because the company he worked for went bankrupt. He has been unable to find a new job but has a job interview in 10 days' time. His wife is now working full time, so the family finances are OK. They have two grown children who no longer live at home.

He denies any significant medical illness except for high blood pressure, just diagnosed last year. His family history is negative for illness, with the exception of alcoholism. His mother is a recovering alcoholic who was treated at an inpatient facility and is maintaining her sobriety. Ms. Dee, the admitting nurse, asks Mr. Young questions about his use of alcohol, including quantity, frequency, and withdrawal experiences. In general, he denies any significant alcohol involvement. Ms. Dee shares with him the fact that the disease of alcoholism runs in families. She asks Mr. Young whether (1) he knows this and (2) if it concerns him with regard to his own drinking. Mr. Young says that he knows and that he does not want to think about it.

Ms. Dee then speaks with Mrs. Young about the events of the day. Ms. Dee states that she spoke with Mr. Young and that she is concerned that he might have an alcohol problem. Ms. Dee shares the impressions that led her to that tentative conclusion and asks Mrs. Young to describe her husband's involvement with alcohol. Mrs. Young's shoulders slump; she sighs and says, "I have spent the entire day talking to a counselor at the local treatment center to see if I can get him in. He won't admit that he has a problem. " Mrs. Young then recounts a 6-year history of steadily

CASE STUDY: WORKING WITH A PERSON DEPENDENT ON ALCOHOL (Continued)

increasing alcohol use. She says that for a while she could not admit to herself that her husband was an excessive drinker. "He tried to hide it, but gradually I knew. I could tell from little changes that he was intoxicated. I couldn't believe it was happening because he had been through the same thing with his mother and we'd always had such a good relationship. I thought I knew him. Actually, I guess I did when he was a working man. Being unemployed and unable to find a job has really floored him. And now he's even going to job interviews intoxicated."

Mrs. Young recounts how her husband's drinking worsened dramatically with unemployment and how she tried ridding their home of liquor, only to find bottles hidden in their mobile home one day when she went to clean it. She describes her feelings, which are like an emotional roller coaster—elated and hopeful when he seems to be doing OK; dejected and desperate on other occasions, such as the time that she found the alcohol in their mobile home. Mrs. Young hates going to work for fear of what he might do while she is gone. She says she is terrified that one day her husband will crack up the car and kill himself, because he often drives when intoxicated. Ms. Dee discusses with Mrs. Young her own involvement as part of the family system. Options for Mrs. Young and her husband are discussed.

Meanwhile, the physician in the emergency department has examined Mr. Young. The diagnosis is radial nerve palsy. Mr. Young most likely passed out while lying on his arm. Because Mr. Young was intoxicated, he had not felt the signals that his nerves sent out to warn him to move (numbness, tingling). Mr. Young continued to lie in this position for so long that the resultant cutting off of circulation was sufficient to cause some temporary nerve damage.

Mr. Young's BAL is 0.31 mg%. This is three times the legal limit in many states of intoxication (0.1 mg%). Even though he has a BAL of 0.31 mg%, Mr. Young is alert and oriented, not slurring his speech or giving any other outward signs of intoxication. The difference between Mr. Young's BAL and his behavior indicates the development of tolerance, a symptom of physical dependence (see Table 25–1).

ASSESSMENT

Ms. Dee organizes her data into objective and subjective components.

OBJECTIVE DATA

- Drives when intoxicated
- Nerve damage owing to having passed out while lying on arm
- Increased alcohol use during stress of unemployment
- Capacity to obtain employment impaired by alcohol use
- Disruption in marital relationship caused by alcohol use
- Unable to see effect of his drinking
- Family history of alcoholism
- BAL three times the legal limit of intoxication; has developed tolerance

SUBJECTIVE DATA

- Denies he has an alcohol problem

NURSING DIAGNOSIS

From the data, the nurse formulates the following nursing diagnosis:

Ineffective individual coping related to alcohol use, as evidenced by

- Increased alcohol use during stressful period of unemployment
- Capacity to obtain employment impaired by alcohol use
- Disruption in marital relationship caused by alcohol use
- Unable to see effect of his drinking on his life functioning

Continued on following page

CASE STUDY: WORKING WITH A PERSON DEPENDENT ON ALCOHOL (Continued)

PLANNING

PLANNING OUTCOME CRITERIA

It is decided to allow Mr. Young to sober up in the emergency department because it is difficult to discuss goals when the client is intoxicated. When the client is sober, the nurse establishes goals with the client that are realistic, appropriate, and measurable.

NURSING DIAGNOSIS	LONG-TERM OUTCOME	SHORT-TERM GOALS
1. **Ineffective individual coping** related to alcohol use	1. Client will abstain from alcohol.	1a. Client will identify the role of alcohol in his life and his risk for alcoholism, given his family history. 1b. Client will agree to remain sober until his job interview 10 days hence. To assist in this effort, he agrees to ▪ Obtain an appointment at a community alcohol center. ▪ Attend at least one AA meeting/day. ▪ Call his sponsor when he feels the need for a drink. 1c. Client will state two alternative behaviors to engage in when he experiences the urge to drink. 1d. Client will name two ways to begin to rebuild trust in his relationship with his wife.

NURSE'S FEELINGS AND SELF-ASSESSMENT

The denial the alcoholic client exhibits often results in rejection by nurses, who feel that the alcoholic causes his or her own problems. Nurses generally feel sympathetic toward spouses and other family members but have a sense of helplessness about ability to effect change.

Feelings of rejection, sympathy, and helplessness impair the nurse's ability to facilitate change. True, some alcoholic persons do maintain their denial and effectively resist intervention, but many others welcome the opportunity to begin to learn different ways of coping with life problems. Before dismissing alcoholic clients as "not wanting help" or being "the only ones that can change things," nurses need to ask themselves if they have done all that they can in an attempt to engage the client in the change process.

Ms. Dee has seen many clients with the disease of alcoholism make radical changes in their lives, and she has learned to view alcoholism as a treatable disease. She is aware also that it is the client who makes the changes, and she no longer feels responsible when a client is not ready to make that change.

CASE STUDY: WORKING WITH A PERSON DEPENDENT ON ALCOHOL (Continued)

INTERVENTION

Ms. Dee suggests that Mrs. Young attend Al-Anon meetings and gives her information on where she can find groups in her area. She also urges Mrs. Young to discuss what is going on with her grown children and tells her about the problems that adult children of alcoholics often experience. She encourages Mrs. Young to let her children know of support groups they could go to if they feel the need.

Ms. Dee also urges Mrs. Young *not* to go in the car with her husband if he is driving while intoxicated. Ms. Dee states that she should not protect him from the results of his drinking (e.g., bail him out of jail if he is arrested for driving while intoxicated or make excuses for him). Ms. Dee adds that Al-Anon could offer crucial support for Mrs. Young and could assist her in minimizing her enabling behaviors, which family members often exhibit.

Ms. Dee outlines an initial care plan for Mr. Young (Nursing Care Plan 25–1). Attending AA is a central part of the treatment program, along with a variety of other interventions, like skills training, education, medical intervention, family counseling, and evaluation for naltrexone therapy.

EVALUATION

Mr. Young's willingness to become actively involved in planning short-term goals is evidence that the goals are realistic and appropriate. In this case, the main opportunity for evaluating the short-term goals is when and if Mr. Young calls back to report on steps he has taken to meet those goals. At that time, he should be supported and applauded for the progress he has made and encouraged to "keep up the good work. " Other referrals may be given if indicated.

Mr. Young does continue with AA. His denial persists, but he is highly motivated to keep his marriage. He gradually accepts a variety of referrals; as time progresses, he finds that the positive feedback and support from others increases his self-esteem, decreases his feelings of isolation, and reinforces his long-term goal of sobriety.

NURSING CARE PLAN 25–1 A PERSON WITH ALCOHOLISM: MR. YOUNG

NURSING DIAGNOSIS

Ineffective Individual Coping: related to alcohol use

Supporting Data

- Alcohol use increases in response to the stress of job loss, lowered role status.
- Alcohol use has impaired client's capacity to obtain employment.
- Alcohol use is causing disruptions in relationship with wife.
- Family history of alcoholism exists.

Outcome Criteria: Client will abstain from alcohol.

SHORT-TERM GOAL	INTERVENTION	RATIONALE	EVALUATION
1. Client will identify the role of alcohol in his life and his risk for alcoholism, given his family history.	1a. Point out relationship between no job and increased alcohol use. 1b. Provide information on the disease of alcoholism. 1c. Point out the factors placing person at risk for alcoholism. 1d. Communicate concern, empathy, nonjudgmental acceptance, warmth.	1a. Use assessment data to clarify behavior patterns. 1b. Stressing alcoholism as a disease can lower guilt and help increase self-esteem. 1c. Children with alcoholic parents are at a greater risk for developing alcoholism themselves. 1d. Helps establish a therapeutic relationship based on understanding and provides an atmosphere of openness and support. Helps client maintain self-esteem.	*GOAL MET* Client listens to nurse—admits that going to job interviews intoxicated would lower the chance of getting a job. States that he felt so down that he needed alcohol to feel OK.
2. Client will remain sober from now until his job interview (10 days)	2a. Refer to AA. 2b. Refer to local resources for an appointment with an alcohol counselor. 2c. List other available supports (e.g., friends, family).	2a–c. Much support and encouragement are needed for making major life changes, e.g., stopping drinking. A variety of support systems help decrease feelings of alienation and isolation.	*GOAL MET* Client calls the emergency department to report on carrying out the plan; states that potential employer wants him back for second interview.
3. Client will state two alternative behaviors that he can exercise when experiencing the urge to drink by (date).	3a. Evaluate client's situation by using a crisis intervention model, i.e., assessing precipitating events, support systems, and coping skills.	3a. Identifies high-risk situations and opportunities for change.	*GOAL MET* After 3 weeks, client states that he has attended AA every day. He is learning to identify situations that trigger the urge to drink and is learning new coping behaviors.

Continued on following page

NURSING CARE PLAN 25–1 A PERSON WITH ALCOHOLISM: MR. YOUNG *(Continued)*

SHORT-TERM GOAL	INTERVENTION	RATIONALE	EVALUATION
	3b. Explore alternative coping skills. Skills training may be needed (e.g., assertion, socialization, problem solving)	3b. Behavior change is a learning process. Relapse prevention can be practiced.	After 5 weeks, client has a slip and drinks for 2 days; he decides to try disulfiram.
	3c. Encourage participation in AA, group therapy, or other appropriate modalities.	3c. Provides support and minimizes feelings of isolation while client is learning new skills.	
	3d. Referral to a physician for complete physical examination; possible disulfiram (Antabuse) therapy.	3d. Disulfiram may help provide the external control needed during early months of sobriety; because it can cause physiological crises when taken with alcohol, a physical examination is needed.	
4. Client will name two ways to begin to rebuild trust in his relationship with his wife by (date).	4. Referral to a marital counselor.	4. Alcoholism is a "family illness" that adversely affects those close to the alcoholic.	*GOAL MET* Wife has been attending Al-Anon for 6 weeks, three times per week, after finding a group that she feels comfortable with. Client and wife decide to start couples therapy in 2 weeks.

SUMMARY

Substance use and dependence occur on a continuum, and the development of addiction and dependence is a time-related phenomenon. Various theories attempt to explain why some people develop a substance abuse problem and others do not. Because no clear consensus exists about the nature of alcoholism and other drugs, notions about treatment are also inconsistent. The more closely clinics are matched to a range of treatment alternatives, the greater the likelihood that sobriety or drug-free behavior will be achieved and overall life functioning will be improved.

Nurses encounter people with alcohol and drug problems in all areas of practice and thus must be prepared for assessing, planning, implementing, and evaluating nursing care of their clients. Assessment strategies are outlined in this chapter for determining severity of illness, levels of anxiety, and coping styles, as well as physiological and psychosocial changes. Some nursing diagnoses applicable to alcoholic clients include ineffective denial, risk for injury, hopelessness, risk for infection, altered family process, risk for self-harm, and many more.

Planning nursing care is important in setting mutually agreed-on goals as well as in fitting the treatment modality to the individual client. Principles and specific examples of psychotherapeutic interventions include behavior therapy; individual, group, family, and marital therapy; and self-help groups, such as AA. Some somatic treatments are helpful, as are outpatient and employer-assisted programs. Whatever techniques are used, the nurse must make clear to the client what expectations are reasonable. Issues common in early treatment are discussed, as are some general approaches to relapse prevention.

Nurses and other health care workers are at an even higher risk for chemical dependency than non–health care workers. Specific interventions and guidelines can help protect clients who are under an impaired nurse's care and can save the nurse's future livelihood—if not the impaired nurse's life.

REFERENCES

Alexander, D. E., Gwyther, R. E. (1995). Alcoholism in adolescents and their families. *Pediatric Clinics of North America*, 42(1):217.

American Psychiatric Association (1994). *Diagnostic and statistical manual of mental disorders* (4th ed.). Washington, DC: American Psychiatric Association.

Bell, K. (1992). Identifying the substance abuser in clinical practice. *Orthopaedic Nursing*, 11(2): 29.

Bird, R. D., and Makela, E. H. (1994). Alcohol withdrawal: What is the benzodiazepine of choice? *Annals of Pharmacotherapy*, 28:67.

Bohn, M. J. (1993). Alcoholism. *Psychiatric Clinics of North America*, 16(4):679.

Bradshaw, J. (1988). *Bradshaw on the family: Healing the shame that binds you.* Deerfield Beach, FL: Health Communications.

Brown, R. L. (1992). Identification and office management of alcohol and drug disorders. In M. F. Fleming, K. L. Barry (Eds.), *Addictive disorders*. St. Louis: Mosby–Year Book.

Cadoret, R. J., et al. (1995). Adoption study demonstrating two genetic pathways to drug abuse. *Archives of General Psychiatry*, 52:42.

Caplehorn, J. R., and Ross, M. W. (1995). Methadone maintenance and the likelihood of risky needle-sharing. *International Journal of Addiction*, 30(6):685.

DeJong, W. (1994). Relapse prevention: An emerging technology for promoting long-term drug abstinence. *International Journal of Addiction*, 29(6):681.

Ewing, J. A. (1984). Detecting alcoholism: The CAGE Questionnaire. *JAMA*, 252(14):1905.

Fink, L., Williams, J., and Stanley, R. (1996). Nurses referred to a peer assistance program for alcohol and drug problems. *Archives of Psychiatric Nursing*, 10(5):319.

Hansen, W. B., and Rose, L. A. (1995). Recreational use of inhalant drugs by adolescents: a challenge for family physicians. *Family Medicine*, 27(6):383.

Hughes, J. R., Higgins, S. T., and Bickel, W. K. (1994). Common errors in the pharmacologic treatment of drug dependence and withdrawal. *Comprehensive Therapy*, 20(2):89.

Jarvis, M. A. E., and Schnoll, S. H. (1994). Methadone treatment during pregnancy. *Journal of Psychoactive Drugs*, 26(2):155.

Jerrell, J. M., and Ridgely, M. S. (1995). Comparative effectiveness of three approaches to serving people with severe mental illness and substance abuse disorders. *Journal of Nervous and Mental Disease*, 183(9):566.

Mayfield, D., McLeod, G., and Hall, P. (1974). The CAGE questionnaire: Validation of a new alcoholism screening instrument. *American Journal of Psychiatry*, 131:1121.

Madden, J. S. (1993). Alcohol and depression. *British Journal of Hospital Medicine*, 50(5):261.

Mudd, S. A., et al. (1994). Alcohol withdrawal and related nursing care in older adults. *Journal Gerontological Nursing*, 20(10):17.

Mynatt, S. (1996). A model of contributing risk factors to chemical dependency in nurses. *Journal of Psychosocial Nursing*, 34(7):13.

National Institute on Drug Abuse (1994). National survey results on drug use from the Monitoring the Future Study, 1975–1993 (NIH 94-3809). Washington, DC:.

National Institute on Drug Abuse Clinical Report Series (1994a). Mental health assessment and diagnosis of substance abusers (NIH Publication No. 94–3846). Washington, DC:.

National Institute on Drug Abuse Clinical Report Series (1994b). Relapse prevention (NIH Publication No. 94-3845). Washington, DC:.

National Institute on Drug Abuse Conference Highlights (1993). NIDA Second National Conference on Drug Abuse Research and Practice 1993. (NIH Publication No. 94–3729). Washington, DC:.

National Institute on Drug Abuse Research Report Series (1994c). Inhalant abuse (NIH Publication No. 94–3818). Washington, DC: U. S. Department of Health and Human Services.

O'Connor, L. E., and Weiss, J. (1993). Individual psychotherapy for addicted clients: An application of control mastery theory. *Journal of Psychoactive Drugs*, 25(4):283.

O'Connor, P. G., Samet, J. H., and Stein, M. D. (1994). Management of hospitalized intravenous drug users: Role of the internist. *American Journal of Medicine*, 96:551.

Ries, R. (1994). Assessment and treatment of patients with coexisting mental illness and alcohol and other drug abuse (DHHS Publication No. [SMA] 94–2078). Washington, DC: U. S. Department of Health and Human Services.

Riley, J. A. (1994). Dual diagnosis. *Nursing Clinics of North America*, 29(1):29.

Swift, R. M. (1995). Effect of naltrexone on human alcohol consumption. *Journal of Clinical Psychiatry*, 56(Suppl. 7):24.

Thomas, H. (1993). Psychiatric symptoms in cannabis users. *British Journal of Psychiatry*, 163:141.

U. S. Department of Health and Human Services (1993). Eighth special report to the U. S. Congress on alcohol and health (NIH Publication No. 94-3699). Washington, DC: National Institutes of Health.

Volpkalli, J. R., et al. (1995). Naltrexone in the treatment of alcoholism: Predicting response to naltrexone. *Journal of Clinical Psychiatry*, 55(7):39.

Wallace, B. C. (1993). Cross-cultural counseling with the chemically dependent: Preparing for service delivery within a culture of violence. *Journal of Psychoactive Drugs*, 25(1):9.

Whitefield, C. (1988). Our most common addiction. *Wellness Associates Journal*, 1:6.

Wilson, S. (1994). Can you spot an alcoholic patient? *RN*, 57(1):46.

Ziedonis, D. M., et al. (1994). Psychiatric comorbidity in white and African-American cocaine addicts seeking substance abuse treatment. *Hospital and Community Psychiatry*, 45(1):43.

FURTHER READING

Albanese, M. J., et al. (1994). Comparison of measures used to determine substance abuse in an inpatient psychiatric population. *American Journal of Psychiatry*, 151(7):1077.

Brennan, S. J. (1991). Recognizing and assisting the impaired nurse: Recommendations for nurse managers. *Nursing Forum*, 26(2):12.

Brown, B. S., and Needle, R. H. (1994). Modifying the process of treatment to meet the threat of AIDS. *International Journal of Addiction*, 29(13):1739.

Comtois, K. A., Ries, R., and Armstrong, H. E. (1994). Case manager ratings of the clinical status of dually diagnosed outpatients. *Hospital and Community Psychiatry*, 45(6):568.

Donovan, D. M., and Marlatt, G. A. (1993). Recent developments in alcoholism behavioral treatment. *Recent Developments in Alcoholism*, 11:397.

Elangovan, N., et al. (1993). Substance abuse among patients presenting at an inner-city psychiatric emergency room. *Hospital and Community Psychiatry*, 44(8):782.

Foote, J., et al. (1994). An enhanced positive reinforcement model for the severely impaired cocaine abuser. *Journal of Substance Abuse Treatment*, 11(6):525.

Hagman, G. (1994). Methadone maintenance counseling. *Journal of Substance Abuse Treatment*, 11(5):405.

Johnson, J. G., et al. (1995). Psychiatric comorbidity, health status, and functional impairment associated with alcohol abuse and dependence in primary care patients: Findings of the PRIME MD-1000 study. *Journal of Consulting and Clinical Psychology*, 63(1):133.

McCartney, J. (1994). Understanding and helping the children of problem drinkers: A systems-psychodynamic perspective. *Journal of Substance Abuse Treatment*, 11(2):155.

McCrady, B. S. (1994). Alcoholics Anonymous and behavior therapy: Can habits be treated as diseases? Can diseases be treated as habits? *Journal of Consulting and Clinical Psychology*, 62(6):1159.

Moos, R. H, Pettit, B., and Gruver, V. A. (1995). Characteristics and outcomes of three models of community residential care for abuse patients. *Journal of Substance Abuse*, 7(1):99.

National Nurses' Society on Addictions (1995). Outpatient detoxification: Guidelines for nurses. *Perspectives in Addictions Nursing*, 6(2):8.

Rawsom, R. A., et al. (1994). Cocaine abuse among methadone maintenance patients: Are there effective treatment strategies? *Journal of Psychoactive Drugs*, 26(2):129.

Ross, H. E., et al. (1994). Diagnosing comorbidity in substance abusers. *Journal of Nervous and Mental Disease*, 182(10):556.

Slywka, S., and Hart, L. L. (1993). Fluoxetine in alcoholism. *Annals of Pharmacotherapy*, 27:1066.

Swindle, R. W., et al. (1995). Inpatient treatment for substance abuse patients with psychiatric disorders: A national study of determinants of readmission. *Journal of Substance Abuse*, 7(1):79.

Tims, F. M., Leukefeld, C. G. (Eds.) (1993). Cocaine treatment: Research and clinical perspectives (NIDA Research Monograph 135, NIH Publication No. 93-3639). Rockville, MD: U. S. Department of Health and Human Services.

SELF-STUDY AND CRITICAL THINKING

True or false

Place T (true) or F (false) next to each statement.

1. ________ Therapeutic communities are the treatment modalities of choice for individuals who have a long history of antisocial behavior and a poor record in methadone maintenance programs.
2. ________ Outpatient drug-free programs are the treatment modalities of choice for persons who have a job and an intact family or who are polydrug abusers.

Short answer

3. List four general goals that a substance-dependent person should meet in order to begin improving the quality of his or her life.
   A. ________
   B. ________
   C. ________
   D. ________
4. List six actions you might take if you were supervising a chemically dependent employee.
   A. ________
   B. ________
   C. ________
   D. ________
   E. ________
   F. ________

Identify two possible nursing diagnoses for a person with alcohol problems and formulate two short-term goals (measurable and realistic) for each diagnosis.

5. Nursing Diagnosis 1: ________
   Short-term goal 1a: ________
   Short-term goal 1b: ________
6. Nursing Diagnosis 2: ________
   Short-term goal 2a: ________
   Short-term goal 2b: ________

Short answer

7. Name six principles of counseling interventions with a substance-dependent client.
   A. ________
   B. ________
   C. ________
   D. ________
   E. ________
   F. ________

8. Name two issues a therapist needs to address when treating a substance-dependent client.

   A. ______________________________
   B. ______________________________

9. Name five therapeutic modalities used with substance-dependent clients.

   A. ______________________________
   B. ______________________________
   C. ______________________________
   D. ______________________________
   E. ______________________________

10. Name four treatment outcomes that indicate effective recovery from substance abuse.

   A. ______________________________
   B. ______________________________
   C. ______________________________
   D. ______________________________

Matching

Indicate withdrawal (W), intoxication (I), or overdose (O).

11. __________ Unsteady gait, slurred speech, drowsiness
12. __________ Tachycardia, marked insomnia, diaphoresis, irritability
13. __________ Coma, shock, convulsions, respiratory or cardiovascular depression
14. __________ Impaired social or occupational functioning, impaired judgment or memory

Indicate cocaine (C), amphetamine (A), or both (B).

15. __________ Overdose can result in respiratory depression or arrest, hyperpyrexia, seizures, cardiac shock or arrest, and death.
16. __________ Short-acting; tolerance builds rapidly.
17. __________ Long-term users have a runny nose due to erosion of nasal septum.
18. __________ Intoxication includes grandiosity, paranoia, impaired judgment, tactile or other hallucinations, and psychosis.
19. __________ Medical management and nursing care are vital in severe overdose.

Match the following phenomena of an alcoholic person with a predictable defensive style.

20. ________ Not acknowledging certain life difficulties
21. ________ Influenced by emotions—doing what feels good
22. ________ Gets others to do things for person, take care of person
23. ________ Structured, restricted choices
24. ___A___ "It takes one to know one"

A. Projection
B. Rationalization
C. All-or-none thinking instills guilt in others
D. Obsessional focusing
E. Manipulation
F. Preference for nonanalytical thinking
G. Denial

Multiple choice

Choose the answer that most accurately completes the statement.

25. In intervening with an intoxicated client, it is useful to first
    A. Let him or her sober up first.
    B. Decide on goals immediately, while the client is still in a good mood.
    C. Gain compliance by sharing your drinking habits with the client.
    D. Ask what other drugs the client might be taking.

26. Ms. Turk, a highly successful editor, has been taking cocaine intranasally for 4 years and started freebasing 2 months ago. For the past week, she has been locked in her apartment and has taken $8000 worth of cocaine. She is unconscious when brought to the hospital. Nursing measures include all the following *except*
    A. Monitor vital signs every 15 minutes.
    B. Maintain a patent airway; give oxygen when indicated by physician.
    C. Observe for seizures and hyperpyrexia.
    D. Give ammonium chloride.

27. After the drug is out of Ms. Turk's system, she is most likely to experience
    A. Hyperactivity and diaphoresis.
    B. Anxiety and depression.
    C. Marked insomnia and coarse, hard hands.
    D. Increased sexual impulses and euphoria.

28. Ms. Turk is admitted to the inpatient treatment unit. As an adjunct to group and individual therapy, the nurse could work with Ms. Turk on all the following *except*
    A. Educating Ms. Turk about the psychological actions of the drug, its dangers, and the latest research.
    B. Exploring strengths and activities that Ms. Turk enjoyed before becoming involved with the drug.
    C. Teaching Ms. Turk the indicators for, and the side effects and action of, prescribed medications to ease withdrawal (e. g., antidepressants).
    D. Assuming an authoritarian leadership role, because Ms. Turk is now so dependent.

29. You know your teaching has been effective when a client states, "I know that as long as I take disulfiram (Antabuse), I need to avoid. . . "

    A. All aged cheeses and meat extracts.
    B. Bright sunlight and wear sunscreen.
    C. Driving a car and heavy machinery.
    D. Cough medicines, mouthwash, and after-shave lotions.

Short answer

30. A 32-year-old heroin addict is admitted to the hospital for cellulitis to the right hand caused by "skin-popping." She does not want her husband to know how she got the cellulitis. With regard to her substance dependency, which of the following is the most appropriate goal for her hospitalization? Discuss the pros and cons of each choice.

    A. Ignore it and focus on the cellulitis only.
    B. Determine her average daily drug use and provide nearly the same in the hospital by substituting morphine or methadone.
    C. Begin detoxification.
    D. Arrange an intervention so that she can get help.

31. What do the letters in the acronym CAGE stand for?

    C ____________ A ____________ G ____________ E ____________

32. Name two goals of relapse prevention.

    A. ______________________________
    B. ______________________________

33. Describe two nursing actions important for a person with a substance abuse diagnosis.

    A. ______________________________
    B. ______________________________

34. Describe two *different* nursing actions important for a person with a substance dependence diagnosis.

    A. ______________________________
    B. ______________________________

35. What are two ways you would know if a client had developed tolerance to his or her drug of choice?

    A. ______________________________
    B. ______________________________

36. What are two ways of determining whether your client is experiencing intoxication or withdrawal?

    A. ______________________________
    B. ______________________________

Critical thinking

37. Write a paragraph regarding your possible reactions to a drug-dependent client to whom you are assigned.

    A. Would your response differ, depending on the substance, e. g., alcohol versus heroin; marijuana versus cocaine? Give a reason for your answer.
    B. Would your response be different if the substance-dependent person were a professional colleague? Please state why or why not.

26

People with Eating Disorders

KATHLEEN IBRAHIM

OUTLINE

KEY TERMS AND CONCEPTS

The key terms and concepts listed here also appear in bold where they are defined or discussed in this chapter.

Anorexia nervosa
Bulimia nervosa
Binge/purge cycle
Binge eating disorder
Ideal body weight
Cognitive distortions

OBJECTIVES

After studying this chapter, the reader will be able to

1. Differentiate between the four theories of eating disorders discussed in this chapter.
2. Compare and contrast the signs and symptoms of anorexia nervosa with those of bulimia nervosa.
3. Identify three life-threatening conditions stated in terms of nursing diagnoses for a client with an eating disorder.
4. Develop three realistic outcome criteria for (a) a client with anorexia and (b) a client with bulimia nervosa.
5. Recognize which therapeutic interventions are appropriate for the acute phase of anorexia and which are appropriate for the long-term phase of treatment.
6. Explain the basic premise of cognitive-behavioral therapy in the treatment of anorexia nervosa.
7. Describe at least seven group dynamics or themes seen in families with a member who has an eating disorder.
8. After reading the chapter, try to empathize and describe in your own words the possible thoughts and feelings of a young anorectic girl during the acute phase of her illness.

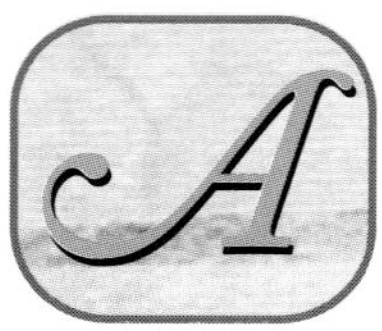

Anorexia nervosa has existed for centuries, but the condition was first described as a defined medical illness in 1689 by Thomas Morton. In 1874, Sir William Gull labeled the illness **anorexia nervosa,** and over the next hundred years, it has evolved to assume its current prominence as a diagnostic entity. Bruch (1973) documented the antecedent psychological factors in the development of anorexia nervosa and subsequently challenged the traditional psychoanalytic explanation and treatment of the disorder.

In 1979, Russell described a clinical entity that was a new version of anorexia nervosa, and in 1980, *bulimia,* as a separate diagnosis, entered the *Diagnostic and Statistical Manual of Mental Disorders,* third edition (DSM-III) (APA 1980) for the first time. Although purging was not necessary for a diagnosis of bulimia in DSM-III, in 1987 DSM-III (revised) (APA 1987) required that purging or inappropriate compensatory behaviors be present for the diagnosis now called *bulimia nervosa.* With increasing frequency, clinical cases of anorexia and bulimia nervosa have been described and diagnosed, evolving into the current *Diagnostic and statistical manual of mental disorders,* fourth edition (DSM-IV) (APA 1994) criteria for eating disorders.

Increasingly, some anorectic individuals have been unable to maintain thinness without resorting to binge eating and/or purging. Formerly, two diagnoses—anorexia nervosa and bulimia nervosa—were given to episodes of binge eating and purging that developed during the course of anorexia nervosa. In DSM-IV, anorexia nervosa is now subtyped to further define the illness according to food restricting or binge eating/purging behaviors. Bulimia nervosa is further subtyped to indicate purging and nonpurging behaviors. Eating disorders that do not meet full criteria for anorexia nervosa or bulimia nervosa are classified as **eating disorder not otherwise specified** (NOS). Binge eating disorder—binge eating without compensatory behavior—is an entity that is mentioned in the DSM-IV appendix as requiring further study. Currently, such a clinical entity would be classified as eating disorder NOS (APA 1994). Figure 26–1 provides diagnostic criteria for eating disorders.

THEORY

Neurobiological/Neuroendocrine Theories

Several conceptual models of the cause of eating disorders exist. The coexistence (comorbidity) of eating disorders and depression has received considerable focus in the literature. The symptoms of undereating and overeating in eating disorders parallel the primary symptoms of melancholic and atypical depression. Devlin and Walsh (1989) proposed hypothetical relationships: the eating disorder either causes a depression or is a variant of a depressive disorder. Another relationship they hypothesized is one of common biopsychosocial vulnerabilities that lead to depression and/or eating disorders. Further, these authors noted the increased frequency of depression in biological relatives of clients with eating disorders. In some cases, major depressive disorder predated the eating disorder; in other cases, it developed after treatment of the eating disorder. In depression, as in eating disorders, complex interrelationships of altered neurotransmitters exist, as well as aberrant patterns involving multiple systems and pathways. However, Devlin and Walsh (1989) also cautioned against assuming similar pathological features in eating disorders and depression based on the treatment response to antidepressant medication in the two groups.

ANOREXIA NERVOSA

A. Refusal to maintain body weight over a minimum normal weight for age and height, e.g., weight loss leading to maintenance of body weight less than 85% of that expected, or failure to make expected weight gain during period of growth, leading to body weight less than 85% of that expected.

B. Intense fear of gaining weight or becoming fat, even though underweight.

C. Disturbance in the way in which one's body weight or shape is experienced, undue influence of body weight or shape on self-evaluation, or denial of the seriousness of the current low body weight.
In females, postmenarcheal amenorrhea, i.e., the absence of at least three consecutive menstrual cycles. (A woman is considered to have amenorrhea if her periods occur only after hormone, e.g., estrogen administration.)

Specify type:
Binge eating/purging type: During the episode of anorexia nervosa, the person engages in recurrent episodes of binge eating or purging behaviors.

Restricting type: During the episode of anorexia nervosa, the person does *not* engage in recurrent episodes of binge eating or purging behaviors.

BULIMIA NERVOSA

A. Recurrent episodes of binge eating. An episode of binge eating is characterized by both of the following:
(1) Eating in a discrete period (e.g., within any 2-hour period) an amount of food that is definitely larger than most people would eat during a similar period and under similar circumstances.
(2) A sense of lack of control over eating during the episode (e.g., a feeling that one cannot stop eating or control what or how much one is eating).

B. Recurrent inappropriate compensatory behavior to prevent weight gain such as self-induced vomiting; misuse of laxatives, diuretics, enemas, or other medications; fasting; or excessive exercise.

C. The binge eating and inappropriate compensatory behavior both occur on average at least twice a week for 3 months.

D. Self-evaluation is unduly influenced by body shape and weight.

E. The disturbance does not occur exclusively during episodes of anorexia nervosa.

Specify type:
Purging type: During the current episode of bulimia nervosa, the person has regularly engaged in self-induced vomiting or the misuse of laxatives, diuretics, or enemas.

Nonpurging type: During the current episode of bulimia nervosa, the person has used other inappropriate compensatory behaviors, such as fasting or excessive exercise, but has not regularly engaged in self-induced vomiting or the misuse of laxatives, diuretics, or enemas.

EATING DISORDER NOT OTHERWISE SPECIFIED (NOS)

The eating disorder not otherwise specified category is for disorders of eating that do not meet the criteria for any specific eating disorder. Examples include

1. For females, all the criteria for anorexia nervosa are met except that the individual has regular menses.
2. All the criteria for anorexia nervosa are met except that despite significant weight loss, the individual's current weight is in the normal range.
3. All the criteria for bulimia nervosa are met except that the binge eating and inappropriate compensatory mechanisms occur at a frequency of less than twice a week for a duration of less than 3 months.
4. The regular use of inappropriate compensatory behavior by an individual of normal body weight after eating small amounts of food (e.g., self-induced vomiting after the consumption of two cookies).
5. Repeatedly chewing and spitting out, but not swallowing, large amounts of food.
6. Binge eating disorder: recurrent episodes of binge eating in the absence of the regular use of inappropriate compensatory behaviors characteristic of bulimia nervosa.

Figure 26–1 Diagnostic criteria for eating disorders. (Adapted from American Psychiatric Association (1994). *Diagnostic and statistical manual of mental disorders (DSM-IV)* (4th ed.). Washington, DC: American Psychiatric Association. Reprinted with permission. Copyright 1994 American Psychiatric Association.)

Similar neuroendocrine abnormalities have been noted in both diagnostic entities, and neuroendocrine abnormalities have been much researched and documented in eating disorders (Hsu 1990; Irwin 1993a). Whether the relationships are causal or result from starvation or abnormal eating behaviors is not clear. Abnormalities of the hypothalamic-pituitary-adrenal axis are similar to those in major depression in anorexia nervosa, and the abnormalities of the hypothalamic-pituitary-thyroid axis appear to be the result of starvation in anorexia, but similar to those abnormalities of the hypothalamic-pituitary-adrenal axis seen in major depression and bulimia nervosa. Cholecystokinin, an intestinal hormone, is present at low levels in bulimic persons; and endogenous opioids, gastrointestinal hormones, and vasopressin have received attention, but the findings are not clear. The aforementioned findings represent the biological abnormalities observed in people with eating disorders and may help to explain the drive toward dieting, hunger, preoccupation with food, and tendency toward binge eating (Devlin et al. 1990).

Psychological Theories

Anorexia nervosa results in amenorrhea and physiological changes, which interfere with the development of an age-appropriate sexual role. Psychoanalytic theorists long believed that conflict over one's sexual role was primary for anorectic persons (Bruch 1985). Bruch's work with anorectic women failed to prove these theoretical assumptions but postulated developmental factors that led to anorexia nervosa.

According to Bruch, girls who go on to have anorexia experience themselves as ineffectual, passive, and unable to assert their will. Misguided efforts to separate and establish an autonomous adult existence leads to self-starvation and a distorted sense of being special and powerful. People with anorexia are anxious about losing control over their eating and do not accurately experience hunger or satiety. These sensations result in a feeling of powerlessness and in a lack of ability to identify what they need. Defiance regarding eating occurs in an effort to define oneself, but it represents a futile endeavor to establish independence. The inauthentic identity has a veneer of competence, while underneath, the individual has panic about losing control and feeling ineffectual.

Some eating disorder models postulate an affect regulation mechanism. Hsu (1990) stated that "affective overcontrol and intolerance, lack of self-direction, and personal effectiveness" are maladaptive responses to the developmental tasks of adolescence. Bruch (1985) described anorectic females who feel powerless and attempt to regulate their anxiety and feelings of effectiveness by controlling their eating, and, in so doing, achieve a societal ideal. Some individuals learn to control their dysphoria by binge eating and to numb their negative feelings by eating. These behaviors contribute to the avoidance of experiencing underlying negative emotions, which become replaced by the distress over binge eating and purging (Hsu 1990). Affective instability and poor impulse control are consistently associated with bulimia. Current findings of mothers and daughters (Pike 1991) suggest a possible connection. Mothers of daughters with eating disorders had a longer dieting history and had a higher incidence of eating disorder compared with mothers of daughters who were not eating disordered.

It is a popular notion that sexual abuse is causal in the development of eating disorders, and frequently, clinicians expect to uncover a history of such abuse. Welch and Fairburn (1994) noted that sexual abuse is a risk factor for the development of a psychiatric disorder, including bulimia nervosa, but it is not specific to bulimia. Pope and Hudson (1992) reviewed controlled retrospective studies of sexual abuse in individuals with eating disorders, uncontrolled studies, and studies of sexual abuse in the general population. They determined that sexual abuse does not constitute a specific risk factor for bulimia nervosa.

Sociocultural Models

Western sociocultural models emphasize the middle-class and upper-middle-class societal values of thinness as mediating the development of eating disorders. Although the numbers of individuals who are overweight continue to increase, individuals with eating disorders have internalized the societal ideal to be thin as a compelling force. Wooley (1995) observed that the feminist perspective is to assist women to resist a pathogenic culture. The Western ideal for women who are at risk is to be competent in traditional and nontraditional ways. For these women, being a mother and homemaker as well as a career woman may be experienced as a conflict. Bemporad (1996) noted that eating disorders do not flourish in male-dominated societies, where women are forced into a stereotypical nurturing role; rather, the incidence of eating disorders has risen in a society in which women have a choice in social roles. In developing countries where dieting has recently become popular, eating disorders, formerly uncommon, are on the rise (Hsu 1990). This surge in dieting is linked to the increased incidence of eating disorders.

Hsu (1990) noted that the characteristics of men with eating disorders are similar to those of women with eating disorders. In a study of college men, Olivardia and colleagues (1995) noted that men with eating disorders had characteristics similar to those of women with eating disorders but were different from men without eating disorders.

Although many women are no longer living with their family of origin, the ties may be more intense than seem apparent. Minuchin (1974) has written extensively of family processes of psychosomatic families and the defining elements that result in a particular expression. The interrelated functional elements are enmeshment, overprotectiveness, rigidity, lack of conflict resolution, and the symptom—the eating behavior—as the regulator of the family system. Chapter 28 provides more details on Minuchin's elements in psychosomatic families. The effectiveness of the client in regulating family stability reinforces both the symptom and the particular family organization.

Biopsychosocial Theories

Numerous hypotheses and studies are providing new data on eating disorders. Currently, an integrated biopsychosocial model is applied to the understanding and treatment of eating disorders. One study that looked for genetic factors found a 56% concordance rate in monozygotic twins for anorexia nervosa (Holland 1984).

The genetic vulnerability that might be responsible for the development of anorexia nervosa might lead to poor affect, poor impulse control, or an underlying neurotransmitter dysfunction. A family history of affective disorder and alcohol abuse was found to be common in monozygotic sets of twin pairs, in which one of the pair was diagnosed with bulimia nervosa. Kendler and colleagues (1991) found a 22.9% concordance rate for bulimia in monozygotic twins and an 8.7% rate in dizygotic twins. Hsu (1990) suggested that "significant psychiatric symptoms, such as depression, social anxiety and phobia, and obsessive-compulsive features" may contribute along with the dieting to the development of an eating disorder. Thiel and associates (1995) found a significant incidence of obsessive-compulsive disorder in a sample of anorectic clients and bulimic clients, who had obsessions and compulsions that were unrelated to eating behaviors.

According to Hsu (1990), "dieting provides the entree into an eating disorder" in the context of adolescent turmoil. However, this is not the only trigger; other mediating factors are subsumed into a biopsychosocial model. Obviously, eating disorders do not develop in all dieters, but certain risk factors increase the potential for such development. All of the previously cited theories postulate factors that could contribute to the risk of developing an eating disorder.

Crisp (1980) has long maintained that the development of anorexia nervosa results in the desired avoidance of the sexual role. Hsu (1990) described that females in Western countries experienced adolescent turmoil as unhappiness significantly more than their male counterparts. This same finding was true of Japanese females, who expressed lower self-esteem than males (Lerner et al. 1980).

Physical attractiveness and its importance in the female have been demonstrated in many studies to be correlated with self-esteem. Depression was also correlated with estimation of body size; those of normal weight who overestimate their size were more depressed than those who did not perceive themselves as fat (Kandel and Davies 1982).

Several researchers (Bruch 1985; Crisp 1980; Selvini-Palazzoli 1985) have highlighted the conflict the female faces in establishing an identity. The adolescent female is expected to be both nurturing and competitive and to combine these extremes into a consistent female identity. No clear guidelines exist for the adolescent female, and the expectations may seem conflicting.

A comprehensive, biopsychosocial theory would subsume all of the aforementioned contributing factors, with specific risk factors playing more of a role in the development of an eating disorder in certain individuals.

All important, however, is the experienced event of dieting. The perception of being overweight is the most immediate cause for dieting that predisposes an individual to an eating disorder. Hsu (1990) postulated that once aberrant eating behaviors are established, they are reinforced through positive and negative factors, and the eating disorder becomes self-perpetuating. According to Fairburn and Cooper (1989), most of the problematic behaviors of anorexia nervosa and bulimia nervosa occur as a result of the overvalued ideas regarding weight, shape, and body image. Box 26–1 provides a description of dysfunctional thoughts that people with eating disorders might hold.

BOX 26–1 COGNITIVE DISTORTIONS

Overgeneralization: A single event affects unrelated situations.

- "He didn't ask me out. It must be because I'm fat."
- "I was happy when I wore a size 6. I must get back to that weight."

All-or-nothing thinking: Absolute, extreme reasoning in mutually exclusive terms of black or white, good or bad.

- "If I have one popsicle, I must eat five."
- "If I allow myself to gain weight, I'll blow up like a balloon."

Catastrophizing: Magnifying the consequences of an event.

- "If I gain weight, my weekend will be ruined."
- "When people say I look better, I know they think I'm fat."

Personalization: Overinterpretation of events as having personal significance.

- "I know everybody is watching me eat."
- "I think people won't like me unless I'm thin."

Emotional reasoning: Subjective emotions determine reality.

- "I know I'm fat because I feel fat."
- "When I'm thin, I feel powerful."

Adapted from Garner, D., and Bemis, K. (1982). A cognitive-behavioral approach to anorexia nervosa. *Cognitive Therapy and Research,* 6:123–150.

ANOREXIA NERVOSA

Anorectic individuals often enter the health care system by being admitted to an intensive care unit with electrolyte imbalance. This condition may be due to the fact that the restrictive anorectic subtype is receding in incidence, and the purging subtype is becoming more common.

Box 26–2 identifies some criteria for hospital admission for a client with an eating disorder.

Assessment

The nurse assessing the anorectic client observes a severely underweight male or female who may have fine,

BOX 26–2 CRITERIA FOR INPATIENT ADMISSION OF A PERSON WITH AN EATING DISORDER

- Weight < 75%; < 60% compelling
- Rapid decline in weight
- Life-threatening physiological problem, e.g., electrolyte imbalance, infections
- Suicidal or severely out of control (self-mutilating or abusing, using large amounts of laxatives, emetics, diuretics, or street drugs)
- Hypothermia due to loss of subcutaneous tissue
- Inability to gain weight repeatedly with outpatient treatment

Adapted from Fairburn, C. G., and Cooper, P. J. (1989). Eating disorders. In K. Hawton, P. M. Salkovskis, J. Kirk, and D. M. Clark (Eds.), *Cognitive behaviour therapy for psychiatric problems* (pp. 277–314). New York: Oxford University Press.

downy hair growth of the face and back with mottled, cool skin of the extremities, and low blood pressure, pulse, and temperature readings, consistent with a malnourished, dehydrated state. Table 26–1 lists the signs and symptoms of anorexia and bulimia.

▶ On admission to an eating disorder unit for inpatient treatment of anorexia nervosa, Tina, a 16-year-old young woman at 60% of ideal body weight, appears cachectic. She presents with a fine lanugo over most of her body and prominent parotid glands. She is further assessed to be hypotensive (86/50 mm Hg) and dehydrated, and she has a low serum potassium level and dysrhythmias that appear on an electrocardiogram. A decision is made to transfer her to the intensive care unit until she is medically stabilized. As an intravenous catheter is inserted, her severe weight phobia and fear of fat are underscored when she cries, "There's not going to be sugar in the IV?" The nurse responds, "I hear how frightened you are. We need to do what's necessary to get you past this crisis."

As with any comprehensive psychiatric nursing assessment, a complete evaluation of biopsychosocial function is mandatory. The areas to be covered include the client's perception of the problem, the eating habits and history of dieting, the methods used to achieve control (restricting, purging, exercising), the value attached to a specific shape and weight, the client's interpersonal and social functioning, and an assessment of mental status with psychological and physiological parameters (Fairburn and Cooper 1989). Table 26–2, a comprehensive nursing assessment, and Table 26–3, the body shape questionnaire, provide some useful assessment tools for people with eating disorders.

Nursing Diagnosis

Altered nutrition: less than body requirements is usually the most compelling nursing diagnosis initially for individuals with anorexia. Altered nutrition: less than body requirements generates further nursing diagnoses, for example, **decreased cardiac output** and **risk for injury (electrolyte imbalance),** which would have first priority when problems are addressed. Other nursing diagnoses include **body image disturbance, anxiety, low self-esteem, knowledge deficit, ineffective individual coping, powerlessness,** and **hopelessness.**

Planning

In order to evaluate the effectiveness of treatment, outcome criteria are established to measure treatment results. The objectives that guide the treatment plan lead to the expected outcomes. Some common outcome criteria for clients with anorexia nervosa follow:

- The client will normalize eating patterns, as evidenced by eating 75% of three meals/day plus two snacks.
- The client will achieve 85% to 90% of ideal body weight.
- The client will demonstrate improved self-acceptance, as evidenced by both verbal and behavioral data.
- The client will have less distorted perceptions of body image.
- The client will demonstrate behaviors and interests that are appropriate to age.
- The client will participate in long-term treatment to prevent relapse.

Implementation

Many anorectic persons are able to contain their illness and compartmentalize it in order to achieve personal goals. The focus of the therapeutic interventions is guided by the intensity of the disordered eating and the impact on the life of the anorectic person. Although a range of treatment modalities from psychoanalysis to nutrition counseling has been applied to anorexia nervosa, cognitive therapy has shown improved outcomes (Fairburn and Cooper 1989).

Acute Care: Inpatient Treatment

The type of treatment for anorexia nervosa is partly determined by the severity of the weight loss. Anorectic individuals whose weight is below 75% of **ideal body weight,** according to Metropolitan Life Insurance Company height and weight tables (1983), are considered to be medically unstable (Hsu 1990). Admission to an inpatient unit may be necessary to reverse the downward spiral of dietary

TABLE 26–1 SIGNS AND SYMPTOMS OF ANOREXIA AND BULIMIA

DISORDER	CAUSAL RELATIONSHIPS
Restrictive anorexia	
Low weight	Caloric restriction, excessive exercising
Amenorrhea	Low weight
Low T_3, T_4 levels	Starvation
CT scan, EEG changes	Starvation
Cardiovascular abnormalities	Starvation, dehydration
▸ Hypotension	Electrolyte imbalance
▸ Bradycardia	
▸ Heart failure	
Impaired renal function	
Dehydration, hypokalemia	
Yellow skin	Hypercarotenemia
Lanugo	Starvation
Anemia, pancytopenia	Starvation
Decreased bone density	Estrogen deficiency, low calcium intake
Cold extremities	Starvation
Peripheral edema	Hypoalbuminemia and on refeeding
Muscle weakening	Starvation, electrolyte imbalance
Constipation	Starvation
Bulimia nervosa	
Normal to slightly low weight	Excessive caloric intake with purging, excessive exercising
Electrolyte imbalance	Purging: vomiting, laxative, diuretic use
▸ Hypokalemia	
▸ Hyponatremia	
Cardiovascular abnormalities	Electrolyte imbalance
▸ Cardiomyopathy	
▸ ECG changes	
Dental caries, erosion	Vomiting
Parotid swelling	Vomiting
Gastric dilatation, rupture	Binge eating
Calluses, scars on hand	Self-induced vomiting
Peripheral edema	Rebound fluid especially if diuretic
Muscle weakening	Electrolyte imbalance

Adapted from American Psychiatric Association (1994), *Diagnostic and statistical manual of mental disorders* (4th ed.). Washington, DC: American Psychiatric Association. Reprinted with permission. Copyright 1994 American Psychiatric Association; and Hsu, L. K. G. (1990). *Eating disorders.* New York: Guilford Press.

T_3, triiodothyronine; T_4, thyroxine; EEG, electroencephalographic; CT, computed tomographic; ECG, electrocardiographic.

restriction and weight loss. Indeed, anorexia nervosa is a chronic illness requiring both inpatient and outpatient management, with therapeutic interventions that include individual, group, and family therapy and psychopharmacological therapy during different phases of the illness. The nature of the treatment is determined both by the intensity of the symptoms, which may vary over time, and the experienced disruption of one's life. The mainstay of treatment, however, is outpatient therapy.

In the current health care climate, reimbursement for inpatient treatment is limited. Brief hospitalization can address only acute complications, such as electrolyte imbalance, dysrhythmias, limited weight restoration, and acute psychiatric symptoms.

A potentially catastrophic treatment complication is the *refeeding syndrome*, in which the demands that a repleted circulatory system places on a nutritionally depleted cardiac mass result in cardiovascular collapse (Mehler 1996).

Another acute symptom targeted on the acute inpatient unit is depression. The more persistent symptoms that attend undernutrition and fear of weight gain with distorted body image would more likely to be addressed on an outpatient basis.

General inpatient psychiatric units, although providing excellent care for most psychiatric disorders, are not structured to address the requirements of acute treatment of anorectic clients in the weight-restoration phase.

TABLE 26–2 COMPREHENSIVE NURSING ASSESSMENT

ASSESSMENT	POTENTIAL RESPONSES
Client's perception of problem	Anorectic client may complain of severe fatigue with resultant physical limitations, e.g., inability to exercise at usual extreme level, as the only real difficulty. Does not view self as emaciated. Experiences binge eating and purging behaviors as distressing, shameful.
Assess history of dieting, weight	May report history of being overweight at 11 or 12 years of age. Began restricting calories; weight began spiraling downward.
Eating habits	May eat only one "meal" a day. "Good" foods and "bad" foods exist. Often a strict vegetarian. Strict avoidance of fat. Clients who binge report trigger foods, e.g., french fries, or a particular situation, e.g., watching television. May eat alone or in secret. May hide food. Total preoccupation with food. May feel eating is out of control. May enjoy preparing food for others but does not partake. Avoids buffet-style dining.
Methods used to control weight	May severely restrict only. Frequently exercises excessively. May induce vomiting, use laxatives, and/or diuretics.
Attitudes toward weight and shape	Weight and shape at the core of identity, determines self-worth. An overwhelming fear of being fat, extreme pursuit of thinness. A particular weight has value, may become very anxious as he or she approaches the 100-lb mark, going from two-digit to three-digit weight. Frequently a value in being a particular dress size. Thinks particular body part, e.g., thighs, are enormous and does not like them to touch or spread out when sitting down.
Mental status examination	May be anxious or irritable, with depressed mood. May have impaired cognition, particularly at very low weight. May be extremely obsessive-compulsive. May have passive or active suicidal ideation.
History of psychiatric illness	May report many treatment attempts with subsequent relapse. May report physical and/or sexual abuse. May have prior hospitalization. May also meet criteria for personality disorder. May have family history of depression, substance abuse.
Interpersonal, social, vocational history	May have enmeshed family relationships. May have chaotic, unstable relationships. May be socially isolated. May be in a high-risk profession for eating disorders, e.g., ballet dancing, modeling, sports/physical training. Reports others have expressed concern about weight or eating habits.
Physical examination	Determine weight and height. If weight is $<$ 75% of ideal body weight, client is considered medically unstable. Often presents with bradycardia, hypotension, hypothermia. May have arrythmia noted on electrocardiogram. May have cachectic appearance with lanugo. May have parotid swelling with dental erosion. Abnormal laboratory findings include anemia, leukopenia, abnormal electrolyte levels, especially low potassium.

Ideally, before the client is discharged from an acute care setting, a comprehensive outpatient treatment plan is arranged (see Acute Care: Outpatient Treatment).

MILIEU THERAPY (BASIC LEVEL). Clients who are admitted to an inpatient unit designed to treat eating disorders participate in a treatment program that consists of an interdisciplinary team and a combination of therapeutic modalities. These modalities are designed to normalize eating patterns and to begin to address the issues raised by the illness. The milieu of an eating disorder unit is purposefully organized to assist the client to establish more adaptive behavioral patterns, including normalization of eating. The highly structured milieu includes precise meal times, adherence to the selected menu, observation during and after meals, and regularly scheduled weighings. Groups are led by nurses and other interdisciplinary team members and are tailored to issues of clients with eating disorders. Client privileges are correlated with weight gain and treatment plan compliance.

THERAPY (BASIC AND ADVANCED LEVELS). The nurse on an inpatient unit may have multiple roles: primary nurse (basic level), group leader (basic level), and psychotherapist (advanced practice). Interventions include teaching, counseling, and psychotherapeutic functions. The initial focus depends on the results of a comprehensive assessment. Any acute psychiatric symptoms, such as suicidal ideation, must be immediately addressed. At the same time, the anorectic client begins a weight-restoration program that allows for incremental weight gain. Based on height, a treatment goal is set at 90% of ideal body weight, the weight at which most women are able to menstruate.

Establishing a therapeutic alliance with the anorectic client is difficult because the compelling force of the illness runs counter to therapeutic interventions. As clients

TABLE 26–3 THE BODY SHAPE QUESTIONNAIRE

We would like to know how you have been feeling about your appearance over the PAST FOUR WEEKS. Please read the questions and circle the appropriate number to the right. Please answer all the questions.

Over the Past Four Weeks:	Never	Rarely	Sometimes	Often	Very Often	Always
1. Has feeling bored made you brood about your shape?	1	2	3	4	5	6
2. Have you ever been so worried about your shape that you have been feeling you ought to diet?	1	2	3	4	5	6
3. Have you ever thought that your thighs, hips, or bottom are too large for the rest of you?	1	2	3	4	5	6
4. Have you ever been afraid that you might become fat (or fatter)?	1	2	3	4	5	6
5. Have you ever worried about your flesh being not firm enough?	1	2	3	4	5	6
6. Has feeling full (e.g., after eating a large meal) made you feel fat?	1	2	3	4	5	6
7. Have you ever felt so bad about your shape that you have cried?	1	2	3	4	5	6
8. Have you avoided running because your flesh might wobble?	1	2	3	4	5	6
9. Has being with thin women made you feel self-conscious about your shape?	1	2	3	4	5	6
10. Have you worried about thighs spreading out when sitting down.	1	2	3	4	5	6
11. Has eating even a small amount of food made you feel fat?	1	2	3	4	5	6
12. Have you noticed the shape of other women and felt that your own shape compared unfavorably?	1	2	3	4	5	6
13. Has thinking about your shape interfered with your ability to concentrate (e.g., while watching TV, reading, listening to conversation)?	1	2	3	4	5	6
14. Has being naked, such as when taking a bath, made you feel fat?	1	2	3	4	5	6
15. Have you avoided wearing clothes which make you particularly aware of the shape of your body?	1	2	3	4	5	6
16. Have you ever imagined cutting off fleshy areas of your body?	1	2	3	4	5	6
17. Has eating sweets, cakes, or other high-calorie food made you feel fat?	1	2	3	4	5	6
18. Have you not gone out to social occasions (e.g., parties) because you have felt bad about your shape?	1	2	3	4	5	6
19. Have you felt excessively large and rounded?	1	2	3	4	5	6
20. Have you felt ashamed of your body?	1	2	3	4	5	6
21. Has worry about your shape made you diet?	1	2	3	4	5	6
22. Have you felt the happiest about your shape when your stomach has been empty?	1	2	3	4	5	6
23. Have you thought that you are the shape you are because of lack of self-control?	1	2	3	4	5	6
24. Have you worried about other people seeing rolls of flesh around your waist and stomach?	1	2	3	4	5	6
25. Have you felt that it is not fair that other women are thinner than you?	1	2	3	4	5	6
26. Have you vomited in order to feel thinner?	1	2	3	4	5	6
27. When in company have you worried about taking up too much room (e.g., sitting on a sofa or a bus seat)?	1	2	3	4	5	6
28. Have you worried about your flesh being dumpy?	1	2	3	4	5	6
29. Has seeing your reflection (e.g., in a mirror or shop window) made you feel bad about your shape?	1	2	3	4	5	6
30. Have you pinched areas of your body to see how much fat there is?	1	2	3	4	5	6

Continued

TABLE 26–3 THE BODY SHAPE QUESTIONNAIRE *(Continued)*

We would like to know how you have been feeling about your appearance over the PAST FOUR WEEKS. Please read the questions and circle the appropriate number to the right. Please answer all the questions.

Over the Past Four Weeks:	Never	Rarely	Sometimes	Often	Very Often	Always
31. Have you avoided situations where people could see your body (e.g., communal changing rooms or swimming baths)?	1	2	3	4	5	6
32. Have you taken laxatives to feel thinner?	1	2	3	4	5	6
33. Have you been particularly self-conscious about your shape when in the company of other people?	1	2	3	4	5	6
34. Has worry about your shape made you feel you ought to exercise?	1	2	3	4	5	6

From Cooper, P. J., Cooper, Z., Fairburn, C. G., and Taylor, M. J. (1987). The Development and Validation of the Body Shape Questionnaire. *International Journal of Eating Disorders*, 6(4):485–494.

begin to refeed, they ideally begin to participate in the milieu therapy, attending individual psychotherapy and group therapy sessions as well as nutritional counseling. The **cognitive distortions** mentioned earlier perpetuate the illness and must be confronted consistently by all members of the interdisciplinary team. While the eating behavior is targeted, the underlying emotions of anxiety, dysphoria, and low self-esteem and the feelings of lack of control are also addressed.

▸ In a multifamily group on an inpatient unit, Mrs. Demi (who last saw her anorectic daughter, before she had gained 40 pounds) is asked by the group leader how she regards her daughter. Mrs. Demi replies, "She looks healthy." Her daughter responds with an angry, sullen look. She ultimately verbalizes that comments about her "healthy" appearance are experienced as "You look fat." In the multifamily group, there is a commonly expressed view that the illness "is not about weight," but that thinness conferred a feeling of being special, and being at a normal weight (healthy) meant that special status was lost.

Table 26–4 identifies some other dynamics that surface in the multifamily group.

TABLE 26–4 GROUP DYNAMICS AND THEMES IN THE MULTIFAMILY GROUP

PHENOMENON	EXAMPLE
Concrete formulation	Parent uses a mechanical metaphor, denying emotional feelings. "An engine needs fuel to run."
Lack of ownership of problem	Client states she would be okay if only family would stop scrutinizing her behavior.
Lack of trust	Client complains others do not trust her. Client behaves in a manner that provokes questions from others (extended period of time in bathroom). Later, she asserts that others do not trust her.
Shifting coalitions	Client allies with mother against father then switches. Parent(s) initially allied with treatment team now takes up client's part against group leader(s). The excluded person is out of the loop of communication.
Avoiding shame	Client tries to control the flow of communication within the group to deny underlying feelings.
Proxy phenomenon	Parent and client from different families initially find it easier to communicate than to speak to own family member.
Reenactment of family dynamics	Client behaves toward group members and team leader(s), recreating family patterns of communication.
Competition with mother	Client expresses wish to please mother and yet outdo her.
Mixed messages	Parent compliments daughter's healthy appearance; the daughter feels criticized: "It feels like you're saying I'm fat."
Lack of perceived support	Client is frequently unable to use support from others, instead experiencing negative feedback.

Adapted from Ibrahim, K., and Rosedale, M. (1994). Perspectives in multiple family group therapy with eating disordered patient. Paper presented at the meeting of the Society for Education and Research in Psychiatric Nursing, Rockville, MD, November 1994.

HEALTH TEACHING (BASIC LEVEL). Self-care activities are an important part of the treatment plan. These activities include learning more constructive coping skills, improving social skills, and developing problem-solving and decision-making skills. The skills become the focus of both therapy sessions and supervised shopping trips. As the client approaches the goal weight, he or she is encouraged to expand the repertoire to include eating out in a restaurant, preparing a meal, and eating forbidden foods. The following vignette exemplifies some of the issues that may complicate discharge.

▸ Alice, a 35-year-old woman with a long history of refractoriness to treatment for anorexia, wants to leave the hospital on reaching 75% of her ideal body weight (regarded as the minimum weight at which an individual may be considered medically stable). Discharge is feasible for this client only if her mother agrees to take Alice home. Initially, the mother allied herself with the treatment team and refused to go along with Alice's decision to leave at this low weight. The mother relents when Alice becomes threatening and angry, saying "I won't love you anymore." Although the mother fears for Alice's life, the perceived emotional abandonment and separation from her seems more real and threatening. The hastily arranged discharge plan for outpatient follow-up includes a counseling referral for this mother.

Discharge planning is a critical component in treatment and, as the aforementioned example demonstrates, can be complex. Often, family members benefit from counseling. The discharge planning process must address living arrangements, school, and work, as well as feasibility of an independent financial status, applications for entitlements (if needed), and follow-up outpatient treatment.

PSYCHOBIOLOGICAL INTERVENTIONS. As with most other psychiatric diagnoses, psychopharmacological treatment has become a common component of the successful treatment of eating disorders. The success of tricyclic antidepressants in the treatment of anorexia is not convincing; however, further studies are needed. The selective serotonin reuptake inhibitors (SSRIs), such as fluoxetine (Prozac), are promising pharmacologic agents that have been shown to improve the rate of weight gain and reduce the occurrence of relapse in anorexia nervosa (Walsh and Devlin 1995).

Acute Care: Outpatient Treatment

In the current climate of health care reform, with managed care and critical pathways that define treatment options, acute treatment of anorexia nervosa now occurs increasingly in an outpatient setting. As stated earlier, anorexia nervosa requires both inpatient and outpatient management composed of various therapeutic interventions, including individual, group, and family therapy and psychopharmacological therapy at different phases of the illness. The mainstay of treatment, however, has been outpatient therapy.

PSYCHOTHERAPY (ADVANCED PRACTICE). Whether in a partial hospitalization program, community mental health center, psychiatric home care program, or the more traditional outpatient treatment consisting of individual, group, or family therapy, the goals of treatment remain the same: weight restoration with normalization of eating habits and beginning treatment of psychological, interpersonal, and social issues that are integral to the experience of the client. In the acute, weight-restoration phase, the focus of the therapeutic interventions are almost wholly determined by the client's medically unstable weight. Attention to the underlying psychodynamic conflict is not feasible at this stage; a cognitive-behavioral approach to treatment is required at this time. Box 26–3 illustrates how cognitive therapy works.

Like the general psychiatric inpatient units, many existing day programs and partial hospitalization programs are not set up to care for the anorectic client in the weight-restoration phase. However, outpatient partial hospitalization programs designed to treat eating disorders are structured to achieve outcomes comparable with those of inpatient eating disorder units. Formerly, many therapists contracted with anorectic clients regarding the terms of treatment; outpatient treatment could continue only if the client maintained an agreed-on weight. If weight loss below the goal weight occurred, other treatment arrange-

BOX 26–3 HOW COGNITIVE-BEHAVIORAL THERAPY WORKS

The overall goal is to modify conscious processes, perceptions, and attitudes that maintain behavior. In clients with eating disorders the goal is to challenge dysfunctional thoughts and values about shape and weight. These thoughts and values support behaviors such as severe dieting, vomiting, use of laxatives and diuretics, excessive exercising, and an extreme preoccupation with one's body shape and weight. This treatment uses a therapeutic approach called cognitive restructuring, which incorporates problem-solving and self-regulation techniques. Cognitive restructuring has four basic steps, which are preliminary to changing behavior. They are

1. Identification of dysfunctional thoughts.
2. Examination of these thoughts.
3. Identification of underlying dysfunctional beliefs and values.
4. Examination of these beliefs and values.

Adapted from Beck, A., Rush, A., Shaw, B., and Emery, G. (1979). *Cognitive therapy of depression.* New York: Guilford Press.

ments had to be made until the client returned to the goal weight. The highly structured approach to clients whose weight is below 75% of ideal body weight is necessary, even for therapists who are psychodynamically oriented. Techniques such as assisting the client with a daily meal plan, reviewing a journal of meals and dietary intake maintained by the client, and providing for weighing weekly (ideally 2 to 3 times a week) are essential if the client is to reach a medically stable weight.

One alternative to the traditional acute treatment of anorexia nervosa is being developed. The alternative is a *psychiatric home care program* for clients who meet the criteria for inpatient admission (with the exception of acute suicidal risk). Critical pathways for clients with eating disorders are being developed with outcomes that compare with those of a 3-month hospitalization. A comprehensive, multidisciplinary treatment approach includes a complete biopsychosocial assessment with laboratory and diagnostic tests. The psychiatric home care nurse/clinical specialist both coordinates and provides care. This is a unique role for the psychiatric nurse that allows for a wide range of interventions. Behavioral strategies include psychoeducation about the eating disorder, meal planning, relaxation techniques, and cognitive-behavioral therapy to address the distorted perceptions and values regarding eating, body shape, and weight. The psychiatric home care nurse plans the frequency and duration of the home visits, with the expected objectives to be accomplished by the client at predicted intervals. Issues of food preparation, including shopping for food, may be arranged for by a family member or a home health attendant. The psychiatric home care nurse must be innovative in the approach to the client with an eating disorder. Such nontraditional nursing interventions as eating a meal and shopping for food with the client are crucial (Rosedale 1996).

Long-Term Treatment

THERAPY. Clients with a diagnosis of anorexia nervosa are at various stages according to the percentage of ideal body weight that has been achieved, the extent to which self-worth is defined by shape and weight, and the amount of disruption of their personal life. Clinical specialists and nurse practitioners in an advanced-practice model are providers of long-term follow-up treatment of anorectic clients, often in collaboration with other mental health professionals. Long-term treatment includes a variety of modalities to ensure a successful outcome (e.g., individual therapy, family therapy, group therapy, and psychopharmacological treatment).

Types of groups available to the client with anorexia nervosa include a recovery model (Overeaters Anonymous), anorexia and bulimia groups, women's groups, and traditional psychotherapy groups. Anorexia and bulimia groups typically have a regular multifamily group session.

In long-term treatment, the underlying issues affecting the client's illness and personal goals can be addressed. In addition to weight maintenance, the overriding goal for the client is to achieve a sense of self-worth and self-acceptance that is not exclusively based on appearance. Clients need assistance to find satisfaction in other areas of their lives (e.g., interpersonal, social, vocational). The combination of individual, group, and family therapy (especially for the younger client) provides the anorectic client with the greatest chance for a successful outcome.

Clients with anorexia nervosa have failed to achieve a sense of independence. Some clients report that the disordered eating behavior is a way to obtain nurturance and to cope with loneliness. They may even admit that these behaviors were unsuccessful in meeting those needs. Families often report feeling powerless in the face of behavior that is mystifying. Clients are often unable to experience compliments as support and therefore are unable to internalize the support. They often seek attention from others but feel scrutinized when they receive it. Clients want their families to care for and about them but are afraid that they do not care. Reasonable expressions of caring are not experienced as such. When others do respond in an attempt to show love and support, it is not internalized as a good feeling. The following two vignettes demonstrate this phenomenon.

- In a family session, a grandmother says to Gina (her 18-year-old anorectic granddaughter), "Gina, you're young, you're smart, you're beautiful. You can do anything." When the client does not react to the statement by feeling praised, the grandmother looks bewildered. After exploring what Gina is feeling, it becomes clear that such statements result in her feeling guilty and more ineffectual since she does not perceive herself as either beautiful or smart but feels that she should be acting both smart and beautiful.
- In a group setting, Terri's mother tells a poignant story of concern for her anorectic daughter. She describes lying awake at night, afraid that in the morning she would find her daughter dead. Although it seems to the group that this expressed sentiment is genuine, the daughter appears to be unmoved. It is later pointed out by the group and the group leader that although Terri often verbalizes that her mother does not care, she is actually unable to receive expressions of concern for her health as caring.

Often, families and significant others are seeking a way to communicate with the anorectic client. Much miscommunication occurs between the client and others. This confusion of thoughts and feelings leads to the client's inability to validate perceptions. Consequently, families experience the tension of saying or doing the wrong thing and then feeling responsible if a setback occurs. Psychiatric nurse clinicians have an important role in assisting families and significant others to develop strategies for improved communication and to search for ways to be comfortably supportive to the client. The following vignette demonstrates a young anorectic client's awareness of how she has been communicating and a breakthrough in her treatment.

▶ Harriet, an anorectic client, has made significant strides in her treatment and comes to recognize that her emotions are being expressed through her eating behaviors. In the presence of her family, she says, "It's up to me. Only I can do it." This is said with fierce pride.

The issue of control, which is commonly expressed in clients with eating disorders, is highlighted in this exchange. Harriet and other clients like her frequently find it difficult to ask for appropriate help.

Evaluation

The process of evaluation is ongoing, and short-term and intermediate goals revised as necessary to achieve the treatment outcomes established. These goals are the daily guides to reaching successful outcomes and must be continually re-evaluated for their appropriateness.

Text continued on page 815

CASE STUDY: A YOUNG WOMAN WITH ANOREXIA NERVOSA

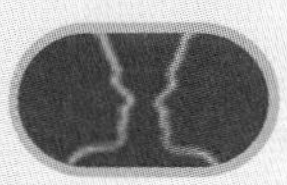

Cindy is a 20-year-old woman who is brought to the inpatient eating disorder unit of a psychiatric research hospital by two older brothers, who support her on either side. She is profoundly weak, holding her head up with her hands.

ASSESSMENT

Cindy gives a history of being a good student in elementary and high school. She delayed plans to attend college to care for her mother, who was very ill. The family further reports that Cindy began to attend exclusively to her mother and the household, totally neglecting herself and becoming extremely perfectionistic about her responsibilities. Although she had always been of normal weight with no prior eating problems, she began to restrict her food intake while spending an inordinate amount of time planning and preparing meals for others in the household. She rarely ate meals with the family and became increasingly socially isolated as she grew thinner.

On admission to the unit, her height and weight are taken: at 62 inches (5′2″) and 58 pounds, her weight is 50% of her ideal body weight. A complete physical examination reveals her to be extremely hypotensive (74/50 mm Hg), bradycardic (54 beats/min), and anemic (hemoglobin, 9 g/dl). Other laboratory test results are abnormal as well, reflecting her extreme malnutrition. She is immediately placed on therapeutic bed rest to conserve energy and calories, and an intravenous line is started to increase her hydration.

Cindy presents her problem as being one of extreme fatigue and needing to have more energy. She does not acknowledge that her extreme fasting has created the illness. When informed that the treatment would commence with prescription of a dietary supplement to provide nutrition, she does not object.

As Cindy slowly begins to furnish a history of her eating pattern, she states that more recently, she would begin the day with some water and half a piece of toast. During the day, she might have a piece of fruit. Her only "meal" is dinner, which consists of a very small quantity of turkey breast and carrots. She is ultimately unable to eat with others and avoids mealtimes. She eats in isolation. Her thoughts throughout the day are preoccupied with food. She maintains her extremely low weight both by exercising and restricting food intake. Ultimately, she is too lethargic to exercise and maintains her extremely low weight entirely by restricting her food intake. She denies having a history of binge eating or purging. Cindy does not acknowledge that she is too thin, insisting instead that she is too fatigued. She speaks about examining her body daily for evidence of fat. When she sits down, she does not like her thighs to touch. Cindy's affect is constricted, and she reports that her mood is depressed. She denies having suicidal thoughts. She is oriented in all spheres, with good attention and memory. Her thinking is concrete when explaining a proverb.

Continued on following page

This is Cindy's first hospitalization and her first treatment for anorexia nervosa. She denies having a history of substance abuse or depression before her weight loss. She reports having no history of physical or sexual abuse.

Cindy is the youngest of 12 children, with a 10-year difference between her and her next oldest sibling. Cindy's father died 2 years ago. Around that time, her 68-year-old mother became very ill. Cindy considers herself an only child because of the difference in ages between her and her siblings and because she lives alone with her mother at a great distance from the rest of the family. Since she began taking care of her mother, she has become socially isolated, which is further complicated by the development of anorexia. She has not maintained contact with high school friends in the past year. Currently, she says "I do not know what I want to be when I grow up."

NURSING DIAGNOSES

The first two nursing diagnoses formulated for Cindy are **altered nutrition** and **body image disturbance.**

PLANNING AND INTERVENTION

Initial measures are taken in order to address Cindy's unstable physiological state (e.g., restoring fluid and electrolyte balance, increasing red blood cell count, preventing hypothermia, and stabilizing vital signs). As Cindy begins the weight-restoration phase of treatment, she is placed on an 1800-calorie diet but is unable to eat and spends most of the mealtime poking at her food. A liquid supplement is prescribed, which is the exclusive source of her nutritional intake for several weeks, after which she slowly begins to eat solid food. As she gains weight, she can frequently be found doing jumping jacks in her room or speed walking down the corridors of the unit. Nursing Care Plan 26–1 provides an intervention for a client with anorexia nervosa.

NURSING CARE PLAN 26–1 A CLIENT WITH ANOREXIA NERVOSA

NURSING DIAGNOSIS

Altered Nutrition: Less Than Body Requirement: related to restricting caloric intake, secondary to extreme fear of weight gain

Supporting Data

- 58 lb (50% of ideal body weight)
- Cachectic appearance, pale with fine lanugo, BP, 74/50 mm Hg, pulse, 54, barely palpable
- Depressed mood
- Denies being underweight: "I need treatment because I get fatigued so easily."
- Anemia (HGB, 9 g/dl)

Outcome Criteria: Client will reach 75% of ideal body weight—92 lb—by discharge*

SHORT-TERM GOAL	INTERVENTION	RATIONALE	EVALUATION
1. Client will gain a minimum of 1/2 lb at each weigh-in (Mon-Wed-Fri).	1a. Acknowledge the emotional and physical difficulty the client is experiencing. Use client's extreme fatigue to engage her cooperation in the treatment plan.	1a. A first priority is to establish a therapeutic alliance.	WEEK 1: Client increases caloric intake with liquid supplement only. Client unable to eat solid food. Client does not gain weight.
	1b. Weigh the client daily for the first	1b. These measures ensure weight is accu-	Client remains hypotensive, bradycardic, anemic

NURSING CARE PLAN 26–1 A CLIENT WITH ANOREXIA NERVOSA *(Continued)*

SHORT-TERM GOAL	INTERVENTION	RATIONALE	EVALUATION
	seven days; then three times a week. Client should be weighed in bra and panties only. There should be no oral intake, including a drink of water, before the early AM weight. Do not negotiate the weight with the client nor reweigh the client. The client may choose not to look at the scale or request that she not be told the weight.	rate. Morning weigh-in procedure is a high-anxiety time. Knowledge of the weight increasing induces feelings of being out of control, especially during initial phase of refeeding.	(HGB=9 g/dl). WEEK 2: Client gains 2 lb drinking liquid supplement—minimal solid food. Client remains hypotensive, bradycardic (HGB=10 g/dl). WEEK 3: Client gains 3 lb drinking liquid supplement. Client selects meal plan but is unable to eat most of solid food.
	1c. Vital signs TID until stable, then daily. Repeat ECG and laboratory tests until stable.	1c. As client begins to increase in weight, cardiovascular status improves to within normal range and monitoring is less frequent.	Client's BP=84/60 mm Hg, pulse=68, regular; HGB=11 g/dl.
	1d. Provide a pleasant, calm atmosphere at mealtimes. Clients should be told the specific times and duration (usually a half hour) of meals.	1d. Mealtimes become episodes of high anxiety, and knowledge of regulations decreases tension in the milieu, particularly when the client has given up so much control by entering treatment.	WEEKS 4–6: Client gains an average of 2½ lb/week. Client samples more of solid food selected from meal plan. Client's BP=90/60 mm Hg; pulse=68, regular; HGB=11.5 g/dl.
	1e. Administer liquid supplement as ordered.	1e. Client may be unable to eat solid food at first.	WEEK 7: Client weighs 71 lb (almost 60% of ideal body weight); calories are mostly from liquid supplement.
	1f. Observe client during meals to prevent hiding or throwing away of food for at least 1 hour after meals and snacks to prevent purging.	1f, g. The compelling force of the illness is such that these behaviors are difficult to stop. A power struggle between staff and client may emerge in which the client appears to comply but defies the rules (appearing to eat but throwing away food).	Client selects balanced meals, eating more varied, solid food: turkey, carrots, lettuce, fruit. Client's HGB=12.5 g/dl, maintains normal range of BP and pulse. Client continues to increase participation in social aspects of eating.
	1g. Encourage client to try to eat some solid food. Preparation of client's meals should be guided by likes and dislikes list, as client is unable to make own selections to complete menu.		

Continued on following page

NURSING CARE PLAN 26–1 A CLIENT WITH ANOREXIA NERVOSA *(Continued)*

SHORT-TERM GOAL	INTERVENTION	RATIONALE	EVALUATION
	1h. Be empathetic with client's struggle to give up control of her eating and her weight as she is expected to make minimum weight gain on a regular basis.	1h. The client is expected to gain at least a half pound on a specific schedule, usually three times a week (Mon-Wed-Fri).	WEEKS 8–12: Client gains an average of 2 lb/week and weighs 82 lb (approx. 68% of ideal body weight). Client is eating more varied solid food, but most caloric intake is still from liquid supplement. Client maintains normal vital signs and HGB levels. Client maintains social interaction during mealtimes and snacks.
	1i. Monitor client's weight gain. A weight gain of 3 to 5 lb/week is medically acceptable.	1i. Weight gain of over 5 lb in a week may result in pulmonary edema.	
	1j. Provide teaching regarding healthy eating as the basis of a healthy life style.	1j. Enforces healthy aspects of eating, e.g., increased energy, rather than gaining weight.	
	1k. Continue to provide a supportive, empathetic approach as client continues in weight restoration.	1k. Eating regularly for the anorectic client, even within the framework of restoring health, is extremely difficult.	WEEK 13: Client has reached medically stable weight at the end of 16th week—92 lb (75% of ideal body weight). Client continues to eat more solid food with relatively less liquid supplement. Client is not able to engage in planned exercise program until client reaches 85% of ideal body weight.
	1l. Use a cognitive-behavioral approach to client's expressed fears regarding weight gain. Identify and examine dysfunctional thoughts, identify and examine values and beliefs that maintain these thoughts.	1l. Confronting the dysfunctional thoughts and beliefs is crucial to changing eating behaviors.	
	1m. As client approaches her target weight, there should be encouragement to make her own choices for menu selection.	1m. The client can assume more control of her meals, which is empowering for the anorectic client.	
	1n. Emphasize social nature of eating. Encourage conversation that does not have the theme of food during mealtimes.	1n. Eating as a social activity, shared with others and participating in conversation, serves both as a distraction from obses-	

NURSING CARE PLAN 26–1 A CLIENT WITH ANOREXIA NERVOSA *(Continued)*

SHORT-TERM GOAL	INTERVENTION	RATIONALE	EVALUATION
		sional preoccupations and as a pleasurable event.	
	1o. The weight maintenance phase of treatment challenges the client. This is the ideal time to address more of the issues underlying the client's attitude toward weight and shape.	1o. At a healthier weight, the client is cognitively better prepared to examine emotional conflicts and themes.	
	1p. Focus on the client's strengths, including her good work in normalizing her weight and eating habits.	1p. The client who is beginning to normalize weight and eating behaviors has achieved a major accomplishment, of which she should be proud. Explores non-eating activities as a source of gratification.	
	1q. Provide for a planned exercise program when the client reaches target weight.	1q. The client experiences a strong drive to exercise; this measure accommodates this drive by planning a reasonable amount.	
	1r. Encourage the client to apply all the knowlledge, skills, and gains made from the various individual, family, and group therapy sessions.	1r. The client has been receiving intensive therapy and education, which have provided tools and techniques that are useful in maintaining healthy behaviors.	

NURSING DIAGNOSIS

Body Image Disturbance: related to client's belief of being overweight (although emaciated) and fear of being fat

Supporting Data

- Denies being extremely underweight
- Examines body daily for evidence of fat
- Measures circumference of thighs after eating

Outcome Criteria: Client will display a realistic perception of body size and shape.

SHORT-TERM GOAL	INTERVENTION	RATIONALE	EVALUATION
1. Client will challenge dysfunctional thoughts and beliefs about weight.	1a. Establish a therapeutic alliance with the client.	1a. Anorectic clients are initially unwilling to give up their disordered eating behaviors, which are egosyntonic.	WEEK 1: Client is unable to begin journal. Client is unable to meet other goals.

Continued on following page

NURSING CARE PLAN 26–1 A CLIENT WITH ANOREXIA NERVOSA *(Continued)*

SHORT-TERM GOAL	INTERVENTION	RATIONALE	EVALUATION
	1b. Challenge the client's fears gently, particularly in the early stage of treatment at such a low weight, regarding size and shape.	1b. At 60% of ideal body weight, cognition is often impaired, making rational thought more difficult. The client is unable to accurately perceive her emaciated body.	WEEKS 2–3: Client is able to record a few thoughts in journal. Client is still unable to meet other goals.
	1c. Give feedback about the client's low weight and resultant impaired health.	1c. Focuses on health and benefits of increased energy.	WEEK 4: Client is able to record more thoughts and beliefs in journal. Client is unable to meet other goals.
	1d. Challenge the client's perceptions and beliefs in a systematic manner that will assist the client to modify thinking.	1d, e. As the client gains weight, she is able to do more productive cognitive and emotional work. The client's self-image is part of a distorted system in which thinness is viewed as special.	
	1e. Provide feedback and encouragement when the client expresses less distorted thoughts and ideas.		WEEK 5: Client begins to challenge thoughts and beliefs recorded in journal. Client is unable to verbalize more realistic perception of body or accept statements that she is looking healthier.
	1f. Assist the client to distinguish between thoughts and feelings. Statements such as, "I feel fat" should be challenged and reframed.	1f. It is important for the client to distinguish between feelings and facts. The client often speaks of feelings as if they are reality.	WEEKS 6–8: Client continues to maintain journal and challenge automatic thoughts and beliefs. Client still perceives self as fat. Client is able to accept statements that she looks healthier.
	1g. Discuss the reactions of others, particularly family and significant others, to client as she proceeds in treatment.	1g, h. Reactions of others often become triggers for dysphoric reactions and distorted perceptions. Relationships with others, while not casual, are the context in which the eating disorder exists and thrives. Families and significant others need assistance in how to communicate and share a relationship with the anorectic client.	
	1h. Educate family regarding the client's illness and encourage attendance at family and group therapy sessions.		WEEKS 9–12: Client is able to do more work in challenging thoughts and beliefs. Client is more accepting of compliments. Client continues to see herself as fat but feels healthier.

NURSING CARE PLAN 26–1 A CLIENT WITH ANOREXIA NERVOSA *(Continued)*

SHORT-TERM GOAL	INTERVENTION	RATIONALE	EVALUATION
			WEEK 13 Client meeting all goals except perception of body image, which she accepts as healthy but prefers to be thinner.

**At 75% of ideal body weight, a client may be considered medically stable, and treatment might continue as an outpatient. In this example, the client is in a research facility that allows for long-term inpatient treatment, allowing the client to remain hospitalized until reaching 90% of ideal body weight.*

TID, three times a day; ECG, electrocardiogram; BP, blood pressure; HGB, hemoglobin.

BULIMIA NERVOSA

Although *boulimos* was known in ancient Greece and described by Hippocrates as a sick hunger, in the 1940s this phenomenon began to be more widely known, along with purging, as part of the behaviors of some anorectic persons. Bruch (1985) described the person who resorts to compensatory behaviors when he or she is unable to maintain rigid control of eating as the "me too" anorectic. According to Bruch, the early anorectic person originated the illness all on his or her own and maintained it passionately, bearing little resemblance to the person with the binge eating and/or purging type of eating disorder that emerged. Increasingly, in addition to those with anorexia nervosa, individuals of normal weight were also binge eating and purging. Russell (1985) addressed the "me too," copycat phenomenon and cited instances in which an individual had symptoms after reading of the disorder or being questioned by a physician. Another group of individuals who were obese were also binge eating but without purging or other compensatory behaviors (Stunkard 1993).

Bulimia as a diagnosis first entered DSM-III in 1980, but without purging or inappropriate compensatory behaviors as a criterion. The diagnosis became **bulimia nervosa** with the addition of the preceding criterion in 1987. Currently, in DSM-IV (APA 1994), it is further subtyped as purging or nonpurging type (see Fig. 26– 1).

Assessment

Clients with bulimia nervosa may not initially appear to be physically or emotionally ill. They are often at or slightly below ideal body weight. However, as the assessment continues and the nurse makes further observations, the physical and emotional problems of the client become apparent. On inspection, the client demonstrates enlargement of the parotid glands with dental erosion and caries if the client has been inducing vomiting. The history disclosed is often one of chaotic relationships, both family and interpersonal, with unstable patterns in vocational and social functioning. Table 26–5 compares and contrasts bulimia with anorexia.

◗ Jenny is being admitted to an inpatient eating disorder unit. During the initial assessment, the nurse wonders if Jenny is actually in need of hospitalization. The nurse is struck by how well the client presents, appearing healthy looking, well dressed, and articulate. As Jenny continues to relate her history, she tells of restricting her intake all day until early evening, when she buys her food and begins to binge as she is shopping. She arrives home and immediately induces vomiting. For the remainder of the evening and into the early morning hours, she "zones out" while watching television and binge eating. Periodically, she goes to the bathroom to vomit. She does this about 15 times during the evening. The nurse admitting Jenny to the unit reminds her of the goals of the hospitalization, including interrupting the binge/purge cycle and normalizing eating. The nurse further explains to Jenny that she has the support of the eating disorder treatment team and the milieu of the unit to assist her toward recovery.

Nursing Diagnosis

The assessment of the client with bulimia nervosa yields nursing diagnoses that result from the disordered eating and weight control behaviors. Problems resulting from purging are a first priority because electrolyte and fluid balance and cardiac function are affected. Common nursing diagnoses include decreased cardiac output, potential for injury (electrolyte imbalance), body image disturbance, and powerlessness.

TABLE 26–5 COMPARISON OF CHARACTERISTICS OF ANOREXIA AND BULIMIA

ANOREXIA—RESTRICTING TYPE	BULIMIA
Prevalence	
About 0.5%–1.0% for presentations that meet full criteria. Those who are subthreshold for the disorder (Eating Disorder NOS) are more common.	About 1%–3% among adolescent and young adult females. The disorder in males is about one tenth that in females.
Appearance	
Below 85% of ideal body weight	Normal weight range, may be slightly above or below
Onset of Illness	
Early adolescence with peaks at 14 and 17 years of age	Late adolescence, early adult
Physical Signs	
Thin, emaciated Amenorrhea Slight yellowing of skin Bradycardia Hypotension, hypothermia Peripheral edema	Enlarged parotid glands Dental erosion, caries Calluses on dorsum of hands Electrolyte imbalance, especially hypokalemia Fluid retention
Familial Patterns	
Increased incidence of mood disorders—1st degree relatives	Increased incidence of mood disorders, substance abuse, dependence—1st degree relatives
Personality Traits	
Perfectionism Social isolation	Poor impulse control Low self-esteem
Insight into Illness	
Denies seriousness of illness, eating disordered behaviors are ego-syntonic	Aware of illness, disturbed behaviors are ego-dystonic

From American Psychiatric Association (1994). *Diagnostic and statistical manual of mental disorders* (4th ed.). Washington, DC: American Psychiatric Association. Reprinted with permission. Copyright 1994 American Psychiatric Association.

Planning

The effectiveness of treatment interventions is evaluated against established outcome criteria. Some common outcomes for clients with bulimia follow:

- The client will refrain from binge eating.
- The client will exercise within normal limits.
- The client will abstain from purging.
- The client will state that he or she wants to live.
- The client will remain safe.

Implementation

Acute Care: Inpatient Treatment

The criteria for inpatient admission of a client with bulimia nervosa are included in the criteria for inpatient admission of a client with an eating disorder. Like the client with anorexia nervosa, the client with bulimia may be treated for life-threatening complications (i.e., gastric rupture [rare], electrolyte imbalance, cardiac dysrhythmias) in an acute care unit of a hospital. If the client is admitted to a general inpatient psychiatric unit for acute suicidal risk, again only the acute psychiatric manifestations are addressed short term (see Table 26–1 for physical signs and symptoms of anorexia and bulimia).

▶ Iris weighs 85% of her ideal body weight. She has a history of diuretic abuse, and she became very edematous when she stopped their use and entered treatment. Iris could not tolerate the weight gain and the accompanying edema, despite education about the edema's being related to the use of diuretics and thus transient, and that it would resolve after normalization of eating habits and discontinuation of the diuretics. She restarted the diuretics, perpetuating the cycle of fluid retention and the risk of kidney damage. The nurse empathizes with the inability to tolerate the feelings of anxiety and dread that the client experiences because of her markedly swollen extremities.

Ideally, clients who are this severe are referred to an inpatient eating disorder unit for comprehensive treatment of their illness. Inpatient units designed to treat eating disorders are especially structured to interrupt the cycle of binge eating and purging and to normalize eating habits. Therapy is begun to examine the underlying conflicts and the distorted perceptions of shape and weight that maintain the illness. Evaluation for treatment of comorbid disorders, such as major depression and substance abuse, is also addressed. In most cases of substance dependence, the treatment of the eating disorder must occur after the substance dependence is treated.

MILIEU THERAPY (BASIC LEVEL). The highly structured milieu of an inpatient eating disorder unit has as its primary goals the interruption of the **binge/purge cycle** and the prevention of the disordered eating behaviors. Interventions such as observation during and after meals to prevent purging, normalization of eating patterns, and appropriate exercise are integral elements of such a unit. The interdisciplinary team of the unit uses a comprehensive treatment approach to address the emotional and behavioral problems that arise when the client is no longer binge eating or purging. The underlying feelings have been masked by the disordered eating behaviors, and the interruption of the binge/purge pattern brings these psychodynamic issues to the fore.

PSYCHOTHERAPY (ADVANCED PRACTICE). Central to the treatment approach of bulimia nervosa is the emphasis on educating clients and helping them avoid dieting and restricting of caloric intake, particularly for many hours, which sets up the response to binge eat and then compensate by purging or excessively exercising. While the client is attending individual, group, and family therapy sessions, it is hoped that the binge/purge cycle will be interrupted and the normalization of eating and meal planning can begin.

HEALTH TEACHING (BASIC LEVEL). The client is now ready to enter the second phase of treatment, in which there are carefully planned challenges to the client's newly developed skills. For instance, the client is expected to have a meal while "on pass" outside the hospital or to plan an overnight pass with meals at home. On return to the unit, the client shares the experience.

On discharge from the hospital, the client is referred for long-term care to solidify the goals that have been achieved and to treat both the attitudes and the perceptions that maintain the eating disorder and the psychodynamic issues that attend the illness.

Long-Term Treatment

THERAPY (ADVANCED PRACTICE). Clients with bulimia nervosa, because of possible coexisting depression, substance abuse, and personality disorders, are often in various therapies. Although the specific eating-disordered behaviors may not be targeted specifically in some therapies, it is those very behaviors that are responsible for much of the client's emotional distress. Therefore, it is imperative that dysfunctional attitudes and perceptions of weight and shape be a primary focus of the therapy. When the client does not indulge in these bulimic behaviors, issues of self-worth and interpersonal functioning become more prominent. The psychodynamic issues can be addressed by numerous psychotherapeutic approaches, but cognitive-behavioral therapy is most effective in the acute phase of bulimic behaviors. Compared with the food-restricting anorectic client, the client with bulimia nervosa often more readily establishes a therapeutic alliance with the advanced practice nurse because the eating-disordered behaviors are so ego-dystonic.

▶ Patty, a 23-year-old client with a 6-year history of bulimia nervosa, struggles with issues of self-esteem. She expresses much guilt about "letting her father down" in the past by engaging in drinking alcohol excessively and binge eating and purging. She is determined that this time she is not going to fail at treatment. After her initial success in stopping the aforementioned behaviors, she says defiantly, "I'm doing this for me." Patty experiences her behavior as either pleasing or disappointing to others. She begins to realize that her feeling of self-worth is very much dependent on how others see her and that she needs to develop a better sense of herself.

PSYCHOBIOLOGICAL INTERVENTIONS (BASIC LEVEL). Walsh and Devlin (1995) noted that antidepressant medication has been used extensively in the treatment of bulimia, although when compared with cognitive-behavioral therapy, the superiority of medication has not been established. The (SSRIs), such as fluoxetine, have proved to be particularly useful because their side effects are well tolerated. Walsh and Devlin further noted that a combination of psychopharmacology and cognitive behavior therapy may be more effective than either therapy alone.

Evaluation

Evaluation of treatment effectiveness is ongoing, and goals are revised as necessary to reach the desired outcomes.

CASE STUDY: A WOMAN WITH BULIMIA NERVOSA

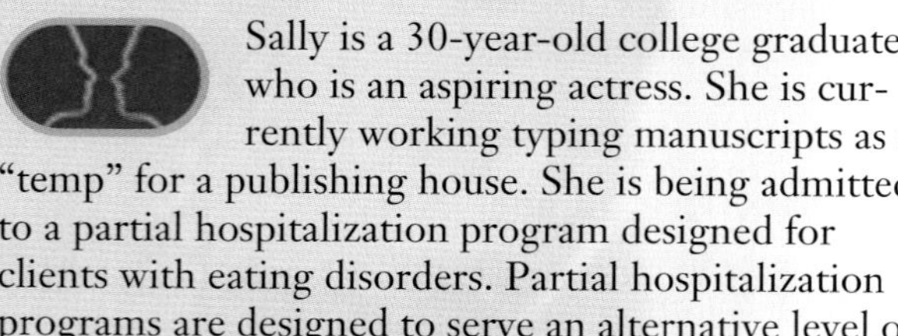

Sally is a 30-year-old college graduate who is an aspiring actress. She is currently working typing manuscripts as a "temp" for a publishing house. She is being admitted to a partial hospitalization program designed for clients with eating disorders. Partial hospitalization programs are designed to serve an alternative level of care (subacute care, transition from hospital to community) and to accommodate different levels of client functioning (working clients, clients requiring more structure and support than traditional outpatient therapy provides). Services vary from 2 to 5 days a week for several hours a day. Some programs have evening hours to further address the needs of working clients.

ASSESSMENT

Sally states that on returning home after her first semester at college, her mother met her at the airport and greeted her with "You better go on a diet." Sally began to diet, fasting for most of the day and then beginning to eat in the evening. She quickly developed a pattern of fasting and binge eating at dinner, followed by vomiting. Her unstructured, chaotic life style contributed to her impulsivity and bulimic behaviors.

Sally's weight is approximately normal; at 65 inches (5′5″) and 127 pounds, her weight is at 95% of ideal body weight. Physical examination reveals a blood pressure of 120/80 mm Hg sitting and 90/60 mm Hg standing; her pulse is 70 sitting and 96 standing. Her parotid glands are enlarged. There is considerable dental erosion present. Laboratory tests reveal a potassium level of 2.7 mmol/L (normal range, 3.3–5.5 mmol/L). Her electrocardiogram is abnormal, consistent with hypokalemia.

Sally has a dread of being fat, and the thought of not being slim makes her very anxious. She states that she cannot stop the cycle of binge eating and purging that causes her to feel guilty and ashamed. Sally fasts for most of the day, and then, once she begins to eat, she feels compelled to binge and then vomit. She finds this pattern to be particularly true if she eats certain foods, such as french fries. The cycle of binge eating and vomiting occurs at least 5 times a day. Sally works odd hours, doing her manuscript typing mostly at night. Because she works alone and can avoid being observed, she binge eats while doing her work and ultimately purges by inducing vomiting. Sally maintains her weight through vomiting and exercising for several hours daily at a gym. She reports that she has used laxatives and over-the-counter diuretics only a couple of times in the past. Sally thinks that her current weight, which is 96% of her ideal body weight, is "OK. If I gain an ounce, I'll be fat." She regards her slim figure as crucial to her success. Sally's affect is appropriate to her mood, which is anxious. She denies having suicidal ideation currently, although she has recently felt passively suicidal. The remainder of the mental status examination is normal.

Sally gives a history of being hospitalized for depression for 4 weeks at the age of 19. At that time, she was treated with an antidepressant and continued in outpatient treatment for about 6 months. She reports that her eating disorder was never diagnosed at that time. She also gives a history of intermittent marijuana and alcohol abuse but is not currently using. She stated her mother is in therapy and is being treated with Prozac.

Sally is raised in an upper-middle-class family with highly successful parents and siblings who all resided 3000 miles away. Of the five children in her family, she is the only one who does not have a career or an intimate relationship, both of which she

CASE STUDY: A WOMAN WITH BULIMIA NERVOSA (Continued)

very much wants. Sally states that her mother frequently uses her as a confidante in inappropriate ways. For instance, she shares with Sally that she is having an affair with her business partner. Sally regards her father as unapproachable and distant but feels guilty about not telling him about her mother's affair. Sally graduated from college but never had a job that was appropriate to her education, settling for temporary work. She maintains that she needs the kind of job that is flexible and at off hours so that she can be available to attend acting and dance classes and auditions.

It is not clear how assiduously Sally pursues acting. She reports that she has never actually had an acting job. It becomes apparent that the aspiring actress is mostly a fantasy, with no real substance. In reality, her unstructured life style contributes to her impulsivity and her bulimic behaviors.

NURSING DIAGNOSES

Risk for injury (electrolyte imbalance) and **powerlessness.** Nursing Care Plan 26–2 provides interventions for a client with bulimia.

NURSING CARE PLAN 26–2 A CLIENT WITH BULIMIA

NURSING DIAGNOSIS

Risk for Injury: related to low potassium and other physical changes secondary to binge eating and purging

Supporting Data

- Potassium level of 2.7 mmol/L
- Abnormal electrocardiogram
- Enlarged parotid glands
- Dental erosion, caries
- History of binge eating/purging

Outcome Criteria: Client will demonstrate ability to regulate eating patterns in the absence of untoward signs and symptoms.

SHORT-TERM GOAL	INTERVENTION	RATIONALE	EVALUATION
1. Client will identify signs and symptoms of low potassium (K^+) level and K^+ level will remain within the normal limits throughout hospitalization.	1a. Educate the client regarding the ill effects of self-induced vomiting, low K^+ level, dental erosion. 1b. Educate the client about binge/purge cycle and its self-perpetuating nature. 1c. Teach the client that fasting sets one up to binge eat.	1a. Health teaching is crucial to treatment. The client needs to be reminded of the benefits of normalization of eating behavior. 1b, c. The compulsive nature of the binge/purge cycle is maintained by the cycle of restricting, hunger, bingeing, purging accompanied by feelings of guilt, and then repeating the cycle over and over.	WEEK 1: Client begins to select balanced meals. Client demonstrates knowledge of untoward effects of vomiting and of K^+ deficiency. Client begins to demonstrate understanding of repetitive nature of binge/purge cycle. WEEK 2: Client begins to challenge dysfunctional thoughts and beliefs that maintain

Continued on following page

NURSING CARE PLAN 26–2 A CLIENT WITH BULIMIA (Continued)

Short-Term Goal	Intervention	Rationale	Evaluation
	1d. Explore ideas about trigger foods.	1d. Trigger foods are foods that provide the stimulus for a binge: french fries, donuts.	bulimic behaviors. Client continues to plan nutritionally balanced meals, including dinner at home.
	1e. Challenge dysfunctional thoughts and beliefs about "forbidden" foods.	1e. The client also has a list of "forbidden foods," which cause excessive weight gain or cannot be eaten in normal amounts, e.g., ice cream, cake.	Client begins to sample "forbidden foods" and discuss thoughts and attitudes about same.
	1f. Teach the client to plan and eat regularly scheduled, balanced meals.	1f. Planning and structuring meals helps to ensure success in maintaining abstinence from binge/purge activity.	WEEK 3: Client discusses triggers to binge and resultant behavior. Client continues to challenge dysfunctional thoughts and beliefs in individual and group sessions. Client plans meals, including "forbidden foods." WEEK 4: Client reports no binge/purge behaviors at day program or outside. Client demonstrates understanding of repetitive nature of binge/purge cycle. Client continues to challenge dysfunctional thoughts and beliefs.

NURSING DIAGNOSIS

Powerlessness: related to uncontrollable binge eating and purging

Supporting Data

- Inability to stop binge/purge cycle.
- Guilt over uncontrollable behavior.
- Distorted perceptions and beliefs regarding eating and self-image.
- "If I gain an ounce, I'll feel fat. Being thin is crucial to my success."

Outcome Criteria: Client will demonstrate control of eating.

Short-Term Goal	Intervention	Rationale	Evaluation
1. Client will not binge/purge during day program hours (8 AM to 3 PM)	1a. Explore the client's experience of out-of-control eating.	1a. Listening in an empathetic manner to the client describing the repetitive, uncontrollable experience	WEEK 1: Client reports no bingeing but purges two times at the day program. Client discusses pattern of

NURSING CARE PLAN 26–2 A CLIENT WITH BULIMIA *(Continued)*

SHORT-TERM GOAL	INTERVENTION	RATIONALE	EVALUATION
		of the binge/purge cycle establishes a therapeutic alliance.	eating before admission. Client begins journal recording of dysfunctional thoughts and beliefs.
	1b. Reinforce the effects of fasting on the pattern of eating.	1b. Restriction of dietary intake in a bulimic individual sets up a binge.	Client begins to select meals.
	1c. Educate the client about the need for structured, planned meals.	1c. Structuring and scheduling mealtimes assist the client in overcoming the chaotic and impulsive context in which the bulimia has thrived.	Client exercises for 2 hours in the evening. WEEK 2: Client reports no bingeing or purging while at the day program. Client continues to share journal and challenge automatic thoughts. Client selects meals. Client reports continuing to exercise excessively at home.
	1d. Challenge dysfunctional thoughts and beliefs in a systematic manner. 1e. Encourage the client to keep a journal of thoughts and feelings and the context in which they occur.	1d, e. The binge/purge cycle is maintained by automatic thoughts and beliefs, which must be examined and challenged. A journal is an excellent way to illuminate these dysfunctional thoughts and underlying assumptions.	WEEK 3: Client reports no binge/purge behavior at day program, but it occurs one time at home over the weekend. Client continues to record in journal. Client continues to challenge automatic thoughts. Client begins to demonstrate understanding of negative triggers to bulimic behavior.
	1f. Examine the logic of a specific thought and feeling and the behavior that resulted.	1f. Client must acknowledge that there is no logical connection between an untoward event (i.e., criticism, broken date) and a binge.	Client reports reducing amount of exercise.
	1g. Teach the client to challenge automatic thoughts. 1h. Assist the client to apply more constructive problem-solving techniques when confronted with problematic situations. 1i. Teach the client that	1g-j. Bulimia is a chronic illness. The client must do "homework" on her own to maintain healthy behaviors. The client should record in her journal the analysis of her thoughts and beliefs in the decision involved in using	WEEK 4: Client reports non–binge/purge behavior. Client identifies negative triggers and reports more constructive responses. Client reports adhering to structured meal schedule. Client reports appropriate exercise program.

Continued on following page

NURSING CARE PLAN 26–2 A CLIENT WITH BULIMIA *(Continued)*

SHORT-TERM GOAL	INTERVENTION	RATIONALE	EVALUATION
	the distorted perceptions of weight and shape maintain the binge eating and inappropriate compensatory behaviors, i.e., purging, excessive exercising.	more constructive responses. The client's life is organized in large measure around her disordered eating behaviors and needs to be examined and restructured to prevent the binge/purge cycle and to provide a new focus.	
	1j. Assist the client to examine her current life style and how it impacts on her illness.		
	1k. Encourage the client to apply new skills learned in individual and group therapy in communications with others, particularly family.	1k. The outcome of techniques that have been learned should be evaluated in terms of the client's relationships, and what is working should be reinforced.	
	1l. Provide reinforcement of the client's successes: normalization of eating, not purging, exercising more appropriately.	1l, m. The compelling force of the illness is always a threat to the client's returning to dysfunctional behaviors. The client needs the support of the therapeutic relationship.	
	1m. Teach the client that a lapse is not a relapse. One slip in loss of control does not eliminate all positive accomplishments.		

EATING DISORDER NOT OTHERWISE SPECIFIED: BINGE EATING DISORDER

Binge eating disorder as a variant of compulsive overeating is presented here both to remain within the framework of the third edition of this text and to bring obesity caused by compulsive overeating up to date. Although considerable controversy exists over whether this proposed diagnosis constitutes a separate eating disorder, 20% to 30% of obese individuals seeking treatment report binge eating as a pattern of overeating (Marcus 1995). In the DSM-IV appendix, research criteria are listed for further study of binge eating disorder (Fig. 26–2). Because there are no compensatory behaviors (purging, exercise) to attempt to control weight in this disorder, it is currently diagnosed as *eating disorder NOS.*

In the United States, approximately 25% of the population is considered to be overweight (Williamson 1993), despite the national epidemic of attempting to live a healthier life style. This fact, in part, has led to the approval of dexfenfluramine (Redux), an appetite suppressant, for the treatment of obesity (1996). The reasons for obesity are varied, and the most appropriate treatment decision considers the degree of overweight, associated illness, duration of being overweight, and heredity factors. The greater the above-mentioned factors, the greater the need for professional intervention (Brownell and Wadden 1991). See Table 26–6 for matching classification of obesity with treatment.

In the World Health Organization's *ICD-10 classification of mental and behavioral disorders*, overeating associated with other psychological disturbances, including obesity due to overeating as a reaction to a distressing event, is classified as an atypical eating disorder (World Health Organization 1992). However, obesity due to eating disturbances secondary to medical and psychiatric conditions is not classified as an eating disorder according to DSM-IV criteria.

Overeating is frequently noted as a symptom of an affective disorder (i.e., atypical depression). Higher rates of affective and personality disorders were found among binge eaters (Marcus 1990). Binge eaters reported a history of major depression significantly more than non–binge eaters. They further reported that disordered eating occurred during negative mood states and that they experienced binge eating as soothing or serving the function of mood regulation. Although dieting is almost always an antecedent of binge eating in bulimia nervosa, in approximately 50% of a sample of obese binge eaters, no attempt to restrict dietary intake occurred (Marcus 1992).

An effective program for obese binge eaters must integrate modification of the disordered eating and the depressive symptoms with the ultimate goal of a more appropriate weight for the individual.

Text continued on page 828

Binge Eating Disorder (Compulsive Overeating)

A. Recurrent episodes of binge eating. An episode of binge eating is characterized by both of the following:
   1. Eating, in a discrete period (e.g., within any 2-hour period), an amount of food that is definitely larger than most people would eat in a similar period under similar circumstances.
   2. A sense of lack of control over eating during the episode (e.g., a feeling that one cannot stop eating or control what or how much one is eating).

B. The binge-eating episodes are associated with three (or more) of the following:
   1. Eating much more rapidly than normal
   2. Eating until feeling uncomfortably full
   3. Eating large amounts of food when not feeling physically hungry
   4. Eating alone because of being embarrassed by how much one is eating
   5. Feeling disgusted with oneself, depressed, or very guilty after overeating

C. Marked distress regarding binge eating is present.

D. The binge eating occurs, on average, at least 2 days a week for 6 months.

   Note: the method of determining frequency differs from that used for bulimia nervosa; future research should address whether the preferred method of setting a frequency threshold is counting the number of days on which binges occur or counting the number of episodes of binge eating.

E. The binge eating is not associated with the regular use of inappropriate compensatory behaviors (e.g., purging, fasting, excessive exercise) and does not occur exclusively during the course of anorexia nervosa or bulimia nervosa.

Figure 26–2 Research criteria for binge eating disorder. (Adapted from American Psychiatric Association (1994). *Diagnostic and statistical manual of mental disorders (DSM-IV)* (4th ed.). Washington, DC: American Psychiatric Association. Reprinted with permission. Copyright 1994 American Psychiatric Association.)

TABLE 26–6 CONCEPTUAL SCHEME FOR SELECTING TREATMENT FOR OVERWEIGHT INDIVIDUALS

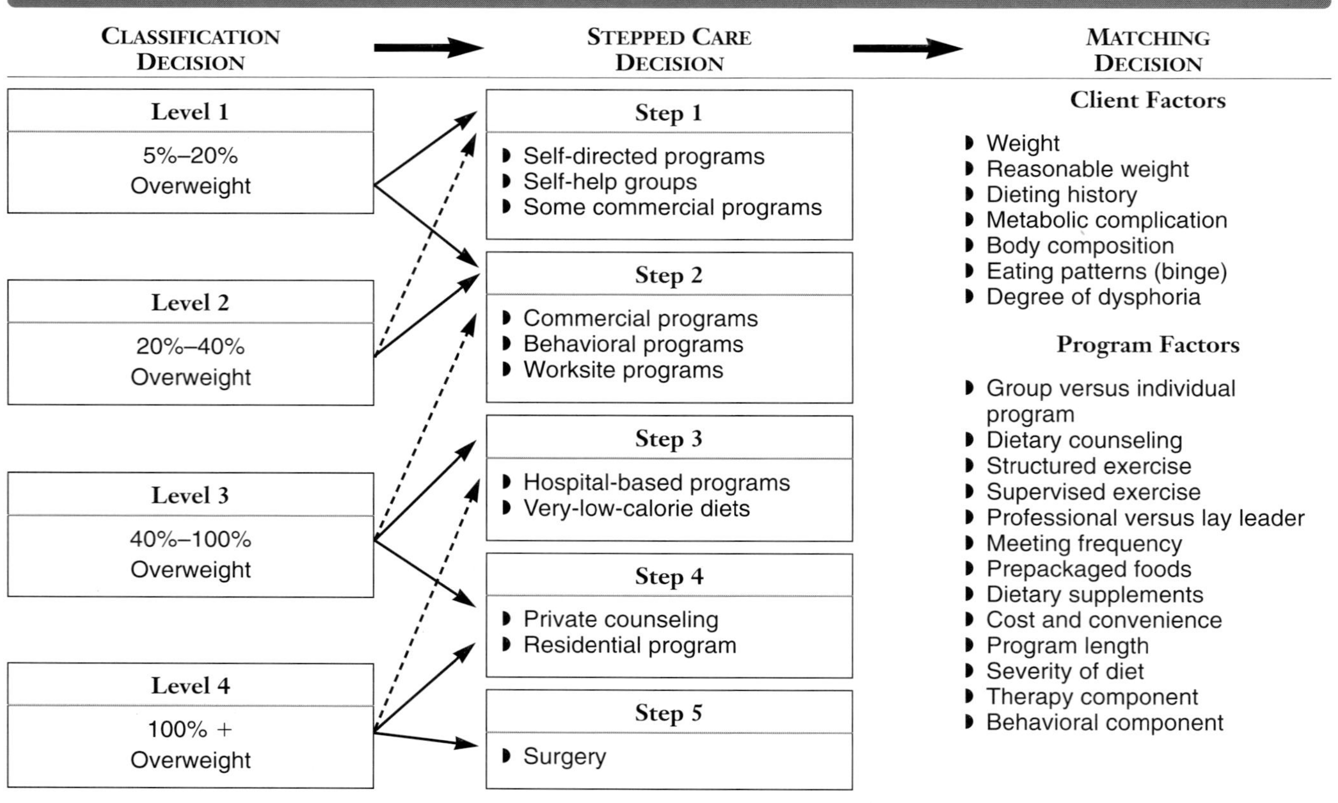

Adapted from Brownell, K. D., and Wadden, D. A. (1991). The heterogeneity of obesity: Fitting treatments to individuals. *Behavior Therapy*, 22. 163–177. © 1991 by Association for Advancement of Behavior Therapy. Reprinted by permission of the publisher.

CASE STUDY: A YOUNG WOMAN WITH AN EATING DISORDER NOT OTHERWISE SPECIFIED

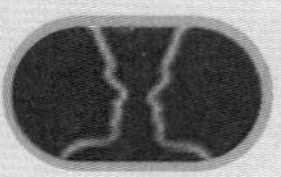

Phyllis is a 25-year-old schoolteacher who gives a history of overeating since the age of 10 years. She seeks treatment at a community mental health center because she has recently felt more depressed.

ASSESSMENT

Phyllis gives a history of being overweight since the age of 6 years. At the age of 10, she began to overeat in a more serious fashion. She reports that her overeating was related to her dysphoric mood, which is frequently associated with a perceived rejection. While attending a prestigious university, she began to binge eat several times a week but did not attempt to compensate by exercising or purging. Phyllis became very depressed in her third year of college and made a suicide attempt with 20 extra-strength acetaminophen tablets. She subsequently went into treatment with a psychiatrist, who diagnosed depression and prescribed fluoxetine, 60 mg daily. She subsequently stopped treatment because she continued to binge eat compulsively, although her mood was less dysphoric while she was taking fluoxetine.

Phyllis's weight is 200 pounds at a height of 61 inches (5′1″), placing her at 180% of ideal body weight. Her physical examination is otherwise unremarkable.

One of the reasons Phyllis gives for the increase in her depressive symptoms is her upcoming position as a first-grade teacher at an exclusive private school, a school she attended as a child. She speaks of the promise she once displayed as a child and

CASE STUDY: A YOUNG WOMAN WITH AN EATING DISORDER NOT OTHERWISE SPECIFIED (Continued)

of the low opinion she currently has of herself and her accomplishments. She expresses having a lot of conflict about teaching what she calls "rich brats." She further states that the youngsters represent a promise for the future of which she is envious. "I once displayed that promise and look at me now."

Phyllis describes her appetite as voracious: "I'll eat anything in sight." She describes her eating pattern as constant if food is available. She states that she feels herself to be out of control in the presence of food. She reports eating a variety of foods, including nutritious ones, but in excess. Her attempts to restrict her intake have always been unsuccessful. She reports that Weight Watchers, Overeaters Anonymous, and dieting on her own have never had even minimal success. She denies using laxatives, diuretics, or self-induced vomiting. Phyllis feels guilty about being overweight and describes the envy and hostility she feels toward women who are slender. She is dressed neatly in loose, baggy clothing. Her affect is agitated with a depressed mood. She maintains good eye contact during the interview. She denies having an active suicidal plan but does admit to wishing that she would not wake up in the morning.

Phyllis gives a history of depression with a serious suicide attempt. Treatment with fluoxetine improves her mood only slightly. She denies having a history of substance abuse. She reports no physical or sexual abuse. She states that her father has a drinking problem.

Phyllis is an only child of highly successful parents. She describes parents who are achievement oriented and who have high expectations for Phyllis. "My parents seem confident that I can do anything, but I'm not so sure. I feel I never measure up." She is currently living with her parents, a temporary arrangement until she begins teaching in 2 months. She has few close friends and tends to isolate herself. She states that she is interested in music, art, and reading but frequently is inactive and uninvolved.

NURSING DIAGNOSIS

Altered nutrition: more than body requirements and **low self-esteem.** Nursing Care Plan 26–3 provides outcome criteria, interventions, and evaluation for Phyllis's care. The length of long-term follow-up, along with the effectiveness of the interventions for Phyllis, must be measured against the outcome criteria for normalizing eating patterns, acceptable weight loss, and mood stabilization.

NURSING CARE PLAN 26–3 A CLIENT WHO IS OBESE

NURSING DIAGNOSIS

Altered Nutrition: **more than body requirement**—180% of ideal body weight related to overeating, including episodes of bingeing

Supporting Data

- 200 lb (180% of ideal body weight)
- Uncontrollable eating pattern.
- "I'll eat anything in sight."

Outcome Criteria: Client will normalize eating pattern and achieve a specific target date according to a predetermined plan.

Continued on following page

NURSING CARE PLAN 26–3 A CLIENT WHO IS OBESE *(Continued)*

SHORT-TERM GOAL	INTERVENTION	RATIONALE	EVALUATION
1. Client will learn coping strategies that result in adhering to a structured meal schedule.	1a. The clinical nurse specialist can use many techniques of cognitive behavioral therapy in addressing the issues of overweight and disordered eating. The client should begin a journal.	1a. Cognitive-behavioral techniques can be useful in addressing automatic behaviors. Recording what and where one eats begins to identify patterns that can be modified.	WEEK 1: Client selects a meal plan with structured times and places; begins journal and maintains it consistently. Client begins to relate feelings around eating.
	1b. Teach the client to structure and plan ahead for times and places where she will have her meals and snacks for the day.	1b. Organization and structure can allow for a different choice.	WEEK 2: Client is able to adhere to structured meal schedule approximately 25%. Client expresses the struggle and feelings of tension around implementing structured meal schedule—some modifications are made to allow the client to be more successful.
	1c. Teach the client not to abstain from eating for longer periods of time than planned in order to avoid rebound binge eating.	1c, d. Extended periods of abstinence, restrictive dietary intake, or very-low-calorie diet can result in rebound overeating.	Client shares contents of journal, which she consistently maintains.
	1d. Review the nutritional content of dietary intake to ensure a balanced diet.		Client reports weight is unchanged; client was unable to change pattern of exercise.
	1e. Review the journal with the client to identify areas for improvement in adhering to the treatment plan.	1e. The journal is an important tool in modifying eating behaviors.	WEEK 3: Client is adhering to schedule 50% of the time.
	1f. Explore with the client the thoughts and feelings she is experiencing about this new regimen.	1f, g. The nurse must be empathetic and supportive of the client's experience, which is one of struggle accompanied by feelings of tension. The nurse should explore the thoughts and beliefs accompanying the eating behavior.	Client shares journal entries and relates thoughts and feelings around eating. Client reports 1/2-lb weight loss. Client is beginning to walk for a half an hour as part of her daily routine.
	1g. Identify thoughts and beliefs and underlying assumptions that reinforce disordered eating patterns.		

NURSING CARE PLAN 26–3 A CLIENT WHO IS OBESE *(Continued)*

SHORT-TERM GOAL	INTERVENTION	RATIONALE	EVALUATION
	1h. Establish a once-a-week schedule of weighing.	1h. There may be minimal or no weight reduction, leading to discouragement.	WEEK 4: Client continues to adhere to structured schedule approximately 75% of the time. Client walks regularly, experiencing a better sense of well-being. Client thinks she is up to the challenge of continuing the plan to normalize her eating pattern and increase her energy expenditure. Client's weight is 196 lb (−4 lb); she acknowledges that progress has and will continue to be slow.

NURSING DIAGNOSIS

Low self-esteem: related to feelings of inadequacy, loss of control over eating

Supporting Data

- Feelings of envy and hostility secondary to being obese.
- Depressed mood with passive suicidal ideation.
- "I feel I never measure up."
- Inability to control her disordered eating behavior.

Outcome Criteria: Client will report improved feelings of self-worth and confidence.

SHORT-TERM GOAL	INTERVENTION	RATIONALE	EVALUATION
1. Client will demonstrate a number of coping techniques to cope with negative feelings.	1a. The clinical nurse specialist can provide a combination of supportive psychotherapeutic and cognitive-behavioral techniques to assist the client to work through her depressed feelings and develop a more positive self-image. 1b. Teach the client to maintain a journal of activities and feelings. 1c. Review the journal with the client to identify triggers for negative feelings and negative reactions, i.e., disordered eating.	1a. Cognitive-behavioral strategies can supply the client with tools and techniques to begin to modify her behavior, along with a supportive, psychotherapeutic relationship in which the client can express her feelings. 1b, c. The use of a journal is crucial in tracking the disordered eating behavior and in placing it in an emotional context.	WEEK 1: Client is maintaining a journal, identifying negative triggers to dysphoric responses. WEEK 2: Client demonstrates reframing techniques. Client demonstrates knowledge of relaxation techniques. Client continues to share contents of journal.

Continued on following page

NURSING CARE PLAN 26–3 A CLIENT WHO IS OBESE *(Continued)*

SHORT-TERM GOAL	INTERVENTION	RATIONALE	EVALUATION
	1d. Teach the client reframing techniques to allow for a more constructive response to identified triggers.	1d. Reframing can allow the client to perceive differently and to construct a different behavioral response.	WEEK 3: Client agrees to antidepressant. Client reports using reframing and relaxation techniques to cope with negative triggers and feelings.
	1e. Explore the possibilities for anticipating triggers and plan for more constructive responses.	1e. The journal can be a most useful tool in tracking stimuli that elicit dysphoric reactions and in allowing for more constructive choices.	WEEK 4: Client continues to meet short-term goals.
	1f. Teach the client relaxation techniques to cope with anxiety.	1f. Relaxation techniques allow the client to focus more constructively.	WEEK 8: Client reports slight improvement in mood. Client feels more confident in her abilities.
	1g. Assess the client's mental status for improvement or worsening of depressive symptoms.	1g. Assessment of mental status is ongoing. The client is at risk for suicidal and self-destructive behaviors.	
	1h. Consider pharmacological intervention, such as fluoxetine, in conjunction with cognitive-behavioral psychotherapy.	1h. The combination of an antidepressant with psychotherapy is often more effective than either alone. Fluoxetine or another selective serotonin reuptake inhibitor (SSRI) would be the antidepressant of choice, particularly with an overweight client.	

SUMMARY

Many theoretical models help explain, at least in part, the origins of eating disorders. For example, neurobiological theories identify an association between eating disorders and depression and neuroendocrine abnormalities. Psychological theories explore issues of control in anorexia and affective instability and poor impulse control in bulimia. Sociocultural models look at both our present societal ideal of being thin and the feminine ideal in general. Interestingly, males with eating disorders share many of the characteristics of women with eating disorders. Biopsychosocial theories explore genetic vulnerabilities that may predispose people toward eating disorders.

Anorexia nervosa can be a life-threatening eating disorder in young women and, less frequently, in men. Findings include severe underweight; low blood pressure, pulse, and temperature; and dehydration. Critical symptoms may include low serum potassium level and dysrhythmias. Altered nutrition: less than body requirements is a primary nursing diagnosis, and decreased cardiac output, risk for injury, body image disturbance, and powerlessness are other important considerations. Having the client achieve 85% to 90% of ideal body weight and normalizing eating patterns are among some of the main targeted outcome criteria. Initially, anorexia may be treated in an *inpatient treatment setting*, where milieu therapy, psychotherapy (cognitive), self-care skills, and psychobiological interventions can be implemented.

Because of short hospital stays, *acute care: outpatient treatment* is needed, where psychotherapy and psychopharmacology continue. Long-term treatment aims to help clients maintain healthy weight and includes treatment modalities such as individual therapy, family therapy, group therapy, and psychopharmacology.

Bulimia nervosa clients are often at or slightly below ideal body weight. On assessment, the client may have clear physical and emotional problems. For example, the client may have enlargement of the parotid glands and dental erosion and caries if she has induced vomiting. Often, the family life and personal life styles of these clients are unstable. Nursing diagnoses can include decreased cardiac output, potential for injury (electrolyte imbalance), body image disturbance, and powerlessness. Among the outcome criteria for these clients is helping the client refrain from binge eating and purging and remain safe. Acute care may be necessary when life-threatening complications are present, such as gastric rupture (rare), electrolyte imbalance, and cardiac dysrhythmias. Within the highly structured milieu of the inpatient eating disorder unit, the goal of interventions is to interrupt the binge/purge cycle. Psychotherapy as well as self-care skill training are included. *Long-term treatment* focuses on therapy aimed at intervening with any coexisting depression, substance abuse, and or personality disorders that are causing the client distress and interfering with the client's quality of life. Self-worth and interpersonal functioning eventually become issues that are useful for the client to target.

Eating disorders NOS include a variety of patterns, and in this chapter, obesity due to binge eating disorder was examined. Approximately 25% of Americans are overweight, despite the emphasis in the media on leading healthier lives. It is also true that binge eaters report a history of major depression significantly more often than non–binge eaters. An effective program for obese binge eaters must integrate modification of the disordered eating and the depressive symptoms with the ultimate goal of a more appropriate weight for the individual.

REFERENCES

American Psychiatric Association (1980). *Diagnostic and statistical manual of mental disorders* (3rd ed.). Washington, DC: American Psychiatric Association.

American Psychiatric Association (1987). *Diagnostic and statistical manual of mental disorders* (3rd ed., revised). Washington, DC: American Psychiatric Association.

American Psychiatric Association (1994). *Diagnostic and statistical manual of mental disorders* (4th ed.). Washington, DC: American Psychiatric Association.

Beck, A., Rush, A., Shaw, B., and Emery, G. (1979). *Cognitive therapy of depression.* New York: Guilford Press.

Bemporad, J. (1996). Self-starvation through the ages: Reflections on the pre-history of anorexia nervosa. *International Journal of Eating Disorders,* 19(3):217–237.

Brownell, K. D., and Wadden, T. A. (1991). The heterogeneity of obesity: Fitting treatments to individuals. *Behavior Therapy,* 22(2):153–177.

Bruch, H. (1973). *Eating disorders: Obesity, anorexia, and the person within.* New York: Basic Books.

Bruch, H. (1985). Four decades of eating disorders. In D. M. Garner and P. E. Garfinkel (Eds.), *Handbook of psychotherapy for anorexia nervosa and bulimia* (pp. 7–18). New York: Guilford Press.

Crisp, A. H. (1980). *Anorexia nervosa: Let Me Be.* New York: Academic Press.

Devlin, M. J., and Walsh, B. T. (1989). Eating disorders and depression. *Psychiatric Annals,* 19(9):473–476.

Devlin, M. J., et al. (1990). Metabolic abnormalities in bulimia nervosa. *Archives of General Psychiatry,* 47(2):144–148.

Drug facts and comparisons (pp. 239c–240a). (1996). St. Louis: Facts and Comparisons.

Fairburn, C. G., and Cooper, P. J. (1989). Eating disorders. In K. Hawton, P. M. Salkovskis, J. Kirk, and D. M. Clark (Eds.), *Cognitive behaviour therapy for psychiatric problems* (pp. 277–314). New York: Oxford University Press.

Garner, D., and Bemis, K. (1982). A cognitive-behavioral approach to anorexia nervosa. *Cognitive Therapy and Research,* 6:123–150.

Holland, A. J., et al. (1984). Anorexia nervosa: A study of 34 twin pairs and one set of triplets. *British Journal of Psychiatry,* 145:414–418.

Hsu, L. K. G. (1990). *Eating disorders.* New York: Guilford Press.

Ibrahim, K., and Rosedale, M. (1994). Perspectives in multiple family group therapy with eating disordered patient. Paper presented at the meeting of the Society for Education and Research in Psychiatric Nursing, Rockville, MD, November 1994.

Irwin, E. G. (1993a). A focused overview of anorexia nervosa and bulimia: I. Etiological issues. *Archives of Psychiatric Nursing,* 7(6):342–346.

Kandel, D. B., and Davies, M. (1982). Epidemiology of depressive mood in adolescents. *Archives of General Psychiatry,* 39:1205–1212.

Kendler, K., et al. (1991). The genetic epidemiology of bulimia nervosa. *American Journal of Psychiatry,* 148(12):1627–1637.

Lerner, R. M., et al. (1980). Self-concept, self-esteem, and body attitudes among Japanese male and female adolescents. *Child Development,* 51:847–855.

Marcus, M. D. (1995). Binge eating and obesity. In K. D. Brownell and C. G. Fairburn (Eds.), *Eating disorders and obesity: A comprehensive handbook* (pp. 441–444). New York: Guilford Press.

Marcus, M. D., Smith, D., Santelli, R., and Kaye, W. (1992). Characterization of eating disordered behavior in obese binge eaters. *International Journal of Eating Disorders,* 12(3):249–255.

Marcus, M. D., et al. (1990). Psychiatric disorders among obese binge eaters. *International Journal of Eating Disorders,* 9(1):69–77.

Mehler, P. S. (1996). Eating disorders: 1. Anorexia nervosa. *Hospital Practice (Office Edition),* 31(1):109–113, 117.

Metropolitan Life Insurance Company (1983). 1983 Height and weight tables. *Statistical Bulletin,* 64(1):3–9.

Minuchin, S. (1974). *Families and family therapy.* Cambridge, MA: Harvard University Press.

Olivardia, R., Pope, G., Mangweth, B., and Hudson, J. (1995). Eating disorders in college men. *American Journal of Psychiatry,* 152(9):1279–1285.

Pike, K. (1991). Mothers, daughters, and disordered eating. *Journal of Abnormal Psychology,* 1200(2):198–204.

Pope, H. G., and Hudson, J. I. (1992). Is childhood sexual abuse a risk factor for bulimia nervosa? *American Journal of Psychiatry,* 149(4):455–463.

Rosedale, M. (1996). *Eating disorders critical pathway.* New York: US Home Care.

Russell, G. (1979). Bulimia nervosa: An ominous variant of anorexia nervosa. *Psychological Medicine,* 9:429–448.

Russell, G. (1985). The changing nature of anorexia nervosa. *Journal of Psychiatric Research,* 19:101–109.

Stunkard, A. (1993). A history of binge eating. In C. G. Fairburn and G. T. Wilson (Eds.), *Binge eating: Nature, assessment, and treatment* (pp. 15–34). New York: Guilford Press.

Thiel, A., et al. (1995). Obsessive-compulsive disorder among patients with anorexia nervosa and bulimia nervosa. *American Journal of Psychiatry,* 152(1):72–75.

Walsh, B. T., and Devlin, M. (1995). Eating disorders. *Child and Adolescent Psychiatric Clinics of North America,* 4(2):343–357.

Welch, S. L., and Fairburn, C. G. (1994). Sexual abuse and bulimia nervosa: Three integrated case control comparisons. *American Journal of Psychiatry,* 151(3):402–407.

Williamson, D. F. (1993). Descriptive epidemiology of body weight and weight change in U.S. adults. *Annals of Internal Medicine,* 19(7):646–649.

Wooley, S. C. (1995). Feminist influences on the treatment of eating disorders. In K. D. Brownell and C. G. Fairburn (Eds.), *Eating disorders and obesity: A comprehensive handbook* (pp. 294– 298). New York: Guilford Press.

World Health Organization (1992). *ICD-10 Classification of mental and behavioral disorders: Clinical descriptions and diagnostic guidelines* (pp. 176–181). Geneva: World Health Organization.

FURTHER READING

Bruch, H. (1978). *The golden cage.* New York: Vintage.

Fairburn, C. G., and Wilson, G. T. (Eds.) (1993). *Binge eating: Nature, assessment, and treatment.* New York: Guilford Press.

Fontaine, K. L. (1991). The conspiracy of culture: Women's issues in body size. *Nursing Clinics of North America,* 26(3):669–676.

Gordon, R. A. (1990). *Anorexia and bulimia: Anatomy of a social epidemic.* Cambridge, MA: Basil Blackwell.

Heatherton, T., Nichols, P., Mahamedi, F., and Keel, P. (1995). Body weight, dieting, and eating disorder symptoms among college students, 1982–1992. *American Journal of Psychiatry,* 152(11):1623–1629.

Irwin, E. G. (1993b). A focused overview of anorexia nervosa and bulimia: II. Challenges to the practice of psychiatric nursing. *Archives of Psychiatric Nursing*, 7(6):347–352.

Love, C. C., and Seaton, H. (1991). Eating disorders: Highlights of nursing assessment and therapeutics. *Nursing Clinics of North America*, 26(3):677–692.

McGowan, A., and Whitbread, J. (1996). Out of control: The most effective way to help the binge-eating patient. *Journal of Psychosocial Nursing*, 34(1):30–37.

Selvini-Palazzoli, M. (1985). Anorexia nervosa: A syndrome of the affluent society. *Transcultural Psychiatric Research Review*, 22:199–205.

Smith, D. E., Marcus, M. D., and Kaye, W. (1992). Cognitive-behavioral treatment of obese binge eaters. *International Journal of Eating Disorders*, 12(3):257–262.

Stein, K. (1996). The self-schema model: A theoretical approach to the self-concept in eating disorders. *Archives of General Psychiatric Nursing*, 10(2):96–109.

SELF-STUDY AND CRITICAL THINKING

Multiple choice

1. Which statement best describes the personality traits of clients with anorexia nervosa and bulimia nervosa?

   A. Food-restricting anorectic clients and nonpurging bulimic clients are most alike.
   B. Purging anorectic clients and normal-weight, purging bulimic clients are most alike.
   C. Binge eating/purging anorectic clients and slightly overweight, nonpurging bulimic clients are most alike.
   D. None of the above.

2. A client with anorexia nervosa may have edema of the lower extremities during the weight-restoration phase because

   A. This is an expected occurrence during refeeding.
   B. This is evidence of compromised kidney function.
   C. This is evidence of poor cardiac function.
   D. All of the above.

3. Which of the following clients with eating disorders would be at risk for a low potassium level?

   A. A restricting anorectic
   B. A purging anorectic
   C. A binge eating, nonpurging bulimic
   D. All of the above

4. Which of the following statements is the most accurate?

   A. Self-induced vomiting is an effective (although pathological) method of weight reduction.
   B. Excessive exercise puts one at risk to binge eat.
   C. Severely restricting one's food intake for many hours is a setup for a client with an eating disorder to binge eat.
   D. All of the above.

5. Which of the following statements is descriptive of cognitive-behavioral therapeutic technique?

   A. Problem-solving techniques are a form of cognitive-behavioral therapy.
   B. Relaxation training is a form of cognitive-behavioral therapy.
   C. Assertiveness training is a form of cognitive-behavioral therapy.
   D. All of the above.

6. Antidepressants may be useful in the treatment of clients with eating disorders in which clinical situation?

   A. To treat comorbid depressive symptoms
   B. To effect a more rapid weight gain in anorexia nervosa
   C. To reduce the incidence of binge eating and purging
   D. All of the above

Critical thinking

7. What is the interrelationship of eating disorders and mood disorders?
8. Are anorexia nervosa and bulimia nervosa a variant of one eating disorder? Explain why or why not.
9. Is "normal" dieting on a behavioral continuum with eating disorders?
10. What are at least three acute concerns for a client who is (a) extremely anorectic, (b) severely bulimic, (c) binge-purging obese? Discuss appropriate interventions for each of the above acute concerns.

UNIT SEVEN

Mental Health Issues: Special Populations

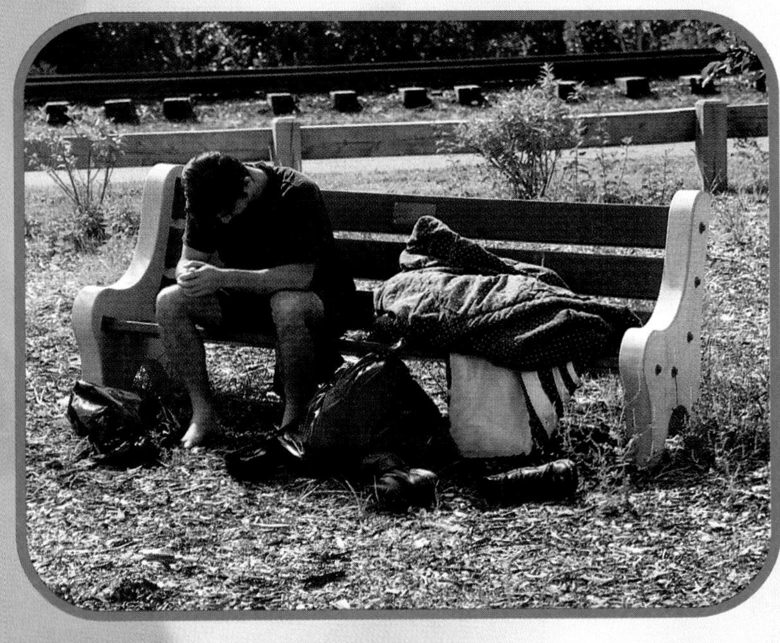

Let us not look back in anger, nor forward in fear, but around us in awareness.

JAMES THURBER

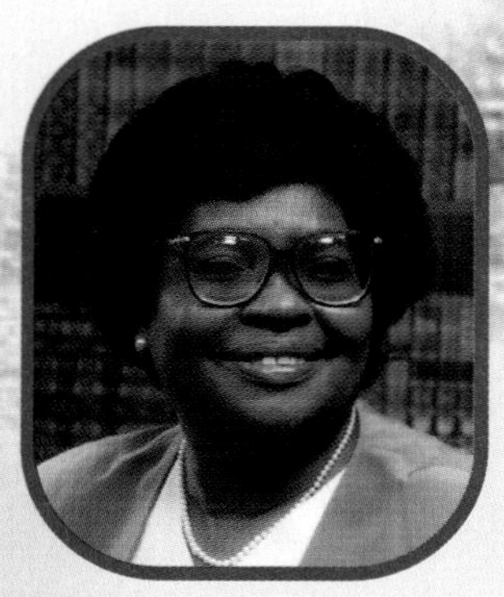

A Nurse Speaks

Rosie Gooden Taylor

I teach a psychiatric nursing practicum to two groups of baccalaureate students in a clinical setting, which demonstrates an excellent model of collaboration of disciplines in providing continuity of care in the mental health setting. Students are invited and encouraged to actively participate in all aspects of care during their 7-week rotation in the center, known as Mental Health Connections. The range of client care offered encompasses admission through individual follow-up in community settings.

Program facilities are operated under the joint auspices of Dallas County Mental Health and Mental Retardation Centers (DCMHMRC) and University of Texas Southwestern Medical School (UTSWMS) to serve Dallas County residents who utilize the public sector to meet their mental health service needs. Program areas include (1) acute inpatient care, (2) day treatment center, (3) transitional residential program, (4) extend team, and (5) supported housing. Assumptions inherent in the philosophy of care contribute to the success and positive outcomes of the program. These assumptions include respect for the rights, dignity, and autonomy of the client; focus on relief of symptoms; development of the skills and independence of the client; family involvement; recognition of cultural differences; and the need for personalized case management services that connect the client with needed human services (Feiner 1995).

In the inpatient setting, clients are admitted or readmitted to a specifically designated multidisciplinary team composed of an attending psychiatrist, several RNs, a psychologist, a social worker (case worker), a chemical dependency counselor, an activity therapist, and several therapy technicians. These team members remain consistent for the client during his or her stay and for any subsequent admissions that may be necessary. The service makes every effort to readmit relapsing patients who have previously been treated in the program. Care is provided and outcomes are evaluated through interdisciplinary treatment planning and implementation. The program emphasizes the inclusion of client support systems (family members, social networks, and community resources) in providing and evaluating care and outcomes.

Because a significant percentage of the population (75%) experiences chemical dependence in addition to major mental illness, relapse prevention concepts are applied as a major component of the program both for mental illness and for chemical dependency (Feiner 1995). These concepts are incorporated through classes, therapy groups, individual counseling, and outside Alcoholics Anonymous (AA) and Narcotics Anonymous (NA) groups, when appropriate. Teaching, rather than process group, is the center of the clinical program, and staff nurses are the core teachers and trainers. Clients are taught about their illnesses, medications, relapse signs, and social skills. Psychosocial rehabilitation, another aspect of the treatment program, is incorporated to facilitate the client's maximal potential for reintegrating into a functional and healthful life style within personal limitations. During the discharge planning process, staff, including psychiatrists, psychiatric residents, RNs, nursing students, and other members of the team, make home visits in order to understand the client's environment and its impact upon teaching and referral needs.

The day treatment center is an outpatient rehabilitation program that operates 5 days a week for 5 or 6 hours a day. Clients are referred from the inpatient program and other agencies within the DCMHMRC system for the purpose of gaining focused skills and guidance in specific functional areas. The program also seeks to provide services to assist the client toward normalized community living. Psychosocial skills, life skills, and intensive casework are provided. These skills are taught in the program through classes, in the client's home environment, on the job, or in the social environment, as indicated by the client's needs. Family involvement is facilitated in all phases of treatment through individual education and/or counseling sessions. Structured programs include a quarterly all-day family education workshop and weekly family education groups that discuss family coping skills and community resources.

The transitional residence (TR) program operates on a 24-hour basis and consists of four apartment clusters within a general apartment complex. These residential services are designated as short-term and are available to the client for approximately 6 months, as the client develops skills to facilitate increased independence. Additional space is maintained within the TR for transient situational crises that may be experienced by clients and to offer respite for families. The clients receive mobility training and learn to travel approximately 6 miles, by public transportation if necessary, to participate in the day treatment program. Social work staff and psychosocial technicians function as case coordinators and work directly with clients during their transitional residence experience. Specific functions include assistance with meeting vocational, housing, educational, or psychosocial rehabilitation needs. Residents may be in training programs, attending school, or working in paid or volunteer positions.

Extend team is an outreach team coordinated by an RN and includes the inpatient attending psychiatrist, a chemical dependency counselor, case manager, an additional RN, and two life skills trainers. This team may be considered a hospital-based assertive community treatment team, whose key objective is early interruption of relapse. Clients visited by the extend team are typically those who are living in independent settings but require monitoring for stability, maintenance of independent functioning, or adherence to medication or follow-up schedules.

The following case of Ms. Lindy demonstrates how the team functions:

Ms. Lindy is a 40-year-old woman who was diagnosed with schizoaffective disorder at age 20. During the past 15 years she has become estranged from her family and has had multiple hospitalizations at both private and state facilities for acute exacerbation of psychotic symptoms. Most of the hospitalizations have been initiated through involuntary commitment by the mental illness court system and ranged from 7 to 30 days. Periods of stable functioning have been brief and sporadic because minimal self-care skills and environmental stressors added increased risk factors. Ms. Lindy was admitted for inpatient care at a mental health clinic following her most recent commitment. Treatment lasted for 45 days and included pharmacotherapy, milieu therapy, and supportive psychotherapy. Skills in activities of daily living (ADLs) were taught, reinforced, and monitored to increase Ms. Lindy's level of independence and to determine the level of support that would be required after discharge. She attended weekly medication management groups and received individual instruction on medications she would require after discharge. Her understanding and knowledge were monitored and evaluated through regular assessment at each medication administration. Before discharge, Ms. Lindy was provided with a weekly medication organizer and was supervised in the preparation of prescribed medications. Feedback was provided on accuracy as well as the degree of supervision the client would require during the next phase of treatment. Ms. Lindy was discharged from inpatient treatment to the day treatment and TR programs. While participating in day treatment and TR programs, Ms. Lindy received daily supervision by a TR staff member in self-administration of her medications until staff were assured of her competence, safety, and adherence. Continuity of teaching was assumed by the RN in day treatment, who regularly monitored adherence, evaluated understanding of medication issues, and assessed for effects of medications. Classes at day treatment included, among others, information to help Ms. Lindy identify situations that increased her risk for relapse of illness, cues that might signal relapse, and classes to increase and reinforce skills in ADLs and social and recreational skills. Field trips were incorporated to apply the information learned. Ms. Lindy worked closely with a case manager who involved her in vocational testing to determine her interests and skills, and she is currently training for transitional employment. With support, she continues to increase independent living skills. The guidance and supervision of a skills trainer at the TR program have enabled Ms. Lindy to assume responsibility for planning and preparing her own meals, and she is gaining independence in traveling within the city by public transportation in order to accomplish necessary tasks. With continued progress, it is anticipated that Ms. Lindy will "graduate" from day treatment and TR program to supported or independent housing and will be monitored on a regular basis by the extend team.

REFERENCE

Feiner, J. S. (1995). A comprehensive approach to the care of persons with major mental illness and psychiatric disability. *Community Psychiatrist*, 9:1.

27

The Severely and Persistently Mentally Ill

ANN COWLEY HERZOG
PEGGY H. MILLER

OUTLINE

KEY TERMS AND CONCEPTS

The key term and concept listed here also appears in bold where it is defined or discussed in this chapter.

severely and persistently mentally ill

OBJECTIVES

After studying this chapter, the reader will be able to

1. Explain what is meant by the term *severe and persistent mental illness.*
2. Discuss effective nursing strategies for clients with severe and persistent mental illness with regard to the following: (a) medication, (b) psychosocial rehabilitation, and (c) psychotherapy.
3. Describe the reciprocal relationship between the family and the mentally ill member.
4. Identify specific issues regarding physical illness in the population of the severely and persistently mentally ill.
5. Distinguish between the roles of the psychiatric advanced practice nurse and the basic level nurse when caring for the severely and persistently mentally ill.
6. Explain the role of the case manager in the care of severely and persistently mentally ill people.
7. Identify and describe the unique problems of four subcategories of the homeless population.
8. Develop a plan of care for a severely and persistently mentally ill person.

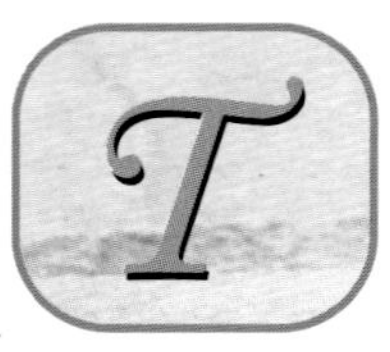

The term *chronic mental illness* refers to a phenomenon whereby mental illness extends in time beyond the acute stage into a long-term stage that is marked by persistent impairment of functioning. Almost all mental illnesses are chronic, with remissions and exacerbations of varying lengths. This decrease in functioning pervades the person's abilities to perform in all, or nearly all, aspects of daily living. Skill deficits range from an inability to prepare meals to an inability to cope with everyday stressors. Currently, the preferred term for those who have chronic mental illness is the **severely and persistently mentally ill.** The older term, *chronic mental illness*, has a more negative connotation that connotes inevitable and progressive deterioration, which in fact is not always the case. Grob (1994) states that the seriously mentally ill include individuals with quite different disorders, prognoses, and needs, whose outcomes vary considerably over time. Often the severity and course of the illness are influenced by poverty, racism, and substance abuse.

The severely and persistently mentally ill population is at risk for multiple physical, emotional, and social problems. Indeed, the person with a mental illness often has impairments in well-being and functioning that exceed those in people with chronic physical problems (Hays et al. 1995).

DEMOGRAPHICS

Precise calculation of the extent of severe and persistent mental illness in the United States is difficult. Before de-institutionalization, the mentally disabled population was easier to quantify. People with severe mental illness were hospitalized, sometimes for the remainder of their lives. With the move to community-based mental health centers, and after changes within the population itself, there is no way to tabulate this group accurately. However, it is estimated that two thirds of those with major mental illness have persistent physical and emotional problems (Worley et al. 1990).

Chronicity can occur in persons of any gender, age, culture, or geographic location. However, this population includes two subgroups with unique characteristics: (1) those old enough to have experienced institutionalization (before approximately 1975) and (2) those young enough to have been hospitalized only during acute exacerbations of their disorders.

Older Populations

Before the move in 1975 to de-institutionalize the severely and persistently mentally ill, psychiatric hospitals were the long-term residences for many people. Medical paternalism was a pervasive philosophical stance at that time. The health care approach to the severely mentally ill person was that of making all their decisions. The daily institutional routine left little room for a person to exercise what social and problem-solving skills remained. Much of a person's behavior became a combination of the disease process and the decreased sense of self that resulted from the lack of autonomy.

Marian was a resident at a facility for the severely and persistently impaired during her adolescence and young adulthood. On discharge, she moved to a community home, where she spent long periods sitting in front of the living room window. Marian did not ask to go out into the garden she watched for so many hours. Indeed, she rarely asked for anything, including snacks or recreational activities. The caregivers worked with Marian for several months to get her to recognize her needs of the moment and then to articulate or act on them. There was a major celebration the day that she walked into the kitchen and made a peanut butter sandwich of her own volition. Some of the dependency caused by the institutionalization was being positively altered.

Younger Populations

People young enough never to have been institutionalized may not have the problems of passivity and lack of autonomy that long-term hospitalization causes. However, lack of experience with formal treatment may contribute to the person's not truly believing that there is a problem. Denial, often coupled with the use of recreational drugs that further impair already faulty judgment and impulse control, put severely ill young adults at particular risk for many additional problems, including brushes with the law and frequent loss of employment after short periods.

In addition, an increasingly large proportion of the general population is coming of age in families affected by mental health issues such as depression, violence, addictions, and chronic mental illness. As these children develop, their world view may be distorted. Frequently, social interaction and coping skills are compromised. In the presence of major stressors, many youths who are vulnerable may develop their own problems with mental illness. This sets the stage for their own persistent long-term mental illness.

▶ Joshua, 26 years old, has had several short hospitalizations for treatment of schizophrenia. Between admissions, he lives in unstable short-term settings, varying from rooming houses to his car. He no longer lives with his mother or siblings; his mother has been imprisoned for drug dealing and his siblings are in foster homes. He has been jailed several times for misdemeanors such as shoplifting and creating a public nuisance (e.g., loud arguments in stores). He has difficulty finding and keeping jobs as a laborer.

DEVELOPING A SEVERE AND PERSISTENT MENTAL ILLNESS

Severe and persistent mental illness has much in common with persistent long-term physical illness. The original problem sets in motion an erosion of basic coping mechanisms and compensatory processes. As the disorder extends beyond the acute stage, more and more of the neighboring systems are involved. For example, with chronic congestive heart failure the lungs and kidneys begin to deteriorate. However, the disability of severe and persistent mental illness may go much further in destroying a person's quality of life. In the case of an illness such as schizophrenia, a person's thought processes, ability to maintain contact with others, and ability to stay employed frequently deteriorate. For example, a person may have difficulty thinking clearly about even ordinary things such as self-care and relations with others. This causes the person's interactions to be perceived as bizarre, unsatisfying, and anxiety provoking by both self and others. In turn, the person, friends, and even family members will hesitate to seek out interactions. Problematic communications escalate the tensions in relationships and erode the person's self-image. In the case of a business relationship between supervisor and employee, the person's ability to remain productive and employed is endangered. These stressors strain an already vulnerable person and can precipitate further deterioration in function.

Another similarity between physical illness and mental illness is the unpredictability of the disease course. Not knowing when the problem will exacerbate contributes additional stress. There is a major deficit in adequate coping mechanisms for stress in those with a severe and persistent mental disorder. The fear of relapse and avoidance of stress can cause a withdrawal from life that eventually heightens the person's social isolation and apathy, just as is the case with a physical dysfunction such as incontinence.

Exacerbations may decrease in frequency and intensity through careful attention to both the history of the disease itself and awareness of daily functioning. Assessment in these areas requires thorough and regular evaluation by an interdisciplinary psychiatric team (nurse, physician, social worker, occupational therapist). In this way, subtle impairments may be noted before the onslaught of more dramatic deterioration. As in the aphorism "A stitch in time saves nine," assessing an early symptom or sign and initiating treatment can decrease the severity of the exacerbation and the accompanying disruption of the person's life.

Rehabilitation is a critically important concept for people with severe and persistent mental illness. Through rehabilitation, disabilities and inabilities resulting from long-term mental illness can be attended to, in the hope that they may be lessened or eradicated. Just as in medical-surgical nursing, the best mental health rehabilitation begins on the first day of acute care and continues after discharge from the facility. This can take place in a variety of community centers and programs.

The Role and Care of the Family

The movement toward de-institutionalization resulted in families of the severely mentally ill becoming the "institution of choice" (Parker 1993). The intention to provide assistance to the client in the community fell woefully short of its goal, and the family became the primary source of support and care. Most families were given this responsibility without adequate knowledge or preparation to meet the multiple, complex demands of this role. Historically, the impact of mental illness on the family has been given little attention. At times, the family has even been blamed for actually causing the mental illness (Peternelj-Taylor and Hartley 1993). We are slowly beginning to understand the overwhelming impact a mentally ill member has on the family unit. Dealing with a family member who has a mental illness is a major crisis for the family that pervades all aspects of family life. It is important that professionals not only recognize the problems facing the family but also identify the strengths from which the family can plan support.

There seems to be no question that a burden does exist for the family caring for a severe mentally ill member at home. Family life can become disorganized, household routines are upset, and family members fear unexpected psychotic episodes (Loukissa 1995). Extreme degrees of stress are often experienced by families attempting to cope with a family member who is disorganized in thinking and unpredictable in behaviors. Economic and human burdens mount, along with increased responsibilities. Research on these stresses and the strain on family members did not begin until the 1960s, when the effect of specific client behaviors and the impact of short hospitalizations on the family were studied (Grad and Sainsbury 1993). Today, research is focused on caregiver characteristics such as kinship and gender. There is also greater awareness of the importance of exploring social support and educating the family about all aspects of their ill member's disease and care.

An examination of the issues of family burden makes clear the need to give adequate care and attention to caregivers. Often the family becomes the most accurate source of information for use in diagnosis and client management. Cooperative planning and respect for family members are essential in providing individualized client care as well as support for the caregivers. In this way, clients can develop coping skills to assist them throughout the lengthy and unpredictable course of the disease.

An important need of families caring for the severely and persistently mentally ill is education to help them understand the disease process. Families need to be prepared to meet the many concerns related to safety, communication, medication compliance, and symptom and behavior management. This should include written instruction and supportive follow-up by phone or home visits. Resources for respite and day care should also be made available when appropriate. "Providing families with knowledge and information has been associated with a decrease in fear, anxiety, and confusion—and helps them cope with the illness and all its ramifications" (Peternelj-Taylor and Hartley 1993). Refer to Chapter 22 for more information on psychoeducational groups and multiple family groups for families with a severely and persistently ill member.

The need to provide multiple types of support for families cannot be overstressed. Without ties to family, the confusion, alienation, poverty, and lack of coping and communication skills can lead to another person's joining the ranks of the homeless: girls and boys, men and women, the elderly, and even entire families.

INTERVENTION STRATEGIES

Many of the intervention strategies used to treat long-term mental illness are the same as those used for acute conditions. However, with severe and persistent mental illness, basic intervention strategies often require special considerations.

Psychobiological Interventions (Basic Level)

Antipsychotic drugs are a significant part of the treatment of many people with severe and persistent mental illnesses. Despite serious side effects, these drugs are very effective in reducing or removing delusions and hallucinations for most clients. However, the standard antipsychotic agents are not effective in treating many of the negative signs and symptoms (e.g., withdrawal and apathy) of some disorders (e.g., schizophrenia) (see Chapter 22). The use of antipsychotics is only one step in providing a basis for treatment. Other psychopharmacological drugs that are important in helping individuals maintain some stability, but which require careful monitoring, are the antidepressants and mood stabilizers.

Problems are inherent in the use of medications in a community setting, and they increase proportionally with the number of medications taken. Such problems include issues of compliance and the occurrence of side effects and adverse reactions. The cognitive impairment caused by long-term mental illness makes it difficult for the client to take the medication as prescribed. Side effects that make medication usage unpalatable to the client further decrease compliance. Adverse reactions may go unnoticed and become dangerous, or may even progress to cause permanent damage.

Adequate monitoring of efficacy by a community-based health care provider is difficult. Often a psychiatric social worker is the primary contact. Because the physical issues of pharmacotherapeutics are often subtle, they are frequently missed until they have mushroomed and caused dramatic problems. For example, constant smacking of the lips by an individual may be assessed by a nonmedical person as a manifestation of agitation and anxiety and not as an early sign of tardive dyskinesia (TD). Neuroleptic malignant syndrome, agranulocytosis, and liver dysfunction may also result from the use of medications. Without early detection and treatment, a person is at high risk for possible permanent impairment or even death. For this reason, it is imperative for the person with a severe and persistent mental illness to see a psychiatric nurse or physician regularly for monitoring of medications and possible side effects. This can take place in any community-based facility or even at home through a home health care agency.

Careful health teaching is imperative both for the person who takes medication and for family members. Health teaching can increase the probability of proper administration of the drugs and observance for therapeutic effects, and can create an early warning system for both side effects and noncompliance.

Health Teaching (Basic Level)

During rehabilitation, it is important to view the person as capable of positive change. With this approach, skills training and the building of self-esteem can begin. Teaching emphasizes the skills necessary for basic everyday life, such as interpersonal, problem-solving, communication, and vocational skills. When clients are able to master certain basic skills, get their needs met more effectively through communication, increase their social support system, and learn important job skills, a sense of hopefulness and empowerment often follows. These skills can aid many people with long-term mental problems to lead more satisfying and productive lives. Such skills can also help clients become more involved with the people and opportunities around them and can help prevent the downward shift to the least desirable of all sequelae, isolation and homelessness.

Families also need health teaching and to learn skills to help them cope with their own stresses, feelings, and need for information. To help families care for a severely and persistently mentally ill loved one, family members need guidance and counseling to gain access to resources and to learn and improve existing coping skills.

Case Management (Basic Level)

Whether as a broker of services or as a therapist, the case manager can provide entrance into the system of care. Severely and persistently mentally ill people often have many needs that span many different categories. One major problem is their frequent inability to "access or accept services that may help them to attain and maintain a maximum level of independence or a reasonable quality of life" (Melzer et al. 1991). Casually made multiple referrals can be beyond the coping capabilities of the chronically mentally ill. With one person coordinating services, help can be more efficient. In addition, the basic needs of the person (food, shelter, clothing) are more likely to be addressed (Lapierre and Padgett 1992).

However, case management needs to be more than simple coordination of services. The person needing the assistance must be identified, brought into the system, assessed for immediate needs, and given the opportunity to receive needed interventions. Interventions must then be reevaluated and monitored for their efficacy. Throughout this process, the effective case manager functions as a caring person with a "positive, empathetic understanding of the client" (Repper et al. 1994). Ideally, this helpfulness and connectedness by the case manager will provide a role model for the client in achieving interpersonal and problem-solving skills. This is important for a severely and persistently ill person with disaffiliation; furthermore, quality relationships between health care providers and clients also depend on trust and openness.

Families need the help of case managers. They need assistance to weather the storms of crisis and to become "partners in rehabilitation, which will frequently reduce relapse and recidivism" (Bernheim 1990).

RESOURCES

Although the trend in health care is based on the concept of a national network of strong, community-based health care centers that work to maintain a client's ability to function independently out of the hospital setting, the reality has yet to be realized. Today, both large state hospitals and small private institutions still house and care for the many severely mentally ill who are unable to live on their own, either temporarily or for an extended period. Most often, improvements seen in a client's behavior in the hospital setting do not last long after the client has been discharged into the community. One of the main reasons for this inability to maintain more effective behaviors is the failure to take prescribed medications, which leads to the "revolving door syndrome." Severely and long-term mentally ill persons need appropriate resources as well as medication to be able to function in the community. A well-coordinated, comprehensive, and cost-effective system of care that is individualized and available to all in need is the ideal situation. Chapter 9 discusses many community programs that provide services to the severely mentally ill.

The goal of these programs is to provide broad community mental health services that will prevent psychiatric hospitalization, maintain stability in a community setting, and achieve the highest possible level of functioning. Adult outpatient services provide evaluation for possible psychiatric hospitalization, both voluntary and involuntary; initiate mental health treatment when necessary; respond to crisis calls and walk-in requests for services; and coordinate psychiatric emergency responses with hospitals, police, and other community service providers. Day care services are designed to provide alternatives to 24-hour care and to supplement other modes of treatment and residential services. Case managers serve as coordinators to ensure the integration and cooperation of the various elements of the system and to act as advocates for the clients in the system.

A variety of services are focused on the mentally ill who are also diagnosed with alcohol-related problems. Regional outpatient clinics provide therapeutic and rehabilitative services for alcoholics and drug abusers and their families. Services include medical and psychosocial assessment, detoxification, crisis intervention, and monitored disulfiram (Antabuse) administration. Similar services are available for mentally ill persons who abuse drugs, including direct treatment, referral, community education, and crisis intervention. Some communities have a specialized methadone program for addicts who wish to completely detoxify from heroin or to receive a long-term maintenance dose of methadone. Some communities also provide a perinatal program for substance abusers who are either pregnant or have lost custody of their children as a result of their substance abuse.

Community mental health services are designed to provide outreach and case management for the persistently and seriously mentally disabled who are also homeless. Client participation in the program is voluntary. State and county moneys fund these programs, which operate through three components: outreach programs, short-term housing, and multiservice centers. Shelter beds and multiservices are contracted out to private service providers. Liaison is maintained with law enforcement and with governmental and nonprofit agencies that provide services to the homeless. Services are delivered in an individualized, self-enabling manner based on a philosophy that respects each individual's dignity, privacy, and right to refuse treatment. This service approach allows the client to achieve the highest level of independence and self-sufficiency possible.

Community outreach programs send professional and nonprofessional workers into streets, parks, temporary shelters, bus stations, beaches, and anywhere else the mentally ill may be found. A team approach is used to gain access to clients and to connect them with the various services available to meet their needs. A trusting relationship must be established and maintained between the outreach worker and the client before communication can develop. In this way, the client's needs may best be considered and met. Outreach services provide liaison with community services and case management to provide assistance in obtaining benefits (e.g., general relief, food stamps, Social Security), mental health services, medical treatment, and transportation. The role of the outreach worker is to be an advocate in all areas of client need, to foster client independence, and to terminate outreach services when appropriate.

Temporary shelters do not provide the ideal living situation but are usually a safe and supportive environment for individuals who have no other option. The mentally ill do need a place to live, even if it is temporary. A life can go either way in a public shelter. A person may become more chronically entrenched or may take steps toward improving quality of life. Often, the longer people stay in a shelter setting, the less likely are they to emerge from it.

Multiservice centers collaborate with the outreach unit in implementing individualized service plans for the persistently mentally ill. They supply hot meals, laundry and shower facilities, clothing, social activities, transportation to and from shelters, access to a telephone, and a mailing address for the individual.

For example, at the Weingart Center in Los Angeles, the various programs and services available to the mentally ill who are homeless include Screening and Referral/High Risk Homeless, Short-Term Action Integration Referral Service (STAIRS), Testing Living Center (TLC), Recuperative Care, and the Specialized Shelter Program for severely and persistently mentally ill homeless individuals. These special programs for the mentally ill are funded through the County of Los Angeles Department of Mental Health. The Weingart Center provides basic living support in the form of short-term transitional housing, food, clothing, hygiene supplies, and limited supervision for homeless adults who are also chronically mentally ill and considered to be vulnerable on the streets. This temporary housing program provides the staff with an opportunity to stabilize clients' conditions by the use of medications, to resolve benefit problems, and to provide placement in more permanent housing. A study by Murray and Baier (1995) found that by using a transitional residential program, 48% of the residents who were formerly homeless and severely and persistently mentally ill were able to maintain permanent housing and a disability pension or a job.

▸ Carl, a 36-year-old man, is admitted to the Specialized Shelter Program in March. He has recently moved from Salt Lake City, Utah, where he resided with his sister. Carl is diagnosed as a paranoid schizophrenic and is also mildly developmentally disabled. He is a pleasant man who wants to stay in Los Angeles because of the mild climate. He has never been homeless before but finds himself without funds to rent an apartment. Because Carl is an affable person who is eager to please, he is very easy to manipulate, which increases his vulnerability on the streets. His mental health case manager requests close monitoring via shelter placement. With the support of his case manager and the Specialized Shelter Program, Carl realizes his goals to move into a hotel, where he can be taught additional independent living skills, and to obtain his own apartment eventually.

Johnson (1990) cites housing as the first need of the mentally ill once they are discharged from a hospital setting. Families are not always able to provide shelter, and there is no hope of recovering from any illness on the streets. These people also need a place where they can belong—a refuge or haven. The severely and persistently mentally ill also require aggressive outreach programs and a mental health program that creates and adjusts its services to the limited abilities of its clients. These people need ready access to hospitals and permission to regress, and also frequently require training in living skills, including personal hygiene and grooming, shopping, budgeting, traveling, and social skills. Next, the mentally ill need work to occupy their time and give them an idea of what it is like to live in the real world. The severely and persistently mentally ill deserve treatment free of condescension for as long as they need it. A lifetime disability requires long-term access (Johnson 1990).

CARE THROUGH THE NURSING PROCESS

Nurses come into contact with people, both homeless and domiciled, who have persistent mental illness in a number of settings, including the hospital emergency department, community health programs, outreach programs, and mobile units.

Most nurses have many of the skills necessary to care for this population. However, nurses with advanced education are prepared to work in expanded roles. Psychiatric clinical nurse specialists and nurse practitioners have additional talents. The advanced practice of such nurses comes from advanced preparation in various aspects of nursing. The clinical nurse specialist graduated from a program of study that emphasized leadership, the change process, and research in addition to clinical work with clients. Nurse practitioners undergo many of the same courses as clinical nurse specialists, but their curriculum stresses advanced assessment skills and treatment courses to prepare for an additional licensure examination. In some states, the nurse practitioner can furnish medications (similar to prescribing). Nurse practitioners tend to work in outpatient locations such as clinics. In many states, there is only the advanced practice nurse, who is clinically certified and may work in either an inpatient or outpatient setting with prescriptive authority, if granted by that state.

Both advanced practice and basic level nurses can make a positive difference in the quality of care available to people with severe and persistent mental illness.

Assessment

Information regarding the "where" and "what" of home is important for both current and discharge planning. Because of problems with thought processes and communication, the person may not be able to describe clearly what is wrong. The nurse can obtain some vital clues from assessing hygiene status, signs of injury or violence (e.g., scars, bruises, abrasions), appropriateness of clothing, evidence of poor nutrition, and untended infections (including tuberculosis) or infestations (e.g., lice, scabies). Frequently, during the taking of the nursing history, clients may be vague about sleeping, eating, and other activities. It may be necessary to question them directly about living arrangements.

As discussed, homelessness is not an uncommon side effect of severe and persistent mental illness. Although homelessness alone is not grounds for admission to an inpatient facility, it may be a prime motivator for a client to come to an emergency department. The warm, dry, relatively safe hospital with plenty of food ("three hots and a cot"), when weighed against living on the street with minimal or no resources, may not be such a bad alternative. Indeed, such behavior could be interpreted as reasonable and adaptive.

Nursing Diagnosis

Nursing diagnoses are the matrix on which the plan of care rests. Great care must be taken to ensure that the definitions and defining characteristics of the nursing diagnoses are actually drawn from the nurses' data and client's perspective, and do not consist of hackneyed phrases. For example, **noncompliance** is not defined as the client's refusal to follow medical advice but as "the state in which an individual . . . *desires* to comply but is prevented from doing so by factors that deter adherence to health-related advice given by health professionals" (Carpenito 1995). Box 27–1 lists possible nursing diagnoses applicable to a severely and persistently mentally ill homeless person.

BOX 27–1 NURSING DIAGNOSES: THE SEVERELY AND PERSISTENTLY MENTALLY ILL

Adjustment, impaired
Anxiety
Comfort, alteration
Coping, ineffective individual/family
Denial, ineffective
Deficit, fluid volume
Health maintenance, alteration in
Hopelessness
Ineffective management of therapeutic regimen
Injury, risk for
Infection, risk for
Nutrition, alteration: less than body requirements
Powerlessness
Post-trauma response
Self-care deficit
Sleep pattern disturbance
Thought process, alteration in
Self-esteem, chronic low
Self-mutilation, risk for
Skin/tissue integrity, impaired
Social interaction, impaired
Social isolation
Verbal communication, impaired

Planning

The assessment data often show patterns or cues that revolve around basic issues: independence in self-care (hygiene, nutrition, health care) and difficulties in relationships with others. Other problems, such as TD or risk of self-harm, may widen the constellation of concerns. Various areas of concerns are evaluated with regard to *realistic* and measurable outcomes, and specific outcome criteria are formulated.

Intervention

The duality of severe psychosocial and physical needs may strain the health care provider's available resources, especially those of time and talent. Complicated physical interventions can be an additional burden on the nurse already busy with groups and activities, and a client with significant psychosocial dysfunction may compound the problems for the nurse attempting to care for several people with physical needs. Many psychiatric mental health nurses find ample opportunity to perfect their communication and therapeutic skills but may have had far less need for "medical-surgical–type" skills in the past. Conversely, the nurse in the medical-surgical setting may be proficient at applying complicated dressings and energy conservation techniques but less adept at using common psychological strategies. A nurse equally expert in both these areas is ideally suited to working with this population.

People with severe and persistent mental illness are increasingly requiring attention to physical problems. Worley and colleagues (1990) report that significant physical illness occurs in this group at a higher rate than in the general population. This is compounded by the special gerontological implications of people who are growing older. Thus, the psychiatric nurse must have regular updates of medical-surgical nursing information, in addition to keeping current with psychosocial topics. The medical-surgical nurse must be similarly prepared. It does not follow that people with a severe and persistent mental illness will never be admitted to a general unit for an appendectomy or an exacerbation of congestive heart failure.

However, the expectation that all nurses should be expert in all areas of nursing is not realistic. Colleagues with different specialties can be consulted. A quick conversation can make a big difference in the quality of care provided to a client. Resources of information not regularly used should be readily available. Reference books and access to staff education materials from other units can help jog a memory or suggest something novel. Electronic media such as CD-ROMs and the Internet (World Wide Web) can also quickly yield current data on a variety of medical, surgical, and psychosocial topics.

Access to medical records for a transient population poses special problems. Computer-based medical records available through the use of database strategies may provide more secure and reliable client information in the future (see Chapter 1) (Church and Barnett 1994).

The nurse's delivery of care to the severely and persistently mentally ill person can be viewed in terms of the nine roles of the professional nurse, as defined by Kozier and associates (1995): care provider, communicator/helper, teacher, counselor, client advocate, change agent, leader, manager, and researcher (Table 27–1). The nurse may embody one role at a time, or several simultaneously. All these functions are applicable to both psychosocial and physical concerns and are accomplished through the nursing process.

Basic psychosocial needs do not change simply because the person has developed a long-term illness. However, ways in which health care workers meet these needs must be adapted in order to connect with those in need. Chronic disaffiliation makes more problematic the first

TABLE 27–1 ROLES OF THE PROFESSIONAL NURSE

Role	Description
1. Care provider	Provides comfort and support; facilitates normal health/healing processes; safeguards against injury and complications
2. Communicator/helper	Develops the person's database and disseminates information to other members of the health care team
3. Teacher	Instructs on health problems and ways to change behavior
4. Counselor	Facilitates interrelationships and personal growth through guided insight and support
5. Client advocate	Works with a central purpose of the person's rights and needs
6. Change agent	Facilitates modifications in the person, family, or organization to provide for higher-level wellness
7. Leader	Influences others with the goal of increasing effectiveness of care, improving health status, or providing additional resources
8. Manager	Interacts within the organization to achieve optimal nursing care for patients and families
9. Researcher	Bases clinical practice on scientific studies and participates in the research process, perhaps through data collection

From Kozier, B., Erb, G., Blais, K., and Wilkinson, J. M. (1995). *Fundamentals of nursing: Concepts, process, and practice* (5th ed.). Menlo Park, CA: Addison-Wesley. Copyright © 1995 by Addison-Wesley Publishing Company.

step in caring for a client's health care needs (i.e., establishing a rapport).

Care Provider

Fear, anxiety, and distrust are pervasive in the lives of severely and persistently mentally ill persons. These people have a decreased ability to deal successfully with stressors. In addition, they commonly have significant physical problems that require attention.

◗ Susie is brought to a community psychiatric hospital by the police when local shopkeepers complain about her frequent bizarre behavior. She screams that the red traffic light at the corner is making the worms in her head angry. At first, the nurse can only attempt to make Susie feel less threatened in this new environment by providing plenty of physical distance and making no demands. The room is cleared of any objects that Susie could use to hurt herself or others.

◗ Later, as Susie begins to trust a little more, the nurse coaxes her into eating a hot meal. Still later, Susie agrees to take her first dose of medications. Before she falls asleep that night, Susie takes the blankets off the bed and curls up in the corner of her room to sleep for a few hours. In the morning, Susie will not shower, but the nurse is able to persuade her to wash from the basin. The nurse also convinces her that it would be OK to attend to an infected wound on Susie's hand. Later that morning, after another dose of medications, Susie is calm enough to consider attending a group therapy session. There, the nurse is able both to begin connecting Susie to her peers and to help her with her altered thought processes.

Communicator/Helper

The health care team, including nurses and physicians as well as social workers, activity therapists, and others, relied on the nurses' assessment data. Only nurses observed Susie's functioning and were available for interventions 24 hours a day. The admitting nurse suggested getting Susie involved in the art therapy group. All staff members addressed discharge planning from the first day of Susie's admission. At their suggestion, before discharge, the psychiatrist changed Susie's antipsychotic agent, oral fluphenazine hydrochloride (Prolixin), to fluphenazine decanoate (Prolixin Decanoate). This long-acting (2- to 4-week) decanoate preparation can facilitate Susie's maintenance of an adequate serum level of the antipsychotic drug. This was important, because Susie's compliance with her drug regimen was doubtful once she was discharged. Susie was also referred to a case manager and a transitional community center. The team met with her family to assess their needs and to include them in the discharge planning.

Teacher

The nurses leading various groups and activities addressed some of Susie's problems. One of these was that Susie needed to continue her medications after discharge. She would also need help in improving her independence in activities of daily living (ADLs). An evening shift nurse continued the health teaching started during a day session. Throughout her stay, Susie saw how the nurses behaved toward her, toward her peers, and toward other health care workers. These interactions gave her a model of alternative methods of relating to others.

Counselor

The staff wanted to help Susie deal with people in a more productive and satisfying manner. The team developed a plan whereby groups and one-to-one sessions would best address that need. Also, Susie's family attended a few special groups just for significant others, where they addressed their own needs. Under the nurses' guidance, Susie's parents entered into long-term therapy to deal with some unique issues.

Client Advocate

"Advocacy involves concern for and defined actions in behalf of another person . . . to bring about a change" (Kozier et al. 1995). Although nurses do not have the role of client advocate exclusive of any other helping professional, it is very much a part of professional practice.

◗ Jaqui is admitted one morning. She suffers from depression and has not eaten properly for some months. With much coaxing, the nurse is able to entice her to eat about 25% of her lunch. At supper, Jaqui just stares at her hot dog and french fries. When the nurse tries to tempt her to take a bite, she insists that she "would be sinning if I ate that thing. It's got pork in it." The nurse calls the dietary department to order a more acceptable entrée, but the dietary aide says that they are very busy and don't have the time to make a special plate for her. He suggests giving her peanut butter and crackers out of the unit pantry, and in the morning the dietitian will make rounds. The nurse continues to state the need for a substitute dinner until she convinces the aide of the client's right to a meal that does not offend her cultural beliefs.

Change Agent

Through the use of the nursing process, the nurse pursues change in the person's health status. In Jaqui's case, the nurses ensured that the care plan addressed **hopelessness, alteration in nutrition: less than body re-**

quirements, and **altered family processes** on the problem list. Through attention to varied facets of the person, higher-level wellness can be approached holistically and change can be meaningful.

Leader

When the nurses took the time to encourage Jaqui to eat or obtain a new dinner tray, they manifested their leadership. Other staff were influenced by their vision or quality, person-centered care.

Manager

The charge nurse met with the nurse manager of the area the next day to discuss the difficulty of obtaining the dinner tray. Together they brainstormed ways to avoid a similar incident in the future. The nurse manager then met with the supervisor of the dietary department. Among other strategies implemented, an educational program was provided to the dietary workers to help them learn about special cultural aspects of food preferences. In this way, the organization itself was addressed.

Researcher

Although the nursing staff of the units where Susie and Jaqui were hospitalized did not develop and conduct their own research projects, they were good consumers of nursing research. Because of their reading of current studies, they knew of recent successes in milieu therapy in transitional community centers. For that reason, they suggested a referral for Susie.

Evaluation

The goals of intervention are client centered; therefore, the final evaluation is based on (1) the client's satisfaction with the new health status and (2) the health care team's estimation of improvement. Achieving these goals may take much longer than current funding from private insurance or governmental plans allows. Therefore, referrals and plans for continued care are often essential to success. Although resources are available for the persistently mentally ill, local community programs vary widely.

The problems of the severely and persistently mentally ill are becoming even more widespread and complex. Nurses, in conjunction with their health care facilities and with other supportive groups, could be instrumental in developing more assistance alternatives. Client advocacy remains a primary function of the professional nurse in all settings, as emphasized in the Chapter 1 and throughout this book. Refer to the case study later in this chapter for an example of a nurse's work with a person who has a severe and persistent mental illness.

HOMELESS IN AMERICA

Intense debate continues concerning the number of homeless people in the United States. A study by Link and associates (1994) found that the combined lifetime and 5-year prevalence of all types of homelessness was 14%. This finding underlines the significance of the problem of homelessness. The Interagency Council on the Homeless (1994), Department of Housing and Urban Development, has updated its statistics to include children. They estimate that between 4.95 and 9.32 million people (with a mean of 7 million) experienced homelessness in the late 1980s.

A 1996 review of 50 cities found that, in virtually every city, the official estimated number of homeless people greatly exceeded the numbers of emergency shelters and transitional housing (National Law Center on Homelessness and Poverty 1996). Moreover, there are few or no shelters in rural areas of the United States despite significant levels of homelessness (Aron and Fitchen 1996). Research indicates that families, single mothers, and children make up the largest group of people who are homeless in rural areas (Vissing 1996). Homelessness among Native Americans and migrant workers is also largely a rural phenomenon.

There is a high turnover in the homeless population, suggesting that many more people experience homelessness than was previously thought, and that many of these people are homeless for a relatively short time and need support to tide them over in a crisis. Refer to Box 27–2 for one person's story. Unfortunately, many other people have complex long-term mental and physical problems that require more time and extensive support to help them maintain some level of quality in their lives.

About 40% to 50% of the homeless abuse alcohol, and 10% to 15% abuse drugs. The average age of the homeless population has dropped from the late 40s and 50s to the early 30s. Homeless families account for over 40% of this population, and it is estimated that there are 750,000 to 1 million children in homeless families. The number of adolescents living on their own ranges between 100,000 and 400,000, and people over 60 years of age account for approximately 10% of the homeless population (Damrosch and Strasser 1988; Ryan 1989).

There is a consensus, however, that there is no single solution for this complex problem. Homelessness does not confine itself to a particular race, age, or sex, and it is more than a lack of a place to live. The homeless also lack food, appropriate clothing, access to health care and social services, and educational opportunities (Riesdorf-Ostrow 1989).

BOX 27–2 ONE STORY

Stories keep us excited here at the Task Force. As I was returning a call Tuesday from a local restaurant, I asked the manager if she could donate something to our shelter. She gladly described to me the 70-person feast they would donate for the overflow shelter the following night.

"Thank you," I told her. "You'll never know how glad these cold and hungry people will be to get this food."

I heard a chuckle and the manager said, "Oh yes I will. What you don't know is that my husband and I came to the Task Force looking for shelter and help about a year ago. You all helped us so much that we got housing and jobs, and now I'm the manager here and he has a good job."

"You've made my holiday," I said. And she went on to say, "You don't know how wonderful you all have been. I thank God for you every day. And I'm just delighted to be in a position to give some little something back."

From Beaty, A. (1996). *Task Force for the Homeless: Reflections of 1996.* Atlanta, GA: Task Force for the Homeless.

Factors contributing to homelessness are many. The high rates of unemployment and underemployment and the reductions in public support programs and low-cost housing are a few sources of the homeless problem today. The current trend toward cutting aid to our most vulnerable populations, if carried forward, will only intensify the problem. De-institutionalization of the mentally ill from mental institutions into the community is another undisputed cause (see Chapters 1 and 9). A study by Cohen (1994) found that the numbers of homeless persons, including those who are mentally ill, primarily reflect structural factors such as the availability of low-cost housing and public benefits. Multiple factors have contributed to de-institutionalization's side effect of homelessness. New drugs and treatments that control symptoms have made it possible for the mentally ill to live in the community. On the other hand, being homeless and living in a shelter may result in an emotional crisis that could exacerbate a mental disorder (Johnson 1990). There is a strong relationship between life without a home and mental disorder. Life on the street or in a shelter, whether temporary or not, can have a very negative influence on a person's self-esteem. Homelessness on top of a fragile mental status could be all that is necessary to provoke a crisis or exacerbate an existing mental disorder. People found wandering the streets in a daze and talking to themselves have often been taken to hospitals and labeled with an unwarranted psychiatric diagnosis; their response to a life of hardship and the loss of a home should not be unexpected.

Another factor currently contributing to homelessness is the issue of domestic violence. Battered women who live in poverty are often forced to choose between abusive relationships and homelessness. For example, a study in Michigan showed that 60% of battered women who returned to violent partners did so because of the lack of affordable housing (Appel 1990). It is clear that homelessness is often the result of a complex set of circumstances that push people into poverty and force impossible choices among food, shelter, and other basic needs.

To deal with this problem, we must ask ourselves the question: Why do homeless persons remain on the street? The Interagency Council on the Homeless (1991) reported that some remain street dwellers owing to a lack of available shelter beds. Others exhibit characteristics or behaviors that many shelters will not tolerate, such as specific psychiatric symptoms, intoxication, or aggressive acting out behavior. Some homeless persons *choose* not to use shelters, citing dangerous, dirty, crowded, or noisy conditions. Still others resent the rules and requirements enforced by the shelters. Finally, there are persons who either shun contact with others or who have developed a workable support and survival system outside the shelters. In describing the problem, it is necessary to discuss some of the subgroups that make up the homeless population.

Subcategories of Homelessness

Subgroups of the homeless addressed in this section are (1) the severely and persistently mentally ill; (2) long-term substance abusers; (3) age-related populations, including families with children, adolescents, and the elderly; and (4) those with communicable diseases.

The Severely and Persistently Mentally Ill

The severely and persistently mentally ill are well represented in each of these subgroups. As mentioned, de-institutionalization has left many mentally ill persons without shelter. Community mental health centers that were intended to provide inpatient and outpatient care, day care, outreach services, emergency treatment, consultation, and educational services, as well as specific services for children, adolescents, and the elderly, failed in large part because of lack of funds (review Chapters 1 and 9). As a result, many of the long-term mentally ill received no social or medical support. Unfortunately, mental health authorities are reluctant to make homelessness a "mental health problem" because this might result in the re-institutionalization of people in this population (Riesdorf-Ostrow 1989).

The severely and persistently mentally ill homeless population consists of men and women who may have primary DSM-IV (*Diagnostic and statistical manual of mental disorders*, fourth edition) diagnoses, including psychotic disorders (schizophrenia, bipolar and depression disorders), personality disorders (borderline, dependent, antisocial), cognitive impairments, and numerous others. For example, homeless people are more likely to have a diagnosis of schizophrenia, five times more likely to be diagnosed with a major depressive disorder, and three times more likely to have a primary diagnosis of alcoholism than a general population sample (Leshner 1992).

Characteristics common to this population include fragile ego development; extreme suspiciousness; vulnerability to stress; and impairments in thinking, perception, attention span, and concentration. Pathological defenses against anxiety are evidenced by frequent incidences of suicide, substance dependence, retreat to psychosis, and violence. Martell and associates (1995) found violent crimes to be 40% higher among the homeless mentally ill than among domiciled mentally ill.

Mentally ill young adults also demonstrate tremendous deficits in their ability to form satisfactory interpersonal relationships, their social skills, and their competence in performing ADLs (Brunger 1986). As mentioned, the severely and persistently mentally ill population experiences major problems with money management, transportation, compliance with medication regimens, meal preparation, and articulating their needs for other basic services. As a result, the persistently mentally ill in the community frequently live impoverished lives devoid of basic services that were available in state hospitals and other institutions.

Long-Term Substance Abusers

Chronic substance abusers may become homeless as a result of their addictions, which interfere with getting and keeping a job. Disaffiliation from family and friends may bring the abuser to a life on the streets. A study by Drake and Wallach (1989) showed that substance abuse added to the problems of disruptive, disinhibited, and noncompliant behaviors in clients dually diagnosed with substance abuse and chronic mental illness. These clients are younger, more often male, and less able to manage their lives in the community by maintaining regular meals, adequate finances, and stable housing. They are also less able to comply with the rules in available living situations, such as boarding homes, and are often evicted or choose to leave. Homeless persons with substance abuse problems are at high risk for human immunodeficiency virus (HIV) infection and are more likely to have serious health problems and severe mental illness, to be arrested, to be victimized on the streets, and to suffer an early death (Williams 1992).

Age-Related Populations

Homelessness can occur during any of the developmental stages of life. Therefore, age-related populations to be considered include families with children, adolescents, and the elderly.

FAMILIES WITH CHILDREN. It is a disturbing fact that women and children have been the fastest-growing subpopulation of homeless since the mid-1980s (Thrasher and Mowbray 1995). A survey of 30 U.S. cities found that families with children account for 39% of the homeless population (Waxman 1994). This is a consequence of a cut in welfare programs, specifically Aid to Families with Dependent Children (AFDC), and reductions in food stamp and affordable housing programs that seem destined to increase in the new age of welfare cuts and health care reform. The problem becomes much more complex if a parent is diagnosed with a severe and persistent mental illness (Norton and Ridenour 1995).

ADOLESCENTS. Adolescents find themselves homeless as a result of running away from home or being thrown out by their families. One study (Bassuk 1987) found that more than half of these youths had left home by 13 years of age and since that time had averaged nine moves a year. These adolescents come from chaotic families, most have a parent with a criminal history or a substance abuse problem, and one half have been physically abused (Bassuk 1987). There is no question that the great majority of runaway youths have been the victims of persistent, extreme abuse experienced at a young age (Janus et al. 1995).

THE ELDERLY. An increasing number of elderly people are finding themselves at risk for homelessness at a time when the demand for low-income housing is larger than the supply and the federal allocations for public housing have been severely cut. It is predicted that persons over 60 years of age will be the next group hit hard by homelessness. A single medical emergency or tragic incident could place many older persons living near the poverty level at risk for homelessness.

Populations with Communicable Diseases

The homeless population is vulnerable to a variety of diseases and conditions, which for the most part go untreated. Dental problems and undernourishment are pervasive among this population. Many homeless persons are infected with sexually transmitted diseases. However, the two medical conditions that warrant the most immediate concern for many is the rise of tuberculosis and HIV infection among the homeless (St. Lawrence and Brasfield 1995).

Tuberculosis has become increasingly common since the early 1990s. This increase has been facilitated by the growing number of clients with concurrent HIV infection, by cases due to multiple-drug resistant strains, by incomplete tuberculosis therapy among homeless and noncompliant clients, and by some cases in immigrants from other countries where tuberculosis prevalence is high (McGowan and Blumberg 1995). Barclay and associates (1995) identify several factors that complicate the diagnosis and treatment of tuberculosis in the homeless:

alcoholism, substance abuse, and psychiatric illness. They cite an urgent need for appropriate screening, prevention, and treatment undertaken in collaboration with local health departments.

HIV infection among homeless adults and runaway youths is a serious mental health problem. Homeless persons have an increased risk of HIV infection because they are more apt to be involved in high-risk behaviors such as drug use, sexual contact with a person at risk for HIV, and the exchange of drugs for sex (Allen et al. 1994). A study by Kipke and associates (1995) in a sample of street youths found that 58% had injected a drug within the last 30 days. Allen and associates urge that HIV prevention and treatment be integrated into comprehensive health and medical programs serving homeless populations. Lebow and associates (1995) in their study of people with AIDS found that the homeless population had a significantly higher diagnosis of *Mycobacterium tuberculosis* infection and esophageal candidiasis than did the people with AIDS who were not homeless.

The Process of Homelessness

Some people have a brief episode of homelessness as the result of a sudden crisis such as unemployment, eviction, or domestic upheaval. Many, however, experience homelessness as a situation that exists for a significant length of time. Disaffiliation, arrested social development, conflicts with employers, being on welfare, psychosexual difficulty, limited insight, and self-mutilation are life experiences that thousands of homeless men and women share across the United States. Bassuk (1984) found that 74% of shelter residents had no family relations and that 73% had no friends. Both figures jump to 90% for homeless persons who also had psychiatric histories. The study concluded that chronic homelessness is often the final stage in a lifelong series of crises and missed opportunities, the culmination of a gradual disengagement from supportive relationships and institutions.

Many long-term homeless people are treated by a variety of hospitals and clinics, and over time they may be given various psychiatric diagnoses. This does not necessarily indicate psychiatric confusion or a lack of communication among treatment facilities, but rather supports the fact that treating the chronically homeless person is a complex proposition. A look at the hospital records indicates that, although a person presents with an array of symptoms that warrant a specific diagnosis, the person does not stay in one place long enough to allow any sort of diagnostic fine tuning to take place. Before a more accurate diagnosis can be developed, more prolonged care must be used to establish a therapeutic alliance. Because persons who suffer from homelessness as a life style problem are severely and actively disaffiliated and estranged from themselves, others, and their environment, 1 or 2 hours, or even one or two sessions, are not enough to develop the necessary therapeutic alliance. Jezewski (1995) mentions specific barriers that complicate the ability of health care workers to stay connected with this population. These barriers include lack of health insurance, insensitivity of health care providers toward homeless persons, stigmatization, cultural barriers, and communication breakdown.

Complicating this already complex picture is the unfortunate occurrence of caseload transfers or the introduction of new or replacement treatment staff. Inconsistent staffing and use of registry personnel also compounds the issue, making it difficult to coordinate the multiple problems presented by the homeless person. Even though a homeless person may be involved in effective treatment, a new therapeutic alliance must be established if a new staff person takes over all or part of the client's treatment, which prolongs therapy.

Future Directions

If the problem is clearly defined, there may be a solution. That is, if *de*-institutionalization is considered the primary cause, *re*-institutionalization will be seen as the solution. If the lack of low-cost housing is considered the main cause, a housing solution will be sought. Unfortunately, such a complex problem cannot be corrected by any single solution. The Center for Mental Health Services (1995) reported some key findings on five projects that were completed to test the effectiveness of a variety of approaches to providing mental health treatment, housing, and related services to homeless adults with severe mental illness. It was found that these individuals can be reached by the service system, will accept and benefit from mental health services, and can remain in community-based housing with the appropriate help. In addition, improving the integration of existing services and entitlement programs will not only alleviate human suffering but also reduce the costs of institutionalization and hospitalization.

Carol Johnson, director of the homeless services for the Massachusetts Department of Mental Health, has stated, "Mental health issues are an integral part of the experience of homelessness. . . . You can't separate homelessness, mental illness and bureaucratic structures. . . . The opposite of homelessness is community, not shelter" (J.O.C. 1988).

There are great opportunities for nursing within the wide range of services for the mentally ill who are homeless. Carter and associates (1994) advocate the development of nurse-managed free clinics as an effective means of servicing the needs of the homeless and indigent in an atmosphere of support and concern. Aiken (1987) suggests the following strategies for nurses in assisting the mentally ill:

1. Consolidating authority and accountability in the fiscal management of clinical programs

2. Rooting authority in local government, where local officials can manage broad-based programs
3. Developing new service settings to include group homes, foster homes, mobile clinics, and the streets
4. Creating outreach programs much like the public health nursing model, in which nurses meet clients in the home, on the streets, and on the job
5. Reforming financial methods of reimbursement
6. Attracting professionals to public sector careers
7. Joining the national public debate about homelessness and the severely and persistently mentally ill

In these ways, nursing can assume a key role in delivering services and providing care to the severely and persistently mentally ill who are homeless.

CASE STUDY: A PERSON WITH SEVERE AND PERSISTENT MENTAL ILLNESS

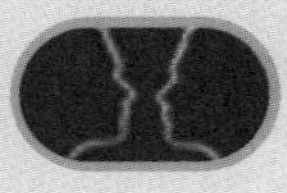

Evelyn is a 42-year-old woman who was originally diagnosed with schizophrenia approximately 20 years ago. During the last two decades, she has been hospitalized several times in acute care psychiatric facilities. Her last admitting diagnosis was borderline personality disorder. Evelyn married for the first time at age 20 and was divorced a few years later. She has been divorced and remarried and has had more informal relationships several times since. She has a 10-year-old daughter, Marie. Evelyn states that she doesn't have any friends: "There just aren't any people who want to be friendly."

During her last separation and divorce, which took place 2 years ago, Evelyn's clinical presentation became more exaggerated. She had worked intermittently up to that time as a temporary clerical worker through a local personnel agency. However, her overreactions to office stress and her manipulating behaviors became so pronounced that she was fired.

Evelyn and Marie live in a dirty motel room. Marie is in and out of foster care homes. She attends school occasionally but says she hates it "because the kids are so mean and I'm so stupid." She can read on a first-grade level.

Evelyn is seeking admission because "there's a man down the street who says he's going to hurt me. There are a lot of nasty, mean people out there. You just can't get away from them. You've got to let me in!" Although the weather is cold and rainy, she wears no coat. Both her clothes and her body are dirty. She has a large leg ulcer and says, "My leg gets real tired sometimes. I don't remember when my leg got sore like that."

In addition to her psychiatric difficulties, Evelyn has medical problems: a large weeping ulcer (5 cm, stage 3) on a swollen left ankle (4+/4+ to midcalf), high blood pressure (right arm, 154/96; left arm, 160/98), and a serum glucose level of 263. The nurse is unable to get Evelyn to undress because of her agitation. The nurse does, however, feel protruding bones under Evelyn's clothes. Evelyn's skin is dry and flaky, with multiple scars, abrasions, and bruises. Her feet are calloused and cracked. Her heart rate is 98 and her respiration rate 22. She refuses to have her temperature taken. She tells the nurse, "I'm so tired and hungry."

ASSESSMENT

The nurse assessed the following:

OBJECTIVE DATA

1. Several psychiatric admissions over 20 years
2. Multiple short-term relationships with men
3. Difficulty maintaining relationships with others
4. Has a 10-year-old daughter
5. Jobless and underhoused for 2 years
6. Poor hygiene
7. Clothes inappropriate for weather
8. Large leg ulcer, hypertension, hyperglycemia
9. Undernourished
10. Multiple signs of past injuries
11. Difficulty keeping focused during intake interview

SUBJECTIVE DATA

1. "A man . . . says he's going to hurt me."
2. "I'm so tired and hungry."
3. "Marie is in school today. I got scared and couldn't wait for her."
4. "My leg gets real tired sometimes."
5. "There are a lot of nasty, mean people out there. You just can't get away from them."
6. "I don't remember when my leg got sore like that."

CASE STUDY: A PERSON WITH SEVERE AND PERSISTENT MENTAL ILLNESS (Continued)

NURSING DIAGNOSIS

The following nursing diagnoses were formulated:

1. **Altered thought processes** related to psychiatric dysfunction as evidenced by distractibility and cognitive defects.
   - "A man says he's going to hurt me."
   - Difficulty staying focused
   - "I don't remember when my leg got sore like that."
   - Inability to obtain and retain a job
   - Inability to provide a clean home for self and daughter (Marie)
   - No preparation for Marie's care during the hospitalization
2. **Ineffective family coping: disabling** related to psychiatric dysfunction and poverty, as evidenced by neglect of daughter.
   - Jobless and underhoused for 2 years
   - Motel room dirty
   - Marie's infrequent school attendance and poor academic function
   - Evelyn's not being where Marie expects to find her after school
   - No preparation for Marie's care during the hospitalization
3. **Impaired tissue integrity** related to venous stasis and impaired cellular function, as evidenced by large ulcer on left ankle.
   - 5-cm, stage 3 ulcer
   - 4+/4+ edema to midcalf on left leg
   - "My leg gets real tired sometimes."

Other nursing diagnoses that deserve attention are

1. **Self-care deficit: hygiene** related to homelessness and decreased cognitive function and poverty, as evidenced by dirty, torn clothing and dirty hair/skin.
2. **Altered nutrition: less than body requirements** related to impaired glucose metabolism and poverty, as evidenced by emaciation.
3. **Risk for injury** related to decreased cognitive function and hyperglycemia.

PLANNING

PLANNING OUTCOME CRITERIA

DIAGNOSES	OUTCOME CRITERIA	SHORT-TERM GOALS
1. **Altered thought processes** related to psychiatric dysfunction and hyperglycemia, as evidenced by distractibility and cognitive defects.	1. Evelyn will demonstrate improved thought processes during this admission, as evidenced by decreased distractibility and increased ability to problem-solve care for herself and her daughter.	1a. Evelyn will demonstrate ability to concentrate on learning and/or therapy activities for at least 10 minutes. 1b. Evelyn will identify three appropriate actions that can be taken to decrease anxiety in the event of stress. 1c. Evelyn will demonstrate ability to plan and execute three aspects of self-care.

Continued on following page

CASE STUDY: A PERSON WITH SEVERE AND PERSISTENT MENTAL ILLNESS *(Continued)*

DIAGNOSES	OUTCOME CRITERIA	SHORT-TERM GOALS
2. **Ineffective family coping: disabling** related to psychiatric dysfunction and poverty, as evidenced by neglect of daughter.	2. Evelyn will demonstrate improved nurturing behavior toward daughter by discharge, as evidenced by awareness of how to access support for basic needs and education, as well as specified nurturing behaviors.	2a. Evelyn will verbalize an appropriate plan for care of Marie during Evelyn's hospitalization. 2b. Evelyn will discuss with social worker how to access benefits and programs for Marie's support and education by discharge. 2c. Evelyn will demonstrate nurturing behaviors toward Marie during visits throughout this hospitalization.
3. **Impaired tissue integrity** related to venous stasis and impaired cellular function, as evidenced by large ulcer on left ankle.	3. Evelyn's ulcer will decrease from 5 cm to 1 cm by discharge.	3a. Evelyn's ulcer will no longer exude serosanguineous drainage. 3b. Evelyn's ulcer will be free from infection.

NURSES' FEELINGS AND SELF-ASSESSMENT

Most nurses become skilled in dealing with both the medical and psychosocial needs of the hospital's population. Through close work with case managers and social workers, help can often be made available after discharge. However, dealing with child neglect and abuse is often difficult for nursing staff. Neglected and abused children do not learn or experience healthy bonding, and they do not develop effective social skills, problem-solving techniques, competencies necessary for employment, self-esteem, and many other skills needed to succeed in life. To care adequately for Evelyn, and indirectly for Marie, the staff realized that the social worker would be an important resource person, providing access and referrals to meet some of this family's needs.

INTERVENTION

Initially, during the first few hours, the focus was on lowering Evelyn's anxiety so that she would accept needed care. Meeting some of her physiological needs (e.g., food, euglycemia) gave the staff the opportunity to make contact with Evelyn. The social worker, Mr. Todd, was contacted and informed that Marie would return from school and not be able to find her mother. Mr. Todd located Marie at school and explained the problem. He then brought her to the hospital to see Evelyn before taking her to an emergency foster home. This activity was necessary not only to protect Marie but also to emphasize to Evelyn how important such interventions were to Marie's well-being.

CASE STUDY: A PERSON WITH SEVERE AND PERSISTENT MENTAL ILLNESS *(Continued)*

EVALUATION

Evelyn's psychosocial and medical health improved slowly during the short admission. Her ability to think increased modestly. Her leg ulcer began to show signs of granulation. The edema decreased to 1/4+ and remained at ankle level. Her serum glucose level remained between 140 and 180. Evelyn articulated plans for job training and living at a halfway house during the training period. She also talked about keeping Marie in a stable foster care home until she was working and had a proper home for the two of them. Evelyn agreed to continuing parenting classes through the child welfare agency. However, Marie was demonstrating various acting out behaviors both in the foster home and at school. She stated, "My mother loves me and I want to be with her now. The way we lived was just fine." Her therapist felt considerable resistance from her.

SUMMARY

Severe and persistent mental illness is a complex problem that affects an increasing number of Americans today. The number of persistently and severely mentally ill persons within the community is escalating. Chronic disaffiliation from society, friends, and family weakens the support system so important to persons with long-term mental illness. Families, when present, bear a tremendous burden and increased stress on financial, emotional, and physical systems. This burden affects the functioning of the individual and of family members, disrupts family functioning, and can limit the resources sought by the mentally ill family member.

Interventions include careful use of medication, rehabilitation programs, therapy, and case management. Evaluation of the effectiveness of these interventions is imperative for effective long-term care.

Nurses can take advantage of the many opportunities for assisting the severely and persistently mentally ill, and play an important role in providing care and services. The nine roles of the nurse were illustrated and applied to case studies. Some selected nursing diagnoses in the care of the severely and persistently mentally ill were also presented. Each step of the nursing process was used to provide a systematic method of addressing both the psychosocial and physical needs of a severely and persistently mentally ill person. Evelyn's story helps to illustrate the complex needs of a homeless person with a severe and persistent mental illness.

Available resources for the persistently mentally ill do not meet all the needs of this population. Community mental health services provide much support in the form of community outreach programs, multiservice centers, and transitional care shelters. Shelter and ongoing assistance are the first of many needs to arise upon discharge from the hospital. These resources must be available on an ongoing basis to meet the complex and diverse needs of this population. Services must be adjusted to the specific needs of each individual. Unfortunately, there is no single solution to this complex problem.

REFERENCES

Aiken, L. (1987). Unmet needs of the chronically mentally ill: Will nursing respond? *Image: Journal of Nursing Scholarship*, 19(3):121.

Allen, D. M., et al. (1994). HIV infection among homeless adults and runaway youth. AIDS United States, 1989–1992. Field Services Branch. *AIDS*, 8(11):1593.

Appel, M. (1990). *From emergency shelter to permanent housing: The obstacles to safe, decent, affordable housing encountered by battered women*. Ann Arbor, MI.

Aron, L. Y., and Fitchen, J. M. (1996). *Rural homelessness: A synopsis in homelessness in America*. Washington, DC: Oryx Press.

Barclay, D. M., Richardson, J. P., and Fredman, L. (1995). Tuberculosis in the homeless. *Archives of Family Medicine*, 4(6):541.

Bassuk, E. L. (1984). The homeless problem. *Scientific American*, 251(1):40.

Bassuk, E. L. (1987). Homelessness. *Harvard Medical School of Mental Health*, 3(7):4.

Bernheim, K. (1990). Promoting family involvement in community residences for chronically mentally ill persons. *Hospital and Community Psychiatry*, 41:668.

Brunger, J. B. (1986). The young chronic client in mental health today. *Nursing Clinics of North America*, 21(3):451.

Carpenito, L. J. (1995). *Nursing diagnosis: Application to clinical practice* (6th ed.). Menlo Park, CA: J. B. Lippincott.

Carter, K. F., Green, R. D., Green, L., and Dufour, L. T. (1994). Health needs of homeless clients accessing nursing care at a free clinic. *Journal of Community Health Nursing*, 11(3):139.

Center for Mental Health Services (1995). *Making a difference—interim status report of the McKinney demonstration program for homeless adults with serious mental illness*. Rockville, MD: Center for Mental Health Services.

Church, H. C., and Barnett, G. O. (1994). Client-server, distributed database strategies in a health-care system for a homeless population. *Journal of American Medical Informatics Association*, 1(2):186.

Cohen, C. L. (1994). Down and out in New York and London: A cross-national comparison of homelessness. *Hospital and Community Psychiatry*, 45(8):769.

Damrosch, S., and Strasser, J. A. (1988). The homeless elderly in America. *Gerontological Nursing*, 14(10):26.

Drake, R. E., and Wallach, M. A. (1989). Substance abuse among the chronic mentally ill. *Hospital and Community Psychiatry*, 40(10):1041.

Grad, J., and Sainsbury, P. (1993). Mental illness and the family. *Lancet*, (1):544.

Grob, G. N. (1994). Mad, homeless and unwanted. A history of the care of the chronic mentally ill in America. *Psychiatric Clinics of North America*, 17(3):541.

Hays, R. D., et al. (1995). Functioning and well-being outcomes of patients with depression compared with chronic general medical illnesses. *Archives of General Psychiatry*, 52(1):11.

Interagency Council on the Homeless (1991). *Reaching out—A guide for service providers*. Washington, DC: Department of Housing and Urban Development.

Interagency Council on the Homeless (1994). *Priority: Home! The federal plan to break the cycle of homelessness*. Gaithersburg, MD: Department of Housing and Urban Development.

Janus, M. D., et al. (1995). Physical abuse in Canadian runaway adolescents. *Child Abuse and Neglect*, 19(4):433.

Jezewski, M. A. (1995) Staying connected: The core of facilitating health care for homeless persons. *Public Health Nursing*, 12(3):203.

J.O.C. (1988). Building a sense of community cooperation among agencies key to helping the homeless. *Psychiatric News*, 23(8):29.

Johnson, A. B. (1990). *Out of bedlam: The truth about deinstitutionalization.* New York: Basic Books.

Kipke, M. D., et al. (1995). Street youth in Los Angeles. Profile of a group at high risk for human immunodeficiency virus infection. *Archives of Pediatric and Adolescent Medicine*, 149(5):513.

Kozier, B., Erb, G., Blais, K., and Wilkinson, J. M. (1995). *Fundamentals of nursing: Concepts, process, and practice* (5th ed.). Menlo Park, CA: Addison-Wesley.

Lapierre, E. D., and Padgett, J. (1992). What does a nurse need to know and do to maintain an effective level of case management? *Journal of Psychosocial Nursing and Mental Health Services*, 30(3):35.

Lebow, J. M., et al. (1995). AIDS among the homeless of Boston: A cohort study. *Journal of Acquired Immune Deficiency Syndromes and Human Retrovirology*, 8(3):292.

Leshner, A. (1992). *Outcasts on Main Street: Report from the Federal Task Force on homelessness and severe mental illness.* Rockville, MD: National Institute of Mental Health.

Link, B. B., et al. (1994). Lifetime and five-year prevalence of homelessness in the United States. *American Journal of Public Health*, 84(12):1907.

Loukissa, D. A. (1995). Family burden in chronic mental illness: A review of research studies. *Journal of Advanced Nursing*, 21:248.

Martell, D. A., Rosner, R., and Harmon, R. B. (1995). Base-rate estimates of criminal behavior by homeless mentally ill persons in New York City. *Psychiatric Services*, 46(6):596.

McGowan, J. E., and Blumberg, H. M. (1995). Inner-city tuberculosis in the USA. *Journal of Hospital Infection*, June, 30 Suppl.:282.

Melzer, D., et al. (1991). Community care for patients with schizophrenia one year after hospital discharge. *British Medical Journal*, 303:1023.

Murray, R. L., and Baier, M. (1995). Evaluation of a transitional residential program for homeless chronically mentally ill people. *Journal of Psychiatric and Mental Health Nursing*, 2(1):3.

National Law Center on Homelessness and Poverty (1996). *Mean sweeps: A report on anti-homeless laws, litigation and alternatives in 50 United States cities.* Washington, DC: National Law Center on Homelessness and Poverty.

Norton, D., and Ridenour, N. (1995). Homeless women and children: The challenge of health promotion. *Nurse Practitioner Forum*, 6(1):29.

Parker, B. A. (1993). Living with mental illness: The family as caregiver. *Journal of Psychosocial Nursing*, 31(3):19.

Peternelj-Taylor, C. A., and Hartley, V. L. (1993). Living with mental illness: Professional-family collaboration. *Journal of Psychosocial Nursing*, 31(3):23.

Repper, J., Ford, R., and Cooke, A. (1994). How can nurses build trusting relationships with people who have severe and long-term mental health problems? Experiences of case managers and their clients. *Journal of Advanced Nursing*, 19:1096.

Riesdorf-Ostrow, W. (1989). The homeless chronically mentally ill. Deinstitutionalization: A public policy perspective. *Journal of Psychosocial Nursing*, 27(6):4.

Ryan, M. T. (1989). Providing shelter. *Journal of Psychosocial Nursing*, 27(6):15.

St. Lawrence, J. S., and Brasfield, T. L. (1995). HIV risk behavior among homeless adults. *AIDS Education and Prevention*, 7(1):22.

Thrasher, S. P., and Mowbray, C. T. (1995). A strengths perspective: An ethnographic study of homeless women with children. *Health and Social Work*, 20(2):93.

Vissing, Y. (1996). *Out of sight, out of mind: Homeless children and families in small town America.* Lexington, KY: University Press of Kentucky.

Waxman, L. (1994). *A status report on hunger and homelessness in America's cities.* Washington, DC: United States Conference of Mayors.

Williams, L. (1992). *Addiction on the street: Substance abuse and homelessness in America.* Washington, DC: National Coalition for the Homeless.

Worley, N. K., Drago, L., and Hadley, T. (1990). Improving the physical health–mental health interface for the chronically mentally ill: Could nurse case managers make a difference? *Archives of Psychiatric Nursing*, 4(2):108.

SELF-STUDY AND CRITICAL THINKING

Multiple choice questions

1. As a result of de-institutionalization, the primary source of care for the severely and persistently mentally ill shifted to the

   A. Home health agencies.
   B. Community-based outpatient programs.
   C. Reorganized inpatient facilities.
   D. Family.

2. Important areas to be emphasized by the nurse in educating families of the severely and persistently mentally ill include

   A. Coping skills to assist the family in dealing with the increased stress of caring for a family member at home.
   B. Knowledge regarding the disease process and treatment strategies.
   C. Safety issues and behavior management.
   D. Available resources for respite and day care.
   E. All of the above.

3. The cornerstone of treatment for successfully maintaining the severely and persistently mentally ill within the community is

   A. Intense psychotherapy.
   B. Referrals to appropriate community resources.
   C. Compliance with neuroleptic medication regimens.
   D. Support and respite for the family.

4. Mr. L. is very withdrawn upon admission and his nurse includes the diagnosis *impaired social interaction* in his care plan. Which of the following behaviors indicates the highest level of achievement of the goal "Mr. L. will improve social interaction as evidenced by participation in group sessions"?

   A. He said hello to all staff and peers as he entered the day room.
   B. He sat next to Mr. S. in group and smiled at him.
   C. Although Mr. L. had never done so before, he agreed to help prepare snacks for the evening party to celebrate a holiday.
   D. When the therapist worked with the group on life problems, Mr. L. said "How sad" after Mr. S. shared that his father had died last night.

5. Late one evening, the community mental health clinic nurse assesses a client's behaviors. Which one of the following would be least likely to warrant immediate consultation with the physician?

   A. New-onset frequent chewing movement
   B. Severe resting tremor
   C. Markedly increased liver function tests (LFTs)
   D. Complaints of dry mouth

6. Maggie is a 38-year-old homeless woman with an 18-year history of schizophrenia. She has not been seen by a physician or nurse practitioner for over a year. She comes to the hospital with complaints such as "I've got to get rid of this devil in me. He's growing bigger and bigger every day" and "Turn off the TV. It's just a brisablink." She is 8½ months' pregnant and has an upper respiratory infection. Which of the following would have the highest priority and warrant the most immediate interventions?

   A. Antenatal examination and care as well as close observation during hospitalization
   B. Job training and use of resources for sheltered employment
   C. Psychotherapy to explore the underlying emotional dynamics of Maggie's problems
   D. Social services consult for foster care and parenting classes

Critical thinking

7. Discuss the advantages of case management for the severely and persistently mentally ill person with at least two classmates.

8. Identify three burdens that families struggle with when caring for their severely and persistently mentally ill member. What are some potential interventions for these areas?

9. Write about four nursing considerations that you believe are most important when working with family members of a persistently mentally ill client.

10. Formulate a plan of care for the following client. Prioritize the nursing diagnoses, goals, and key interventions.

    Tim is 39 years old and was first diagnosed with schizophrenia 15 years ago. He has had several acute psychiatric hospitalizations since then. Over the years, he has been intermittently employed as a day laborer, but he has not worked at all for nearly 2 years. He lives on and off with his mother. Tim was admitted a few hours ago. He is agitated, suspicious, dirty, and emaciated. He paces the halls, occasionally leaning against the wall and closing his eyes for a moment.

Formulate two nursing diagnoses and one outcome criterion and one short-term goal for each nursing diagnosis. Formulate a plan of action (intervention) and give the rationale for at least three interventions.

1. Nursing Diagnosis

____

____

OUTCOME CRITERIA	SHORT-TERM GOAL
______	______
______	______
______	______

INTERVENTION	RATIONALE
1. ______	1. ______
______	______
2. ______	2. ______
______	______
3. ______	3. ______
______	______
4. ______	4. ______
______	______

2. Nursing Diagnosis

____

____

OUTCOME CRITERIA	SHORT-TERM GOAL
______	______
______	______
______	______

INTERVENTION	RATIONALE
1. ______	1. ______
______	______
2. ______	2. ______
______	______
3. ______	3. ______
______	______
4. ______	4. ______
______	______

28

Psychosocial Issues of People with Physical Illness

MICHELLE CONANT DAN-EL

OUTLINE

KEY TERMS AND CONCEPTS

The key terms and concepts listed here also appear in bold where they are defined or discussed in this chapter.

"worried well"
psychosomatic
psychophysiological disorders
psychological factors affecting medical condition
somatization
body language
conversion
hypochondriasis
malingering
pain-prone
accident-prone
surgery-prone
primary gain of illness
secondary gain of illness
enmeshment
overprotectiveness
rigidity
lack of conflict resolution
general adaptation syndrome
neurotransmitters
alternative healing
therapeutic touch
coping styles
psychiatric nurse liaison

OBJECTIVES

After studying this chapter, the reader will be able to

1. Describe behaviors associated with the most common emotional and psychological responses to physical illness.
2. Discuss the connections between mind and body in terms of the body's responses to stress, using leading stress theories.
3. Discuss the potential uses and rationale of therapeutic touch, relaxation training, and teaching coping skills by nurses.
4. Perform a holistic (psycho-social-spiritual) nursing assessment.
5. Apply knowledge of psychiatric disorders to clients in nonpsychiatric settings.
6. Identify situations in which consultation with a psychiatric nursing liaison is useful.
7. Apply theories of grieving to clients experiencing physical losses.

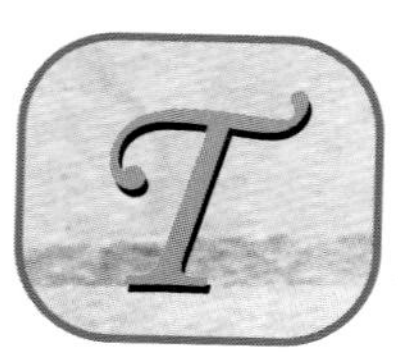

The nurse's view of the individual as a complex blend of many parts has contributed to the multifaceted role of professional nurses. Because other health care professionals have a more specific focus for their practice, nurses have taken on the task of case management, which mandates that nurses maintain a holistic view of the individual. Nurses who care for people with physical illnesses who are receiving physical treatments need to maintain a holistic view that involves an awareness of psycho-social-cultural and spiritual issues (Dossey et al 1995). Further challenging nurses is the plethora of new, alternative therapies that focus on the need for a harmonious relationship between the mind and the body (Dossey et al 1995). People are pursuing these therapies because they are becoming better-educated consumers of the health care system and are demanding that providers treat them as whole persons rather than just as a diagnosis.

Nurses practice in a variety of health care settings and intervene for a wide range of human responses. In this chapter, theories from other chapters of this text are applied to several situations encountered by nurses in emergency departments, inpatient units, nursing homes, and client homes, among others. It is not possible to address every type of situation since each individual is unique, but by using Figures 28–1 and 28–2 as guides, it is possible to see patterns that emerge in persons who experience similar losses. Figure 28–1 looks at commonalities among people with physical illness, and Figure 28–2 identifies commonalities in people who have had surgery or a treatment procedure.

A mentally healthy person who experiences psycho-social-cultural-spiritual problems as a result of a situational crisis is sometimes referred to as one of the **"worried well."** Usually, some time-limited crisis intervention or brief supportive counseling is sufficient to bolster their already adequate coping skills until the crisis is past. However, when the situational crisis is a persistent life-threatening or disabling disease, or when a permanent change occurs in the person's situation, long-term interventions may be required.

It is often the nurse who observes and assesses these problems, makes the appropriate referrals, and monitors the client's overall progress. The psychiatric nurse liaison is an important support for nurses who care for clients with psychosocial problems. In addition to helping the nurse identify a nursing diagnosis and recommending interventions, the nurse liaison can support the staff by helping them to deal with their feelings of frustration, hopelessness, sadness, or fear that may be elicited by these clients.

PSYCHOLOGICAL RESPONSES TO PHYSICAL ILLNESS

Among the most common emotional and psychological responses to physical illness are depression, fear, denial, anxiety, anger, withdrawal, apathy, regression, dependency, and self-centeredness.

Anxiety accompanies every illness, especially when pain, disability, hospitalization, economic loss, or fear of death is present. Verbalizing is an effective outlet for anxiety, but the ability to verbalize may be compromised by cultural expectations, disability, or lack of a listener. Helplessness often accompanies anxiety in the person who feels a loss of control over events, such as when awaiting surgery and undergoing invasive treatments. In this case, defense mechanisms may be used with greater frequency, or compulsive behaviors may surface. Self-centeredness, characterized by unreasonable requests of caregivers, may also be a cover for feelings of inadequacy or worthlessness.

At 27, Ted tests positive for human immunodeficiency virus (HIV). During the posttest counseling session at

PHYSICAL ILLNESS	LOSSES—REAL OR PERCEIVED
Alopecia Alzheimer's disease HIV disease Severe burns Cancer COPD Post CVA Hemophilia Post MI Crohn's disease Multiple sclerosis Diabetes mellitus Parkinson's disease AIDS dementia	▸ Active life style ▸ Self-esteem ▸ Change in socioeconomic status ▸ Productive role in family ▸ Decision-making power ▸ Ability to think rationally ▸ Ability to communicate clearly ▸ Ability to enjoy previous range of activities ▸ Feeling of security ▸ Previous future goals ▸ Friends

RELATED NURSING DIAGNOSIS		ETIOLOGY		MEASURABLE/ OBSERVABLE SIGNS/SYMPTOMS
Caregiver role strain, risk for	→	Psychological or cognitive problems in care receiver	→	Stress or nervousness in relationship with care receiver
Communication; impaired verbal	→	▸ Decrease in circulation to brain ▸ Psychosis	→	▸ Refusal/inability to speak ▸ Loose association/ flight of ideas
Coping; ineffective family, compromised or disabling Coping; ineffective individual	→	▸ Family disorganization and role changes ▸ Highly ambivalent family relationships ▸ Inadequate coping method	→	▸ Intolerance/rejection ▸ Abandonment ▸ Hostility/aggression ▸ Agitation ▸ Inappropriate use of defense mechanisms ▸ Destructive behavior to self and others
Decisional conflict re: institutionalization of family member	→	▸ Perceived threat to value system ▸ Disagreement among family members	→	▸ Vacillation/delayed decision making ▸ Increased stress on family members
Disuse syndrome, risk for	→	▸ Fear of creating pain ▸ Fear of injury	→	▸ Further deterioration of body systems
Family process altered	→	Situational crisis	→	▸ Family system unable to meet physical/spiritual needs of members
Grieving; anticipatory or dysfunctional	→	▸ Perceived potential loss of 1. Significant other 2. Physiopsychosocial well-being 3. Personal possessions ▸ Chronic fatal illness ▸ Thwarted response to a loss ▸ Lack of resolution of previous loss	→	▸ Denial of potential loss ▸ Guilt ▸ Sorrow ▸ Anger ▸ Choked feelings ▸ Altered sleep/eating/sexual patterns ▸ Developmental regression ▸ Labile mood ▸ Poor concentration
Health maintenance: altered	→	▸ Perceptual/cognitive impairment ▸ Lack of gross/fine motor skills	→	▸ Lack of adaptive behaviors ▸ Lack of support system

Figure 28–1 Commonalities among people with physical illness. HIV, human immunodeficiency disease; COPD, chronic obstructive pulmonary disease; CVA, cerebrovascular accident; MI, myocardial infarction.

the health department by the public health nurse, Ted is given information regarding the virus and referrals. The nurse notes that Ted is having difficulty focusing on details and needs to have information repeated several times as he writes copious notes. The nurse gives Ted the opportunity to explore feelings, but Ted has difficulty in this area because he was raised to believe that dealing with crisis alone is a strength. Ted is also experiencing a great deal of denial in this initial period of loss (see the discussion about the stages of death and dying in Chapter 20). For these reasons, the nurse anticipates the most common and immediate concerns that might be facing a person who has just discovered that he is HIV positive and gently leads Ted into discussing those concerns over a period of several weeks, with the use of reflective statements and silence. This approach gives Ted the opportunity to verbalize his anxieties in a safe environment.

SURGERY/ TREATMENT PROCEDURE	LOSSES—REAL OR PERCEIVED	RELATED NURSING DIAGNOSIS	ETIOLOGY	MEASURABLE/ OBSERVABLE SIGNS/SYMPTOMS
Respirator/ventilator Hemodialysis, peritoneal dialysis Chemotherapy Colostomy/nephrostomy Mastectomy Amputation Radical neck/facial surgery Hysterectomy Prostatectomy Transsexual surgery Posttransplant (hepatic-renal-cardiac)	▸ Control of bodily functions ▸ Independence, self-determination ▸ Health/life ▸ Physical attractiveness ▸ Sexual role ▸ Positive body image ▸ Reproductive power ▸ Positive self-regard ▸ Decreased stimulation in daily activity ▸ Loss of valued beliefs	Ineffective management of therapeutic regimen →	▸ Impaired cognitive or emotional functioning ▸ Mistrust of regimen/provider ▸ Family patterns of health care →	▸ Acceleration of symptoms ▸ Verbalized feelings of hopelessness in client and caregiver
		Impaired home maintenance management →	▸ Insufficient family organization and planning ▸ Inadequate support systems →	▸ Exhaustion and tension in family members ▸ Increased arguments
		Impaired physical mobility →	▸ Depression or severe anxiety ▸ Decreased strength or endurance ▸ Pain or discomfort ▸ Perceptual or cognitive impairment →	▸ Reluctance to attempt movement ▸ Limited range of motion ▸ Inability to move purposely
		Social isolation → Altered sexuality pattern →	▸ Need to plan life around treatment ▸ Need to spend several hours/day in treatment ▸ Need for machines (respirator/ventilation) ▸ Alteration in physical appearance ▸ Unaccepted social values ▸ Inability to engage in satisfying personal relationships →	▸ Sad, dull affect ▸ Withdrawn/preoccupied ▸ Hostile voice and behavior ▸ Exists in subculture ▸ Insecurity in public ▸ Limitations or changes in sexual patterns
		Spiritual distress →	▸ Challenged belief and value system ▸ Separation from religious and cultural ties →	▸ Anger toward God ▸ Questions meaning of life/death/suffering
		Body image disturbance →	▸ Deformity from surgery ▸ Physical changes from aesthetic or transgender surgery ▸ Phantom limb pain ▸ Hair loss from chemotherapy ▸ Emaciation from "wasting syndrome" →	▸ Refusal to be seen by others ▸ Verbalization of shame of appearance ▸ Preoccupation with body parts ▸ Refusal to engage in sexual behavior
		Fear (of death) →	▸ Real or imagined prognosis →	▸ Signs of any or all stages of death and dying

Figure 28–2 Commonalities among people who have undergone surgery/treatment procedures.

SURGERY/ TREATMENT PROCEDURE	LOSSES—REAL OR PERCEIVED	RELATED NURSING DIAGNOSIS	ETIOLOGY	MEASURABLE/ OBSERVABLE SIGNS/SYMPTOMS
Respirator/ventilator Hemodialysis, peritoneal dialysis Chemotherapy Colostomy/nephrostomy Mastectomy Amputation Radical neck/facial surgery Hysterectomy Prostatectomy Transsexual surgery Posttransplant (hepatic-renal-cardiac)	◗ Control of bodily functions ◗ Independence, self-determination ◗ Health/life ◗ Physical attractiveness ◗ Sexual role ◗ Positive body image ◗ Reproductive power ◗ Positive self-regard ◗ Decreased stimulation in daily activity ◗ Loss of valued beliefs	Powerlessness →	◗ "Out of control" bodily changes ◗ Treatments or effects of surgery ◗ Loss of options or fewer alternatives ◗ Dependency on machines or treatment for survival or pain relief →	◗ Verbalization of hopelessness ◗ Passivity ◗ Dependence resulting in anger/irritability ◗ Apathy ◗ Does not participate in treatment
		Anxiety →	◗ Threat of death ◗ Situational crisis ◗ Unmet needs ◗ Threat to self-concept →	◗ Tearfulness ◗ Complaints of fatigue ◗ Anger
		Diversional activity deficit →	◗ Lack of stimuli in environment ◗ Prolonged hospitalization ◗ Frequent, time-consuming treatments →	◗ Boredom ◗ Restlessness ◗ Verbalization of missing usual hobbies

Figure 28–2 *(Continued)* Commonalities among people who have undergone surgery/treatment procedures.

NURSING DIAGNOSIS

Anxiety related to	◗ Threat of death ◗ Change in health status ◗ Interpersonal transmission and contagiousness ◗ Threat to self-concept
Manifested by	◗ Difficulty concentrating ◗ Inability to verbalize feelings

Some persons who are experiencing a major depressive episode (see Chapter 20) use somatic complaints to mask the symptoms commonly found with the diagnosis of depression. For example, insomnia and anorexia may be indicative of depression or chronic pain. Vague and generalized physical complaints may be a way of seeking relief for feelings of depression. Fatigue may be attributed to any one of several physical conditions when it is actually a low-energy level of depression. Unfortunately, some depressed people may be more comfortable with a physical diagnosis, and so they approach health care providers to seek treatment for such diagnoses. A study of "somatizers" referred for psychiatric consultation found that 45% had a major depression (Katon 1984).

Another problem in recognizing major depression concerns persons with neurological diseases (Table 28–1). Poor concentration, memory loss, apathy, and difficulty making decisions are characteristics often seen in some neurological disorders as well as in major clinical depression or dysthymic disorder (Robinson and Asnis 1989). Many medications as well as medical disorders may create or exacerbate a clinical depression. Medications that may trigger depression include some antihypertensives, corticosteroids, narcotics, and hormonal agents (e.g., estrogen, progesterone). Medical disorders related to depression include cardiovascular disease, viral infections,

Table 28–1 NEUROLOGICAL DISORDERS/ DEPRESSION

NEUROLOGICAL DISORDERS (FREQUENCY OF DEPRESSION)	SIGNS OF DEPRESSION OR NEUROLOGICAL DISORDER
Epilepsy (30%–60%) Stroke (50%) Trauma (30%) Tumors (20%) Multiple sclerosis (30%) Parkinson's disease (40%) Huntington's disease (35%) Wilson's disease (20%) HIV encephalopathy (30%) Alzheimer's disease (40%) Vascular dementia (40%) Lewy body disease (20%)	Memory loss Apathy Anhedonia Poor concentration Sleep disturbance Reduced energy Low self-esteem Feelings of hopelessness Guilt Psychomotor retardation Hypophonia Agitation Irritability Suicidal ideation Psychosis Mania Tearfulness

Modified from Cummings, J. L. (1994). Depression in neurological diseases. *Psychiatric Annals*, 24(10):525–531.
HIV, human immunodeficiency virus.

neoplastic disease, neurological conditions, and rheumatoid arthritis.

Furthermore, aphasia or dementia makes it difficult for the person to communicate feelings of hopelessness, guilt, or low self-esteem that are commonly experienced with depression. Lability of affect (e.g., tearfulness mingled with periods of elation) is commonly seen with some cases of cognitive impairment disorders but could cause the person to be mislabeled as being clinically depressed. Sometimes, the use of antidepressants is recommended in order to see if a change in mental status occurs before a diagnosis can be made.

◗ Emma, a 64-year-old woman, had a cardiovascular accident that left her with global aphasia. She has been experiencing frequent and prolonged periods of tearfulness, alternating with periods of loud screaming and physical assault on the caregivers in the nursing home. She appears "wide-eyed" and apprehensive toward strangers. The clinical nurse specialist, who acts as a psychiatric liaison to the nursing home staff, has found it difficult to assess Emma for depression because her sleep and nutrition patterns are adequate and unchanged and Emma cannot be tested by use of standard cognitive tests. The clinical nurse specialist recommends a trial of antidepressants as well as a major tranquilizer combined with close study of the patterns of Emma's behavior to assess for changes in the environment that might relieve her extreme mood swings. The staff is made aware of Emma's need for a consistent activity schedule and monitoring of vital signs as well as frequent reorientation to her surroundings.

NURSING DIAGNOSIS

Fear related to	◗ Language barrier ◗ Loss of physical support
Manifested by	◗ Attack behavior ◗ Wide-eyed appearance ◗ Aggressiveness

Responses to being dependent might be exhibited as inability to accept warmth, nurturing, or tenderness from caregivers or as refusal to accept treatment or medical advice. This reaction is strongest in those who have unmet dependency needs or who have had negative experiences when help was sought in the past. Anger at caregivers may mask acute embarrassment over being in a dependent position by one who needs to project an independent image.

Others find themselves becoming fearful of not having dependency needs met and do not express any negative feelings to caregivers. These people need to be "good" clients for fear that they will be abandoned if perceived to be difficult. Any anxiety or anger they suppress may be exhibited through increased somatic complaints.

◗ Lillian is a 47-year-old woman who is being treated with hemodialysis and has been complaining of frequent tension headaches and occasional stomach upsets before her treatment appointments. The hemodialysis nurse has always been impressed by Lillian's patience and compliant attitude in spite of her debilitating illness, which has robbed her of a "normal" family life. For this reason, the nurse suspects that Lillian's physical complaints could be a way for her to deal with other emotions, so the nurse makes a point of spending more time with Lillian to allow her to talk about her frustrations. Lillian expresses anger and some feelings of hopelessness. She resents others who are "healthy," including the people who care for her. Frequent opportunities to verbalize these feelings gradually result in the lessening of her somatic complaints and decrease her sense of powerlessness and isolation.

NURSING DIAGNOSIS

Denial related to	◗ Fear of alienating caregivers
Manifested by	◗ Increased somatization ◗ Overcompliant behavior ◗ Denied admission of invalidism

As an unconscious defense mechanism, denial is a common response to physical illness. The person may believe that the pain is "really nothing" (even though it is severe and lasts for long periods) or may minimize dramatic bodily changes. Even after hearing a diagnosis with a poor prognosis, the person in denial may hear only the more positive or hopeful message and may block out the negative. This is a protective measure used by the person and is necessary in the early stages of loss but can interfere with treatment if it continues for too long. When a person minimizes physical complaints, the nursing staff may unwittingly collude with the person in the denial by not performing a complete assessment and accept the person's subjective statements at face value.

◗ After a car accident, Carol is being assessed by the triage nurse in the emergency department for possible injuries. She complains of a "slight headache and dizziness" but denies having any other pain or symptoms. Carol is preoccupied with seeing that her 2-year-old son, who was also in the car, is being examined, so she denies her own need for medical attention. Carol's blood pressure is 86/50 mm Hg, and her body posture indicates that she is guarding her abdomen. These observations are reported to the examining physician immediately, because they indicate possible internal bleeding and danger of shock. Carol is eventually taken to the operating room to stop the bleeding.

NURSING DIAGNOSIS

Denial related to	▸ Need to reduce anxiety
Manifested by	▸ Delay in perceiving physical distress ▸ Minimization of symptoms

These examples of psychological responses to physical illness reflect but a few of the many possible responses the nurse can expect to encounter in practice in a variety of health care settings. Application of psychiatric nursing concepts to the behaviors of persons who are experiencing the stress of a physical illness requires a careful study of these concepts as well as listening and observation skills.

PHYSICAL ILLNESS AS A PSYCHOLOGICAL RESPONSE

For more than 100 years, the term **psychosomatic** has been used to describe some physical conditions that are thought to be stress related. The specific type of stress, the personality style, the psychological make-up, and the environmental factors that combine to create psychosomatic disorders are still being studied and debated. The term psychosomatic was updated to **psychophysiological disorders** in DSM-II. With DSM-III, a substantial change in terminology occurred. DSM-III developed a category called *psychological factors affecting physical conditions.* This category has been retained in DSM-IV. Figure 28–3 provides DSM-IV diagnostic criteria for **psychological factors affecting medical conditions.** Psychological or behavioral factors play a role in the symptoms or treatment of almost every general medical condition. However, this DSM-IV category applies to those conditions in which psychological factors have a clinically significant effect on the course or the outcome of the disease (APA 1994). Psychological or behavioral factors can affect almost any major disease (e.g., cardiovascular conditions, gastrointestinal conditions, neoplastic conditions, neurological, and pulmonary, renal, and rheumatological conditions).

Somatization is a physiological manifestation of a person's emotions. It may be a physical complaint occurring at a time when feelings are conscious, such as severe headaches during periods of acute grief. It may also be a defense against conscious awareness of emotional conflict, such as chronic back pain whenever a particular conflict is surfacing. An example of one type of conflict is dependence versus independence. Somatization is experienced by everyone to some degree. An example of this is seen with the fight-or-flight response, discussed in Chapter 13, which is experienced during periods of high anxiety. These responses include perspiration, pallor, palpitations, or tremors. When physical responses are a primary reaction to emotional situations and occur with enough intensity over a long duration, they may lead to permanent organic changes. We call these changes *psychophysiological disorders.* Some common idiomatic expressions of mind-body interactions are

- "That turns my stomach."
- "He is a pain in the neck."
- "My heart is breaking."
- "I feel empty inside."

Even the term **body language** was coined to describe the ability of the person to display emotions to the astute observer through various body movements and postures. Conversion, hypochondriasis, and malingering, discussed in Chapter 18, are all phenomena that involve the body in some way. **Conversion** is the channeling of anxiety into a physical symptom that has no organic basis and for which the individual does not usually display appropriate concern or distress. **Hypochondriasis** is the preoccupation with an imagined illness for which no observable symptoms or organic changes exist. **Malingering** is deliberately falsification of an illness for a definite purpose.

Example of conversion	Mary became blind after witnessing an accident in which a good friend died.
Example of hypochondriasis	John sought treatment from several physicians for cancer, although he exhibited no objective or observable signs of an illness and does not have a significant family history of cancer.
Example of malingering	Sam sought frequent admissions to psychiatric units, informing the staff that he hears voices telling him to kill himself. He knows that he will be admitted if he states this to the admitting physician, and he needs a record of hospital admissions to receive disability payments.

Some maladaptive coping patterns that are manifested over a long time but are exhibited more as behavioral patterns or styles than symptoms are pain-proneness, accident-proneness, and surgery-proneness. The underlying dynamic involved in clients who manifest these tendencies is the presence of strong dependency needs and early learning experiences that reinforced these patterns in spite of the loss of quality of life.

Underlying guilt and need to self-punish may be a part of the person's unconscious. In conversion and hypochondriasis, the psychological influences are unconscious, and the fact that they are unconscious reinforces their power. Intervention is aimed at awareness of unconscious conflicts and needs during long-term treatment. Relaxation techniques are taught so that the client can interrupt these patterns. Cognitive and behavioral approaches may also be used. Malingering, on the other hand, is conscious and

Psychological Factors Affecting Medical Conditions

A. A general medical condition (coded on Axis III) is present.

B. Psychological factors adversely affect the general medical condition in one of the following ways:
1. The factors have influenced the course of the general medical condition as shown by a close temporal association between the psychological factors and the development or exacerbation of, or delayed recovery from, the general medical condition
2. The factors interfere with the treatment of the general medical condition
3. The factors constitute additional health risks for the individual
4. Stress-related physiological responses precipitate or exacerbate symptoms of the general medical condition

Choose the name on the basis of the nature of the psychological factors (if more than one factor is present, indicate the most prominent):

Mental Disorder Affecting . . . *[Indicate the General Medical Condition]* (e.g., an Axis I disorder such as major depressive disorder delaying recovery from a myocardial infarction)

Psychological Symptoms Affecting . . . *[Indicate the General Medical Condition]* (e.g., depressive symptoms delaying recovery from surgery; anxiety exacerbating asthma)

Personality Traits or Coping Style Affecting . . . *[Indicate the General Medical Condition]* (e.g., pathological denial of the need for surgery in a patient with cancer; hostile, pressured behavior contributing to cardiovascular disease)

Maladaptive Health Behaviors Affecting . . . *[Indicate the General Medical Condition]* (e.g., overeating; lack of exercise; unsafe sex)

Stress-Related Physiological Response Affecting . . . *[Indicate the General Medical Condition]* (e.g., stress-related exacerbations of ulcer, hypertension, arrhythmia, or tension headache)

Other Unspecified Psychological Factors Affecting . . . *[Indicate the General Medical Condition]* (e.g., interpersonal, cultural, or religious factors)

Figure 28–3 DSM-IV criteria for psychological factors affecting medical conditions. (From American Psychiatric Association (1994). *Diagnostic and statistical manual of mental disorders (DSM-IV)* (4th ed.). Washington, DC: American Psychiatric Association. Reprinted with permission. Copyright 1994 American Psychiatric Association.)

is used to manipulate and extract some sort of gain (often monetary).

The **pain-prone** person, or one who experiences psychogenic pain, tends to have a history of complaints of pain in the absence of illness. The pain may serve as punishment for guilt regarding repressed hostility. It also serves the function of eliciting nurturance from others in the form of pain relief. These persons tend to avoid or deny conflicts and unpleasant emotions and are lacking in insight. Verbalizing painful emotions is a first step toward breaking the cycle of experiencing physical pain to avoid emotional pain.

- Laura, age 34, has been hospitalized for chronic back pain, from which she has experienced only brief periods of relief by using pain medications and frequent chiropractic visits. The source of her pain has never been identified, in spite of the extensive diagnostic testing and visits to specialists.
- During a psychosocial assessment by the psychiatric nurse liaison, Laura describes a pattern of frequent corporal punishment by her mother. As a child, when Laura would cry loudly after a spanking, her mother would hold her until she felt better. Otherwise, she describes her mother's interaction as being distant or uninvolved.

The **accident-prone** person has been described as one who has a pattern of accidents that are actually self-inflicted injuries because the need to self-punish is present, although unconscious. A conflict involving aggression and a need for dependency seems to be present. The client may also have a wish to escape a life situation in an acceptable manner, rather than with an overt refusal. It is an abdication of responsibility. Accident-prone people are thought to be impulsive and have a low tolerance for frustration and impaired control over anger.

▶ Over the past 3 years, Dan has been involved in six auto accidents, the last being the most serious. The local emergency department staff sees the pattern and refers Dan to the crisis unit for a psychosocial evaluation. Dan is found to be suffering from feelings of depression with occasional thoughts of "dying," but he denies having any active suicidal ideation. Dan's "accidents" began shortly after the birth of his son, and Dan expresses concern about his ability to handle his responsibilities as a father and manager of a local supermarket because of his injuries.

Surgery-prone persons undergo numerous operations for the same symptoms, with unsatisfactory results. In the short term, the client has symptom relief, but until the underlying dynamics are addressed, new symptoms requiring more surgery appear. The dynamics of surgery-proneness may involve a masochistic need to suffer for unconscious guilt. Often, the client has a family history of frequent illnesses with surgical intervention. Surgery-prone persons are able to repeat this cycle by persistently demanding surgery of physicians who are unaware of this syndrome.

▶ Pat, a 30-year-old woman, complains of pain and diarrhea that have lasted for several months. A series of tests does not reveal any organic cause, but exploratory surgery is performed. A few months after the operation, Pat complains that her symptoms are worse, and she is scheduled for a subtotal gastrectomy. For 2 years after the surgery, Pat's symptoms grow worse in spite of special diet and medication. The underlying dynamics of Pat's physical complaints and surgery-seeking behavior come to light when she is evaluated by a crisis nurse after a suicide attempt.

The **primary gain** of a psychosomatic disorder is anxiety reduction or control by keeping the source of the anxiety suppressed or repressed. **Secondary gains** are unconsciously sought and can vary with the individual. Secondary gains include getting out of responsibilities, manipulating people in the environment, and getting attention. When obtained, secondary gains reinforce the use of somatization and becomes stronger. Refer to Chapter 18.

▶ Mary, aged 34, develops ulcerative colitis shortly after her marriage. Psychoanalytic theory explains this as an unconscious expression of her dependency needs. In response to Mary's illness, her husband has curtailed his activities outside the home in order to spend more time with his wife, who is often in severe pain. Mary now experiences the secondary gains of controlling her husband's actions and having her dependency needs met. Mary is not aware of the functions served by her colitis.

Minuchin (1978), a renowned family therapist, identified four characteristics of a *psychosomatic family.* This is a family in which repression and somatization are frequently used as defense mechanisms and reinforced by the family system. These characteristics are **enmeshment, overprotectiveness, rigidity,** and **lack of conflict resolution.** Refer to Chapter 11.

Enmeshed families have poorly differentiated boundaries and intense family interactions and are characterized by excessive intrusiveness and lack of privacy for its members. Examples of this would be opening other people's mail, failing to knock on doors before entering, or lack of locks on bathroom doors.

Overprotectiveness impedes the development of independence and individuation, which leads to feelings of powerlessness. Overprotective families shield children from unpleasant realities or make decisions for others in order to "spare" them any anxieties. The hallmark of *rigid* families is the need to avoid change or to maintain the status quo for fear of "losing control." One way of avoiding change is to avoid conflict or to ignore conflict. Because of this stance taken by the family, conflict resolution is not learned. An example of this might be to deny marital problems for fear of eventual divorce.

A psychosomatic disorder in one member may serve a secondary gain for the family, such as regulating the family system.

▶ Lisa, a 14-year-old high school student, develops anorexia nervosa at a time when her parents are facing a marital crisis. The decision to separate is postponed until "Lisa's problem" can be resolved. In this way, Lisa's parents find a secondary gain from her anorexia by using it to avoid conflict resolution.

Stress is an energy that a *stressor* or stimulus creates in an organism and that can result in a variety of responses. Some of these responses may result in psychosomatic disorders. Stressors may be internal, such as conflicts and needs, or external. Both internal and external stressors operate simultaneously. An example of this is a person who has a dependence-independence conflict and has experienced the loss of a significant relationship in which the basic dependency needs were met. When both types of stressors converge to create physiological responses that lead to physical illness, the illness is called psychosomatic.

Stress has been defined by Selye, in his **general adaptation syndrome,** as a phenomenon that, combined with hormonal changes, results in disease. Selye believed that a specific stressor could not be linked to a specific response (see Chapter 13).

Another area of research in the field of psychosomatic medicine involves chemical substances in the central nervous system known as **neurotransmitters.** At least 30 known neurotransmitters exist, and understanding the effects of stress on these chemicals will shed light on the impact of emotional stress on the body. As described in Chapter 3, neurotransmitters act as a bridge between the mind and body by relaying information between neurons. Different parts of the brain contain specific types of neurons with specific functions, and they release specific neurotransmitters. The messages determine brain functioning, which, in turn, determines body movement, feelings, and thinking. It is also being speculated that these substances could explain problems with the immune system.

Jenkins (1984) proposed that five variables exist that must be taken into account in order to understand psychosomatic illness completely. He believed that simple cause and effect between two variables was only one piece of the puzzle. These variables are (Table 28–2)

- Adaptive capacity.
- Stressor.
- Alarm reaction.
- Defensive reaction.
- Pathological reaction.

Nursing interventions for psychosomatic disorders are aimed at relieving physical symptoms while reducing

TABLE 28–2 INTERACTION OF STRESS AND THE ORGANISM

LEVEL	ADAPTIVE CAPACITY	STRESSORS	ALARM REACTION	DEFENSIVE REACTION	PATHOLOGICAL END-STATE
Biological	State of physique, nutrition, vigor Natural or acquired immunities	Deprivation of biological needs Excess inputs of physical or biological agents	Arousal—hunger, thirst, pain, fatigue Changes in physiological function	General adaptation syndrome Physiological compensation Shifts in metabolism Changes in pain threshold	Deficiency diseases "Exhaustion" Addictions Chronic dysfunction Structural damage
Psychological	Resourcefulness, problem-solving ability Ego strength Flexibility Social skills	Perceptions and interpretations of danger, threat, loss, disappointment, frustration, or sense of failure or hopelessness Loss of self-acceptance Threat to security	Feelings of deprivation—boredom, grief, sadness Feelings of anxiety, pressure, guilt Fear of danger	Ego defenses—denial, repression, projection Defensive neuroses Perceptual defenses—wishes, fantasies, motives Planning Problem solving	Despair, apathy Chronic personality pattern disturbances Psychoses Chronic affective disorders Meaninglessness
Interpersonal	Primary relationships including family Network of social supports	Social isolation Lack of acceptance Insults, punishments, rejections Changes in social groups, especially losses	Antagonism, conflict, suspicion Withdrawal Feelings of rejection, punishment	Defensive, rigid social relating Avoidance Assuming sick role Aggressiveness "Acting out" Enlisting social supports	Chronic exploitation Becoming an outcast Imprisonment Permanent disruption of interpersonal ties Chronic failure to fulfill roles
Sociocultural	Values Norms and practices "Therapeutic" social institutions Systems of knowledge and technology	Cultural change Role conflict Status incongruity Value conflicts with important others Forced change in life situation	Communication of concern and alarm Expressive behavior of crowds Mobilization of social structures	Culturally prescribed defenses—scapegoating, prejudice Explanatory ideologies Legal and moral systems Use of curers and institutions	Alienation, anomie Breakdown of social order Disintegration of the cultural systems of values and norms

Modified from Jenkins, D. (1984). A model depicting the interaction of stress and the organism. In P. D. Barry, (Ed.), *Psychosocial nursing assessment and intervention* (p. 106). Philadelphia: J. B. Lippincott.

stress. Since these disorders cause actual organ damage and may be life threatening, symptom reduction is the primary target for intervention. These interventions have traditionally been based on the practices of modern Western medicine. A growing interest in ancient healing practices from other cultures, particularly from the East, has provided a plethora of holistic adjunct and alternatives. Continued nursing research into these forms of **alternative healing** are taking place in many health care settings. One form of alternative healing that is practiced by nurses is **therapeutic touch.** Barnett and Chambers (1996) presented sound rationales for the inclusion of adjunct and alternative forms of healing in the treatment of psychosomatic disorders:

> When we view the human being as a dynamic energy system, we realize that health is not a static goal. As current research suggests that the world we see is more than just matter, and the body is more than just a collection of functioning parts, there is increased curiosity about subtle energy and the role it plays in healing. With increasing interest in the mind's influence on bodily health, credible medical experts (such as Herbert Benson, Joan Borysenko, Deepak Chopra, Barbara and Larry Dossey, David Eisenberg, Richard Gerber, Jon Kabat-Zinn, Ted Kaptchuk, Christine Northrup, Mehmet Oz, Bernie Siegel, and Andrew Weil) are leading the efforts to articulate a new way of viewing the mind/body relationship. Alternative medicine, a topic once confined to health-food stores and new-age venues, is now the subject of television and radio shows and books on the best-seller lists.
>
> Several leading causes of death, including heart disease, stroke, and cancer, are largely preventable by changing behaviors. However, due to a scientific paradigm that has traditionally applied surgical and pharmaceutical "solutions" to health problems, modern medicine has, to date, inadequately addressed lifestyle-related illnesses. Only recently have physicians begun to recognize that there are other important determinants of health.
>
> The importance of relationship is beginning to be spoken about by some visionaries in the health-care field. And recent research findings have strongly suggested that psychosocial factors play a much more significant role in health than has ever been previously understood. Slowly it is being recognized that the way we think and feel—whether we feel cared for and nurtured and have a sense of meaning in life—has an effect on the course of the disease.

Treatment and intervention for psychosomatic disorders occur on two levels because these disorders are physical but are affected by psychological factors. Physiological symptoms vary with each disorder and each individual, and a discussion of this is not within the scope of this chapter. Table 28–3 provides a list of common diseases that can be exacerbated by stress. The table includes the hypothesized personality traits that were once thought to be common to each disorder, but this hypothesis was subsequently not backed up by research. Also included in this table are the biological correlates, common precipatory factors, and nonmedical therapies. Nursing interventions that address the psychological issues underlying these disorders often address

- Behavioral changes.
- Anxiety levels.
- Cognitive changes.

The desired outcome is a reduction of physical symptoms to a manageable level in the short term and a basic change that will enable the individual to deal with emotion in a healthier way in the long term.

Relaxation training can be accomplished through progressive relaxation, meditation or yoga, hypnosis, biofeedback, or autogenic training. The purpose of relaxation training is to lower anxiety levels; this leads to a reduction of somatic complaints (see Chapter 13).

Teaching **coping styles** involves changing the way a person thinks about stressors in order to change the way a person responds to stress. Weisman (1984) identified both effective and not so effective coping styles seen in people with medical problems:

1. Seek information; get guidance.*
2. Share concern; find consolation.*
3. Laugh it off; change emotional tone.
4. Forget it happened; put it out of your mind.
5. Keep busy; distract yourself.*
6. Confront the issue; act accordingly.*
7. Redefine; take a more sanguine view.*
8. Resign yourself; make the best of what cannot be changed.
9. Do something, anything, perhaps exceeding good judgment.
10. Review alternatives; examine consequences.
11. Get away from it all; find an escape, somehow.†
12. Conform, comply; do what is expected or advised.*
13. Blame or shame someone, something.†
14. Give vent; feel emotional release.
15. Deny as much as possible.†

By reorganizing the specific coping styles and learning alternatives, people can become more flexible in the way they approach everyday stress.

In 1978, Minuchin described a cognitive and behavioral technique that involves five steps toward increasing stress tolerance. These steps are

1. Teaching individuals to identify cognitive patterning that increases stress.
2. Teaching them to monitor these thoughts
3. Teaching more effective ways of thinking.
4. Practicing new behaviors, such as more effective communication (role playing).
5. Applying new behaviors to real-life situations.

*Seen most in healthy copers.
†Seen most in poor copers.

TABLE 28–3 COMMON DISEASES EXACERBATED BY STRESS

Hypothesized Personality Traits	Incidence	Genetic and Biological Correlates	Common Precipitating Factors	Useful Therapies Other Than Medical Management
Migraine and Vascular Headaches				
Is obsessive, controlling, perfectionistic; suppresses anger. Excessive self-demands, highly competitive.	15%–20% of all men, 20%–30% of women between puberty and menopause Begins in mornings or on weekends Lasts a few hours to a few days	Two thirds have family history.	Can be brought on by foods (e.g., monosodium glutamate, tyramine, chocolate), fluctuating levels of estrogen. Often in unilateral, temporal, or frontal areas. May include prodromata (nausea, vomiting and photophobia).	Prodromal stage treated most effectively with ergotamine or analgesics.
Tension Headaches and Muscular Contractions				
People with type A characteristics, e.g., tense, high strung, and competitive.	Occurs in 80% of population when under stress Begins at the end of the workday or early evening		Associated with anxiety and depression. Begins suboccipitally; usually bilateral.	Psychotherapy usually prescribed for chronic tension headaches. Learning to cope or avoiding tension-creating situations or people. Relaxation techniques helpful for some.
Respiratory—Bronchial Asthma				
No one personality type identified. Some asthmatic children have poor impulse control, are babyish, overly polite, and emotionally explosive; boys—passively dependent, timid, and immature; girls—try to be self-sufficient, often chronically depressed.	Usually occurs in younger children Usually occurs in people 40 years and older	*Extrinsic:* **usually** in 30%–50% of younger children, immunoglobulin E–type antibody formation to specific antibodies as a predisposition. 1. Runs in families. 2. Occurrence is seasonal. 3. Allergens play a part. *Intrinsic:* **often** marked by sensitivity to drugs, intense emotions, exercise, or weather changes.		Children—removal from home can radically alter attacks in some children. Others—need for steroids is lessened when removed from home environment. Others—have attacks in home environment only, e.g., not in schools.
Cardiovascular—Essential Hypertension				
Anecdotal accounts: longs for approval, superficially easygoing, suppresses rage and suspicion. Hard driving and conscientious.	Higher in males until age 60	Family history of cardiac disease and hypertension.	Life changes and traumatic life events. Stressful jobs, e.g., air traffic controller. Hypothesized to be found more in areas of social stress and conflict.	Behavioral biofeedback, stress reduction techniques, meditation, yoga, hypnosis. However, *pharmacological treatment is considered primary.*

TABLE 28-3 COMMON DISEASES EXACERBATED BY STRESS *(Continued)*

Hypothesized Personality Traits	Incidence	Genetic and Biological Correlates	Common Precipitating Factors	Useful Therapies Other Than Medical Management
		Cardiovascular—Coronary Heart Disease		
Type A personality traits. Time urgency—difficulty doing nothing, always harried. Excessive competitiveness and hostility—always plays to win, general distrust of others' motives (e.g., altruism), authoritarian.	Higher in males until age 60 Higher in white population than in black population	Family history of cardiac disease a risk factor. Other risk factors include hypertension, increased serum lipid levels, obesity, sedentary life style, and cigarette smoking.	Often, myocardial infarction (MI) occurs after sudden stress preceded by a period of losses, frustration, and disappointments.	Progressive relaxation, auto hypnosis, meditation, biofeedback; behavior modification; support groups for type A personalities; prescribed program of physical exercise (prophylaxis against post-MI depression). When indicated, anxiolytics (benzodiazepines) and antidepressants are prescribed.
		Gastrointestinal—Peptic Ulcer		
Ambitious, independent. Regressive, overly dependent, repressed.	Occurs in 12% of men, 6% of women (more prevalent in industrialized societies)	Elevated pepsinogen level identified as an autosomal recessive trait. Both peptic and duodenal ulcers cluster in families, but separately from each other.	Periods of social tension and increased life stress. After losses—often after menopause.	Biofeedback can alter gastric acidity; behavioral approaches are used to reduce stress.
		Gastrointestinal—Ulcerative Colitis		
Compulsive personality traits; neatness, orderliness, cleanliness; punctuality; hyperintellectualism; obstinacy, humorlessness; timidity; inhibition of feelings (especially anger); extreme sensitivity to real or imagined hurts.	Occurs equally in men and women Develops in second and third decades of life and around age 50 High in Jewish population Higher in whites than in blacks	Possible autoimmune response. Runs in families; no genetic marker found.	Centered on losses, especially key relationships. Narcissistic loss—client thinks he or she has failed, feels hurt or humiliated, unable to please others he or she depends on.	Psychotherapy; treating issues of separation, loss, rejection, dependency.
		Cancer		
Suppression of emotions, e.g., anger; easy to please and unaggressive; stoic, self-sacrificing; inhibited; self-effacing; rigid; may appear strong, puts others' needs first, conscientious.	Men—most common in lung, prostrate, colon, and rectum Women—most common in breast, uterus, colon, and rectum Death rates higher in men (especially black men) than in women	Genetic evidence suggests dysfunction of cellular profusion. Familial patterns—breast cancer, colorectal cancer, stomach cancer, melanoma.	Prolonged and intensive stress. Stressful life events, e.g., separation from or loss of significant other 2 years before diagnosis. Feelings of hopelessness, helplessness, and despair (depression) may precede the diagnosis of cancer.	Relaxation, e.g., meditation, autogenic training, self-hypnosis. Visualization. Psychological counseling.

Any of these techniques may be combined with pharmacotherapy. The long-term use of antianxiety medications (see Chapter 17) is to be avoided, as they can be habit forming and can result in physical and psychological dependency; however, they are useful for reducing anxiety to a manageable level so that other approaches can be used.

Nursing is concerned with the whole person and with both the inner and the outer reality of the individual. The techniques discussed in this chapter are the focus of the nurse engaged in psychiatric mental health nursing practice, and all nurses must also be aware that stressors may be reduced by collaboration with other professionals or with the client's family, friends, or co-workers to create a less stressful work or home environment.

HOLISTIC ASSESSMENT OF CLIENTS WITH A PHYSICAL ILLNESS

The assessment presented in this chapter can be completed in approximately 30 minutes, depending on the ability of the person to cooperate in the interview. It may be accomplished in more than one session, if time is limited and, as with any interview dealing with personal issues, should be conducted in private and in a relaxed atmosphere. Persons in physical discomfort are dealing with added anxiety, and it may be necessary to conduct the interview after the pain or discomfort is relieved. An unstructured approach is often less anxiety provoking and allows for the expression of feelings so that nursing intervention can be accomplished during the assessment. Regardless of the individual situation, the psychosocial goal of any interaction with clients who have a physical illness is anxiety reduction. Since intervention begins with the first nurse-client contact, the initial assessment should be conducted with that goal as a priority. Chapter 7 describes effective interviewing techniques.

Any assessment begins with a history, which can be elicited from the client, significant others, or a chart, if one exists.

PSYCHOSOCIAL HISTORY

Systems/resources

Social
- Family
- Friends
- Religious affiliations
- Leisure activities
- Home environment
- Work environment
- Educational background

Physical
- Major illness
- Treatments
- Hospitalizations

Family
- Effects of client's illness,treatments, and recovery on family in the past

Addictions/mental health
- Past emotional problems
- Past compulsions/ addictions
- Family's health patterns
- Client's perception of past problems or insight
- Effective treatments
- Obstacles to health or recovery

Current problem
- Explore with the client the period of time from the first awareness of symptoms and ask for a complete description of the life stressors present at that time. Review any life stressors present in the year preceding the onset of the first symptoms. List the ways in which the client attempted to cope with the symptoms and the success of these attempts.

Neurovegetative functioning
- Appetite, sleep, bowel, and sexual patterns

Compulsive behaviors/addictions
- Smoking, working, spending, gambling, drinking, substance abuse, and so on

Feelings about "being a client" or "being ill"
- Effect on life style, relationships, self-concept—any "gains" from sick role

Spiritual state
- Meaning and purpose of life and inner strength
- Spiritual connections with others

The client's mental status (Chapters 6 and 23) should be assessed during each contact and includes

- Orientation and level of awareness.
- Appearance and behavior.
- Speech and communication.
- Mood.
- Thought process.
- Perception.
- Insight and judgment.

It is important to note the time of day and any factors that may effect the client's current mental status (e.g., pain, hunger, fatigue).

SPECIAL PROBLEMS

Any type of treatment or procedure that is intended to treat a physical illness and that creates a major permanent change is accompanied by feelings of loss (see Fig. 28–2). The dynamics involved in coping with these feelings are similar to those operating in the person who is dealing with their own death or the death of a loved one. The person must grieve this loss, just as the dying person must work through the confusion and darkness until a degree of acceptance and relative peace is achieved. Negotiating the loss of physical well-being involves movement through feelings of frustration, vulnerability, and sadness to become a "whole" person once again. This journey encompasses spiritual as well as emotional changes and, as such, requires a spiritual assessment of the client as well as a focus on psychosocial issues.

Even though the procedures may extend or promote life, they often take their toll on the client's physical state because of the high degree of anxiety they evoke. Education regarding the specific treatment and facilitation of problem solving and coping skills by the nurse have been shown to positively affect the client's recovery. Focusing on the client's strengths and reinforcing existing coping skills (e.g., prayer, hobbies, relaxation techniques) are important nursing interventions before and after the procedures.

THE CLIENT WITH A MENTAL ILLNESS IN A MEDICAL-SURGICAL SETTING

Persons who are hospitalized or attending an outpatient clinic for a physical illness are subjected to anxiety-provoking situations or stimuli in the form of treatments, waiting for attention by health care providers, or experiencing physical symptoms. For the person who is also experiencing acute psychiatric symptoms, this anxiety is compounded and requires special planning of nursing interventions. Table 28–4 is a supplement to the information found in other chapters in this book and is intended as an example of the application of psychiatric nursing concepts to the care of persons with a dual diagnosis that is both psychiatric and physical.

THE CHALLENGE TO THE HIV-POSITIVE PERSON

The psychosocial issues of HIV infection are sometimes overwhelming to both nurses and their clients. The "related concepts" column of Figure 28–1 can be used to address the most common human responses of the HIV-positive person.

The psychological impact of hearing that one has been infected with HIV or the fear that one may test positive for the virus in the future because of past behaviors has led to a new focus by health care professionals who work with populations seeking HIV testing. The nurse now has the role of counselor, which requires an extreme sensitivity to the personality style and coping style of the individual as well as an appreciation of the ramifications of the decision to be tested. The reaction to hearing of a positive test result may be so devastating to the person that face-to-face counseling must be given before the test is performed and again after the results are received. Even receiving a negative test result, if it is not accompanied by adequate health education, can produce a false sense of security and negative health behaviors. Tough questions like "Who should be tested?" or "Should HIV-positive women become pregnant?" are being addressed by mental health professionals in many settings, and position statements are being formalized by professional associations and other committees. The controversial "end of life" issues, including the nurse's response to persons who request assisted suicide, are confronting nurses in the community who are caring for persons with HIV illnesses. A guideline for interventions for some common issues faced by people with HIV infection is shown in Table 28–5.

Human immunodeficiency virus encephalopathy (acquired immunodeficiency virus dementia) and the central nervous system infections of cryptococcosis and toxoplasmosis have created a need for psychiatric instruction for emotionally and physically depleted caretakers. The fact that many young people are HIV positive has contributed to the devastation that society experiences as the lives of children and young adults are ended before they can realize their goals. The middle-aged population, who are often both caretakers for their children and for their parents, have special needs for support and respite.

HUMAN RIGHTS ADVOCACY FOR STIGMATIZED PERSONS

Some consumers of health care and some health care providers have voiced the need for examination of human rights abuses of persons stigmatized by the health care system. These people include those who have a mental illness, those who are HIV positive, and those who have been the recipient of transgender surgery or treatments. These are abuses that can result in inadequate care, leading to undue stress, worsening of physical illness, or even death. By assuming that persons with certain illnesses are "bad," "disgusting," or even just "unusual," health care workers fail to acknowledge and understand that the psychosocial issues of these people are similar to those of others and that the same nursing interventions for anger, anxiety, or grief are applicable. (Some of these interventions are discussed in the tables and vignettes in this chapter.) Examples of human rights abuse include

- Neglect in fully investigating somatic complaints made by emergency department clients with a history of psychiatric illness.
- Avoidance of contact with, or refusal to care for, persons who are stigmatized, which results in worsening illness or death.
- Hasty labeling with a psychiatric diagnosis and prescription of antipsychotics for persons who have the normal emotional responses (e.g., sadness, anger) to chronic physical illness.
- Inappropriate psychiatric admissions of persons who are on medical units or in nursing homes based on the financial need of the institution or on staff's inability to manage emotional responses to physical illness or the aging process.

TABLE 28–4 MENTAL DISORDERS, INTERVENTIONS, AND RESPONSES

RELEVANT CONCEPTS FOR PLANNING NURSING INTERVENTIONS	EXAMPLE	NURSING RESPONSE
	Schizophrenia	
▸ Motor activity that appears "clumsy" or bizarre may either be caused by side effects of medications or be a feature of the illness.	▸ Client holds arms stiffly at side while walking.	▸ Assess anxiety level and muscle rigidity and perform AIMS test.
▸ There may be an inability to learn or carry out goal-directed activities.	▸ Client repeats instructions of the nurse but appears confused when expected to demonstrate activity, e.g., self-administration of insulin.	▸ Caregiver in the home must learn to supervise client in glucose testing and self-administration of insulin.
▸ Bodily complaints may be expressed in a delusional or illogical manner.	▸ Client complains of feet being "cut off."	▸ Assess complaint carefully, using clarification of vague or symbolic descriptions by patients.
▸ Overly familiar gestures of inconsistent behavior on the part of the staff may generate anxiety for the patient or be misinterpreted.	▸ Busy nurse did not speak to the client so he refused treatment, saying that the nurse wants to "harm" him.	▸ Be consistent in behavior with client and be aware of body language. Keep routine of care on schedule.
▸ Judgment is often poor when the person is in acute distress.	▸ Client who is sedated and unsteady on her feet does not return to bed when directed by staff.	▸ Ensure that basic physiological and safety needs are monitored closely.
▸ Behavior may be very withdrawn, and the client may be almost mute. Staff could be misled by this and believe that the behavior indicates fatigue.	▸ Client does not discuss symptoms freely or give a full history during the physical assessment.	▸ Ask client direct, simple questions and allow more time than usual for the client to respond.
	Depression	
▸ Irritability or agitation may accompany frustrations, which seem minor.	▸ Client throws dinner tray on the floor because the "food is cold."	▸ Maintain accepting attitude toward the client and encourage verbalization of frustration.
▸ Appetite and sleep disturbances are common.	▸ Client leaves most food on the tray and is sleeping whenever the staff enters the room.	▸ Use food supplements and encourage food from home if appropriate. Monitor hours slept in 24 hr and offer diversions that help client maintain a more normal schedule for sleep.
▸ There is often indifference to events that normally elicit an emotion.	▸ Client does not exhibit pleasure at seeing visitors or does not seem disturbed by unpleasant procedures.	▸ Do not withdraw from client even though he or she may seem apathetic to staff interaction. Approach client frequently for brief interactions.
▸ Danger of suicide is increased when the person's energy level increases. A lift in mood or an attitude of resignation may indicate that a decision is to be made.	▸ Client who had been very withdrawn and quiet is becoming more verbal and interested in surroundings.	▸ Increase frequency of observation and make environment "safe." Assess for suicidal ideation and for any plans client has for the future. Report changes to entire treatment team.
▸ Clinical manifestations of anxiety often mimic symptoms of some physical disorders.	▸ Client complains of chest pain, palpitations, and dizziness and is perspiring profusely.	▸ Encourage slow, regular breathing while monitoring vital signs. Assess for physical illness before deciding it is anxiety.
	Anxiety Disorder	
▸ The greater the person's anxiety, the more narrow the person's perceptual field—this makes learning difficult.	▸ Client is not able to concentrate on the details he is being told by the nurse about his new medication.	▸ Speak in a low, slow manner and for anxiety to decrease before teaching.
▸ Anxiety responds to interventions that are chemical as well as interpersonal.	▸ Client reports that she is feeling "out of control" and as if "something awful is going to happen."	▸ Reduce caffeine in client's diet, use antianxiety medication as needed, and teach relaxation techniques.
▸ Obsessive preoccupation increases when a person is alone and not engaged in some activity.	▸ Client is unable to sleep because of unwanted and intrusive worries.	▸ Teach the client to focus on pleasant images or deep breathing. Use medication in evening.

From Lewis, S., et al. (1989). *Manual of psychosocial nursing interventions.* Philadelphia: W. B. Saunders.
AIMS, Abnormal Involuntary Movement Scale. See Chapters 3 and 22 for a copy of the scale.

TABLE 28–5 COMMON ISSUES FACED BY PEOPLE WITH HIV AND INTERVENTION GUIDELINES

INTERVENTION	RATIONALE
Nursing Diagnosis: Social isolation related to HIV, as evidenced by feelings of rejection	
1. Assess social supports: Who are the individuals in the client's network? Are they reliable and available? Does the client feel they are supportive?	1. Social support can buffer the effects of physical and psychological stress.
2. Determine which local agencies and resources would be useful and available to the client. For example, ◗ National AIDS Coalition Hotline (1-800-342-AIDS) ◗ People with AIDS Coalition Hotline (1-800-828-3280)	2. Clients are often unaware of where they can get specific help and emotional support.
3. Encourage and facilitate verbal expression of client's concerns, questions, and fears.	3. When others show genuine concern for the client's experience, his or her anxiety may decrease, along with feelings of alienation.
Nursing Diagnosis: Decisional conflict related to sharing diagnosis with others, as evidenced by fear of rejection	
1. Assist and support client in sharing information with significant others regarding his or her HIV-positive status. For example, role play what client wants to say to family, lover, and close friends.	1. Many people want their family and close friends to know of their HIV status. Role-playing helps the client become comfortable in disclosing diagnosis.
2. Assess if the client wants others, e.g., employer and casual friends, to know diagnosis.	2. Dentist and general practitioner need to know HIV status. Telling employer and casual friends may be risky. Potential for losing job is real.
Nursing Diagnosis: Moderate to severe anxiety related to feelings of helplessness, as evidenced by feeling loss of control of one's life	
1. Encourage PWA to participate in determining goals and decision making regarding his or her care.	1. Promotes a sense of control and may reduce anxiety.
2a. Provide accurate information about procedures, tests, transmission, and hospital routines. If nurse is unsure, he or she should contact the infectious disease department in hospital of the local health department for up-to-date information.	2a. People often misinterpret the rationale or the reason for procedures and tests. Up-to-date information can reduce anxiety.
2b. Continue to discuss transmission and ways to avoid infecting others.	2b. When anxiety is high, retention of information is diminished.
3. Clarify misperceptions.	3. Helps reduce anxiety, thereby facilitating retention of information.
4. Maintain continuity of nursing care throughout each phase of hospitalization.	4. Continuity helps the PWA maintain trust with the nurse and his or her environment.
Nursing Diagnosis: Ineffective coping related to crisis of HIV, as evidenced by anger or denial	
1. Assess for maladaptive coping strategies, e.g., prolonged denial.	1. Prolonged denial interferes with client's accepting diagnosis and obtaining treatment.
2. Avoid false reassurances, e.g., implying that the cure for HIV disease may be at hand.	2. Stories of PWAs who have adjusted to their diagnoses successfully encourage realistic hope.
3. Help the PWA deal with his or her anger. The nurse can ◗ Assess reason for client's anger ◗ Avoid personalizing client's verbal abuse ◗ Encourage realizations that will assist the PWA in resolving some of his or her angry feelings ◗ Use peers to discuss personal feelings and frustrations and give a clear perspective.	3. Anger is an expected response; however, excess hostility that alienates all support networks is maladaptive. The client's anger often comes from lack of control over situation, fear or isolation, or fear of losing employment.

Data from McGrough, K. N. (1990). Assessing social support of people with AIDS. *Oncology Nursing Forum*, 17(1):31; Nyamathi A., Van Servellen, G., (1989). Maladaptive coping in critically ill patients with acquired immune deficiency syndrome: Nursing assessment. *Heart and Lung*, 18(2):113.

AIDS, acquired immunodeficiency syndrome; HIV, human immunodeficiency syndrome; PWA, person with AIDS.

These situations may occur more frequently in the cases of persons who lack family support or the personal resources to advocate for themselves (e.g., those from the lower socioeconomic class, newly arrived immigrants, those living "unacceptable" alternative life styles).

Cynthia Bruce was critically injured in a car accident on Monday, August 7, at 50th and C Streets, SE. The accident occurred at approximately 3:30 p.m. Numerous witnesses report that when the Fire Department personnel working on Cynthia discovered she was biologically a male, they temporarily stopped treatment and made disparaging remarks and jokes about the victim. Cynthia was apparently semiconscious during this time. Cynthia died a short time later at D.C. General Hospital. (*Renaissance News & Views*, Vol. 9, No. 9, September 1995.)

The key to increasing awareness of human rights issues in mental health care may be the integration of these concepts in nursing curricula. However, humanitarian values are often sown early in life, and nurses hesitate to confront employers regarding accepted practices that violate human rights. A committee composed of nurses who do not experience a conflict of interest while in the role of client advocates as well as other hospital employees could be formed to review such cases in order to make recommendations to the hospital administration. In this age of managed care and cuts in hospital budgets, human rights is one of nursing's greatest challenges.

PSYCHIATRIC LIAISON NURSING

Psychiatric liaison nursing is a relatively new subspecialty of psychiatric nursing that was initiated in the early 1960s. Usually, the **psychiatric nurse liaison** is a Master's-prepared nurse with a background in psychiatric and medical-surgical nursing. A psychiatric nurse liaison functions as a nursing consultant in managing psychosocial concerns and as a clinician in helping the client deal more effectively with physical and emotional problems. Throughout the five steps of the nursing process (assessing, diagnosing, planning, intervening, and evaluating), a psychiatric nurse liaison assists the nursing and medical staff in caring for hospitalized, medically ill clients who are presenting management problems or who have problems that impede client care. Therefore, the psychiatric nurse liaison is a resource for the nursing staff who feel unable to intervene therapeutically with a client.

The psychiatric nurse liaison first meets with the nurse who initiated the consultation. The liaison nurse then reviews the medical records, talks with the physicians, and interviews the client. After interviewing the client, the liaison nurse discusses the assessment and suggestions with the referring nurse. If a psychiatric consultation is warranted, the psychiatric nurse liaison initiates the consultation by contacting the client's medical doctor. A case conference is sometimes needed to enhance communication and consistency in the care of a particular client.

SUMMARY

Just as physical illness is accompanied by emotional responses, so are the emotions often expressed through physical symptoms. It was the purpose of this chapter to explore this interconnection between the psyche and the body as it applies to the nursing process. The holistic philosophy of nursing dictates that all nurses, regardless of their roles or specialties, maintain a view of clients as having complex needs as well as strengths. Applying the theories and concepts of psychiatric mental health nursing to the care of all clients not only is a challenge to nurses but also is required by today's health care consumer. Illness disrupts the lives of clients and their families on many levels. By understanding these dynamics, the nurse promotes health.

A growing concern for clients is the state of their spiritual life. Including this dimension, the holistic nursing assessment allows nurses to see inner strengths in their clients that might be overlooked by a more traditional approach. Interventions coming from this holistic perspective may be more creative as Eastern and Western approaches are united. Self-assessment allows nurses to explore their own inner strengths and how to use them in their professional lives in the service of clients who challenge nurses most—those who confront nurses with conflicting values, life styles, and beliefs. It is incumbent on nurses not only to care for clients but also to advocate for them in this ever-changing health care system so that their psycho-social-spiritual needs are not overlooked (see Box 28–1 on pp. 875–876).

REFERENCES

American Psychiatric Association (1980). *Diagnostic and statistical manual of mental disorders* (3rd ed.). Washington, DC: American Psychiatric Association.
American Psychiatric Association (1994). *Diagnostic and statistical manual of mental disorders* (4th ed.). Washington, DC: American Psychiatric Association.
Barnett, L., and Chambers, M. (1996). *Reike: Energy medicine*. Rochester, VT: Healing Arts Press.
Barry, P. (1984). *Psychosocial assessment and intervention*. Philadelphia: J. B. Lippincott.
Cummings, J. L. (1994). Depression in neurological diseases. *Psychiatric Annals*, 24(10):525–531.
Dossey, B. et al. (1995). *Holistic nursing: A handbook for practice*. Gaithersburg, MD: Aspen Publishers.
Jenkins, D. (1984). A model depicting the interaction of stress and the organism. In P. D. Barry (Ed.), *Psychosocial nursing assessment and intervention*. Philadelphia: J. B. Lippincott.
Katon, W. (1984). Depression: Relationship to somatization and chronic medical illness. *Journal of Clinical Psychology*, 45:4–11.
Lewis, S., et al. (1989). *Manual of psychosocial nursing interventions*. Philadelphia: W. B. Saunders.
Minuchin, S. (1978) *Psychosomatic families: Anorexia nervosa in context*. Cambridge, MA: Harvard University Press.
Robinson, E. P., and Asnis, G. M. (1989). Major depression: Masks, misconceptions, and nosologic ambiguities. *Psychiatric Annals*, 19(7):360–364.
Selye, H. (1974) *Stress without distress*. Philadelphia: J. B. Lippincott.
Weisman, A. (1984). The coping capacity: On the nature of being mortal. New York: Human Sciences Press.

BOX 28–1 INFORMATION GUIDE FOR PERSONS WITH PHYSICAL ILLNESS AND PSYCHOSOCIAL PROBLEMS

ALZHEIMER'S DISEASE

- *Alzheimer's Disease and Related Disorders Association*
  70 East Lake Street
  Chicago, IL 60601
  (312) 853-3060
- *National Institute on Aging*
  9000 Rockville Pike
  Bethesda, MD 20205
  (301) 496-9265
- *The Alzheimer's Foundation*
  877 South Harvard
  M/C-114
  Tulsa, OK 74137
  (918) 631-3665

AMYTROPHIC LATERAL SCLEROSIS (ALS)

- *The ALS Association*
  21021 Ventura Blvd #321
  Woodland Hills, CA 91364
  (818) 340-7500

BIRTH DEFECTS

- *March of Dimes Birth Defects Foundation*
  Provides referrals to local chapters for counseling as well as information and counseling on prenatal care, nutrition, exercise, and birth defects.
  1275 Mamaroneck Avenue
  White Plains, NY 10605
  (914) 428-7100

BRAIN TUMORS

- *Association for Brain Tumor Research*
  2720 River Road, Suite 146
  Des Plaines, IL 60018
  (708) 827-9910

CANCER

- *American Cancer Society*
  Education regarding early detection, free seminars on nutrition, tobacco control, and skin, breast, cervical, and ovarian cancer. Referrals for free or low-cost mammograms and health screenings for breast, ovarian, and cervical cancer, "Reach to Recovery," a one-to-one support program.
  1-800-227-2345 (ACS-2345)
- *Cancer Care, Inc.*
  Provides individual, group, and family counseling plus Special Outreach programs for: older adults, people with AIDS, cancer survivors, African American and Hispanic outreach. Provides services for children and adolescents. Handles referrals on a nationwide basis.
  New York City Central Offices:
  1180 Avenue of the Americas
  New York, NY 10035
  (212) 221-3300
  Long Island Main Office:
  20 Crossways Park North
  Woodbury, NY 11797-2007
  (516) 364-8130
  New Jersey Main Office:
  241 Millburn Avenue
  Millburn, NJ 07041
  (201) 379-7500
  Connecticut Office:
  120 East Avenue
  Norwalk, CT 06851
  (203) 854-9911

CEREBRAL PALSY

- *American Academy for Cerebral Palsy and Developmental Medicine*
  (708) 698-1635

DISEASES OF THE LUNG

- *American Lung Association*
  1-800-LUNG-USA
  (1-800-586-4872) See telephone white pages for local offices.

DOWN SYNDROME

- *Down Syndrome Congress*
  1605 Chantilly Drive, Suite 250
  Atlanta, GA 30324
  1-800-232-6372

EPILEPSY

- *Epilepsy Foundation of America*
  451 Garden City Drive
  Landover, MD 20785
  (301) 459-3700

GUILLAIN-BARRÉ SYNDROME

- *Guillain-Barré Syndrome Foundation International*
  P.O. Box 262
  Wynnewood, PA 19096
  (215) 667-0131

HEADACHE

- *National Headache Foundation*
  5252 North Western Avenue
  Chicago, IL 60625

HEAD INJURY

- *The National Head Injury Foundation*
  333 Turnpike Road
  Southboro, MA 01772
  (617) 485-9950

HEREDITARY DISEASES

- *Hereditary Disease Foundation*
  1427 7th Street, Suite 2
  Santa Monica, CA 90401
  (213) 458-4183

HIGH BLOOD PRESSURE

- *American Heart Association*
  Support groups, low-cost blood pressure, and cholesterol screening. Provides information and referrals
  (800) 242-8721 (AHA-USA1)

HIV INFECTION

- *New York State Aids Information*
  AIDS Drug Assistance Program
  (English and Spanish)
  1-800-542-2437
  General Information and Referral:
  1-800-541-AIDS
- *New York State Division for Women*
  AIDS Hotline:
  1-800-541-AIDS

HUNTINGTON'S DISEASE

- *Huntington's Disease Society of America*
  140 West 22nd Street, 6th Floor
  New York, NY 10011-2420
  (212) 242-1968
- *Huntington's Disease Society of Canada*
  Box 333
  Cambridge, Ontario
  CANADA N1R 5T8

HYDROCEPHALUS

- *National Hydrocephalus Foundation*
  Rt. 1, Box 210A
  River Road
  Joliet, IL 60436

MENTAL RETARDATION

- *Learning Disabilities Association of America*
  4156 Library Road
  Pittsburgh, PA 15234
  (412) 341-1515

Continued

BOX 28–1 INFORMATION GUIDE FOR PERSONS WITH PHYSICAL ILLNESS AND PSYCHOSOCIAL PROBLEMS *(Continued)*

MIGRAINE

- *National Migraine Foundation*
  5252 North Western Avenue
  Chicago, IL 60625

MULTIPLE SCLEROSIS

- *National Multiple Sclerosis Society*
  205 East 42nd Street
  New York, NY 10017-5706
  (212) 986-3240

MUSCULAR DYSTROPHY

- *Muscular Dystrophy Association*
  810 Seventh Avenue
  New York, NY 10019
  (212) 586-0808

MYASTHENIA GRAVIS

- *The Myasthenia Gravis Foundation*
  National Office
  52 West Jackson Blvd, Suite 909
  Chicago, IL 60604
  (312) 427-6252

NARCOLEPSY

- *American Narcolepsy Association*
  P.O. Box 1187
  San Carlos, CA 94070
  (415) 591-7979

PAIN

- *Chronic Pain Outreach*
  822 Wycliff Court
  Manassas, VA 22110
  (703) 368-7357
- *National Chronic Pain Outreach Association, Inc.*
  4922 Hampden Lane
  Bethesda, MD 20814
  (301) 652-4948

PARKINSON'S DISEASE

- *American Parkinson Disease Association*
  116 John Street
  Suite 417
  New York, NY 10038
- *National Parkinson Foundation*
  1501 NW Ninth Avenue
  Miami, FL 33136
- *Parkinson's Disease Foundation*
  Wm. Black Medical Building
  640 West 168th Street
  New York, NY 10032
- *Parkinson's Educational Program*
  1800 Park Newport #302
  Newport Beach, CA 92660
  (714) 640-0218
- *United Parkinson Foundation*
  360 West Superior Street
  Chicago, IL 60610
  (312) 664-2344

SEXUAL DYSFUNCTION

- *Sexual Dysfunction Program*
  Univ. of MN School of Medicine
  2630 University Ave., SE
  Minneapolis, MN 55414
  (612) 627-4360

SPINAL INJURIES

- *American Paralysis Association*
  500 Morris Avenue
  Springfield, NJ 07081
  (800) 225-0292
- *National Spinal Cord Injury Association*
  600 West Cummings Park
  Suite 2000
  Woburn, MA 01801
- *Paralyzed Veterans of America*
  801 18th Street, NW
  Washington, DC 20006
  (202) 872-1300
- *Spinal Cord Society*
  Wendell Road
  Fergus Falls, MN 56537
  (218) 739-5252

STROKE

- *American Heart Association*
  7320 Greenville Avenue
  Dallas, TX 75231
  (214) 750-5300
- *American Occupational Therapy Association*
  1383 Piccard Drive
  Box 1725
  Rockville, MD 20850
- *National Stroke Association*
  300 East Hampden Ave., Suite 240
  Englewood, CO 80110-2622
  (303) 762-9922
- *NINDS*
  Building 31, Room 8A-16
  Bethesda, MD 20205
  (301) 496-5751

TARDIVE DYSTONIA

- *Tardive Dyskinesia/Tardive Dystonia National Association*
  4244 University Way, Northeast
  Post Office Box 45732
  Seattle, WA 98145-0732
  (206) 522-3166

TAY-SACHS DISEASE

- *National Tay-Sachs and Allied Diseases Associations, Inc.*
  385 Elliot Street
  Newton, MA 02164
  (617) 964-5508

TOURETTE SYNDROME

- *Tourette Syndrome Association*
  42-40 Bell Boulevard
  Bayside, NY 11361
  1-800-237-0717
- *Tourette Syndrome Foundation of Canada*
  173 Owen Boulevard
  Willowdale, Ontario
  CANADA M2P 1GB

TREMOR

- *International Tremor Foundation*
  360 West Superior Street
  Chicago, IL 60610
  (312) 664-2344

WOMEN'S HEALTH

- *New Jersey Hospital Association*
  NJ Osteoporosis Resource Manual available. Complete statewide listings.
  760 Alexander Road
  Princeton, NJ 08543
  (609) 275-4000
- *New York State Division for Women*
  Hotline: 1-800-877-8077
- *New York City Dept. of Health*
  The Women's Healthline:
  (212) 230-1111
- *After Breast Cancer Surgery YM-YWHA of Bergen County*
  605 Pascack Road
  Washington Township, NJ 07675
  (201) 666-6610
- *Planned Parenthood Federation of America*
  Breast examinations and self-examination instruction. Referrals for infertility testing. Fees are on a sliding scale based on income. Callers are directed to their local chapter.
  (800) 230-7526 (PLAN)

AIDS, acquired immunodeficiency syndrome; HIV, human immunodeficiency virus.

SELF-STUDY AND CRITICAL THINKING

Multiple choice

1. The following is a spiritual self-assessment. Check the answers that apply to you. They are statements that may be used in performing a spiritual assessment of clients.

   A. I believe that life has value, meaning, and direction.
      Often Sometimes Seldom
   B. I feel a connection with the universe.
      Often Sometimes Seldom
   C. I believe in a power greater than myself.
      Often Sometimes Seldom
   D. I believe that my actions make a difference.
      Often Sometimes Seldom
   E. I believe that my actions express my true self.
      Often Sometimes Seldom

2. After a miscarriage in her third month of pregnancy, Ellen began experiencing severe headaches. She denied any strong feelings of disappointment about the loss, saying that she and her husband "would just try again. " The headaches, which persisted for several weeks, could be an example of

   A. Malingering.
   B. Somatization.
   C. Conversion reaction.
   D. Primary gain.

3. John's family members call each other several times each week to discuss the intimate problems they are experiencing with their spouses. This includes John's mother, who confided in him regarding his father's "sexual" problems. Minuchin (1978) would say that John's family is

   A. Rigid.
   B. Overprotective.
   C. Enmeshed.
   D. Open.

4. Whenever Susan hears about problems with her work from her instructor, she denies that the feedback is important. This is an example of

   A. Problem solving.
   B. A coping style.
   C. Reaction formation.
   D. A behavioral change.

5. Mrs. Peters, during her psychosocial assessment, reported that she became angry whenever it was time for her dialysis treatment. The hemodialysis nurse understood her anger as

   A. A normal response to loss.
   B. An organic change.
   C. A flaw in Mrs. Peters' personality.
   D. A psychiatric disorder.

6. Mary is a 27-year-old woman who is HIV positive and asymptomatic. She tells the clinic nurse that she wishes to become pregnant while she is "still healthy." The nurse should first

   A. Give Mary information about HIV infection.
   B. Encourage Mary to seek counseling.
   C. Explore her initial feelings upon hearing this from Mary.
   D. Change the subject and hope that Mary will forget about it.

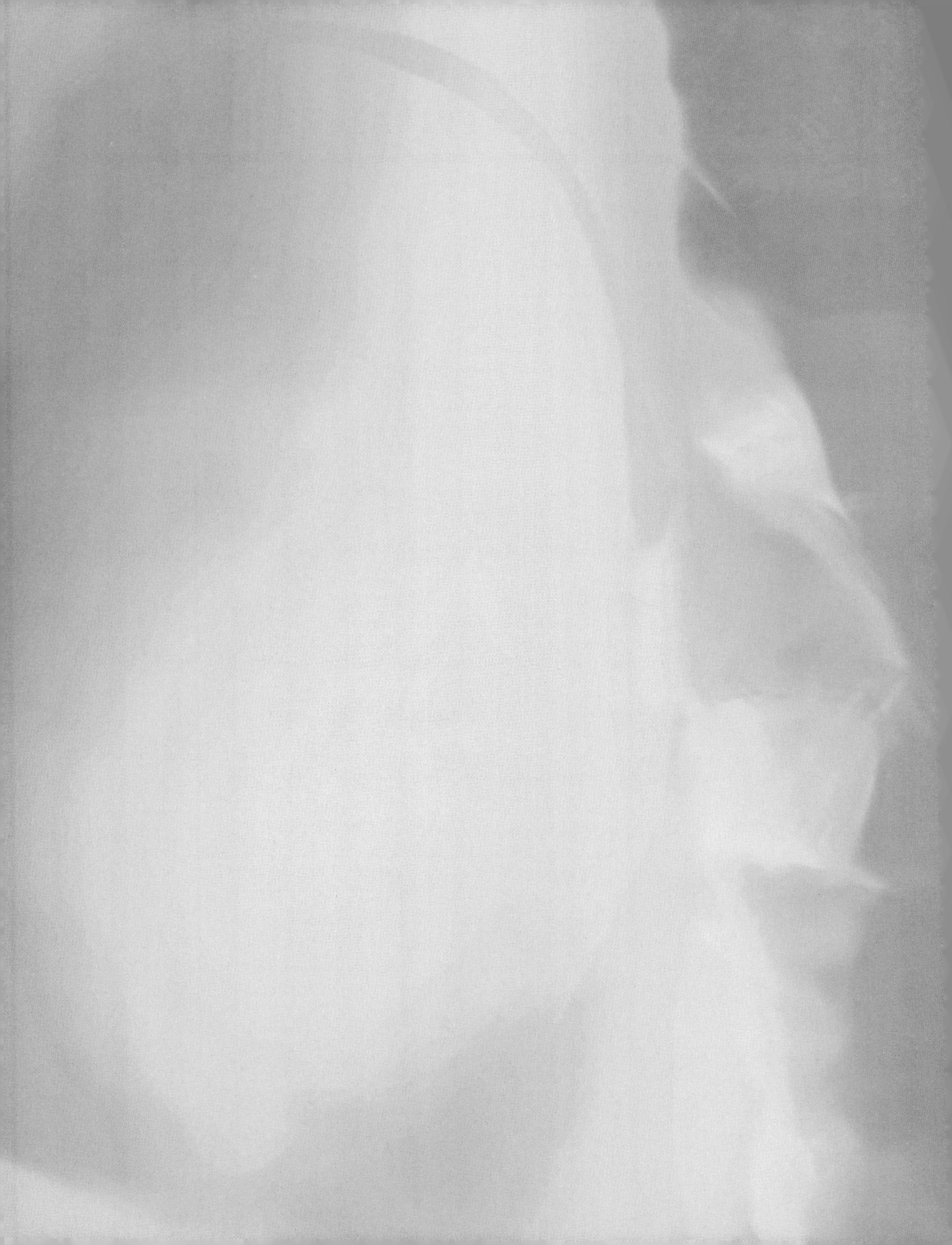

Unit Eight

Mental Health Issues Along the Life Span

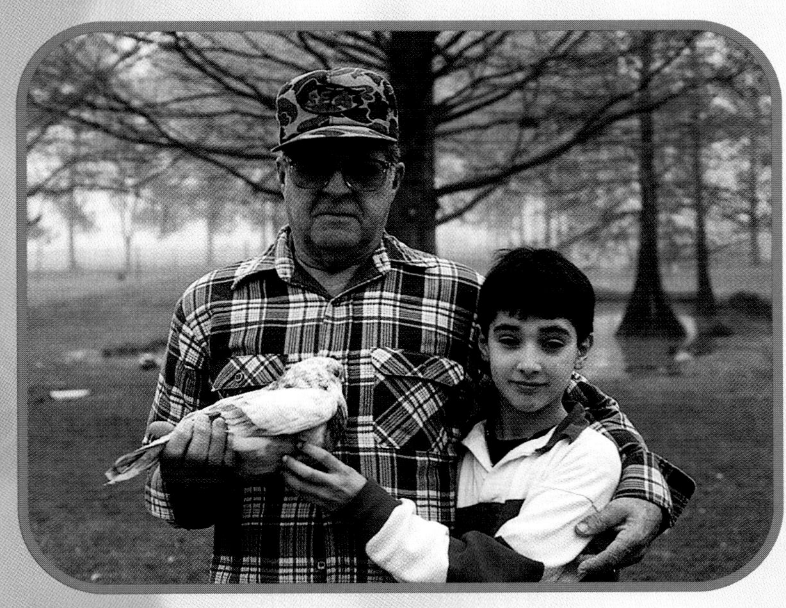

Children have never been very good at listening to their elders, but they have never failed to imitate them.

James Baldwin

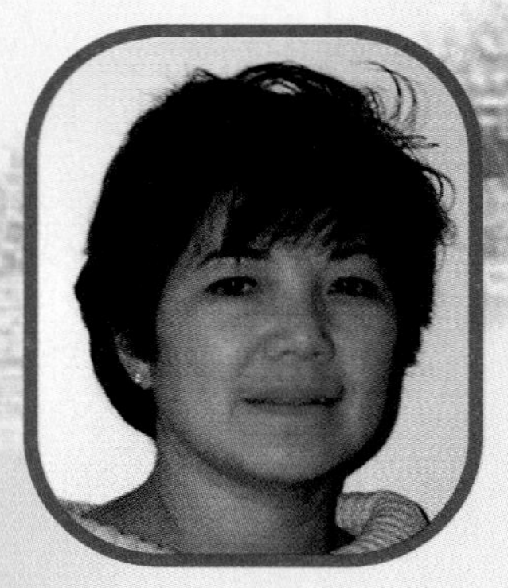

A Nurse Speaks

Kem B. Louie

The caring for the mental health needs of elderly Asian Americans in the United States presents a major challenge for nurses. It is estimated that by the year 2030, 25% of the U.S. population will be over the age of 65. Nurses need knowledge in the areas of mental health and mental illness; care of the elderly; and cultural traditions, values, and practices.

Asian Americans and Pacific Islanders (AAPIs) compose 2.9% of the total U.S. population; 73% are located in the states of California, Hawaii, and New York while 3% are located in Illinois, New Jersey, Texas, and Washington. Asian American and Pacific Islanders include more than 20 diverse subgroups such as Chinese, Filipino, Japanese, Asian Indian, Korean, Vietnamese, Cambodian, Hmong, Thai, Hawaiian, Samoan, Tongan, Polynesian, Micronesian, and Guamanian. Each subgroup has its own language, values, beliefs, and practices. Other characteristics of this diverse group are that 70% are foreign born, and a majority are monolingual.

Ethnicity is important in understanding the mental health of elderly. What is maladaptive in one culture may not be maladaptive in another culture. In general, in Asian cultures, it is not appropriate to share feelings with people outside the family. Mental illness or psychological difficulties are considered a stigma that brings shame to the family. The family and close friends try to care for the elderly person at home for as long as they can before he or she is seen in a mental health facility.

The lack of knowledge and understanding of the specific cultural values and beliefs can lead to therapists overdiagnosing or underdiagnosing AAPIs. What follows is an example of *underdiagnosing:* A frail-looking elderly Japanese woman was brought to the clinic by her neighbor; she had recently lost her husband of 45 years. She showed no emotion and was not talkative when interviewed. The therapist knew that Asians do not generally express their emotions and are quiet, and therefore concluded that the elderly woman was behaving within the cultural norm. The client might actually be presenting with clinical depression. An example of *overdiagnosing:* An elderly Chinese man was seen by his physician in a nursing home. The resident insisted on worshiping his ancestors where he would be able to light candles and incense. The physician referred the resident to a psychiatrist for possible diagnosis of religious delusions. The resident was practicing within his religion and not delusional.

AAPI groups view mental health and mental illness differently from Westerners. For example, an elderly Filipina woman was brought into the emergency room by the police. She told the interviewer that she wanted to die since she was unable to care for her grandchildren because of her severe osteoporosis. The interviewer suggested that she hire a babysitter and that she deserved to relax in her old age. Some of the AAPI groups define mental health as the ability to perform roles such as taking care of the family.

Somatization is a common behavioral response to psychological difficulties and feelings of depression among AAPIs. Somatic problems do not carry the stigma or negative consequences of emotional problems, and it is thought that this reflects the holistic view of health. For example, an elderly Korean man was brought to the clinic because of chronic complaints of abdominal pain. The results showed mild gastric acidity. His family had recently moved to another state because of job relocation and he refused to move away with them because there would not be any other Korean people to talk to in the other state. Further assessments were necessary to determine whether he was experiencing depression. Culturally relevant interventions include having health providers who speak the language, involving the family, offering short-term problem-focused solutions, and networking with the AAPI community and organizations.

29

Children and Adolescents

CHERRILL W. COLSON

OUTLINE

KEY TERMS AND CONCEPTS

The key terms and concepts listed here also appear in bold where they are defined or discussed in this chapter.

temperament
anomie
resilient child
mental status assessment
assessment/monitoring clinical pathway
pervasive developmental disorder (PDD)
attention deficit hyperactivity disorder
conduct disorder
oppositional defiant disorder
separation anxiety disorder
social phobia
posttraumatic stress disorder
Tourette's disorder
adjustment disorder
therapeutic holding
life space interview
play therapy
therapeutic games
bibliotherapy

OBJECTIVES

After studying this chapter, the reader will be able to

1. Discuss key events in the evolution of child psychiatry and child psychiatric nursing.
2. Differentiate among the roles of child psychiatric nurses.
3. Describe the predisposing factors that put children and adolescents at risk for psychiatric disorders.
4. Define mental health in children and adolescents.
5. Identify the characteristics of resilience.
6. Compile a holistic assessment of a child or adolescent using guidelines from the chapter.
7. Describe the clinical features of at least three child and adolescent psychiatric disorders, including related nursing diagnoses.
8. Compare and contrast treatment modalities for children and adolescents.
9. Formulate three nursing diagnoses stating client outcomes with corresponding interventions for at least three child and adolescent psychiatric disorders.
10. Suggest areas in child and adolescent mental health that need to be researched by nurses.

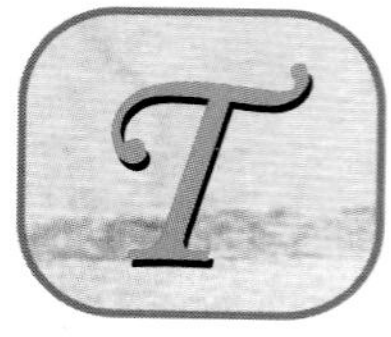

Thirty-seven million children in the United States live in poverty and 10 million are without health insurance (Fulginiti 1991). Between 12% and 22% of all U.S. children are in need of some form of mental health services, and approximately 50% of these affected children are handicapped or severely disturbed (USDHHS 1991). Public recognition of these problems has been longstanding, but the development and funding of child and adolescent services have always been slow.

The etiology of mental illness in children and adolescents encompasses multiple factors. Distinguishing among the genetic, organic, and environmental causes of mental illness makes diagnosis difficult. Increasing numbers of children are born with, or develop, disordered brain function related to malnutrition, human immunodeficiency virus (HIV), fetal alcohol syndrome (FAS), drug addiction, and child abuse. (See Chapter 25 for issues related to substance abuse.) Younger children are far more difficult to diagnose than older children. Pediatricians and parents often have to wait to see whether some "symptoms" are a result of developmental lag that will eventually be corrected, or something more serious. Therefore, early intervention may be delayed during these periods. Emotionally disturbed children often meet the criteria for more than one diagnostic category. For example, 60% of children with attention deficit hyperactivity disorder (ADHD) have a coexisting diagnosis of oppositional defiant disorder, 45% have conduct disorder, and 25% to 50% have learning disabilities (Institute of Medicine 1989). Multiple services are needed for dual or coexisting diagnoses, such as when depression and suicidal ideation coexist with substance abuse, conduct disorders, or ADHD.

Mental illness can become severe and persistent without effective early intervention. Children with conduct disorder may go on to develop an antisocial personality and end up in the criminal justice system. Children raised by a depressed mother have a 30% to 50% chance of developing emotional problems (Cox 1988). One resultant emotional problem is "learned helplessness," which leaves the child anxious or apathetic and unable to learn how to master the environment. Another result may be the child's inability to make an emotional attachment when the depressed mother is emotionally unavailable.

Abused and neglected children are at great risk for developing emotional, intellectual, and social handicaps as a result of their traumatic experiences (Children's Defense Fund 1990). Abused children are also at risk for identifying with the aggressor and becoming the "neighborhood bully," becoming an abuser in adulthood, or developing dysfunctional behavior patterns in close interpersonal relationships. See Chapter 15 for information about child abuse.

Meeting the mental health needs of children and adolescents is a challenge as their needs increase and funding resources diminish (Killeen 1990). The scope of the nurse's responsibility for assessment and early intervention in the mental health problems of youths and their families continues to increase. This chapter describes the evolution of child psychiatry and child psychiatric nursing, assessment and interventions for selected mental disorders in children and adolescents, and available treatment modalities.

EVOLUTION OF CHILD PSYCHIATRY

The evolution of child and adolescent psychiatry is brief in comparison with adult psychiatry. For centuries, children were seen as miniature adults and subjected to the same treatment for mental illness, either being left to wander or confined with adults to asylums and jails. The first documented psychological treatment of a child occurred in the late 1700s when Itard, a Frenchman, attempted to civilize a young boy who had been raised by wolves. The history of child psychiatry in America may have begun in 1848 when one of Itard's students was instrumental in establishing the first training school for mentally retarded children. The significant events that influenced the evolution of child and adolescent psychiatry are listed in Box 29–1.

CHILD PSYCHIATRIC NURSING

History

Nurses had no role in the early treatment of mentally ill children. When nurses became involved in custodial care, they acted as surrogate parents, structured the child's milieu, and assisted with somatic therapies. As psychiatric treatment became more dynamic and less custodial, the nurse's value in establishing therapeutic relationships with the disturbed children was recognized.

Nurses sought graduate education to be better prepared for this new psychotherapeutic role.

Boston University opened the first clinical specialist graduate program in child psychiatric nursing in 1954. By 1969, there were seven programs in the United States, and the number doubled over the two next decades. Cuts to education and the restructuring of graduate curricula to meet the demand for nurse practitioners led to the closing of many of these clinical specialist programs. The events that shaped child psychiatric nursing as a discipline are described in Box 29–2.

Philosophy

Child psychiatric nursing is based on the following beliefs about the growth of children and adolescents: (1) every child has a potential for growth, (2) the potential may be fostered in various ways, (3) the growth pattern will have periods of progression and regression, and (4) healthy growth occurs when the child is helped to move from dependence to autonomy (Chisholm 1968).

The knowledge base for child psychiatric nursing includes the biopsychosocial theories of human behavior, treatment modalities and techniques, and the therapeutic use of self.

Roles of the Child Psychiatric Nurse

The first roles the child psychiatric nurse generalist assumed were parental surrogate, socializing agent, teacher, counselor, manager of a therapeutic milieu, and member of a multidisciplinary team (Christ et al. 1965; Middleton and Pothier 1970). More recently, the combined child and adult *Standards of psychiatric-mental health nursing practice* of the American Nurses' Association (ANA 1994) identified the basic level functions as

Box 29–1 SIGNIFICANT EVENTS IN CHILD AND ADOLESCENT PSYCHIATRY

1848–1900

- Concern about increasing numbers of abused, orphaned, and abandoned children led to public and private actions.
- Increasing numbers of school dropouts and juvenile delinquents led to studies that blamed faulty or absent parenting.
- 1896, first clinic for emotionally disturbed children established at the University of Pennsylvania.

1900–1920

- Studies of disturbed youth identified the need for "emotional cushioning" by placement in foster and residential care.
- 1905, infant and childhood forms of schizophrenia described.
- 1909, first psychiatric clinic to serve the juvenile court system established in Chicago.
- 1909, Clifford Beer's Mental Hygiene Movement had as its slogan "The Prevention of Insanity and Delinquency."
- 1920, nine states had special education classes for the retarded.

1920–1940

- 1921, child guidance movement started with Boston Habit Clinic to treat "everyday problems of the everyday child."
- By 1930, 500 child guidance clinics established to work with parents and schools on changing detrimental attitudes.
- 1924, American Orthopsychiatric Association, founded a multidisciplinary organization to foster child mental health.
- Child psychology courses instituted in medical school, social work, and teacher education programs.
- Child psychiatric clinics established in pediatric hospitals.

1940–1960

- 1943, Leo Kanner described "infantile autism" and "symbiotic infantile psychosis" as childhood disorders.
- Benjamin Spock integrated emotional aspects of child care into parenting, relaxing the rigid attitudes about habit training.
- Child psychiatric units began using nurses in milieu therapy.
- Drug therapy: amphetamines for hyperactivity, antidepressants for enuresis, major tranquilizers for the severely disturbed and retarded.
- 1952, DSM-I listed childhood schizophrenia as a diagnosis.
- 1953, American Academy of Child Psychiatry established.
- 1955, Joint Commission on Mental Health identified need for child and adolescent psychiatric services.

1960–1980

- 1963, Community Mental Health Act passed to establish centers for education, prevention, screening, and intervention for all ages.
- 1965, Head Start Programs founded to ameliorate the effects of poverty.
- Family therapy approach introduced.
- 1970, Children's Defense League established to advocate on all issues relating to youth.
- 1975, Project on the Classification of Exceptional Children resulted in Public Law 94–142 mandating public education for all physically and mentally handicapped children.
- 1978, President's Commission on infant, child, and adolescent mental health resulted in Mental Health System Act (1980).

1980–1990

- 1980, DSM-III defined "pervasive developmental disorders."
- Mental health services remained fragmented.
- Dramatic increase in inpatient child and adolescent admissions related to increase in acting out behaviors, increase in private treatment centers, and availability of third-party payment.
- School-based primary prevention and outreach programs piloted.

1990–PRESENT

- 1994, DSM-IV redefined "pervasive developmental disorders."
- Problems with health care reform and budget cuts affected child and adolescent services.
- Inpatient brief treatment changed from months to weeks as Managed Care put limits on psychiatric treatment.

- Health promotion and health maintenance.
- Intake screening and evaluation.
- Care management/provision of a therapeutic environment.
- Monitoring of psychobiological regimens.
- Health teaching.
- Crisis intervention/counseling.
- Outreach activities.

Nurses who have master's preparation in child psychiatric nursing and advanced practice certification are able to carry out further interventions (ANA 1994):

- Psychotherapy with individuals, groups, and families
- Psychobiological interventions (prescriptive authority)
- Clinical supervision/consultation
- Consultation-liaison

The prescriptive authority for pharmacological agents is a change in advanced practice that has influenced many

BOX 29–2 EVENTS IN THE EVOLUTION OF CHILD PSYCHIATRIC NURSING

1900–1930	Nurses were not involved in the child guidance movement. Custodial care was left to attendants.
1930–1940	Nurses became involved with somatic treatments, managing the milieu and surrogate parenting.
1950–1960	The therapeutic role of nurses was being recognized.
1954	First graduate program in child psychiatric nursing opened at Boston University.
1956	Professional Nurse Traineeship Program (1957–1972) funded graduate education for nurses.
1968	Work Conference: Nursing in Child Psychiatry set philosophy, roles, and conceptual framework.
1971	Advocates for Child Psychiatric Nursing (ACPN) established as a professional organization.
1972	Claire Fagin published *Nursing in child psychiatry.*
1979	American Nurses' Association (ANA) certification available for child psychiatric nurses as generalist or clinical specialist.
1985	ACPN collaborated with ANA in developing *Standards of child and adolescent psychiatric–mental health nursing.*
1988	*Journal of Child and Adolescent Psychiatric and Mental Health Nursing* began publication.
1991	National Workshop: Child Psychiatric Nursing made recommendations concerning education, service, and research.
1993	ACPN changed its name to Association of Child and Adolescent Psychiatric Nurses (ACAPN).
1995	Nurse practitioner graduate programs began replacing clinical specialist programs in psychiatric nursing.

psychiatric graduate programs to include nurse practitioner skills.

Current Issues

Inpatient child and adolescent psychiatric nursing is changing dramatically. There was a substantial increase in the number of children and adolescents treated in inpatient facilities during the 1980s owing to the availability of third-party reimbursement, an increase in psychiatric beds, competition among providers, few treatment alternatives to hospitalization, and the increasing social problems of drugs and violence (Carbray and Rogers Pitula 1991). Now, in response to managed care directives and budget cuts, inpatient psychiatric care has been modified to brief treatment and staffing has been reduced. This change means that the child psychiatric nurse must work with more acutely ill clients in a shorter time period, making it more difficult to achieve a therapeutic alliance and to bring about lasting behavioral changes (Delaney 1992).

In addition to there being more acutely ill inpatients, the kinds of childhood disorders seen in the inpatient population have changed. In urban areas, most children have a diagnosis of conduct disorder, and fewer than one third come from an intact family (Jemerin and Phillims 1988). These children have been referred to as "functional orphans" because adequate parenting was never available. The lack of a family support system limits the nurse's ability to work with caregivers on parenting issues and to ensure that the gains made in treatment are sustained. Case management for aftercare and disposition becomes difficult to coordinate because multiple community agencies are involved with the children, which provides more opportunity for the client to "fall through the cracks."

The development of clinical pathways is changing nursing care. In the past, multidisciplinary treatment plans were structured on the child's problems, expected outcomes, and therapeutic interventions. Now, brief treatment requires assessment, stabilization, and discharge planning to be quick and systematic, which has led to the development of clinical pathways to guide care from admission through discharge (McGihon 1994). The pathways are standardized plans with target dates that identify diagnostic studies, assessments, observation and safety precautions, therapeutic activity schedules, patient education, medications, referrals, and behavioral goals and outcomes. Clinical pathways for child psychiatric disorders are in their infancy, although specific diagnostic and treatment protocols for eating disorders have existed for some time. Because the pathways are generic in nature, they do not address the child's individual needs or the nurse's interpersonal therapeutic process. A current challenge for nursing is to develop clinical pathways for child and adolescent disorders that integrate the therapeutic process into the clinical pathway.

Psychiatric care is moving from inpatient facilities into the community. To secure a role in community care, nurses need to continue to increase their recognition by the public and the policymakers as experts in the mental health problems of children and adolescents (Killeen 1990).

Currently, mental health nurses are becoming an integral part of home care and hospice teams, proving their ability to work with children and adolescents in the home. Advanced practice nurses and nurse clinical specialists are establishing school-based primary prevention and treatment programs for children and adolescents (Conley and Kendall 1989; Lamb and Puskar 1991; Korczynski 1989). Therapeutic work is being carried out in nontraditional settings such as homeless and battered women's shelters (Gilbert 1988).

THEORY

Predisposing Risk Factors

There are numerous neurobiological and psychosocial factors that put children and adolescents at risk for emotional and mental disorders. A child's vulnerability to risk factors is the result of a complex interaction among the child's constitutional endowment, trauma, disease, and interpersonal experiences (Anthony and Cohler 1987). The degree of vulnerability changes over time. The plasticity of the growing child and the presence of positive environmental factors enable the child to continue learning and adapting, which in turn decreases the vulnerability to mental disorders.

Genetic

Heredity factors have been implicated in a number of mental disorders, including bipolar disorders, schizophrenia, anxiety, alcoholism, and attention-deficit problems. Vulnerability to these disorders exists even when the child is not being raised by the natural parents (Barker 1995). Since not all vulnerable children develop mental disorders, it is assumed that constitutional resilience and a supportive environment play a role in keeping the disorder from developing. According to the *Diagnostic and statistical manual of mental disorders*, fourth edition (DSM-IV) (APA 1994), some disorders have a direct genetic link, such as the mental retardation in Tay-Sachs disease, phenylketonuria, and fragile X syndrome. These conditions will be manifested whenever the gene is passed to the child.

Biochemical

Alterations in neurotransmitters play a role in the etiology of child and adolescent disorders.

Decreases in norepinephrine and serotonin levels are related to depression and suicide; elevated levels are related to mania. Acetylcholine is important for cognition and memory, and low levels of acetylcholine, norepinephrine, and serotonin may be a factor in ADHD (Zametkin 1989).

Elevated testosterone levels in aggressive behavior have been studied and may have a role in mediating how the child responds to environmental stresses (Lewis 1994).

Prenatal and Postnatal

Adverse environmental factors affect the developing child and contribute to the onset of disordered brain function and other pathologic conditions. Prenatal factors involve exposure to drugs (e.g., medications, illegal drugs, alcohol), other toxins, infections, fetal malnutrition, and prematurity.

Postnatal factors include birth hypoxia, lead poisoning, central nervous system (CNS) infections, and brain injuries due to accidents or abuse. These insults can result in hyperactivity, learning disorders, attention deficits, aggressive behavior, impulsivity, and mental retardation (APA 1994).

Temperament

Temperament, according to Thomas and Chess (1977), is the style of behavior the child habitually uses to cope with the demands of and expectations from the environment. Temperament is a constitutional factor and is thought to be genetically determined. It may be modified by the parent-infant relationship, with positive or negative results. In the case of the "difficult-child" temperament, if the caregiver is unable to respond positively to the child, there is a risk of insecure attachment, developmental problems, and future mental disorders.

Psychosocial Developmental Factors

The psychodynamics of child and adolescent disorders need to be considered in the context of developmental theory. (See Chapter 2 for personality theories.) According to Freud's psychoanalytic theory, the child who fails to gain control of aggressive id impulses by developing effective ego and superego functions will develop antisocial behavior. This diagnosis in a child is now called a *conduct disorder*. These children also experience low self-esteem, because their underdeveloped superegos cannot provide them with praise, and much of their behavior brings negative feedback. The child with an overpunitive superego will experience chronic guilt, self-doubt, and low self-esteem. As a result, the child may become inhibited, obsessive-compulsive, or depressed.

In Bowlby's (1969) attachment theory, the child who does not have a positive bonding experience with the caregiver never gains a feeling of trust or personal validation. This child will have problems in forming interpersonal relationships, either being chronically anxious and depressed, or never attaching and developing bonds of affection. Erikson (1963) described the same results from failure to develop basic trust but believed that issues of trust can be reworked during later developmental stages.

The separation/individuation process, which takes place during the child's first 3 years of life, can be disrupted, causing an arrest in personality development (Mahler et al. 1979). The incomplete or immature personality is thought to be the cause of severe and persistent depression, separation anxiety, and borderline and antisocial personality disorders.

Once the child has mastered the transition from home to school, the grade-school years are relatively free of emotional upheavals, provided that there are no major losses, traumatic events, or academic failures. When the child approaches adolescence, the separation/individuation process is reworked as the child begins to question parental values and redefines the emotional distance in the parent-child relationship. At this point, a child can become rebellious as a way to separate. If the child suffers a major loss or damage to self-esteem, he or she may develop clinging and dependent behavior, depression, and school phobia (e.g., adjustment disorder, separation anxiety disorder) or may act out the emotions in risk-taking behaviors, aggression, and truancy.

The formation of an identity is the major developmental task of adolescence. Identity confusion (identity crisis) can result from ambivalence about strivings for independence versus dependence, the loss of a parental role model, and the breakdown of the parent-child alliance. Another problem in formulating an identity results from the rejection of parental values and the adolescent's failure to establish his or her own values and goals. The youth is left with feelings of **anomie** (lack of purpose), apathy, alienation, and personal distress. These feelings are then expressed in depression and suicide behaviors. The risk-taking and acting out behaviors of the adolescent in response to these developmental and environmental stresses are thought to "mask" depression. (See Chapter 20 for symptoms of masked depression.) The acting out and suicidal behaviors are major factors in the hospitalization of adolescents.

Social/Environmental Factors

External factors in the environment put stress on children and adolescents and shape their development. Rutter (1987) identified the following familial risk factors as correlating with child psychiatric disorders: (1) severe marital discord, (2) low socioeconomic status, (3) large families and overcrowding, (4) parental criminality, (5) maternal psychiatric disorders, and (6) foster care placement. The greater the number of stressors, the greater is the incidence of mental disorders.

The abuse of children and stressful life events are known to relate to the increased incidence of accidental injuries, anxious children, depression, and suicidal behaviors (Kelley 1992). Children are now known to develop posttraumatic stress disorder (PTSD) from the traumatic events in their lives. Physical and sexual abuse of young children puts them at risk for developing a dissociative identity disorder as a defense against the overwhelming anxiety associated with the abuse (see Chapter 18) (Ross 1989).

Cultural/Ethnic Factors

Culture shock and cultural conflicts related to assimilation issues put immigrant children at risk for a variety of problems. Siantz (1993) noted that a disproportionate number of minority children are labeled with mental and learning disorders and suffer from this stigma throughout life. Canino and Spurlock (1994) proposed that the lack of cultural role models can put minority children at risk. Cultural beliefs and values that are at odds with the majority may also put these children at risk. Ogbu (1981) noted differences among minority groups in academic and economic success and related it to differences in three types: autonomous, immigrant, and caste-like minorities. The autonomous groups (e.g., Mormons, Amish, Jews) have successful cultural role models and are not considered oppressed. The immigrant minorities (e.g., Asian Americans) emigrated to improve their social and economic status, valuing hard work and academic achievement. The caste-like minorities (e.g., African Americans, Native Americans, and to some extent Native Hawaiians, Mexican Americans, and Puerto Ricans) have been ascribed an inferior status, leading to the belief that individual effort, academic success, and acculturation will not advance their status. Academic success is perceived as "acting white," and to acculturate to European American norms is considered to be "selling out." These differences in cultural expectations, stresses, and support have a profound effect on the child's development and the risk of mental and emotional problems.

Resilience

Most children who grow up "at risk" are able to develop normally without mental problems. They have a resilience that enables them to handle the stresses of a difficult childhood.

The term *resilience* has been associated with the relationship between the child's constitutional endowment and environmental factors. Studies have shown that the **resilient child** has the following characteristics: (1) a temperament that can adapt to changes in the environment, (2) the ability to form nurturing relationships with other adults when the parent is not available, (3) the ability to distance himself or herself from the emotional chaos of the parent or family, (4) good social intelligence, and (5) the ability to use problem-solving skills (Anthony and Cohler 1987). Other studies have identified the cushioning effects of family stability in the face of poverty and adversity. The nurse's role is to foster these characteristics and environmental supports to keep the at-risk child from developing emotional and mental problems.

ASSESSMENT

Nurses work with youths in a variety of settings. This gives them the opportunity to assess the mental health of children and adolescents and to intervene early with those behaviors that indicate stress and adjustment problems before they become serious mental disorders. Assessment requires knowledge of normal growth and development, abnormal behaviors (minimal and extreme psychopathology), and related etiological factors.

Mental Health vs. Mental Illness

A mentally disturbed child or adolescent is one whose progressive personality development is interfered with, or arrested by, a variety of biopyschosocial factors, resulting in impairments in the capacities expected for his or her age and physical and cognitive endowment. In comparison, a mentally healthy child or adolescent's personality development progresses with only minor regressions as the individual masters developmental tasks and learns to love, work, and play with satisfaction (Box 29–3).

Assessment Data

The type of data collected to assess mental health depends on the setting, the severity of the presenting problem, and the availability of resources. The nurse is often the first health professional to have contact with the child and needs to be aware of the types of data that can be collected. Box 29–4 identifies assessment data for the history of the present illness, medical history, developmental history, family history, developmental assessment, mental status assessment, and neurological assessment. Agency policies determine which data are collected and how they are documented, but the nurse in a primary care setting makes an independent judgment about what and how to assess based on the child's presenting problem and the situation. In all cases, a physical examination is part of a complete work-up for serious mental problems.

BOX 29–3 CHARACTERISTICS OF A MENTALLY HEALTHY YOUTH

- Trusts others and sees his or her world as safe and supportive
- Can correctly interpret reality (reality test) and make accurate perceptions of the environment
- Has a positive, realistic self-concept and identity
- Copes with anxiety and stress using age-appropriate behavior
- Can learn and master developmental tasks
- Expresses self in spontaneous and creative ways
- Develops and maintains satisfying relationships

Data Collection

Methods of collecting data include interviewing, screening, testing (neurological, psychological, intelligence), observing, and interacting with the child and adolescent. Histories are taken from parents, caregivers, the child (when appropriate), the adolescent, and other family members.

Structured questionnaires and behavior checklists can be completed by parents and teachers. A genogram can be used to document family composition, history, and relationships. (See Chapter 11 for an example of a genogram.) Numerous assessment tools are available, and with training, nurses can learn to use them effectively.

The observation/interaction part of a mental health assessment begins with a semistructured interview in which the child or adolescent is asked about life at home with parents and siblings, and life at school with teachers and peers. Since the interview is not structured, children are free to describe their current problems, even giving information about their own developmental history. Play activities such as games, drawings, puppets, and free play are used for younger children who cannot respond to a direct approach. An important part of the first interview is observing interactions among the child, the caregiver, and siblings (if available). Whenever possible, the child is observed in situations involving interactions with peers.

Developmental Assessment

The developmental assessment provides information about the child's current maturational level, which, when compared with the child's chronological age, identifies developmental lags and deficits.

One popular assessment tool that provides this comparison is the Denver II Developmental Screening Test for infants and children up to 6 years of age.

Mental Status Assessment

The **mental status assessment** in children is similar to adult assessment except that the developmental level is considered. The developmental and mental status assessments have many areas in common, and for this reason any observation/interaction will provide data for both assessments.

This assessment provides information about the child's mental state at the time of the examination, which identifies problems with thinking, feeling, and behaving. The mental status assessment categories are general appearance, activity level, speech, coordination/motor function, affect, manner of relating, intellectual function, thought processes and content, and characteristics of

BOX 29–4 TYPES OF ASSESSMENT DATA

HISTORY OF PRESENT ILLNESS
- Chief complaint
- Development and duration of problems
- Help sought and tried
- Effect of problem on child's life at home and school
- Effect of problem on family and sibling's life

DEVELOPMENTAL HISTORY
- Pregnancy, birth, neonatal data
- Developmental milestones
- Description of eating, sleeping, elimination habits, and routines
- Attachment behaviors
- Types of play
- Social skills and friendships
- Sexual activity

DEVELOPMENTAL ASSESSMENT
- Psychomotor
- Language
- Cognitive
- Interpersonal-social
- Academic achievement
- Behavior (response to stress, changes in environment)
- Problem-solving and coping skills (impulse control, delay of gratification)
- Energy level and motivation

NEUROLOGICAL ASSESSMENT
- Cerebral functions
- Cerebellar functions
- Sensory functions
- Reflexes
- Cranial nerves

(Functions can be observed in developmental assessment and while playing games involving a specific ability, e.g., "Simon says, touch your nose").

MEDICAL HISTORY
- Review of body systems
- Trauma, hospitalization, operations and child's response
- Illnesses or injuries affecting central nervous system
- Medications (past and current)
- Allergies

FAMILY HISTORY
- Illnesses in related family members (e.g., seizures, mental disorders, mental retardation, hyperactivity, drug and alcohol abuse, diabetes, cancer)
- Background of family members (occupation, education, social activities, religion)
- Family relationship (separation, divorce, deaths, contact with extended family, support system)

MENTAL STATUS ASSESSMENT
- General appearance
- Activity level
- Coordination/motor function
- Affect
- Speech
- Manner of relating
- Intellectual functions
- Thought processes and content
- Characteristics of child's play

play. Box 29–5 gives the criteria for the mental status assessment categories.

Psychopathology

Abnormal findings in the developmental and mental status assessment are related to stress, adjustment problems, or more serious disorders. Pediatricians no longer automatically say "It's just a stage. He'll grow out of it." Although many children will outgrow the difficulty, nurses need to evaluate which behaviors indicate stress and minor regressions and which indicate more serious psychopathology. The child's stress behaviors and minor regressions can usually be handled by the nurse working with the parents. More serious psychopathology needs to be evaluated by the clinical nurse specialist in collaboration with workers in other mental health disciplines. A long-used helpful tool for distinguishing between minimal and severe psychopathology is Senn and Solnit's (1968) behavioral outline (Table 29–1). Some psychiatric terminology in this outline, such as *neurosis*, has changed since the mid-1960s, but child behaviors have not.

Suicide Risk

The number of suicidal children and adolescents increases each year. Because the nurse is often the first health professional to have contact with the child or adolescent, the nurse needs to know how to assess suicidal ideation and risk. Pfeffer (1986) defines suicidal behavior in children as ". . . any self-destructive behavior that has the intent to hurt oneself seriously or to cause death." Some children do make idle threats about killing themselves. However, any child who expresses the wish to die

BOX 29–5 CHILD AND ADOLESCENT MENTAL STATUS ASSESSMENT

GENERAL APPEARANCE
- Size—height and weight
- General health and nutrition
- Dress and grooming
- Distinguishing characteristics
- Gestures and mannerisms
- Looks/acts younger or older than chronological age

SPEECH
- Rate, rhythm, intonation
- Pitch and modulation
- Vocabulary and grammar appropriate to age
- Mute, hesitant, talkative
- Articulation problems
- Other expressive problems
- Unusual characteristics (pronoun reversal, echolalia, gender confusion, neologisms)

AFFECT
- Predominant emotion
- Kinds of feelings expressed
- Feelings appropriate to situation
- Range and stability of feelings
- Intensity of feelings
- Unusual characteristics (apathy, sulking, oppositional behavior)

INTELLECTUAL FUNCTION
- Fund of general information
- Ability to communicate (follow directions, answer questions)
- Memory
- Creativity
- Sense of humor
- Social awareness
- Learning and problem solving
- Conscience (sense of right and wrong, acceptance of guilt and limits)

CHARACTERISTICS OF CHILD'S PLAY
- Age-appropriate use of toys
- Themes of play
- Imagination and pretend play
- Role and gender play
- Age-appropriate play with peers
- Relationships with peers (empathy, sharing, waiting for turns, best friends)

ACTIVITY LEVEL
- Hyperactivity, hypoactivity
- Tics, other body movements
- Autoerotic and self-comforting movements (thumb sucking, ear/hair pulling, masturbation)

COORDINATION/MOTOR FUNCTION
- Posture
- Gait
- Balance
- Gross motor movement
- Fine motor movement
- Writing and drawing skills
- Unusual characteristics (bizarre postures, tiptoe walking, hand flapping, head banging, hand biting)

MANNER OF RELATING
- Eye contact
- Ability to separate from caregiver, to be independent
- Attitude toward interviewer
- Behavior during interview (ability to have fun/play, low frustration tolerance, impulsive, aggressive)

THOUGHT PROCESSES AND CONTENT
- Orientation
- Attention span
- Self-concept and body image
- Sex role, gender identity
- Ego-defense mechanisms
- Perceptual distortions (hallucinations, illusions)
- Preoccupations, concerns, unusual ideas
- Fantasies and dreams

Adapted from Goodman, J. D., and Sours, J. (1987). *The child mental status examination* (2nd ed.). New York: Basic Books.

needs to be carefully listened to in order to determine the cause of the distress and the risk of suicide. Box 29–6 identifies the areas to explore when assessing a child's suicidal risk. The areas are also applicable for assessing adolescents, but additional questions are asked about acting out behaviors and about listening to music or reading books with morbid themes.

Assessing lethality in a child's or young adolescent's suicide plan is complicated by a distorted concept of death, immature ego functions, and a lack of understanding of lethality. A child might think a few aspirins will cause death and the adult knows it will not, yet the child might be highly suicidal. Another child might believe that jumping off a bridge is not fatal and make threats

TABLE 29–1 BEHAVIORS THAT INDICATE PSYCHOPATHOLOGY

MINIMAL PSYCHOPATHOLOGY	EXTREME PSYCHOPATHOLOGY
Birth to 6 Months	
Feeding and digestive problems Sleep disturbances Excessive sucking activity Excessive crying Excessive irritability Hypertonicity Difficult to comfort	Lethargy (depression) Marasmus Cannot be comforted Unresponsive Infantile autism Developmental arrest
6 to 18 Months	
Excessive crying, anger, irritability Low frustration tolerance Excessive negativism Finicky eater Sleep disturbances Digestive problems Elimination problems Noticeable motility patterns (e.g., fingering, rocking) Delayed development	Tantrums and convulsive disorders Apathy, immobility, withdrawal Extreme finger sucking, rocking, head banging No interest in objects, environment, or play Anorexia Megacolon Inexpressive of feeling No social discrimination No tie to mother, wary of all adults Infantile autism Failure to thrive Arrested development
18 Months to 5 Years	
Poor motor coordination Persistent speech problems Timidity toward people and experiences Fears and night terrors Problems with eating, sleeping, eliminating, toileting, weaning Irritability, crying, temper tantrums Partial return to infantile manners Inability to leave mother without panic Fear of strangers Breath-holding spells Lack of interest in other children	Extreme lethargy, passivity, or hypermotility Little or no speech, noncommunicative No response or relationship to people, symbiotic clinging to mother Somatic ills: vomiting, constipation, diarrhea, megacolon, rash, tics Autism, childhood psychosis Excessive enuresis, soiling fears Complete infantile behavior Play inhibited and nonconceptualized Absence or excess of autoerotic activity Obsessive-compulsive behavior: ritual-bound mannerisms Impulsive destructive behavior
5 to 12 Years	
Anxiety and oversensitivity to new experiences (school, relationships, separation) Lack of attentiveness: learning difficulties, disinterest Acting out, lying, stealing, temper tantrums, inappropriate social behavior Regressive behavior (wetting, soiling, crying, fears [common earlier fears, e.g., the dark, someone under the bed]) Appearance of compulsive mannerisms (tics, rituals) Somatic illness: eating and sleeping problems, aches, pains, digestive upsets Fear of illness and body injury Difficulties and rivalry with peers, siblings, adults; constant fighting Destructive tendencies, strong temper tantrums Inability or unwillingness to do things for self Moodiness and withdrawal, few friends or personal relationships	Extreme withdrawal, apathy, depression, grief, self-destructive tendencies Complete failure to learn Speech difficulties, especially stuttering Extreme and uncontrollable antisocial behavior (aggression, destruction, chronic lying, stealing, intentional cruelty to animals) Severe obsessive-compulsive behavior (phobias, fantasies, rituals) Inability to distinguish reality from fantasy Excessive sexual exhibitionism, eroticism, sexual assault on others Extreme somatic illness: failure to thrive, anorexia, obesity, hypochondriasis, abnormal menses Complete absence or deterioration of personal and peer relationships

Table continued on following page

TABLE 29–1 BEHAVIORS THAT INDICATE PSYCHOPATHOLOGY *(Continued)*

MINIMAL PSYCHOPATHOLOGY	EXTREME PSYCHOPATHOLOGY
12 to 15 Years	
Apprehensions, fears, guilt, and anxiety regarding sex, health, and education Defiant, negative, impulsive, or depressed behavior Frequent somatic or hypochondriacal complaints, or denial of ordinary illness Learning irregular or deficient Sexual preoccupation Poor or absent personal relationships with adults or peers Immaturity or precocious behavior Unwillingness to assume responsibility of greater autonomy Inability to substitute or postpone gratifications	Complete withdrawal into self, extreme depression Acts of delinquency, asceticism, ritualism, overconformity Neuroses, phobias, persistent anxiety, compulsion, inhibition or constrictive behavior Persistent hypochondriases Sex aberrations Somatic illness: anorexia, colitis Complete inability to socialize or work (e.g., learning) Psychoses

From Senn, M. J., and Solnit, A. J. (1968). *Problems in child behavior and development.* Philadelphia: Lea & Febiger.

BOX 29–6 ASSESSING SUICIDAL RISK IN CHILDREN

Ask the child questions pertaining to the following areas:

1. **Suicidal fantasies or actions:**
   Ever had thoughts about, or the desire to, hurt or kill self?
   Ever made threats, or tried to, hurt or kill self?
2. **Concepts of what would happen:**
   What would happen if you tried to hurt or kill self?
   Do you think you would be injured, would die?
3. **Circumstances at the time of suicidal behavior:**
   What was happening at the time of the thought, the attempt?
   What was happening before the thoughts, the attempt?
   Was anyone with you at the time?
4. **Previous experience with suicidal behavior:**
   Have you ever thought of killing or tried to kill yourself before?
   Do you know anyone who thought about killing, tried to kill, or killed himself?
   (Explore the child's perceptions of the event.)
5. **Motivation for suicidal behavior:**
   Why did you want to kill yourself; why did you try?
   Did you want to get even with someone, frighten someone?
   Did you want someone to rescue you?
   How are you feeling (hopeless, rejected, unloved, guilty)?
   Do you have frightening thoughts, hear voices saying kill self?
6. **Experience and concepts of death:**
   What happens when people die; where do they go?
   How often do you think or dream about dying?
   Did you know someone who died? (Explore the event.)
   When do you think you will die; what will happen?
7. **Depression and other affects:**
   Feelings of sadness, anger, guilt, rejection
   Description of behaviors—fighting, crying, lack of concentration, fatigue,
   changes in eating and sleeping patterns, problems with peers, withdrawn, isolated
8. **Family and environmental situations:**
   School performance, worries about school failure and parents' reaction
   Major changes—new home, school, siblings, stepparents
   Losses—death, divorce, separation from parents, separation of parents, illness
   Family history of marital conflicts, depression, or suicide

Adapted from Pfeffer, C. R. (1986). *The Suicidal Child.* New York: The Guilford Press.

when in fact he or she does not want to die. Early intervention is important, and parents need to understand that suicidal behavior must be evaluated by mental health professionals.

Cultural Influences

Psychiatric professionals are beginning to recognize the importance of culture in evaluating psychiatric disorders (Canino and Spurlock, 1994) and in working with families (McGoldrick et al. 1982). DSM-IV identifies culture-bound syndromes of mental illness that are not diagnostic categories in Western medicine. Canino and Spurlock (1994) use the term "culture-specific syndromes" to mean the same thing. Sensitivity to cultural influences in mental illness is a necessity in order to avoid stereotyping behavior and clouding assessment. However, overidentification with children from one's own cultural background causes a loss of objectivity (Canino and Spurlock, 1994).

The nurse considers the influence of culture on the child's behavior, thoughts, and emotions. The lack of eye contact when relating to adults is characteristic of respect in African and Caribbean children. The Native American child is taught to withhold the expression of feelings, especially anger, both verbally and nonverbally. The Japanese child learns to play using polite, social manners in interactions, whereas other cultures encourage aggressive retaliation when one is bullied by another.

In assessing speech, the characteristics and the content are considered. For example, the Navajo child's speech is slow and methodical, with pauses that could lead the nurse to believe the child has finished the sentence. The African American child is expected to be verbal, following the oral tradition in which there are multiparty conversations and children are encouraged to demonstrate their wit in outperforming peers. The Hawaiian child, whose speech pattern overlaps another's speech, might be considered rude. Nonstandard English dialects make speech difficult for the outsider to assess and can contribute to stereotyping. The child's bilingual ability always needs evaluation, because proficiency in interpersonal communication does not guarantee academic success. Whenever possible, children should be interviewed in their native language to obtain a more accurate description of their problems.

In evaluating children's cognition, it is important to know whether their beliefs are in keeping with their culture's belief system or are bizarre and indicative of disturbed thought processes. For example, the belief in witchcraft or in communicating with the spirits of the dead might not be pathological if the child is from a Caribbean culture. Folk medicine practices are also considered when evaluating the child. Cambodian refugees, who believe that illness is caused by a bad wind, will rub their child's skin with oil and a heated coin ("kos khyal") in order to raise red welts through which the bad wind escapes (Frye and McGill 1993). In Western culture, these red welts would be mistaken for child abuse. (See Chapter 5 for folk beliefs.)

Canino and Spurlock (1994) identify some culture-specific syndromes that appear in children or adolescents (Table 29–2). Their list is by no means inclusive; a more complete understanding of the child's particular culture and the degree of acculturation of child and family is needed.

Assessment Clinical Pathway

Coursen-Antinone and Anderson (1996) report using an **assessment/monitoring clinical pathway** for the first 5 days of the child's hospitalization (Clinical Pathway 29–1). The pathway identifies (1) types of physical, mental, and behavior assessments/tests; (2) restrictions and precautions; (3) daily tasks for social worker, occupational therapist, and child life worker; (4) patient teaching; and (5) discharge planning. Other sections of the pathway include evaluation of outcomes, goals, and clinical notes. The nurse's role is not specifically identified on the pathway, although nursing staff participate in many of the assessments and interventions that take place for

Text continued on page 901

TABLE 29–2 CULTURAL SYNDROMES IN MENTAL ILLNESS

SYNDROME	CULTURE	BEHAVIORS
Ataque	Puerto Rican Haitian Bahamian West Indian	Falling out, blacking out, bizarre seizure pattern, usually psychogenic, cannot move or speak but is able to hear, can have hallucinations and violent behavior
Taijin Kyotosho	Japanese	Adolescents and young adults exhibit intense fear that bodily parts or functions displease, embarrass, or offend others
Irijua	Peruvian	After birth of a sibling, sadness, hypersensitivity, anorexia, and weight loss.
Mal de Ojo (evil eye)	Mediterranean and elsewhere	Fitful sleep, crying, nausea, vomiting, diarrhea, fever caused by the fixed stare of an adult

Data from Canino, I. A., and Spurlock, J. (1994). *Culturally diverse children and adolescents: Assessment, diagnosis, and treatment.* New York: Guilford Press.

CLINICAL PATHWAY 29–1

THE JOHNS HOPKINS HOSPITAL

DEPARTMENT OF PEDIATRICS

PSYCHIATRY (Child/Adolescent)

ASSESSMENT/MONITORING

CRITICAL PATHWAY

Attending: ______

Resident: ______

Primary Nurse: ______

Social Worker: ______

TARGET BEHAVIORS:

______

______

______

______

for addressograph plate

	DAY 1	DAY 2	DAY 3	DAY 4	DAY 5	COMMENTS
MONITORING/ASSESSMENT	Adm. Hx. & Physical					
	Contraband Search					
	Assess:					
	Mood, Affect, Irritability					
	Attention Span, Distractibility, Impulsivity,					
	Aggression (Verbal/Physical)					
	MMSE/CDI/Connors					
	Substance Abuse					
	Interactions: Peers, Staff, & Family					
	Monitor: Sleep Pattern ADL's & Energy Level (EL)					
	Quiet room use					
MEDS	Assess: History of Med use & Drug allergies	Assess need for Medications				
ACTIVITY	Unit Restricted × 48 hr					
	Restrictions & Precautions (RP)					
	Level 1 (NA) × 48 hrs					

CLINICAL PATHWAY 29–1 *(Continued)*

		DAY 1	DAY 2	DAY 3	DAY 4	DAY 5	COMMENTS
TESTS		U/A-Tox Screen-HCG PPD	Admission Blood Work: M-M-CBC-RPR-EKG	Read PPD			
DIET		Assess for: Food Allergies Nutritional status & Restrictions					
CONSULTS/REFERRAL	SW	Social Work - assessment initiated	Social Work- assessment continues Schedule family session	Social Work - assessment continues	Social Work - assessment continues Family Session	Assessment completed Goals identified Services and counseling continue	
	CL	Discuss group activities with patient & family. Initiate CL Evaluation School - establish educational goals Begin CL Group	Pt. begins educational program & continues child life program Initiate contact with home school	Patient continues participating in education & child life program assessment	Patient continues participating in education & child life program assessment Finish CL Assessment	Patient continues participating in education & child life program assessment Begin school return planning on D/C	
	OT	Initiate interview evaluation with patient if possible Discuss groups with patient and family Pt. will attend groups Observe patient	Complete initial evaluation and treatment plan Identify if OT services are currently being received Pt. will attend groups Begin assessing motor, visual, selfcare functioning	Attend OT groups as indicated Continue assessment Pt. will attend groups	Attend OT groups as indicated Continue assessment Pt. will attend groups	Attend OT groups as indicated Continue assessment and evaluation as indicated Pt. will attend groups	
	MISC	Assess for Psychological Testing					
PATIENT TEACHING		Provide overview to family re: -Behavior management system used on unit; -Explain rules, time outs; -Begin discussion of discharge needs.	First family visit Family Teaching: . . . . . Initiate parent handbook Pt. demonstrates understanding of behavior system	Family visits or contract	Family visits/mtg	Family visits/mtg	

Continued on following page

CLINICAL PATHWAY 29–1 *(Continued)*

	DAY 1	DAY 2	DAY 3	DAY 4	DAY 5	COMMENTS
DISCHARGE PLANNING	Begin D/C needs assessment Meet with family/pt if possible Arrange first meeting Family Goals/Expectations: . . . . . Patient Goals:	Social work initiates discharge planning assessment	Discharge planning continues w/family & community agencies Continue D/C planning needs	Discharge planning continues w/family & community agencies Patient Goals for Home:	Discharge planning continues w/family & community agencies Family D/C Goals/ Expectations:	
EVALUATION OF OUTCOMES	Mood: ___ & pt ___ rated)	Mood: (Staff ___ & pt ___ rated)	Mood: (Staff ___ & pt ___ rated)	Mood: (Staff ___ & pt ___ rated)	Mood: (Staff ___ & pt ___ rated)	
	Sleep - # of hrs ________	Sleep - # of hrs ________	Sleep - # of hrs ________	Sleep - # of hrs ________	Sleep - # of hrs ________	
	Meals: _____ % Breakfast _____ % Lunch _____ % Dinner	Meals: _____ % Breakfast _____ % Lunch _____ % Dinner	Meals: _____ % Breakfast _____ % Lunch _____ % Dinner	Meals: _____ % Breakfast _____ % Lunch _____ % Dinner	Meals: _____ % Breakfast _____ % Lunch _____ % Dinner	
	MMSE ☐ Yes ☐ No ☐ N/A	Conners ☐ Yes ☐ No ☐ N/A	Conners ☐ Yes ☐ No ☐ N/A	Conners ☐ Yes ☐ No ☐ N/A	Conners ☐ Yes ☐ No ☐ N/A	
		CDI ☐ Yes ☐ No ☐ N/A	CDI ☐ Yes ☐ No ☐ N/A	CDI ☐ Yes ☐ No ☐ N/A	CDI ☐ Yes ☐ No ☐ N/A	
	Substance Abuse Consult ☐ Yes ☐ No ☐ N/A				Substance Abuse Consult complete ☐ Yes ☐ No ☐ N/A	
	Family meeting scheduled Date: ____________	Family Visit ☐ Yes ☐ No	Family Visit ☐ Yes ☐ No	Family meeting completed ☐ Yes ☐ No Family Visit ☐ Yes ☐ No	Has achieved level 2 or 3 four out of six days ☐ Yes ☐ No Family Visit ☐ Yes ☐ No	
		Medications Indicated ☐ Yes ☐ No	Medications Indicated ☐ Yes ☐ No	Medications Indicated ☐ Yes ☐ No	Medications Indicated ☐ Yes ☐ No	
	Family goals: 1. ____________ 2. ____________	Family contacted by ☐ Resident/ ☐ SW/ ☐ Nurse ☐ Yes ☐ No	Family goals continued: 1. ____________ 2. ____________	Family contacted by ☐ Resident/ ☐ SW/ ☐ Nurse ☐ Yes ☐ No	Family Goals Completed 1. ☐ Yes ☐ No 2. ☐ Yes ☐ No	

CLINICAL PATHWAY 29–1 *(Continued)*

	DAY 1	DAY 2	DAY 3	DAY 4	DAY 5	COMMENTS
EVALUATION OF OUTCOMES	Patient goals assessed 1. ________ 2. ________ 3. ________	Family contacted by school ☐ Yes ☐ No ☐ N/A	Patient goals evaluated ☐ Yes ☐ No	Organizes and is independent in ADL's 50% ☐ Yes ☐ No	Patient goals completed 1. ☐ Yes ☐ No 2. ☐ Yes ☐ No 3. ☐ Yes ☐ No	
		School contacted by teacher ☐ Yes ☐ No ☐ N/A	Attends groups ≥50% without difficulties ☐ Yes ☐ No	Attends groups ≥75% without difficulties ☐ Yes ☐ No	Affect full range 50% ☐ Yes ☐ No	
	Quiet room used ☐ Yes ☐ No	Quiet room used ☐ Yes ☐ No	Quiet room used ☐ Yes ☐ No	Quiet room used ☐ Yes ☐ No	Quiet room used ☐ Yes ☐ No	
	Discharge Planning Initiated ☐ Yes ☐ No	SE Observed ☐ Yes ☐ No		W/assistance, structures time 50% ☐ Yes ☐ No	Patient thinks before acting 50% ☐ Yes ☐ No	
	Physical Exam WNL ☐ Yes ☐ No	Admission Blood Work Completed ☐ Yes ☐ No	Patient takes time-out 50% of time with staff redirection ☐ Yes ☐ No	Follows directions 50% ☐ Yes ☐ No	Patient and staff mood rating ► 5 ► 50% ☐ Yes ☐ No	
	Physician contacted Referral Agency ☐ Yes ☐ No		Physician contacted Referral Agency ☐ Yes ☐ No	No physical, verbal aggression 50% ☐ Yes ☐ No	Physician contacted Referral Agency ☐ Yes ☐ No	
	Psychological testing done within past year ☐ Yes ☐ No	☐ SW/ ☐ OT/ ☐ CL/ ☐ SL/ assessment begun		☐ SW/ ☐ OT/ ☐ CL/ ☐ SL/ assessment completed	Medication/illness teaching completed ☐ Yes ☐ No	Does the patient meet criteria for the following Critical Paths?
	Precautions initiated ☐ CO ☐ EP ☐ Other		Precautions Continued ☐ CO ☐ EP ☐ Other	Psychological testing indicated and begun ☐ Yes ☐ No ☐ N/A	Positive peer, staff and family interactions 50% ☐ Yes ☐ No	Yes No Affective ☐ ☐ ADHD ☐ ☐
	PPD Done ☐ Yes ☐ No		PPD read ☐ Yes ☐ No	Settles at bedtime 50% ☐ Yes ☐ No	Discharge planning completed ☐ Yes ☐ No	Poor Impulse ☐ ☐ Thought Disorder ☐ ☐
Signature/ Title	Night P	P	P	P	P	P
	Day A	A	A	A	A	A
	Evening					

DEPT OF PEDIATRICS PSYCHIATRY POOR IMPULSE CONTROL CRITICAL PATHWAY

Continued on following page

CLINICAL PATHWAY 29–1 *(Continued)*

	DAY 1	DAY 2	DAY 3	DAY 4	DAY 5	COMMENTS
PATIENT PLAN/GOALS						
FAMILY NOTES						
REPORT NOTES/PASS ON INFO						
Signature/ Time	Night P	P	P	P	P	P
	Day A	A	A	A	A	A
	Evening					

Reprinted with permission from Anderson, K., Antinone K. C., Capozzoli, J., and Hamil, L. (1995) *Critical pathway, assessment and monitoring.* The Johns Hopkins Hospital, Department of Pediatrics Psychiatry (Child/Adolescent), Baltimore, MD.

hospitalized children and adolescents. The assessment/monitoring pathway is followed by a clinical pathway specific to an identified problem (e.g., affective disorder, thought disorder, poor impulse control, ADHD).

CHILD AND ADOLESCENT PSYCHIATRIC DISORDERS

Before specific psychiatric disorders were identified, disturbed children were thought to be either imbeciles (mentally retarded) or feeble-minded (mentally ill owing to a "weak" mind). In the late 1800s, when Kraepelin began to classify mental illness according to constellations of symptoms, mental illness was considered an organic process related to a disease or a structural abnormality in the brain. With the personality development theories of Freud, Sullivan, and Erikson, the focus shifted to the influence of nurturance and the environment as the cause of mental problems.

Thus, when Kanner (1943) first identified the clinical features of infantile autism, he attributed the etiology to a cold, distant mother-child relationship. Symbiotic infantile psychosis was attributed to an overprotective mother who did not allow for psychological differentiation, leaving the child stuck in the symbiotic phase of Mahler's separation/individuation process (Mahler et al. 1979).

By the 1960s, studies on the etiology of child and adolescent disorders focused on dysfunctional communication patterns and dysfunctional family processes. There is one disorder whose proposed etiology has not changed significantly for 100 years and that is disturbance in conduct that continues to be attributed to the lack of nurturance and guidance in a hostile environment. Today, as research tools and brain imaging become more sophisticated, interest has shifted to identifying biological factors and etiologies for many childhood disorders.

Pervasive Developmental Disorders

The diagnostic categories for severe childhood disorders have been periodically revised as differential diagnoses have evolved. Originally called infantile autism, symbiotic psychosis, atypical psychosis, or childhood schizophrenia (Kanner 1972), most of these disorders now fall under the classification of **pervasive developmental disorder (PDD).** The exception is schizophrenia, which has a childhood onset that is very rare and can be distinguished from PDD by its later onset and its associated delusions and hallucinations (APA 1994).

PDDs are characterized by severe and pervasive impairment in reciprocal social interaction and communication skills, usually accompanied by stereotyped behavior, interests, and activities (APA 1994). Mental retardation is present in 75% to 80% of cases. The latest diagnostic refinement in DSM-IV identifies the four subtypes as autistic, Asperger's, Rett's, and childhood disintegrative disorders.

Autistic Disorder

Autistic disorder is usually observed before 3 years of age, and the prognosis is related to the child's overall intellectual level and the development of social and language skills (APA 1994).

Some children show improvement as they develop, but puberty can be a turning point for either improvement or further deterioration. Cognitive function and social skills can decline or improve independently of each other. The prevalence rate is 2 to 5 in 10,000, and the male-to-female ratio is 4:1 or 5:1. Autism is more common in siblings than in the general population. A small percentage of autistic children go on to develop seizure disorders and/or schizophrenia.

Most cases have no clearly identifiable etiology, although genetic factors play a dominant role. In monozygotic twins, the concordance rate for autism is between 36% and 95.7% (Folstein and Rutter 1987). The single-gene theory is associated with fragile X syndrome, tuberous sclerosis, and phenylketonuria. Other factors include higher maternal age, maternal use of medications during pregnancy, anoxia at birth, and maternal rubella.

Autism is viewed as a behavioral syndrome resulting from abnormal brain function. Problems with left hemisphere functions (e.g., language, logic, reasoning) are evident, whereas music and visual-spatial activities can be enhanced, such as in savant syndrome. There have been children who were severely autistic but who were able to paint, play an instrument, or do mathematical computations phenomenally and brilliantly well. These children represent a deviant form of autism called *savant syndrome*. The movie *The Rain Man* with Dustin Hoffman depicted such an individual. The abnormality in brain function involves hemispheric specialization, arousal, and neurotransmitters (Dalton and Howell 1989). Dopamine levels are elevated, and administration of a dopamine antagonist (haloperidol [Haldol]) appears to control some autistic behaviors. Serotonin levels are also elevated in one third of autistic individuals. Fenfluramine (Pondimin), which lowers serotonin levels, has been found to improve both autistic behaviors and IQ. The opiate excess theory explains the diminished response to pain that has been observed in autistics who are self-mutilators.

Autism is first noticed by the mother or caretaker when the infant fails to be interested in others or to be socially responsive with eye contact and facial expressions. The autistic infant or child seems indifferent to, or has an aversion to, affection and physical contact. Later, the child may treat adults as interchangeable objects or may cling to one person. Odd responses to sensory input may be present, such as being oversensitive to or ignoring sounds.

The development of intellectual skills is uneven, and impairments are noted in both verbal and nonverbal communication. Language characteristics may be any of the following: (1) delayed or totally absent, (2) delayed or immediate echolalia, (3) unusual vocalizations (e.g., babbling, clicking), (4) immature grammatical structures and pronoun reversal, (5) inability to name objects, and (6) idiosyncratic words with private meanings. Speech can be monotonous or may have a singsong quality. There is a failure to develop imaginative play, and the child does not develop friendships or play cooperatively with other children.

Abnormalities in mood and emotions include (1) labile moods, (2) an absence of emotions, (3) excessive fearfulness, (4) lack of fear in dangerous situations, and (5) inappropriate affect (e.g., continuous giddiness). Self-injurious behaviors (e.g., head banging, finger or hand biting, hair pulling) may develop. Abnormalities of posture, gait, and motor behaviors are evident in the following: (1) poor coordination, (2) tiptoe walking, (3) peculiar hand movements (e.g., flapping, clapping), and (4) stereotyped body movements (e.g., rocking, dipping, swaying, spinning). The child develops a restricted repertoire of activities and interests, often manifested by fascination with making objects move (e.g., turning toy truck wheels, pouring sand or water, waving a piece of string) and exclusive interests in objects such as buttons or body parts. Changes in daily routines or in the child's physical environment can cause catastrophic reactions. The DSM-IV diagnostic criteria for autistic disorder are presented in Figure 29–1.

Asperger's Disorder

This disorder differs from autistic disorder. The exact prevalence rate is unknown; it affects more males than females. The cause is also unknown, although there appears to be a familial pattern. Like autism, restricted and repetitive patterns of behavior and idiosyncratic interests (e.g., fascination with remembering train schedules or dates) may develop. The distinguishing characteristics of Asperger's disorder are as follows:

- Recognized later than autistic disorder
- No significant delays in cognitive and language development
- No significant delays in self-help skills
- Severe and sustained impairment in social interactions
- Development of restricted, repetitive patterns of behavior
- Interests and activities resembling autistic disorder
- Sometimes delayed motor milestones, with clumsiness noted in preschool
- Social interaction problems more noticeable when the child enters school

Autistic Disorder

A. A total of six (or more) items from (1), (2), and (3), with at least two from (1), and one each from (2) and (3).

1. Qualitative impairment in social interaction, as manifested by at least two of the following:
   a. Marked impairment in the use of multiple nonverbal behaviors such as eye-to-eye gaze, facial expression, body postures, and gestures to regulate social interaction
   b. Failure to develop peer relationships appropriate to development level
   c. Lack of spontaneous seeking to share enjoyment, interests, or achievements with other people (e.g., by lack of showing, bringing, or pointing out objects of interest)
   d. Lack of social or emotional reciprocity

2. Qualitative impairments in communication as manifested by at least one of the following:
   a. Delay in, or total lack of, the development of spoken language (not accompanied by an attempt to compensate through alternative modes of communication such as gesture or mime)
   b. In individuals with adequate speech, marked impairments in the ability to initiate or sustain a conversation with others
   c. Stereotyped and repetitive use of language or idiosyncratic language
   d. Lack of varied, spontaneous make-believe play or social imitative play appropriate to developmental level

3. Restricted, repetitive, and stereotyped patterns of behavior, interests, and activities, as manifested by at least one of the following:
   a. Encompassing preoccupation with one or more stereotyped and restricted patterns of interest abnormal in either intensity or focus
   b. Apparently inflexible adherence to specific, nonfunctional routines or rituals
   c. Stereotyped and repetitive motor mannerisms (e.g., hand or finger flapping or twisting, or complex whole-body movements)
   d. Persistent preoccupation with parts of objects

B. Delays or abnormal functioning in at least one of the following areas, with onset prior to 3 years of age: (1) social interaction, (2) language as used in social communication, or (3) symbolic or imaginative play.

C. The disturbance is not better accounted for by Rett's disorder or childhood disintegrative disorder.

Figure 29–1 DSM-IV Pervasive Developmental Disorder: Autistic Disorder. (Adapted from American Psychiatric Association (1994). *Diagnostic and statistical manual of mental disorders* (4th ed.). Washington, DC: American Psychiatric Association. Reprinted with permission. Copyright 1994 American Psychiatric Association.)

- Problems with empathy and modulating social relationships that may continue into adulthood

Rett's Disorder

This disorder differs from autistic and Asperger's disorders in that it has been observed only in females, with the onset before 4 years of age (APA 1994). The exact cause is unknown, but the disorder has been associated with electroencephalographic abnormalities, seizure disorder, and severe or profound mental retardation. The distinguishing characteristics of Rett's disorder are as follows:

- Development of multiple deficits after a normal prenatal and postnatal period of development
- Head circumference normal at birth, but growth rate slowing between 5 and 48 months of age
- Persistent and progressive loss of previously acquired hand skills between 5 and 30 months of age
- Development of stereotyped hand movements (e.g., hand wringing, hand washing)
- Problems with coordination of gait and trunk movements
- Severe psychomotor retardation
- Severe problems with expressive and receptive language
- Loss of interest in social interactions (although this interest may return later in childhood or adolescence)

Childhood Disintegrative Disorder

This rare disorder occurs in both sexes but is more common in males (APA 1994). The age of onset is between 2 and 10 years, with most cases occurring between 3 and 4 years of age.

The onset can be abrupt or insidious and the cause is unknown, although it is thought to be related to an insult to the CNS. The distinguishing characteristics for childhood disintegrative disorder are

- Marked regression in multiple areas of function after at least 2 years of normal development.
- Loss of previously acquired skills in at least two areas: communication, social relationships, play, adaptive behavior, bowel/bladder control, motor skills.
- Deficits in communication and social interactions (same as in autistic disorder).
- Stereotyped behaviors (same as in autistic disorder).
- Loss of skills reaching a plateau, which may be followed by limited improvement.

NURSING DIAGNOSES. NANDA diagnoses include the following:

Growth and development altered
Impaired social interactions
Impaired verbal communication
Personal identity disturbance
Self-care deficit (feeding, bathing, dressing, toileting)
Self-mutilation

Other behaviors not specifically addressed by NANDA categories include the following:

Anger
Aggressive behaviors
Abnormal, stereotypic body movements
Bizarre behaviors
Clinging and dependent behaviors
Low frustration tolerance
Poor impulse control
Ritualistic behaviors

INTERVENTIONS. The goals for working with children who have PDD focus on helping them reach full potential by developing communication and social interaction skills, appropriate emotional responses (including empathy), and intellectual and problem-solving skills; and by decreasing bizarre and self-destructive behaviors. Children are treated in therapeutic nursery schools and day programs, their education mandated under the Children with Disabilities Act. Treatment plans include working with parents, who are taught how to modify the child's behavior and to foster the development of skills when the child is home. Pharmacological agents such as haloperidol and fenfluramine are being used with some success.

Nursing interventions for impaired verbal communication and social interaction and self-mutilative behaviors are described in Nursing Care Plan 29–1 for a child with autistic disorder.

Attention-Deficit and Disruptive Behavior Disorders

Attention-Deficit/Hyperactivity Disorder

Children with **attention-deficit/hyperactivity disorder** (ADHD) show an inappropriate degree of inattention, impulsiveness, and hyperactivity (APA 1994). ADHD occurs in different cultures and is difficult to diagnose before 4 years of age. ADHD is more common in males, with the male-to-female ratio ranging from 4:1 to 9:1, depending on the population studied. It is also more common in first-degree biological relatives of children with ADHD. The prevalence rate for schoolchildren is 3% to 5%. The three subtypes of ADHD are (1) predominantly inattention, (2) predominantly hyperactivity, and (3) combined type. The child who has the inattention or hyperactivity subtype can go on to develop the combined type.

The exact cause of ADHD has eluded researchers for over 50 years. There are no laboratory tests or definitive

NURSING CARE PLAN 29–1 A CHILD WITH AUTISTIC DISORDER

NURSING DIAGNOSIS: *Impaired verbal communication*

OUTCOME CRITERIA	INTERVENTION	RATIONALE
1. Expresses interest in communicating with eye contact and gestures in 1:1 relationship	1a. Use 1:1 attention to engage the child in a therapeutic alliance beginning with non-verbal play.	1a. The nurse enters the child's world in a nonthreatening manner to form a trusting relationship.
	1b. Recognize subtle cues indicating the child is attending to nurse's actions.	1b. The cues that indicate the child is paying attention are subtle and difficult to recognize (e.g., glancing out of the corner of the eye).
2. Attempts to use single words and short phrases appropriately.	2a. Verbalize for the child what is happening and what the child might be experiencing.	2a. Naming objects and describing action, thoughts, and feelings help the child use symbolic language.
	2b. Encourage vocalizations with sound games and songs.	2b. Children learn through play.
	2c. Identify desired behaviors and rewards (e.g., hugs, treats, points).	2c. Behavior that is rewarded will increase in frequency.
3. Identifies self and others by name and proper pronoun.	3a. Use names frequently and encourage the use of correct pronouns (e.g., I, me, he).	3a. Problems with self-identification and pronoun reversal are common in PPD.
	3b. Foster ego development by reinforcing self-identity and ego boundaries through drawing, stories, and play activities.	3b. Development of ego functions are impaired in this disorder.
4. Increases verbalizations with parents and siblings.	4. Teach parents how to facilitate speech development in order to continue the behavior modification when visiting the child and after discharge.	4. Education and emotional support helps parents take a more therapeutic role at home and at time of discharge.

NURSING DIAGNOSIS: *Impaired social interactions*

OUTCOME CRITERIA	INTERVENTION	RATIONALE
1. Develops a trusting relationship and seeks out nurse for activities/ADLs, and for comfort when in distress.	1. Use 1:1 attention to engage the child in a therapeutic alliance; provide ego support in ADLs and activities; recognize emotional distress; provide comfort.	1. Trust is a basic attitude needed for social interactions, making emotional attachments and for separation/individuation tasks.
2. Makes attempts to interact and engage in play with peers.	2. Set up play situations with peers; role model social skills; reward attempts to interact and play with peers.	2. Learning occurs through imitation, modeling, feedback, and reinforcement.
3. Shows sensitivity and concern for feelings of others, including interest, empathy, sharing, and cooperation.	3. Facilitate superego development by role modeling empathy and sharing in activities with child's peers; reward appropriate affect development.	3. Autistic children have deficits in the development of empathy and the expression of appropriate affect.

NURSING CARE PLAN 29–1 A CHILD WITH AUTISTIC DISORDER *(Continued)*

NURSING DIAGNOSIS: *Risk for self-mutilation*

OUTCOME CRITERIA	INTERVENTION	RATIONALE
1. Will not injure self with self-mutilative behavior.	1a. Observe for increasing anxiety; determine emotional and situational triggers.	1a. Behavioral cues signal increasing anxiety.
	1b. Intervene early; provide ego support for reality testing and impulse control.	1b. Support is needed for an underdeveloped ego.
	1c. If the child does not respond well to verbal controls, use therapeutic holding.	1c. Holding reassures that an adult is in control, and feelings of security can become feelings of comfort and affection.
2. Will seek out nurse instead of expressing tension in self-mutilative behavior.	2. Help the child connect feelings to behavior. Substitute more appropriate behavior for the expression of feelings (e.g., throwing a soft toy).	2. The child gains insight into feelings, behavior, and better ways to cope with and express tension.

PPD, pervasive personality disorder; ADLs, activities of daily living.

changes in neurotransmitters that differentiate ADHD from other disorders. From 1937 the disorder was treated with CNS stimulants for their supposed "paradoxical effect," but this notion is no longer accepted. Although the fundamental cognitive defect responsible for ADHD remains unclear, brain imaging techniques have shown that children with ADHD have reduced blood flow in the striatal region of the brain, and administration of methylphenidate (Ritalin) increases blood flow and improves behavior. Other factors associated with ADHD are child abuse, neglect, foster home placements, lead poisoning, encephalitis, drug exposure in utero, low birth weight, and mental retardation. Children with ADHD are often dually diagnosed as having *oppositional defiant disorder* or *conduct disorder*. They also have a higher incidence of disorders involving mood, anxiety, learning, and communication. ADHD is often associated with Tourette's disorder and precedes its onset.

ADHD in the preschool child manifests itself as excessive gross motor activity that is less pronounced as the child matures. The disorder is most often picked up when the child has difficulty making the adjustment to elementary school and exhibits excessive fidgeting, restlessness, talkativeness, impulsivity, and difficulty sticking to and completing tasks. The symptoms worsen in situations requiring sustained attention. The attention problems and the hyperactivity contribute to a low frustration tolerance, temper outbursts, labile moods, poor school performance, rejection by peers, and low self-esteem. Some children exhibit enuresis and encopresis. In most cases of ADHD the symptoms lessen in late adolescence and early adulthood.

The DSM-IV criteria for ADHD are listed in Figure 29–2.

NURSING DIAGNOSES. NANDA diagnoses include the following:

Growth and development altered
Impaired social interaction
Self-esteem disturbance
Social isolation
Noncompliance

Others not specifically identified by NANDA categories include the following:

Aggressive behaviors
Attention seeking
Intrusive behaviors
Low frustration tolerance
Poor impulse control
Short attention span
Poor school performance

INTERVENTIONS. The interventions for ADHD are behavior modification and pharmacological agents for the disruptive/impulsive behaviors, special education programs for the attention difficulties, and psychotherapy/play therapy for the emotional problems that de-

Attention-Deficit/Hyperactivity Disorder (ADHD)

A. Either (1) or (2):

1. Six (or more) symptoms of inattention persisting for at least 6 months that are maladaptive and inconsistent with developmental level

Inattention

a. Fails to give close attention to details or makes careless mistakes
b. Has difficulty sustaining attention in tasks or play
c. Does not seem to listen when spoken to directly
d. Does not follow through and fails to finish tasks
e. Has difficulty organizing tasks and activities
f. Avoids or dislikes tasks requiring sustained attention
g. Loses things necessary for tasks or activities
h. Is easily distracted by extraneous stimuli
i. Is forgetful in daily activities

2. Six (or more) symptoms of hyperactivity-impulsivity persisting for at least 6 months that are maladaptive and inconsistent with developmental level

Hyperactivity

a. Fidgets with hands or feet, or squirms in seat
b. Leaves seat in classroom when expected to remain seated
c. Runs and climbs excessively in inappropriate situations
d. Has difficulty in playing or engaging in leisure activities quietly
e. Acts as if "driven by a motor," constantly "on the go"
f. Talks excessively

Impulsivity

g. Blurts out answers before question is completed
h. Has difficulty waiting for turn
i. Interrupts and intrudes on others' conversation and games

B. Some hyperactive-impulsive or inattentive symptoms were present before 7 years of age.

C. Some impairment from the symptoms is present in two or more settings (school, work, or home).

D. There must be clear evidence of clinically significant impairment in social, academic, or occupational functioning.

E. The symptoms are not part of other psychiatric disorders.

Figure 29–2 DSM-IV Attention-Deficit/Hyperactivity Disorder. (Adapted from American Psychiatric Association (1994). *Diagnostic and statistical manual of mental disorders* (4th ed.). Washington, DC: American Psychiatric Association. Reprinted with permission. Copyright 1994 American Psychiatric Association.)

velop as a result of the disorder. Methylphenidate (Ritalin) is the most widely used psychostimulant because of its safety and simplicity of use (Table 29–3) (Scahill and Lynch 1994b). Much of the work is with parents, who are the key players in carrying out the treatment plan, using behavior modification techniques at home, monitoring the medication and its effects, collaborating with the teacher to foster academic success, and setting up a home environment that promotes the achievement of normal developmental tasks.

NURSING CARE PLAN 29–2 A CHILD OR ADOLESCENT WITH ATTENTION DEFICIT/HYPERACTIVITY DISORDER

NURSING DIAGNOSIS: *Self-esteem disturbance (low self-esteem)*

OUTCOME CRITERIA	INTERVENTION	RATIONALE
1. Demonstrates increased self-esteem by verbalizing positive feelings about self and accomplishments.	1a. Help the child set realistic goals; set up situations that bring success; give genuine praise for accomplishments.	1a. Avoid "set-ups" for failure from unrealistic goals. Success teaches better than failure, and praise reinforces the behavior.
	1b. Use a behavior modification program if additional motivation is needed.	1b. A system of rewards will increase motivation.
2. Uses less attention-seeking behaviors to meet self-esteem needs.	2. Give positive attention for age-appropriate behaviors before attention seeking begins; give extra attention when indicated.	2. Reinforce adaptive behaviors before maladaptive ones are needed to gain attention.
3. Shows increased confidence in peer relationships by being willing to help others and share attention.	3. Help the child find a special friend who will be able to give attention; use peer group to provide opportunities for positive experiences and positive feedback.	3. Self-esteem comes from respect by peers and affection from a special friend.

NURSING DIAGNOSIS: *Impaired social interactions*

OUTCOME CRITERIA	INTERVENTION	RATIONALE
1. Demonstrates increased ability to participate in groups and 1:1 play activities without being intrusive, bossy, provocative, or aggressive.	1a. Identify the desired behaviors and observe for them so that positive feedback can be given immediately.	1a. Describing expected behavior is more effective than telling children what they cannot do.
	1b. Role model appropriate behaviors.	1b. Demonstrations are more effective than verbal instructions.
	1c. Use the techniques for handling disruptive behaviors; use "antiseptic bouncing" or "time out" as needed.	1c. Start with the least attention to the disruptive behavior to avoid reinforcing it.
	1d. Use situations that develop as learning experiences to develop more mature behavior and better adaptive coping (e.g., "life-space interview").	1d. Ventilation of feelings, reality testing, problem solving, and testing new behaviors are necessary for psychosocial development.
	2a. Use therapeutic play to teach social skills (e.g., puppets, role play, "mutual story telling," therapeutic games).	2a. Therapeutic play allows the child to try social skills in fantasy play and in real life situations with peers.
	2b. Support the child's efforts to use new social skills by "coaching," praising, and processing the results with the child.	2b. Verbal encouragement to control impulses and try new behavior supports the child's ego development.

Continued on following page

NURSING CARE PLAN 29–2 A CHILD OR ADOLESCENT WITH ATTENTION DEFICIT/HYPERACTIVITY DISORDER *(Continued)*

NURSING DIAGNOSIS: *Impulsive behavior with low frustration tolerance*

OUTCOME CRITERIA	INTERVENTION	RATIONALE
1. Demonstrates an increased ability to delay gratification.	1. Gratify wishes in a reasonable amount of time; keep anxiety/frustration from escalating by using verbal interventions and redirection of activities; increase waiting time gradually.	1. Ego support keeps the anxiety and frustration manageable. Performing other activities while waiting decreases anxiety.
2. Demonstrates attempts to control acting out impulses by seeking out staff, and using techniques that encourage thinking before acting.	2a. Contract or use behavior modification to help the child to use the nurse for external control of behavior.	2a. External controls are needed until internal controls are developed.
	2b. Teach techniques that the child can use to think before acting (e.g., count to ten).	2b. Cognitive control of emotions is necessary to curb impulsive behavior. Psychostimulants are used to increase cognitive function.
3. Expresses feelings of anger and frustration verbally in age-appropriate behaviors rather than acting them out.	3a. Give the child a chance to express feelings without being rejected.	3a. A child needs to know that feelings are OK.
	3b. Use the Quiet Room with staff support if feelings have overwhelmed the child's ability to continue in the activity.	3b. Privacy and emotional support provide an opportunity to work on difficult feelings.
	3c. Help the child connect feelings to the current situation and the acting out behavior.	3c. Understanding the connection between feelings and behavior is necessary for developing internal control.
	3d. Help the child develop problem-solving and conflict resolution skills by 1:1 interventions, therapeutic play, and role modeling.	3d. More mature coping skills are required as the child learns to control the impulses and feelings.

NURSING DIAGNOSIS: *Altered parenting*

OUTCOME CRITERIA	INTERVENTION	RATIONALE
1. Parents will participate in the child's therapeutic program.	1. Use empathy to form a therapeutic alliance and explore the impact of ADHD on family life; assess parents' knowledge of ADHD and give needed information; assess the family's support system.	1. Problem identification and analysis of learning needs is necessary before intervention begins.
2. Parents will set realistic goals for behavior at home.	2a. Discuss how to make a safe home environment.	2a. The home environment needs to provide support by being comfortable and break-proof and by allowing for moderate levels of activity.

NURSING CARE PLAN 29–2 A CHILD OR ADOLESCENT WITH ATTENTION DEFICIT/HYPERACTIVITY DISORDER *(Continued)*

OUTCOME CRITERIA	INTERVENTION	RATIONALE
	2b. Discuss realistic behavioral goals; how to set goals and evaluate outcomes.	2b. Mutual goal setting increases parents' participation, motivation, and satisfaction.
3. Parents will use a systematic approach to managing the child's behavior.	3. Teach behavior modification techniques and give parents support as they learn to apply them.	3–4. Education and follow-up support is the key to a successful treatment program for ADHD.
4. Parents will follow the medication regimen wisely.	4. Give educational information about medications that enable parents to monitor their effectiveness and side effects.	
5. Parents will develop a support system and use available resources to advocate for the child's educational needs.	5. Refer parents to a local chapter of an ADHD parents' group; facilitate collaboration between parents and the school system; serve as a child/parent advocate with other agencies.	5. Parental self-help groups can provide a unique support system and valuable information on ways to obtain child services.

Nursing interventions for disturbances in self-esteem, social interactions, and impulsive behaviors are described in Nursing Care Plan 29–2 for the child with ADHD. In addition, nursing interventions for work with parents include the following:

- Assess parents' knowledge of ADHD and give needed information.
- Explore the impact of ADHD on family life.
- Assess the family's support system.
- Discuss how to make home a safe environment.
- Discuss realistic behavioral goals and how to set them.
- Teach behavior modification techniques.
- Give parents support as they learn to apply techniques.
- Give educational information about medications.
- Refer parents to a local chapter of an ADHD parents' group.
- Be a child/parent advocate with the educational system.

Conduct Disorder

Conduct disorder is characterized by a persistent pattern of behavior in which the rights of others and age-appropriate societal norms or rules are violated (APA 1994). Misconduct is classified into four types:

1. Aggressive conduct that causes or threatens harms to other people and animals
2. Destruction of property (destroyed property or fire setting)
3. Deceitfulness or theft
4. Serious violation of rules

The prevalence of conduct disorder for youths under age 18 is 9% for boys and 2% for girls, making it the largest single category of mental disorders in children and adolescents. Predisposing factors are ADHD, oppositional child behaviors, parental rejection, inconsistent parenting with harsh discipline, early institutional living,

TABLE 29–3 STIMULANT DRUGS USED IN THE TREATMENT OF ATTENTION-DEFICIT HYPERACTIVITY DISORDER

DRUG	DAILY DOSE RANGE	SERUM HALF-LIFE	DAILY DOSE SCHEDULES
Methylphenidate (Ritalin)	5–60 mg	2–5 hr	2–3 doses
Dextroamphetamine (Dexedrine)	2.5–40 mg	6–8 hr	2 doses
Pemoline (Cylert)	18.75–112.5 mg	8–12 hr	1 dose

Data from: Scahill, L. and Lynch, K. A. (1994). Pharmacology notes: The use of methylphenidate in children with attention-deficit/hyperactivity disorder. *Journal of Child and Adolescent Psychiatric Nursing*, 7 (4):44–47. Reprinted with permission, Nursecom, Inc.

frequent shifting of parental figures, large family size, absence of father or alcoholic father, antisocial and drug-dependent family members, and association with a delinquent group.

Kernberg and Chazan (1991) describe four etiological views of conduct disorder. The first is ego psychology, which attributes the disorder to major developmental impairments in cognitive function, impulse control, judgment, modulation of affect, and tolerance of anxiety and frustration. The child has a core feeling of being unloved and unlovable, and often provokes rejection to get attention, even though the attention is negative. The second view is derived from attachment theory, which attributes the disorder to an insecure attachment to a significant caretaker's causing ongoing distortions in the child's relationships with others. The third view relates to temperament theory and attributes the disturbance in conduct and relationships to the "difficult child" pattern and the misfit between child and parental characteristics. Learning theory, in which the disturbed conduct has been modeled and reinforced by significant persons in the child's environment, is the basis for the fourth view. This last-named view becomes an important theoretical approach in the treatment of this disorder.

Conduct disorder, which develops in childhood before 10 years of age, is more often seen in males and manifests as physical aggression toward others, with little empathy or concern for other persons and a lack of guilt or remorse. These children frequently misperceive the intentions of others as hostile and believe their aggressive responses are justified. They have little loyalty and blame peers for their misdeeds. Although children with conduct disorder try to project a "tough" image, they have low self-esteem, low frustration tolerance, irritability, and temper outbursts. These children are more likely to develop antisocial personality disorder than those who develop the disorder in adolescence.

The adolescent-onset type of conduct disorder demonstrates less aggressive behaviors and more normal peer relationships. These youths tend to act out their misconduct with their peer group (e.g., early-onset sexual behavior, smoking, drinking, substance abuse, risk-taking behaviors).

The male-to-female ratio is not as high as for the childhood-onset disorder.

Complications associated with conduct disorder are academic failures related to below-average reading/verbal skills and learning disabilities, school suspensions and dropouts, juvenile delinquency, and the need for the juvenile court system to assume responsibility for youths who cannot be managed by their parents. Psychiatric disorders that frequently coexist with conduct disorder are anxiety, depression, ADHD, and learning disabilities.

The outcome for children with conduct disorder is poor and they account for a large percentage of inpatient admissions and institutional placements (Harnett 1989). Studies indicate that the antisocial behaviors persist into adulthood and often result in the diagnosis of antisocial personality disorder. The DSM-IV criteria for conduct disorder are listed in Figure 29–3.

NURSING DIAGNOSES. NANDA diagnoses include the following:

Defensive coping
Impaired adjustment
Impaired social interactions
Ineffective individual coping
Self-esteem disturbance
Violence directed at others

Other behaviors not specifically addressed by NANDA categories include the following:

Anger/hostility
Aggressive behaviors

Conduct Disorder

A. A repetitive and persistent pattern of behavior in which the basic rights of others or major age-appropriate societal norms or rules are violated, manifested by three (or more) of the following behaviors in the past 3 months and at least one behavior present in the past 6 months.

Aggression to People and Animals
1. Often bullies, threatens, and intimidates others
2. Often initiates physical fights
3. Has used a weapon that could cause serious injury (e.g., bat, brick, broken bottle, knife, gun)
4. Has been physically cruel to others
5. Has been physically cruel to animals
6. Has stolen while confronting a victim
7. Has forced someone into sexual activity

Destruction of Property
8. Has deliberately set fires intending to cause damage
9. Has deliberately destroyed another's property

Deceitfulness or Theft
10. Has broken into a house, building, or car
11. Often lies to obtain goods or favors
12. Has stolen items of nontrivial value (shoplifting)

Serious Violations or Rules
13. Often stays out at night despite parental prohibitions beginning before 13 years of age
14. Has run away from home at least twice, or once for a lengthy period of time
15. Often truant from school beginning before 13 years of age

B. The disturbance in behavior causes clinically significant impairments in social, academic, or occupational functioning.

Figure 29–3 DSM-IV Conduct Disorder. (Adapted from American Psychiatric Association (1994). *Diagnostic and statistical manual of mental disorders* (4th ed.). Washington, DC: American Psychiatric Association. Reprinted with permission. Copyright 1994 American Psychiatric Association.)

Disregard for social norms or rules
Lack of remorse
Low frustration tolerance
Poor impulse control
Poor school performance
Violence toward property

INTERVENTIONS. The focus of treatment is on correcting the child's faulty ego development, which involves developing more mature and adaptive coping mechanisms. This process is gradual and cannot be accomplished during short-term hospitalization. However, inpatient hospitalization is often needed for crisis intervention, evaluation, treatment planning, and transfer to long-term residential treatment.

To control aggressive behaviors, a large variety of pharmacological agents have been tried, including antipsychotics, lithium carbonate, anticonvulsants, antidepressants, and beta-adrenergic blockers. Cognitive-behavioral therapy is used to change the pattern of misconduct by fostering the development of internal controls, both cognitive and emotional. Problem solving, conflict resolution, empathy, and social interaction skills are important components of the treatment program. Families are involved in therapy and are given support in parenting skills designed to help them provide nurturance and set consistent limits. When families are abusive, drug dependent, or highly disorganized, the child will benefit by an out-of-home placement. See Nursing Care Plan 29–3 for children or adolescents with conduct disorder.

Oppositional Defiant Disorder

Oppositional defiant disorder is a recurrent pattern of negativistic, disobedient, hostile, defiant behavior toward authority figures without serious violations of the basic rights of others (APA 1994). The child exhibits persistent stubbornness and argumentativeness, persistent testing of limits, an unwillingness to give in or negotiate, and a refusal to accept blame for misdeeds. This behavior is evident at home but may not be elsewhere. These children and adolescents do not see themselves as defiant; instead they feel they are responding to unreasonable demands or situations.

This disorder is usually evident before 8 years of age and is more common in males (until puberty, when the rates are equal). According to DSM-IV, oppositional defiant disorder has at least four of the following characteristics persisting for 6 or more months:

- Often loses temper
- Often argues with adults
- Often actively defies or refuses to comply
- Deliberately annoys people
- Blames others for his or her mistakes
- Is easily annoyed by others
- Is often angry and resentful
- Is often spiteful or vindictive

NURSING DIAGNOSES. Any of the diagnoses under conduct disorder could be applicable, with the exception of violence.

INTERVENTION. Youths with this disorder are generally treated on an outpatient basis. Much of the focus is on parenting issues, using individual, group, or family therapy.

Anxiety Disorders

Separation Anxiety Disorder

Children and adolescents with **separation anxiety disorder** become excessively anxious when separated from, or anticipating a separation from, their home or parental figures (APA 1994). Their misery at being away from home makes them refuse to attend school or camp or to visit or sleep at a friend's house. They may exhibit "clinging" behavior, even "shadowing" the parent around the house. These children often have difficulty falling asleep without an adult present, may have nightmares, and go to the parent's room when they awaken during the night. The severe anxiety can also result in stomachaches, headaches, nausea, and vomiting. Their behavior is described as demanding and intrusive. A depressed mood often accompanies the anxiety.

Separation anxiety disorder may develop after a significant stress, such as the death of a relative or pet, illness, or a move or change in schools. The onset can be any time between preschool years and age 18. The prevalence of the disorder in children is estimated to be 4%, with equal numbers of males and females treated. However, epidemiological studies show a higher incidence of the disorder in females. Separation anxiety disorder is more common in first-degree biological relatives, and the incidence may be related to having a mother with panic disorder. The DSM-IV characteristics of separation anxiety disorder are

- Excessive distress when separated or anticipating separation from home or parental figures.
- Excessive worries about being lost or kidnapped or that parental figures will be harmed.
- Fear of being home alone or in situations without other significant adults.
- Refusal to sleep unless near a parental figure and refusal to sleep away from home.
- Refusal to attend school or other activities without a parental figure.
- Physical symptoms as a response to anxiety.

NURSING DIAGNOSES. NANDA diagnoses include the following:

Adjustment impaired
Anxiety/fear

NURSING CARE PLAN 29–3 A CHILD OR ADOLESCENT WITH CONDUCT DISORDER

NURSING DIAGNOSIS: *Violence directed at others*

OUTCOME CRITERIA	INTERVENTION	RATIONALE
1. Forms a trusting relationship with the primary nurse.	1. Use a 1:1 relationship to engage the child in a therapeutic alliance.	1. The development of trust has often been disrupted in this disorder.
2. Will not hurt other persons or property by acting out hostile, aggressive impulses.	2a. Use 1:1 or appropriate level of observation; monitor rising levels of anxiety; determine situational and emotional triggers.	2a. External controls are needed for ego support and to prevent acts of aggression/violence.
	2b. Intervene early to calm the child and defuse the potential incident; use techniques for managing disruptive behavior (see Box 29–9).	2b. Learning can take place before the child loses control; new ways to cope can be discussed and role modeled.
	2c. Set clear, consistent limits in a calm, nonjudgmental manner; remind the child of the consequences of acting out; avoid power struggles.	2c. A child gains a sense of security with clear limits and calm adults who follow through on a consistent basis.
	2d. Use strategic removal if the child cannot respond to limits (e.g., time out, Quiet Room, therapeutic holding).	2d. Removal allows the child to express feelings and discuss problems without losing face in front of peers.
	2e. Process the incident with the child to make it a learning experience (e.g., "life space interview," role playing, role modeling).	2e. Reality testing, problem solving, and testing new behavior are necessary for ego development and psychosocial growth.
	2f. Use medication if indicated to reduce anxiety and aggression.	2f. A variety of medications are effective in a child who experiences behavioral dyscontrol.
3. Seeks out staff and verbalizes frustrations and anxiety rather than acting them out.	3. Use a behavior modification program that rewards the individual for seeking help with handling feelings and controlling impulses to act out.	3. Rewarding the child's efforts to seek help increases the behavior.
4. Channels aggression into constructive activities and age-appropriate competitive games.	4. Redirect the expression of feelings into nondestructive, age-appropriate behaviors; channel excess energy into physical activities.	4. Learning how to modulate the expression of feelings and use anger constructively is essential for self-control.
5. Demonstrates a beginning sense of empathy for others and remorse for misdeeds.	5a. Help the child see how the acting out hurts others; appeal to the child's sense of "fairness" for all, including the target of the child's actions.	5a. These children are insensitive to the feelings of others but can understand the concept of "fairness" and generalize it to other persons.
	5b. Encourage the feelings of empathy for others and the remorse for misdeeds.	5b. Superego development is a therapeutic goal with these children.

NURSING CARE PLAN 29–3 A CHILD OR ADOLESCENT WITH CONDUCT DISORDER *(Continued)*

NURSING DIAGNOSIS: *Self-esteem disturbance (low self-esteem)*

OUTCOME CRITERIA	INTERVENTION	RATIONALE
1. Demonstrates increased self-esteem by verbalizing positive feelings about self and accomplishments.	1a. Help the child set realistic goals; set up situations that bring success; give genuine praise for accomplishments.	1a. These children often have a need to control by manipulation and intimidation. Realistic goals will avoid this.
	1b. Give "unconditional positive regard" and reinforce the child's self-worth without reinforcing negative behaviors.	1b. These children often set up situations in which their behavior brings rejection.
2. Uses less manipulative behaviors and more mature methods to get self-esteem needs met.	2a. Recognize and intervene in attempts to use manipulative behavior; help the child identify needs and express them in a direct way.	2a. The child who can identify needs will use more direct communication in getting them met and have better control of the environment.
	2b. Use a behavior modification program to limit manipulative behaviors and reward adaptive behaviors.	2b. Give positive attention to the adaptive behaviors rather than negative attention to the manipulation.
3. Demonstrates self-confidence in controlling impulses and expressing emotions.	3. Consistently recognize the child's self-control in difficult situations; encourage the expression of a complete range of emotional affect appropriate to the situation.	3. Self-control needs to become a source of pride (superego function). The child needs to be in touch with all emotions and not fear that their expression is a sign of weakness.
4. Shows pride in being able to help others.	4. Take advantage of or set up situations in which the child can use his or her expertise to help others.	4. Altruism is a needed attitude in this disorder, and its development will increase self-esteem.

NURSING DIAGNOSIS: *Impaired social interaction*

OUTCOME CRITERIA	INTERVENTION	RATIONALE
1. Demonstrates an increased ability to participate in group and 1:1 activities without attempts to intimidate or manipulate others.	1. Monitor behavior for manipulation and intimidation of peers; intervene early; provide alternative ways to handle the situation.	1. Appropriate social behaviors can be learned from positive and negative feedback. Early intervention prevents rejection by peers.
2. Uses age-appropriate skills in play activities and friendships.	2. Use therapeutic play to teach social skills such as sharing, cooperation, realistic competition, and manners (e.g., role playing, "mutual story telling," therapeutic games).	2. Learning new ways to interact with peers allows for the development of friendship and brings satisfaction.
3. Develops a genuine, equal status friendship with a peer.	3. Help the child find and develop that special friendship; set up 1:1 situations; be available for problem-solving peer relationship conflicts; role model friendship behaviors.	3. Developing trust in a peer is an important step in personality development and success in social skills.

Growth and development impaired
Impaired social interactions
Ineffective individual coping
Sleep pattern disturbances

Other behaviors not specifically addressed by NANDA categories include the following:

Clinging/dependent behaviors
School refusal
Physical symptoms of anxiety (stomachache, headache, nausea and vomiting)

INTERVENTIONS. Children and adolescents with the disorder are given individual, group, or family therapy on an outpatient basis. The focus is on issues of separation/individuation, with behavior modification used to reinforce self-control behaviors. Children who refuse to start primary school are introduced gradually, with parents present for support part of the day. For adolescents who develop school phobia, the goal is to return them to the classroom at the earliest possible date and to give parents support in setting limits on truancy. Issues that precipitated the school phobia are worked on in individual or group therapy. The most commonly used pharmacological agents for the anxiety and depression are antihistamines, anxiolytics, and antidepressants (Gittelman 1986).

Social Phobia

Children who develop **social phobia** may become excessively timid, freeze, become mute, cry and cling to a familiar person, or even have tantrums in unfamiliar social situations (APA 1994). They frequently refuse to play and stay on the periphery of activities. These children are usually unable to avoid the feared situation and unable to identify the cause of their anxiety. When the onset is early in childhood, the ability to achieve an expected level of function is impaired. Adolescent onset results in a decline in social and academic performance.

Obsessive-Compulsive Disorder

The behavioral manifestations of obsessive-compulsive disorder (OCD) in childhood and adolescence are similar to adult behaviors (e.g., washing, checking, touching rituals). The child does not recognize the behaviors as being ego-dystonic. However, the parents seek help when they see the child's concentration and school performance decline. Onset is 6 to 15 years of age for males and 20 to 29 years of age for females.

Posttraumatic Stress Disorder

Posttraumatic stress disorder (PTSD) can occur at any age and has now been recognized in children. Rather than reliving the traumatic event, younger children with PTSD have dreams about the event that turn into generalized nightmares (APA 1994). The content of the nightmares will be monsters, threats to self or others, and rescue of others. The child may also relive the trauma by repetitively playing out the event. Other symptoms may be dependent and regressive behaviors, separation anxiety, extreme fear and avoidance of events that remind the child of the trauma, and physical complaints such as headache and stomachache. (See Chapter 17 for a discussion of PTSD.)

Mood Disorders

It was once believed that children did not suffer from the same type of depression that adults did and that a child's sadness in reaction to an event or situation would be short-lived. Now, with increasing suicide rates in childhood and suicide the third leading cause of death in adolescence, depression is being treated with psychotherapy and medication rather than letting it run its course (Valente 1989). (See Chapter 20 for depressive disorders.) Symptoms of depression may differ between children and adolescents: somatic complaints, irritability, and social withdrawal are more common in childhood; psychomotor retardation, hypersomnia, and delusions are more evident in adolescence (APA 1994). The acting out behaviors of adolescents, once considered symptoms of a "masked depression," can be related to depression or to the beginning of a bipolar disorder. The signs of depression in both children and adolescents are listed in Box 29–7.

Factors associated with child and adolescent depression are physical and sexual abuse, neglect, homelessness, marital discord, death, divorce, separation of parents, separation from parents, learning disabilities, chronic illness, conflicts with family or peers, and rejection by family or peers.

The complications of depression are school failure and dropping out, drug and alcohol abuse, sexual promiscuity, pregnancy, running away, illegal and antisocial behavior, and suicide.

NURSING DIAGNOSES. NANDA diagnoses include the following:

Adjustment impaired
Grieving
Hopelessness
Impaired social interaction
Loneliness
Self-esteem disturbance
Social isolation
Violence, risk directed at self

INTERVENTION. Suicidal children and adolescents are hospitalized for evaluation and treatment with psychotherapy and antidepressants and/or mood stabilizers. Individual, group, and family therapies are used to relieve the distress; correct self-appraisals and improve self-

BOX 29–7 SIGNS OF DEPRESSION IN CHILDREN AND ADOLESCENTS

MOOD/AFFECT CHANGES
Apathy
Anhedonia
Anger
Sadness/crying
Irritability
Guilt
Decreased self-esteem
Decreased spontaneity
Monotone speech

COGNITIVE CHANGES
Apathy
Boredom
Decreased concentration
Loss of interest in school
Decreased school performance
Decreased creativity
Loss of interest in activities
Preoccupation with illness
Preoccupation with death
Thoughts of dying
Suicidal ideation
Suicidal threats

PHYSICAL CHANGES
Loss of energy
Insomnia/hypersomnia
Nightmares
Appetite changes
Weight loss/gain
Physical complaints (head, stomach, leg aches)

SOCIAL BEHAVIORAL CHANGES
Isolation (self-imposed or rejection by peers)
Change in friends
Loss of girl/boyfriend
Risk taking
Drug/alcohol use
Running away/truancy
Misuse of sex
Decrease in after-school activity and playtime
Interest in morbid music and literature
Suicidal gestures/attempts

esteem; and promote problem-solving and adaptive coping skills. Tricyclic antidepressants (TCAs) are still used but only with careful monitoring for cardiac effects. Newer atypical antidepressants in the form of selective serotonin reuptake inhibitors (SSRIs)—sertraline (Zoloft) and fluoxetine (Prozac)—are now being used for children and adolescents.

Tourette's Disorder

Tourette's disorder involves motor and verbal tics that cause marked distress and significant impairment in social and occupational function (APA 1994). Tics may appear as early as 2 years of age, but the average age of onset for motor tics is 7 years. Motor tics usually involve the head but can also involve the torso or limbs, and they change in location, frequency, and severity over time. In one half of the cases the first symptom is a single tic, most often eye blinking. Other motor tics are tongue protrusion, touching, squatting, hopping, skipping, retracing steps, and twirling when walking. Vocal tics include words and sounds (barks, grunts, yelps, clicks, snorts, sniffs, coughs). Coprolalia (uttering obscenities) is present in less than 10% of cases. The duration of the disorder is usually lifelong, but there can be periods of remission, and the symptoms often diminish during adolescence or sometimes disappear by early adulthood.

Tourette's disorder affects 4 to 5 individuals per 10,000 and is 1.5 to 3 times more common in males. There is a familial pattern in about 90% of cases. Vulnerability is transmitted in an autosomal dominant pattern, with 70% of females and 99% of males who have inherited the gene developing the disorder. "Nongenetic" Tourette's disorder often coexists with PDD or a seizure disorder.

Symptoms associated with Tourette's disorder are obsessions, compulsions, hyperactivity, distractibility, and impulsivity. In addition, the child or adolescent with tics has low self-esteem from feeling ashamed, self-conscious, and rejected by peers. The fear of having tic behavior in public situations causes the individual to limit activities severely. CNS stimulants increase the severity of the tics, and therefore children with coexisting ADHD must have their medication carefully monitored. The DSM-IV characteristics for Tourette's disorder are

- Multiple motor and one or more vocal tics, which do not have to occur concurrently.
- Tics occurring many times a day, nearly every day, for more than 1 year.
- Tics causing marked distress, or significant impairment in important areas of function (e.g., school, occupation).

NURSING DIAGNOSES. NANDA diagnoses include the following:

Anxiety
Adjustment impaired
Impaired social interaction

Self-esteem disturbance
Social isolation
Loneliness

Other behaviors not specifically addressed by NANDA categories include the following:

Abnormal body movements and vocalizations (tics)
Bizarre patterns of body movement
Obsessive-compulsive behaviors
Impaired school performance

INTERVENTIONS. The focus of treatment is on helping the child, family, and school understand and cope with the tic behaviors. This disorder is treated on an outpatient basis unless there are severe tics and/or obsessive-compulsive behaviors that impair school performance. In the latter event, inpatient or day hospitalization is needed for a complete evaluation and pharmacological intervention.

Adjustment Disorder

This is a residual category used for emotional responses to an identifiable stressor that do not meet the criteria for a DSM-IV, Axis I psychiatric disorder (APA 1994). **Adjustment disorder** is a frequently used category for children and adolescents whose problems are not severe enough to require hospitalization, but who are showing a decreased performance at school and temporary changes in social relationships. The disorder begins within 3 months of the stress and lasts no longer than 6 months after the stress has ceased. The subtypes are classified according to the presenting symptoms: adjustment disorder (1) with anxiety, (2) with mixed anxiety and depressed mood, (3) with disturbance of conduct, (4) with mixed disturbance of emotions and conduct, and (5) unspecified.

Feeding and Eating Disorders

Three such disorders are pica, rumination disorder, and feeding and eating disorder of infancy or early childhood (APA 1994). Pica is the persistent eating of nonnutritive substances, although there is no aversion to eating food. Infants and toddlers may eat paint, plaster, string, or cloth.

Older children may eat sand, pebbles, insects, or even animal droppings. This behavior is frequently associated with mental retardation. Rumination disorder is the repeated regurgitation and rechewing of food without apparent nausea, retching, or gastrointestinal problems. This disorder may occur with developmental delays between 3 and 12 months of age. It occurs later in mentally retarded children. In the feeding and eating disorder, the infant or child fails to eat adequate amounts of food, despite availability, and there is no medical condition or mental retardation. The individual fails to gain weight or has a significant weight loss, which then contributes to developmental delays. Chapter 26 addresses anorexia, bulimia, and compulsive eating.

PLANNING

Planning Outcome Criteria

Claire Fagin's (1972) classic child psychiatric nursing textbook describes the purpose of the nurse's therapeutic interventions and treatment goals (expected outcomes) for the child. Fagin notes that the nurse always uses verbal communication skills, but more often in working with children the communication is through a series of activities. Children are dependent on adults, and therefore the nurse manipulates the child's environment to foster growth, development, and learning (either in the home or in the treatment setting). The purposes of nursing interventions identified by Fagin (1972) are

- To assist children with new learning regarding themselves and their world.
- To assist the child and family with relearning of roles and relationships, and expectations.
- To assist in restoring those aspects of living that show deprivations.

The therapeutic outcome criteria for the child are

- To learn through individual and group relationships.
- To develop a self-identity that includes greater body image integrity and greater interpersonal competence.
- To restore or relearn missing or distorted developmental functions.

The purposes of nursing intervention and the child's therapeutic goals serve as the basis for planning nursing care. The interventions are implemented through the use of the various treatment modalities described in the next section.

INTERVENTIONS

The forms of treatment described in this section can be used in a variety of settings: inpatient, residential, outpatient, day treatment, and outreach programs. Many of the modalities involve the normal activities of a child's day, such as activities of daily living (ADLs), learning activities, multiple forms of play and recreational activities, and interactions with adults and peers.

Family Therapy

Children and adolescents are part of a family, and that family needs to be included in the treatment of the client.

In the past, children who were treated in long-term facilities had limited contact with parents. This approach changed as family dynamics were viewed as an etiological factor in the child's disorder and family therapy was developed as a treatment modality. Goren (1992) notes that the literature on child psychiatry continues to blame parents for the child's pathology rather than focusing on making a therapeutic alliance with parents. Goren advocates involving parents in treatment decisions and in designing a plan that considers potential parental competencies and family organization. To ensure optimal outcomes in treating troubled and vulnerable children and adolescents, it is vital to involve and educate the family in the treatment process. The family remains the integral part of the supportive and educative system for the child or adolescent.

In addition to therapy with a single family, multiple family therapy is being used in inpatient settings (Bender 1992). This modality engages families as co-therapists for other families in working through problems of daily life. During the process the families learn to (1) like and respect others, (2) accept shortcomings and capitalize on strengths, (3) develop insight and improve judgment, (4) use new information, and (5) develop lasting and satisfying relationships.

Milieu Therapy

Milieu therapy remains the philosophical basis for structuring inpatient, residential, and day treatment programs. According to both the *Standards of child and adolescent psychiatric and mental health nursing practice* (ANA 1985) and the same organization's combined adult and child standards of practice (1994), the nurse collaborates with other health care providers in structuring and maintaining a therapeutic environment, which facilitates the individual's growth and positive behavioral change. Critchley (1991) describes a traditional psychiatric nurse's role in inpatient settings as ". . . a role model for being a milieu team member and for using therapeutically the everyday life events in the milieu" (p. 253).

Three major goals of a therapeutic milieu are to

1. Provide physical and psychological security.
2. Promote growth and mastery of developmental tasks.
3. Ameliorate psychiatric disorders.

The physical milieu is designed to provide a safe, comfortable place to live, play, and learn, with areas for private time as well as group activity. Inpatient, residential, and day programs may have a gym, an outdoor playground, a swimming pool, a garden, cooking and other recreational facilities, and even pets. No matter what physical facilities exist, the essential parts of a therapeutic milieu are the multidisciplinary team and the therapeutic activities. The unit's schedule structures the activities, such as getting up, grooming/dressing, eating, resting, school, therapy sessions, play time, group activities and "outings," and family and home visits. This structure provides a needed sense of security for the disturbed youth. The multidisciplinary team shares a philosophy of how to provide psychological security, promote personal growth, work with the behavioral symptoms, and ameliorate the causes of the mental disorder. The youth's behavior, emotions, and cognitive processes are the focus of the therapeutic interventions in the milieu. Therapy is a combination of cognitive and behavioral approaches. The therapeutic factors operating in the milieu's structure, activities, and interactions with staff are listed in Box 29–8.

Activities of Daily Living

ADLs are recognized as part of the therapeutic milieu in the standards for psychiatric nursing practice, and are to be used in goal-directed ways to foster growth and well-being (ANA 1994). The child's problems with ADLs are identified and individual interventions planned. The following vignette shows how ADLs are used to promote adaptive behaviors and mastery of developmental tasks.

▶ Betty Jean, a 4-year-old who has grown up as a "wild child" because of neglect by an alcoholic mother, spends mealtimes trying to flip the food out of her spoon and turn over her plate, while squealing "Betty Jean flip the food . . . flip the food." She requires one-to-one intervention during mealtimes to control her behavior and to provide her a role model for proper eating skills.

BOX 29–8 THERAPEUTIC FACTORS IN THE MILIEU

- "Holding environment" with roles, boundaries, and limits
- Reduction in stressors
- Situations for expression of feelings without fear of rejection or retaliation
- Available emotional support and comfort
- Assistance with reality testing and support for weak or missing ego functions
- Interventions in impulsive/aggressive and inappropriate behaviors
- Opportunities for learning and testing new adaptive behaviors and mastering developmental tasks
- Consistent, constructive feedback
- Reinforcement of positive behaviors and development of self-esteem
- Corrective emotional experiences
- Role models for making healthy identifications and positive attachments
- Opportunities to develop better peer relationships and be influenced by positive peer pressure
- Opportunities to be spontaneous and creative
- Experiences leading to identity formation

Behavior Modification

Behavior modification is based on the principle that behavior which is rewarded will more likely be repeated. Developmentally appropriate behaviors are normally rewarded with praise by a significant adult in the child's life, so modifying behavior in this manner is a standard parenting technique *(operant conditioning)*. Behavior modification is easy to learn and does not require an understanding of the child's psychopathology. It is necessary only to identify the desired behavior and the reward and to apply the process systematically. To extinguish undesirable behavior, either the behavior is ignored or, if it is too disruptive, limits having specified consequences are set.

Although there is an individualized treatment plan for each child or adolescent, most treatment settings use a behavior modification program, such as token economy, to motivate and reward age-appropriate behaviors. One popular method is the point and level system, with points awarded for desired behaviors and with increasing levels of privileges that can be earned. The point value for specific behaviors and the privileges for each level are spelled out on a large memo board. Each child's status and acquired points for the day are recorded. A more permanent copy is kept in the child's nursing records. Older children and adolescents can be made responsible for keeping their own daily point sheet, and for requesting points for appropriate behaviors. Points are given for age-appropriate behaviors (e.g., getting up/dressed, attending school/activities on time without disruptive behaviors, demonstrating social skills). The child who works on individual behavioral goals (e.g., seeking out staff for help in problem solving) is also rewarded with points.

Points are collected and used to obtain a specific reward (token economy program). A unit might require the child to earn a certain number of points in order to move from one privilege level to the next. Another unit might reward the child with a visit to the "point store" at the end of the week to pick out a toy. The level system defines privileges, with the lowest level confining the child to the unit for all activities. Each level has increasing privileges (e.g., going off the unit with a staff member, later bedtime on weekends). At the highest level, the privilege might be to go off the unit unescorted.

Peterson and colleagues (1994) describe a behavior modification program for an inpatient unit that includes "hold assignments" for acting out. For example, an adolescent who refuses to attend a therapy session is given the "hold assignment" of going to the session within the next 10 minutes, and his or her privilege level is put "on hold." In those 10 minutes the staff help the adolescent explore feelings and resolve the resistance to attending the therapy session. If the adolescent does not complete the "hold assignment," privileges are dropped one level, and if three "hold assignments" are given in a 24-hour period, privileges are also dropped one level. The authors report this program to be effective in changing behavior and reducing the need to use mechanical restraints by 82% within the first 6 months of operation.

Modifying Disruptive Behavior

Managing and modifying disruptive behaviors in group activities and in the therapeutic milieu is a real challenge for the nurse. If the disruptive behavior is not interrupted early, the contagion effect will derail the group activity and cause chaos on the unit. Intervention techniques for working with disruptive behaviors are rarely described in the nursing literature. Delaney (1994) advocates taking a proactive approach by increasing the structure of a group activity, using all available resources (e.g., increasing staff presence), and anticipating the contagious effects with "antiseptic bouncing" of a disruptive child from the activity. Box 29–9 describes a series of classic intervention techniques developed by Redl and Wineman (1957) that modify disruptive behaviors and prevent the contagion effect.

Removal and Restraint

Seclusion

Controversy over the use of seclusion in dealing with children continues, there being no clear evidence that it is therapeutic (Walsh and Randell 1995). Child and adolescent units may have a seclusion room, but its use is limited because youths who are out of control can become self-destructive.

Seclusion is most frequently used for noncompliant behaviors that might have been managed in other ways before the behavior escalated. Seclusion may bring about superficial compliance, but it has little to do with real behavioral change (Goren 1991). The child perceives seclusion as punishment, and the experience of being overpowered by adults is terrifying for a child who has been abused.

Quiet Room

Instead of seclusion, a unit may have an unlocked Quiet Room for the child who needs to be removed from the situation for either self-control or staff control (Joshi et al. 1988). Other approaches include the Feelings Room, which is carpeted and supplied with soft objects that can be punched or thrown (Samenfeld 1991), and the Freedom Room, which contains a large ball for throwing or kicking (Herrmann 1982). The child is encouraged to express freely and work through feelings of anger, frustration, and sadness in private and with staff support. When a child has difficulty being in touch with or expressing feelings, staff can provide practice sessions and act as role models.

BOX 29-9 TECHNIQUES FOR MANAGING DISRUPTIVE BEHAVIORS

- **Planned ignoring:** evaluate surface behavior and intervene when the intensity is becoming too great.
- **Use of signals or gestures:** use a word, a gesture, or eye contact to remind the child to use self-control.
- **Physical distance and touch control:** move closer to the child for a calming effect, maybe put an arm around the child.
- **Increased involvement in the activity:** redirect the child's attention to the activity and away from a distracting behavior by asking a question.
- **Additional affection:** ignore the provocative content of the behavior and give the child emotional support for the current problem.
- **Use of humor:** use well-timed kidding as a diversion to help the child save face and relieve feelings of guilt or fear.
- **Direct appeals:** appeal to the child's developing self-control, "Please, . . . not now."
- **Extra assistance:** give early help to the child who "blows up" and is easily frustrated when trying to achieve a goal; do not overuse this technique.
- **Clarification as intervention:** help the child understand the situation and his or her own motivation for the behavior.
- **Restructuring:** change the activity in ways that will lower the stimulation or the frustration; e.g., shorten a story or change to a physical activity.
- **Regrouping:** Use total or partial changes in the group's composition to reduce conflict and contagious behaviors.
- **Strategic removal:** remove a child who is disrupting or acting dangerously, but consider whether this gives the child too much status or makes the child a scapegoat.
- **Physical restraint:** use "therapeutic holding" to control, to give comforts, and to assure children that they are protected from their own impulses to act out.
- **Setting limits and giving permission:** use sharp, clear statements about which behavior is not allowed and give permission for the behavior that is expected.
- **Promises and rewards:** use very carefully and very infrequently to avoid situations in which the child bargains for a reward.
- **Threats and punishment:** use very carefully: the child needs to internalize the frustration generated by the punishment and use it to control impulses rather than externalize the frustration in further acting out.

Data from Redl, F., and Wineman, D. (1957). *The aggressive child.* New York: Free Press. Adapted with the permission of The Free Press, a division of Simon & Schuster.

Time Out

Time out from the group or unit activity is another method for intervening in disruptive or inappropriate behaviors (Gallagher et al. 1988). Time-out procedures are designed so that staff can be consistent in their interventions. Time out may require going to a designated room or sitting on the periphery of an activity until the child gains self-control and reviews the episode with a staff member. The child's individual behavioral goals are considered in setting limits on behavior and using time out.

Therapeutic Holding

At times a child's behavior is so destructive that physical restraint is needed. Although a mechanical restraint such as a helmet for head banging may be used, **therapeutic holding** is a long-established practice for the control of destructive behaviors (Redl and Weinman 1957; Miller et al. 1989). This intervention requires prompt, firm, nonretaliatory protective restraint that is gently and continuously personal in order to lead to a reduction in the child's distress, greater relaxation, a return of self-control, and trust in the staff (Langley Porter Neuropsychiatric Institute 1965). One technique, the basket hold, involves one nurse holding the child from behind by the wrists, while the child's arms are crossed over the torso. The nurse can immobilize the child's legs if necessary by sitting and crossing one or both of the nurse's legs over the child's legs.

Throughout the episode the nurse talks to the child in a reassuring manner, providing comfort, and keeping the child's self-esteem intact (Klotz 1982). Another holding/restraining technique involves placing the child in a prone position on a mat or blanket. One nurse holds the child's head, turned to the side to prevent head banging or biting, while the second nurse straddles the child's buttocks and legs and restrains the child's arms next to the hips. A small pillow is placed between the nurse's back and the child's feet for protection from kicks (Barlow 1989). For each restraint situation to be therapeutic, the nurse reviews the event with the child after the restraint is released. This review of the event and a discussion of alternate ways to cope foster learning and self-control.

Cognitive/Behavioral Therapy

Fritz Redl's **life space interview** (1966) is a 1:1 intervention technique for working with aggressive and disturbed youths. In this intervention, the adult assumes a mediating role between the child and his or her daily life experiences and uses them to provide "emotional first aid" on the spot and/or to help the child work through issues that are causing emotional and behavioral problems.

Stressful life events can happen at any point during the child's day, and prompt 1:1 intervention from a caring adult is part of the therapy. Redl considered these interventions as important as individual therapy sessions and an absolute necessity in milieu therapy. The therapeutic goals for the life space interview are as follows:

- Reality "rub-in": help the child achieve a clear understanding of how the stressful situation developed and what the child's role was.
- Symptom estrangement: help the child see that the secondary gain from a behavioral symptom (acting out) is meager and that problem solving brings better results.
- Massaging numb value areas: help the child recognize the value of "fairness" and how it applies equally to all.
- New tool salesmanship: help the child select and try new adaptive behaviors in recurring problem situations.
- Manipulation of self-boundaries: help the child maintain self-boundaries to keep from being "sucked into" another child's emotional state or acting out behavior.

Although the life space interview techniques were developed for use with aggressive children, the concept of intervening in the child's stressful daily life events to give "emotional first aid" and help the child resolve issues and cope effectively is standard practice for professionals working with children. The nurse uses this concept in teaching parenting skills.

Play Therapy

Play is the "work of childhood" and the way a child learns to master impulses and adapt to the environment. Play is the language of childhood and the communication medium for assessing developmental and emotional status, determining diagnosis, and instituting therapeutic interventions. Melanie Klein (1955) and Anna Freud (1965) were the first to use play as a therapeutic tool in their psychoanalysis of children in the 1920s and 1930s. Axline (1969) identified the guiding principles of play therapy, which are still used by mental health professionals:

- Accept the child as he or she is and follow the child's lead.
- Establish a warm, friendly relationship that helps the child express feelings completely.
- Recognize the child's feelings and reflect them back, so the child can gain insight into the behavior.
- Accept the child's ability to solve personal problems.
- Set limits only to provide reality and security.

There are many forms of play therapy used individually or in groups. The term **play therapy** usually refers to a 1:1 session the therapist has with a child in a playroom. Most playrooms are equipped with art supplies, clay/playdough, dolls/doll houses, hand puppets, toy telephones, building materials (blocks), and trucks/cars. The dolls, puppets, and doll house provide the child an opportunity to act out conflicts and situations involving the family, work through feelings, and develop more adaptive ways to cope. The following vignette shows how play therapy can help a child cope with a significant loss.

- Jennie, a 6-year-old, began having nightmares and refusing to go to school after her babysitter grandmother died. Her parents did not let her attend the funeral, thinking it would upset her. Jennie became fearful and preoccupied with the events surrounding the death. In play sessions she repeatedly used dolls to act out her grandmother's hospitalization, death, and funeral. She then pretended to bury the grandmother in a small, coffin-like box. The parents had told Jennie that grandma had gone to heaven. Jennie demonstrated the concept by removing "Grandma" from the box and placing her high up on a bookshelf in the playroom looking down on the rest of the doll family.

Dramatic Play

Psychodrama, now more commonly referred to as theater, is a treatment modality that uses dramatic techniques to act out emotional problems, examine subjective experience, develop new perspectives, and try out new behaviors. This modality may be used with groups of verbal children and adolescents. If they are psychotic, reality-based role plays are substituted for fantasies.

Dramatic play, less formal than psychodrama, is used in many settings with one or more children.

Hand puppets and puppet shows are a favorite way to act out problems and solutions. Uninhibited children and adolescents enjoy acting roles in dramas that they have created spontaneously or scripted. The dramas can be videotaped so that the nurse can review the experience and facilitate new learning with the group. A favorite type of dramatic play for children is "dress up," and a box of clothes is all that is needed. It is normally unstructured, and the staff observe the activity and intervene only if behavior becomes destructive.

Mutual storytelling is a psychodramatic technique developed by Gardner (1971) to help young children express themselves verbally. The child is asked to make up a story; it cannot be a known fairy tale, movie, or TV show. The story must have a beginning, a middle, and an ending. At the end of the story, the child is asked to give a lesson or the moral of the story. The nurse determines the psychodynamic meaning of the story and selects one or two of its important themes. Using the same characters and a similar setting, the nurse retells the story providing healthier resolutions, adaptations, and values. The lesson of the story is also reformulated to help the child become consciously aware of the better resolution. If the child has trouble starting a story, the nurse can assist by beginning the story with "Once upon a time in a faraway land there lived a . . ." and then point to the child to continue. After the child has identified the main characters, the nurse may need to keep prompting the child with comments such as "and then . . ." until the story is completed. The story can be audio- or videotaped, which increases the child's motivation to participate and allows for a review to reinforce the learning.

Therapeutic Games

Children enjoy games, so this treatment modality is ideal for children who have difficulty talking about their feelings and problems. Playing a game with the child facilitates the development of a therapeutic alliance and provides an opportunity for conversation. The game might be as simple as checkers, but **therapeutic games** are more effective in eliciting children's fears and fantasies.

Gardner (1979) developed a series of therapeutic games for children, two of which, "Board of Objects" and "Bag of Toys," can be used for children 4 to 8 years of age. The game pieces consist of small figures of people, animals, and various objects, which are placed on a checker board or in a bag. The players roll a pair of dice with one side of each die colored red. If the red side lands face up, the player selects an object. To get a reward chip, the player must say something about the object; if the player tells a story about the object, he or she gets two reward chips. The child's statement or story can be used in a therapeutic interchange (e.g., to communicate empathy or make a statement suggesting a more adaptive way to cope with a difficult situation). In the end, the player with the most chips wins (usually the child).

A board game appropriate for latency and preadolescent children is Gardner's (1986) "Talking, Feeling, and Doing Game." The player throws the dice and advances his playing piece along a pathway of different-colored squares. Depending on the color landed upon, the player draws a "talking," "feeling," or "doing" card, which gives instructions or asks a question. A reward chip is given when the player responds appropriately. For example, a "feeling" card might read: "All the girls in the class were invited to a birthday party except one. How did she feel?" If this game is played with more than one child, the nurse can elicit additional responses and engage the whole group in the therapeutic interchange. The nurse may "stack the deck" to make sure that cards relating to the child's problem(s) will be selected.

Bibliotherapy

Bibliotherapy involves using children's literature to help the child express feelings in a supportive environment, gain insight into feelings and behavior, and learn new ways to cope with difficult situations (Cohen 1987). While children listen to a story, they unconsciously identify with the characters and experience a catharsis of feelings. The books selected by the nurse should reflect the situations or feelings the child is experiencing. It is important to assess not only the needs of the child but also the readiness for the particular topic and the child's level of understanding. A children's librarian has access to a large collection of stories and knows which books are specifically written to help children deal with a particular subject. Whenever possible, the nurse consults with the family to make sure the books do not violate their belief system. A choice of several books is offered and a book is never forced upon the child.

Therapeutic Drawings

Children love to draw and paint and will spontaneously express themselves in art work. The drawings capture the thoughts, feelings, and tensions the child may not be able to express verbally, is unaware of, or is denying. Children do not have to draw themselves. In drawing any human figure, the child leaves an imprint of the inner self, revealing personality traits, relationships with others, attitudes/values from the family and cultural group, behavioral self-characteristics, and perceived strengths or weaknesses (Klepsch and Logie 1982). Drawings are most reliable after the child is able to create objective representations of what is seen (usually between 5 and 7 years of age). Drawings are less reliable when the child has cognitive impairments. To use this modality, the nurse needs to be familiar with the expected drawing capabilities for the child's developmental level.

Therapeutic drawing may be used in play therapy with individuals or groups. The drawing activity can be (1) entirely spontaneous (e.g., giving drawing materials with no instructions); (2) free drawing in response to a stimulus (e.g., drawing characters in a story); (3) copying figures (e.g., geometric figures); (4) drawing self, family members, and significant others; or (5) drawing self and others in action (e.g., child and family doing something together). The use of this modality involves observing children while they draw, asking questions about the picture, and looking for messages in what has been drawn. "Color Your Life" is an example of a free drawing technique used to help a child get in touch with feelings by having the child pair colors and feelings and answer questions while coloring on a blank piece of paper (Raynor and Manderino 1989).

Often the child draws or is asked to draw human figures. The following characteristics of human figures are general indicators of a child's emotions, and not necessarily indicative of psychopathology (Klepsch and Logie 1982):

- Size of figures: very large (aggression, poor impulse control), very small (shyness, insecurity)
- Emphases and exaggeration of body parts: large heads (desire to be smarter), large mouths (speech problems), large arms (desire for strength and power)

- Omissions of body parts: hands (trauma, insecurity), arms (inadequacy), legs (lack of support), feet (insecure, helpless), mouth (difficulty relating to others)
- Facial expressions: mood and affect
- Integration of body parts: scattered or disorganized parts indicate cognitive and/or psychological problems

Drawing can be used in working with children and families. In the following vignette, the art therapist and the nurse used a family art session to identify family dynamics and begin interventions.

- Melvin, a highly intelligent 15-year-old with obsessive-compulsive behaviors and severe insecurity, lives with his parents and younger sister. In the art session, each family member is given paper on an easel and asked to draw themselves and the other members of the family. Melvin draws his parents and sister as all the same size and standing together shoulder to shoulder. He draws himself as a tiny figure in a box that appears to be suspended in space. When questioned, he reports feeling as though he were trapped in a falling elevator and disconnected from the family.
- The family is surprised that he feels isolated (he was a normal size in their drawings). After completing a series of drawings and discussing them, the family is asked to draw a joint picture that requires them to work together. The picture they draw shows a smiling family standing by a house near a tree and a fence. The picture clearly demonstrates how the family does view Melvin as separate and different, for although he is standing beside the family, he is placed behind the fence. This observation is discussed, and as an intervention the family is given the task of finding ways to make Melvin feel included.

Music Therapy

Music is found in every culture and has a history of being used to calm and heal individuals. Music as therapy brings about changes in both the physiology of the body systems and in social interactions. Music therapy may incorporate recorded music, songs, movement and music, song writing, or use of an instrument to create music. Children love simple noise-making instruments, which may be used for the expression of feelings, for the development of coordination and rhythm, and as an opportunity for social interactions. Music is also used on inpatient units to create a relaxing mood for rest periods and at bedtime.

Adolescents especially like to use music to express moods and feelings, and they appear more sensitive to its message than other age groups. Weidinger and Demi (1991) found that adolescents who listen to music with negative lyrics and themes have more dysfunctional psychosocial behavior than those who listen to other types of music. Whether this is the cause and effect or a correlational finding is unknown. The music preferences of the adolescent need to be assessed, and the lyrics and themes can be used as content in individual or group therapy.

Movement/Dance Therapy

Movement/dance therapy is one of the oldest expressive therapies with concepts dating back to the ancient Greeks. Movement is a direct expression of the self that helps the child get in touch with feelings and thoughts, work off tensions, develop greater body awareness, improve or correct a distorted body image, improve coordination, and increase social interactions. The type of movement used with children can be as simple as a game of "Follow the Leader" or it can be creative, free form movements to the mood of the music. For older children and adolescents, more formal classes in exercise, karate, or the latest dance craze may be of interest.

Recreational Therapy

Recreational activities generally take place off the unit and are conducted by a recreational therapist with assistance from the nursing staff. Activities can be organized around a game that teaches psychomotor and social skills, or they can be individual activities (e.g., riding a bike, learning to swim). Special field trips and "outings" give children the opportunity to do what other children are doing and to act appropriately in public situations. The communicated expectation is that the children's behavior will be within normal limits, and this becomes a self-fulfilling prophesy leading to increased self-control and self-esteem.

Group dynamics play a part in the therapeutic process, and the leader works to develop cohesiveness in the group activity. McGinnis (1989) used a gardening project with children who had behavior disorders to provide practice in teamwork, delay of gratification, and dealing with issues of life and death.

Group Therapy

Group therapy for younger children takes the form of play; for grade-school children, it combines playing and talking about the activity. These groups help children learn social skills by taking turns and sharing with their peers. For adolescents, group therapy involves more talking, and focuses largely on peer relationships and specific problems (West and Evans 1992). The difficulty in using groups with children and adolescents lies in the contagious effect of disruptive behavior.

There is a wealth of information in the nursing literature about how to use group therapy with children and adolescents. Groups have been used effectively to deal with specific issues in the child's life (e.g., bereavement and loss, physical and sexual abuse, substance abuse, sexuality and dating, teenage pregnancy, chronic illnesses, depression, suicidal ideation). The mental health promotion and prevention activities, which nurses are now carrying out in school-based clinics, involve working with multiple groups (e.g., students, teachers, parents, community leaders). See Chapter 10.

Pharmacological Therapy

The first drug prescribed to treat children was amphetamine (for hyperactivity) in 1937; it was followed by methylphenidate in the 1950s. As the phenothiazines developed in the 1950s and 1960s, they were used for children with aggressive, self-mutilative, and disordered behaviors.

By the 1970s, TCAs were used for nocturnal enuresis, attention-deficit disorders, obsessive-compulsive behavior, and separation anxiety. After lithium was approved by the Food and Drug Administration for bipolar disorders in adults, it was found to be effective in attenuating child and adolescent aggression and stabilizing moods. Anticonvulsants were also being used as mood stabilizers. Lithium and many of the drugs currently in use are not approved for children under 12 years of age. A research priority in the 1990s "Decade of the Brain" is to study the effectiveness of drugs in child and adolescent disorders as well as the long-term effects on development.

Central Nervous System Stimulants

Studies indicate that as many as 6% of elementary school children are on CNS stimulants for ADHD, and 75% of the prescriptions have been written by pediatricians (Scahill and Lynch 1994b). The large numbers of children being treated and the possibility that some of the drugs have been indiscriminately prescribed carry implications for nursing practice. These children and parents will appear at some point for health care and the nurse will need to know the drugs' clinical characteristics in order to work with the parents to monitor and evaluate progress.

The three psychostimulants used with ADHD are methylphenidate (Ritalin), pemoline (Cylert), and dextroamphetamine (Dexedrine). Methylphenidate remains the most popular CNS stimulant, making up 90% of the prescriptions, because it is safe and simple to use. It is a short-acting drug (1 to 4 hours) that is given in multiple doses throughout the day. A physical examination is completed and a behavioral baseline established before a drug trial is started. A baseline is determined by parents and teachers, who fill out behavioral rating scales. These scales will also be used at intervals to determine drug effectiveness. The usual starting dose for methylphenidate is 5 mg in the morning. After 4 to 7 days, a noontime dose can be introduced. A third dose may be needed in the evening when the child is doing homework. The most common side effects are insomnia, loss of appetite, irritability, nervousness, and tachycardia. If these effects persist, the dose can be lowered. The drug should be taken with meals so that it will not affect appetite. Height and weight are monitored for evidence of growth retardation. If a rebound effect occurs (increased hyperactivity), the dosage can be lowered or a third late-afternoon dose can be added. If the child becomes "overfocused" and preoccupied, the dose should be lowered. Drug holidays, such as weekends and summer vacations, are worked out with the parents and prescribing physician. Because of the short half-life of methylphenidate, stopping and restarting the drug causes no problems (see Table 29–3).

Antidepressants

TCAs were first used for nocturnal enuresis in the early 1960s and were gradually expanded to include ADHD, obsessive-compulsive behaviors, separation anxiety, and school phobia (Scahill and Lynch 1994b). Their effectiveness with child and adolescent depression has not been conclusively proved in clinical trials. The TCA clomipramine (Anafranil) has proved effective for obsessive-compulsive and tic disorders in children (Scahill and Lynch 1996).

The TCAs are used with great caution since a report of cardiac arrests in children was associated with the TCA desipramine (Norpramin). The potential risks of cardiac arrhythmias and seizures need to be explained to the family. An electrocardiogram (ECG) is taken before a drug trial and ECG changes are monitored throughout treatment. TCAs are contraindicated if there is a family history of arrhythmias or syncope. The hepatic metabolism of TCAs is more rapid in children, who may require an adult dose and a longer time period for the drug to be effective. Multiple daily dosing is recommended to avoid side effects from peak serum levels and withdrawal symptoms from the rapid metabolism. The therapeutic window for plasma levels in prepubescent children ranges between 125 and 250 ng/ml, but in adolescents and young adults there is no relationship between the plasma level and the effectiveness of the drug (Laraia 1996).

The SSRIs (fluoxetine, paroxetine [Paxil], and sertraline) are better tolerated than the TCAs and have become the drugs of choice for children and adolescents. Monoamine oxidase inhibitors are not used with children and rarely with adolescents because of the dietary restrictions. (See Chapter 20 for additional information on antidepressants.)

Antipsychotics

The low-potency phenothiazines, chlorpromazine (Thorazine) and thioridazine (Mellaril), were the first to be used to control aggressive, self-destructive behaviors. However, these are too sedating and have troublesome side effects. The newer high-potency antipsychotics fluphenazine (Prolixin) and haloperidol are less sedating and may increase concentration, but they carry a high incidence of extrapyramidal side effects. Since antipsychotic drugs are thought to impair learning, their use is reserved for psychotic symptoms and selected disorders.

Risperidone (Risperdal) is being used to control the flashbacks and aggression in PTSD and the aggressive behaviors in PDDs and conduct disorders. From anecdotal reports, risperidone appears to be less effective with adolescents. There is a problem with weight gain because risperidone increases the appetite. Clozapine (Clozaril) is not used with children but is proving effective with older adolescents who have not responded to other antipsychotic drugs.

Haloperidol and pimozide (Orap) are used to treat the tics exhibited in Tourette's disorder. Haloperidol has also shown some success in controlling autistic behaviors. (See Chapter 22 for additional information on antipsychotic drugs.)

Mood Stabilizers

Lithium is being used successfully in children 7 years of age and older and adolescents to stabilize moods and reduce aggressive outbursts. Children and adolescents may need higher doses of lithium than adults to achieve therapeutic blood levels because their renal clearance level is higher. Lithium is also being used to augment the TCAs and SSRIs in treatment-resistant children and adolescents. The anticonvulsant drugs carbamazepine (Tegretol) and valproic acid (Depakene and Depakote) are being used to stabilize moods and control aggressive outbursts. (See Chapter 21 for additional information on mood stabilizers.)

Other Drug Classifications

The antihypertensive drugs are being used to control aggression and explosive behavior.

Propranolol (Inderal) is being used for the rage reactions in conduct disorder, PTSD, and other organic brain dysfunctions (Sims 1990). Clonidine (Catapres) is used frequently for the disordered and impulsive behaviors of ADHD and conduct disorder. Another antihypertensive drug, guanfacine (Tenex), is being tried for ADHD when clonidine does not work. Clonidine is also being used to control tics in Tourette's disorder, and for the inattention, impulsivity, and hyperactivity of ADHD (Scahill and Lynch 1996). The family needs to be taught how to monitor side effects and blood pressure for children and adolescents on these drugs.

The anorexigenic drug fenfluramine is being used for autistic children with elevated serotonin levels.

A variety of antianxiety drugs are used; however, treatment goals often involve having the child or adolescent learn how to handle anxiety and frustration. Drugs such as lorazepam (Ativan) and alprazolam (Xanax) are being used less with adolescents because of their potential for addiction and misuse. When prn medication is needed, diphenhydramine hydrochloride (Benadryl) is often the drug of choice.

RESEARCH ISSUES

The research role of the child psychiatric nurse has been recognized as a result of the National Advisory Mental Health Council's *National Plan for Research on Child and Adolescent Mental Disorders* (1990). Child psychiatric nursing is identified in the plan as one of the four core mental health disciplines; the role is described as follows:

> This discipline offers a unique research perspective on the mental disorders of the young. Researchers in child psychiatric nursing focus on both children and their families. Research on improving the delivery of clinical services is a natural area of interest, as is the study of the delivery systems through which such care is offered. Also of interest are programs designed to promote early detection of and intervention for developmental problems, especially for children with serious disorders who need prolonged medical care, including premature and/or addicted newborn babies. (p. 35)

McBride (1992), one of the nursing contributors to the National Plan, urges nurses to identify gaps in nursing knowledge and set a research agenda. McBride suggests that child psychiatric nurses research the following areas:

- Factors that put children/adolescents at risk for emotional and behavioral problems
- Factors that influence judgments about emotional and behavioral problems in children/adolescents
- The effect of the parents' mental illness on their perceptions of their children's behavior
- The reliability of assessing mental status in young children
- Interventions to limit dysfunction among children subjected to abuse, neglect, and social disadvantage
- The special mental health needs of children with chronic physical illness
- The effectiveness of various approaches in supporting families of children who have severe mental disorders
- The development of innovative services to meet the needs of children with mental disorders and their families (home care, respite care, mobile crises for schools)

The body of nursing knowledge for child psychiatry is growing rapidly. Since beginning publication in 1988, the *Journal of Child and Adolescent Psychiatric Nursing* has presented research and clinical reports addressing many of the areas McBride noted. Box 29–10 gives examples of this research.

BOX 29-10 EXAMPLES OF CHILD AND ADOLESCENT PSYCHIATRIC NURSING RESEARCH

From *Journal of Child and Adolescent Psychiatric and Mental Health Nursing:*

Factors that put children and adolescents at risk for disorders:

Kelley, S. (1992). Child maltreatment, stressful life events, and behavior problems in school-aged children in residential treatment. Vol. 5, No. 2:5–15

Siantz, M. L. (1993). The stigma of mental illness on children of color. Vol. 6 No. 4:10–17

Interventions to limit dysfunction in abused or neglected youths:

Bennett, C. (1993). Sexually abused boys: Awareness, assessment, and intervention. Vol. 6 No. 2:29–35

Houch, G., and King, M. (1993). Cognitive functioning, and behavioral and emotional adjustment in maltreated children post-intervention. Vol. 6 No. 2:5–17

Mental health needs of the physically ill child or adolescent:

Austin, J. (1989). Comparison of child adaptation to epilepsy and asthma. Vol. 2, No. 4:139–144

Martinson, I., and Bossert E. (1994). The psychological status of children with cancer. Vol. 7, No. 2:16–23

McClowry, S. (1991). Behavioral disturbances among medically hospitalized school-age children. Vol. 4, No. 2:62–67

Family interventions and family support:

Rosenwald, E., and Demi, A. (1993). A primary prevention group for latency age children dealing with adoption issues. Vol. 6, No. 1:15–21

Williams-Burgess, C., Vines, S., and Ditullio, M. (1995). The parent baby venture program: Prevention of child abuse. Vol. 8 No. 3:15–23

Innovative services for children and adolescents:

Conley, J., and Kendal, J. (1989) A school-based primary prevention group for children with alterations in health status. Vol. 2 No 3:123–128

Niznik, K. (1994). The nurse's role in school-based mental health promotion: Easing the transition into adolescence. Vol. 7, No. 1:5–8

Wagner, J., Melragon, B, and Menke, E. (1993). Homeless children: Interdisciplinary drug prevention intervention. Vol. 6, No. 1:23–30

EVALUATION

Nursing care plans for autistic disorder, ADHD, and conduct disorder were presented in the section on child and adolescent psychiatric disorders. Each disorder has a series of nursing diagnoses and outcome criteria corresponding to the most problematic behaviors usually exhibited by children or adolescents with these disorders.

Frequent evaluation of these outcome criteria help the multidisciplinary team to assess the value of specific intervention strategies and to alter or add intervention strategies. Since these care plans are generic in nature, they do not address all the needs of an individual. Thus, the nursing interventions and treatment modalities are most effective when tailored to address the child's or adolescent's unique needs, psychodynamics, interests, and manner of relating.

SUMMARY

Between 12% and 22% of children and adolescents are estimated to have emotional problems, and only a small percentage of these youths actually receive treatment. The mentally disturbed child or adolescent is one whose progressive personality development is interfered with or arrested by a variety of factors resulting in impairments in the capacities expected for age and physical and cognitive endowment. Risk factors known to contribute to the development of mental and emotional problems in children and adolescents include genetic, biochemical, pre- and postnatal, temperament, psychosocial development, social/environmental, and cultural factors. However, not all at-risk children develop problems, and the characteristics of resilient children have been identified as an adaptable temperament, ability to form nurturing relationships with surrogate parental figures, ability to distance the self from emotional chaos in parent and family, and good social intelligence and problem-solving skills.

The most commonly diagnosed child psychiatric disorders are ADHD, adjustment reactions, conduct and oppositional disorders, separation anxiety disorder, and mood disorder (depression). The PDDs are rare.

The field of child psychiatry is new to the twentieth century, and child psychiatric nursing evolved gradually as the therapeutic value of nurses' relationships with children in custodial care became recognized. Nurses sought to further develop this role through graduate education. In 1954 the first graduate program in child psychiatric nursing was opened. Advocates for Child Psychiatric Nursing, the professional organization for this nursing specialty, was established in 1971, and the first ANA certification of child psychiatric nurses took place in 1979. The ANA's *Standards of child and adolescent psychiatric and mental health nursing practice* were published in 1985.

The philosophy of child psychiatric nursing holds that every child has the potential for growth and that healthy growth occurs when the child is helped to move from dependency to autonomy, taking into account normal periods of regression. Child psychiatric nurses use this philosophy in a variety of clinical settings when providing assessments and interventions for children, adolescents, and their families. The child psychiatric nurse uses a wide range of treatment modalities, including milieu therapy, behavior modification, cognitive-behavioral therapy, therapeutic play, group and family therapy, and pharmacological agents.

Child and adolescent psychiatric nurses are increasingly becoming aware of the need to involve and educate the family in the treatment process. The family remains the integral part of the supportive and educative system of the child and adolescent.

Child psychiatric nursing is changing as inpatient stays become brief; treatment protocols (clinical pathways) are established; care settings move into the community (school-based clinics); and multiple pharmacological agents are used with increasing frequently.

REFERENCES

American Nurses' Association (1985). *Standards of child and adolescent psychiatric and mental health nursing practice.* St. Louis, MO: American Nurses' Association.

American Nurses' Association (1994). *Statement on psychiatric–mental health clinical nursing practice and standards of psychiatric–mental health clinical nursing practice.* Washington, DC: American Nurses' Association.

American Psychiatric Association (1994). *Diagnostic and statistical manual of mental disorders* (4th ed.). Washington, DC: American Psychiatric Association.

Anthony, J. E., and Cohler, B. J. (1987). *The invulnerable child.* New York: Guilford Press.

Axline, V. (1969). *Play therapy.* New York: Ballantine Books.

Barker, P. (1995). *Basic child psychiatry* (6th ed.). Cambridge, MA: Blackwell Science.

Barkley, R. (1990). *Attention deficit hyperactivity disorder: A handbook for diagnosis and treatment.* New York: Guilford Press.

Barlow, D. (1989). Therapeutic holding: Effective intervention with the aggressive child. *Journal of Psychosocial Nursing and Mental Health Services,* 27(1):10–14.

Bender, P. A. (1992). Multiple family therapy for adolescents. *Journal of Child and Adolescent Psychiatric Nursing,* 5(1):27–31.

Bowlby, J. (1969). *Attachment and loss.* Vol. 1. *Attachment.* New York: Basic Books.

Canino, I. A., and Spurlock, J. (1994). *Culturally diverse children and adolescents: Assessment, diagnosis, and treatment.* New York: Guilford Press.

Carbray, J. A., and Rogers Pitula, C. (1991). Trends in adolescent psychiatric hospitalization. *Journal of Child and Adolescent Psychiatric Nursing,* 4(2):68–71.

Children's Defense Fund (1990). *Children 1990: A report card, briefing book, and action primer.* Washington, DC: Children's Defense Fund.

Chisholm, M. M. (Ed.) (1968). *Work conference: Nursing in child psychiatry* (monograph). Boston: Boston University School of Nursing.

Christ, A., Critchley, D., Larson, M., and Brown, M. (1965). The role of the nurse in child psychiatry. *Nursing Outlook,* 13(1):30–32.

Cohen, L. J. (1987). Bibliotherapy. *Journal of Psychosocial Nursing,* 25(10):20–24.

Conley, J. F., and Kendall, J. (1989). A school-based primary prevention group for children with alterations in health status. *Journal of Child and Adolescent Psychiatric Nursing,* 2(3):123–128.

Coursen-Antinone, L., and Anderson, K. (1996). *Critical pathways: The way to the future.* Paper presented at the Association of Child and Adolescent Psychiatric Nurses National Conference, San Diego, September 1996.

Cox, A. D. (1988). Maternal depression and impact on children's development. *Archives of Disease in Childhood,* 63:90–95.

Critchley, D. (1991). Nursing's contributions to a psychiatric inpatient treatment milieu for children and adolescents. In R. L. Hendren and I. N. Berlin (Eds.), *Psychiatric inpatient care of children and adolescents* (pp. 250–263). New York: John Wiley.

Dalton, S. T., and Howell, C. C. (1989). Autism: Psychobiological perspectives. *Journal of Child and Adolescent Psychiatric Nursing,* 2(3):92–96.

Delaney, K. R. (1994). Calming an escalated psychiatric milieu. *Journal of Child and Adolescent Psychiatric Nursing,* 7(3):5–13.

Delaney, K. R. (1992). Nursing in child psychiatric milieus: Part I: What nurses do. *Journal of Child and Adolescent Psychiatric Nursing,* 5(1):10–14.

Erikson, E. H. (1963). *Childhood and society* (2nd ed.). New York: W. W. Norton.

Fagin, C. M. (1972). *Nursing in child psychiatry.* St. Louis: C.V. Mosby.

Folstein, S. E., and Rutter, M. L. (1987). Autism: Familial aggregation and genetic implications. In E. Schopler and G. H. Mesibov (Eds.), *Neurobiological issues in autism* (pp. 83–105). New York: Plenum Press.

Freud, A. (1965). *Normality and pathology in childhood: Assessments of development.* New York: International Universities Press.

Frye, B. A., and McGill, D. (1993). Cambodian refugee adolescents: Cultural factors and mental health nursing. *Journal of Child and Adolescent Psychiatric Nursing,* 6(4):24–31.

Fulginiti, J. (1991). Far from the ideal: The plight of poor children in the United States (editorial). *American Journal of Diseases of Children,* 145:489–490.

Gallagher, M., Mittelstadt, P., and Slater, B. (1988). Establishing time out procedures in a day treatment facility for young children. *Residential Treatment of Children and Youth,* 5(4):59–69.

Gardner, R. A. (1971). *Therapeutic communication with children: The mutual storytelling technique.* New York: Jason Aronson.

Gardner, R. A. (1979). Helping children cooperate in therapy. In J. D. Noshpitz and S. I. Harrison (Eds.), *Basic handbook of child psychiatry: Therapeutic interventions* (pp. 414–432). New York: Basic Books.

Gardner, R. A. (1986). The talking, feeling and doing game. In C. E. Schaefer and S. E. Reid (Eds.), *Game play: Therapeutic use of childhood games* (pp. 41–72). New York: John Wiley.

Gilbert, C. M. (1988). Children in women's shelters: A group intervention using art. *Journal of Child and Adolescent Psychiatric Nursing,* 1(1):7–13.

Gittelman, R. (1986). *Anxiety disorders of childhood.* New York: Gilford Press.

Goodman, J. D., and Sours, J. (1987). *The child mental status examination* (2nd ed.). New York: Basic Books.

Goren, S. (1991). What are the considerations for the use of seclusion and restraint with children and adolescents? (letter to the editor). *Journal of Psychosocial Nursing and Mental Health Services,* 29(2):32–33.

Goren, S. (1992). Practicing in partnership with families in the inpatient setting. *Journal of Child and Adolescent Psychiatric Nursing,* 5(3):43–46.

Harnett, N. E. (1989). Conduct disorder in childhood and adolescence: An update. *Journal of Child and Adolescent Psychiatric Nursing,* 2(2):74–76.

Herrmann, C. (1982). The freedom room. In J. Schulman and M. Irwin (Eds.), *Psychiatric hospitalization of children* (pp. 151–159). Springfield, IL: Charles C Thomas.

Institute of Medicine (1989). *Research on children and adolescents with mental, behavioral, and developmental disorders.* Washington, DC: National Academy Press.

Jemerin, J. M., and Phillims, I. (1988). Changes in inpatient child psychiatry: Consequences and recommendations. *Journal of the American Academy of Child and Adolescent Psychiatry,* 27:397–403.

Joshi, P., Capozzoli, J., and Coyle, J. (1988). Use of a quiet room on an inpatient unit. *Journal of the American Academy of Child and Adolescent Psychiatry,* 27:642–644.

Kanner, L. (1943). Autistic disturbances of affective contact. *Nervous Child,* 2:217–250.

Kanner, L. (1972). *Child psychiatry* (4th ed.). Springfield, IL: Charles C Thomas.

Kelley, S. J. (1992). Child maltreatment, stressful life events, and behavior problems in school-aged children in residential treatment. *Journal of Child and Adolescent Pychiatric and Mental Health Nursing,* 5(2):5–13.

Kernberg, P. F., and Chazan, S. E. (1991). *Children with conduct disorders.* New York: Basic Books.

Killeen, M. R. (1990). Challenges and choices in child and adolescent mental health–psychiatric nursing. *Journal of Child and Adolescent Psychiatric Nursing,* 3(4):113–119.

Klein, M. (1955). The psychoanalytic play technique. *American Journal of Orthopsychiatry,* 25:223–237.

Klepsch, M., and Logie, L. (1982). *Children draw and tell.* New York: Brunner/Mazel.

Klotz, N. (producer/director) (1982). *The anger within* (film). Available from NAK 1 Productions, P.O. Box 39108, Washington, DC 20016.

Korczynski, J. (1989). Socialization groups in a school outreach program. *Journal of Child and Adolescent Psychiatric Nursing,* 2(4):166–167.

Lamb, J., and Puskar, K. R. (1991). School-based adolescent mental health project survey of depression, suicidal ideation and anger. *Journal of Child and Adolescent Psychiatric Nursing,* 4(3):101–104.

Langley Porter Neuropsychiatric Institute (1965). *Guidelines for child psychiatric unit.* San Francisco: Langley Porter Neuropsychiatric Institute.

Laraia, M. T. (1996). Current approaches to the psychopharmacologic treatment of depression in children and adolescents. *Journal of Child and Adolescent Psychiatric Nursing,* 9(1):15–26.

Lewis, D. (1994). Etiology of aggressive conduct disorder. *Child and Adolescent Psychiatric Clinics of North America,* 3:303–320.

Mahler, M. S., Pine, F., and Bergman, A. (1979). *The psychological birth of the human infant: Symbiosis and individuation.* New York: Basic Books.

McBride, A. (1992). Commentary: Nurses develop a plan for research on child and adolescent mental disorders. *Journal of Child and Adolescent Psychiatric and Mental Health Nursing,* 5(1):41–43.

McGihon, N. N. (1994). Health care reforms: Clinical implications for inpatient psychiatric nursing. *Journal of Psychosocial Nursing and Mental Health Services,* 32(11):31–33, 42–43.

McGinnis, M. (1989). Gardening as therapy for children with behavioral disorders. *Journal of Child and Adolescent Psychiatric Nursing,* 2(3):87–91.

McGoldrick, M., Pearce, J., and Giordano, J. (1982). *Ethnicity and family therapy.* New York: Guilford Press.

Middleton, A., and Pothier, P. (1970). The nurse in child psychiatry: An overview. *Nursing Outlook,* 18(5):52–56.

Miller, D., Walker, M., and Friedman, D. (1989). The use of a holding technique to control the violent behavior of seriously disturbed adolescents. *Hospital and Community Psychiatry,* 40:520–524.

National Advisory Mental Health Council. (1990). National plan for research on child and adolescent mental disorders (DHHS Publication No. (ADM) 90-1683. Rockville, MD: National Institute for Mental Health.

Ogbu, J. U. (1981). Origins of human competence: A cultural ecological perspective. *Child Development,* 52:413–429.

Peterson, E. J., Gray, K. A., and Weinstein, S. R. (1994). A look at adolescent treatment in a time of change. *Journal of Child and Adolescent Psychiatric Nursing*, 7(2):5–15.

Pfeffer, C. R. (1986). *The suicidal child.* New York: Guildofrd Press.

Raynor, C. M., and Manderino, M. A. (1989). Color your life: An assessment and treatment strategy for children. *Journal of Child and Adolescent Psychiatric Nursing* 2(2):48–51.

Redl, F. (1966). *When we deal with children.* New York: Free Press.

Redl, F., and Wineman, D. (1957). *The aggressive child.* New York: Free Press.

Ross, C. (1989). *Multiple personality disorder: Diagnosis, clinical features, and treatment.* New York: John Wiley.

Rutter, M. (1987). Psychosocial resilience and protective mechanisms. *American Journal of Orthopsychiatry*, 57:316–339.

Samenfeld, L. G. (1991). The feelings room. *Journal of Child and Adolescent Psychiatric Nursing*, 4(2):80–81.

Scahill, L., and Lynch, K. A. (1994a). Pharmacology notes: Tricyclic antidepressants: Cardiac effects and clinical implications. *Journal of Child and Adolescent Psychiatric Nursing*, 7(1):37–39.

Scahill, L., and Lynch, K. (1994b). Pharmacology notes: The use of methylphenidate in attention-deficit/hyperactivity disorder. *Journal of Child and Adolescent Psychiatric Nursing*, 7(4):44–47.

Scahill, L., and Lynch, K. A. (1996). Contemporary approaches to pharmacotherapy in Tourette's syndrome and obsessive-compulsive disorder. *Journal of Child and Adolescent Psychiatric Nursing*, 9(1):27–43.

Senn, M. J., and Solnit, A. J. (1968). *Problems in child behavior and development.* Philadelphia: Lea & Febiger.

Siantz, M. L. (1993). The stigma of mental illness on the children of color. *Journal of Child and Adolescent Psychiatric Nursing*, 6(4):10–17.

Sims, J. (1990). Pediatric psychopharmacologic uses of propranolol: Review and case illustrations. *Journal of Child and Adolescent Psychiatric Nursing*, 3(1):18–24.

Thomas, A., and Chess, S. (1977). *Temperament and development.* New York: Brunner/Mazel.

U.S. Department of Health and Human Services (1991). *Implementation of the national plan for research on child and adolescent mental disorders* (PA-91-46). Rockville, MD: National Institute of Mental Health.

Valente, S. M. (1989). Adolescent suicide: Assessment and intervention. *Journal of Child and Adolescent Psychiatric Nursing*, 2(1):34–39.

Walsh, E., and Randell, B. P. (1995). Seclusion and restraint: What we need to know. *Journal of Child and Adolescent Psychiatric Nursing*, 8(1):28–40.

Weidinger, C. K., and Demi, A. S. (1991). Music listening preferences and preadmission dysfunctional psychosocial behaviors of adolescents hospitalized on an in-patient psychiatric unit. *Journal of Child and Adolescent Psychiatric Nursing*, 4(1):3–8.

West, P., and Evans, C. L. (1992). *Psychiatric and mental health nursing with children and adolescents.* Gaithersburg, MD: Aspen.

Zametkin, A. (1989). The neurobiology of attention-deficit hyperactivity disorder: A synopsis. *Psychiatric Annals*, 19:584–586.

Further Reading

Finke, L. M., and Siantz, M. L. (1993). National workshop: Implementation of practice with severely mentally and emotionally disturbed children and adolescents. *Journal of Child and Adolescent Psychiatric Nursing*, 6(1):31–32, 37.

Scahill, L., and Lynch, K. A. (1995). Pharmacology notes: Pharmacologic treatment of children and adolescent with obsessive-compulsive disorder. *Journal of Child and Adolescent Psychiatric Nursing*, 8(4):36–40.

SELF-STUDY AND CRITICAL THINKING

Short sentence completion

1. Identify four characteristics of a mentally healthy youth:

   A. __________
   B. __________
   C. __________
   D. __________

2. For each of the following categories, identify one factor that puts the infant, child, or adolescent at risk for developing a mental disorder:

   Genetic __________
   Biological __________
   Developmental __________
   Social/environmental __________
   Cultural __________

3. Describe two characteristics of a resilient child:

   A. form nurturing relationships
   B. good social intelligence

4. Identify six types of data used in assessing children and adolescents:

   A. medical hx
   B. mental
   C. family
   D. developmental
   E. mental status
   F. neuro

Matching

5. Distinguish between behaviors indicating minimal (M) psychopathology and those indicating extreme (E) psychopathology:

4-year-old

__M__ Fears and night terrors
__E__ Lethargy and inhibited play
__M__ Poor motor coordination
__E__ Impulsive, destructive behavior
__M__ Breath-holding spells
__E__ Little or no speech

12-year-old

__E__ Acts of delinquency
__M__ Frequent somatic complaints
__M__ Fears related to sex
__E__ Anorexia
__E__ Phobias and persistent anxiety
__M__ Poor peer relationships

6. Match the following mental disorders with their behavioral characteristics:

__F__ ADHD
__E__ Separation anxiety
__C__ PDD
__B__ Tourette's
__D__ Conduct disorder
__A__ Adjustment reaction

A. Regressive behavior since the arrival of a new sibling.
B. Abnormal movements that increase in frequency under stress.
C. Unresponsiveness to caregiver.
D. Destructiveness toward persons or property.
E. Fear of visiting a friend's home.
F. Impulsive, intrusive, and demanding behavior.

Fill in assessment data

7. List four signs of depression for each of the following assessment areas:

Mood/Affect Changes

A. ______
B. ______
C. ______
D. ______

Physical Changes

A. ______
B. ______
C. ______
D. ______

Cognitive Changes

A. ______
B. ______
C. ______
D. ______

Social/Behavioral Changes

A. ______
B. ______
C. ______
D. ______

Matching

8. Match the age group to the appropriate treatment modality. More than one age group can be used.

Preschool 3–5 School Age 6–9 Preadolescent 10–12 Adolescent 13–17

Music therapy ______
Therapeutic drawings of figures in action ______
Therapeutic games:
Board of objects ______
Talking, feeling, doing ______

Puppet play ____________________
Mutual story telling ____________________
Recreational group ____________________
Psychodrama ____________________
Bibliotherapy ____________________

Fill in pharmacologic data

9. Identify which medications are being used for the following mental disorders:

   A. Autistic disorder antipsychotic
   B. Mood disorder (depression) antidepr Tricyclic SSRI
   C. ADHD Ritalin
   D. Tourette's disorder Haloperidol
   E. Separation anxiety antihistamine anxiolytics
   F. Conduct disorder antipsychotic

10. What are three universal goals for nursing interventions with children and adolescents?

    A. ____________________
    B. ____________________
    C. ____________________

Critical thinking

11. Describe what would be included in an orientation for parents and children to an inpatient or day treatment program.

12. Discuss how the therapeutic factors inherent in the milieu can be used in planning care for a child or adolescent.

13. What individual dynamics are considered when making decisions about using "therapeutic holding" to control aggressive and violent behaviors?

14. What is the most therapeutic way to handle sexual curiosity on a child's inpatient or day treatment program?

15. What suggestions should parents be given about how to make their home environment safer and less stressful for their child with ADHD?

16. What can the nurse do to make therapeutic contact with a child who has PDD and likes to spend quiet times smearing saliva and chewed-up candy and paper on various objects?

30

Adult Relationships and Sexuality

CARLA E. RANDALL

OUTLINE

KEY TERMS AND CONCEPTS

The key terms and concepts listed here also appear in bold where they are defined or discussed in this chapter.

sexual response patterns
fetishism
pedophilia
exhibitionism
voyeurism
transvestitism
sexual sadism and masochism (S/M)
frotteurism
sexually transmitted diseases (STDs)

OBJECTIVES

After studying this chapter, the reader will be able to

1. Explain three reasons why nurses need to be able to discuss topics related to sexuality, sexual behavior, and sexual conduct in relation to working with clients.
2. Role play with a classmate how a nurse, from a different culture than the client, would respond to one overt and one subtle concern regarding side effects from a prescribed medication related to the client's sexual relationship(s).
3. Incorporate into a medication teaching plan possible side effects that might interfere with a client's sexual response/behavior.
4. Role play how to assess in a nonthreatening manner a client's sexual satisfaction in an acute care setting, an outpatient setting, a home setting, and a long-term facility.
5. Teach a classmate the normal sexual response of males and three normal types of sexual responses of females.
6. Discuss two sexual dysfunctions for a man and two for a woman, identifying the particular phase of the sexual response the dysfunction presents.
7. Describe gender identity disorders and medical interventions for them.
8. Discuss sexual addiction and give examples of assessment questions that might be used to assess for this addiction.
9. Compare and contrast the symptoms of four STDs and their treatments.
10. Teach a client general "safe sex" information, including how to correctly use a condom whether the partner is male or female.

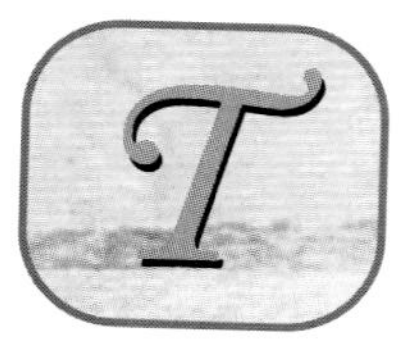

This chapter explores issues and raises questions (as well as making some suggestions) about how nurses can move into the twenty-first century, aware and open to the changing times in which they practice—regardless of, or perhaps in spite of, their own personal beliefs or biases regarding sex, sexuality, and relationships. Throughout the chapter, you will be asked to grapple with various issues, situations, and dilemmas.

Not all issues or questions are, or should be, answered directly in this chapter. This is because you know more than you think you know about relationships. You are currently in numerous adult relationships. Every day you utilize the skills being addressed in this chapter. It is hoped that the issues raised here will cause you to think, challenge many of your basic beliefs, and make you reexamine the automatic assumptions you make about people and the situations in which you find yourself. Remembering that you have experiences from which to draw, you are being presented with a new opportunity to grow and learn.

In an informal survey carried out by this author of fifteen nursing home, home health care, and acute care nurses, not one nurse spoke of a planned nursing approach to assessing client relationships and sexual satisfaction, yet, judging from the media, sex is the activity that consumes us. Isn't it interesting that what we are told about ourselves, and how we actually spend our time, differ greatly in our society? Keeping this dichotomy in mind, as well as the growing focus on morality, a nursing textbook needs to focus on how nursing can incorporate acceptance of various ways of adult living in the world. At the core of all psychosocial developmental stages are sexuality and relationships, and in the context of relationships it is especially important to note the prominent role culture plays for ourselves and those we "nurse." It would serve nursing well to address these topics with open and caring dialogue.

Fundamental to all actions taken by the nurse should be some sort of theoretical framework. All developmental theorists have concerned themselves with the importance of sexuality and the personal struggles that individuals have with sexuality and relationships. Choosing any of the developmental process theories to determine the placement of sex and relationships on a hierarchy or continuum, you can easily see how important sex and relationships are in the healthy development of individuals. Whether it be Maslow's (1970) hierarchy of needs, Piaget's (1962, 1963) theory of cognitive development, Mahler's (1975, 1980) separation-individuation process, Sullivan's (1953) interpersonal developmental schema, Erikson's (1963) stages of psychosocial development, or Gilligan's (1982) challenge to Kohlberg's (1969) stages of moral development, each of them at their core describes an individual's relationship with others and implies that a significant component of those relationships is sexual. For example, Maslow's hierarchy of basic needs categorizes the importance of sex and relationships to humans as a physiological need and places it at the base of the pyramid. Not only is sex and sexuality considered to be at the foundation of human needs, but it is also the only need that is repeatedly expressed throughout the pyramid. Freud places the importance of sex and relationships at the very core of his developmental theory. Further on in this chapter we will discuss how culture affects relationships and sexual intimacy issues for nurses.

ESTABLISHING RAPPORT

Today, nurses come into the home to do a dressing change, to assess suicidal ideation, to administer antibiotics, or to teach the client or family to carry out procedures previously not considered possible in the home. This "invasion," while offering the comforts of home for the client and family, can also create isolation and silence for the client and family unless the nurse is clearly "available." The nurse has to be able to see beyond personal preconceptions of the client's environment and be open to possibilities not necessarily easily visible. For example, what about the client who is receiving antibiotics that must be refrigerated? Does the client have a refrigerator or have access to one? It is essential that the nurse assess for adequate resources; more important, the nurse must do this in a way that communicates care and understanding rather than condescension and arrogance. Clients who are thoughtlessly belittled because of economic status, or made to feel "less than human" in their current situation, will be unwilling to share intimate details of life. It is essential that, no matter what the current circumstances, the nurse communicate acceptance and understanding while managing the client's needs to the greatest potential.

Numerous nursing theories talk about seeing clients in their totality (Rogers 1970, 1980), maximizing potential (King 1971, 1978, 1981), adaptation needs of clients and their families (Roy 1976, 1980), or self-care (Orem 1985). Theorists speak of the inclusion of sexuality and relationships, but little has been done to examine how the nurse is prepared to assist the client in these endeavors. Much of a client's intimate life is deferred or is completely unaddressed in a nursing assessment. How many of you have been told that trust is at the heart of a client's sharing deeper concerns? How many of you have asked questions about a client's intimate life? How many of you have wondered how to establish trust with a new client? What would you do if someone did share something of alarming concern? What you might consider alarming and what a client might consider alarming may well be very different things.

▶ Chuck has been placed on glyburide (Micronase), a common medication for treatment of diabetes. Does anyone tell Chuck that a common side effect of this medication is impotence? Even if someone does happen to mention impotence as a side effect, does anyone give Chuck and his partner support as they explore the consequences for their relationship? Who is concerned when Chuck and his partner are being intimate and Chuck is unable to have or maintain an erection? Who is available for Chuck or Chuck's partner to discuss this loss? What if there are other concerns about Chuck's health? Perhaps Chuck's partner begins to believe that he or she is the reason for the impotence and is unable to verbalize that fear to Chuck or someone else? The whole relationship can be called into question over something that is a direct cause of the medication used to "maintain" Chuck's health.

Keep in mind that it is the client who generally determines what is alarming. For example, a client who has been married for 30 years and has had sex regularly now mentions that for the past 3 months there has been no sex. This is alarming. Or a client shares with you in a history that her son just "came out" as a gay man and the client doesn't know how to help him. This is alarming. How about the 80-year-old woman who reports having thought that she was done having periods but says that for the past couple of months she has been bleeding off and on? This is alarming.

In each of these examples the nurse is asked to utilize good communication skills and clarify the problem with the client. The best way to do this is to seek clarification by re-asking the question: "So you've been having 'periods' for the past 2 months after not having them for years?" or "Your son recently 'came out' to you as being gay and you would like to know how to help him. In what ways do you believe he needs help?" Keep in mind that you need to explore with clients what help they are seeking. The woman with the gay son may be asking for spiritual guidance, a support group for parents, or reassurance that she has done nothing wrong as a mother. You, as the nurse, are asked to move beyond your own sense of "right," "wrong," or "help" to discover what it is the client or family needs in terms of assistance, information, support, or referral source that will help them in their adaptation to this new situation.

▶ Mabel and Clarence, who have enjoyed sexual activities well into their eighties, now find themselves worried about Medicaid/Medicare cutbacks and how they are going to meet expenses and also maintain their current level of health. The stress of these worries may very well cause distance between the two, which in turn may lead one of them to drink a little more than usual to numb the pain of the worries. With increase of alcohol consumption there is a decrease in sexual drive. Compound this with other presenting health problems and this couple's intimate life is in crisis. What once was satisfying and stress-relieving behavior now becomes a situation of isolation and disappointment.

How does the nurse in this situation intervene to help Mabel and Clarence? Try the following exercise.

CRITICAL THINKING EXERCISE 30–1

Break into small groups of four and practice. One of you play the part of the nurse, one the part of Mabel, another the part of Clarence, and the fourth person the silent role of observer. How does the nurse approach this situation? Is it best to work 1:1 with Mabel and Clarence or is it best to talk with them together? What focus does the nurse need to have in this conversation? Does the nurse ever address the issues of sex directly? Does the nurse refer the couple to a medical social worker, a drug and alcohol treatment center, a counselor? How would the nurse address each of these referrals if it is determined that the referral is an appropriate one? How did it feel to you to be Mabel, or Clarence? Did you feel comforted, supported, listened to, or brushed off as the nurse responded? As an observer, what did you notice about this interaction?

EFFECTS OF MEDICAL TREATMENT ON SEXUALITY

Both procedures performed and medications prescribed to preserve a person's health may be beneficial while still leaving clients with permanent sexually related disabilities as well as unspoken worries and fears. Think about the woman who has a breast removed because of cancer, or a teenager who has ulcerative colitis and has had a permanent colostomy at age 16. How do we, as nurses, set about assisting these clients, or their significant others (now or in the future), in dealing with the consequences of these life-saving interventions, especially in their most intimate relationships? How do we come to terms with what it would be like for us to have had this experience?

Side effects of even simple prescribed medications may seriously affect a client's ability to function sexually. Many medications given as "everyday" treatment for acute and chronic illnesses have side effects that can drastically affect intimate relationships. Refer to Table 30–1 for a list of drugs that may induce sexual dysfunction. These side effects may be minor and easily correctable (e.g., the use of water-soluble lubricants for someone taking medications that have an anticholinergic effect and decrease vaginal secretions). Other side effects may have more impact: decreased responsiveness, decreased libido, or impotence.

Consider the possible side effects for a client who has hypertension and is taking propranolol (Inderal). A common side effect is drowsiness, which may be only annoying, but which may have drastic consequences in a relationship if the individuals involved are not clear in their communication. The partner may assume from the client's drowsiness a disinterest in sexual contact; this may not be the case. The client may be able to perform activities of daily living (ADLs), but the energy needed for sexual contact may simply be too much at this time. Nevertheless, the partner's conclusion that sexual intimacy is no longer desired by the client may have crisis-producing effects. It would be helpful in this situation for the nurse to explain the side effects, and offer support and understanding to both the client and partner. The nurse can encourage open dialogue between the partners and suggest that they explore new ways of being intimate. The nurse might also suggest that the client look into other ways of decreasing blood pressure (e.g., biofeedback, regular exercise, diet changes, relaxation, counseling) under the supervision of a physician. The nurse could suggest that the couple set up specific "dates" when the client is more fully rested and is under less everyday stress, and also suggest that the partner try to be supportive rather than taking the outcome of the interaction as a personal triumph or failure. The nurse could also suggest that if the symptoms persist and the couple is unable to develop a satisfying new way of interacting sexually, it may be necessary to seek a different medication from the physician. Try the following exercise.

CRITICAL THINKING EXERCISE 30–2

Describe how you would interact with an individual who has a diagnosis of depression, is taking a tricyclic antidepressant such as imipramine or desipramine, and reports not being interested in his or her usual activities. How would you approach finding out if this includes sexual activity?

Table 30–2 suggests strategies the nurse can use to facilitate communication. Remember that you need to make these questions your own, and that they should be asked from a standpoint of seeking understanding of the client's situation.

It is important for the nurse to be at ease when assessing the client's sexual satisfaction. Sexuality needs to be seen as an acceptable subject for discussion. For those clients who initially cannot bring themselves to volunteer information, permission needs to be given to open up a discussion later. There are several ways to do this. For example, questions about sex should be included on any self-administered intake history questionnaire used by the institution. The questions can be as simple as "Sexual difficulties—yes or no?" or "Sex is entirely satisfactory—yes or no?" These one-liner questions sometimes open the door for further discussion or follow-up education. Another approach is to ask about satisfaction or difficulties on a scale of 1 to 5. Keep in mind that these first questions are intended to gain a general sense of the client's situation.

TABLE 30–1 SOME DRUG-INDUCED SEXUAL DYSFUNCTION

DRUG	INDUCED SEXUAL DYSFUNCTION
▶ Alcohol	Decreased libido; gynecomastia; interferes with sperm production
▶ Amitriptyline (Elavil)	Loss of libido; impotence; no ejaculation
▶ Anticholinergic tricyclic antidepressants (desipramine hydrochloride [Norpramin], imipramine [Tofranil])	Block dilation of arterial supply to corpus cavernosum and corpus spongiosum (penis erectile tissue unable to acquire fluid to expand—necessary for erection)
▶ Barbiturates (e.g., amobarbital sodium, phenobarbital, secobarbital)	Decreased libido; impotence
▶ Chlorpromazine (Thorazine)	Decreased libido; impotence; no ejaculation
▶ Cimetidine (Tagamet)	Antiandrogen (inhibits hormone that promotes male characteristics)
▶ CNS depressants (e.g., benzodiazepines)	Impotence; decreased libido
▶ Diazepam (Valium)	Decreased libido; delayed ejaculation; retarded or no orgasm in women
▶ Digoxin (Lanoxin)	Interferes with libido
▶ Hydralazine (Apresoline)	Impotence; priapism (abnormal erection of penis)
▶ Indomethacin (Indocin)	Interferes with libido
▶ Levodopa (L-dopa)	Increased libido
▶ Lithium (Eskalith, Lithonate)	Decreased libido; impotence
▶ Marijuana	Decreased libido; gynecomastia; interferes with sperm production
▶ Methyldopa (Aldomet)	Elevated serum prolactin levels; decreased libido; impotence; impaired ejaculation
▶ Metronidazole (Flagyl)	Interferes with libido
▶ Opiates (morphine)	Increased prolactin levels (results in growth of breast tissue and lactation)
▶ Phenothiazide antipsychotics Trifluoperazine (Stelazine) Fluphenazine (Prolixin) Perphenazine (Trilafon)	Block dilation of arterial supply to corpus cavernosum and corpus spongiosum
▶ Phenytoin (Dilantin)	Interferes with libido
▶ Propranolol (Inderal)	Loss of libido; impotence
▶ Ranitidine (Zantac)	Loss of libido; impotence
▶ Spironolactone (Aldactone)	Gynecomastia; decreased libido
▶ Thiazide diuretics (hydrochlorothiazide)	Impotence
▶ Thioridazine (Mellaril)	Impotence; priapism; delayed, decreased, painful, retrograde, or no ejaculation
▶ Tobacco	Affects small peripheral vasculature, documented by statistically significant abnormal penile brachial index values
▶ Verapamil (Calan, Isoptin)	Impotence

In taking a verbal history, a more direct approach may be taken. When possible, it is best to have clients fully clothed, which helps them feel less "exposed." It may be helpful to include questions about sexuality and relationships right along with other aspects of the history (e.g., when asking questions about menstrual cycles, bowel movements, or vaginal infections). This naturally leads into questions about sexual practices and performance, use of contraception, "safe sex" teaching needs, and any specific concerns of the client.

There are several general, open-ended questions that you can use routinely. The first is "How satisfactory is your sexual functioning?" This question is appropriate for every sexually active client. Avoiding the word *intercourse* signals that nothing is assumed about the sexual activities of the client. This may help the client feel comfortable in disclosing accurate personal information. You may also say "Many people have unanswered questions or need information about sexual functioning. What questions do you have about sex?" This opens up the conversation for the person to ask his or her questions and directs the path of teaching-learning opportunities.

Questions for assessing risk factors associated with sexual behaviors may include the following: "Do you always engage in 'safe sex' practices? What does that entail for you?" "Since beginning regular sexual activity, how many different partners have you had?" "Have you or your sexual partner(s) ever used intravenous drugs?" If the answers indicate no problems or concerns, you can simply leave the door open for clients to bring up any concerns they may have in the future. If there are concerns, there needs to be some kind of follow-up, either with you or with the appropriate health care professional.

TABLE 30–2 STATEMENTS THAT FACILITATE COMMUNICATION

SITUATION BEING EXPLORED	FACILITATING STATEMENT
Giving rationale for question	As a nurse, I'm concerned about all aspects of your health. Many individuals have concerns about sexual matters, especially when they are sick or when they are having other health problems.
Giving statements of "generality" or "normality"	Most people are hesitant to discuss . . . . Many people worry about feelings . . . . Many people have concerns about . . . .
Identifying sexual dysfunction	Most people have difficulties at some time during their sexual relationships. Have you had any problems?
Obtaining information from an unmarried individual	The degree to which unmarried persons have sexual outlets varies considerably. Some have sexual partners, others have none, some relieve sexual tension through masturbation, others need no outlet at all. What has been your pattern?
Identifying sexual myths	While growing up, most of us have heard some sexual myths or half-truths that continue to puzzle us. Are there any that come to mind?
Identifying feelings about masturbation	Many of us grown-ups have heard various stories about masturbation and what problems it supposedly causes. This can create worry even into adulthood. What have you heard?
Determining whether homosexuality is a source of conflict	What is your attitude toward your homosexual orientation?
Identifying older individuals' concern about sexual functioning	Many people, as they get older, believe or worry that this signals the end of their sex life. Much misinformation surrounds this myth. What is your understanding about sexuality during the later years? How has the passage of time affected your sexuality (sex life)?
Obtaining and giving information (miscellaneous areas)	Frequently, people have questions about . . . . What questions do you have about . . . . What would you like to know about . . . ?
Closing the history	Is there anything further in the area of sexuality that you would like to bring up now? I hope that if questions or concerns do come to mind in the future, we'll be able to discuss them.

Adapted from Green, R. (1975). *Human sexuality: a health practitioner's text.* Baltimore: Williams & Wilkins.

CLIENT ASSESSMENT

Nurses are often the first to hear of concerns regarding sexuality that are affecting the mental health of clients. Changing family situations, sexual development and desires, and physical diseases are all issues that many people have difficulty discussing. Nurses can often encourage discussion by being aware of the importance of these concerns and by being receptive when clients make seemingly casual references to issues that are really of vital concern to them. Nurses can both encourage questions and offer opportunities for teaching-learning situations to come to the surface.

Where do you begin an assessment of a client's intimate life? How do you ask questions about relationships and sexual satisfaction? This area of nursing is often met with uneasiness and a degree of embarrassment. Do you recall the first couple of interactions you had with a client? Remember when you first began learning about nursing assessments? In general, the questions were probably a little awkward and not something you easily became comfortable asking. Likewise, asking individuals about their sexual relationships will be awkward at first. Keep in mind there are some things that will help make this easier. First and foremost, this is about your assessment of the client, made in order to develop an overall picture of the individual so that you can provide him or her with optimal nursing care. It is not about your personal needs or desires. It is about your professional responsibility to provide holistic nursing care. You will learn to approach this with understanding and purpose. Keep in mind that it will require practice.

Hogan (1980) suggests that the nurse have an introductory statement prepared. For example, "As a nurse I am concerned about all aspects of your health. However, we often neglect helping clients in what may be a very important part of their lives—their sexual needs. I'm going to ask you some questions in this area." Try the following exercise.

CRITICAL THINKING EXERCISE 30–3

Divide into pairs and practice initiating a conversation that will assess the client's satisfaction with her or his sexual relationships. Use Table 30–2 as a guide. After coming up with three or four ways of beginning this assessment, stop. Combine two or three pair groups into one larger group and discuss what was particularly difficult about this exercise. Identify what approaches worked best for you as the nurse and for you as the client. Discuss why this was so for you.

Factors that will play a part in your ability to connect with the client and correctly assess the situation are multifaceted. Keep in mind that all the things you identified as factors for your current world view also contribute to the client's world view, even though the client's response may be quite different from yours.

Be sure that you are looking beyond the immediate moment when assessing a client. Place the client in the context of a whole life. If you are working in an outpatient area, imagine the client's world at home. If this is an acute setting, try to create a picture of this client before the incident that brought her or him into the hospital. If you are seeing the client at home, imagine the individual's life outside the four walls.

Probably one of the first questions asked of an individual during an assessment is something about marital status. Usually the question is "Are you married?" While this is a perfectly acceptable question, it does limit the sort of response available from the client. "Are you married?" or "What is your marital status?" is an example of a closed question. You have asked the client to respond with one word. This provides only limited information. What if this individual lives with someone and is having an intimate relationship but is not married? How does he or she answer your questions? What if the person you are speaking with is lesbian or gay or bisexual? How do these clients answer in a way that identifies who is important in their life? And how do they convey to you how they want this person involved in their health care? Think for a few minutes about how you could ask a question that gets more directly to issues you are really asking when you routinely ask "Are you married?" Practice asking each other these questions and see what sort of answers you can give that move beyond the limited one-word answers.

There are all types of adult relationships. Some of these are more common and socially acceptable than others, but regardless of this, you as a nurse caring for individuals must allow them to state personal choices without judgment and comment. The type of relationship these adults are in should not affect the quality of nursing care you provide. They could be in a traditional marriage, single, in a premarital relationship, in an open marriage, divorced, in a multi-partner relationship, in a remarried/blended family, a single parent, or in a lesbian/gay relationship. So, since you need to know who is important to this client, and how this person or persons interacts with the client, it might be better for you to ask questions that get at what you need to know.

Deevey (1993) acknowledges the complications that gays and lesbians have in sharing their life style with others, especially health care providers. Table 30–3 offers suggestions to lesbian women for responding to the various reactions of people who are threatened by alternative sexual life styles.

Then, of course, there are concerns about the client's past. How does a history of incest, sexual abuse, or battering play a part in the development and maintenance of intimate relationships? How do these experiences help or hinder clients' ability, or desire, to share information about their lives? Not all your clients will have had these experiences, but research indicates that a surprising number of people, both women and men, have been or currently are victims of such experiences. Federal Bureau of Investigation (FBI) statistics indicate that every 15 seconds a woman is beaten and every 6 minutes a woman is brutally raped (Brownmiller 1993). One in three women is sexually assaulted during her lifetime. One fifth to one half of American women were sexually abused as children, and nearly one third of female homicide victims are killed by their husbands or boyfriends (Boston Women's Health Book Collective 1992).

Keep in mind that clients' fears, hesitations, embarrassment, emotional pain, and confusion should play a crucial part in how you approach them, even in the most routine of questions. It is your responsibility as a professional to develop ways of asking questions that help place clients at ease and allow them to share with you what they are ready to confide at that moment. Remember that this may be a time to begin brainstorming possible referrals if it becomes evident that the information being discussed is beyond your scope of practice or timing in this given situation.

SEXUALITY

Although Freud's writings are challenged today, he is acknowledged for introducing ideas and theories that brought the complexity of sex and sexuality into scientific research. Sexuality is now viewed as an integral part of human behavior throughout the life cycle. Some form of sexuality is addressed by all the major growth and development theorists. Before Freud, little was known, let alone researched, regarding the sexual development of children. Now, we are aware of the importance of adults' reactions as a child passes through various stages of self-esteem and sexual development. Early experiences in emotional relating have important consequences in later years. A positive and accepting attitude by parents and caregivers provides a background for satisfactory adult relationships.

Human Sexual Response

The most extensive research on sexual response is that of the team of William Masters and Virginia Johnson (1966, 1970, 1979). Their extensive research in the mid-1960s has had a profound impact on the field of sexology and on the development of sex therapy techniques. Masters and Johnson discovered that there is one **sexual response**

TABLE 30–3 HOMOPHOBIC REACTIONS TO LESBIAN SELF-DISCLOSURE

REACTION	PRIVATE RESPONSE	PUBLIC RESPONSE
"You're a sinner."	The God-Hates-You Attack	"I respect your religious beliefs, but I insist that you treat me with respect."
"You're fired."	The Financial-Ruin Attack	"This is a very emotional topic. Let's discuss it when we've both had a chance to think about this."
"Your mother/father was cold/sick/weak and caused you to be a lesbian."	The Child-of-Bad-Parents Attack	"We don't really know what causes either heterosexual or homosexual orientation. About 10% of all people are gay and lesbian, whatever their family background."
"You're an ugly woman who couldn't get a man."	The Body-Image Attack	"Stereotypes about lesbians often include physical unattractiveness, man hating, or lack of heterosexual experience, but none of these stereotypes are true."
"You should be ashamed—you bring danger/humiliation to this family/profession/neighborhood/nation."	The Guilt-Trip Attack	"I am proud and happy to be a lesbian. I'd be glad to answer your questions about lesbian culture."
"I'll report you to the authorities. They'll take away your child."	The Unfit-Mother Attack	"I am confident that I am a good parent to my child. She/he benefits from the courage and wisdom I have gained in dealing with my oppression as a lesbian."
"A patient complained to the head nurse that you asked him if he is gay. Why did you do that?"	The Professional-Integrity Attack	"I believe each patient should be asked about sexual orientation to make clear that we offer good care to *all* patients."
"I'll tell your partner's parents/employer/grandmother."	The Attack on the Closeted Partner	"You can threaten me with scandal, but blackmail is illegal, and I will sue you."
"Are you the little boy or the little girl?"	The Lesbians-as-Pseudoheterosexuals Attack	(Some questions I don't dignify with an answer.)
"It's OK with me if you're a lesbian, so long as you keep your hands off my neck."	The Predatory-Lesbian Attack	"We lesbians make pretty clear distinctions between courting and friendship with women. I think you'll continue to feel safe with me."
"You mean all this time you didn't tell me? Why don't you trust me?"	The Lesbians-Are-Liars Attack	"Try to imagine for the next 48 hours that you are a lesbian. It takes courage and compromise to survive in a hostile environment."
"You're so comfortable talking about lesbian issues, I can't believe you get angry or scared about homophobia."	The Looks-So-Easy Attack	"I do accept myself. But the world is still hostile and violent toward gay and lesbian people. I never can predict if I'll be safe in a new situation."
"There's no reason to do research on lesbian women, no need to provide special services. You have convinced me that lesbian women are no different from other women."	The Denial-of-Difference Attack	"It's true that lesbian women are not 'different' in the sense of being emotionally disturbed or sinful or criminal. But the prejudice against us causes minority stress and has generated a hidden lesbian culture that few straight people know about."
"When you get AIDS, I'll take care of you."	The So-Much-to-Learn Attack	"Lesbian women are actually the lowest-risk population for AIDS, but I appreciate your support."
"You're disgusting and sick."	The Blatant Attack	"I see you have a problem. I'd be glad to recommend a good therapist."
"I never met one before."	The Honest-Truth Response—one I respect	"Well, you're in luck. If you want to know more about gay and lesbian culture, I love to answer questions. I've been asked all kinds of things, so don't be shy."

Adapted from Deevey, S. (1993). Lesbian self-disclosure strategies for success. *Journal of Psychosocial Nursing*, 31(4):25.

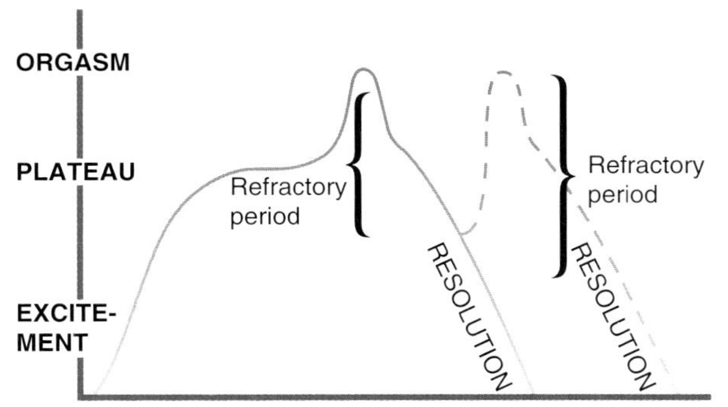

Figure 30–1 Male sexual response cycle. (Redrawn from Masters, W. H., and Johnson, V. E. (1966). *Human sexual response*. Boston: Little, Brown.)

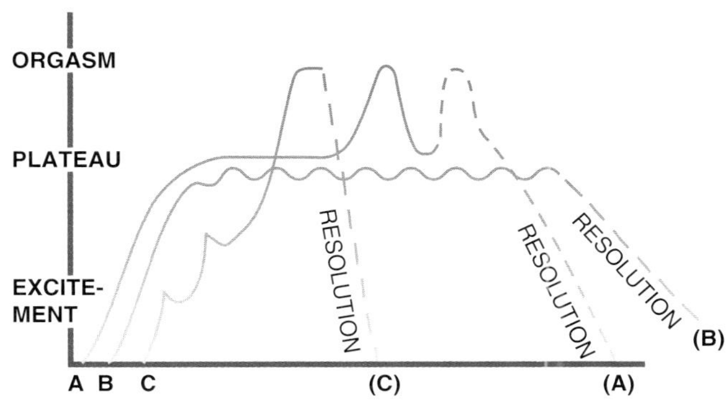

Figure 30–2 Female sexual response cycle. (Redrawn from Masters, W. H., and Johnson, V. E. (1966). *Human sexual response*. Boston: Little, Brown.)

pattern for males (Fig. 30–1) and three patterns for females (Fig. 30–2). They recorded the sexual responses of both men and women by observing over 10,000 sexual cycles during intercourse and masturbation. From this they determined that, during sexual intercourse, individuals experience four stages and have specific physical responses in each stage (Table 30–4).

The information obtained from this research has both educational and therapeutic value. Indeed, one of the primary motives for conducting these studies was to help people experiencing some kind of sexual dysfunction. Through research, Masters and Johnson have been able to develop specific techniques to deal with various male and female sexual dysfunctions.

TABLE 30–4 PHYSIOLOGICAL RESPONSES TO SEXUAL EXCITEMENT

PHASE	MALE	FEMALE
Excitement	Erotic feelings	Erotic feelings
	Erection of penis Testes elevate toward perineum Nipples become erect	Vaginal lubrication Swelling of breasts and labia Tenting of cervix and uterus Nipples become erect Clitoris begins to enlarge
	In both men and women, the blood pressure and pulse begin to elevate; "sex flush" (reddening of the skin) may appear.	
Plateau	*Continuation of the excitement phase for both men and women*	
	Penis increases in diameter Glans may darken Testes elevate tightly against perineum Preejaculatory fluid is secreted from Cowper's gland	Clitoris retracts under clitoral hood Bartholin's gland secretes mucoid substance
	Both men and women experience increase in myotonia, which leads to voluntary and involuntary contractions of arms, legs, neck, rectum, and buttocks. Heart rate, blood pressure, and respiratory and muscular tension increase throughout this phase.	
Orgasm		
	Prostate seminal vesicles and ampullae contract rhythmically Semen flows into distended urethral meatus Urethral contractions Expulsion of semen	Involuntary rhythmic contractions of orgasmic platform and uterus Whole body warmth Throbbing sensation in pelvis
	Vital signs for both men and women peak. Respiration around 40/min, heart rate 110–180 beats/min, systolic blood pressure increases 30–100 mm Hg, diastolic blood pressure increases 20–50 mm Hg.	
Resolution	*For both men and women, there is release of muscular tension and return of organs and tissue to an unstimulated state.*	

Data from Masters, W. H., and Johnson, V. E. (1966). *Human sexual response*. Boston: Little, Brown; Smeltzer, S. C., and Bare, B. G. (1992). *Brunner*

Sexual Disorders

The concept of what is "normal" in adult relationships and sexuality is related to values and religious beliefs, in addition to physical responses, and is shown to cover a wide spectrum of human behavior.

Keeping in mind the range of normal, it is necessary when studying sexual disorders and dysfunctions that abnormalities be considered those things that cause the *client* discomfort, pain, or interference with a healthy adult sexual response. It is necessary that a nurse be familiar with both the terms and the symptoms of disorders. Without additional education, a nurse is limited in the type of therapeutic interactions that can be used to assist a client in making a significant change. It is appropriate that the basic-level nurse be able to identify alterations in normal sexuality and relationships and gain confidence about when to refer the client for additional assistance.

The *Diagnostic and statistical manual of mental disorders*, fourth edition (DSM-IV) (APA 1994) classifies sexual disorders in four categories: sexual dysfunctions, gender identity disorders, paraphilias, and sexual disorder not otherwise specified (NOS).

Sexual Dysfunctions

Sexual dysfunctions include sexual desire disorders, sexual arousal disorders, orgasmic disorders, sexual pain disorders, sexual dysfunction due to a general medical condition, and substance-related sexual dysfunction. General characteristics of a sexual dysfunction include a "disturbance in the processes that characterize the sexual response cycle or by pain associated with sexual intercourse" (APA 1994).

When working with a person who has a sexual dysfunction, it is important to note that an individual's ethnic, cultural, religious, and social backgrounds play a significant role and may influence sexual desire, expectations, and attitudes about performance (APA 1994).

Orgasmic Disorders

Orgasmic disorder is a persistent or recurrent delay in, or absence of, orgasm after a normal sexual excitement phase. Orgasmic disorder in females is referred to as *female orgasmic disorder* and is the most commonly presented female problem. Some women are not interested in orgasm, but many are very interested in being able to enjoy sex fully.

Male orgasmic disorder entails persistent or recurrent delay in, or absence of, orgasm after a normal sexual excitement phase (DSM-IV). Most commonly, it takes the form of inability to reach coital orgasm during intercourse, although manual or oral stimulation by a partner can bring the man to orgasm.

Premature ejaculation used to be the most commonly presented sexual difficulty of males, but the effective therapeutic techniques used for this problem have relegated it to second place, behind inhibited desire. There are many ways to define what is premature. Some have suggested that any ejaculation occurring before the partner is satisfied is premature. Others suggest that ejaculation occurring more than 50% of the time before the man wishes it is premature. DSM-IV defines this disorder as "persistent or recurrent ejaculation with minimal sexual stimulation before, on, or shortly after penetration and before the person wishes it." The usual duration of coitus is between 4 and 7 minutes, so anything less than maintaining a 2-minute erection could be considered premature.

Premature ejaculation is not uncommon in young males who learn to delay orgasm with sexual experience and aging. In older men who have experienced a period of adequate sexual functioning, premature ejaculation may occur after decreased frequency of sexual activity, intense performance anxiety with a new partner, or loss of ejaculatory control related to difficulty achieving or maintaining erections.

Sexual Desire Disorders

Among the sexual desire disorders are hypoactive sexual desire disorder and sexual aversion disorder. For the diagnosis of disorder, both of these conditions must include (a) that it causes the person marked distress or interpersonal difficulty and (b) that the disorder is not caused by another Axis 1 disorder.

A diagnosis of *hypoactive sexual desire disorder* is made when a person has a persistent or recurrent deficit or absence of sexual fantasies and desire for sexual activity. Onset can be in puberty, but more commonly it develops in adulthood. Often the individual has had adequate sexual interest, but in the face of stressful life events or interpersonal difficulties sexual desire is lost. This loss may be continuous or episodic. Differential diagnosis includes ruling out the effect of a substance (medication/drug of abuse) or a general medical condition that contributes to the individual's sexual loss.

Sexual aversion disorder is characterized by aversion to and active avoidance of genital sexual contact with a sexual partner. A person with this disorder might experience anxiety, fear, or disgust when confronted by the opportunity for a sexual encounter with a partner. The continuum ranges from lack of pleasure to extreme psychological distress.

Sexual Arousal Disorders

Female sexual arousal disorder may be accompanied by a sexual desire disorder and/or a female orgasmic disorder. Women with this disorder have a persistent or recurrent inability to attain, or to maintain until the completion of

TABLE 30–5 FEMALE SEXUAL DYSFUNCTION

PROBLEM	PHASE	MAJOR SYMPTOM
Inhibited desire	Arousal	No lubrication, little interest
Orgasmic dysfunction	Orgasmic	Inability to have orgasm most of the time
Dyspareunia	Any phase	Pain experienced before, during, or after intercourse
Vaginismus	Orgasmic if vaginal penetration	Involuntary, painful spasms when vaginal penetration is attempted

sexual activity, adequate lubrication and swelling response related to sexual excitement.

In *male erectile disorder*, most erectile difficulties are associated with sexual anxiety, fear of failure, concerns about sexual performance, and a decreased subjective sense of sexual excitement and pleasure. Most cases of acquired erectile disorder remit spontaneously 15% to 30% of the time (DSM-IV). The type of partner or the intensity or quality of the relationship may also affect a man's ability to have an erection. Simply stated, male erectile disorder is the persistent or recurrent inability to attain, or to maintain until completion of sexual activity, an adequate erection (DSM-IV).

Sexual Pain Disorders

This disorder is found in both males and females and consists of genital pain associated with sexual intercourse. Symptoms range from mild discomfort to sharp pain and there may be a chronic course.

Vaginismus is the persistent and recurrent involuntary contraction of the peritoneal muscles surrounding the outer third of the vagina when vaginal penetration with a penis, finger, tampon, or speculum is attempted. Some women may experience vaginismus in the anticipation of vaginal insertion. A woman, however, may still experience desire and pleasure and be brought to orgasm if penetration is not attempted or anticipated. The disorder is found mostly in young women and especially if there is a history of being sexually abused or traumatized, and in females with negative attitudes toward sex.

Refer to Tables 30–5 and 30–6 for an overview of female and male sexual problems.

Biological Causes of Sexual Dysfunction

It is believed that there are biological causes of sexual dysfunction in only 20% or less of presenting cases. Biological causes include general illness (e.g., influenza, colds, fatigue) and those of more severe and persistent origin (e.g., diabetes, hepatitis, multiple sclerosis). Hormonal disorders in which medications cause a decrease in androgen levels, such as hypopituitary problems and the feminizing effects of testicular tumors, may also cause sexual dysfunction. Alcohol and drug use (e.g., cocaine, heroin) decreases sexual drive. Hypertensive drugs and the phenothiazines (e.g., Prolixin, Trilafon, Mellaril) affect sexual performance in some clients. Many of the SSRIs and other antidepressants may also cause sexual difficulties for some individuals. Refer to Table 30–1 for a list of drug-induced sexual dysfunctions and common physical manifestations.

Other physical conditions that can cause pain during sex include arthritis, back pain, obesity, vaginal infection, and late stages of pregnancy. Age can be a factor in sexual dysfunction. Postmenopausal women may need additional lubrication, and older men may find they do not ejaculate as frequently as they did when they were

TABLE 30–6 MALE SEXUAL DYSFUNCTION

PROBLEM	PHASE	MAJOR SYMPTOM
Inhibited desire	Arousal-excitement	No erection, no sexual interest
Erective incapacity	Arousal-excitement	No or partial erection 50% of the time
Premature ejaculation	Orgasmic	Ejaculation before the man wishes 50% of the time
Orgasmic dysfunction	Orgasmic	Inability to ejaculate following normal sexual excitement phase
Dyspareunia	Any phase	Pain experienced before, during, or after intercourse

younger. Also, if a partner is lost through death or divorce and the remaining partner has no sexual activity for a period of years, it may be difficult to regain sexual function. Age in itself does not cause dysfunction; many people report active and satisfactory sex lives well into their eighties and nineties.

Psychological causes of sexual dysfunction for all individuals can be attributed to the following:

- Ignorance regarding which actions are stimulating for oneself or one's partner
- Anxiety due to fear of failure
- Partner's or self's demand for performance or an excessive need to please the partner
- Perceptual and intellectual defenses that get in the way of eroticism, such as "not feeling"
- Allowing judgmental thoughts to intervene and becoming engrossed in self-observation instead of participation
- Poor relationship choices that can result in partner rejection, lack of trust, power struggles, and sexual sabotage that virtually guarantee that sex will not be rewarding

TREATMENT. Various schools of psychology have taken different approaches to the causes and treatment of sexual problems. Therapies, regardless of theoretical base, rely heavily on the research of sexologists such as Masters and Johnson (1970) and Helen Singer Kaplan (1979). Individual practitioners who have had special training (nurses, social workers, psychologists) adopt a theoretical framework and treatment plan that fits their values and beliefs and their own style of therapy.

Typical sexual counseling consists of a general history, a complete physical examination (to rule out any organic causes), and a thorough sexual history. The sexual history should focus on specific details about what the individual or couple actually do sexually, identifying both physical and emotional components. The therapist will also want to determine which stage of the response cycle is impaired. Communication patterns and expectations should be assessed so that the therapist can determine whether the primary focus is one of sexual behaviors or some other psychosocial area. Sometimes what is presented as a sexual difficulty may be a reflection of distress throughout the relationship.

Therapeutic intervention generally required in all cases of dysfunction includes anxiety reduction and a certain amount of "permission giving." The attitude that it is all right to enjoy sex is vital for successful treatment. Couples are urged to discuss their sexual needs and desires openly and to take turns in giving and receiving pleasure with one another.

For therapy for sexual dysfunctions to be successful, it must be focused on the construction of a sound and healthy relationship. If a healthy and mutually respectful relationship is not present, it may be necessary to focus on building one before following with therapy focused on the sexual problems.

Gender Identity Disorder

Gender, the physical fact of maleness or femaleness, is usually the first thing known about a person. Social groups prescribe different role models for males and females. Boys and girls are treated differently from birth, ranging from areas such as choice of toys and clothing to the amount of handling and cuddling each receives.

Children become aware early in life of the psychological and physiological differences between the sexes, and most are firmly committed to the societal expectations for their gender as early as 18 months of age. In rare cases in which gender was misassigned at birth owing to physical abnormality or in which accidental damage has been suffered, it is considered almost impossible to reassign a child to the opposite sex after 18 months of age. By then, the sense of gender identity, of being male or female, is too firmly rooted to change.

For most people, the private sense they have of themselves as being male or female matches their physical make-up. Most children enter adolescence aware that they are to be a man or a woman and, regardless of heterosexual or homosexual preferences, they are satisfied with their gender identity.

Some people do not have this match between biological gender and psychological gender identity. These individuals have early and persistent feelings that they are trapped in a body with the wrong genitals. In reality, they believe they are and were always meant to be of the opposite sex. There are no recent studies on the prevalance of gender identity disorder, but data from smaller European countries with access to total population statistics suggest that 1 per 30,000 males and 1 per 100,000 females seek sex-reassignment surgery (DSM-IV, p. 535).

Little is known about the origins of gender identity disorder, but childhood patterns seem to be fairly consistent. As early as 2 and 4 years of age some children may have cross-gender interests and activities. However, only a small percentage of children who display gender identity disorder characteristics will continue these characteristics into adolescence or adulthood. Typically, children who become transsexual relate better to the other sex. Boys prefer female friends and activities and cross-dress whenever possible. Girls imitate what they consider to be masculine behavior and refuse to be involved in activities usually assigned to females.

At puberty, the individual is greatly dismayed at the physical changes taking place; this is not true for most homosexuals or transvestites. About 75% of boys who had a childhood history of gender identity disorder report a homosexual or bisexual orientation. The remainder report a heterosexual orientation (DSM-IV). The corresponding percentages for women is not known. People with gender identity disorder continue to prefer the opposite-sex behavioral style into adulthood; often, they come to desire sexual reassignment as they find partners whom they wish to live with or marry. These individuals never consider themselves to be homosexual. The biological female who falls in love with a woman believes herself actually to be a man who loves that woman. Thus, a desire for congruity in gender identity and physiology becomes important for many (Green and Blanchard 1995).

Adults with gender identity disorder seek various solutions when they suffer from gender dysphoria. Some people seek to have help in suppressing their cross-gender feelings, others want more information, and others come for surgery resulting in sex reassignment. When gender dysphoria is severe and intractable, sex reassignment may be the best solution (Green and Blanchard 1995).

Hormone therapy is usually the first step (males taking estrogen and females taking androgen). Hormones help develop the bodily characteristics desired: for example, hips and breasts in the biological male, and body hair and lack of menstruation in the biological female.

Most clinics in North America and Western Europe require their clients to live in the cross-gender role for 1 to 2 years before surgery (Green and Blanchard 1995). This includes going to work or attending school, to help the client determine if he or she can interact successfully with members of society in the cross-gender mode (Green and Blanchard 1995). Legal and social arrangements are made: name change on various documents, and new employment if it is necessary to leave a former job owing to discrimination. Relationship issues, such as what to tell parents, children, and former spouses need to be resolved. Only after it appears that a successful outcome is likely is the second step, surgery performed.

Professionals debate the value of sex-change surgery, and conflicting studies make the issue unclear. Some transsexuals appear to live happy and productive lives without undergoing this expensive and painful surgery, whereas others seem unable to function without it. However, outcome studies, although not conclusive, tend to support the conclusion that postoperative improvements in social integration, sexual adjustment, and psychological health can be attributed to surgical intervention (Green and Blanchard 1995).

Paraphilias

The essential features of paraphilias are recurrent and intense sexually arousing fantasies, sexual urges, or behaviors, generally involving inanimate objects, the suffering or humiliation of oneself or one's partner, or the use of children or other nonconsenting persons (APA 1994). Certainly history, culture, and experience play a role in what is considered paraphilia. Currently the following are considered unusual enough to be called paraphilias: fetishism, pedophilia, exhibitionism, voyeurism, transvestitism, sexual sadism and masochism, and frotteurism. All paraphilias include (1) presence for at least 6 months and (2) the fantasies, sexual urges, or behaviors causing significant distress or impairment, in social, occupational, or other areas of functioning.

Fetishism is the presence of intense sexually arousing fantasies, sexual urges, or behaviors involving the use of inanimate objects (e.g., female undergarments).

Pedophilia involves sexual activity with a prepubescent child (generally 13 years or younger). Because of the illegal nature of pedophilia, its incidence is unknown. The person is at least 16 years old and at least 5 years older than the child. A typical profile of a pedophiliac is that of a somewhat conservative, married male. When pedophilia involves family members, it is called *incest;* most incestuous behavior occurs between father or stepfather and daughter.

Exhibitionism is the intentional display of the genitals in a public place. Sometimes the individual masturbates while exposing himself. Although illegal, it seems to be done more for shock value than as a preamble to sexual assault or rape. It has been suggested that this behavior is triggered by stress; the usual perpetrators are sedate, middle-class males.

Voyeurism is the viewing by stealth of other people in intimate situations (e.g., naked in the process of disrobing or engaging in sexual activity). Voyeurs are also called "peeping toms." Voyeurism is considered one of the paraphilias only when the "peeping" becomes compulsive and preferable to other sexual activity. The voyeur is almost always a heterosexual male who wishes no contact with those on whom he is spying. Often the man is described as shy, socially unskilled, and without close friends.

Transvestitism involves sexual satisfaction by means of dressing in the clothing of the opposite gender. This behavior is related to fetishism but often goes beyond the use of one particular object. Usually this behavior develops early in life. Unlike gender identity disorders, there are no sexual orientation issues, and transvestites do not desire a sex change. Usually heterosexual, many transvestites cross-dress only in specific sexual situations, and often receive the cooperation and support of their partners.

Sexual sadism and masochism (S/M) are two related paraphilias involving the giving (sadism) and receiving (masochism) of psychological and/or physical pain or domination to achieve sexual gratification. Much of what may be labeled as S/M falls outside the definition as outlined by DSM-IV. Masters and Johnson (1979) reported that S/M fantasies are frequent among both homosexuals and heterosexuals.

Frotteurism involves touching, rubbing against, or fondling an unfamiliar woman to achieve sexual satisfaction. This behavior usually occurs in busy public places where he can escape after touching his victim.

OTHER PARAPHILIAS. There are numerous other nonstandard sexual behaviors that some people engage in as either a part of or a major source of pleasure. As with the other paraphilias discussed, they may or may not cause a problem for the participant, depending on the availability of consenting partners and the societal norms at the time.

Some other sexual behaviors include zoophilia, or sexual contact with animals; coprophilia, klismaphilia, and urophilia, which are associated with feces, enemas, and urine, respectively; necrophilia, in which a corpse is desired; and telephone scatophilia, in which obscene language is used to a stranger over the phone.

Many of the people involved in nonstandard sexual practices find no need for therapy because their sexual activities are carried out with a consenting adult partner and neither involve illegal actions nor are physically or emotionally harmful to either partner. If, however, the person is experiencing relationship difficulties, wishes to change the sexual behaviors, becomes involved in illegal activity, or is physically or emotionally harming others or being harmed, therapy is indicated.

The usual treatment design for working with paraphilias is cognitive and behavioral therapy. An attempt is made to help the person learn a new sexual response pattern that will eliminate the need for the activity that is causing the problem. Techniques range from positive reinforcement for appropriate object choices to aversion techniques, in which mild electric shocks may be used for inappropriate choices. Other treatment modalities include psychodynamic techniques designed to help the client understand the origin of the paraphilia. Psychotropic agents may also be used in those practices that are acutely or dangerously compulsive. No matter what the treatment employed (pharmacological, cognitive, behavioral, dynamic, or combinations of those) it is unlikely to be effective unless extended over a very long period (Meyer 1995).

Sexual Addictions

Although not specifically outlined in DSM-IV, sexual addiction has surfaced in the 1990s as a matter of legitimate concern. Kasl (1989) reports that there have been Sex Addicts Anonymous groups (modeled after the Alcoholics Anonymous 12-step program) since 1978, the first ones beginning in Minneapolis. Kasl, describing sexual addictions, says "For some people, sex and relationships become the primary way of attempting to fill their emptiness. Paradoxically, in the process they get hungrier and hungrier, and often more angry or hopeless, because sex does not quiet the nameless yearning. Still, since they don't know what else to do, . . . they intensify their attachment to a relationship and it becomes addictive. At this point, all aspects of their lives are affected—work, friendships, health, and peace of mind."

In her book *Women, sex, and addiction*, Kasl (1989) devotes an entire chapter (Chapter 8) to questions that explore whether sex is an addiction. Some of these include the following:

- Do you feel compelled to have frequent sex, either with a partner or by masturbating?
- Are you bewildered about your sexual behavior?
- Do you have a pattern of unsuccessful love relationships in spite of longing for a permanent relationship?
- Is your life full of chaos and drama?
- Do sex and romance usually involve alcohol, drugs, or compulsive eating or not eating?
- Do you usually feel remorse or shame after having a sexual encounter? Do you feel as if you need to get away after you've had sex?
- In order to please your partner, do you engage in activities that feel repulsive or uncomfortable to you?

As with any addiction, it is important that individuals seek out a community where they can feel understood; practice being in honest, loving, caring environments; and stop the behavior that is causing harm to themselves and those around them. This may be effected through formal counseling, support groups, or friends. As a nurse, it is important for you to be aware of what community resources are available and how to assist a client in tapping into those resources.

Sexually Transmitted Diseases

Sexually transmitted diseases (STDs) range from merely annoying to life threatening. Some are easily treatable, while others have no known treatment; once infected, the individual is infected for life (Table 30–7). It is estimated that one of every three Americans will contract an STD in their lifetime. Therefore, it is essential that the nurse be able to discuss in specific terms what STDs are, how they are transmitted, how to assess a client for STDs, and when and how to make an appropriate referral for treatment.

Physical assessment for STDs is not discussed in this chapter. Emphasis here is on interviewing techniques and communication. It is important here to review how you can approach a client in this perhaps embarrassing circumstance and have your approach be experienced by the client as a genuine inquiry about health rather than an unwanted intrusion. It is essential that nurses be able to talk openly about sexual activities and know how to set boundaries. You have been given the professional task of assisting clients with their health using a holistic rather than a merely disease-oriented focus. How do you determine the need for further assessment for the presence of

TABLE 30–7 SEXUALLY TRANSMITTED DISEASES

DISEASE	AGENT
	Bacteria
Gastroenteritis	*Shigella, Salmonella*
Genital tuberculosis	*Mycobacterium tuberculosis*
Gonorrhea	*Neisseria gonorrhoeae*
Nongonococcal urethritis	*Ureaplasma* (prev. *Mycoplasma*) *urealyticum*
Nongonococcal urethritis, cervicitis	*Chlamydia trachomatis* (serotypes D–K)
Nonspecific vaginitis	*Gardnerella* (prev. *Corynebacterium* or *Haemophilus*) *vaginalis*
Syphilis	*Treponema pallidum*
	Fungi
Vaginitis; balanitis	*Candida* species
	Parasites
Amebiasis	*Entamoeba histolytica*
Giardiasis	*Giardia lamblia*
Trichomonas vaginitis	*Trichomonas vaginalis*
Scabies	*Sarcoptes scabiei*
Vaginitis (pinworm)	*Enterobius vermicularis*
	Viruses
AIDS	Human immunodeficiency virus
Cytomegalovirus mononucleosis	Cytomegalovirus
Genital warts	Papillomavirus
Hepatitis B (serum hepatitis)	Hepatitis B virus
Herpes genitalis	Herpes simplex virus

an STD? The place to begin is with yourself. You need to be at ease asking these personal questions or you will get very little information from your client. By being direct and professional in your approach, you will be able to set boundaries that clearly communicate to clients that these questions are limited to their health status and nothing beyond that. It is important to practice letting clients know that you are not interested in them sexually and that questions regarding sex, sexual relationships, and intimate behavior are about seeing them in their totality rather than as a disease or complaint.

Because of the potential for life-threatening consequences for clients who engage in unprotected sex, nurses must be prepared to teach clients how to practice "safe sex" and to have readily available referrals for someone who has questions beyond what is comfortable for you to discuss.

Routinely, nurses need to ask about the use of dental dams and condoms and about multiple partners, being careful not to make assumptions about the fidelity of partners. Clients should be referred for human immunodeficiency virus (HIV) testing, or testing for other STDs, if there is a reason to suspect exposure.

Acquired Immunodeficiency Syndrome

It is not possible to discuss adult sexual relationships today without a serious look at the impact of acquired immunodeficiency syndrome (AIDS). Conservative estimates are that 1 in every 250 Americans is infected with the virus (AHCPR 1994). Depending on an individual's life situation, the percentage may be considerably higher. AIDS/HIV infection was the fourth leading cause of death among women aged 25 to 44 in the United States in 1994, according to the Centers for Disease Control and Prevention (AHCPR 1994). In the United States, the incidence of AIDS is increasing more rapidly among women than among men (MMWR 1995). This may be due to the change in establishing the diagnosis of AIDS. Before 1993, many of the symptoms with which women presented were determined to be AIDS related and diagnosed as ARC (AIDS-related complex). These individuals were not given the diagnosis of AIDS, nor counted among the statistics of those with AIDS. Most notable were the symptoms of dementia and neurological deficiencies that affect women disproportionately. Since this 1993 revision of what constitutes the diagnosis of AIDS, there has been a sharp increase in women diagnosed with the disease. It is reported that 1 in every 10 gay or bisexual males under the age of 25 is infected, and 1 in 5 of all chronic drug users; if there is involvement in sex for drugs, the individual is almost certain to come into contact with the virus. These are alarming statistics that have an impact on physical and psychosocial care.

How does AIDS/HIV affect your practice as a nurse? If you are not able to make a sizable list, it might serve you well to get together with classmates and discuss the impact beyond the obvious (e.g., wearing gloves, using pocket masks for cardiopulmonary resuscitation (CPR), practicing needle safety). How do you view AIDS/HIV clients? What kinds of questions do you ask? What kinds of equipment do you use in AIDS health care? How do you handle blood donation? What questions do AIDS clients ask you? Should there be mandatory testing of health care providers? Do you have a sense of personal safety as a nurse? Do you get tested?

Because HIV-infected individuals may remain asymptomatic for 10 years or more, nurses will come in contact with individuals who are HIV positive and unaware of it. This means that you will be working with clients who were infected years ago and are just now becoming ill. For the sake of generations to come, it is to be hoped that awareness of AIDS is altering how adults interact with one another.

You might want to make an informal survey of friends, family, and colleagues to see how much AIDS has influenced how they interact sexually with others. How has AIDS affected your relationships with others? Are you currently taking precautions 100% of the time when you are sexually active?

Unless you have been discussing sex all your life, you will probably feel a little uncomfortable when you first begin to discuss topics that involve sexual behaviors. Because AIDS has had such an impact on health care in general, it would seem a disservice to finish this chapter without discussing ways of talking openly about "safe sex" (the quotation marks are a reminder that there is no universally safe sexual practice; however, some practices are considerably safer than complete lack of protection).

Teaching basic "safe sex" practices needs to be a matter of habit for nurses as we move into the twenty-first century. "Safe sex" practices have been shown to substantially decrease the spread of STDs.

The basics include how to put on and remove a condom correctly. The expiration date of the condom needs to be checked to ensure maximal protection. Condom use affords good protection for those having sex with male partners, but remember that sex with female partners needs to be practiced safely also. Dental dams, as well as condoms, can be used by those who participate in oral sex with women. Dental dams are not as readily available as condoms, but it is possible to cut off the end of a condom and slit it open, creating a rectangular piece of latex that can be placed over the vulva and vaginal opening so that the partner performing oral sex will remain safe from possible exposure. Even in sexual situations, whenever bodily fluids come into contact with another person, gloves should be worn to provide additional protection from possible infection through a break in the skin.

Teaching "safe sex" practices can be done without knowing the gender of the client's partner(s). It is probably best to make a habit of including "safe sex" practices in your teaching whether the client's partner or partners are female or male, or both. This way you will be providing education that, while perhaps not directly helpful to the client, will give valuable information the client may subsequently share with friends or family.

Without a doubt, AIDS has had an impact on people and their intimate relationships. How do you, as a nurse, support the choices that clients make regarding their lives and teach them how to remain safe? What about the schizophrenic client who is sexually active, or the mentally retarded individual who has recently awakened to her or his sexuality in a group home, or the middle-aged individual who has recently separated from a spouse, or the elderly person who voices a concern about sexual contact after the spouse has died? Giving clients the number of the National AIDS Hotline (1-800-342-AIDS) may encourage them to obtain information they need if they are not comfortable asking health care personnel.

Other Sexually Transmitted Diseases

Any disease that can be contracted by sexual contact can be classified as an STD (see Table 30–7). Symptoms vary, depending on the STD and the duration of the disease. When doing a nursing assessment, it is important to note whether the client has discharges, ulcers, or nodules. Although diagnostic tests are required for an accurate diagnosis, Box 30–1 groups STDs by manifesting symptoms that can guide you during your assessment. If *any* symptoms are noted, they should be brought to the primary caregiver's attention immediately.

BOX 30–1 MANIFESTATIONS OF SEXUALLY TRANSMISSIBLE DISEASES

Diseases manifested by discharges
- Gonorrhea
- Nongonococcal urethritis

Diseases manifested by nodules
- Genital warts
- Secondary syphilis

Diseases manifested by ulcers
- Syphilis
- Herpes simplex
- Chancroid

HERPES. Another STD is herpes simplex virus (*Herpesvirus hominis*). The incidence of reported cases continues to increase in the United States (Fig. 30–3). Each year as many as 500,000 new cases of genital herpes are estimated to occur (NIAID 1992). There is no permanent cure, although the drug acyclovir has been effective in reducing the frequency and duration of outbreaks. Herpes is most often found in the 15- to 30-year-old age group.

Herpes genitalis is an infection resulting in rupture of vesicles that cause painful ulcers. Systemic symptoms include fever, malaise, and inguinal node enlargement. Symptoms occur within approximately 2 to 10 days of exposure and last an average of 2 to 3 weeks (NIAID 1992). The ulcers are usually present on the medial aspects of the labia minora, clitoris, vagina, urethra, and cervix in women and in the urinary passage in men. The first attack tends to be the most severe, and about 66% of herpes victims do not have any more outbreaks, although the virus does remain in the system. One third of the victims have recurring infections, which are contagious as long as the symptoms are present.

Other side effects of herpes can include keratitis, if the virus is transferred to the eyes. Psychological effects can also be profound, with some people losing all sexual desire because of fear of contracting or spreading the disease. Among some single adults, the question "Are you healthy?" has become part of the dating procedure, so that the herpes client is left feeling most undesirable.

Health care professionals can do a great deal to educate the public about the prevention of herpes. Persons experiencing an outbreak can be taught to avoid sexual activity. Mothers can be encouraged to have their babies delivered by cesarean section if an outbreak occurs. Washing of hands and towels and sheets can help prevent the spread of the virus.

CHLAMYDIA. Chlamydial infections are the most prevalent of all STDs. From 1984 to 1994, reported rates increased dramatically from 3.2 to 188.4 cases per 100,000 population. Reported rates for women exceed those for men. About 80% of women have no observable symptoms and are diagnosed only when a partner is diagnosed. Symptoms can include genital discharge, burning during urination, and pain in the lower abdomen or testicle. Undetected chlamydial infection can cause sterility in women. These infections are treated with antibiotics, and intercourse should be avoided until treatment is completed.

GENITAL WARTS. Genital warts, which are caused by a virus, affect almost 2 million Americans. Not always visible, the warts are often soft and flat and can grow and itch. If not treated medically, they can block openings of the vagina, anus, or throat and can lead to cancer of the cervix, vulva, or penis.

HEPATITIS B. Each year an estimated 300,000 persons in the United States become infected with the hepatitis B virus (HBV) (NIAID 1997). HBV is most commonly transmitted by sharing needles, high-risk sexual behaviors, from mothers to newborns, and in the health care setting. When there are symptoms, they can include fatigue, headache, dark urine, light stools, and jaundice. This disease is very contagious and can easily be passed during intimate sexual encounters as well as during more casual contact. A vaccine is available to protect health care workers and those in relationships with infected people. About 90% of adults recover completely from hepatitis B, but severe liver disease and even death can occur from lack of treatment.

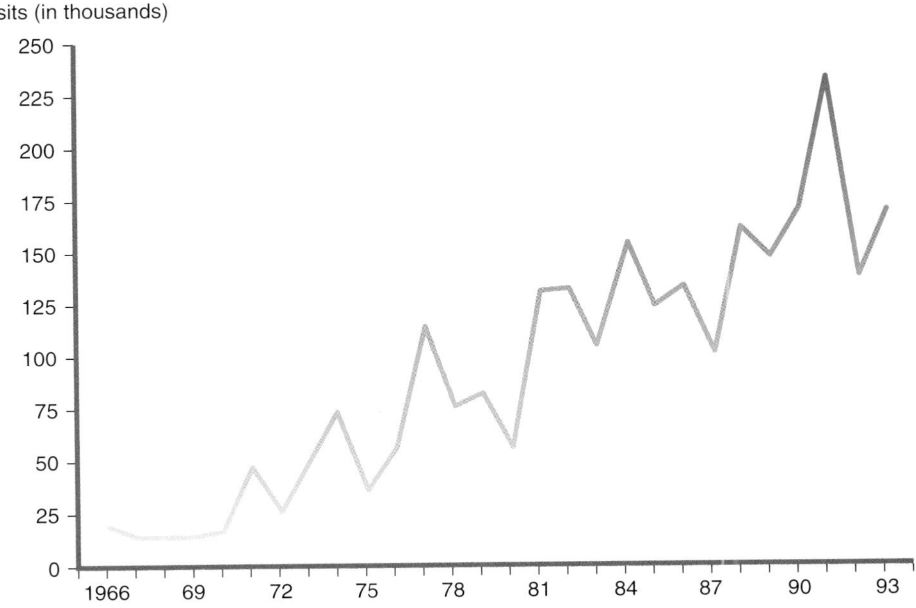

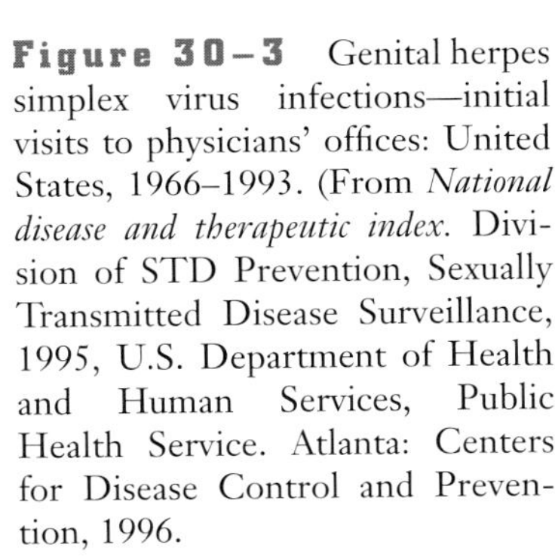
Figure 30–3 Genital herpes simplex virus infections—initial visits to physicians' offices: United States, 1966–1993. (From *National disease and therapeutic index*. Division of STD Prevention, Sexually Transmitted Disease Surveillance, 1995, U.S. Department of Health and Human Services, Public Health Service. Atlanta: Centers for Disease Control and Prevention, 1996.

GONORRHEA. Gonorrhea is one of the most common STDs. It is a bacterial infection (*Neisseria gonorrhoeae*) that enters the body through warm, moist areas such as the genitals or mouth. Males tend to experience discharge and pain when urinating; about 50% to 75% of females have less obvious early indications and may be asymptomatic, whereas others may experience painful urination and discharge. Sterility can be caused by untreated gonorrhea in both men and women.

Because the early stages are not obvious in women, it is likely that the disease will not be treated, and secondary infections such as pelvic inflammatory disease can occur. A baby born to an infected mother will become blind if the bacteria enters the eyes. Therefore, all newborns' eyes are treated with tetracycline or silver nitrate to prevent possible blindness. Although the overall rates of gonorrhea declined between 1975 and 1994, the rates increased in women, among black adolescents (ages 15 to 19), and in some midwestern states between 1993 and 1994 (CDC 1995).

Early diagnosis of gonorrhea is important. Treatment is relatively simple with effective antibiotics. There has been a recent increase in strains that are resistant to the more commonly prescribed antibiotics. Use of condoms, washing of the genitals, and visual inspection of a partner's genitals can help prevent the spread of this and other STDs.

SYPHILIS. Syphilis, caused by the spirochete *Treponema pallidum*, remains a serious STD. Penicillin or other antibiotics can cure the disease at any stage, although damage that has already been caused by the disease cannot be reversed.

In 1994, 20,627 cases of primary and secondary syphilis were reported to the CDC—the fewest cases reported since 1977. Rates remain high in the South, in about half of America's largest cities, and in black adolescents and are 3.5 times higher in Hispanics than in whites. It seems that race and ethnicity in the United States serve as risk markers that correlate with other more fundamental determinants of health status such as poverty, access to quality care, and health care–seeking behaviors (CDC 1995).

Syphilis appears to have existed for many centuries in all parts of the world. It is a severe and persistent infection that can be transmitted via the mouth, genitals, anus, or any small lesion. It travels through the bloodstream to all parts of the body and can take many years to develop into a serious and life-threatening illness.

In its *primary stage*, syphilis can be detected by darkfield examination after the incubation period of 10 to 90 days. The only symptom is a painless sore called a *chancre*, which usually appears near the mouth, anus, or genitals within a week to several months after infection. The chancre grows for 1 to 8 weeks and generally is open at the top, with a band of hard tissue around the base. Because it is painless, and in females may be growing internally, this sore is often undetected or ignored. If it is not treated at this stage, the chancre will heal in 3 to 9 weeks, and the disease goes on to the second stage.

The *second stage* lasts between 2 and 10 weeks while the disease spreads, with sores or lesions appearing on the vulva, mouth and pharynx, and axilla and under the breasts. During this stage, systemic symptoms may occur, such as fever, sore throat, and headache. All these symptoms disappear even without treatment, and the disease can still be unknown to its victim.

The *third*, or *latent*, *stage* of syphilis can last for decades. No longer contagious, except to a child born of a carrier parent, the disease nonetheless may attack various parts of the body, including the circulatory and nervous systems.

Only in the *fourth*, or *late*, *stage* of syphilis does its presence become obvious. Serious illness, blindness, and mental and cardiovascular problems can all be present.

Treatment of syphilis in the primary and secondary stages is with penicillin G benzathine. Clients allergic to penicillin may be given erythromycin.

SUMMARY

Because of the nature of nursing practice, it is possible for the nurse to begin a dialogue about sexual satisfaction as part of the nursing assessment, whether in an acute or a long-term care facility or as a community health nurse. It is essential that the nurse be open to the client's situation rather than placing personal values in the way.

Nurses are in contact with literally thousands of people, none of whom are exactly the same. How people express themselves in relationships varies from person to person and from culture to culture. It is important that the nurse have done enough personal research to feel comfortable talking with individuals about basic sexual exploration, "safe sex," and evaluation of satisfaction in relationships. It is equally important that the nurse provide a warm and caring environment when discussing results of diagnostic tests and listen carefully to the client's response.

REFERENCES

Agency for Health Care Policy and Research (1994). *Evaluation and management of early HIV infection: Clinical practice guideline.* Pub. No. 94–0572. Rockville, MD: Agency for Health Care Policy and Research, Public Health Service, U. S. Department of Health and Human Services.

American Psychiatric Association (1994). *Diagnostic and statistical manual of mental disorders* (4th ed.) (DSM-IV). Washington, DC: American Psychiatric Association.

Boston Women's Health Book Collective (1992). *The new our bodies, ourselves.* New York: Simon & Schuster.

Brownmiller, S. (1993). *Against our will: Men, women and rape.* New York: Simon & Schuster.

Deevey, S. (1993). Lesbian self-disclosure strategies for success. *Journal of Psychosocial Nursing,* 31(4):25.

Erikson, E. H. (1963). *Childhood and society.* New York: W. W. Norton.

Freud, S. (1961). *The standard edition of the complete psychological works of Sigmund Freud,* translated and edited by James Strachey. London: Hogarth Press.

Gilligan, C. (1982). *In a different voice.* Cambridge: Harvard University Press.
Green, R., and Blanchard, R. (1995). Gender identity disorder. In H.I. Kaplan and B.J. Sadock (Eds.), *Comprehensive textbook of psychiatry* (6th ed.), Vol I. Baltimore: Williams & Wilkins.
Heyward, C. (1995). *Staying power.* Cleveland: Pilgrim Press.
Hogan, R. (1980). *A nursing perspective.* New York: Appleton-Century-Crofts.
Kantrowitz, B. (1994). Dissent on the hard drive. *Newsweek* June 27, 1995, 123(26):59.
Kaplan, H. S. (1979). *Disorders of sexual desire.* New York: Simon & Schuster.
Kasl, C. D. (1989). *Women, sex, and addiction.* New York: Harper & Row.
King, I. M. (1971). *Toward a theory for nursing: General concepts of human behavior.* New York: John Wiley.
King, I. M. (1978). The "why" of theory development. In *Theory development: What, why, how?* New York: National League for Nursing.
King, I. M. (1981). *A theory for nursing: Systems, concepts, process.* New York: John Wiley.
Kohlberg, L. (1969). The cognitive-developmental approach to socialization. In D. Goslin (Ed.), *Handbook of socialization.* Chicago: Rand McNally.
Library Journal (1995). October 15, 1995, 120(17):36.
Mahler, M. (1980). The rapprochement subphase of the separation-individuation process. In R. R. Lax, S. Bach and J. A. Burland (Eds.), *Rapprochement.* New York: Aronson.
Mahler, M. (1975). *The psychological birth of the human infant: Symbiosis and individuation.* New York: Basic Books.
Maslow, A. H. (1970). *Motivation and personality.* New York: Harper & Row.
Masters, W. H., and Johnson, V. E. (1966). *Human sexual response.* Boston: Little, Brown.
Masters, W. H., and Johnson, V. E. (1970). *Human sexual inadequacy.* Boston: Little, Brown.
Masters W. H., and Johnson, V. E. (1979). *Homosexuality in perspective.* Boston: Little, Brown.
Meyer, J. K. (1995). Paraphilias. In H. I. Kaplan and B. J. Sadock (Eds.), *Comprehensive textbook of psychiatry* (6th ed.) Vol I. Baltimore: Williams & Wilkins.
Morbidity and Mortality Weekly Report (1995). Update: AIDS among women—United States, 1994. *MMWR,* 44(5):1.
National Institute of Allergies and Infectious Diseases (1997). *Hepatitis fact sheet.* Washington, D.C.: National Institute for Health.
National Institute of Allergies and Infectious Diseases (1992). *Herpes fact sheet.* Washington, D.C.: National Institute of Allergies and Infectious Diseases.
Orem, D. E. (1985). *Nursing: Concepts of practice.* New York: McGraw-Hill.
Piaget, J. (1962). The stages of the intellectual development of the child. *Bulletin of the Menninger Clinic,* 26(4103):120.
Piaget, J. (1963). *The child's conception of the world.* New York: Littlefield, Adams.
Rogers, M. E. (1970). *An introduction to the theoretical basis of nursing.* Philadelphia: F. A. Davis.
Rogers, M. E. (1980). Nursing: A science of unitary man. In J. P. Riehl and C. Roy (Eds.), *Conceptual models for nursing practice* (2nd ed.). New York: Appleton-Century-Crofts.
Roy, C. (1976). *Introduction to nursing: An adaptation model.* Englewood Cliffs, NJ: Prentice-Hall.
Roy, C. (1980). The Roy adaptation model. In J. P. Riehl and C. Roy (Eds.), *Conceptual models for nursing practice* (2nd ed.). New York: Appleton-Century-Crofts.
Sullivan, H. S. (1953). In H. S. Perry (Ed.), *Interpersonal theory of psychiatry.* New York: W. W. Norton.

FURTHER READING

American Libraries (1994). *American Libraries,* 24(4):272.
Bradley, J. C., and Edinberg, M. A. (1990). *Communication in the nursing context* (3rd ed.). New York: Appleton & Lange.
Bradshaw, J. (1988). *Bradshaw on: The family: Healing the shame that binds you.* Deerfield Beach, FL: Health Communications.
Centers for Disease Control and Prevention (1995). Surveillance for sexually transmitted diseases. *Morbidity and Mortality Weekly Report,* 45(55-3):1.
Cermak, T. L. (1986). Diagnostic criteria for codependency. *Journal of Psychoactive Drugs,* 18(1):15.
Cohen, M. S. (1995). Prevention of HIV and STDs. *Postgraduate Medicine,* 98(3):63.
Economist (1995). Suffer little children. September 23, 333, 334, p. 24.
Felstein, I. (1986). *Understanding sexual medicine.* Lancaster, England: MTP Press.
Kniffel, L. (1995). In the name of the children. *American Libraries,* 26(8):24.
Markarian, M. F. (1986). Surgical approach to musculoskeletal system dysfunction. In C. R. Kneisl and S. W. Ames (Eds.), *Adult health nursing.* Reading, MA: Addison-Wesley.
McCausland, L. H. (1986). Surgical approach to musculoskeletal system dysfunction. In C. R. Kneisl and S. W. Ames (Eds.), *Adult health nursing.* Reading, MA: Addison-Wesley.
Schaef, A. W. (1986). *Co-dependence: Misunderstood—mistreated.* San Francisco: Harper & Row.
Smeltzer, S. C., and Bare, B. G. (1992). *Brunner and Suddarth's textbook of medical-surgical nursing* (7th ed.). Philadelphia: J. B. Lippincott.
Snow, C., and Willard, D. (1989). *I'm dying to take care of you: Nurses and codependence: Breaking the cycles.* Redmond, WA: Professional Counselor Books.
Stier, F. L. (1986). The nursing process for clients with major blood vessel dysfunction. In C. R. Kneisl and S. W. Ames (Eds.), *Adult health nursing.* Reading, MA: Addison-Wesley.
Suarez, L. (1994). Pap smear and mammogram screening in Mexican-American women: The effects of acculturation. *American Journal of Public Health,* 84(5):742.
Sundeen, S. J., Stuart, G. W., Rankin, E. A., and Choeh, S. A. (1989). *Nurse-client interaction* (4th ed.). St. Louis: C. V. Mosby.
Whitefield, C. (1988). Co-dependence: Our most common addiction. *Wellness Associates Journal,* Spring:1.

SELF-STUDY AND CRITICAL THINKING

Multiple choice

Circle the one answer that is most correct for each of the following questions:

1. Nurses take an interest in the client's sexual history because

   A. It is interesting.
   B. It is required by the professional standards of nursing.
   C. Sexuality is part of a holistic approach to nursing practice.
   D. It helps the physician make a more accurate diagnosis.

2. In conversation with a client you learn that she is upset with her husband, who keeps "pushing himself on her for sex." You would

   A. Refer her to a domestic violence advocate immediately, as this is a possible abuse situation.
   B. Ask her to share more about what happens with her and her husband.
   C. Tell her that her lack of interest in sex is related to medications she is taking.
   D. Do nothing, as men have a higher sex drive than women and this is normal behavior.

3. All the following medications *except* one have possible side effects that could have a negative impact on clients' sexual response/behavior. Which one does not have a possible negative impact?

   A. Alcohol
   B. Amitriptyline (Elavil)
   C. Ranitidine (Zantac)
   D. Chlorpromazine (Thorazine)
   E. Folic acid

4. You are assessing a client who has recently been admitted to the unit you work on. Which of the following responses would you make to the statement made by the client, "I don't want to tell you anything about my sexual behaviors."

   A. That's fine, George. I'm only asking because it is on the admission form. I'll just write that you would prefer not to respond.
   B. I can imagine that it is difficult to talk to someone you don't know about something so private. I'll check in with you later after we've gotten to know each other a little better.
   C. Yeah, I wouldn't want to answer a question about what I do either. I don't know why they even put it on this form.
   D. Well, it is your right not to answer questions. I'll just write down that you said "no comment."

5. Vaginismus is sexual dysfunction that occurs in which phase of female sexual response?

   A. Arousal/excitement phase
   B. Refractory period
   C. Plateau phase
   D. Orgasmic phase

6. Sexually transmissible diseases that present with ulcers include

   A. Gonorrhea and nongonococcal urethritis.
   B. Genital warts and secondary syphilis.
   C. AIDS, hepatitis, and shingles.
   D. Syphilis, herpes simplex, and chancroid.

Match the following words to the example or definition.

7. ________ fetishism
8. ________ frotteurism
9. ________ masochism
10. ________ pedophilia
11. ________ scatophilia
12. ________ voyeurism

A. Having to have a pair of black lacy underwear present to find sexual gratification.
B. Having sex with a child.
C. Intentional display of one's genitals in public.
D. "Peeping tom" behavior.
E. Enjoyment of giving pain in a sexual encounter.
F. Enjoyment of receiving pain in a sexual encounter.
G. Sexual activity involving feces.
H. Sexual activity involving enemas.
I. Sex in which obscene language is used.
J. Sexual gratification obtained by rubbing up against a stranger.

Critical thinking

13. Arrange to obtain some condoms for this exercise. Break into small groups of three or four. Practice teaching "safe sex" skills using one of the group members as the client. After practicing among yourselves, use role play techniques to teach "safe sex" methods to

    A. A group member role playing a medical-surgical client.
    B. A group member who is role playing a 15-year-old male.
    C. A person of your same gender. Teach this person how to practice using "safe sex" techniques with a member of the same gender.

Describe how you used different teaching methods to teach the various clients with whom you were working. Was one "client" easier or more difficult to teach? What other information do you need to teach "safe sex" effectively?

14. In groups of three or four, discuss how to phrase questions to clients when assessing a client's knowledge of STDs. Try role playing the following three situations. Take turns in different roles: nurse, client, and partner of a client. Have the observers give feedback and helpful suggestions.
15. You walk into a client's room and are aware that the client is masturbating. How would you respond?
16. During a home visit, a client who has been started on an antipsychotic medication tells you that sex doesn't interest him or her anymore. How could you address this issue? What are the options you could offer to the client? What other members of the health team might be contacted?
17. Kate is a 39-year-old woman who just learned that her husband of 19 years had an affair. She has come in to have a blood test for AIDS, syphilis, and gonorrhea because her husband was diagnosed with gonorrhea last week and has to contact his sexual partners for follow-up testing and treatment. Upon meeting you, Kate says "I'm not all that sure that I need to have these tests done. I mean, my husband only did this once and I don't understand all the fuss." You, as the nurse, need to respond to her statement.

31

The Elderly

SALLY K. HOLZAPFEL

OUTLINE

KEY TERMS AND CONCEPTS

The key terms and concepts listed here also appear in bold where they are defined or discussed in this chapter.

ageism
Social Dysfunction Rating Scale
Zung's Self-Rating Depression Scale
remotivation therapy
reminiscing therapy
group psychotherapy
day care programs
physical restraints
chemical restraints
Omnibus Budget Reconciliation Act (OBRA)
Patient Self-Determination Act (PSDA)
living will
directive to physician
durable power of attorney for health care (DPAHC)
medical futility
hospice philosophy
withholding hydration

OBJECTIVES

After studying this chapter, the reader will be able to

1. Discuss five myths on aging.
2. Compare the purpose, format, and desired outcomes among the following group treatments: remotivation, reminiscing, and psychotherapy.
3. List two characteristics of physical and chemical restraints.
4. List two institutional requirements of the Patient Self-Determination Act.
5. List three differences between living wills, directives to physicians, and durable power of attorney for health care.
6. Recognize guidelines a nurse can employ in approaching issues of life and death with a client.
7. Discuss ways in which the nurse can assist families of dying clients.
8. Summarize the concept of a hospice program.
9. Identify the elderly group at highest risk for suicide.
10. Describe the characteristics of two types of elderly alcohol abusers.

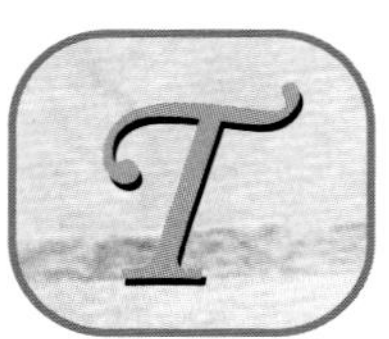

The growing number of elderly people and their proportion in the general population of the United States have had a significant impact on the country's economy and its health and social services. Since the turn of the twentieth century, the population aged 65 or over has increased 11-fold compared with those under 65 (which population tripled). By the year 2040, the United States will have more individuals over 65 than people under 20 years of age (Bureau of the Census 1995). Among the elderly, the fastest-growing age groups are the minorities, the poor, and those aged 85 and over. By the year 2030, the minority population will make up 25% (up from 13% in 1995) of all aged (Bureau of the Census 1995; Harper 1995).

As the population is living longer, chronic illness and disability have become major threats to the health of the elderly. Almost one third of all older persons consider their health only fair to poor. This is a significantly higher percentage than in persons under age 65, among whom only 10% hold this view (Harper 1995).

At least 80% of all individuals over age 65 have at least one chronic condition; many elderly people have more than one. The likelihood of developing one or more chronic illnesses increases notably with age: individuals 75 years of age and older are the most prone to chronic illnesses and functional disabilities. Chronic illness is responsible for more than 70% of all deaths. After age 85, there is a one-in-three chance of developing dementia, immobility, incontinence, or other age-related disabilities (Walsh 1992).

According to the Bureau of the Census (1995), today's life expectancy at birth is 72 years for men and 79 years for women, with an average of 76 years for both sexes. Upon reaching age 65, the elderly, on average, can expect to live 17 more years. The death rate for men at every age is higher than for women. Elderly women outnumber elderly men in a ratio of 3:2. At age 85 and over, this ratio increases to 5:2.

As a general rule, women outlive men. Since husbands more often predecease their spouses, they have their wives' assistance and support when their health starts to fail. On the other hand, many older women do not have this support because of the earlier death of their husbands (Bureau of the Census 1995). Women's greater longevity has significant ramifications for society at large and for the health care profession in particular. Not only do women form the largest bloc among the elderly, they also utilize health care services more than men, and seek such services earlier, and even for minor conditions (Sapp and Bliesmer 1995).

Generally, a distinction should be made between the needs of persons in the age group 85 and older (the "old-old") and the elderly who have not yet reached that age. There are noticeable differences between individuals in their sixties and people in their eighties. While the younger group is relatively healthy, the older group is much more vulnerable, frail, and at risk for visual problems, cognitive impairment, and falls. They also have more limited economic resources and community supports, and are more affected by the chronic diseases and disorders of aging (Ebersole and Hess 1994).

Burnside (1988) identifies specific facts about mental health and the aged:

1. Mental illness is more prevalent among the elderly than among younger persons.
2. Psychosis increases significantly after age 65.
3. Suicide occurs more frequently among the elderly than in any other age group.
4. Dementia is the fourth leading cause of death among the elderly.
5. Fifteen percent of the elderly have chronic physical problems that can result in negative psychological responses.

The most common type of dementia, affecting up to 11% of the population aged 65, is Alzheimer's disease. Of the elderly with severe intellectual impairments, about one half are diagnosed with Alzheimer's disease. The course of this disease may run from 1 to 15 years, with death usually occurring because of respiratory complications, urinary tract infection, pressure ulcers, or iatrogenic disorders (Ebersole and Hess 1994). See Chapter 23 for a discussion of Alzheimer's disease.

The continued increase in the aged population is having a significant impact on the utilization and cost of health care services. Per capita health care expenses for the elderly are nearly four times higher than those for the rest of the population (Sapp and Bliesmer 1995). Questions of appropriate care and issues about health care delivery, in particular managed care, need to be addressed. An important concern is whether nursing will be able to operate under managed care. Since the aged population is expected to grow proportionately as we move into the twenty-first century (as is managed care), nursing, to maintain its professional identity with its unique skills and expertise, will have to adjust to these developments and identify new strategies and approaches.

THE ROLE OF THE NURSE

Nurses have made a substantial contribution to the care and health promotion of the elderly. However, questions arise as to whether nurses in training are given enough information and sufficient exposure to the elderly not only to develop an interest in them but also to gain a better understanding of the elderly and the aging process. Adequate theory and principles are needed to provide safe and excellent care for the elderly. Any lack of specific information necessary for a student nurse to make sound decisions in regard to elderly clients is in part a result of the following:

- Negative faculty attitudes toward the old
- Lack of exposure to and lack of clinical emphasis on older persons
- Negative student attitudes toward the elderly because of information based on myths and stereotypes
- Unfamiliarity with gerontological information and resources

The negative view frequently held by nurses (as well as the general population) toward the elderly is part of the phenomenon of ageism.

Ageism

Ageism has been defined as a bias against older people because of their age; it is a system of destructive, erroneous beliefs. In essence, ageism reflects a dislike by the young of the old, depicting the disparaging effect of society's attitudes toward the elderly. This age prejudice is based on the notion that aging makes people increasingly unattractive, unintelligent, asexual, unemployable, and senile (Atchley 1994).

Ageism is not limited to the way the young may look at the old; it also includes older people's views, which tend to be critical about themselves and their peers. Indeed, the attitudes of the elderly toward their peers, particularly those with mental disabilities, are often more negative than the views held by the young (although this is not always the case). The threat of social contagion by association with the frail and infirm may simply be too strong to bear. Age proximity raises feelings of vulnerability (Ebersole and Hess 1990). This may explain why older persons often do not like to be referred to as "old." By seeing themselves as "young" rather than "old," they adjust better to their advancing years (Hogstel 1990).

Ageism differs from other forms of discrimination in that it cuts across gender, race, religion, and national origin. Old age does not award a desirable status or membership in a sought-after club; rather, it is a social category with negative connotations (Matthews 1979). According to Butler (1975):

> Ageism is manifested in a wide range of phenomena, both on individual and institutional levels—stereotypes and myths, outright disdain and dislike, or simply subtle avoidance of contact; discriminatory practices in housing, employment, and services of all kinds; epithets, cartoons, and jokes.

The results of ageism can be observed throughout every level of society; even health care providers are not immune to its effects. Negative values can surface in a myriad of ways in the health care system. Financial and political support for programs for the elderly is difficult to obtain; their needs are addressed only after those of younger, albeit smaller, population groups. The Grey Panthers and American Association of Retired Persons (AARP) are, however, powerful lobbying groups that are fighting to change this trend.

Health care personnel do not always share medical information, recommendations, and opportunities with the elderly. A study of over 200 cardiac patients finds that, compared with younger persons, those over 60 years of age receive considerably less information on available resources, practices to reduce the risk of future problems, and health management measures (USDHHS 1990). Another study shows that only about one half of all physicians believe that the older adult should receive maximal evaluation and treatment for an acute illness (USDHHS 1990). This reluctance to provide information and treatment also applies to mental health. The elderly are often not considered suitable to receive this care in the belief that providing such resources would be wasteful (Moak 1990).

Health care workers who deal on a daily basis with the confused, ill, and frail older adult may tend to develop a somewhat negative and biased view of the elderly. Their attitudes often reflect society's values, which are characterized by negativism and stereotyping. The rendering of medical care to aged clients has been burdened with pessimism, defeatism, and professional aversion. Such thinking can be found among professionals as well as among ancillary personnel working in nursing homes and other institutional settings (Adelson et al. 1982).

Most health professionals, including physicians and nurses, prefer to work with children or young adults rather than to specialize in geriatrics (Gomez et al. 1985; Green 1981). Younger caregivers, in particular, may feel the prejudice of ageism and experience *gerontophobia*, the fear of growing old (Burnside 1988).

Other factors affecting the health care worker's approach are the clients' social conduct and level of functional independence. Nursing assistants, which as a group are likely to have the closest daily contact with the elderly, have expressed negative feelings about caring for extremely dependent clients. Independence in self-care and pleasing conduct by the client elicit more positive feelings on the part of the health care worker; conversely, socially unacceptable behaviors provoke unfavorable attitudes (Elliot and Hybertson 1982).

Positive attitudes toward the elderly and their care need to be instilled during basic nursing education and should be included in the curriculum. Existing misconceptions about the elderly and possible negative views held by the health care provider should be discussed. Nursing personnel need to be made aware that their own actions may augment the very behaviors they dislike in the elderly. A better understanding of the aging process, and the ability to differentiate between normal and abnormal (e.g., dementia vs. normal aging), are necessary for a productive and positive interaction between nursing caregivers and their aging clients.

To overcome existing misconceptions about the elderly and to improve their care, educational programs are recommended and should provide (1) information about the aging process, (2) discussion of attitudes relating to the care of the elderly, (3) sensitization of participants to their clients' needs, and (4) exploration of the dynamics of nurse/staff-client interactions.

Such programs, designed to prepare nurses to function more effectively and be more receptive to work with the elderly, should help to increase the numbers of nurses wanting to work with the elderly. In addition, since the implementation of managed care makes employment opportunities in the acute care setting more limited, nurses will look for professional work in other areas.

In defining one of the objectives of nursing care of the elderly, Preston (1986) comments:

> We must resist the ease of paternalism, which weakens our relationship with the elderly. We must endeavor to study them and their particular problems as vigorously as we study diseases. And we should love them, for that is the only way we can love ourselves when we take their places.

Table 31–1 presents a quiz on the facts and myths about aging.

TABLE 31–1 QUIZ: FACTS AND MYTHS ABOUT AGING

T	F	1. Most adults past the age of 65 are demented.
T	F	2. The senses of vision, hearing, touch, taste, and smell all decline with age.
T	F	3. Muscular strength decreases with age.
T	F	4. Sexual interest declines with age.
T	F	5. For the older adult, regular sexual expressions are important to maintain sexual capacity and effective sexual performance.
T	F	6. At least 50% of restorative sleep is lost as a result of the aging process.
T	F	7. As a group, the elderly are major consumers of prescription drugs.
T	F	8. Older adults are not able to learn new tasks.
T	F	9. The elderly have a high incidence of depression.
T	F	10. As individuals age, they become more rigid in their thinking and set in their ways.
T	F	11. The aged are well off and no longer impoverished.
T	F	12. Many individuals experience difficulty when they retire.
T	F	13. The elderly are prone to become victims of crime.
T	F	14. Most elderly people are infirm and require help with daily activities.
T	F	15. Older individuals are more dependable and have fewer accidents than younger persons.
T	F	16. Most older adults are socially isolated and lonely.
T	F	17. Medicaid is a federally assisted program providing health care benefits to anyone over the age of 65.
T	F	18. The term *ageism* reflects society's positive views toward the elderly.
T	F	19. Widowers are more likely to remarry than widows.
T	F	20. Older widows appear to adjust better than younger ones.

Answers at end of chapter

Generalist vs. Gerontological Nursing Practice

Some elements of nursing practice remain the same between generalist nursing practice and gerontological nursing practice. For example:

1. Goals of nursing
2. Generic nursing process and methods
3. Professional practice roles:
   - Standards of practice
   - Code of ethics
   - Accountability to clients

Four levels of nursing personnel are involved in the care of the elderly (Table 31–2). Nurses who care for the elderly need to have specific knowledge of aging and the interaction of health, aging, and illness, as well as knowledge and skill to modify and implement nursing methods. Box 31–1 outlines gerontological nursing skills.

Psychiatric nurse specialists who work with the elderly experiencing mental health problems also need to know about normal aging and interactions between aging and illness, which are discussed in most medical-surgical nursing components of the nursing curriculum. Ronsman (1987) provides an overview of the nursing process in the care of elderly clients (Table 31–3).

UNIQUE ASSESSMENT STRATEGIES

Nurses who work with the elderly benefit from specific knowledge about normal aging, drug interactions, and chronic diseases. Those who work with elderly clients who have mental health problems also need to have special skills (e.g., interviewing, assessing, knowing effective treatment modalities). Lekan-Rutledge (1988) outlines approaches to the elderly person during the initial assessment. Because examination and interviews can produce anxiety in the elderly, and because the initial interview is often in unfamiliar surroundings, the guidelines in Table 31–4 are useful no matter what the setting or purpose of the interview.

Because effective coping, problem-solving, and adaptive behaviors are necessary for healthy social function-

TABLE 31–2 NURSES PREPARED TO CARE FOR THE ELDERLY

LEVELS OF NURSING PRACTITIONERS INVOLVED IN CARE OF THE AGED

Practitioner	Function	Education Preparation
1. Nursing assistant, also known as patient care assistant (PCA), nurses' aide (NA)	Assists professional nurse in patient care tasks	Certified through taking short courses at technical colleges or through inservice training; competency-based evaluation must be passed
2. Licensed practical nurse (LPN) or licensed vocational nurse (LVN)	Assists professional nurse in patient care tasks	Technical college or vocational high school preparation; must pass licensure examination and maintain licensure to practice
3. Registered nurse (RN)	Practices professional nursing with patients/clients in any health care setting	Multiple levels of entry, including Associate degree (ADN) in 2-year program Diploma (3-year hospital-based program) Baccalaureate degree (BSN), 4-year university-based program Nursing doctorate (ND), 4-year program after college degree in another field State licensure required for all levels of entry
4. Advanced Level Nurse Practitioners (clinical specialists, nurse practitioners, administrators of nursing services for the aged)	Performs "medical" acts such as management of chronic disease, prescription of medicines, diagnosis of disease	Multiple levels of entry, including Certificate programs open to any RN regardless of level of preparation and master's level programs; all are RNs certified jointly by state boards of nursing and medicine
Clinical specialist	Advanced practitioner of nursing, clinical teacher	Master's degree (MSN, MN), also are RNs
Nurse scientist/gerontologist	Nurse research and/or nurse educator	Doctor of Nursing Science (DNSc) or Doctor of Philosophy (PhD) in nursing or other field (psychology, sociology, physiology, anthropology), public health, epidemiology

From Matteson, M. A., McConnell, E. S., and Linton, A. D. (1997). *Gerontological nursing: Concepts and practice* (2nd ed.) (p. 42). Philadelphia: W. B. Saunders.

BOX 31–1 SKILLS FOR GERONTOLOGICAL NURSING

Gerontological nurses should be skillful in applying generic nursing methods to care of the aged and be able to do the following:

- Use research findings from gerontology as well as from nursing and the biomedical and behavioral sciences to inform nursing practice.
- Interact with individuals who have sensory loss.
- Perform multidimensional assessment of the elderly person by using existing standardized tools and individualized approaches.
- Implement rehabilitative nursing techniques.
- Help clients integrate past life with present.
- Include the older person and family members in developing goals for nursing care, even if the individual has significant communication or cognitive impairments.
- Modify the environment to maximize the older person's ability to function independently.
- Provide excellent palliative, supportive, and spiritual care for those who are dying.
- Give counsel to the grieving.
- Consider ethical dilemmas encountered by old people, their kin, and their health care providers.
- Help families and communities overcome hostilities toward the elderly.
- Participate in professional activities designed to improve health care for the elderly.
- Supervise the efforts of paraprofessional and lay caregivers in providing nursing care to the aged.
- Teach paraprofessional and lay caregivers and old people about the impact of the aging process and the disease process on self-care abilities and requisites of older persons.
- Teach paraprofessional and lay caregivers and old people about techniques to achieve self-care objectives.
- Establish developmentally appropriate criteria for evaluation and nursing care.

Adapted from Matteson, M. A., and McConnell, E. S. (eds.). (1988). *Gerontological nursing: Concepts and practice* (pp. 37–38). Philadelphia: W. B. Saunders.

ing, the degree of social dysfunction needs to be assessed. The **Social Dysfunction Rating Scale** (Table 31–5) is widely used for this purpose.

Depression and substance abuse among the elderly are both major health problems. Because depression and substance abuse affect each other, a special scale for detecting the presence of depression among the elderly has been devised. **Zung's Self-Rating Depression Scale** is one of the most widely used (Table 31–6). Clients rate themselves, unless illiterate or having vision problems. The score is derived by dividing the sum of the 20 items by 80 (the maximum score) (Lekan-Rutledge 1988). Scores above 0.38, or a raw score of 50 and over, signify depression requiring hospital treatment (Zung 1965).

UNIQUE INTERVENTION STRATEGIES

Pfeiffer (1978) emphasizes that most older persons are well. Those who do manifest mental problems are treatable and responsive. Pfeiffer stresses that psychotherapeutic approaches need to be simplified and modified for older clients. Certain psychotherapeutic techniques are useful for the elderly client:

1. Using crisis intervention techniques (see Chapter 14)
2. Understanding empathetically
3. Encouraging ventilation of feelings
4. Reestablishing emotional equilibrium when anxiety is moderate to severe
5. Explaining alternative solutions

Burnside (1988) offers specific guidelines for caring for an elderly client, urging nurses to pace themselves, *not* to move quickly, rush, or joggle the client. She suggests that nurses "truly listen" and make the *quality* of their time important, not the quantity. Burnside's instructions for one-to-one relationships and interviews are found in Box 31–2.

Inpatient Settings

When clients are institutionalized, group therapy is an economical way to provide therapeutic intervention. **Remotivation therapy, reminiscing therapy,** and **group psychotherapy** are three modalities often led by nurses who have special training or education. Table 31–7 outlines the purpose, format, and desired outcomes for each type of group. Box 31–3 gives an example of a remotivation therapy session.

Community-Based Programs

The hazards of institutionalization are numerous and include increased mortality, decreased social opportunity, and "learned helplessness." Community-based programs are an alternative whose purpose is to promote the elder's

TABLE 31–3 THE NURSING PROCESS IN THE CARE OF THE ELDERLY CLIENT

	Assessment	Nursing Diagnosis	Establishing Goals	Intervention	Evaluation
1. **Physiological needs:** Food/fluid Shelter/warmth Air Rest/Sleep Avoidance of pain Sex	Usual and present nutritional, elimination, sleep, and sexuality patterns Physical activity exercise pattern Emotional pain and discomfort Physical health Medications	**Altered patterns of urinary elimination** **Altered nutrition** Dehydration **Constipation** **Sleep pattern disturbance** **Sexual dysfunction** **Knowledge deficits** Medications or physical illnesses that may cause depression **Chronic pain**	Establishing and maintaining adequate biological functioning in areas of sleep, nutrition, and elimination Relief from emotional pain and discomfort Elimination of drug- or disease-induced depression	Assist with ADLs Support self-care abilities Encourage to start a physical activity regimen Teach side effects of antidepressants Treat medical problems under poor control Change medications that may cause depression	Feelings of physical satiation Homeostasis Optimal physical health
2. **Safety and security needs:** Feel free from danger Need for a predictable, lawful, orderly world Need to feel in control	Home environment assessment Mental status examination Assessment of visual acuity and hearing Knowledge of disease process Physical mobility Suicide potential	**Ineffective individual coping** **Powerlessness** **Risk for self-harm** **Risk for injury** **Sensory/perceptual alterations** **Impaired physical mobility** **Self-care deficit** **Impaired memory** **Chronic confusion** **Impaired environmental interpretation syndrome**	Establishment of predictability and structure in environment Maintenance of a safe environment Realistic understanding of disease course and expected outcome Reversal of treatable confusion	ECT, hospitalization, antidepressant medications for the severely depressed Avoid relocations when possible Correct environmenttal hazards Encourage a structured daily routine Instruct about disease course and prognosis	Feeling in control of one's disease and optimistic about the future Confidence in the future Feelings of safety, peace, security, protection, lack of danger and threat
3. **Need for love, belonging, and affection:** Need for contact and intimacy Need for friends Need for feeling of having a place and "belonging" Need for interactions with others	Family relationships and members Friends who are supportive Recent losses Present and past social interactions	Disruption in significant relationships **Social isolation** Lack of contact with, or absence of, significant others **Impaired social interactions** **Ineffective community coping** **Caregiver role strain**	Maintenance of significant relationships with family and friends Establishment of community support system Resumption of previous level of social activity	Encourage social interactions that have been enjoyed in the past Encourage interactions with family members, friends, and health caregivers Provide reassuring, supportive atmosphere	Feelings of loving and being loved, of being one of a group, of acceptance

Table continued on following page

TABLE 31–3 THE NURSING PROCESS IN THE CARE OF THE ELDERLY CLIENT *(Continued)*

	Assessment	Nursing Diagnosis	Establishing Goals	Intervention	Evaluation
4. **Need for esteem and self-respect:** Need for achievement, mastery, and competence Need for reputation or prestige, appreciation, and dignity Need for love of self	Amount of pleasurable pursuits Emotional or mood assessment Role patterns Coping-stress-tolerance pattern Attitude about self, the world, the future	**Disturbance in self-esteem** Loss of significant roles Unrealistic self-expectations **Anxiety** Life style change Dependency on others **Altered family functioning: alcoholism**	Acceptance of realistic limitations Establishment of appropriate roles Achievement of self-acceptance Acceptance of ownership of consequences of one's own behavior	Teach problem-solving skills Cognitive therapy Promote self-care Counseling Behavior therapy Relaxation techniques	Feelings of self-confidence, worth, strength, capability, and adequacy; of being useful and necessary in the world
5. **Need for self-actualization:** Need for beauty Need for self-expression Need for new situations and stimulation	Occupation, job history Value-belief patterns	Loss of zest for life **Spiritual distress** **Grieving** **Dysfunctional grieving**	Expression of self through meaningful recreational activities Exploring new interests	Encourage a nonrestrictive environment Provide beauty in environment Read to the sick or hard of hearing Music	Autonomy Freshness of appreciation Creativeness Spontaneity Feelings of self-fulfillment

ADLs, activities of daily living; ECT, electroconvulsive therapy.
Adapted from Ronsman, K. (1987). Therapy for depression. *Journal of Gerontological Nursing*, 13(12):21; NANDA (1994). *Nursing diagnoses: Definitions and classification* 1997–1998. Philadelphia: NANDA.

TABLE 31–4 GUIDELINES FOR THE FIRST INTERVIEW

APPROACH	PROCESS COMMENTS
1. Approach the client: note appearance, posture, spontaneous activity, grooming, hygiene, comfort, presence of others, facial expression, attentiveness, interest.	1. Cues gathered about musculoskeletal, neurological, genitourinary, gastrointestinal, cardiovascular, and pulmonary systems; cognitive and emotional function; senses; and social support.
2. Address the client by name. Introduce self: "My name is . . . I prefer to be called . . . What do you like to be called?	2. Hearing. Ability to respond to social situation and to cues about cognitive and affective function.
3. Offer to shake hands or grasp the client by the hand.	3. Neuromuscular function, strength, skin temperature, and texture.
4. Establish eye contact; ask about visual ability and use of glasses. Position self in full view of client. Adjust lighting for brightness, but avoid glare.	4. Assess vision.
5. Ask the client about any hearing difficulties and if the client can hear you clearly. Ask about the use of hearing aid, lip reading, better hearing in one ear than the other.	5. Cues about hearing and cognitive function.
"How are you feeling today?" If a clinic visit, "What brings you here today?" or "Is anything troubling you lately?" Probe specifically with open-ended questions, e.g., "Oh, you're hurting, tell me more about that."	Self-assessment of health, symptoms assessment, cognitive and verbal function, communication skills, optimism, and emotional response.
"What would you like help with today?" Note the issues identified and the order of concerns.	Cues about client's priorities, expectations, response to health, or social problems or concerns.
6. Summarize the interaction so far. "Mrs. J., we have approximately 45 minutes together to address your concerns. I think that will give us time to deal with the concerns you have voiced. I would like to proceed now by asking you a few more questions and then do the following exam procedures for these reasons."	6. Establish trust, contract for and set mutual expectations for the encounter, prioritize concerns, and validate inferences with the client.

From Matteson, M. A., and McConnell, E. S. (eds.) (1988). *Gerontological nursing: Concepts and practices* (p. 80). Philadelphia: W. B. Saunders.

TABLE 31–5 NURSING ASSESSMENT: SOCIAL DYSFUNCTION RATING SCALE

Directions: Score each of the items as follows:
1. Not present 2. Very Mild 3. Mild 4. Moderate 5. Severe 6. Very Severe

Self-esteem

1. _____ Low self-concept (feelings of inadequacy, not measuring up to self-ideal)
2. _____ Goallessness (lack of inner motivation and sense of future orientation)
3. _____ Lack of a satisfying philosophy or meaning of life (a conceptual framework for integrating past and present experiences)
4. _____ Self-health concern (preoccupation with physical health or somatic concerns)

Interpersonal system

5. _____ Emotional withdrawal (degree of deficiency in relating to others)
6. _____ Hostility (degree of aggression toward others)
7. _____ Manipulation (exploiting of environment or controlling at others' expense)
8. _____ Overdependency (degree of parasitic attachment to others)
9. _____ Anxiety (degree of feeling of uneasiness or impending doom)
10. _____ Suspiciousness (degree of distrust or paranoid ideation)

Performance system

11. _____ Lack of satisfying relationships with significant persons (spouse, children, kin, or significant persons serving in a family role)
12. _____ Lack of friends or social contacts
13. _____ Expressed need for more friends or social contacts
14. _____ Lack of work (remunerative or nonremunerative, productive work activities that normally give a sense of usefulness, status, or confidence
15. _____ Lack of satisfaction from work
16. _____ Lack of leisure time activities
17. _____ Expressed need for more leisure, self-enhancing, and satisfying activities
18. _____ Lack of participation in community activities

Continued

TABLE 31–5 NURSING ASSESSMENT: SOCIAL DYSFUNCTION RATING SCALE *cont.*

19. ______ Lack of interest in community affairs and activities that influence others
20. ______ Financial insecurity
21. ______ Adaptive rigidity (lack of complex coping patterns to stress)

PATIENT: ______________________ RATER: ______________ DATE: ______________

From Linn, M. W., et al. (1969). A social dysfunction rating scale. *Journal of Psychiatric Research*, 6:299. Copyright 1969, with kind permission from Elsevier Science Ltd., The Boulevard, Langford Lane, Kidlington 0X5 1GB, United Kingdom.

independent functioning and reduce the stress on the family system. **Day care programs** are one of these.

As a result of the negative view and rising costs of institutionalization, interest in day care programs is increasing. When individuals and their families cannot afford the expense of a nursing home, they may look at a day care facility as an acceptable solution.

The concept of day care is not new. It started in England in the early 1940s and was introduced in the United States about a decade later. Essentially, there are three types of day care programs: (1) social day care, (2) adult day health or medical treatment model, and (3) maintenance model. In each of the three variations, the elderly are being taken care of during the day while staying in a home environment at night. The boundaries of these programs blend and overlap.

Social day care affords the participants the opportunity for recreation and social interaction. Nursing, medical, or rehabilitative care is usually not provided. This is the more common type of day care and is less expensive to operate. Generally, the clients are older adults who need socialization or continued physical activities, or individuals with mild dementia or physical frailty (Buckwalter et al. 1995; Nikolassy 1995).

The *adult day health* or *medical treatment model* goes beyond meeting recreational and social needs: it provides services such as medical interventions, psychiatric nursing, and rehabilitation for the high-risk elderly, and psy-

TABLE 31–6 NURSING ASSESSMENT: ZUNG'S SELF-RATING DEPRESSION SCALE*

	NONE OR LITTLE OF THE TIME	SOME OF THE TIME	A GOOD PART OF THE TIME	MOST OR ALL OF THE TIME
1. I feel down-hearted, blue, and sad.	1	2	3	4
2. Morning is when I feel the best.	4	3	2	1
3. I have crying spells or feel like it.	1	2	3	4
4. I have trouble sleeping through the night.	1	2	3	4
5. I eat as much as I used to.	4	3	2	1
6. I enjoy looking at, talking to, and being with attractive women/men.	4	3	2	1
7. I notice that I am losing weight.	1	2	3	4
8. I have trouble with constipation.	1	2	3	4
9. My heart beats faster than usual.	1	2	3	4
10. I get tired for no reason.	1	2	3	4
11. My mind is as clear as it used to be.	4	3	2	1
12. I find it easy to do the things I used to do.	4	3	2	1
13. I am restless and can't keep still.	1	2	3	4
14. I feel hopeful about the future.	4	3	2	1
15. I am more irritable than usual.	1	2	3	4
16. I find it easy to make decisions.	4	3	2	1
17. I feel that I am useful and needed.	4	3	2	1
18. My life is pretty full.	4	3	2	1
19. I feel that others would be better off if I were dead.	1	2	3	4
20. I still enjoy the things I used to do.	4	3	2	1

*A raw score of 50 or above is associated with depression requiring hospital treatment.
From Zung, W. K. (1965). A self-rating depression scale. *Archives of General Psychiatry*, 12:63. Copyright 1965, American Medical Association.

BOX 31–2 HELPFUL INTERVIEW TECHNIQUES WITH THE ELDERLY

1. **Select a setting** that provides privacy for the interview.
2. Make certain that the **client is physically comfortable.**
3. Ask the client what name he or she prefers to be called and then use it often.
4. **Touch may be effective** in getting the client's attention.
5. **Assess the client's mental status,** e.g., look for any deficits in recent or remote memory and determine if any mental confusion exists. Be aware of *all* medications that the client is taking and their effects, any side effects, and possible drug interactions. A patient taking many medications can be confused.
6. **Ascertain the status of the client's sight and hearing faculties.** If the client has a hearing aid or glasses, or both, make certain they are being worn.
7. **Lighting in the interview setting is important,** as the older adult needs three times more light to see than the teenager. Do not allow sunlight or bright lights to shine directly into the client's face, as the older adult's eyes are very sensitive to glare.
8. **Sit close to and speak directly to any clients who have hearing deficits.** Maintain direct eye contact with the client when sitting or standing not more than 5 feet away. When speaking, do *not* exaggerate lip movements; this action distorts the mouth and what is being said. Talk in a moderate voice with a slower than normal rate of speech. Do *not* shout; this action accentuates the vowel sounds and obscures the consonants, which are already hard for the elderly person to hear.
9. **Observe the client for any signs of fatigue.** Gauge his or her attention span and keep the interview short if necessary.
10. **Pace the interview,** slowing it, if necessary, to match the client's needs. At the same time, allow the client enough time to think and respond to any questions, instructions, or discussions.
11. Try to include the client in all decisions.
12. Explain clearly to the client all the possible options from which to choose when making a decision. (Remember that choices may be more limited for the aged.)
13. When possible, **use reminiscing strategies to keep obtaining information.** Stimulate memory chains by attempting to recall patterns of association that will improve the client's recollection.
14. If the client verbalizes low self-esteem or negative views of aging, pick up on his or her strengths and point them out.
15. **Give instructions to the client slowly and clearly; print them in letters large enough to be read later, when the client's anxiety level may be lower.** If you are using handouts, make sure the type is large enough for the client to read.
16. **Make an appointment for the next meeting.** The client should understand what is expected both of the interviewer and of the client before the next meeting.
17. If possible, **include family members** in part of the interview for added input, clarification, support, and reinforcement.
18. **Be an advocate** for the elderly.

Adapted from Burnside, I. (1988). *Nursing and the aged. A self-care approach* (pp. 194–209). New York: McGraw-Hill.

chosocial interventions for the frail aged. Qualified personnel (nurses, pharmacists, physicians, physiotherapists, occupational therapists, social workers) are available, forming a broad base of support necessary for such care. This program, which requires physician referral, aims to prevent or slow down any mental, physical, or social deterioration and thus seeks to maximize the older adult's full potential regardless of disease or condition. If clients reach their full potential, they can be discharged from the program (Buckwalter et al. 1995).

The *maintenance day care* program assists clients at high risk for institutionalization. Placement is usually upon physician referral. An interdisciplinary team, including a psychiatrist, plans the care. Clients' condition does not require the full medical attention or rehabilitation provided by the medical model. The client mix includes frail persons with dementia and those with persistent and severe psychiatric disorders (e.g., schizophrenia, personality disorders) (Buckwalter et al. 1995). The program's emphasis is on maintaining clients' functional abilities. Although the inevitable cognitive decline cannot be prevented, clients' quality of life is enhanced and psychosocial dysfunction decreases. The restlessness, anxiety, and agitation that frequently occur in the demented client are kept to a minimum (Ebersole and Hess 1990). Discharge from this program is most often to an increased level of care such as found in an inpatient hospital or nursing home (Steingart 1991).

All three models are meant to provide a safe, supportive, and nonthreatening environment and play a vital function for older adults and their families. The programs permit the elderly to continue their present living arrangements and maintain their social ties to the community. This service relieves families of the burden of 24-

TABLE 31–7 USEFUL GROUP MODALITIES FOR ELDERLY CLIENTS

REMOTIVATION THERAPY	REMINISCING THERAPY (LIFE REVIEW)	PSYCHOTHERAPY
	Purpose of Group	
▶ Resocialize *regressed* and *apathetic* clients. ▶ Reawaken interest in their environment.	▶ Share memories of the past ▶ Increase self-esteem. ▶ Increase socialization. ▶ Increase awareness of the uniqueness of each participant.	▶ Alleviate psychiatric symptoms. ▶ Increase ability to interact with others in a group. ▶ Increase self-esteem. ▶ Increase ability to make decisions and function more independently.
	Format	
▶ Groups are made up of 10–15 clients. ▶ Meetings are held once or twice a week. ▶ Meetings are highly structured in a classroom-like setting. ▶ Group uses props. ▶ Each session discusses a particular topic. ▶ See Box 31–3 for the five basic steps used in each session.	▶ Groups are made up of 6–8 people. ▶ Meetings are held once or twice weekly for 1 hour. ▶ Topics include holidays, major life events, birthdays, travel, and food.	▶ Group size is 6–12 members. ▶ Group members should share similar a. Problems. b. Mental status. c. Needs. d. Sexual integration. ▶ Group meets at regularly scheduled times (number of times a week, duration of session) and place.
	Desired Outcomes	
▶ Increases participant's sense of reality. ▶ Offers practice of health roles. ▶ Realizes more objective self-image.	▶ Alleviates depression in institutionalized elderly. ▶ Through the process of reorganization and reintegration provides avenue by which elderly can a. Achieve a new sense of identity. b. Achieve a positive self-concept.	▶ Decreases sense of isolation. ▶ Facilitates development of new roles and reestablishes former roles. ▶ Provides information for other group members. ▶ Provides group support for effecting changes and increasing self-esteem.

Data from Matteson, M. A., and McConnell, E. S. (eds.). (1988). *Gerontological nursing: Concepts and practice.* Philadelphia: W. B. Saunders.

hour daily care for their elderly dependents. If institutionalization becomes necessary, day care staff can work with elderly clients and their families to assess the present situation and make recommendations for placement.

Payment for these programs depends on the facility and its funding source. Services may be paid for privately or by a federal or state governmental agency, according to their eligibility requirements. Most social day care centers derive their funding from clients, donations, and fundraising. Many of the medical models are funded through private insurance or Medicaid. Because of these sources, they are highly regulated and impose strict admission requirements.

ISSUES THAT AFFECT THE MENTAL HEALTH OF SOME ELDERLY

The issues chosen here for discussion are five of the most prevalent problems for many elderly:

1. *Use of restraints* in the elderly comes into the forefront with changes in federal law.
2. *Death and dying* of the elderly pose complex legal and ethical issues for the elderly client, the family, doctors, and nurses.
3. *AIDS and the elderly.*
4. *Suicide* is a growing phenomenon among the elderly.
5. *Alcoholism* is a "neglected disease" affecting both the physical and the mental health of some elderly people.

Elder abuse, another serious problem for many elderly people, is addressed in Chapter 15.

Restraints

The use of restraints in the elderly is an issue of ethical and legal interest. Restraints can be both physical and chemical. **Physical restraints** are any manual method or mechanical device, material, or equipment that inhibits free movement (Hogstel 1995; National Citizens' Coalition for Nursing Home Reform 1991). **Chemical restraints** are drugs given for the very specific purpose of inhibiting a specific behavior or movement (Hogstel 1995).

PHYSICAL RESTRAINTS. According to a Health Care Financing Administration (HCFA) report on state

BOX 31–3 EXAMPLE OF A REMOTIVATION SESSION (BODIES OF WATER)

STEP 1: CLIMATE OF ACCEPTANCE

The leaders personally welcomed each participant as he or she arrived at the group session. After the leaders introduced themselves, each group member made a self-introduction. The leader used a calendar to orient the members to the date and time of the current remotivation session. The theme for session 4 was introduced by the leader as "bodies of water—rivers, lakes, and oceans." All group members had some familiarity with bodies of water because of their residence in Seattle.

STEP 2: CREATING A BRIDGE TO REALITY

The world globe was used as a visual aid to stimulate discussion on bodies of water. The leader asked questions, such as "How are bodies of water formed from glaciers?" Pictures of glaciers, rivers, and lakes were shown.

The leader read poems about tide pools, sea shells, and fishing written by anonymous grade school children. Discussion was stimulated by the leader asking, "What can we do at the ocean?" Visual aids and props were provided for direct sensory stimulation. Some examples of these aids and props included (1) different types of sea shells, (2) fishing tackle and bait, (3) suntan lotion, (4) sun hat, and (5) sunglasses.

A poem by an anonymous author about fishing was read to the group. This was followed by recorded music with lyrics about fishing experiences.

STEP 3: SHARING THE WORLD WE LIVE IN

Group discussion focused on jobs related to bodies of water. Topics the participants discussed in regard to self or others included crabbing, clamming, shrimping, and fishing. Visual aids were provided to stimulate further discussions of past-related experiences involving bodies of water. Pictures of river-rafting, canoeing, scuba diving, and sailing were shared.

STEP 4: AN APPRECIATION OF THE WORK OF THE WORLD

This time was used for the members to think about work in relation to others. More experiences in past-related work roles as well as hobbies and pastimes were discussed. The group then participated in singing a familiar old song, "Love Letters in the Sand," written in 1931 by J. Fred Coots and revived in 1957 when sung by Pat Boone.

STEP 5: CLIMATE OF APPRECIATION

The group members were thanked individually by the leaders for coming to the group and sharing their experiences. The following remotivation session theme and meeting date were announced prior to terminating the session.

GROUP RESPONSE TO SESSION 4

Most members of the group appeared to enjoy discussing their experiences in relation to bodies of water. Many members recalled fishing and boating experiences. Other members expressed interest in this topic by their nonverbal participation in touching and smelling some physical props and observation of visual aids. All but two participants touched the seashells and smelled the fish eggs. One lady in the group stood up and modeled the sun hat and glasses, while a man demonstrated how to reel in the line on a fishing pole. Several participants remarked on how beautiful the pictures of the glaciers were. All but a couple of group members sang to the recorded lyrics on fishing. One member stood up and danced to the music while many others clapped to her movements.

From Janssen, J. A., and Giberson, D. L. (1988). Remotivation therapy. *Journal of Gerontological Nursing,* 14(6):31.

and federal licensure surveys of nursing facilities in the United States, 42% of all nursing home residents are tied at one time or another to their beds or chairs (Stilwell 1991). In hospitals and nursing homes combined, every day more than 500,000 older people are restrained in one way or another (Evans and Strumpf 1989). Furthermore, there is a greater likelihood that, once a resident is physically restrained, he or she will continue to be restrained regularly for an indefinite period (Blakeslee et al. 1991).

There has always been the question whether health care providers have the right to restrain another individual physically. Physical restraints can be a humiliating and demoralizing experience. The elderly have responded to such action with anger, fear, or resignation (Evans and Strumpf 1989).

Health care providers often apply restraint measures to the hospitalized or institutionalized confused elderly because of fear of litigation in case of injury to an unrestrained person. However, such interventions do not necessarily create safer conditions (Masters and Marks 1990). *Clients who are restrained are much more likely to be hurt than those who are not.* Residents in restraint-free facilities have experienced fewer injuries from falls than those in facilities using restraints. Of great concern is the risk of death through strangulation or asphyxiation with their use (Blakeslee et al. 1991).

In addition to these most severe consequences, immobilizing the elderly can result in many physical problems (Brower 1991; Blakeslee et al. 1991):

- Chronic constipation or impaction
- Disrupted vestibular function
- Reduced or impaired circulation
- Incontinence of urine and feces

- Abrasions and skin tears or pressure sores
- Loss of bone mass
- Reduced or impaired circulation
- Reduced metabolic rate
- Electrolyte losses
- Muscle atrophy, decreased tone and strength, and contractures

Any confused behavior exhibited by restrained residents may become intensified through immobilization. Restraints also have a dehumanizing effect on both the caregiver and the resident. Their use is in conflict with the concept of human dignity and individual independence (Blakeslee et al. 1991).

To correct these injustices, the **Omnibus Budget Reconciliation Act (OBRA)** came into law in 1990. Nursing homes are now held accountable to a higher standard of care that focuses on the resident's "highest practicable, physical, mental, and psychosocial well-being," and are directed to support "individual needs and preferences" and to "promote maintenance or enhancement of the quality of life" (National Citizens' Coalition for Nursing Home Reform 1991). The OBRA mandates that each resident has the right to be free from unnecessary drugs and physical restraints and is provided treatment to reduce dependency on chemical and physical intervention (Hogstel 1990).

Restraints may be imposed only (1) to ensure *the physical safety of the resident and/or other residents*, and (2) upon the written order of a physician that *specifies the duration and the circumstances* under which the restraints are to be used (National Citizens' Coalition for Nursing Home Reform 1991). The Food and Drug Administration (FDA) issued a safety alert in 1992 on the potential dangers of restraint devices. The Agency mandated that all physical restraints be labeled with directions informing health care providers of the dangers of physical restraints and the specific usage (Myers 1994; Hogstel 1995). In addition, the FDA advised that patients or their representatives be informed of the contemplated action and its risks and benefits (Stolley 1995).

The federal government has set standards of care for every nursing home receiving Medicare or Medicaid funds. The HCFA has been charged with enforcing these standards through inspections or "surveys." The guidelines (National Citizens' Coalition for Nursing Home Reform 1991) direct HCFA surveyors to evaluate the use of physical restraint and determine whether

- Less-restraining measures were attempted.
- Occupational or physical therapists were consulted.
- The client and family received a complete explanation.
- The device was used only for definite periods as an "enabler" to the resident or for brief periods to provide necessary life-saving treatment.
- Use of restraints was detrimental to the resident's physical, mental, or psychosocial well-being.

CHEMICAL RESTRAINTS. HCFA will investigate to determine whether

- Residents are free from unnecessary drugs.
- Residents are given antipsychotic drugs only to treat a specific condition.
- Residents are given gradual dose reductions, drug holidays, and behavioral programming whenever possible, in lieu of medications.

The guidelines on antipsychotic drugs list certain circumstances for which they can be prescribed, e.g., cognitive impairment disorders, including dementia, with associated psychotic or agitated features (National Citizens' Coalition for Nursing Home Reform 1991), defined by

- Specific behaviors defined quantitatively and objectively that cause residents to present a danger to themselves or to others or actually hinder the staff in its ability to provide care.
- Psychotic symptoms that cause the "resident frightful distress."

After the enactment of OBRA for long-term care institutions, the Joint Commission on the Accreditation of Healthcare Organizations (JCAHO) developed recommendations on the use of physical restraints in acute care facilities. Generally following OBRA's guidelines, JCAHO stipulates as a basis for physical restraints (Myers 1994):

- A physician's order.
- Time-limited application.
- Documentation of alternative approaches.
- Documentation of ongoing observation and assessment of the patient.

Nurses can avoid liability by knowledge of the law, adherence to the policies and procedures of the institution, and use of good nursing judgment. All nursing homes and hospitals should have written restraint procedures and policies available to all health care providers. If restraints are used, the nurse is responsible for the safety of the client during the time of their use. The client should be restrained only for a limited time and for a limited purpose.

Restraints do not enhance resident care. Creative nursing skills and interventions are frequently more beneficial. The necessity of applying restraints "for the resident's safety" can often be avoided when effective communication and planning are used to decrease the client's anxiety and agitation. Nurses should be familiar with alternative methods of client control to produce desirable results. They should be aware of current research findings and support continued research in this sensitive area.

Death and Dying

Life is bounded by two milestones: birth and death. To some, death is the completion of a life process; to others, it is a passage to another life. For all, however, the thoughts and fears of death and its irreversibility have a particular significance.

In the early 1950s, the elderly approaching death found themselves not in the nursing home or hospital but at home, with death usually taking place in familiar surroundings. The individual could thus progress through the dying process in the more intimate home setting.

As a youth-oriented society, Americans tend to view death not as an immediate concern but rather as a remote prospect. By turning their sick over to the medical experts, Americans expect advanced technologies to answer all problems; thus, they insulate themselves from death (Ross 1981). Polls have been conducted on themes of death and prolonging life. When members in a retirement community were asked to assess the extent of intervention they would like should they be dying, the majority desired only comfort care; they were not interested in the life-extending processes. Many wanted to ensure that their wishes were followed by having a written document of such wishes accessible to their physicians (Snow and Atwood 1985). A Louis Harris poll of over 1000 adults found that 86% thought that terminally ill clients should be allowed to tell their physicians to let them die; almost an equal percentage favored withdrawal of feeding tubes, if this were the client's desire (Wallis 1986).

Another group was asked what they would desire if they had severe memory loss, were unable to care for themselves, or had no chance of recovery. A much greater percentage of older persons than younger ones said they would refuse intensive care or tube feeding.

Advances in Technology

Technological advances in medicine have brought about corresponding changes in life-sustaining machinery. Increasing efforts are made to keep alive elderly persons who otherwise would die. Physicians are having a difficult time making decisions affecting the care of their dying clients. The American College of Physicians Committee on Medical Ethics states that physicians have a responsibility to make certain that their hopelessly ill clients die with dignity and with as little suffering as possible (Jenike 1984).

These recommendations are not always easy to follow. As a rule, physicians feel compelled to apply treatment regardless of the client's prognosis, unless the client specifically objects or has a written living will (Kleiman 1985). Preserving life is what nurses and physicians have been educated and trained to do and what they have promised in their professional oaths. Their actions are geared toward sustaining and prolonging life. Withholding treatment from hopelessly ill clients may open physicians to malpractice charges (Kleiman 1985).

Medical technology has frequently outpaced our ability to apply it judiciously (Pinch and Parsons 1992). The lives of those who would have died sooner are often prolonged regardless of their mental capacity. The percentage of elderly people not dying at home but in a hospital or nursing home has been steadily increasing. Today, approximately 80% of all people die in hospitals or nursing homes, often surrounded by life-extending apparatuses (Wallis 1986).

Although technology has resulted in decreased mortality in some areas, prevention of chronic illness has lagged behind. A definite aging population has evolved, which means that physicians, the elderly, and their families are facing more treatment decisions than ever before (Pinch and Parsons 1992). Society has never before faced the problem of so many people living for so long with such severe impairments. No specific cure exists for many of the severe and persistent diseases afflicting the elderly (e.g., senile dementia, stroke, osteoporosis, advanced cancer, rheumatic disease, arteriosclerosis).

Lower mortality rates and increased life expectancy have made death "less visible, less meaningful, and less controllable than it was in the past." For many persons, death has been "transposed, insulated, technologicalized, decontextualized" (Ross 1981). There is a growing concern that death in America is too often controlled by machines rather than by nature. Because of advances in medicine, the ability to extend life may carry "overwhelming emotional hardships, agonizing pain, and devastating financial costs" (Kaufman 1989). In the case of a terminally ill or severely demented client, a point may be reached at which the balance of what is to be "saved," when weighed against the emotional and financial ruin to be suffered by the family, tilts toward the family. The question must be asked, "Should the quality of life become a weightier consideration than mere survival?" (Nelson 1982).

Technology has its price, and financing health care is a quickly escalating concern. Currently, 12.5% of the gross national product is allocated to health care. Cost should not determine ethical decisions, but financial considerations are important if technology is used when it is not desired or when the outcome does not warrant the risks involved (Pinch and Parsons 1992).

Since the 1960s, the public's desire to have a voice in making decisions about its care has been increasing. This interest in client advocacy has been recognized with the passage of the **Patient Self-Determination Act (PSDA)** of 1990.

Although the elderly are becoming better-educated consumers of health care, they are still reluctant to make health care decisions about the extent of medical interventions or to create a living will; instead, they prefer to rely informally on family members to make choices for them (Shawler et al. 1992). Before the passage of the PSDA, only about 10% of the population had some form of written advance directive, and less than 5% of acute care hospitals routinely inquired about the existence of such directives at the time of clients' admission (Boyle 1992).

Patient Self-Determination Act (PSDA) of 1990

In June 1990 the U. S. Supreme Court, in deciding the Nancy Cruzan "right-to-die" case, affirmed the right of a competent person to reject life-sustaining treatment (including hydration and nutrition). The court, however, held that states may ascertain the degree of proof required before a client's wishes set forth in an advance directive are honored. In response to the court's decision, Congress enacted the PSDA (Burke and Walsh 1992).

This act establishes guidelines regarding clients' requests before and during episodes of serious illness. It fosters clearer communication among them, their families, physicians, and health care workers (Smith 1992). Health care institutions that receive federal funds are now required to provide, at the time of admission, written information to each client regarding his or her right to execute "advance health care directives" and to inquire if such directives have been made by the client. The client's admission records should state whether such directives exist (Box 31–4).

Clients use such directives to indicate their preferences for the types of medical care they want or regarding how much treatment they desire to have provided to them. The directives come into effect should physical or mental incapacitation prevent clients from making their health care decisions. These wishes can be communicated through one or more of the following instruments: (1) a living will, (2) a directive to physician, and (3) a durable power of attorney for health care. These documents must be in writing and witnessed; depending on state and institutional provisions, they may require notarization. Preprinted forms, varying from one to several pages, are available through various organizations (e.g., Concern for Dying/Society for Right to Die), hospitals, stationery stores). These directives may be valid for up to 7 years unless state law stipulates a shorter period. The individual must be of age and competent when signing the instrument.

Living wills express clients' wishes about their future medical care. During times of crisis, living wills can influence the course of therapy. The idea originated in the late 1960s as a tool to allow individuals to restrict medical intervention when technology or treatment can no longer advance a reasonable quality of life or chance of recovery (MacKay 1992). Various sample forms are available if the individual does not want to have a lawyer draft his or her own living will.

BOX 31–4 RESPONSIBILITIES OF HEALTH CARE PROVIDERS UNDER THE PATIENT SELF-DETERMINATION ACT OF 1990

Hospitals, skilled nursing facilities, home health agencies, hospice organizations, and health maintenance organizations servicing Medicare and Medicaid clients must

1. Maintain written policies and procedures for providing information to clients for whom they provide care.
2. Give written material to clients concerning their rights under state law to make decisions about medical care, including the right to accept or refuse surgical or medical care and to formulate advance directives and provide for written policies and procedures for the realization of these rights.
3. Document in clients' records whether they have advance directives.
4. Not discriminate in care or other ways against clients who have or have not prepared advance directives.
5. Make sure that policies are in place to ensure compliance with state laws governing advance directives.

The written information should be made available to clients as follows:

1. In hospitals, on admission as an inpatient
2. In skilled nursing facilities, on admission as a resident
3. By home health agencies, on coming under care of the agency
4. By hospice programs, on receiving care from the program
5. For health maintenance organizations, at the time of enrollment

Modified from Schlossberg, C., and Hart, M. A. (1992). Legal perspectives. In M. Burke and M. Walsh (Eds.), *Gerontologic nursing care of the frail elderly* (p. 469). St. Louis: Mosby–Year Book.

The concept of a living will has been adopted nationwide. Corresponding statutes have been enacted in 46 states plus the District of Columbia. These statutes allow individuals to exercise control over their medical care. This applies in particular to decisions regarding life-sustaining treatment in instances of terminal conditions or permanent unconscious conditions (Goeber 1996).

A living will, however, may not offer as much protection as the client might think—there are limitations. Although every state with living will legislation protects the individual's decision as it relates to **terminal** illness, only about one third of the states do not require the individual to be terminally ill in order to refuse medical treatment. These states will also enforce the living will of an individual in a persistent vegetative state (Goeber 1996).

A competent client may alter a living will at any time. The question of wheather an incompetent person can change a living will has to be addressed on a state-by-state basis. Although there may be states (e.g., Iowa) that permit changes in a living will by a person no longer competent, the general rule seems to be that once a person is incompetent, changes are no longer possible.

Health care providers who are present when a client wants to change a living will have an obligation to inform the institution and provide the means to do so in writing. Oral statements are legally binding in most states but should be heard by more than one person (Olson 1997).

Health care providers are obligated to abide by the advanced care directive unless their clients are told beforehand in writing that one or more of the provisions are against the institution's policy (within confinement of applicable state law) (Olson 1997). Care must be taken when acting as witness for a client's living will, since over one third of the states have laws prohibiting the client's physician or employees of a health care facility from acting as witnesses to prevent undue pressure or influence.

Executing a living will may not always guarantee its application. American medicine is still largely ignoring end-of-life decisions. A study conducted in five teaching hospitals in the United States found that physicians often disregard or misunderstand their clients' requests, with the result that a significant number of individuals die against their wishes in intensive care units, isolated and in pain after days or weeks of futile treatment. This study monitored over 9000 critically ill individuals. Significant differences were found between what the clients desired and what they actually received: less than half of all physicians knew when their clients did not want cardiopulmonary resuscitation (CPR); even when there was knowledge, almost half of the do-not-resuscitate (DNR) orders were written only within 2 days of death (SUPPORT Investigations 1995).

Notwithstanding the institution's legal obligation to inquire into the existence of any such directives, the client simply may not be in a condition to respond to such questions at the time of admission. Almost half of all persons admitted to nursing homes may have serious cognitive defects (MacKay 1992). Thus, in many cases, the institution may not become aware of the existence of such a document, and the client's specified wishes may go unheeded. Consequently, it is advisable for anyone having such a document to keep it readily available and not hidden away. It would also be helpful if a family member, a close friend, or the client's physician have copies or access to them.

The living will may designate a person to be contacted in case questions of interpretation arise. In the absence of such designation, the health care provider will follow an affirmative course under the maxim "when not certain, provide treatment."

A further shortcoming of the living will is the lack of specificity when it comes to naming the "heroic" measures the client chooses to relinquish (CPR, mechanical ventilation, surgery). The use of vague terms such as "hopeless" and "extraordinary" may also burden the usefulness of the living will (Rosenthal 1991).

With a **directive to physician,** a physician is appointed by the individual to serve as proxy. This directive must be completed on a prescribed form. Many of the features parallel those of a living will (presence of terminal illness, verification by the physician, competency at time of signing).

The directive to physician can be particularly useful in cases in which a terminally ill individual with no family or close ties to others feels most comfortable with having the physician act as surrogate. The physician must agree in writing to be the client's agent and must also be one of the two physicians who made the original determination that the client is terminally ill (MacKay 1992). Like the living will, the directive to physician can be revoked orally at any time without regard to client competency.

The **durable power of attorney for health care (DPAHC)** differs from the two earlier instruments in that a person (other than a physician) is appointed to act as the client's agent and there is no waiting period for implementation. Furthermore, with the DPAHC, the client must not only be competent and of age when making the appointment but must also be competent to revoke the power. Designating a health care proxy is generally a simple step. No waiting period is necessary for the DPAHC to go into effect. Furthermore, individuals do not have to be terminally ill or incompetent for the person appointed with the health care power of attorney to act on their behalf. No physician's certification is required.

Agents can make decisions for their clients whenever necessary. They need not be relatives but can be anyone whom the client trusts and who is willing to accept the responsibilities. The scope of their authority reaches beyond decisions on withholding interventions or treatment to more general aspects of medical care. The agent becomes the client's advocate in all medical matters and may even prevent the institution from providing services to the client that the agent believes are not wanted.

Health care providers who have backed away from living wills because of frequent ambiguities may find the DPAHC more agreeable. Relying solely on a living will document to make a life-or-death decision can be uncomfortable for the provider. Under the DPAHC, a surrogate is named with whom the health care provider can consult and discuss treatment alternatives (Rosenthal 1991).

Because not all state laws authorize these instruments, they may not be binding in jurisdictions without explicit statutes. In such cases the health care providers would decide whether to accept the advanced directives (Janofsky 1990).

In short, the DPAHC provides the best option for most clients (MacKay 1992). However, some individuals may choose to supplement a DPAHC with a living will, keeping the latter "in reserve" in case of the possible need for clarification of their wishes.

Medical Futility

End-of-life decisions are a matter of concern not only for the client, family, or surrogate but also for the health care provider. Problems may arise when the clients (and more frequently the family or surrogate) express desires that life-prolonging actions be taken while, on the other hand, physicians recommend that treatment be withheld. The concept of **medical futility** is developing as an ethically acceptable rationale to withhold treatment. It has been defined thus (Futility: The Concept and Its Use 1993):

> A treatment is considered medically futile when the treatment affords no benefit weighing the intrusiveness, burdens, and risks against the ultimate outcome.

In applying this concept to clinical practice, the health care provider will consider the beneficial effects of continued therapy or intervention. If treatment is "highly unlikely" to benefit certain clients, it may be deemed "futile" to continue. Critics of this rationale question whether "highly unlikely" to succeed equals "futile" (Edwards 1995).

Although the decision to withhold treatment primarily falls within the domain of the physician, the nurse must be aware of the medical futility concept and should be asked for input. In addition, the facility's Ethics Committee should be involved in the process. Although, upon admission and during their stay, clients should be asked about their end-of-life wishes, physicians often feel uncomfortable dealing with these issues. Virmani and colleagues (1994) found that most physicians who treated critically ill cancer patients never discussed end-of-life treatment decisions with them and were unaware of their clients' wishes in this regard.

Curtis and co-workers (1995), in their study on medical futility rationale and DNR orders, found that the concept of futility is often misunderstood. They recommended the development of guidelines for the evaluation of the quantitative and qualitative elements of medical futility as well as the education of health care providers.

Hospice Care

One alternative to dying in a hospital or nursing home setting is the hospice approach. In its original concept a hospice was a place of shelter and rest for pilgrims or strangers. Today this idea has broadened beyond the physical setting to recognize a program to meet the needs of the dying.

The **hospice philosophy** is characterized by the acceptance of death as a natural conclusion to life, with clients rather than health care providers making the decisions how they want to live and die. Terminally ill clients can remain at home and receive supportive care. The focus is on keeping them comfortable, free of pain, as active as possible, and close to their families. They need not fear being subjected to prolonged medical care against their wishes.

Recently, some health care facilities have set aside "hospice beds" whose occupants are treated in accordance with the hospice philosophy. The hospice approach may constitute for many an acceptable equilibrium between clients' needs and wishes and the emotional and financial strain on their relatives.

Withholding Hydration

Contrary to earlier teaching, hydration is no longer advised when a terminally ill client facing imminent death is dehydrated. Although many nurses have been taught that dehydration causes suffering and that skilled care requires hydration, it is necessary to readjust this thinking (Zerwekh 1993). Research has shown that terminally ill clients in end-stage dehydration experience less discomfort than clients receiving medical hydration at that stage (Taylor 1995; Printz 1992). With respect to food, McCann and colleagues (1994) found that those terminally ill with cancer generally did not experience hunger, and those who did needed only small amounts of food for alleviation.

Hydration needlessly extends the dying process. **Withholding** artificial **hydration** and nutrition from an individual in an irreversible coma does not bring on a destructive state but rather permits an already existing fatal condition to take its natural course. When death is imminent, the moral responsibility to prolong life is outweighed by not unnecessarily burdening the dying process (Taylor 1995).

Nurses' Role in the Decision-Making Process

In the absence of clear instructions or when clients cannot decide for themselves, nurses may be in the best position to know whether "the remaining life is worth the suffering of the client." Not only do they spend more time with the client than the physician (and often even family members), but they also have a broader understanding of the client because of their communication skills and concerns with the sociological and psychological basis of illness and health. Nurses are often involved in decisions about whether to treat clients aggressively or allow them to die without the use of life-support equipment. Box 31–5 offers guidelines relating to issues of life and death (Alford 1986).

In working with the client's family, the nurse should orient family members and significant others about the

BOX 31–5 GUIDELINES RELATING TO ISSUES OF LIFE AND DEATH

1. Understand that it is the client's will, not health, that is all-important.
2. Assess the client for ethicolegal factors, e.g., living wills, guardianship, and competency.
3. Know the state's nursing practice act and understand the state laws and the institution's policies concerning death and the termination of life support systems.
4. Follow the American Nurses' Association (ANA) Code of Ethics and the ANA Standards of Gerontological Nursing.

Data from Alford, D. (1986). Managing ethical and legal dilemmas in the care of the elderly. Presentation at Current Directions in Gerontological Nursing, Bethesda, MD.

ethicolegal policies of the institution and assist them to live with, and understand the concepts of, dying and death. The nurse should explain that the family need not feel morally obligated to provide for all possible medical care when it would only extend the suffering of a loved one. This is especially true when such extraordinary measures do not represent the person's values and beliefs.

Maintaining an open and continuing dialogue among client, family, nurse, and physician is of principal importance. The nurse should serve as an advocate for competent clients in their decision making and should be supportive of the client's surrogate when determinations need to be made.

If no living will exists, any indication that clients might have given in the past about their view toward death and dying should be given consideration with respect to medical care. *Old age alone ought not to be a factor.* Age becomes significant only when it is expressed by the client (e.g., "I'm tired, I'm too old, I want to go") (Gadow 1979).

Each health care institution should have a written policy on "coding" to serve as a guideline for physicians and nurses. Affected clients should have orders in effect for implementation. **The nurse should never accept verbal "no-code" orders from physicians** (Alford 1986).

In addition, each health care facility receiving federal funds must have written policies and procedures and protocols in compliance with the Patient Self-Determination Act of 1990 (PSDA). Such guidelines result in more, not less, involvement and responsibilities for nurses (Shawler et al. 1992). Nurses must prepare themselves for the legal, ethical, and moral issues involved when giving advance directive counseling (Moore 1992). The new law does not specify who must talk with clients about treatment decisions, but in many facilities nurses are being asked to do this.

When this is the case, policy and procedure manuals should outline the nurses' responsibility for discussing "advance directives" with clients and for ensuring that such directives are included in the clients' charts. In some states it is not legal for the caregivers in a facility (especially nursing homes) to assist clients to write advance directive since this is considered a conflict of interest.

Institutions are required to implement the mandates of the PSDA. Although federal law, through the Act, requires institutions to develop corresponding policies and procedures, state law governs the specifics of such guidelines. *Nurses need to be cognizant of their state laws,* such as what advanced directives are permitted and what can be withheld. Nurses should be available to clients and their families to respond to questions on the ramifications of the act and to provide appropriate resources in answering their questions (Boyle 1992).

If the nurse becomes aware that the advance directive of a client is not being carried out, the nurse, as the client's advocate, should intervene on the client's behalf. If the problem is not resolved after the nurse talks with the individual's physician, the nurse should follow the facility's protocol by notifying the appropriate supervisor (Boyle 1992).

Making decisions regarding the treatment of an incapacitated client is never easy. The existence of an advance directive can guide the health care providers in this process. Clear-cut answers will not always be found. However, a conscientious and informed health care provider, together with clear and established written policies and procedures of the institution, will facilitate the process of following the client's wishes (Gobis 1992).

AIDS and the Elderly

Acquired immunodeficiency syndrome (AIDS) not only affects young persons and intravenous drug users but also is present in the older population, accounting for 10% of all reported AIDS cases (CDC 1993). The actual number is likely to be higher, because health care providers may not recognize AIDS as a possible diagnosis and older adults may be hesitant to discuss earlier sexual practices or drug abuse with them (Schuerman 1994).

Blood transfusions are a main cause for the spread of AIDS in the elderly. Fifteen percent of all transfusions are given to persons aged 60 and over (Schuerman 1994). Although today's blood supply is more rigorously monitored, the impact of transfusions in the mid-1980s may manifest itself only now. Consequently, the aged who received blood transfusions before 1985, and their spouses, are particularly at risk. The same applies to the elderly who participated in unprotected sex outside a monogamous relationship (Catina et al. 1989).

Older adults are frequently not considered targets for acquiring human immunodeficiency viruse (HIV) infection and AIDS through sexual activity. However, their sexual behavior should not be underestimated. They have a high degree of interest in sexuality and continued sexual activity when a partner is available. In many cases, sex for the elderly has been reported as even more satisfying than in earlier years (Butler et al. 1991).

Notwithstanding the age of the client, the risk of contracting AIDS looms in the background. The elderly's compromised immune systems make them more susceptible to AIDS than younger persons (Ebersole and Hess 1994). Older women may be at greater risk for getting the virus from an infected partner than older men. Changes in vaginal tissue because of the aging process can lead to breaks in the vaginal mucosa during intercourse, allowing the HIV virus to penetrate. In addition, since pregnancy is no longer a threat, use of condoms in this age group is uncommon. This puts the older woman at greater risk of exposure (Wallace et al. 1993).

Because dementia caused by AIDS and Alzheimer's dementia (AD) can be easily confounded, a careful assessment and work-up is required. The health care provider must be aware that AIDS can occur in the elderly. Early symptoms of AIDS dementia that may mimic AD can be apathy, withdrawal, forgetfulness, and confusion (Sabin 1987). See Table 23-3 in Chapter 23 for the differences between AIDS dementia and AD.

Generally, health care providers have directed their educational efforts in AIDS prevention toward an age group younger than that of the elderly. Consequently, appropriate information may not be reaching the older adult. The nursing and medical community must realize that age does not preclude sexual activity and that a potential exposure of the older adult to AIDS exists. In the recognition that the elderly may fall victim to AIDS, educational programs should address prevention strategies for both the elderly and health care providers, as well as providing information on assessment and treatment of AIDS across the life span.

Suicide

Although suicide is often connected with the young, the suicide rates of the elderly in the United States are the highest of any age group. Suicide is now one of the top ten causes of death among the aged. While the general population's suicide rate is 12 per 100,000, it increases nearly 50% to 17 per 100,000 over age 65. The elderly white male has the highest prevalence of suicide, accounting for 23% of all suicides (Moody 1994; Horne and Blazer 1992). Refer to Chapter 24 on suicide.

One explanation for the high white male suicide rate may lie in changes of occupational status and measures of success in men at the time of retirement and thereafter. Such changes seem to affect white males, as a group, more than other elderly people, including women (Ebersole and Hess 1994). With retirement, a man may lose status, influence, contact with fellow workers, and standing in the community. On the other hand, the older woman retains many of her earlier activities and roles. It remains to be seen whether women and other groups becoming more active in the work force will suffer the same effects upon retirement.

Other factors that can lead to suicide are feelings of hopelessness, uselessness, and despair. For older adults, suicide may be seen as a final gesture of control at a stage when independence is at risk or activities are limited. For this reason, the suicide attempts of the elderly are more likely to succeed. Unlike younger persons, whose suicidal gestures may be intended to draw attention to their problems, those of older adults do not signify a call for help but rather a desire to die (Atchley 1994; Stanley and Beare 1995; Ebersole and Hess 1990). Persistent and terminal illness also contributes to increased suicide rates in the elderly.

Financial need can add to the high suicide rate. Federal reductions in programs like Medicare, Medicaid, and food stamps, along with state-ordered cuts in medical care, cause many elderly Americans to worry about their future. An inverse relationship between economic conditions and suicide rate has been identified (Marshall 1978).

Even though the elderly's suicide rates are high, they are probably underreported. Suicide is often not listed on the death certificate, even if it may be suspected. The numbers also do not reflect those who passively or indirectly commit suicide by abusing alcohol, starving themselves, overdosing or mixing medications, stopping life-sustaining drugs, or simply giving up the will to live (Stanley and Beare 1995).

Assessing Suicide Risk in the Elderly

Other high-risk suicide factors in the elderly are (1) widowhood, (2) illnesses and intractable pain, (3) status change, and (4) losses. Losses may be personal in nature (death of a family member or close friend), economic (loss of earnings or job), or social (loss of prestige or position) (McIntosh 1985; Boxwell 1988). The potential for suicide is intensified by these changes and losses.

Old age has been described as a "season of losses." Frequently, multiple losses accompany the aging process (Osgood 1988). These losses increase stress at a time when the older adult may be the most vulnerable and least resistant to stress, thus precipitating a depressive state. Nevertheless, most older adults are able to function despite their losses. Those who give in may do so because of hopelessness (Boxwell 1988).

The technological advances that extend the lives of older adults sometimes bring a quality of life that is not acceptable to them. Some elderly people may decide that their lives are not worth living under such circumstances and opt for "rational" suicide. In these instances, they may have the tacit support of their children, who may resent the cost and problems involved in keeping their parents alive (Tolchin 1989). Placement in a nursing home can be another catalyst. The fear of this event was highest on a list of reasons given in suicide notes in one study of the elderly (Loebel 1991).

Vigilance against suicide in later life should be maintained. The significant increase in the sheer numbers of elderly people is expected to lead to a doubling in the number of suicides within the next 40 years. These rates are anticipated to swell as baby boomers grow older. Although life expectancy has increased, individuals continue to retire at about the same age. Fears about their livelihood, inflation, and possible collapse of pensions become critical factors. Any cutbacks in medical care will cause anxiety about continuing health care to increase. All these aspects are likely to contribute to an increase in the suicide rate (Blazer et al. 1986).

In assessing suicide risk, the health care provider must examine previous suicidal behavior and understand that the elderly make fewer suicidal gestures than the population at large. An inquiry into the client's idea of the future should also be made.

If suicide is contemplated, there is likely to be a strong determination to succeed, causing the elderly to choose a reliable method. Guns are the most common means of suicide (used by approximately 75% of men and 33% of women) (Suicide Rate Among Elderly Rises 1991). Jumping, hanging, and drowning are also relatively frequent methods. The ratio of attempts to completed suicides among all ages is about 10:1, whereas in those over age 65 the ratio is 10:9 (Richardson et al. 1989).

Depression continues to be the most common factor putting the client at increased risk for suicide. As the most frequent functional psychiatric disorder of later life, it causes between 50% and 70% of late-life suicides (Richardson et al. 1989). Early identification of and treatment for depression are key measures for suicide prevention (Moody 1994).

Right to Suicide

One concern of nursing is the question of whether an elderly individual has the right to commit suicide. Intensifying the ethical and moral dilemma of suicide is the distinction that must be made between suicide and voluntary active euthanasia. Although society frowns on suicide in general, there seems to be a growing recognition that elderly persons with terminal illnesses should be able to take their own lives. If an alert elderly client is confronted with an intractable, lingering, and painful illness, with no hope of relief except for suicide, is the intervention of the health care provider to prevent suicide justifiable? If the determination is made to intervene (e.g., by hospitalization and physical restraint), it could be suggested that the health care provider has placed a higher value on the client's life than the client has (Boxwell 1988).

Although suicide is discussed in Chapter 24, specific factors that concern the elderly are noted here, such as retirement-related difficulties, physical illness, economic problems, loneliness, social isolation, and ageism. Innovative methods to deal with these factors need to be developed for the elderly. Education of the public in general, and health care providers in particular, is necessary to raise the level of awareness of this geriatric problem.

Depression vs. Dementia

Depression is often confused with dementia and not always recognized. This is important for nurses to keep in mind. A careful systematic assessment is therefore necessary to properly identify the illness. Unlike dementia, depression is treatable with medication and other interventions. In the elderly, symptoms of memory loss and other intellectual impairments, or asocial or agitated behavior, may be associated with dementia while actually caused by depression. See Chapter 23 for comparisons between dementia and depression.

In making an assessment, the nurse needs to be familiar with the symptoms of later-life depression (Osgood 1988), which may include one or more of the following:

- Changes in sleep patterns and symptoms of insomnia
- Changes in eating patterns, particularly loss of appetite
- Changes in weight, primarily weight loss
- Excessive fatigue
- Increased concern with bodily functions
- Alterations in mood
- Expression of apprehension and anxiety without any reason
- Low self-esteem, feelings of insignificance or pessimism

A careful evaluation of the cause of the depression is also necessary. Depression can be caused by drugs (e.g., reserpine and other *Rauwolfia* derivatives, steroids, phenothiazines) as well as by metabolic and endocrine disorders such as hepatitis and adrenal and thyroid insufficiency. Chronic health problems may also augment the suicide potential (Osgood 1988).

Antidepressants

In choosing a drug to treat depression in the elderly, primary emphasis should be placed on avoiding possible side effects rather than on efficacy. When starting therapy, low antidepressant dosages are generally recommended, with subsequent slow and gradual increases if needed.

The tricyclic antidepressants (TCAs) were prescribed for many years and continue to be used in the elderly. However, there has always been concern over their various side effects (depending on the nature of the compound). TCAs can cause orthostatic hypotension. Nortriptyline and doxepin are two drugs reported to have low orthostatic effects. TCAs can also increase urinary retention. Desipramine has been shown to produce fewer anticholinergic symptoms and should therefore be the drug of choice for the elderly male with prostatic hypertrophy. Medications with a high degree of sedation, such as doxepin, may be less desirable than desipramine or nortriptyline in the treatment of the elderly with coexisting symptoms of psychomotor retardation or hypersomnolence (Neshkes and Jarvik 1986).

Selective serotonin reuptake inhibitors (SSRIs), a newer category of antidepressants, were developed in the late 1980s. They have been found to be as effective as TCAs, but they have a more tolerable side effect profile and thus appear to be safer for use in the elderly (Lehne 1994; Reynolds 1994). Among the SSRIs on the market for antidepressant use are fluoxetine, paroxetine, and sertraline; other SSRIs are under development.

Generally, the elderly should be treated with lower doses of medication than is prescribed for the population at large. Such lower doses should be gradually increased if and when needed. As a rule, the starting dose should be fluoxetine, 5 mg; paroxetine, 10 mg; and sertraline, 25 mg. It should be noted that 5 mg of fluoxetine is available only in liquid form. Errors and overdosing can occur. Prescribing a 10-mg capsule for *every other day* would be a better alternative. Both fluoxetine and paroxetine can cause symptoms of central nervous system stimulation (e.g., increased awakenings, reduced time in rapid-eye-movement sleep, insomnia) (Lehne 1994). Age does not appear to effect the pharmacokinetics of sertraline. However, the metabolism of fluoxetine and paroxetine in the elderly is impaired, resulting in higher plasma levels (Young and Koda-Kimble 1995). This makes sertraline the preferred antidepressant among the SSRIs for the older population. Generally, SSRIs have lower potential for lethality and are therefore safer than TCAs in overdoses (Reynolds 1994).

The health care provider must realize the importance of the role of antidepressants in treating depression in the elderly. Awareness of their side-effect profile will enable the prescriber to choose the most suitable antidepressant and will help the client comply in long-term treatment. This should result in a reduced suicide rate.

Social networks to reduce suicide potential have not been as successful among older adults as they have been for younger persons (Ebersole and Hess 1990). The elderly with suicidal tendencies infrequently seek help; they have difficulty admitting that they have a weakness. They may be reluctant to turn to others because of the ethical and moral stigma of suicide and suicidal ideation, or the social embarrassment of psychiatric illness. Instead of looking for assistance from the mental health professional, the suicidal geriatric client would rather go to the primary care provider and complain of depressive or somatic manifestations. Primary care providers must therefore acquire sensitive assessment skills for suicidal risk and be knowledgeable about methods of intervention (Boxwell 1988).

Alcoholism

Alcoholism is a significant problem for the older population. More than 10% of all older Americans in the community at large, and 20% of elders who are hospitalized, have serious problems with alcohol (Ebersole and Hess 1994; Ostrander 1992). Unfortunately, most (85%) receive no treatment for this (Parette et al. 1990). There are two major types of abusers: (1) the early-onset alcoholic or "aging alcoholic" and (2) the late-onset alcoholic or "geriatric problem drinker." The aging alcoholic has generally had alcohol problems intermittently throughout life, with a regular alcohol-abuse pattern starting to evolve in late middle age or later. The geriatric problem drinker, on the other hand, has no history of alcohol-related problems but develops an alcohol-abuse pattern in response to the stresses of aging (Egbert 1993; Johnson 1989).

The stressful, or "reactive," factors that precipitate late-onset alcohol abuse are often caused by environmental conditions that may include retirement, widowhood, and loneliness. These stressors in the older adult, who may have retired, may not drive, and may be isolated from family and friends, are often greater than the problems faced by the middle-aged adult, who has to manage a job or career and care for a family and household. Work and family responsibilities may help keep a potential alcoholic from drinking too much. Once these demands are gone and the structure of daily life is disrupted, there is little impetus to remain sober. Older adults who lose a spouse through death, divorce, or legal separation are at the highest risk of becoming late-in-life alcoholics (Kashka and Tweed 1995; Brody 1988).

Alcohol abuse in the elderly may be difficult to identify. This applies in particular when a person is no longer in the familiar surroundings of work or when relatives, family members, friends, and employers are not available to notice changes in behavior and personality attributable to abuse.

Alcohol and Aging

Excessive consumption of alcohol can create particular problems for the elderly. The older adult has an increased biological sensitivity to, or conversely a decreased tolerance for, the effects of alcohol. This diminished resistance, combined with age-related changes such as weakened manual dexterity, balance, and postural flexibility, can increase the likelihood of falls, burns, or other accidents (Valanis et al. 1987).

Some drinkers, as they get older, note changes in their response to alcohol, such as headaches, reduced mental abilities with memory losses or lapses, and feelings of malaise rather than well-being. These problems start to occur at lower levels of consumption than was the case in earlier years. Older persons are likely to drink more frequently but in lesser quantities than younger individuals, who tend to drink larger amounts less often (Gomberg 1980). Thus, the possibility of alcohol abuse in cases of only moderate ingestion by the elderly is not often recognized by the alcoholic's friends or family.

With aging, the body becomes less resilient; healing from injury or infection is slower, and stress is more likely to cause a loss of physiological equilibrium. As the proportion of fatty tissues to lean body mass increases with age, the individual's metabolic rate usually slows down, increasing the amount of time it takes the body to eliminate drugs (Parette et al. 1990).

Alcohol and Medication

The interaction of drugs and alcohol in the elderly can have serious consequences. There is a decreased functioning of the liver enzymes that break down the alcohol, which on a short-term basis has the effect of prolonging the action of many medications, potentiating their effect. On the other hand, chronic ingestion of alcohol enhances the metabolism of many drugs by causing faster turnover of medication.

Older individuals can expect higher blood alcohol levels than younger persons for an equivalent intake of alcohol (Cavanaugh 1993). The effects of alcohol on the brain may be one reason that alcohol abuse sometimes mimics or exacerbates normal changes of aging, because even a moderate intake of alcohol can impair the cognition and coordination skills that are already decreased with age.

Extreme care is required when treating the older alcoholic with medication. Toxicity in the central nervous system from psychoactive drugs increases with aging. Ingestion of antidepressants or tranquilizers can be particularly harmful because their effect is further potentiated by alcohol. The toxicity of other drugs (e.g., acetaminophen) is enhanced by alcohol and by the decrease in age-related clearance (Egbert 1993). The therapeutic use of disulfiram (Antabuse) causes psychological and physiological reactions when alcohol is drunk. This agent is not recommended for the elderly, because many are physically unable to handle these reactions (Lamy 1988). Disulfiram may also cause cardiovascular side effects in older persons.

Alcohol consumption produces a change in sleep patterns, particularly in older adults. Unlike younger persons, the elderly take longer to fall asleep and do not sleep as restfully. Although alcohol may decrease the time it takes to fall asleep, this benefit is offset by frequent awakenings during the night caused by alcohol.

Symptoms of Alcohol Dependence

Health practitioners working with the elderly need to be concerned with, and sensitive to, possible alcohol abuse among their older clients. Signs of alcohol abuse in younger individuals (e.g., alcohol-induced pancreatitis or liver disease, blackouts, major trauma) occur infrequently in older adults. Instead, the elder alcoholic displays vague "geriatric syndromes" of contusions, malnutrition, self-neglect, depression, and falls. Also present may be symptoms of diarrhea, urinary incontinence, a decrease in functional status, "failure to thrive," and apparent dementia (Egbert 1993). Symptoms of poor coordination or visual changes may also mimic the normal aging process while actually being due to excessive drinking. Although confusion and disorientation in an older client is often associated with dementia or Alzheimer's disease, it could be caused by other factors, including alcohol abuse. Assessment of the conditions is necessary to differentiate the normal physiological changes of aging from those due to excessive drinking.

Treatment for the Elderly Alcoholic

Because many elderly people do not live in big families or have work-related contacts, they are less likely to be referred for treatment than are younger drinkers. Too often, by the time the elderly alcoholic comes to the notice of any treatment agencies, the client's support systems and resources are severely decreased or depleted. Declining social, physical, and psychological performances are frequently found in the elderly alcoholic, thus exacerbating the difficulties of loneliness, depression, monotony, accidents, social conflict, loss, and the physiological changes of aging (Burns 1988).

Ageism has deterred the development of treatment programs specially designed for the elderly. Beliefs about the elderly as being too isolated, too embedded in denial of their illness, and too old to function have been detrimental in encouraging health professionals to work with chemically dependent seniors (Lindblom et al. 1992). Another factor that may play a role is that older adults often try to hide alcohol dependence because they consider such abuse sinful or feel they can handle any problems themselves (Ebersole and Hess 1994).

Whenever there is a suspicion or indication that an older adult is abusing alcohol, the health care provider should conduct a screening test. Although commonly used screening tests for alcohol abuse focused on younger individuals, there is now a screening test designed specifically for older patients. This test (MAST-G), which consists of 24 questions and is the geriatric version of the Michigan Alcohol Screening Test (MAST), gives the health care provider a more efficient instrument to assess the elderly (Alcoholism 1993).

Treatment plans for the elderly problem drinker should emphasize social therapies. Elderly alcoholics tend to be more passive than younger alcoholics and may benefit from interpersonal involvement with professional health care personnel. Old people respond easily to emotional and social support (Gulino and Kadin 1986). Family therapy should be encouraged. Group therapy made up of middle-aged and older alcoholics can also be effective.

The older alcoholic who does seek help may be confronted with serious gaps and inadequacies in the health care delivery system (Gulino and Kadin 1986). Substance abuse counselors must therefore be in contact with other agencies providing services to the elderly so that their help can be coordinated. They should be cognizant of the financial and transportation abilities of their elderly clients.

The aging alcoholic is difficult to treat. On the other hand, the prognosis for the geriatric problem drinker—a person who had lived to this point without recourse to alcohol and whose drinking is caused by losses and stress—is excellent. It is important that health care providers recognize this recovery potential. Proper education and awareness of a positive outcome for the geriatric problem drinker could increase the availability of resources; if the prognosis is good, providers and agencies should be more willing to spend resources on treatment. This is valuable knowledge to share with the older client, because restorative outcome is so frequently a self-fulfilling prediction.

Among health care providers, nurses above all are in an excellent position to assess and recognize elderly clients with alcoholic problems, and they can educate the problem drinkers and their families, physicians, and emergency room and other health personnel. It is important for both older persons and practitioners in aging to realize that society's attitudes play a big role in determining how well older people recover. The myths that surround aging become entanglements for alcoholics: they are considered too old to change or are deemed to have earned the right to be left alone to do what they want (Ostrander 1992). The health care provider can overcome these myths by taking an affirmative position that the client, particularly the geriatric problem drinker, can still effectively function and become an active participant in society.

Considering the magnitude of the problems and the likelihood that the numbers of older abusers will continue to increase, efforts need to be intensified to identify the causes and to develop appropriate interventions for treating alcohol dependence among the elderly. If not, such dependence can overwhelm those charged with meeting the health and social service needs of older adults (Parette et al. 1990).

SUMMARY

There are a number of issues that older adults face as they age, and many myths exist that foster negative attitudes. Ageism is found in all levels of society and even among health care providers, thereby affecting the way we render care to our elderly clients.

Nurses who care for the elderly in various settings may function at various levels, such as generalist, nurse practitioner, or clinical specialist in gerontological nursing. All should be knowledgeable about the process of aging and be cognizant of the differences between normal and abnormal aging changes. Nurses working with the mentally ill elderly client should also know about psychotherapeutic approaches to the elderly. Nurses with special training and education may lead remotivation, reminiscing, or psychotherapy groups geared toward the special needs of this population.

Older adults face increasing problems of alcohol and suicide. The OBRA (Omnibus Budget Reconciliation Act) sets guidelines and a philosophy of care for clients to be free from unnecessary drugs and physical restraints. When it comes to dying and death, older adults' wishes and those of their families are frequently ignored. The implementation of the PSDA (Patient Self-Determination Act) of 1990 can afford some clients autonomy and dignity in death.

REFERENCES

Adelson, R., et al. (1982). Behavioral ratings of health professionals' interactions with the geriatric patient. *Gerontologist*, 22(3):227.

Alcoholism (1993). New test designed to screen older patients. *Geriatrics*, 48(4):14.

Alford, D. (1986). *Managing ethical and legal dilemmas in the care of the elderly*. Presentation at Current Directions in Gerontological Nursing, Bethesda, MD.

Atchley, R. (1994). *Social forces and aging*. Belmont, CA: Wadsworth.

Blakeslee, J. A., et al. (1991). Making the transition to restraint-free care. *Journal of Gerontological Nursing*, 17(2):4.

Blazer, D., et al. (1986). Suicide in late life: Review and commentary. *Journal of the American Geriatrics Society*, 34:519.

Boxwell, A. (1988). Geriatric suicide: The preventable death. *Nurse Practitioner*, 13(6):10.

Boyle, L. (1992). Legal implications of the Patient Self-Determination Act. *Nurse Practitioner Forum*, 3(1):12.

Brody, J. (1988). Personal health—The reality of elderly alcoholics and acting to help them. *New York Times*, May 12:B6.

Brower, H. T. (1991). The alternatives to restraints. *Journal of Gerontological Nursing*, 17(2):18.

Buckwalter, K., et al. (1995). Community programs. In M. Hogstel (Ed.), *Geropsychiatric nursing*. St. Louis: Mosby–Year Book.

Bureau of the Census (1995). *Sixty-Five Plus in the United States*. Statistical brief. Washington, DC: U. S. Department of Commerce, Economics, and Statistics Administration.

Burggraf, V., and Stanley, M. (1989). *Nursing the elderly: A care plan approach*. Philadelphia: J. B. Lippincott.

Burke, M., and Walsh, M. (1992). *Gerontologic nursing care of the frail elderly*. St. Louis: Mosby–Year Book.

Burns, B. (1988). Treating recovering alcoholics. *Journal of Gerontological Nursing*, 14(4):18.

Burnside, I. (1988). *Nursing and the aged. A self-care approach*. New York: McGraw-Hill.

Butler, R. (1975). *Why survive? Being old in America*. New York: Harper & Row.

Butler, R., et al. (1991). *Aging and mental health*. New York: Macmillan.

Cadieux, R. (1993). Geriatric psychopharmacology. *Postgraduate Medicine*, 93(4):281.

Caserta, J. (1983). Public policy for long term care. *Geriatric Nursing*, 4(4):244.

Catina, J., et al. (1989). Older Americans and AIDS. Transmission, risks and primary prevention. *Gerontologist* 29(3):373.

Cavanaugh, J. (Ed.)(1993). *Health, adult development and aging.* Belmont, CA: Brooks Cole.

Centers for Disease Control (CDC) (1993). HIV/AIDS Surveillance Report. Atlanta, GA: 5(2):8.

Courtenay, B., and Suharat, M. (1980). *Myths and realities of aging.* Athens, GA: University of Georgia, Georgia Center for Continuing Education.

Curtis, J., et al. (1995). Use of the medical futility rationale in do-not-attempt-resuscitation orders. *Journal of American Medical Society,* 273(2):124.

Ebersole, P., and Hess, P. (Eds.) (1990). *Toward healthy aging human needs and nursing response* (3rd ed.). St. Louis: Mosby–Year Book.

Ebersole, P., and Hess, P. (Eds.) (1994). *Toward healthy aging human needs and nursing response.* (4th ed.). St. Louis: Mosby–Year Book.

Edwards, B. (1995). Physicians won't provide "futile" care. *American Journal of Nursing,* 95(9):56.

Egbert, A. (1993). The older alcoholic: Recognizing the subtle clinical clues. *Geriatrics,* 48(7):63.

Elliot, B., and Hybertson, D. (1982). What is it about the elderly that elicits a negative response? *Journal of Gerontological Nursing,* 8(10):568.

Evans, L., and Strumpf, N. (1989). Tying down the elderly: A review of the literature on physical restraints. *Journal of the American Geriatrics Society,* 37(1):65.

Futility: The Concept and Its Use (1993). Northport Regional Medical Educational Center, National Center for Clinical Ethics. Northport, NY: Department of Veterans Affairs Medical Center.

Gadow, S. (1979). Advocacy nursing and new meanings of aging. *Nursing Clinics of North America,* 14:81.

Gobis, L. (1992). Recent developments in health care law relevant to health care providers. *Nurse Practitioner,* 17(3):77.

Goeber, B. (1996). Who decides if there is "triumph in the ultimate agony"? Constitutional theory and the emerging right to die with dignity. William and Mary Law Review, Winter 37;803.

Gomberg, E. (1980). Drinking and problem drinking among the elderly. Publication #1. *Alcohol, drugs, and aging: Usage and problems.* University of Michigan: Institute of Gerontology.

Gomez, G., et al. (1985). Beginning nursing students can change attitudes about the aged. *Journal of Gerontological Nursing,* 11(1):6.

Green, C. (1981). Fostering positive attitudes toward the elderly: A teaching strategy for attitude change. *Journal of Gerontological Nursing,* 7(3):169.

Gulino, C., and Kadin, M. (1986). Aging and reactive alcoholism. *Geriatric Nursing,* 7(3):148.

Harper, M. (1995). An overview of mental health. In M. Hogstel (Ed.), *Geropsychiatric nursing.* St. Louis: Mosby–Year Book.

Hogstel, M. (1990). *Geriatric nursing.* St. Louis: C.V. Mosby.

Hogstel, M. (1995). *Geropsychiatric nursing* (2nd ed.). St. Louis: Mosby–Year Book.

Horne, A., and Blazer, D. (1992) The prevention of major depression in the elderly. *Clinics in Geriatric Medicine,* 8(1):143.

Janofsky, J. (1990). Assessing competency in the elderly. *Geriatrics,* 45(10):45.

Janssen, J. A., and Giberson, D. L.(1988). Remotivation therapy. *Journal of Gerontological Nursing,* 14(6):31.

Jenike, M. (Ed.) (1984). Ethical considerations in the care of the hopelessly ill patient. *Topics in Geriatrics,* 3(4):13.

Johnson, L. (1989). How to diagnose and treat chemical dependency in the elderly. *Journal of Gerontological Nursing,* 15(12):22.

Kashka, M. S., and Tweed, S. H. (1995). Substance related disorders. In M. Hogstel (Ed.), *Geropsychiatric nursing.* St. Louis: Mosby–Year Book.

Kaufman, I. (1989). Life and death decisions. *New York Times,* October 6, 1989 p. 21.

Kleiman, D. (1985). Uncertainty clouds of dying. *New York Times,* January 18:B1.

Lamy, P. P. (1988). Actions of alcohol and drugs in older people. *Generations,* 12(4):9.

Lehne, R. (1994). *Pharmacology for nursing care.* Philadelphia: W. B. Saunders.

Lekan-Rutledge, D. (1988). Functional assessment. In M. A. Matteson and E. S. McConnell (Eds.), *Gerontological nursing: Concepts and practice.* Philadelphia: W. B. Saunders.

Lindblom, L., et al. (1992). Chemical abuse: An intervention program for the elderly. *Journal of Gerontological Nursing,* 18(4):6.

Linn, M. W., et al. (1969). A social dysfunction rating scale. *Journal of Psychiatric Research,* 6:299.

Loebel, J. P. (1991). Precipitants to elder suicide. *Journal of the American Geriatric Society* 39:407.

MacKay, S. (1992). Durable power of attorney for health care. *Geriatric Nursing,* 13(2):99.

Marshall, J. (1978). Changes in aged white male suicide: 1948–1972. *Gerontologist,* 33:763.

Masters, R., and Marks F. (1990). The use of restraints. *Rehabilitation Nursing,* 15(1):22.

Matteson, M. A., and McConnell, E. S. (1988). *Gerontological nursing: Concepts and practice.* Philadelphia: W. B. Saunders.

Matteson, M. A., McConnell, E. S., and Linton, A. D. (1997). *Gerontological nursing: Concepts and practices* (2nd ed.). Philadelphia: W. B. Saunders.

Matthews, S. (1979). *The social world of old women: Management of self-identity.* Sage Library of Social Research 78. Beverly Hills, CA: Sage Publications.

McCann, R., et al. (1994). Comfort care for terminally ill patients. *Journal of the American Medical Association,* 272(5):1263.

McIntosh, J. (1985). Suicide among the elderly: Levels and trends. *American Journal of Orthopsychiatry,* 55(2):287.

Moak, G. (1990). Improving quality in psychogeriatric treatment. *Psychiatric Clinics of North America,* 13(1):99.

Moody, H. (1994). *Aging concepts and controversies.* Thousand Oaks, CA: Pine Forge Press.

Moore, C. V. (1992). Self-determined advance directives: New issues in primary care. *Nurse Practitioner Forum,* 3(1):10.

Myers, R. (1994). Health legislation update. Restraint free environment for the elderly. *Ostomy Wound Management,* 40(19):12.

National Citizens' Coalition for Nursing Home Reform (1991). *Nursing home reform law: The basics.* Washington, DC: National Citizens' Coalition for Nursing Home Reform.

Nelson, L. (1982). Questions of age. Doctors debate right to stop "heroic" effort to keep elderly alive. *Wall Street Journal,* September 7:20.

Neshkes, R., and Jarvik, L. (1986). Depression in the elderly: Current management concepts. *Geriatrics,* 41(9):51.

Nikolassy, S. (1995). Nurses' role with the elderly in the community. In M. Stanley and P. Beare (Eds.), *Gerontological nursing.* Philadelphia: F. A. Davis.

Olson, M. (1997). *Healing the dying* (pp. 151–155). Albany, NY: Delmarr Publishers.

Osgood, N. (1988). Suicide in the elderly: Clues and prevention. Belle Mead, NJ: *Carrier Foundation Letter No. 133,* April 1988.

Ostrander, N. (1992). Alcoholism and aging—A rural community's response. *Aging Today,* February/March:19.

Palmore, E. (1979). Advantages of aging. *Gerontologist,* 17:220.

Parette, H., et al. (1990). Nursing attitudes toward geriatric alcoholism. *Journal of Gerontological Nursing,* 16(1):26.

Pfeiffer, E. (1978). Sexuality in the aging individual. In R. Solnick (Ed.), *Sexuality and aging.* CA: University of Southern California Press.

Pinch, W. J., and Parsons, M. E. (1992). The patient self-determination act. *Nurse Practitioner Forum,* 3(1):16.

Preston, T. (1986). Ageism undermines relations with elderly. *Medical World News,* December 8:26.

Printz, L. A. (1992). Terminal dehydration, a compassionate treatment. *Archives of Internal Medicine,* 152:697.

Reynolds, C. (1994). Treatment of depression in later life. *American Journal of Medicine,* 97(Suppl. 6A):395.

Richardson, R., Lowenstein, S., and Weissberg, M. (1989). Coping with the suicidal elderly: A physician's guide. *Geriatrics,* 44(9):43.

Ronsman, K. (1987). Therapy for depression. *Journal of Gerontological Nursing,* 13(12):18.

Rosenthal, E. (1991). Filling the gap where a living will won't do. *New York Times,* January 17:B9.

Ross, H. (1981). Society/cultural views regarding death and dying. *Topics in Clinical Nursing,* 3(3):3.

Sabin, J. D. (1987). AIDS: The new "great imitator." *Journal of American Geriatric Society,* 35(5):467.

Sapp, M., and Bliesmer, M. (1995). A health promotion/protection approach to meeting elders' health care needs through public policy and standards of care. In M. Stanley and P. Beare (Eds.), *Gerontological nursing.* Philadelphia: F. A. Davis.

Schlossberg, C., and Hart, M. A. (1992). Legal perspectives. In M. Burke and M. Walsh (Eds.), *Gerontologic nursing care of the frail elderly* (p. 469). St. Louis: Mosby–Year Book.

Schuerman, D. (1994). Clinical concerns. AIDS in the elderly. *Journal of Gerontological Nursing,* 20(7):11.

Shawler, C., et al. (1992). Clinical considerations: Surrogate decision making for hospitalized elders. *Journal of Gerontological Nursing,* 18(6):5.

Smith, D. (1992). Advance directive editorial. *Journal of Enterostomal Therapy,* 19(4):109.

Snow, R., and Atwood, K. (1985). Probable death: Perspectives of the elderly. *Southern Medical Journal,* 78:851.

Stanley, M., and Beare, P. (1995). *Gerontological nursing.* Philadelphia: F. A. Davis.

Steingart, A. (1991). Day programs. In J. Sadovoy et al. (Eds.), *Comprehensive review of psychiatry.* Washington, DC: Am Psychiatry Press.

Stilwell, E. M. (1991). Nurses' education related to the use of restraints. *Journal of Gerontological Nursing,* 17(2):23.

Stolley, J. (1995). Freeing your patients from restraints. *American Journal of Nursing,* 95(2):27.

Suicide Rate Among Elderly Rises, Study Says (1991). *New York Times,* September 19:A25.

SUPPORT Investigators (1995). A controlled trial to improve care for seriously ill hospitalized patients. *Journal of American Medical Association,* 27(20):1591.

Taylor, M. (1995). Benefits of dehydration in terminally ill patients. *Geriatric Nursing,* 16(6): 271.

Tolchin, M. (1989). When long life is too much: Suicide rises among elderly. *New York Times,* July 19:A15.

USDHSS (1990). United States Department of Health and Human Services National Institute on Aging: Special Report on Aging 1990. National Institute of Health. Public Health Service. Bethesda, MD: Government Printing Office.

Valanis, D., et al. (1987). Alcohol use among bereaved and non-bereaved older persons. *Journal of Gerontological Nursing,* 13(5):26.

Virmani, L., et al. (1994). Relationship of advance directives to physician-patient communication. *Archives of Internal Medicine,* 154:909.

Wallace, R., et al. (1993). HIV infection in older patients: When to expect the unexpected. *Geriatrics* 48(6):61.

Wallis, C. (1986). To feed or not to feed? *Time*, March 31:60.
Walsh, M. (1992). The frail elderly population. In M. Burke and M. Walsh (Eds.), *Gerontologic nursing care of the frail elderly*. St. Louis: Mosby–Year Book,
Young, L., and Koda-Kimble, M. (1995). *Applied therapeutics: The clinical use of drug*. Vancouver, WA: Applied Therapeutics.
Zerwekh, J. (1993). Dehydration: A natural analgesic when death is imminent. *Critical Care Specialist*, 1(1):3.
Zung, W. K. (1965). A self-rating depression scale. *Archives of General Psychiatry*, 12:63.

FURTHER READING

American Medical Association (1995). A controlled trial to improve care for seriously ill hospitalized patients. *Journal of the American Medical Association*, 274(20):1591.
Brant, B., and Osgood, N. (1990). The suicidal patient in long-term care institutions. *Journal of Gerontological Nursing*, 16(2):17.
Burke, M., and Walsh, M. (1992).*Gerontologic nursing care of the frail elderly*. St. Louis: Mosby–Year Book.
Ebersole, P., and Hess, P. (Eds.) (1994). *Toward healthy aging human needs and nursing response*. St. Louis: Mosby–Year Book.
Hogstel, M. (1995). *Geropsychiatric nursing*. St. Louis: Mosby–Year Book.
Mellick, E. (1990). Suicide in elderly white men: Development of a profile. Unpublished Master's Thesis. Iowa City: University of Iowa.
Scharnhorst, S. (1992). AIDS dementia complex in the elderly. *Nurse Practitioner*, 17(8):41.

SELF-STUDY AND CRITICAL THINKING

True or false

Place T (true) or F (false) next to each statement. Correct the false statement.

1. ________ The elderly are prone to be crime victims.
2. ________ "Ageism" reflects society's positive view of the elderly.
3. ________ Older adults are able to learn new tasks.
4. ________ Most elderly people are infirm and require help with daily activities.

Matching questions

Match the type of group: R (remotivational), REM (reminiscing), and P (psychotherapy)-with the following descriptions:

5. ________ Shares memories of past events and helps increase esteem and socialization.
6. ________ Can help resocialize regressed and apathetic clients. Structured setting with set agenda.
7. ________ Problems are discussed among people with similar problems; aim is to relieve psychiatric symptoms and solidify functioning.

True or false

Place T (true) or F (false) next to each statement. Correct all false statements.

8. ________ Alcohol provides a beneficial night's sleep.
9. ________ Alcohol effects can mimic the normal changes of aging.
10. ________ Alcohol exacerbates all chronic conditions.
11. ________ Residents in restraint-free facilities experience fewer injuries from falls than those in facilities using restraints.
12. ________ Chemical restraints are devices that inhibit free movement.
13. ________ If restraints are used, the written order of the physician need only specify the duration of their use.

14. __________ The PSDA was passed to assist physicians in making health care decisions about their patients.

15. __________ A living will, a directive to physician, and a durable power of attorney for health care are all forms of advance heath care directives.

16. __________ Among the elderly, the white male has the highest suicide rate.

17. __________ Guns are the most common means of suicide used by the elderly.

18. __________ Acute illnesses are the major threat to an older person's health.

19. __________ Ageism is a bias against older people based on their age.

20. Restraining the elderly is a serious matter. Restraints have led to injuries and even death by strangulation and asphyxiation. Which is the *least* severe consequence of restraining an elderly client?

    A. Reduced or impaired circulation
    B. Reduction in socialization
    C. Loss of bone mass
    D. Muscle atrophy

21. Following OBRA's guidelines, JCAHO stipulates as a basis for physical restraints the following:

    A. They can be used for indefinite periods.
    B. No physician's order is needed.
    C. Documentation of alternative approaches is required before restraints are applied.
    D. Once-a-week observation and assessment of the client.

22. Which statement best describes the hospice philosophy?

    A. Death is a natural conclusion to life, with clients rather than health care providers making the decisions how they want to live and die.
    B. Death takes place in an institution where trained personnel know when the client's time to die has arrived.
    C. Clients turn over to family members the decision of when the client should die.
    D. Death takes place in the community in a setting that clients visit during the day and where they are given excellent nursing care.

23. Each institution should have a written policy on "coding" and all nurses need to be cognizant of their state laws. One true statement regarding the nurse's role in decision making is:

    A. When the nurse becomes aware that the physician is not following the client's advance directive, the nurse should let it drop.
    B. Making decisions regarding the treatment of an incapacitated client is relatively easy and usually clear-cut.
    C. If no living will exists, there is not much that health care professionals can use as a guide for making a decision.
    D. A nurse should never accept a verbal "no-code" order from a physician.

Critical thinking

24. Teach a classmate about alcohol and the elderly. Cover the following:

    A. Discuss the two types of elderly alcohol abuse.
    B. Describe how and why alcohol performs differently in the aged.
    C. Explain the interaction of alcohol and medication in the elderly.
    D. What might you and your classmate assess in your practice for an elderly person with alcohol problems?
    E. Discuss some of the unique considerations when treating elderly clients for alcohol abuse.

25. Mr. Simon, age 85, lives with his family. He has advanced Alzheimer's disease and often has short-lived angry outbursts. Mr. Simon's family wants to keep him at home for as long as possible, but they are overwhelmed with his constant needs. Many well-meaning relatives have suggested that he be placed in a nursing home on a unit specifically designed for Alzheimer's clients.

    Which of the following community placements might be best for Mr. Simon? Explain why.
    A. Social day care
    B. Adult day health (medical model)
    C. Maintenance day care
    D. Community mental health clinic

    Give at least four nursing diagnoses that would be appropriate for Mr. Simon:
    A. ______________________________
    B. ______________________________
    C. ______________________________
    D. ______________________________

    Give at least one nursing diagnosis that would be appropriate for the family:

    ____

    A. From your readings, discuss the different community placements possible for a person with Alzheimer's disease and choose the one you think best for Mr. Simon. Explain your choice.
    B. Identify four main concerns for care you would have for Mr. Simon and state them in the form of a complete nursing diagnosis.
    C. What are some needs of Mr. Simon's family? Identify three possible resources from which a family such as Mr. Simon's would benefit.

TABLE 31–1A ANSWERS: QUIZ: FACTS AND MYTHS OF AGING

1. **False.** 90% of older adults possess a healthy mental ability, 5% exhibit symptoms of chronic mental dysfunction, and another 5% display signs of acute mental impairment (Ebersole and Hess 1994: Courtenay and Suharat 1980).
2. **True.** All the senses decrease with aging. Many of the changes begin slowly when the individual is in his or her mid-forties and increase with aging. (1) Vision: Particularly affected are peripheral vision, visual acuity, adaptation to dark, and accommodation (presbyopia). (2) Hearing: Decreased ability to hear high-frequency sounds with later changes possibly involving middle- and low-frequency sounds (presbycusis); males tend to show hearing loss earlier than women. (3) Taste: The number of functioning taste buds is reduced, which particularly affects the ability to taste sweet and salty flavors. (4) Touch: Simultaneously occurring with age are the loss of receptors and an increased threshold for stimulation; pain and pressure are thus not as easily sensed. (5) Smell: A decline in the number of fibers in the olfactory nerve has been reported, leading to speculation that smell also undergoes age-related changes.
3. **True.** As one ages, muscle fibers atrophy and decrease in number, with fibrous tissue slowly displacing muscle tissue. Overall muscle mass, muscle strength, and muscle movements decrease. The arm and leg muscles, which become particularly flabby and weak, also show these changes. Exercise is important to minimize the loss of muscle tone and strength.
4. **False.** Sexual interest and activity continue to play a pivotal role in providing life satisfaction (Atchley 1994).
5. **True.** Masters and Johnson, in their work on human sexuality, found that regular sexual expressions in the older adult are important for maintained sexual capacity and effective sexual performance (Atchley 1994).
6. **True.** Changes in sleep patterns occur along the entire life span. Restorative sleep declines rapidly with aging and by age 50 is reduced by 50%. It takes the elderly more time to achieve restorative sleep than younger adults, and also with aging, sleep is less effective (Burke and Walsh 1992).
7. **True.** Making up 13% of the population, the elderly accounted for more than 25% of all prescription drugs sold. This is not surprising, since the incidence of chronic diseases among the elderly is high and prescription drugs are often used with chronic disease (Cadieux 1993; Census Bureau 65 Plus in the U.S. 1995).
8. **False.** All age groups can learn. Limited, of course, by any physical limitations, older adults can usually master anything others can do if allowed a little more time. Jobs involving manipulation of objects or symbols or requiring discrete and clear responses are particularly well performed by older people (Atchley 1994; Burggraf and Stanley 1989).
9. **True.** Clinical depressive disorders increase in both prevalence and intensity with age. They may be called the "common cold" of the elderly and are expected to further increase in the years ahead (Ebersole and Hess 1990).
10. **False.** The ability to change and adapt has little to do with one's age but more with one's character.
11. **False.** Although a small number of aged are very well off and many are moderately comfortable, a large segment remains poor. According to government statistics, 12% of older adults live in poverty (Burke and Walsh 1992).
12. **True.** One out of three retirees encounters difficulty adjusting to retirement. Adapting to a diminished income and no longer being in a job-related environment were two of the most frequently listed causes of difficulty (Atchley 1994).
13. **True.** Senior citizens make up 13% of the population but constitute about 30% of the victims of crime. Business and investment frauds rank high on the list of white-collar crimes perpetrated against the elderly. Aged widows are particularly vulnerable (Ebersole and Hess 1994).
14. **False.** Eighty percent of older adults are healthy enough to carry on their normal life styles; 15% have chronic health conditions interfering with their lives; about 5% are institutionalized (Ebersole and Hess 1990).
15. **True.** Older persons are more reliable workers; their accuracy, performance, and stability are better; and the number of accidents is lower except in situations requiring rapid reaction time (Palmore 1979).
16. **False.** Most elderly have relatives, friends, and organizations that are significant to them. About two thirds do not consider loneliness a problem (Ebersole and Hess 1990).
17. **False.** Medicaid is a federally assisted, state-administered program that provides health care benefits to low-income persons. Medicare, on the other hand, provides health insurance basically to individuals 65 and over.
18. **False.** The term *ageism* reflects the negative prejudicial views of older people that pervade our youth-oriented society.
19. **True.** Nearly twice as many widowers wed annually as widows in spite of the fact that older widows outnumber older widowers four times. In addition, half of those widowers who do remarry choose wives under 65 years of age (Atchley 1994).
20. **True.** Sociologists have found that, for the older widow, widowhood is viewed as ordinary with supports available from family, friends, and the community. The younger widow, however, is viewed differently; widowhood is not a normal occurrence. Young women are permitted to play the widow role for only a brief time and are considered to be single rather than widowed. Because they are in the minority, these women feel stigmatized by widowhood. The younger the widow, the more problems she encounters (Atchley 1994).

APPENDIX A

Summary of Contributions to Psychiatric and Mental Health Nursing

SUMMARY OF CONTRIBUTIONS TO PSYCHIATRIC AND MENTAL HEALTH NURSING

PSYCHIATRIC NURSING LEADER	CONTRIBUTION
PRE-1860	
—	Nursing care for the young, ill, and helpless historically has existed as long as the human race. Care was given by family members, relatives, servants, neighbors, members of religious orders or humanitarian societies, or by convalescing patients or prisoners.
1860	
Florence Nightingale	Established Nightingale School at St. Thomas Hospital in London after Crimean War and worked with untrained women caring for soldiers. *Founder of modern-day nursing.*
1860–1880	
—	Emphasized maintaining healthful environment, personal hygiene, cleanliness, and healthful living habits, such as adequate nutrition, exercise, and sleep so that nature could heal. Emphasized kindness toward patients along with custodial care.
Linda Richards	*First graduate nurse and first psychiatric nurse in the United States.* After study under Miss Nightingale, organized nursing services and educational programs in Boston City Hospital and in several state mental hospitals in Illinois.
Dorothea Dix	*Worked to reform psychiatric care in mental hospitals* and to correct overcrowding and the insufficient number of physicians and attendants.
1882	
—	First school to prepare nurses to care for acutely and chronically mentally ill opened at McLean Hospital, Waverly, Massachusetts, through collaboration of Linda Richards and Dr. Edward Cowles.

SUMMARY OF CONTRIBUTIONS TO PSYCHIATRIC AND MENTAL HEALTH NURSING CONTINUED

PSYCHIATRIC NURSING LEADER	CONTRIBUTION
1890–1930	
—	Nurses recognized by some administrative psychiatrists in state and private hospitals for their preparation. Nurses relieved of menial housekeeping chores to engage in physical custodial care of patients. Role primarily to assist physician or carry out procedures for physical care. Few psychological nursing skills. Psychologically concerned with maintaining kind, tolerant attitude and humane treatment.
1920	
Harriet Bailey	*First nurse educator to write a psychiatric nursing text, Nursing Mental Disease,* 1920. She wrote of the importance of a nurse's knowing mental illness and of teaching mental health nursing, and she worked for student experiences in psychiatry. She argued for more holistic care of patients.
1937	
—	The incorporation of psychiatric nursing was recommended by the National League for Nursing for inclusion in basic nursing curriculum.
1946	
—	National Mental Health Act passed, authorizing establishment of National Institute of Mental Health, with funds and programs to train professional psychiatric personnel, conduct psychiatric research, and aid in development of mental health programs at the state level. Provided impetus for psychiatric nursing as a specialty.
1950–1960	
—	Nurse's role included physical care and medications and maintenance of therapeutic milieu. Less emphasis on physical restraints.
Ruth Matheney Mary Topalis	Emphasized importance of milieu therapy and the nurse's using this intervention.
1952	
Hildegard E. Peplau	*Formulated first systematic theoretical framework in psychiatric nursing; presented in Interpersonal Relations in Nursing,* 1952. Emphasized that nursing is an interpersonal process and that psychological techniques and theoretical concepts are essential to nursing practice. Emphasized steps in nurse-patient relationship: 1. Nurse helps patient examine situational factors through observation of behavior. 2. Nurse helps patient describe and analyze behavior. 3. Nurse formulates with patient connections between feelings and behavior. 4. Nurse encourages patient to improve interpersonal competence through testing new behavior. 5. Nurse validates with patient when new behavior is integrated into personality structure. Psychoanalytical, interpersonal, and communication theories used by nurses.

Continued on following page

SUMMARY OF CONTRIBUTIONS TO PSYCHIATRIC AND MENTAL HEALTH NURSING CONTINUED

PSYCHIATRIC NURSING LEADER	CONTRIBUTION
1953	
—	*The Therapeutic Community*, by Maxwell Jones in Great Britain, laid basis for movement in United States toward therapeutic milieu and nurse's role in this therapy.
1956	
—	National Conference on Graduate Education in Psychiatric Nursing introduced concept of psychiatric clinical nurse specialist. Theoreticians begin to differentiate functions based on master's level of preparation in nursing.
1957	
June Mellow	*Introduced second theoretical approach to psychiatric nursing, called Nursing Therapy*, using psychoanalytical theory in one-to-one approach with schizophrenic patient. *Emphasized providing corrective emotional experience rather than investigating pathological processes or interpersonal developmental processes in order to facilitate integration of overwhelmed ego.*
1958	
—	American Nurses' Association established Conference Group on Psychiatric Nursing.
1959	
—	Accredited schools of nursing had to have own psychiatric nursing curriculum and instructor, per National League for Nursing. Could no longer buy services of hospitals to supply education.
1960–1970	
Hildegard E. Peplau Gertrude Ujhely Joyce Travelbee Shirley Burd Loretta Bermosk Joyce Hays Catherine Norris Gertrude Stokes Anne Hargreaves Dorothy Gregg Sheila Rouslin	Nursing leaders emphasized importance of self-awareness and use of self, nurse-patient relationships therapy, therapeutic communication, and psychosocial aspects of general nursing. Peplau formulated the manifestations of anxiety and steps in anxiety intervention, now used by all health care professions. All of these nursing leaders developed various psychological concepts into operational definitions for use in nursing.
1960	
Ida Orlando	*Initiated term* nursing process *and began to delineate its components.* Presented general theoretical framework for all nurse-patient relationships, with focus on client ascertaining meaning of behavior and explaining help needed. Wrote the classic book *The Dynamic Nurse-Patient Relationship*, 1961.
—	Comprehensive Community Mental Health Act passed, 1960; provided impetus for nurses moving from hospital to community setting.

SUMMARY OF CONTRIBUTIONS TO PSYCHIATRIC AND MENTAL HEALTH NURSING CONTINUED

PSYCHIATRIC NURSING LEADER	CONTRIBUTION
1961	
Anne Burgess Donna Aguilera	Engaged in crisis work and short term therapy as well as in long term therapy. *Applied crisis theory to psychiatric nursing.*
Hildegard E. Peplau	Promoted *primary role of nurse as psychotherapist or counselor* rather than as mother surrogate, socializer, or manager.
1960–65	
Sheila Rouslin Suzanne Lego	Opened private practices in psychotherapy.
1967	
—	American Nurses' Association presented Position Paper on Psychiatric Nursing, endorsing role of clinical specialist as therapist in individual, group, family, and milieu therapies.
—	American Nurses' Association, Division in Psychiatric and Mental Health Nursing Practice published first *Statement on Psychiatric Nursing Practice.*
1970–1980	
Sheila Rouslin	*Certification of clinical specialists in psychiatric nursing begun* by Division of Psychiatric Mental Health Nursing, New Jersey State Nurses' Association, *because of her leadership.* Later, certification developed by American Nurses' Association.
Shirley Smoyak	*Client defined as individual, group, family, or community;* nurse defined as family therapist. Expanding role of psychiatric nurse.
Gwen Marram Irene Burnside	*Group and family psychotherapy by graduate-prepared nurses* emphasized by nursing leaders.
Carolyn Clark	*Systems framework was used increasingly* by psychiatric nurses.
—	Change agent, health maintenance, and research roles emphasized in latter half of decade.
Bonnie Bullough	*Legal and ethical aspects of psychiatric care emphasized.*
Madeleine Leininger	*Care of whole person reemphasized. Introduced implications of cultural diversity for mental health services and psychiatric treatment.*
Hector Gonzales Doris Mosley Paulette D'Angi	Practice as autonomous member of team and in independent or private practice increased in latter half of decade. Work with citizens, consumer groups, and consumer organizations increased toward end of decade.
1976	
—	American Nurses' Association Division of Psychiatric and Mental Health Nursing Practice published revised *Statement on Psychiatric and Mental Health Nursing Practice.*

Continued on following page

SUMMARY OF CONTRIBUTIONS TO PSYCHIATRIC AND MENTAL HEALTH NURSING CONTINUED

PSYCHIATRIC NURSING LEADER	CONTRIBUTION
1978	
—	President's Commission Report of 1978 concluded that effects of deinstitutionalization and discharge of patients to community facilities have not worked as expected because of lack of financial, social, medical, and nursing resources and lack of coordination of services.
1980s	
Anne Burgess	*Formulated theory of victimology*, based on extensive studies of adult and child victims of rape and abuse, child victims of neglect, and family violence of incest and battering. *Described rape trauma syndrome, silent rape trauma, and compounded reactions to rape.*
Lee Ann Hoff	*Expanded crisis theory to be used in nursing practice. Contributed to theory of suicidology.* Described battering syndrome after research on battered women and battered elderly.
1982	
—	American Nurses' Association Executive Committee and Standards Committee, Division of Psychiatric and Mental Health Nursing Practice, published *Standards of Psychiatric and Mental Health Nursing Practice.*
1987	
Maxine E. Loomis Anita W. O'Toole Marie Scott Brown Patricia Pothier Patricia West Holly S. Wilson	Began the development of a classification system for Psychiatric and Mental Health Nursing, first published in *Archives of Psychiatric Nursing*, 1(1):16–24, 1987, a new Journal
1994	
Carolyn V. Billings Jean Blackburn Mickie Ceimone Carol Dashiff Kathleen Scharer Anita O'Toole Carole A. Shea	Comprised a Task Force to: • Revise: *A statement on psychiatric–mental health clinical nursing practice* updating the scope and functions for nurses certified at the basic level and those certified at the Advanced Practice level. • Revise: *Standards of psychiatric–mental health clinical nursing practice* describes professional nursing activities that are demonstrated by the nurse through the nursing process for both the Basic Level Certified Psychiatric Nurse and the Advanced Practice Psychiatric Nurse, and *Standards of professional performance.*

Adapted from Murray RB. The nursing process and emotional care. *In* Murray RB, Huelskoetter MMW (eds). Psychiatric Mental Health Nursing—Giving Emotional Care, 3rd ed. Norwalk, CT: Appleton & Lange, 1991, pp 94–97.

APPENDIX B

Psychiatric and Other Nursing Organizations

The American Nurses' Association comprises ANA itself, its 53 constituent state members, three subsidiary organizations, and 13 organizational affiliate members. In addition, ANA established the Nursing Organization Liaison Forum (NOLF), which comprises more than 70 national nursing organizations and serves as a platform for addressing important issues that affect nursing and health care in general.

For more information go to http://www.nursingworld.org/affiil.html

ANA SUBSIDIARIES

- American Academy of Nursing
- American Nurses Credentialing Center
- American Nurses Foundation

ORGANIZATIONAL AFFILIATES

- American Academy of Ambulatory Care Nursing
- American Association of Critical-Care Nurses
- American Association of Nurse Anesthetists
- American Holistic Nurses Association
- American Psychiatric Nurses Association
- American Society of PeriAnesthesia Nurses (ASPAN)
- Association of Operating Room Nurses
- Association of Rehabilitation Nurses
- Association of Women's Health, Obstetric & Neonatal Nurses
- Emergency Nurses Association
- National Association of Orthopaedic Nurses
- National Association of School Nurses, Inc.
- Oncology Nursing Society

NURSING ORGANIZATION LIAISON FORUM (NOLF)

- Academy of Medical-Surgical Nurses
- American Academy of Ambulatory Care Nursing*
- American Assembly for Men in Nursing
- American Association for Continuity of Care
- American Association of Critical-Care Nurses*
- American Association of Neuroscience Nurses
- American Association of Nurse Anesthetists*
- American Association of Nurse Attorneys
- American Association of Occupational Health Nurses
- American Association of Spinal Cord Injury Nurses
- American Heart Association Council on Cardiovascular Nursing
- American Holistic Nurses Association*
- American Medical Informatics Association
- American Nephrology Nurses Association
- American Psychiatric Nurses Association*
- American Public Health Association
- American Radiological Nurses Association
- American Society for Parenteral and Enteral Nutrition
- American Society of Ophthalmic Registered Nurses, Inc.
- American Society of Plastic and Reconstructive Surgical Nurses, Inc.
- American Society of PeriAnesthesia Nurses (ASPAN)*
- American Thoracic Society
- Association for Child & Adolescent Psychiatric Nurses, Inc.
- Association of Black Nursing Faculty in Higher Education, Inc.
- Association of Community Health Nursing Educators
- Association of Occupational Health Professionals
- Association of Nurses in AIDS Care
- Association of Operating Room Nurses, Inc.*
- Association of Pediatric Oncology Nurses
- Association of Rehabilitation Nurses*
- Association of State and Territorial Directors of Nursing

- Association of Women's Health, Obstetric and Neonatal Nurses (formerly NAACOG)*
- Chi Eta Phi Sorority
- Consolidated Association of Nurses in Substance Abuse International
- Council on Graduate Education for Administration in Nursing
- Dermatology Nurses Association
- Developmental Disabilities Nurses Association
- Drug and Alcohol Nursing Association, Inc.
- Emergency Nurses Association*
- Hospice Nurses Association
- International Society of Nurse in Genetics
- Intravenous Nurses Society
- National Association of Directors of Nursing Administration in Long Term Care (NADONA/LTC)
- National Association of Hispanic Nurses
- National Association of Neonatal Nurses
- National Association of Nurse Massage Therapists
- National Association of Nurse Practitioners in Reproductive Health
- National Association of Orthopaedic Nurses*
- National Association of Pediatric Nurse Associates and Practitioners
- National Association of School Nurses, Inc.*
- National Association of State School Nurse Consultants, Inc.
- National Black Nurses Association, Inc.
- National Flight Nurses Association
- National Gerontological Nursing Association
- National League for Nursing
- National Nurses Society on Addictions
- National Nursing Staff Development Organization
- National Organization of Nurse Practitioners Faculties
- National Student Nurses Association
- North American Nursing Diagnosis Association
- Nurses Organization of Veterans Affairs
- Oncology Nursing Society*
- Philippine Nurses Association of America, Inc.
- Respiratory Nursing Society
- Sigma Theta Tau, International, Inc.
- Society for Education and Research in Psychiatric-Mental Health Nursing
- Society for Vascular Nursing
- Society of Gastroenterology Nurses and Associates, Inc.
- Society of Otorhinolaryngology and Head-Neck Nurses, Inc.
- Society of Pediatric Nurses
- Society of Urologic Nurses & Associates, Inc.
- Wound, Ostomy, & Continence Nurses Society

(*denotes Organizational Affiliate members in NOLF)

APPENDIX C

DSM-IV Classification

Multiaxial System

Axis I Clinical disorders
Other conditions that may be a focus of clinical attention
Axis II Personality disorders
Mental retardation
Axis III General medical conditions
Axis IV Psychosocial and environmental problems
Axis V Global assessment of functioning

NOS = Not Otherwise Specified.

An *x* appearing in a diagnostic code indicates that a specific code number is required.

Disorders Usually First Diagnosed in Infancy, Childhood, or Adolescence

Mental Retardation

Note: *These are coded on Axis II.*

317 Mild mental retardation
318.0 Moderate mental retardation
318.1 Severe mental retardation
318.2 Profound mental retardation
319 Mental retardation, severity unspecified

Learning Disorders

315.00 Reading disorder
315.1 Mathematics disorder
315.2 Disorder of written expression
315.9 Learning disorder NOS

Motor Skills Disorder

315.4 Developmental coordination disorder

Communication Disorders

315.31 Expressive language disorder
315.31 Mixed receptive-expressive language disorder
315.39 Phonological disorder
307.0 Stuttering
307.9 Communication disorder NOS

From *Diagnostic and statistical manual of mental disorders* (4th ed.) (DSM-IV). Washington, DC: American Psychiatric Association, 1994.

Pervasive Developmental Disorders

299.00 Autistic disorder
299.80 Rett's disorder
299.10 Childhood disintegrative disorder
299.80 Asperger's disorder
299.80 Pervasive developmental disorder NOS

Attention-deficit and Disruptive Behavior Disorders

314.xx Attention-deficit/hyperactivity disorder
.01 Combined type
.00 Predominantly inattentive type
.01 Predominantly hyperactive-impulsive type
314.9 Attention-deficit/hyperactivity disorder NOS
312.8 Conduct disorder
313.81 Oppositional defiant disorder
312.9 Disruptive behavior disorder NOS

Feeding and Eating Disorders of Infancy or Early Childhood

307.52 Pica
307.53 Rumination disorder
307.59 Feeding disorder of infancy or early childhood

Tic Disorders

307.23 Tourette's disorder
307.22 Chronic motor or vocal tic disorder
307.21 Transient tic disorder
Specify if: single episode/recurrent
307.20 Tic disorder NOS

Elimination Disorders

—.— Encopresis
787.6 With constipation and overflow incontinence
307.7 Without constipation and overflow incontinence
307.6 Enuresis (not due to a general medical condition)

Other Disorders of Infancy, Childhood, or Adolescence

309.21 Separation anxiety disorder
313.23 Selective mutism
313.89 Reactive attachment disorder of infancy or early childhood
307.3 Stereotypic movement disorder
313.9 Disorder of infancy, childhood, or adolescence NOS

Delirium, Dementia, and Amnestic and Other Cognitive Disorders

Delirium

293.0 Delirium due to . . . [*indicate the general medical condition*]
—.— Substance intoxication delirium *(refer to Substance-Related Disorders for substance-specific codes)*
—.— Substance withdrawal delirium *(refer to Substance-Related Disorders for substance-specific codes)*
—.— Delirium due to multiple etiologies *(code each of the specific etiologies)*
780.09 Delirium NOS
290.xx Dementia of the Alzheimer's type, with early onset *(also code on Axis III)*
.10 Uncomplicated
.11 With delirium
.12 With delusions
.13 With depressed mood
290.xx Dementia of the Alzheimer's type, with late onset *(also code on Axis III)*
.0 Uncomplicated
.3 With delirium
.20 With delusions
.21 With depressed mood
290.xx Vascular dementia
.40 Uncomplicated
.41 With delirium
.42 With delusions
.43 With depressed mood
294.9 Dementia due to HIV disease *(also code HIV affecting central nervous system on Axis III)*
294.1 Dementia due to head trauma *(also code on Axis III)*
294.1 Dementia due to Parkinson's disease *(also code on Axis III)*
294.1 Dementia due to Huntington's disease *(also code on Axis III)*
290.10 Dementia due to Pick's disease *(also code on Axis III)*
290.10 Dementia due to Creutzfeldt-Jakob disease *(also code 046.1 Creutzfeldt-Jakob disease on Axis III)*
294.1 Dementia due to . . . *[indicate the general medical condition not listed above] (also code the general medical condition on Axis III)*
—.— Substance-induced persisting dementia
—.— Dementia due to multiple etiologies
294.8 Dementia NOS

Amnestic Disorders

294.0 Amnestic disorder due to . . . *[indicate the general medical condition]*
Specify if: transient-chronic
—.— Substance-induced persisting amnestic disorder
294.8 Amnestic disorder NOS

Other Cognitive Disorders

294.9 Cognitive disorder NOS

Mental Disorders Due to a General Medical Condition Not Elsewhere Classified

239.89 Catatonic disorder due to . . . *[indicate the general medication condition]*
310.1 Personality change due to . . . *[indicate the general medical condition]*
293.9 Mental disorder NOS due to . . . *[indicate the general medical condition]*

Substance-Related Disorders

[a]*The following specifiers may be applied to Substance Dependence:*
With physiological dependence/without physiological dependence
Early full remission/early partial remission
Sustained full remission/sustained partial remission
On agonist therapy/in a controlled environment

The following specifiers apply to Substance-Induced Disorders as noted:
[I]With onset during intoxication/[W]with onset during withdrawal

Alcohol-Related Disorders

Alcohol Use Disorders

303.90 Alcohol dependence[a]
305.00 Alcohol abuse

Alcohol-Induced Disorders

303.00 Alcohol intoxication
291.8 Alcohol withdrawal
291.0 Alcohol intoxication delirium
291.0 Alcohol withdrawal delirium
291.2 Alcohol-induced persisting dementia
291.1 Alcohol-induced persisting amnestic disorder
291.x Alcohol-induced psychotic disorder
.5 With delusions
.3 With hallucinations
291.8 Alcohol-induced mood disorder
291.8 Alcohol-induced anxiety disorder
291.8 Alcohol-induced sexual dysfunction
291.8 Alcohol-induced sleep disorder
291.9 Alcohol-related disorder NOS

Amphetamine (or Amphetamine-Like)–Related Disorders

Amphetamine Use Disorders

304.40 Amphetamine dependence[a]
305.70 Amphetamine abuse

Amphetamine-Induced Disorders

292.89 Amphetamine intoxication
292.0 Amphetamine withdrawal
292.81 Amphetamine intoxication delirium
292.xx Amphetamine-induced psychotic disorder
.11 With delusions[I]
.12 With hallucinations[I]
292.84 Amphetamine-induced mood disorder
292.89 Amphetamine-induced anxiety disorder
292.89 Amphetamine-induced sexual dysfunction
292.89 Amphetamine-induced sleep disorder
292.9 Amphetamine-related disorder NOS

Caffeine-Related Disorders

Caffeine-Induced Disorders

305.90 Caffeine intoxication
292.89 Caffeine-induced anxiety disorder[1]
292.89 Caffeine induced sleep disorder[1]
292.9 Caffeine-related disorder NOS

Cannabis-Related Disorders

Cannabis Use Disorders

304.30 Cannabis dependence
305.20 Cannabis abuse

Cannabis-Induced Disorders

292.89 Cannabis intoxication
292.81 Cannabis intoxication delirium
292.xx Cannabis-induced psychotic disorder
.11 With delusions[1]
.12 With hallucinations[1]
292.89 Cannabis-induced anxiety disorder[1]
292.9 Cannabis-related disorder NOS

Cocaine-Related Disorders

Cocaine Use Disorders

304.20 Cocaine dependence[a]
305.60 Cocaine abuse

Cocaine-Induced Disorders

292.89 Cocaine intoxication
Specify if: with perceptual disturbances
292.0 Cocaine withdrawal
292.81 Cocaine intoxication delirium
292.xx Cocaine-induced psychotic disorder
.11 With delusions[1]
.12 With hallucinations[1]
292.84 Cocaine-induced mood disorder
292.89 Cocaine-induced anxiety disorder
292.89 Cocaine-induced sexual dysfunction[1]
292.89 Cocaine-induced sleep disorder
292.9 Cocaine-related disorder NOS

Hallucinogen-Related Disorders

Hallucinogen Use Disorders

304.50 Hallucinogen dependence[a]
305.30 Hallucinogen abuse

Hallucinogen-Induced Disorders

292.89 Hallucinogen intoxication
292.89 Hallucinogen persisting perception disorder (flashbacks)
292.81 Hallucinogen intoxication delirium
292.xx Hallucinogen-induced psychotic disorder
.11 With delusions[1]
.12 With hallucinations[1]
292.84 Hallucinogen-induced mood disorder[1]
292.89 Hallucinogen-induced anxiety disorder[1]
292.9 Hallucinogen-related disorder NOS

Inhalant-Related Disorders

Inhalant Use Disorders

304.60 Inhalant dependence[a]
305.90 Inhalant abuse

Inhalant-Induced Disorders

292.89 Inhalant intoxication
292.81 Inhalant intoxication delirium
292.82 Inhalant-induced persisting dementia
292.xx Inhalant-induced psychotic disorder
.11 With delusions[1]
.12 With hallucinations[1]
292.84 Inhalant-induced mood disorder[1]
292.89 Inhalant-induced anxiety disorder[1]
292.9 Inhalant-related disorder NOS

Nicotine-Related Disorders

Nicotine Use Disorder

305.10 Nicotine dependence[a]

Nicotine-Induced Disorder

292.0 Nicotine withdrawal
292.9 Nicotine-related disorder NOS

Opioid-Related Disorders

Opioid Use Disorders

304.00 Opioid dependence[a]
305.50 Opioid abuse

Opioid-Induced Disorders

292.89 Opioid intoxication
292.0 Opioid withdrawal
292.81 Opioid intoxication delirium
292.xx Opioid-induced psychotic disorder
.11 With delusions[1]
.12 With hallucinations[1]
292.84 Opioid-induced mood disorder[1]
292.89 Opioid-induced sexual dysfunction[1]
292.89 Opioid-induced sleep disorder
292.9 Opioid-related disorder NOS

Phencyclidine (or Phencyclidine-Like)–Related Disorders

Phencyclidine Use Disorders

304.90 Phencyclidine dependence[a]
305.90 Phencyclidine abuse

Phencyclidine-Induced Disorders

292.89 Phencyclidine intoxication
292.81 Phencyclidine intoxication delirium
292.xx Phencyclidine-induced psychotic disorder
.11 With delusions[1]
.12 With hallucinations[1]
292.84 Phencyclidine-induced mood disorder[1]
292.89 Phencyclidine-induced anxiety disorder[1]
292.9 Phencyclidine-related disorder NOS

Sedative-, Hypnotic-, or Anxiolytic-Related Disorders

Sedative, Hypnotic, or Anxiolytic Use Disorders

304.10 Sedative, hypnotic, or anxiolytic dependence[a]
305.40 Sedative, hypnotic, or anxiolytic abuse

Sedative-, Hypnotic-, or Anxiolytic-Induced Disorders

292.89 Sedative, hypnotic, or anxiolytic intoxication
292.0 Sedative, hypnotic, or anxiolytic withdrawal
Specify if: with perceptual disturbances

292.81 Sedative, hypnotic, or anxiolytic intoxication delirium
292.81 Sedative, hypnotic, or anxiolytic withdrawal delirium
292.82 Sedative-, hypnotic-, or anxiolytic-induced persisting dementia
292.83 Sedative-, hypnotic-, or anxiolytic-induced persisting amnestic disorder
292.xx Sedative-, hypnotic-, or anxiolytic-induced psychotic disorder
.11 With delusions
.12 With hallucinations
292.84 Sedative-, hypnotic-, or anxiolytic-induced mood disorder[I,W]
292.89 Sedative-, hypnotic-, or anxiolytic-induced anxiety disorder[W]
292.89 Sedative-, hypnotic-, or anxiolytic-induced sexual dysfunction[I]
292.89 Sedative-, hypnotic-, or anxiolytic-induced sleep disorder[I,W]
292.9 Sedative-, hypnotic-, or anxiolytic-related disorder NOS

Polysubstance-Related Disorder

304.80 Polysubstance dependence[a]

Other (or Unknown) Substance-Related Disorders

Other (or Unknown) Substance Use Disorders

304.90 Other (or unknown) substance dependence[a]
305.90 Other (or unknown) substance abuse

Other (or Unknown) Substance-Induced Disorders

292.89 Other (or unknown) substance intoxication
292.0 Other (or unknown) substance withdrawal
292.81 Other (or unknown) substance-induced delirium
292.82 Other (or unknown) substance-induced persisting dementia
292.83 Other (or unknown) substance-induced persisting amnestic disorder
292.xx Other (or unknown) substance-induced psychotic disorder
.11 With delusions[I,W]
.12 With hallucinations[I,W]
292.84 Other (or unknown) substance-induced mood disorder[I,W]
292.89 Other (or unknown) substance-induced anxiety disorder[I,W]
292.89 Other (or unknown) substance-induced sexual dysfunction[I]
292.89 Other (or unknown) substance-induced sleep disorder[I,W]
292.9 Other (or unknown) substance-related disorder NOS

Schizophrenia and Other Psychotic Disorders

295.xx Schizophrenia

The following Classification of Longitudinal Course applies to all subtypes of Schizophrenia:

Episodic with interepisode residual symptoms (*specify if:* with prominent negative symptoms)/episodic with no interepisode residual symptoms/continuous (*specify if:* with prominent negative symptoms)

Single episode in partial remission (*specify if:* with prominent negative symptoms)/single episode in full remission

Other or unspecified pattern

.30 Paranoid type
.10 Disorganized type
.20 Catatonic type
.90 Undifferentiated type
.60 Residual type
295.40 Schizophreniform disorder
Specify if: without good prognostic features/with good prognostic features
295.70 Schizoaffective disorder
Specify type: bipolar type/depressive type
297.1 Delusional disorder
Specify type: erotomanic type/grandiose type/jealous type/persecutory type/somatic type/mixed type/unspecified type
298.8 Brief psychotic disorder
Specify if: with marked stressor(s)/without marked stressor(s)/with postpartum onset
297.3 Shared psychotic disorder
293.xx Psychotic disorder due to . . . *[indicate the general medical condition]*
.81 With delusions
.82 With hallucinations
—.— Substance-induced psychotic disorder
Specify if: with onset during intoxication/with onset during withdrawal
298.9 Psychotic disorder NOS

Mood Disorders

Code current state of major depressive disorder or bipolar I disorder in fifth digit:

1 = Mild
2 = Moderate
3 = Severe without psychotic features
4 = Severe with psychotic features
Specify: Mood-congruent psychotic features/mood-incongruent psychotic features
5 = In partial remission
6 = In full remission
0 = Unspecified

The following specifiers apply (for current or most recent episode) to mood disorders as noted:

[a]Severity/psychotic/remission specifiers/[b]chronic/[c]with catatonic features/[d]with melancholic features/[e]with atypical features/[f]with postpartum onset.

The following specifiers apply to mood disorders as noted:

[g]With or without full interepisode recovery/[h]with seasonal pattern/[i]with rapid cycling

Depressive Disorders

296.xx Major depressive disorder
.2x Single episode
.3x Recurrent
300.4 Dysthymic disorder
Specify if: early onset/late onset
Specify: with atypical features
311 Depressive disorder NOS

Bipolar Disorders

296.xx Bipolar I disorder
.0x Single manic episode
.40 Most recent episode hypomanic
.4x Most recent episode manic
.6x Most recent episode mixed
.5x Most recent episode depressed
.7 Most recent episode unspecified
296.89 Bipolar II disorder
Specify (current or most recent episode): hypomanic/depressed
301.13 Cyclothymic disorder
296.80 Bipolar disorder NOS
293.83 Mood disorder due to . . . *[indicate the general medical condition]*
Specify type: with depressive features/with major depressive-like episode/with manic features/with mixed features
—.— Substance-induced mood disorder
Specify type: with depressive features/with manic features/with mixed features
Specify if: with onset during intoxication/with onset during withdrawal
296.90 Mood disorder NOS

Anxiety Disorders

300.01 Panic disorder without agoraphobia
300.21 Panic disorder with agoraphobia
300.22 Agoraphobia without history of panic disorder
300.29 Specific phobia
Specify type: animal type/natural environment type/blood-injection-injury type/situational type/other type
300.23 Social phobia
Specify if: generalized
300.3 Obsessive-compulsive disorder
Specify if: with poor insight
309.81 Posttraumatic stress disorder
Specify if: acute/chronic
Specify if: with delayed onset
308.3 Acute stress disorder
300.02 Generalized anxiety disorder
293.89 Anxiety disorder due to . . . *[indicate the general medical condition]*
Specify if: with generalized anxiety/with panic attacks/with obsessive-compulsive symptoms
—.— Substance-induced anxiety disorder
Specify if: with generalized anxiety/with panic attacks/with obsessive-compulsive symptoms/with phobic symptoms
Specify if: with onset during intoxication/with onset during withdrawal
300.00 Anxiety disorder NOS

Somatoform Disorders

300.81 Somatization disorder
300.81 Undifferentiated somatoform disorder
300.11 Conversion disorder
Specify type: with motor symptom or deficit/with sensory symptom or deficit/with seizures or convulsions/with mixed presentation
307.xx Pain disorder
.80 Associated with psychological factors
.89 Associated with both psychological factors and a general medical condition
Specify if: acute/chronic
300.7 Hypochondriasis
Specify if: with poor insight
300.7 Body dysmorphic disorder
300.81 Somatoform disorder NOS

Factitious Disorders

300.xx Factitious disorder
.16 With predominantly psychological signs and symptoms
.19 With predominantly physical signs and symptoms
.19 With combined psychological and physical signs and symptoms
300.19 Factitious disorder NOS

Dissociative Disorders

300.12 Dissociative amnesia
300.13 Dissociative fugue
300.14 Dissociative identity disorder
300.6 Depersonalization disorder
300.15 Dissociative disorder NOS

Sexual and Gender Identity Disorders

Sexual Dysfunctions

The following specifiers apply to all primary Sexual Dysfunctions:
Lifelong type/acquired type/generalized type/situational type due to psychological factors/due to combined factors

Sexual Desire Disorders

302.71 Hypoactive sexual desire disorder
302.79 Sexual aversion disorder

Sexual Arousal Disorders

302.72 Female sexual arousal disorder
302.72 Male erectile disorder

Orgasmic Disorders

302.73 Female orgasmic disorder
302.74 Male orgasmic disorder
302.75 Premature ejaculation

Sexual Pain Disorders

302.76 Dyspareunia (not due to a general medical condition)
306.51 Vaginismus (not due to a general medical condition)

Sexual Dysfunction Due to a General Medical Condition

625.8 Female hypoactive sexual desire disorder due to . . . *[indicate the general medical condition]*
608.89 Male hypoactive sexual desire disorder due to . . . *[indicate the general medical condition]*
607.84 Male erectile disorder due to . . . *[indicate the general medical condition]*
625.0 Female dyspareunia due to . . . *[indicate the general medical condition]*

608.89 Male dyspareunia due to . . . *[indicate the general medical condition]*
625.8 Other female sexual dysfunction due to . . . *[indicate the general medical condition]*
608.89 Other male sexual dysfunction due to . . . *[indicate the general medical condition]*
—.— Substance-induced sexual dysfunction
302.70 Sexual dysfunction NOS

Paraphilias

302.4 Exhibitionism
302.81 Fetishism
302.89 Frotteurism
302.2 Pedophilia
302.83 Sexual masochism
302.84 Sexual sadism
302.3 Transvestic fetishism
302.82 Voyeurism
302.9 Paraphilia NOS

Gender Identity Disorders

302.xx Gender identity disorder
.6 in children
.85 in adolescents or adults
Specify if: sexually attracted to males/sexually attracted to females/sexually attracted to both/sexually attracted to neither
302.6 Gender identity disorder NOS
302.9 Sexual disorder NOS

Eating Disorders

307.1 Anorexia nervosa
Specify type: restricting type; binge-eating/purging type
307.51 Bulimia nervosa
Specify type: purging type/nonpurging type
307.50 Eating disorder NOS

Sleep Disorders

Primary Sleep Disorders

Dyssomnias

307.42 Primary insomnia
307.44 Primary hypersomnia
Specify if: recurrent
347 Narcolepsy
780.59 Breathing-related sleep disorder
307.45 Circadian rhythm sleep disorder
307.47 Dyssomnia NOS

Parasomnias

307.47 Nightmare disorder
307.46 Sleep terror disorder
307.46 Sleepwalking disorder
307.47 Parasomnia NOS

Sleep Disorders Related to Another Mental Disorder

307.42 Insomnia related to . . . *[indicate the disorder]*
307.44 Hypersomnia related to . . . *[indicate the disorder]*

Other Sleep Disorders

780.xx Sleep disorders due to . . . *[indicate the general medical condition]*
.52 Insomnia type
.54 Hypersomnia type
.59 Parasomnia type
.59 Mixed type
—.— Substance-induced sleep disorder
Specify type: insomnia type/hypersomnia type/parasomnia type/mixed type
Specify if: with onset during intoxication/with onset during withdrawal

Impulse-Control Disorders Not Elsewhere Classified

312.34 Intermittent explosive disorder
312.32 Kleptomania
312.33 Pyromania
312.31 Pathological gambling
312.39 Trichotillomania
312.30 Impulse-control disorder NOS

Adjustment Disorders

309.xx Adjustment disorder
.0 With depressed mood
.24 With anxiety
.28 With mixed anxiety and depressed mood
.3 With disturbance of conduct
.4 With mixed disturbance of emotions and conduct
.9 Unspecified
Specify if: acute/chronic

Personality Disorders

Note: *These are coded on Axis II.*

301.0 Paranoid personality disorder
301.20 Schizoid personality disorder
301.22 Schizotypal personality disorder
301.7 Antisocial personality disorder
301.83 Borderline personality disorder
301.50 Histrionic personality disorder
301.81 Narcissistic personality disorder
301.82 Avoidant personality disorder
301.6 Dependent personality disorder
301.4 Obsessive-compulsive personality disorder
301.9 Personality disorder NOS

Other Conditions That May Be a Focus of Clinical Attention

Psychological Factors Affecting Medical Condition

316 . . . *[Specified psychological factor]* affecting . . . *[indicate the general medical condition]*
Choose name based on nature of factors:
Mental disorder affecting medical condition
Psychological symptoms affecting medical condition
Personality traits or coping style affecting medical condition
Maladaptive health behaviors affecting medical condition

Stress-related physiological response affecting medical condition
Other or unspecified psychological factors affecting medical condition

Medication-Induced Movement Disorders

332.1	Neuroleptic-induced parkinsonism
333.92	Neuroleptic malignant syndrome
333.7	Neuroleptic-induced acute dystonia
333.99	Neuroleptic-induced acute akathisia
333.82	Neuroleptic-induced tardive dyskinesia
333.1	Medication-induced postural tremor
333.90	Medication-induced movement disorder NOS

Other Medication-Induced Disorder

995.2	Adverse effects of medication NOS

Relational Problems

V61.9	Relational problem related to a mental disorder or general medical condition
V61.20	Parent-child relational problem
V61.1	Partner relational problem
V61.8	Sibling relational problem
V62.81	Relational problem NOS

Problems Related to Abuse or Neglect

V61.21	Physical abuse of child
V61.21	Sexual abuse of child
V61.21	Neglect of child
V61.1	Physical abuse of adult
V61.1	Sexual abuse of adult

Additional Conditions That May Be a Focus of Clinical Attention

V15.81	Noncompliance with treatment
V65.2	Malingering
V71.01	Adult antisocial behavior
V71.02	Child or adolescent antisocial behavior
V62.89	Borderline intellectual functioning **Note:** *This is coded on Axis II.*
780.9	Age-related cognitive decline
V62.82	Bereavement
V62.3	Academic problem
V62.2	Occupational problem
313.82	Identity problem
V62.89	Religious or spiritual problem
V62.4	Acculturation problem
V62.89	Phase of life problem

APPENDIX D

Assessment Tool

COMPREHENSIVE NURSING ASSESSMENT TOOL

1. Client History

I. GENERAL HISTORY OF CLIENT

Name ______________________ Age ________ Sex ________
Racial and ethnic data ______________________
Marital status ______________________
Number and ages of children/siblings ______________________
Living arrangements ______________________
Occupation ______________________
Education ______________________
Religious affiliations ______________________

II. PRESENTING PROBLEM

A. Statement in the client's own words of why he or she is hospitalized or seeking help
____
____
____

B. Recent difficulties/alterations in
1. Relationships
2. Usual level of functioning
3. Behavior
4. Perceptions or cognitive abilities

C. Increased feelings of
1. Depression
2. Anxiety
3. Hopelessness
4. Being overwhelmed
5. Suspiciousness
6. Confusion

D. Somatic changes, such as
1. Constipation
2. Insomnia
3. Lethargy
4. Weight loss or gain
5. Palpitations

III. RELEVANT HISTORY—PERSONAL

A. Previous hospitalizations and illnesses ______________________

B. Educational background ______________________

C. Occupational background
1. If employed, where? ______________________
2. How long at that job? ______________________
3. Previous positions and reasons for leaving ______________________
4. Special skills ______________________

D. Social patterns
1. Describe friends ______________________
2. Describe a usual day ______________________

E. Sexual patterns
1. Sexually active? ______
2. Sexual orientation ______
3. Sexual difficulties ______

F. Interests and abilities
1. What does the client do in his or her spare time? ______
2. What is the client good at? ______
3. What gives the client pleasure? ______

G. Substance use and abuse
1. What psychotropic drugs does the client take? ______
How often? ______ How much? ______
2. How many drinks of alcohol does the client take per day? ______
Per week? ______
3. Does the client identify use of drugs as a problem? ______

H. How does the client cope with stress?
1. What does the client do when he or she gets upset? ______
2. Whom can the client talk to? ______
3. What usually helps to relieve stress? ______
4. What did the client try this time? ______

IV. RELEVANT HISTORY—FAMILY

A. Childhood
1. Who was important to the client growing up? ______
2. Was there physical or sexual abuse? ______
3. Did the parents drink or use drugs? ______
4. Who was in the home when the client was growing up? ______

B. Adolescence
1. How would the client describe his or her feelings in adolescence? ______
2. Describe the client's peer group at that time. ______

C. Use of drugs
1. Was there use or abuse of drugs by any family member? ______
Prescription ______ Street ______ By whom? ______
2. What was the effect on the family? ______

D. Family physical or mental problems
1. Who in the family had physical or mental problems? ______
2. Describe the problems. ______
3. How did it affect the family? ______

E. Was there an unusual or outstanding event the client would like to mention? ______

2. Mental and Emotional Status

A. Appearance
Physical handicaps ______
Dress appropriate ______ Sloppy ______
Grooming neat ______ Poor ______
Eye contact held ______ Describe posture ______

B. Behavior **(see Table D–1)**
Restless ______ Agitated ______ Lethargic
Mannerisms ______ Facial expressions ______ Other ______

C. Speech
Clear ______ Mumbled ______ Rapid ______ Slurred ______ Constant ______ Mute or silent ______ Barriers to communications ______ Specify (e.g., client has delusions or is confused, withdrawn, or verbose ______

D. Mood
What mood does the client convey? ______
______

E. Affect
Is the client's affect bland, apathetic, dramatic, bizarre, or appropriate? Describe ______

F. Thought process **(see Table D–2)**
   1. Characteristics
      Describe the characteristics of the person's responses: Flights of ideas ______ Looseness of association ______ Blocking ______ Concrete ______ Confabulation ______
      Describe ______
   2. Cognitive ability
      Proverbs: Concrete ______ Abstract ______
      Serial sevens: How far does the client go? ______ Can the client do simple math? ______
      What seems to be the reason for poor concentration? ______

G. Thought content
   1. Central theme: What is important to the client? ______
      Describe ______
   2. Self-concept: How does the client view him- or herself? ______
      What does the client want to change about him- or herself? ______
   3. Insight? Does the client realistically assess his or her symptoms? ______
      Realistically appraise his or her situation? ______
      Describe ______
   4. Suicidal or homicidal ideation? ______ What is suicide potential? ______ Family history of suicide or homicide attempt or successful completion? ______
      Explain ______

   Preoccupations **(see Table D–3).** Does the client have hallucinations? ______ Delusions ______
   Obsessions ______ Rituals ______ Phobias ______ Grandiosity ______ Religiosity ______
   Worthlessness ______ Describe ______

H. Reality orientation
   Time: ______
   Place: ______
   Person: ______
   Memory: ______

I. Level of anxiety
   Mild Data ______
   Moderate Data ______
   Severe Data ______
   Panic Data ______

TABLE D–1 ABNORMAL MOTOR BEHAVIORS

DEFINITION	EXAMPLE
Echopraxia	
Repeating the movements of another person.	Every time the nurse would move or gesture with her hands, the client would copy her gestures.
Echolalia	
Repeating the speech of another person.	The nurse said to the client, "Tell me your name." The client responded, "Tell me your name, tell me your name."
Waxy Flexibility	
Having one's arms or legs placed in a certain position and holding that same position for hours.	The nurse lifted the client's arm to check the pulse, and the client left his arm extended in the same position.
Parkinson-like Symptoms	
Making masklike faces, drooling, and having shuffling gait, tremors, and muscular rigidity. Seen in people who are on antipsychotic medication, such as phenothiazines.	The nurse noticed that the client's face held no emotion. He walked very stiffly, leaning forward, almost robot-like.
Akathisia	
Displaying motor restlessness, feeling of muscular quivering; at its worst, patient is unable to sit still or lie quietly.	The client's leg kept jiggling up and down when he talked to the nurse. When his feet were still, his arm would jiggle constantly during the interview.
Dyskinesia	
Having distortion of voluntary movements, such as involuntary muscular activity (e.g., tic, spasm, or myoclonus).	The client had a marked facial tic around his mouth, which was distracting to the nurse during the interview.

TABLE D–2 SUMMARY OF ABNORMAL THOUGHT PROCESSES

DEFINITION	EXAMPLE
Tangentiality	
Association disturbance in which the speaker goes off the topic. When it happens frequently and the speaker does not return to the topic, interpersonal communication is destroyed.	The nurse asked the client to talk more about his family. The client continuously left the topic and talked about boats, animals, his apartment, and so forth. Each time the nurse tried to help the client to focus, he would go off on another topic.
Neologisms	
Words a person makes up that have meaning only for the person himself, often part of a delusional system.	"I am afraid to go to the hospital because the *norks* are looking for me there."
Looseness of Association	
Thinking is haphazard, illogical, and confused. Connections in thought are interrupted. Seen mostly in schizophrenic disorders.	"Can't go to the zoo, no money, Oh . . . I have a hat, these members make no sense, man . . . What's the problem?"
Flights of Ideas	
Constant flow of speech in which the person jumps from one topic to another in rapid succession. There is a connection between topics, although it is sometimes hard to identify. Characteristically seen in manic states.	"Say babe, how's it going . . . Going to my sister's to get some money . . . money, honey, you got any bread . . . bread and butter, staff of life, ain't life grand? . . ."
Blocking	
Sudden cessation of a thought in the middle of a sentence. Person is unable to continue his train of thought. Often, sudden new thoughts crop up unrelated to the topic. Can be disturbing to the individual.	"I was going to get a new dress for the . . . I forgot what I was going to say."
Circumstantiality	
Before getting to the point or answering a question, the person gets caught up in in countless details and explanations.	"Where are you going for the weekend, Harry?" "Well I first thought of going to my mother's, but that was before I remembered that she was going to my sister's. My sister is having a picnic. She always has picnics at the beach. The beach that she goes to is large and gets crowded. That's why I don't like that beach. So I decided to go someplace else. I thought of going to my brother's house. He has a large house on a quiet street . . . I finally decided to stay home."
Perseveration	
Involuntary repetition of the same thought, phrase, or motor response to different questions or situations. Associated with brain damage.	N: How are you doing, Harry? H: Fine, nurse, just fine N: Did you go for a walk? H: Fine, nurse, just fine. N: Are you going out today? H: Fine, nurse, just fine.
Confabulation	
Filling in a memory gap with detailed fantasy believed by the teller. The purpose is to maintain self-esteem and is seen in organic conditions, such as Korsakoff's psychosis.	The nurse asked Harry, who spent the weekend at home, what he did that weekend. "Well, I just came back from California after signing a contract with MGM for a film on the life of Roosevelt. We had the most marvelous tour of the studio . . . went to lunch with the director . . ."
Word Salad	
Mixture of words and phrases that have no meaning.	"I am fine . . . apple pie . . . no sale . . . furniture store . . . take it slow . . . cellar door . . ."

TABLE D–3 PREOCCUPATIONS IN THOUGHT CONTENT

DEFINITION	EXAMPLE
Hallucinations	
A sense perception for which no external stimuli exist. Hallucinations can have an organic or a functional etiology.	
Visual: Seeing things that are not there.	During alcohol withdrawal he kept shouting, "I see snakes on the walls."
Auditory: Hearing voices when none are present.	"I keep hearing my mother's voice telling me I am bad. She died a year ago."
Olfactory: Smelling smells that do not exist.	"I smell my stomach rotting."
Tactile: Feeling touch sensations in the absence of stimuli. (Also referred to as haptic.)	A paranoid man feels electrical impulses "from outer space" entering his body and controlling his mind.
Gustatory: Experiencing taste in the absence of stimuli.	A paranoid woman tastes poison in her food while eating at her son's wedding.
Delusions	
A false belief held to be true even with evidence to the contrary. Three common delusions follow:	
Persecution: The thought that one is being singled out for harm by others.	An intern believes that the chief of staff is plotting to kill him to prevent the intern from becoming too powerful.
Grandeur: The false belief that one is a very powerful and important person.	A newly admitted patient told the nurse that he was God, and he was here to save the world.
Jealousy: The false belief that one's mate is going out with other people. The person may take everyday occurrences for "proof."	Sally "knew" that her husband, Jim, was being unfaithful. Even when Sally's brother swore he and Jim really did play pool Friday nights, Sally declared Jim's not being home then was her "proof."
Obsessions	
An idea, impulse, or emotion that a person cannot put out of his or her consciousness. Can be mild or severe.	A young mother, Jane, told the nurse that she was hounded by constant thoughts that something terrible was going to happen to her baby. She knew that this was crazy, but she could not get the thought to stop.
Rituals	
Repetitive actions that people must do over and over until either they are exhausted or anxiety is decreased. Often done to lessen the anxiety triggered by an obsession.	Jane stated to the nurse the only way she could temporarily get these obsessions to cease was to say three "Hail Marys" and knock on wood twice to reassure herself that "nothing terrible was happening."
Phobias	
An intense irrational fear of an object, situation, or place. The fear persists even though the object of the fear is perfectly harmless and the person is aware of the irrationality.	Although she was aware that cats would not harm her, Mary was deathly afraid of cats and refused to visit her sister and friends who had cats.

APPENDIX E

American Self-Help Clearinghouse

SELF-HELP GROUP CLEARINGHOUSES

For help in finding or forming a mutual-aid support group for any type of illness, disability, addiction, loss of a loved one, parenting problem, abuse situation, or other stressful life problem, there are local self-help clearinghouses available to help you. They can advise you if there is any local self-help group near you to meet your need. Most clearinghouses can also help if you are interested in joining with others to start a new group (by providing suggestions, resource materials, local contacts, or training workshops or by publicizing your interest in their newsletters). For a list of all self-help groups on the internet go to **http://www.cmhc.com/selfhelp/**

Alabama	Birmingham area: 205-251-5912 (group information only)
Arizona	800-352-3792 (in Arizona); 602-231-0868
Arkansas	Northeast area: 501-932-5555 (group information only)
California	San Diego: 619-543-0412 San Francisco: 415-772-4357 Sacramento: 916-368-3100 Modesto: 209-558-7454 Davis: 916-756-8181
Connecticut	203-624-6982
Illinois*	312-368-9070, 312-481-8837 Champaign area only: 217-352-0099 Macon Cty: 217-429-HELP
Iowa:	800-952-4777 (in Iowa); 515-576-5870
Kansas	800-445-0116 (in Kansas); 316-689-3843
Massachusetts	413-545-2313
Michigan*	800-777-5556 (in Michigan); 517-484-7373
Missouri	Kansas City: 816-822-7272 St. Louis: 314-773-1399
Nebraska	402-476-9668
New Jersey	800-FOR-MASH (in New Jersey); 201-625-9565
New York	New York City: 212-586-5770 Westchester:** 914-949-0788 ext 237
North Carolina	Mecklenberg area: 704-331-9500
North Dakota	Fargo area: 701-235-SEEK
Ohio	Dayton area: 513-225-3004 Toledo area: 419-475-4449
Oregon	Portland area: 503-222-5555 (group information only)
Pennsylvania	Pittsburgh area: 412-261-5363 Scranton area: 717-961-1234
South Carolina	Midlands area: 803-791-9227
Tennessee	Knoxville area; 423-584-9125 Memphis area: 901-323-8485
Texas*	512-454-3706
Utah	Salt Lake City area: 801-978-3333 (group information only)
Virginia	Tidewater area: 757-340-9380

For international/national group contacts and/or directory:
American Self-Help Clearinghouse: 201-625-7101, TTY 625-9053, and on the World Wide Web at http://www.cmhc.com/selfhelp/
National Self-Help Clearinghouse: 212-354-8525

OTHER HELPFUL INFORMATION HELPLINES IN THE UNITED STATES

- O.D.P.H.P. National Health Information Clearinghouse: 1-800-336-4797 (in U.S.)
- National Organization for Rare Disorders: 1-800-999-NORD (in U.S.)
- Alliance of Genetic Support Groups (genetic illnesses): 1-800-336-GENE (in U.S.)
- National Empowerment Center (for mental health consumer/survivor groups): 1-800-POWER-2-U
- National Mental Health Consumers Self-Help Clearinghouse: 1-800-553-4-Key

SELF-HELP CLEARINGHOUSES IN CANADA

Calgary*	403-262-1117
Nova Scotia	902-466-2011
Toronto*	416-487-4355
Prince Edward Island	902-628-1648
Vancouver	604-733-6186
Winnipeg	204-589-5500 or 633-5955

*Maintains listings of additional local clearinghouses operating within the state/province.

**Call Westchester for information on local clearinghouses in parts of upstate New York.

American Self-Help Clearinghouse • group information 201-625-7101

Adapted with permission from *Self-help sourcebook (6th ed.)* published by the American Self-Help Clearinghouse, Northwest Covenant Medical Center, Denville, NJ 07834-2995, 1997.

APPENDIX F

Drug Information

BENZTROPINE MESYLATE

(Cogentin) ANTIPARKINSONIAN

USES:
1. Treating Parkinson's disease.
2. Treatment of extrapyramidal symptoms (except tardive dyskinesia) due to use of neuroleptic/antipsychotic medications.

ACTION: Cogentin is an anticholinergic agent. This drug increases and prolongs the dopamine activity in the CNS, thereby correcting neurotransmitter imbalances and minimizing involuntary movements.

DOSAGES & ROUTES

	PO	IM/IV
Adult	0.5–2 mg/day initially; gradually increase to 4–6 mg/day. For drug-induced extrapyramidal symptoms, 1–4 mg once or twice a day IM or PO	For acute dystonic reactions, 0.5–2 mg IM or IV
Elderly	Use lower doses	

CONTRAINDICATIONS: Narrow-angle glaucoma, pyloric or duodenal obstruction, peptic ulcers, prostatic hypertrophy, obstructions of the bladder neck, myasthenia gravis, and in children under 3 years of age. Rarely indicated for children.

CAUTIONS: The elderly and clients with cardiac, liver, or kidney disease or hypertension. Also used with caution in clients taking barbiturates or alcohol.

REMARKS: The effects of benztropine are cumulative and may not be evident for 2 or 3 days. After 4 to 6 months of long-term maintenance antipsychotic therapy, antiparkinsonian drugs can be used on an as-necessary basis or withdrawn. Some clients respond best to the medication given every day. Others do better with divided doses. Long-term use of benztropine with a neuroleptic can predispose a patient to tardive dyskinesia.

SIDE EFFECTS

AUTONOMIC: Dry mouth, blurred vision, nausea, restlessness.

CNS: Sedation, vertigo, paresthesias.

CARDIOVASCULAR: Palpitations, tachycardia.

GASTROINTESTINAL: Nausea, vomiting, constipation, paralytic ileus.

GENITOURINARY: Dysuria, urinary retention.

OCULAR: Blurred vision, mydriasis, photophobia.

OTHER: Anhidrosis (abnormal deficiency of sweat).

ADVERSE REACTIONS **CNS**: CNS depression, mild agitation, hallucinations, delirium, toxic psychosis, muscle weakness, ataxia, numbness of the fingers.

NURSING MEASURES:

1. Monitor intake and output. Observe for urinary retention.
2. Give medication after patient voids to reduce possibility of urinary retention.
3. Monitor for constipation; abdominal pain or distention may indicate potential for paralytic ileus.
4. Indications of CNS toxicity (depression or excitement, hallucinations, psychosis, or other) warrant withholding the drug and informing the physician immediately.

INFORM CLIENT:

1. Avoid driving or operating hazardous equipment if drowsiness or dizziness occurs.
2. Tolerance to heat may be reduced owing to diminished ability to sweat. Plan periods of rest in cool places during the day.
3. Stop taking the medication if CNS toxic effects, or difficulty swallowing or speaking, or vomiting occurs. Inform physician immediately.
4. Monitor urinary output and watch for signs of constipation.
5. Consult with physician before using any medication, prescribed or over the counter, once started on benztropine.

BUSPIRONE HYDROCHLORIDE
(BuSpar) ANTIANXIETY AGENT

USES: Management of anxiety disorders.

ACTION: The exact action of buspirone is not clear. It may exert a potent presynaptic dopamine antagonist effect in the CNS, resulting in increased dopamine at the synapses. It may also have an effect on serotonin receptors.

DOSAGES & ROUTES

	PO only
Adult and Elderly	5 mg 2–3 times daily; may increase 5 mg every 3–4 days; maintenance, 15–30 mg/day in 2–3 divided doses; not to exceed 60 mg/day

CONTRAINDICATIONS: In clients with severe renal or hepatic impairment and clients on MAOIs.

CAUTIONS: Renal or hepatic impairment, pregnant or lactating women, elderly or debilitated clients.

REMARKS: The advantages of buspirone (BuSpar) are that it is not sedating, tolerance does not develop, and it is not addicting. The drug has a more favorable side effect profile than do the benzodiazepines.

SIDE EFFECTS: Dizziness, nausea, headache, nervousness, lightheadedness, and excitement, which generally are not major problems. Other less common problems may occur (e.g., blurred vision, tachycardia, palpitations, paresthesia, abdominal distention).

ADVERSE REACTIONS: Overdose may produce severe nausea, vomiting, dizziness, drowsiness, abdominal distention, excessive pupil constriction.

NURSING MEASURES:
1. Offer emotional support to anxious clients.
2. Liver and renal function tests and blood counts should be done regularly for clients on long term therapy.
3. Assist with ambulation and put in place other safety features if dizziness and lightheadedness occur.

INFORM CLIENT AND FAMILY:
1. Teach clients to inform their physicians:
   a. About any medications (prescription or nonprescription), alcohol, or drugs that they are taking.
   b. If they are now or plan to get pregnant.
   c. If they are breast-feeding an infant.
2. Do not drive a car or operate potentially dangerous machinery until they experience how this medication will affect them.
3. Notify physician of difficulty breathing, change in vision, sweating, flushing, or cardiac problems.
4. Improvement may be noted in 7 to 10 days, but it may take 3 to 4 weeks or longer to note therapeutic effects.

CARBAMAZEPINE

(Tegretol, Epitol, Mazepine) — ANTICONVULSANT, ANTINEURALGIC

USES:
1. Management of generalized tonic-clonic seizures (grand mal) and psychomotor seizures.
2. Trigeminal neuralgia.
3. Potential mood stabilizer, particularly in acute mania. Used clinically, but not FDA approved at present for this use.

ACTION: Reduces post-tetanic potentiation at the synapse, preventing repetitive discharge.

DOSAGES & ROUTES
(Seizures)

	PO only (tablets, suspension, and chewable tablets)
Adult	200 mg twice daily, gradually increase until response is attained; maintenance, 800–1200 mg/day
Child (6–12)	100 mg twice daily, gradually increase until response is attained; maintenance, 400–800 mg/day in 3–4 equally divided doses.
	Note: Oral suspensions produce higher peak concentrations. Going from tablets to suspension, give in smaller and more frequent doses.

CONTRAINDICATIONS: History of bone marrow depression, history of hypersensitivity to TCAs.

CAUTIONS: Impaired cardiac, hepatic, and renal function; pregnancy or lactation (crosses placenta, distributed in breast milk, accumulates in fetal tissues).

REMARKS: Monitoring drug levels has increased the safety of anticonvulsant therapy.

SIDE EFFECTS

FREQUENT: Drowsiness, dizziness, nausea and vomiting.

INFREQUENT: Lethargy, visual abnormalities (spots before the eyes, difficulty focusing), dry mouth, headache, urinary frequency or retention, rash.

ADVERSE REACTIONS

HEMATOLOGIC: Blood dyscrasias (e.g., aplastic anemia, agranulocytosis, thrombocytopenia, leukopenia, bone marrow depression).

HEPATIC: Abnormal hepatic function test results; jaundice may be noticed; hepatitis.

CARDIOVASCULAR: Congestive heart failure, edema, aggravation of coronary artery disease, arrhythmias and atrioventricular block, primary thrombophlebitis. Some complications have resulted in fatalities.

CNS: Abrupt withdrawal may precipitate status epilepticus.

NURSING MEASURES:

1. Monitor for therapeutic serum level (3–12 μg/ml).
2. Assess for clinical evidence of early toxic signs (fever, sore throat, mouth ulcerations, easy bruising, unusual bleeding, joint pain).
3. Observe frequently for recurrence of seizure activity.

INFORM CLIENT AND FAMILY:

1. Blood tests should be repeated frequently during the first 3 months of therapy and at monthly intervals thereafter for 2 to 3 years.
2. Do *not* abruptly withdraw medications following long-term use (may precipitate seizures).
3. Avoid tasks that require alertness until response to drug is established.
4. Report visual abnormalities.

CHLORPROMAZINE

(Thorazine, Chlorazine)

ANTIPSYCHOTIC/NEUROLEPTIC

PHENOTHIAZINE

USES:

1. Management of acute psychotic disorders (schizophrenia, manic phase of a bipolar disorder) and to maintain remission of these psychotic disorders.
2. Management of severe behavioral disturbances in (a) children or (b) clients with organic mental disorders.
3. Other: Intractable hiccups, acute intermittent porphyria, tetanus, preoperatively, or to control nausea and vomiting.

ACTION: Blocks postsynaptic dopamine receptors in the cerebral cortex basal ganglia, hypothalamus, limbic system, brain stem, and medulla. Therefore, there is inhibition or alteration of dopamine release, which is thought to be related to the suppression of the clinical manifestations of schizophrenia.

DOSAGES & ROUTES

Hospitalized: Acute Psychotic Disorders

	PO	IM
Adult	Gradually increase over several days to maximum of 400 mg every 4–6 hours	25 mg—may give an additional 25–50 mg in 1 hour if needed

Outpatient: Maintenance Dose

	PO	IM	RECTAL SUPPOSITORY
Adult	10–50 mg twice daily to every 4 hours	25–50 mg 1–4 times daily	50–100 mg 3–4 times daily
Child	0.55 mg/kg every 4–6 hours	None	1.1 mg/kg every 6–8 hours
Elderly	(Debilitated) 25 mg 3 times daily		

CONTRAINDICATIONS: Comatose states, alcohol or barbiturate withdrawal states, bone marrow depression, pregnancy, lactation.

CAUTIONS: Seizure disorders, diabetes, hepatic disease, cardiac disease, glaucoma, prostatic hypertrophy, asthma.

REMARKS: A "low potency" neuroleptic—low neurological symptoms (extrapyramidal symptoms (EPS)—but with high sedation and autonomic side effects (e.g., hypotension, cardiac, allergic). Food or antacids decrease absorption. Liquid preparation is more rapidly absorbed.

SIDE EFFECTS

AUTONOMIC: Dry mouth, nasal congestion, constipation or diarrhea, urinary retention or urinary frequency, inhibition of ejaculation and impotence in men.

CNS: *Extrapyramidal symptoms* (pseudoparkinsonism, akathisia, dystonia). Possible vertigo or insomnia.

CARDIOVASCULAR: Orthostatic hypotension, hypertension, vertigo, EEG changes.

ENDOCRINE: Changes in libido, galactorrhea in women, gynecomastia in men.

OCULAR: Photophobia, blurred vision, aggravation of glaucoma.

OTHER: Weight gain, allergic reactions such as eczema and skin rashes.

ADVERSE REACTIONS

CNS: *Acute dystonias* (e.g., painful neck spasms, torticollis, oculogyric crisis, convulsions). *Tardive dyskinesia* (choreiform movements of the tongue, face, mouth, jaw, and possibly extremities). The elderly and those on the drug for extended periods of time are more susceptible; often the condition is irreversible.

HEMATOLOGIC: Agranulocytosis—stop drug immediately.

HEPATIC: Jaundice; clinical picture resembles hepatitis.

NEUROLEPTIC MALIGNANT SYNDROME (NMS): Rare life-threatening syndrome. Includes severe rigidity, fever, increased white blood cell count, unstable BP, renal failure, tachycardia, tachypnea. Hold all drugs. Immediate administration of dantrolene sodium and bromocriptine is the most successful somatic prescription.

NURSING MEASURES:
1. Take BP lying and standing (withhold if systolic is 90 or below) and notify physician.
2. Hold dose with EPS or jaundice.
3. Check frequently for urinary retention.
4. Check for constipation (avoid impaction).
5. Observe for fever, sore throat, and malaise, and monitor complete blood count, indicating a blood dyscrasia.

INFORM CLIENT:
1. Rise slowly to a sitting position and dangle the legs 5 minutes before standing to minimize orthostatic hypotension.
2. Avoid sun. Use sunscreen when in direct light to avoid skin blotching. Wear long sleeves and hats.
3. Avoid sun. Client may experience severe photosensitivity. Advise wearing sunglasses to minimize photophobia.
4. Avoid use of alcoholic beverages because they enhance CNS depression.
5. Do not operate machinery if drowsiness occurs.

CLOZAPINE
(Clozaril)

ANTIPSYCHOTIC/NEUROLEPTIC

TRICYCLIC DIBENZODIAZEPINE DERIVATIVE

USES: Management of severely ill schizophrenic patients who fail to respond to other antipsychotic therapy.

ACTION: May involve antagonism of dopaminergic, serotoninergic, adrenergic, cholinergic neurotransmitter systems. Exact action unknown.

DOSAGES & ROUTES

	PO only
Adult	Initially, 25 mg 1–2 times daily; may increase by 25–50 mg/day over 2 weeks until 300–450 mg/day achieved; range, 200–600 mg/day; not to exceed 900 mg/day

CONTRAINDICATIONS: Clients who are hypersensitive to tricyclics, have a history of severe granulocytopenia; concurrent administration with other drugs having potential to suppress bone marrow function; clients who are CNS depressed or comatose or have myeloproliferative disorders.

CAUTIONS: Clients with a history of seizures; cardiovascular disease; impaired respiratory, hepatic, or renal function; alcohol withdrawal; urinary retention. Drug has potent anticholinergic effects, and extreme caution is advised for clients with prostatic enlargement or narrow-angle glaucoma. Also use with caution in pregnant or lactating women.

REMARKS: May take 2 to 4 weeks for therapeutic effects or as long as 3 to 6 months. Since 1–2% of people on clozapine develop agranulocytosis, weekly white blood cell (WBC) counts must be done.

SIDE EFFECTS

FREQUENT: Sedation, salivation, tachycardia, dizziness, constipation (in order of frequency).

OCCASIONAL: Hypotension or hypertension, gastrointestinal upset, nausea and vomiting, sweating, dry mouth, weight gain.

RARE: Visual disturbances, diarrhea, rash, urinary abnormalities.

ADVERSE REACTIONS

HEMATOLOGIC: 1–2% of clients develop agranulocytosis; mild leukopenia may develop.

CNS: *Seizures* develop in about 5% of patients on Clozaril and up to 15% of patients on dosages over 550 mg/day.
Neuroleptic malignant syndrome (NMS) has been reported when clozapine is used concurrently with lithium or other CNS-active agents.
Other: Dizziness or vertigo, drowsiness, restlessness, akinesia, agitation.

CARDIOVASCULAR: Severe orthostatic hypotension (with or without syncope); marked tachycardia may occur in 25% of clients.

NURSING MEASURES:

1. Check baseline WBC count before initiating treatment.
2. Check weekly WBC count; hold drug if the count falls below 3000 mm^3 and notify physician.
3. Check BP lying and standing to assess for potential orthostatic hypotension.
4. Observe for signs of agranulocytosis (e.g., sore throat, fever, malaise).
5. Make baseline assessment of behavior, appearance, emotional status, response to environment, speech pattern, and thought content.

INFORM CLIENT AND FAMILY:

1. Teach about the side effects and toxic effects of the drug and the need for a weekly WBC count.
2. Avoid the use of over-the-counter medications, alcohol, or CNS medication because of potential and severe drug interactions.
3. Report immediately the appearance of lethargy, weakness, fever, sore throat, malaise, mucous membrane ulceration, or other possible signs of infection.
4. Refrain from operating machinery, driving, and other tasks that require alertness until response to the drug is established.
5. Inform the physician if pregnancy occurs.
6. Do not breast-feed an infant if Clozaril is being taken.

DIAZEPAM
(Valium)

ANXIOLYTIC (ANTIANXIETY AGENT)

BENZODIAZEPINE

USES:

1. Management of anxiety disorders, for short-term relief of anxiety symptoms.
2. Presurgical sedation to allay anxiety and tension.
3. Alcohol withdrawal.
4. Seizure disorders.
5. Anticonvulsant.
6. Relief of skeletal muscle spasticity.

ACTION: One action of the benzodiazepines is to increase the action of gamma-aminobutyric acid (GABA). The benzodiazepines help GABA open a chloride channel in the postsynaptic membrane of many neurons, thereby reducing the neuron's excitability.

DOSAGES & ROUTES

	PO	IM/IV
Adult	Anxiety: 2–10 mg 2–4 times daily	2–10 mg 2–4 times daily
	Muscle relaxant: 2–10 mg 2–4 times daily	5–10 mg every 3–4 hours
	Convulsions: 2–10 mg 2–4 times daily	5–10 mg at 10-minute intervals
	Alcohol withdrawal: 10 mg 3–4 times daily	10 mg initially, followed by 5–10 mg every 3–4 hours
Elderly	2.5 mg twice daily	Convulsions: 2–5 mg (increase gradually as needed)

CONTRAINDICATIONS: Acute narrow-angle glaucoma, untreated open-angle glaucoma, during or within 14 days of MAOI therapy, depressed or psychotic patients in the absence of anxiety, first-trimester pregnancy, breast-feeding, shock, coma, acute alcohol intoxication.

CAUTIONS: Epilepsy, myasthenia gravis, impaired hepatic or renal function, drug abuse, addiction-prone individuals. Injectable diazepam is used with extreme caution in the elderly, the very ill, and people with chronic obstructive pulmonary disease. May elicit rage reactions in some clients.

REMARKS: The benzodiazepines can produce psychological and physical habituation, dependence, and withdrawal. Therefore, they are recommended for short-term therapy (2–4 weeks). These drugs need to be used with caution in individuals who have histories of addiction. Withdrawal from these drugs should be gradual in order to minimize withdrawal symptoms.

SIDE EFFECTS

CNS: Sedation, vertigo, weakness, ataxia, decreased motor performance, confusion.

OCULAR: Double or blurred vision.

SKIN: Urticaria, rash, photosensitivity.

GASTROINTESTINAL: Change in weight, dry mouth, constipation.

ADVERSE EFFECTS

CNS: Benzodiazepines are CNS depressants. They are fairly safe when used on their own, but when used in combination with other CNS depressants, they can cause death.

CARDIOVASCULAR: Tachycardia to cardiovascular collapse.

METABOLIC: Changes in liver or renal function test results.

INJECTION SITES: Can cause venous thrombosis or phlebitis at injection sites.

NURSING MEASURES:

1. Obtain drug history of prescribed and over-the-counter medications.
2. Periodically monitor blood cell count and liver function test results during prolonged therapy.
3. Assess for unexplained bleeding, petechiae, fever, and so forth.
4. Intramuscular therapy: Aspirate back, administer deep into large muscle mass; inject slowly; rotate injection sites.

INFORM CLIENT:

1. Avoid alcohol or any other CNS depressants (anticonvulsants, antidepressants) while taking a benzodiazepine—can lead to respiratory depression. Check with physician before taking.
2. Avoid driving or operating hazardous machinery if drowsiness or confusion occurs.
3. Avoid abrupt withdrawal of benzodiazepine.

DISULFIRAM
(Antabuse)

ALCOHOL DETERRENT

ALDEHYDE DEHYDROGENASE INHIBITOR

USES: Adjunct treatment for selected clients with chronic alcoholism who want to remain in a state of enforced sobriety. A form of aversion therapy.

ACTION: Inhibits hepatic enzymes from normal metabolic breakdown of alcohol, resulting in high levels.

DOSAGES & ROUTES

	PO only
Adult	Initially, a maximum of 500 mg daily given as a single dose for 1–2 weeks; maintenance, 250 mg daily; not to exceed 500 mg daily.

CONTRAINDICATIONS: Severe heart disease, psychosis, and hypersensitivity to disulfiram.

CAUTIONS: Diabetes, hypothyroidism, epilepsy, cerebral damage, nephritis, hepatic disease, pregnancy.

REMARKS: Clients must abstain from alcohol intake for at least 12 hours before the initial dose of drug is administered.

SIDE EFFECTS: Common side effects experienced during the first 2 weeks of therapy include mild drowsiness, fatigue, headache, metallic or garlic aftertaste, allergic dermatitis, and acne eruptions. Symptoms disappear spontaneously with continued therapy or reduced dosage.

ADVERSE REACTIONS DISULFIRAM-ALCOHOL REACTION Flushing or throbbing in head and neck, throbbing headache, nausea, copious vomiting, diaphoresis, dyspnea, hyperventilation, tachycardia, hypotension, marked uneasiness, vertigo, blurred vision, confusion. Can cause death.

NURSING MEASURES:

1. Client must be able to demonstrate sobriety.
2. Client must be fully aware of drug's action when taken along with alcohol before treatment commences.
3. In severe disulfiram-alcohol reactions, supportive measures to restore BP and treat for shock in a medical facility are vital.

INFORM CLIENT AND FAMILY:

1. Avoid any substances that contain alcohol
   a. *Ingestion:* Elixirs, cough syrups, vinegars, vitamin/mineral tonics; be aware that some sauces, soups, ciders, flavor extracts (vanilla, cherry) and some desserts (flaming, and some cakes and pies) are made with alcohol.
   b. *Topical:* Mouthwash, body lotions, liniments, shaving lotion.
   c. *Inhalation:* Avoid inhaling fumes from substances that may contain alcohol, such as paints, wood stains, varnishes, and "stripping" compounds.
2. Carry a card stating that if they are found disoriented or unconscious, they may be having a disulfiram-alcohol reaction and telling the finder whom to contact for medical care.
3. A disulfiram-alcohol reaction can occur within 5 to 10 minutes after ingestion of alcohol and can last 30–60 minutes or longer.
4. Reaction may occur with alcohol up to 14 days after ingesting disulfiram.

DONEPEZIL HYDROCHLORIDE

(Aricept) CHOLINESTERASE INHIBITOR

USES: Treatment of mild to moderate dementia of the Alzheimer's type

ACTIONS: The cholinergic system deteriorates in Alzheimer's disease. Donepezil inhibits the breakdown of endogenously released acetylcholine.

DOSAGES & ROUTES

Adults and Elderly:	Start with 5 mg daily dose. After 6 weeks may increase to 10 mg daily.

CONTRAINDICATIONS: Hypersensitivity to Donepezil or piperidine derivatives.

CAUTIONS: Cholinesterase inhibitors may increase gastric acid secretion. Therefore, clients should be monitored for gastrointestinal bleeding, especially those at increased risk of developing ulcers (e.g., history of ulcer disease, taking nonsteroidal antiinflammatory medication). Use with caution in clients who have a history of seizures. Prescribe with care to clients with asthma or obstructive pulmonary disease.

SIDE EFFECTS FREQUENT: Nausea, vomiting, diarrhea, insomnia, muscle cramps, fatigue, and anorexia.

ADVERSE REACTIONS: Syncopal episodes have been reported in association with the use of this drug.

NURSING MEASURES

1. Ascertain what other drugs client is taking because donepezil has the potential to interfere with the activity of anticholinergic medications.
2. Discuss with family/friends who is to administer the medication to client, to prevent dosage errors.

INFORM CLIENT AND FAMILY:

1. Take drug in the evening before retiring.
2. Drug may be taken with food.
3. In case of accidental overdose, call a poison control center to determine the latest recommendations for management.

FLUOXETINE HYDROCHLORIDE

(Prozac) ANTIDEPRESSANT

USES:

1. Prozac is an atypical antidepressant medication that is chemically unrelated to TCAs or MAOIs.
2. Has been found effective in clients with bulimia and obsessive-compulsive disorders.

ACTION: Is a potent serotonin reuptake blocker whose use results in an increase in the amount of active serotonin within the synaptic cleft and at the serotonin receptor site. Increased serotonin in these areas appears to modify affective and behavioral disorders.

DOSAGES & ROUTES

Adult	20 mg/day; may reach 40–60 mg in divided doses; do not exceed 80 mg daily
Elderly	Same as for adults
Child	No dosage for children as yet established

CONTRAINDICATIONS: Not to be taken within 14 days of an MAOI. Also, client must wait 5 weeks when going from fluoxetine to an MAOI.

CAUTIONS: Use with clients with concomitant systemic illness has not been studied extensively. Caution should be used with pregnant women or women who are breast-feeding, children, and the elderly. Caution should also be used with clients with liver disease or renal impairment or in a client who has had a recent myocardial infarction.

REMARKS: Fluoxetine, like the TCAs and MAOIs, takes from 2 to 5 weeks to produce an elevation of mood. Advantages of this drug are fewer anticholinergic side effects and a low incidence of cardiovascular effects. However, fluoxetine may impair judgment, thinking, and motor skills.

SIDE EFFECTS **GENERAL:** The most common side effects reported with fluoxetine hydrochloride are nausea, nervousness and anxiety, insomnia, and vertigo. When these side effects are severe, the drug is discontinued. If a rash or urticaria or both develop, the drug should be discontinued. Anorexia may appear in some people.

ADVERSE REACTIONS See Side Effects.

NURSING MEASURES:

1. Fluoxetine hydrochloride is given in the early morning without consideration to meals.
2. Clients who are potentially suicidal are assessed for suicidal thoughts or actions. Carefully observe taking of medication.
3. If client is underweight and experiences anorexia, the physician should be alerted to re-evaluate continuation of medication.

INFORM CLIENT:

1. If rash or urticaria appears, notify physician immediately.
2. Do not drive or operate machinery if drowsiness occurs.
3. Avoid alcoholic beverages.

HALOPERIDOL
(Haldol)

ANTIPSYCHOTIC/NEUROLEPTIC

BUTYROPHENONE

USES:

1. Management of psychotic disorders.
2. Helps control remissions in schizophrenia.
3. Controversial use for children with combative, explosive hyperexcitability.
4. Control of tic and vocal utterances of Tourette's disease.
5. Useful in acute mania and acute and chronic organic psychosis.
6. Management of drug-induced (LSD) psychosis.

ACTION: Blocks the binding of dopamine to the postsynaptic dopamine receptors in the brain.

DOSAGES & ROUTES

	PO	IM
Adult	0.5–2.0 mg 2–3 times daily	(Severe) 3–5 mg every 1–8 hours to control symptoms, then give PO
Child	Not for children under 3 years; for children 3–12 years, 0.05–0.15 mg/kg/ day in 2–3 divided doses	
Elderly	Elderly or debilitated clients may require smaller doses than adults	

CONTRAINDICATIONS: Hypersensitivity, Parkinson's disease, depression, seizures, coma, alcoholism, during lithium therapy.

CAUTIONS: The elderly; clients on anticoagulant therapy; clients with glaucoma, prostatic hypertrophy, urinary retention, asthma, or pregnancy/lactation.

REMARKS: A "high potency" neuroleptic; higher incidence of EPS but lower incidence of sedation and orthostatic hypotension. Haldol Decanoate E or D given intramuscularly can have lasting effects from 1 to 3 weeks.

SIDE EFFECTS **AUTONOMIC**: Dry mouth, nasal congestion, constipation or diarrhea, urinary retention or urinary frequency, inhibition of ejaculation and impotence in men.

CNS: EPS (pseudoparkinsonism, akathisia, dystonia), vertigo, insomnia, headache.

CARDIOVASCULAR: Orthostatic hypotension, hypertension, dizziness, EEG changes.

ENDOCRINE: Changes in libido, galactorrhea in women, gynecomastia in men.

OCULAR: Photophobia, blurred vision, aggravation of glaucoma.

OTHER: Weight gain, allergic reactions such as eczema and skin rashes.

ADVERSE REACTIONS **CNS**: *Acute dystonias* (e.g., painful neck spasms, torticollis, oculogyric crisis, convulsions). *Tardive dyskinesia* (choreiform movements of the tongue, face, mouth, jaw, and possibly extremities). The elderly and those on the drug for extended periods are more susceptible; often irreversible.

HEMATOLOGIC: Agranulocytosis—drug immediately stopped.

HEPATIC: Jaundice; clinical picture resembles hepatitis.

NEUROLEPTIC MALIGNANT SYNDROME (NMS): Occurs within 24–72 hours. Fever, rigidity, renal failure, arrhythmias, and more. Hold drug and give dantrolene sodium or bromocriptine immediately.

NURSING MEASURES:

1. Check for signs of tardive dyskinesia (protrusion of tongue, puffing of cheeks, chewing or puckering of the mouth) and report them to physician immediately.
2. Observe for other signs of EPS and jaundice.
3. Check for orthostatic hypotension (take BP lying and standing). Withhold if systolic is 80 or below.
4. Check frequently for urinary retention.
5. Check for constipation (avoid impaction).
6. Observe for fever, sore throat, and malaise, and monitor complete blood count, indicating a blood dyscrasia.
7. Monitor renal function during long-term therapy.
8. Monitor blood levels every week.

INFORM CLIENT:

1. Rise slowly to a sitting position and dangle the legs 5 minutes before standing to minimize orthostatic hypotension.
2. Use sunscreen when in direct light to avoid skin blotching, and wear sunglasses to prevent photophobia.
3. Avoid the use of alcoholic beverages because they enhance CNS depression.
4. Refrain from operating machinery if drowsiness occurs.

IMIPRAMINE HYDROCHLORIDE

(Tofranil)

ANTIDEPRESSANT

TRICYCLIC

USES:

1. The principal indication for TCAs is the treatment of depression (major, bipolar, or dysthymia).
2. Imipramine is effective in some organic affective disorders and obsessive-compulsive disorders.
3. Imipramine is used as adjunctive treatment in childhood enuresis and in bulimia.
4. Found useful in the treatment of agoraphobia with panic attacks and generalized anxiety disorder.

ACTION: TCAs block the reuptake of norepinephrine and serotonin into their presynaptic neurons.

DOSAGES & ROUTES

	PO	IM
Adult	50 mg/day to start, given in 1–4 divided doses up to 200 mg daily for outpatients. Maintenance level 50–150 mg/day.	Do not exceed 100 mg/day in divided doses
Child	For childhood enuresis, 25 mg before bedtime; for depression in children *over* 12 years, 30–40 mg daily initially	
Elderly	Used with caution—usually start at lower dose. Geriatric clients start on 30–40 mg daily initially	

CONTRAINDICATIONS: Recent myocardial infarction or cardiac disease, severe renal or hepatic impairment. Death may occur if used with a monoamine oxidase inhibitor. However, the two may be cautiously used together in cases of refractory depression. TCAs may also cause fatal cardiac arrhythmias in clients with hyperthyroidism. Use with caution in children and adolescents. Special cautions for the elderly, especially those with cardiac, respiratory, cardiovascular, hepatic, or gastrointestinal diseases.

CAUTIONS: Other cautions include people with renal or hepatic disease, and narrow-angle glaucoma. The potential for suicide must be assessed. TCAs lower the seizure threshold: any client with a seizure disorder needs careful monitoring.

REMARKS:

1. Before receiving TCAs, clients need a thorough physical and cardiac work-up.
2. Patients need to know that mood elevation may not occur for 2 to 4 weeks.

SIDE EFFECTS

ANTICHOLINERGIC: Dry mouth and nasal passages, constipation, urinary hesitancy, esophageal reflux, blurred vision.

CARDIOVASCULAR: Orthostatic hypotension, hypertension, palpitations.

CNS: Tachycardia, vertigo, tinnitus, numbness and tingling of extremities, stimulation.

ENDOCRINE: Galactorrhea, increased or decreased libido, ejaculatory and erectile disturbances, delayed orgasm.

OTHER: Weight gain and impotence, cholestatic jaundice, fatigue.

ADVERSE REACTIONS

AUTONOMIC: Intracardiac conduction slowing.

CARDIOVASCULAR: Myocardial infarction, congestive heart failure, arrhythmias, heart block, cardiotoxicity, cerebrovascular accident, shock.

CNS: Ataxia, neuropathy, EPS, lowered seizure threshold, delirium.

HEMATOLOGIC: Bone marrow depression, agranulocytosis.

PSYCHIATRIC: Hallucinations, shift to hypomania, mania, exacerbation of psychosis.

NURSING MEASURES:

1. Monitor BP (both lying and standing) every 2 to 6 hours when initiating therapy.
2. Observe suicidal clients closely during initial therapy.
3. Supervise drug ingestion to prevent hoarding of drug.
4. Assess for urinary retention.
5. Monitor liver function test results and complete blood count (assess for signs of cholestatic jaundice and agranulocytosis).
6. Small amount of drugs should be dispensed if client is to be discharged.
7. Diabetic clients should be closely monitored especially during early therapy, since hypo- or hyperglycemia may occur in some clients.
8. All clients on TCAs need to be observed for the occurrence of hypomania or manic episodes, urinary retention, orthostatic hypotension, and seizure activity.

INFORM CLIENT:

1. Rise slowly to prevent hypotensive effects.
2. Do not drive or use hazardous machinery if drowsiness or vertigo occurs.
3. Do not use over-the-counter drugs in conjunction with a TCA without a physician's approval.
4. The effects of alcohol and imipramine are potentiated when used together, and alcohol use should be discussed with a physician before taking the drug.
5. One to four weeks may pass before therapeutic effects are experienced.

LITHIUM CARBONATE/CITRATE

(Carbolith, Eskalith, Lithane, Lithizine, Lithonate, Lithobid)

ANTIMANIC

LITHIUM

USES:

1. Primarily used to control, prevent, or diminish manic episodes in people with bipolar depression (manic-depressive psychosis).
2. Used *experimentally* in alcoholism, premenstrual syndrome, drug abuse, phobias, eating disorders, and rage reactions.

ACTION: Lithium is an alkali metal salt that behaves in the body much like a sodium ion. Lithium acts to lower concentrations of norepinephrine and serotonin by inhibiting their release and enhancing their reuptake by neurons. The therapeutic effects, as well as the side effects and toxic effects, of lithium are thought to be related to the partial replacement of sodium by lithium in membrane action.

DOSAGES & ROUTES

	PO
Adult	Acute mania, 600 mg 3 times daily; maintenance dose, 300 mg 3 times daily or 4 times daily
Child	Not labeled for pediatric use
Elderly	Reduce to 600–900 daily to produce low serum concentration of about 0.5 mEq/L

CONTRAINDICATIONS: Pregnancy, nursing mothers, significant cardiovascular or renal disease, schizophrenia, severe debilitation, dehydration, sodium depletion.

CAUTIONS: The elderly, thyroid disease, epilepsy, concomitant use with haloperidol or other antipsychotics, parkinsonism, severe infections, urinary retention, diabetes.

REMARKS: Serum lithium levels must be monitored during drug therapy. The therapeutic range is very narrow, and the potential for toxic effects is high if blood levels are not monitored. During the acute stage, blood levels are raised to 1.0–1.4 mEq/L. Maintenance therapy blood levels run from 0.8–1.2 mEq/L. Side effects and toxic effects are common at higher doses (1.5 mEq/L or more). Before a patient is started on lithium, BUN, T4, T3, and TSH levels should be measured, and an ECG should be done.

SIDE EFFECTS: The major long-term risks of lithium therapy are hypothyroidism and impairment of the kidney's ability to concentrate urine.

Below 1.5 mEq/L: Polyuria, polydipsia, lethargy, fatigue, muscle weakness, headache, mild nausea, fine hand tremor, and inability to concentrate. May experience ankle edema. Symptoms disappear during continued therapy.

ADVERSE AND TOXIC EFFECTS

1.5–2.0 mEq/L: Vomiting, diarrhea, muscle weakness, ataxia, dizziness, slurred speech, confusion.

2.0–2.5 mEq/L: Blurred vision, muscle twitching, severe hypotension, persistent nausea and vomiting. Thyroid toxicity is common.

2.5–3.0 mEq/L or more: Urinary and fecal incontinence, seizures, cardiac arrhythmias, peripheral vascular collapse, death.

NURSING MEASURES:

1. If serum lithium levels are above 1.5 mEq/L or if client has persistent diarrhea, vomiting, excessive sweating in hot weather, infection, or fever, check with physician before giving dose.
2. Check urine specific gravity periodically and teach patient to do so at home (normal: 1.005–1.025).
3. Administer lithium with meals.
4. Ensure that client is well hydrated.

INFORM CLIENT:

1. Drink plenty of liquids (2–3 L/day) during initial therapy and 1–1.5 L/day during remainder of therapy.
2. Know the side effects and toxic effects of lithium therapy and seek out physician immediately if problems arise.
3. Have blood lithium levels measured at regular intervals as directed in order to regulate dosage and prevent toxicity.
4. Maintain a regular diet, thus maintaining average salt intake (6–8 g) required to keep the serum lithium level in the therapeutic range.
5. Avoid alcohol.
6. Be aware that antibiotics (metronidazole and tetracycline) and nonsteroidal anti-inflammatory agents (indomethacin) can increase lithium levels.
7. Know that caffeine can lower lithium levels.

LORAZEPAM

(Ativan)

ANTIANXIETY AGENT

BENZODIAZEPINE

USES:

1. Treatment of anxiety disorders associated with depression.
2. Preoperative sedation
3. Nausea and vomiting associated with chemotherapy for cancer.

ACTIONS: CNS depressant, especially the limbic system and reticular formation. Enhances action of inhibitory neurotransmitter gamma-aminobutyric acid (GABA), producing a calming effect. Can suppress spread of seizure activity and can directly depress motor nerve and muscle function, creating some muscle relaxation.

DOSAGES & ROUTES

	PO
Adult	For anxiety, 2–3 mg daily in 2–3 doses; for insomnia, 2–4 mg at bedtime.
Elderly	For anxiety, 0.5–1 mg daily (may increase gradually); for insomnia, 0.5–1 mg at bedtime.

CONTRAINDICATIONS: Acute narrow-angle glaucoma and alcohol intoxication, pregnant clients or lactating mothers, children under 12.

CAUTIONS: Clients with renal or hepatic dysfunction, elderly or debilitated clients, clients with a history of drug abuse/addictions.

People taking other *CNS depressants (narcotics, barbiturates, alcohol)* may have a synergistic effect, increasing CNS depression. May reduce *Digoxin* excretion, increasing the potential for toxicity.

SIDE EFFECTS: **FREQUENT:** Drowsiness, fatigue, dizziness, incoordination.

OCCASIONAL: Blurred vision, slurred speech, hypotension, headache.

RARE: Paradoxical CNS restlessness, excitement in elderly/debilitated.

ADVERSE REACTIONS: Can have pronounced withdrawal symptoms (seizures, pronounced restlessness, insomnia, abdominal/muscle cramps) with abrupt withdrawal from the drug.

NURSING MEASURES:

1. Assess for history of glaucoma, substance abuse, allergies, past reactions to benzodiazepines, and current list of medications.
2. Before long-term therapy, assess CBC and liver function tests in collaboration with physician.
3. Make sure client has written information about medications covering side effects, doses, precautions, and other information.

INFORM CLIENT AND FAMILY:

1. Avoid tasks that require alertness or motor skills (driving, operating machinery).
2. Do not take over-the-counter medications or new medications without approval from your physician.
3. Do not drink alcohol or take other CNS depressants while taking this medication.
4. Do not stop medication abruptly.

METHYLPHENIDATE

(Ritalin) CENTRAL NERVOUS SYSTEM STIMULANT

USES: Attention deficit disorder (children 6 years and older), narcolepsy, and occasionally for depression in the elderly.

ACTIONS: Direct release of catecholamines into synaptic clefts and thus onto postsynaptic receptor sites; blocks reuptake of catecholamines, thus prolonging their actions; serve as false neurotransmitters.

DOSAGES & ROUTES

	PO
Children	6 years and older usual starting dose is 5 mg twice daily (breakfast and lunch). Most children are maintained on 60 mg/day and should be monitored regularly by prescribing physician.
Adults	Doses may start at 5 mg 2–3 times daily. Dose range for adults is 10 mg/day to not more 60 mg/day (20–40 mg/day is usual).
Elderly	Elderly clients using Ritalin for depression usually are maintained on 2.5–20 mg/day.

CONTRAINDICATIONS: Not to be used for clients with glaucoma, hypertension, heart problems, or a history of Tourette's syndrome. People with a history of seizure disorders may experience an increase in number, duration, or severity of seizures.

CAUTIONS: Can cause growth delay in children. Can interact with other medications, for example, alcohol, antidepressants (MAOIs and TCAs), some over-the-counter medications, health food products containing *ma huang*. Serious problems can also develop if clients are taking any other amphetamine-type or diet drugs.

SIDE EFFECTS

FREQUENT: Nervousness and sleeplessness are most common. Other reactions are loss of appetite, weight loss, nausea, dizziness, heart palpitations, increases in blood pressure, stomach upset, and growth delay in children with prolonged therapy.

OCCASIONAL: Dizziness, dysphoria, joint pain, fever.

ADVERSE REACTIONS: Can increase frequency of seizures in people with seizure disorders; chest pain, dysrhythmias. Can have serious interactions with other medications and over-the-counter preparations.

NURSING MEASURES

1. Take a careful inventory of any other medications client is taking, prescribed and over-the-counter or health food products. Check with pharmacy if there might be a problem with compatibility.
2. Medications are best taken shortly before meals, and not after 12:00 noon or 1:00 PM for children or 6:00 PM for adults, since stimulant effect may keep people awake.

INFORM CLIENT AND FAMILY:

1. Suggest to parents to discuss drug holidays, which can help avoid the side effect of growth delay with their prescribing health care agent (physician, nurse, therapist).
2. Cautions client and family that drug may have serious side effects when mixed with other substances. Have client or family check with physician before taking any over-the-counter medications or other drugs or health food products from other sources.
3. If the child must take this medication during school hours, ask your pharmacist to provide an empty labeled container and place no more than 1 week's worth of medication in the bottle. Be sure the medication is secured with a school official.
4. Once person is stabilized on a dose, Ritalin can be given in extended-release form. These tablets are to be swallowed whole, *never crushed or chewed.*
5. Keep tablets dry, tightly capped, away from direct heat.
6. Keep out of reach of children and pets.

NEFAZODONE

(Serzone)

ANTIDEPRESSANT

SELECTIVE SEROTONIN NOREPINEPHRINE REUPTAKE INHIBITOR (SSNRI)

USES:

1. Treatment of depression

ACTION: Nefazodone and one of its active metabolites exert dual effects on serotoninergic neurotransmission through blockade of serotonin type 2 (5HT2) receptors and inhibition of serotonin uptake. The parent compound (NEF) and another active metabolite also exhibit affinity for the 5-HT1C receptor. Nefazodone lacks anticholinergic or antihistaminic effects but exhibits some affinity for alpha$_1$-adrenergic receptors.

DOSAGES & ROUTES

	PO
Adult	Start on 100–200 mg/day (50–100 mg twice daily), maintenance dose from 300–500 mg/day (150–250 mg twice daily).
Elderly	Start on 50–100 mg/day (25–50 mg twice daily), maintenance dose 150–250 daily (75–175 mg twice daily).

CAUTIONS: During pregnancy this drug should be used only if clearly needed. Lactating women should not nurse their infants while receiving nefazodone. Caution should be used when nefazodone is initiated in people with preexisting hypotension or a labile circulation. Nefazodone should be used with caution on anyone with preexisting liver, kidney, or heart disease or a history of seizures or allergies. As with all antidepressants a suicide assessment is needed and prescriptions should be written for the smallest quantity of tablets consistent with good client management.

CONTRAINDICATIONS: To avoid potentially life-threatening cardiotoxicity, the nonsedating antihistamines *terfenadine (Seldane)* and *astemizole (Hismanal)* should not be taken by clients on nefazodone. Drugs such as *alprazolam* (Xanax) and *triazolam* (Halcion) require dosage reductions when used concomitantly. As with the SSRIs and venlafaxine, nefazodone should not be used in combination with MAOI or within 2 weeks of terminating treatment with MAOI. MAOI should not be introduced until at least 2 weeks after the cessation of nefazodone therapy. Contraindicated in clients with known hypersensitivity to nefazodone, and components of the formulation or other phenylpiperazine antidepressants.

SIDE EFFECTS: **FREQUENT**: Sleepiness, dry mouth, nausea, dizziness (especially when standing), constipation, confusion, incoordination, blurred vision or changes in vision.

INFREQUENT: Irregular heartbeat or skin rash.

ADVERSE REACTIONS **CARDIOVASCULAR**: Sinus bradycardia and first-degree AV block.

GENITOURINARY: Nefazodone is structurally related to trazodone, which has been associated with priapism. *No cases have been reported;* however, a client who presents with a prolonged or inappropriate erection, should discontinue therapy immediately and consult a physician right away.

NURSING MEASURES

1. The drug is given twice daily in divided doses.
2. Clients who are suicidal are observed for suicidal actions if hospitalized; if in the community, they are given the smallest number of tablets consistent with good management.
3. Teach measures for combating orthostatic hypotension in case the client experiences dizziness upon rising.

INFORM CLIENT

1. Do not drive or operate machinery if drowsiness occurs.
2. Drug may take 2–3 weeks before therapeutic effects are noted.
3. Excessive sedation may occur during initial therapy.

OLANZAPINE

(Zyprexa) ATYPICAL ANTIPSYCHOTIC

USES:

1. First-line treatment for schizophrenia, targeting both the positive and the negative symptoms.
2. Other psychotic illness.

DOSAGES & ROUTES

	PO
Adult	Given in 5–10 mg doses once daily, with a target of 10 mg/day (15 mg/day *does not* seem to be more effective than 10 mg/day). Range 5–20 mg/day. Available in 5 mg, 7½ mg, and 10 mg tablets.

ACTION: Olanzapine blocks various serotonin (5-HT2A) receptors and dopamine (D2) receptors. It also antagonizes dopamine D1–D4 receptors, serotonin 5-HT2C and 5HT3 receptors, and the alpha$_1$-adrenergic and H1 histamine receptors.

CAUTIONS: Olanzapine seems to have a good side effect profile and low potential interactions. *Carbamazepine*, may increase olanzapine clearance by 50% at a dose of 200 mg twice daily, and *nicotine* may increase olanzapine clearance by 40% in smokers.

SIDE EFFECTS **FREQUENT:** Psychomotor slowing (somnolence, asthenia), psychomotor activation (agitation, nervousness, insomnia, hostility), and dizziness. Weight gain.

INFREQUENT: At higher doses, anticholinergic effects (constipation, dry mouth, increased appetite). Mild transient dose-related increases in hepatic transaminase and prolactin levels resolve spontaneously and do not require discontinuation of the drug.

PHENELZINE SULFATE

(Nardil)

ANTIDEPRESSANT

MONOAMINE OXIDASE INHIBITOR (MAOI)

USES:

1. MAOIs are used primarily for depression that is refractory to tricyclic antidepressant therapy.
2. MAOIs are particularly effective in atypical depression, agoraphobia, or hypochondriasis.
3. Panic disorders.

ACTION: Antidepressant effect thought to be due to irreversible inhibition of MAO, thereby increasing the concentration of epinephrine, norepinephrine, serotonin, and dopamine within the presynaptic neurons and at the receptor site.

DOSAGES & ROUTES

	PO
Adult	15 mg 3 times daily; increase rapidly to 60 mg daily until therapeutic level is noted
Elderly	Are prone to side effects and in adults older than 60 may be contraindicated
Child	Not used with children

CONTRAINDICATIONS: MAOIs can cause untoward interactions with certain foodstuffs or cold remedies, which may produce hypertensive crises, CVA, or hyperpyrexia states that can lead to coma or death. Therefore, a confused or noncompliant client is at risk with an MAOI.

Other contraindications include people with congestive heart failure, cardiovascular or cerebrovascular disease, impaired renal function, glaucoma, history of severe headaches, or liver disease; elderly or debilitated patients; and people who are pregnant or who have paranoid schizophrenia.

CAUTIONS: Depression accompanying alcoholism or drug addiction, manic-depressive states, suicidal tendencies, agitated clients, and people with chronic brain syndromes or a history of angina pectoris.

REMARKS: Because of the severe interactions of some foodstuffs and medication, clients need comprehensive teaching, teaching aids, and supervision.

High-tyramine foods include beer, red wine, aged cheese, dry sausage, fava beans (Italian green beans), brewer's yeast, smoked fish, any kind of liver, avocados, and bologna. Chocolate and coffee should be used in moderation.

Drugs causing severe medication interactions include meperidine (Demerol), epinephrine, local anesthetics, decongestants, cough medications, diet pills, and most over-the-counter medications.

SIDE EFFECTS **GENERAL:** Constipation, dry mouth, vertigo, orthostatic hypotension, drowsiness or insomnia, weakness, fatigue, weight gain, hypomania, mania, blurred vision, skin rash. Muscle twitching is common.

ADVERSE REACTIONS **HYPERTENSIVE CRISIS**: Intense occipital headache, palpitation, stiff neck, fever, chest pain, bradycardia or tachycardia, intracranial bleeding.

HEPATIC: Jaundice, malaise, right upper quadrant pain, change in color or consistency of stools.

NURSING MEASURES:

1. Monitor BP for orthostatic hypotension every 2 to 4 hours during initial therapy.
2. Assess for other potential signs of hypertensive crises.
3. Observe for marked changes in mood (e.g., hypomania, mania).
4. Monitor intake and output and frequency of stools.
5. Have client dangle legs 5 minutes before standing.
6. Depressed persons are at risk for suicide; continue to monitor and observe for potential suicidal behaviors.

INFORM CLIENT:

1. Inform clients and their families clearly and carefully about foodstuffs and medications to avoid. REVIEW IN DETAIL.
2. Instruct clients taking MAOIs to wear a medical identification tag or bracelet.
3. Caution clients to avoid all over-the-counter drugs unless a physician's approval has been obtained.
4. Caution clients to avoid all alcohol.
5. Encourage clients and their families to go to the emergency room immediately if signs and symptoms of hypertensive crises are suspected. Phentolamine (Regitine) can be given for hypertensive crises.

RISPERIDONE
(Risperdal)

ATYPICAL ANTIPSYCHOTIC

USES: Potent antipsychotic agent, targets negative (withdrawal, apathy, negativism) as well as positive symptoms (hallucinations, delusions, paranoia, hostility) of schizophrenia.

ACTIONS: A potent antagonist at 5HT2A and D2 receptors (serotonin and dopamine).

DOSAGES & ROUTES

	PO	
Adults	Dose range 4–16 mg/day (6 mg/day dose most effective for many)	Tablets only
Elderly	Dose range 1–4 mg/day	Tablets only

CONTRAINDICATIONS: Hypersensitivity to Risperidone.

CAUTIONS: Can cause orthostatic hypotension and tachycardia. Because of these reactions it should be started at low doses (e.g., 0.5 mg in the elderly and 1.0 for adults). Risperidone is associated with dose-related EPS, although often minimal in therapeutic range. Use with caution in clients with a history of seizures.

SIDE EFFECTS: **FREQUENT**: Sedation, insomnia, rhinitis, coughing, back or chest pain, erectile problems in men, weight gain, and decreased sexual interest. Initial dosing especially may cause orthostatic hypotension and tachycardia or syncope. Some clients report anorexia, polyuria/polydipsia and/or an increase in dream activity.

OCCASIONAL: EPS and increases in plasma prolactin can lead to galactorrhea and menstrual disturbances in some women.

ADVERSE REACTIONS: A number of cases of neuroleptic malignant syndrome (NMS) have been reported. Rare cases of priapism have been reported.

NURSING MEASURES

1. Client should know what the medication can do and what it cannot do. This drug can target some of the negative symptoms, and that should be included in client teaching about the drug.
2. Client needs a list of the possible expected side effects and those reactions that would warrant contacting the prescribing nurse, physician, or therapist (e.g., palpitations, erectile or sexual disinterest problems that might threaten compliance, palpitations, or dizziness).
3. Teach clients initially to sit on the side of the bed before getting up in the morning, to avoid dizziness when getting up and potential falls.
4. Check to see if client has had seizures in the past.

INFORM CLIENT AND FAMILY:

1. When starting medication, be careful driving cars, working around machinery, and crossing streets. Medication can make people sleepy and perhaps dizzy, especially initially.
2. Do not suddenly stop taking medication even if there is no immediate return of symptoms. Relapse is a very high risk in the weeks and months after medications have been stopped.
3. Client or family member should notify the doctor if the client is having a sore throat during the first several months of treatment, if NMS appears (client should have a fact sheet on NMS) or if client is going to have general or dental surgery or is experiencing chest pain or tachycardia/palpitations.

SERTRALINE HYDROCHLORIDE

(Zoloft)

ANTIDEPRESSANT

SELECTIVE SEROTONIN REUPTAKE INHIBITOR (SSRI)

ACTION: Enhances serotoninergic activity in the CNS by blocking reuptake of serotonin in neuronal presynaptic membranes. Has only a very weak effect on dopamine and norepinephrine reuptake.

USES:

1. Major depression
2. Obsessive-compulsive disorder (OCD)

DOSAGES & ROUTES

	PO
Adults	Initially 50 mg once daily with morning *or* evening meal. May be increased no sooner than every week up to a maximum of 200 mg/day.
Elderly	Initially 25 mg/day once daily as above. May increase 25 mg every 2–3 days.

CONTRAINDICATIONS: Use within 2 weeks of MAOI. The safety for children and in pregnancy has not been established. Anyone with hypersensitivity to the drug.

CAUTIONS: Severe hepatic or renal insufficiency, elderly and debilitated clients, suicidal clients, and clients with a history of seizures or mania.

DRUG INTERACTIONS: Cimetidine can increase sertraline concentrations. Other drug interactions with sertraline include an increase in diazepam concentrations, a decrease in tolbutamide, and increased bleeding for clients taking warfarin.

SIDE EFFECTS: **FREQUENT:** Dizziness, headache, tremor, insomnia, somnolence, fatigue, agitation, nausea, dry mouth, loose stools/constipation, sexual dysfunction.

OCCASIONAL: Increased sweating, dyspepsia, anorexia, nervousness, rhinitis, abnormal vision.

RARE: Rash, vomiting, frequent urination, palpitations, paresthesia, twitching.

NURSING MEASURES

1. Zoloft is best given in the morning
2. If hospitalized, watch for signs of *cheeking* of medications (i.e., instead of swallowing medications, holding them under the tongue or in the cheek for the purpose of saving them and taking an overdose later).

INFORM CLIENT AND FAMILY

1. Medication may have to be taken 1 to 3 weeks before improvement is noticed, but often the time is much shorter.
2. If client is extremely depressed, client should be given only 1 week's supply at a time.
3. Caution client about premature discontinuation of therapy, which can result in a relapse. In general, medication should continue for at least 6 months to 1 year after symptoms have subsided.
3. Have client and family assess for signs of improvement in symptoms, especially in areas such as depressed mood and loss of interest or pleasure in usual activities.
4. Have client and family watch for signs of suicidal ideation.

TACRINE
(Cognex)

REVERSIBLE CHOLINESTERASE INHIBITOR

USES: Can help mild to moderate dementia in people with Alzheimer's disease. Appears to reverse 6 months of dementia progression.

ACTIONS: Cholinergic system deteriorates in Alzheimer's dementia. Tacrine inhibits breakdown of endogenously released acetylcholine.

DOSAGES & ROUTES

	PO
Adults	40 mg/day (more improvement noticed with 80–160 mg/day). Because of 2–4 hour half-life, needs 4 times daily dosing. Start at 10 mg 4 times daily (40 mg) and continue 6 weeks if tolerated. Every 6 weeks increase *each dose* by 10 mg 4 times daily. If tolerated, go to 160 mg daily.

CONTRAINDICATIONS: Can be hepatotoxic to some clients.

CAUTIONS: Because of elevation in liver enzymes, clients need frequent liver function testing. Other drugs can alter (raise or lower) tacrine levels. Anticholinergic agents can reverse tacrine's effects. Tacrine increases risk of cholinergic agent toxicity. Smoking can lower tacrine levels.

SIDE EFFECTS, FREQUENT: Flulike symptoms without fever; gastrointestinal symptoms (nausea, diarrhea, dyspepsia, anorexia, vomiting).

ADVERSE REACTIONS: Elevation of transaminase (ALT/SGPT). Liver function tests must be done and ALT levels monitored weekly for 6 weeks after each dose increase. Most common reason for dropouts.

NURSING MEASURES

1. Check to see that other medications (and smoking) can alter tacrine levels. Be sure that client has informed prescribing physician and nurse of all medications client is taking.

INFORM CLIENT AND FAMILY:

1. Clients taking tacrine need to have serum transaminases monitored monthly.
2. Remind family to let physician know of any and all medications client is taking, since tacrine levels are easily altered by some medications.
3. This drug is not a panacea but can be very useful in the early stages of dementia.

ZOLPIDEM

(Ambien)

NON-BENZODIAZEPINE SEDATIVE-HYPNOTIC

USES: Short-term treatment of insomnia.

ACTIONS: Zolpidem is thought to bind to the GABA receptors in the CNS, giving the drug sedative, anticonvulsant, and antianxiety properties.

DOSAGES & ROUTES

Adults	10 mg immediately before bedtime.
Elderly	5 mg immediately before bedtime.

CONTRAINDICATIONS: Safety has not been established for pregnancy, lactation, and children under age 18.

CAUTIONS: People with renal or hepatic dysfunction. Clients with history of drug abuse/addictions or depressed and suicidal clients. Elderly or debilitated clients.

SIDE EFFECTS:

FREQUENT: Drowsiness, vertigo, double vision, headache, drugged feeling, euphoria, insomnia, and nausea.

OCCASIONAL: Palpitations, myalgia, sinusitis, rash.

ADVERSE REACTIONS Rarely, doses over 10 mg have been associated with psychotic reactions and amnesia.

NURSING MEASURES:

1. Establish baseline history of sleep pattern.
2. Assess for other medications that the client may be taking that can cause CNS depression, including level of alcohol consumption.
3. Identify other methods client has used to induce sleep.
4. Assess for adverse reactions and side effects.

INFORM CLIENT AND FAMILY:

1. Zolpidem is only for short-term use. Explore other methods of inducing sleep.
2. Do not drive or use machinery once drug has been taken.
3. Take right before sleep.
4. When taking this drug do not take other medications or over-the-counter medications unless approved by physician.
5. Do not consume alcohol while taking this drug.

APPENDIX G

Glossary

Abstract thinking The ability to conceptualize ideas (e.g., finding meaning in proverbs).

Abuse An act of misuse, deceit, or exploitation; wrong or improper use or action toward another, resulting in injury, damage, maltreatment, or corruption.

Accommodation The ability to change one's way of thinking in order to introduce new ideas, objects, or experiences.

Acrophobia Fear of high places.

Acting out behaviors Behaviors that originate on an unconscious level to reduce anxiety and tension. Anxiety is displaced from one situation to another in the form of observable behavioral responses (e.g., anger, crying, or violence).

Activities of daily living For a person with a chronic mental illness, this term refers to the skills necessary to live independently as an adult.

Acute anxiety Anxiety that is precipitated by an imminent loss or a change that threatens an individual's sense of security.

Addiction Addiction incorporates the concepts of loss of control with respect to use of a drug (e.g., alcohol), taking the drug despite related problems, and a tendency to relapse. *Addiction* is an older term that has been replaced by the term *drug dependence.*

Adult Children of Alcoholics (ACOA) A support group for adult children of alcoholics, who often experience similar difficulties and problems in their adult lives as a result of having an alcoholic parent or parents.

Adventitious crises Crises that are not part of everyday life; they are unplanned and accidental. They include natural disasters, national disasters, and crimes of violence such as rapes or muggings.

Affect An objective manifestation of an experience or emotion accompanying an idea or feeling. The observations one would make on assessment. For example, a client may be said to have a flat affect, meaning that there is an absence or a near absence of facial expression. Some people, however, use the term loosely to mean a feeling, emotion, or mood.

Ageism A system of destructive, erroneous beliefs about the elderly; defined as a bias against older people based solely on their age.

Aggression Any verbal or nonverbal (actual or attempted, conscious or unconscious) forceful means to harm or abuse another person or object.

Agnosia Loss of the ability to recognize familiar objects. For example, a person may be unable to identify familiar sounds, such as the ringing of a doorbell (auditory agnosia), or familiar objects, such as a toothbrush or keys (visual agnosia).

Agoraphobia The most serious and the most common phobia for which people seek treatment. It is fear and avoidance of being alone or being in open spaces from which escape might be difficult. At its most severe, a person with agoraphobia may not be able to leave his or her own home.

Agraphia Loss of a previous ability to write, resulting from brain injury or brain disease.

Akathisia Regular rhythmic movements, usually of the lower limbs; constant pacing may also be seen; often noticed in people taking antipsychotic medication.

Akinesia Absence or diminution of voluntary motion. Akinesia is usually accompanied by a parallel reduction in mental activity.

Al-a-Teen A nationwide network for children over 10 years of age who have alcoholic parents.

Al-Anon A support group for spouses and friends of alcoholics.

Alcohol withdrawal delirium An organic mental disorder that occurs 40 to 48 hours after cessation or reduction of long-term heavy alcohol intake and that is considered a medical emergency; often referred to by the older term *delirium tremens (DTs).*

Alcoholic hallucinations Auditory hallucinations reported to occur approximately 48 hours after heavy drinking by alcohol-dependent clients.

Alcoholics Anonymous (AA) A self-help group of recovering alcoholics that provides support and encouragement to those involved in continuing recovery.

Alcoholism The end stage of the continuum that includes addiction to and dependence on the drug alcohol.

Alliance for the Mentally Ill A national support group for families of the mentally ill, with many local and state affiliates; provides educational programs and political action.

Alzheimer's disease A primary cognitive impairment disorder characterized by progressive deterioration of cognitive functioning, with the end result that a person may not recognize once-familiar people, places, and things. The ability to walk and talk is absent in the final stages.

Ambivalence The holding, at the same time, of two opposing emotions, attitudes, ideas, or wishes toward the same person, situation, or object.

Amnesia Loss of memory for events within a specific period of time; may be temporary or permanent.

Anergia Lack of energy; passivity.

Anger An emotional response to the perception of frustration of desires or threat to one's needs.

Anhedonia The inability to experience pleasure.

Anorexia A medical term that signifies a loss of appetite. A person with anorexia nervosa, however, may not have any loss of appetite and often is preoccupied with food and eating. A person with this condition may suppress the desire for food in order to control his or her eating.

Antabuse (disulfiram) A drug given to alcoholics that produces nausea, vomiting, dizziness, flushing, and tachycardia if alcohol is consumed.

Anticholinergic side effects Side effects caused by the use of some medications, e.g., neuroleptics and tricyclics. Symptoms include dry mouth, constipation, urinary retention, blurred vision, and dry mucous membranes.

Anticipatory grief Grief that occurs before an actual loss. During this time, painful feelings may be partially resolved.

Antidepressants Drugs predominantly used to elevate mood in people who are depressed.

Antimanic drugs Drugs used in the treatment of a manic state to lower an elevated and unstable mood and to reduce irritability and aggressiveness.

Antipsychotic drugs (neuroleptics, major tranquilizers) Drugs that have the ability to decrease psychotic, paranoid, and disorganized thinking and positively alter bizarre behaviors; they are thought to reduce the effects of the neurotransmitter dopamine by blocking the dopamine receptors.

Antisocial (sociopathic, psychopathic) These terms are often used interchangeably to refer to a syndrome in which a person lacks the capacity to relate to others. These people do not experience discomfort in inflicting or observing pain in others, and they constantly manipulate others for personal gain. Common behaviors seen in people with this disorder include crimes against society, aggressiveness, inability to feel remorse, untruthfulness and insincerity, unreliability, and failure to follow any life plan.

Anxiety A state of feeling apprehension, uneasiness, uncertainty, or dread resulting from a real or perceived threat whose actual source is unknown or unrecognized.

Anxiolytics (antianxiety drugs, minor tranquilizers) Drugs prescribed usually on a short-term basis to reduce anxiety.

Apathy A state of indifference.

Aphasia Difficulty in the formulation of words; loss of language ability. In extreme cases, a person may be limited to a few words, may babble, or may become mute.

Apraxia Loss of purposeful motor movements. For example, a person may be unable to shave, to dress, or to do other once-familiar and purposeful tasks.

Aristotle (384–322 BC) A philosopher and physician who made significant contributions in the area of clinical observation; observed a continuum in psychological reactions from normal to pathological behaviors.

Assault An intentional act that is designed to make the victim fearful and that produces reasonable apprehension of harm.

Assertiveness training Communications skills that help people ask directly in appropriate (nondemanding, nonthreatening, and nondemeaning) ways for what they want.

Assertiveness Asking for what one wants or acting to get what one wants in a way that respects the rights and feelings of other people.

Assimilation The ability to incorporate new ideas, objects, and experiences into the framework of one's thoughts.

Associative looseness Disturbance of thinking in which ideas shift from one subject to another in an oblique or unrelated manner. When this condition is severe, speech may be incoherent.

Attention-deficit hyperactivity disorder A behavioral disorder usually manifested before the age of 7 that includes overactivity, chronic inattention, and difficulty dealing with multiple stimuli.

Autistic thinking Thoughts, ideas, or desires derived from internal, private stimuli or perceptions that often are incongruent with reality.

Automatic obedience The performance of all simple commands in a robot-like fashion; may be present in catatonia.

Aversion therapy A behavioral technique that uses negative reinforcement or "conditioning" to alter or eliminate an unwanted or negative behavior.

Avolition Lack of motivation.

Axon The part of the neuron that conveys electrical impulses away from the cell body.

Basal ganglia Pockets of integrating gray matter deep within the cerebrum that are involved in the regulation of movement, emotions, and basic drives.

Battering Refers to physical assaults, such as hitting, kicking, biting, throwing, and burning.

Battery The harmful or offensive touching of another's person.

Behavioral modification A treatment modality that focuses on modifying and changing specific observable dysfunctional patterns of behavior by means of stimulus-and-response conditioning. Examples of behavioral therapy techniques include operant conditioning, token economy, systematic desensitization, aversion therapy, and flooding.

Benjamin Rush The Father of American Psychiatry, he wrote the first American textbook of psychiatry in 1812.

Binge-purge cycle An episodic, uncontrolled, rapid ingestion of large quantities of food over a short period of time, often followed by "purging" (vomiting); a characteristic seen in people with bulimia nervosa.

Biofeedback A technique for gaining conscious control over unconscious body functions, such as blood pressure and heartbeat, to achieve relaxation or the relief of stress-related physical symptoms; involves the use of self-monitoring equipment.

Bipolar disorders Mood disorders that include one or more manic episodes and usually one or more depressive episodes.

Bisexuality Sexual attraction toward both males and females, which may be acted on by engaging in both heterosexual and homosexual activities.

Blocking A sudden obstruction or interruption in the spontaneous flow of thinking or speaking that is perceived as an absence or deprivation of thought.

Blurred or diffused boundaries Refers to a blending together of roles, thoughts, and feelings of an individual so that clear distinctions among family members (or others) fail to emerge.

Body image One's internalized sense of self.

Borderline personality disorder Disorder characterized by impulsive and unpredictable behavior and marked shifts in mood. Instability is seen predominantly in the areas of behavior, mood, relationships to others, and images of self.

Boundaries Those functions that maintain a clear distinction among individuals within a family or group and with the outside world. Boundaries may be clear, diffuse, rigid, or inconsistent.

Bulimia An eating disorder characterized by the excessive and uncontrollable intake of large amounts of food (binges), alternating with purging activities such as self-induced vomiting; use of cathartics, diuretics, or both; and self-starvation. These alternating behaviors characterize the eating disorder *bulimia nervosa.*

Case management Duties of a health care worker (e.g., a nurse) that involve assuming responsibility for a client or group of clients—arranging assessments of need, formulating a comprehensive plan of care, arranging for delivery of services to address individual client needs, and assessing and monitoring the services delivered.

Catatonia A state of psychologically induced immobilization at times interrupted by episodes of extreme agitation.

Catecholamines A group of biogenic amines derived from phenylalanine and containing the catechol nucleus. Certain of these amines, such as *epinephrine, norepinephrine,* and *dopamine,* are neurotransmitters and exert an important influence on peripheral and central nervous system activity.

Cathexis A psychoanalytical term used to describe the emotional attachment or bond to an idea, an object, or most commonly, a person.

Character The sum of a person's relatively fixed personality traits and habitual modes of response.

Chemical restraints Drugs given for the specific purpose of inhibiting a specific behavior or movement.

Child abuse—neglect This abuse can be *physical* (e.g., failure to provide medical care), *developmental* (e.g., failure to provide emotional nurturing and cognitive stimulation), *educational* (failure to provide educational opportunities to the child according to the state's education laws), or a combination.

Child abuse—physical battering Physical assaults such as hitting, kicking, biting, throwing, and burning.

Child abuse—physical endangerment The reckless behaviors toward a child that could lead to the child's serious physical injury, such as leaving a young child alone or placing a child in a hazardous environment.

Child abuse—sexual Sexual abuse of children can take many forms. Essentially it is those acts designated to stimulate the child sexually or to use a child for sexual stimulation, either of the perpetrator or of another person.

Chronic anxiety Anxiety that a person has lived with for a long period of time. Chronic anxiety may take the form of chronic fatigue, insomnia, discomfort in daily activities, or discomfort in personal relationships.

Chronic illness The process of progressive deterioration, with a resulting increase in functional impairment, symptoms, and disability over time.

Chronic pain Pain that a client has had for more than 6 months.

Circadian rhythm A 24-hour biological rhythm that influences specific regulatory functions such as the sleep-wake cycle, body temperature, and hormonal and neurotransmitter secretions. The 24-hour biological rhythm is controlled by a "pacemaker" in the brain that sends messages to various systems in the body such as those mentioned above.

Circumstantial speech A pattern of speech characterized by indirectness and delay before the person gets to the point or answers a question; the person gets caught up in countless details and explanations.

Clang association The meaningless rhyming of words, often in a forceful manner.

Clinical (or critical) pathway A written plan or "map" that identifies predetermined times that specific nursing and medical interventions (e.g., diagnostic studies, treatments, activities, medications, teaching, client outcomes, discharge teaching) will be implemented (e.g., day 1 or day 2 for hospital settings, or week 1 or month 2 for community-based settings).

Co-dependent Coping behaviors that prevent individuals from taking care of their own needs and have as their core a preoccupation with the thoughts and feelings of another or others. It usually refers to the dependence of one person on another person who is addicted in one form or another.

Co-therapist A therapist who shares responsibility for therapeutic work, usually work done with groups or with families.

Cognition The act, process, or result of knowing, learning, or understanding.

Cognitive impairment syndromes/disorders A term that refers to disturbances in orientation, memory, intellect, judgment, and affect due to physiological changes in the brain. Delirium and dementia are examples of two cognitive impairment syndromes. An older term is *chronic mental disorders.*

Cognitive rehearsal A technique of having a client imagine each successive step in the sequence leading to the completion of a task, identifying potential "roadblocks" (cognitive, behavioral, or environmental) and planning strategies to deal with them before they produce an unwanted failure experience.

Cognitive therapy A treatment method (particularly useful for depressive disorders) that emphasizes the rearrangement of a person's maladaptive processes of thinking, perceptions, and attitudes.

Community nursing centers (CNCs) Nurse-managed centers that provide direct access to professional nurses who offer holistic, client-centered health services for reimbursement.

Compensation Making up for deficits in one area by excelling in another area in order to raise or maintain self-esteem.

Compulsions Repetitive, seemingly purposeless behaviors performed according to certain rules known to the client in order to temporarily reduce escalating anxiety.

Concrete thinking Thinking characterized by immediate experience rather than abstraction. There is an overemphasis on specific detail as opposed to general and abstract thinking.

Confabulation Filling in a memory gap with a detailed fantasy believed by the teller. The purpose is to maintain self-esteem. This is seen in organic conditions, such as Korsakoff's psychosis.

Confidentiality The ethical responsibility of a health care professional that prohibits the disclosure of privileged information without the patient's informed consent.

Conscious All experiences that are within a person's awareness.

Consensual validation The reality-checking of thoughts, feelings, and actions with others. If a child grows up in an environment in which the chance to validate thoughts, feelings, and behaviors is decreased, the child's ability to perceive reality is greatly impaired.

Conversion The unconscious transfer of anxiety to a physical symptom that has no organic cause.

Coping mechanisms Ways of adjusting to environmental stress without altering one's goals or purposes; they include both conscious and unconscious mechanisms.

Countertransference The tendency of the nurse (therapist, social worker) to displace onto the client feelings that are a response to people in the counselor's past. Strong positive or strong negative reactions to a client may indicate possible countertransferential reactions.

Crisis A temporary state of disequilibrium (high anxiety) in which a person's usual coping mechanisms or problem-solving methods fail. Crisis can result in personality growth or personality disorganization.

Crisis intervention A brief, active, and collaborative therapy that uses an individual's personal coping abilities and resources within the family, health care setting, or community.

Culture The total life style of a people, the social legacy the individual acquires from his or her group, or the environment that is the creation of humankind.

Cunnilingus Oral stimulation of the female genitalia.

Cyclothymia A chronic mood disturbance (of at least 2 years' duration) involving both hypomanic and dysthymic mood swings. Delusions are never present, and these mood swings usually do not warrant hospitalization or grossly impair a person's social, occupational, or interpersonal functioning.

Decode Interpret the meaning of autistic communications, such as in looseness of associations.

Defense mechanisms (DMs) Unconscious intrapsychic processes used to ward off anxiety by preventing conscious awareness of threatening feelings. They can be used in a healthy and a not-so-healthy manner. Examples of defense mechanisms include repression, projection, sublimation, denial, and regression.

Delayed grief A dysfunctional reaction to grief in which a person may not experience the pain of loss; however, that pain is modified by chronic depression, intense preoccupation with body functioning (hypochondriasis), phobic reactions, or acute insomnia.

Delirium An acute, usually reversible brain syndrome with multiple causes (APA 1987).

Delirium tremens (DTs) An older term now replaced by *alcohol withdrawal delirium.*

Delusion A false belief held to be true even with evidence to the contrary (e.g., the false belief that one is being singled out for harm by others).

Dementia An insidious, chronic, often irreversible brain syndrome (APA, 1987).

Dendrite The part of the neuron that conveys electrical impulses toward the cell body.

Denial Escaping of unpleasant realities by ignoring their existence.

Depersonalization A phenomenon whereby a person experiences a sense of unreality or self-estrangement. For example, one may feel that one's extremities have changed, that one is seeing oneself from a distance, or that one is in a dream.

Depressive mood syndrome This term can be defined as "a depressed mood or loss of interest, of at least two weeks' duration, accompanied by several associated symptoms, such as weight loss and difficulty concentrating" (APA 1987).

Derealization The false perception by a person that his or her environment has changed. For example, everything seems bigger or smaller, or familiar objects have become strange and unfamiliar.

Desensitization The reduction of intense reactions to a stimulus (e.g., phobia) by repeated exposure to the stimulus in a weaker or milder form.

Detachment An interpersonal and intrapersonal dissociation from affective expression. Therefore, individuals appear cold, aloof, and distant. This behavior is thought to be learned and is viewed as defensive.

***Diagnostic and statistical manual of mental disorders* (DSM-IV)** Classification of mental disorders that includes descriptions of diagnostic categories. DSM-IV is the most widely accepted system of classifying abnormal behaviors used in the United States today.

Diffused boundaries See *Blurred or diffused boundaries.*

Disorientation Confusion and impaired ability to identify time, place, and person.

Displacement Transfer of emotions associated with a particular person, object, or situation to another person, object, or situation that is nonthreatening.

Dissociation Technique of putting threatening thoughts or feelings out of conscious awareness before they are able to trigger overwhelming and intolerable anxiety; similar to Freud's defense mechanisms of repression.

Dissociative disorders Disorders that involve sudden temporary disturbances or loss of one's normal ability to integrate identity or motor behavior. Psychogenic amnesia and fugue are two examples.

Distractibility Inability to maintain attention; shifting from one area or topic to another with minimal provocation.

Double-bind message A message that contains two contradictory messages given by the same person at the same time, to which the receiver is expected to respond. Constant double-bind situations result in feelings of helplessness, fear, and anxiety in the receiver of the message.

Drug abuse The maladaptive and consistent use of a drug despite social, occupational, psychological, or physical problems exacerbated by the drug; or recurrent use in situations that are physically hazardous, such as driving while intoxicated (APA 1994).

Drug dependence Impaired control of drug use despite adverse consequences, the development of a tolerance to the drug, and the occurrence of withdrawal symptoms when drug intake is reduced or stopped.

Drug interaction The effects of two or more drugs taken simultaneously, producing an alteration in the usual effects of either drug taken alone. The interacting drugs may have a potentiating or an additive effect, and serious side effects may result.

Dual diagnosis A high prevalence for other psychiatric disorders in identified addicts (Talbott et al. 1988). A person with a dual diagnosis is chronically dependent on a drug or alcohol and also has another psychiatric disorder such as a depressive or personality disorder.

Dyskinesia Involuntary muscular activity, such as tic, spasm, or myoclonus.

Dyspareunia Persistent genital pain in either a male or a female before, during, or after sex.

Dysthymia A depression that is mild to moderate in degree and is characterized by a chronic depressive syndrome that is usually present for many years. The depressive mood disturbance is hard to distinguish from the person's usual pattern of functioning, and the person has minimal social or occupational impairment.

Dystonia Muscle spasms of the face, head, neck, and back; usually an acute side effect of neuroleptic (antipsychotic) medication.

Echolalia Mimicking or imitating the speech of another person.

Echopraxia Mimicking or imitating the movements of another person.

Ego One of three psychological processes that make up the Freudian system of personality (id, ego, and superego). The ego is one's "sense of self" and provides such functions as problem-solving, mobilization of defense mechanisms, reality testing, and the capability of functioning independently. The ego is said to be the mediator between one's primitive drives (the id) and internalized parental and social prohibitions (the superego).

Ego boundaries A person's perception of the boundaries between him- or herself and the external environment.

Ego-alien/Ego-dystonic Synonymous terms used to describe symptoms that are unacceptable to the person who has them and not compatible with the person's view of him- or herself (e.g., fear of cats).

Ego-syntonic Symptoms that include behaviors or beliefs that do not seem to bother the person or that seem right to the person. For example, a very paranoid person who wrongly believes that the government is out to get him or her truly believes this thought, and it is consistent with the way this person experiences life.

Egocentric Self-centered.

Electroconvulsive therapy (ECT) An effective treatment for depression that consists of inducing a grand mal seizure by passing an electrical current through electrodes that are applied to the temples. The administration of a muscle relaxant minimizes seizure activity, preventing damage to long bones and cervical vertebrae.

Elopement Escape.

Emotional abuse Essentially, emotional abuse is depriving a child of a nurturing atmosphere in which the child can thrive, learn, and develop. This takes many forms (e.g., terrorizing, demeaning, consistently belittling, withholding warmth).

Empathy The ability of one person to get inside another's world and see things from the other person's perspective and to communicate this understanding to the other person.

Enabling Helping a chemically dependent individual avoid experiencing the consequences of his or her drinking or drug use. It is one component of a person in a co-dependency role.

Endorphins A naturally produced chemical (peptide) with morphine-like action. It is usually found in the brain and associated with the reduction of pain and with feelings of well-being.

Enmeshed boundaries See *Blurred or diffused boundaries.*

Enuresis Nocturnal and daytime involuntary discharge of urine.

Epinephrine (adrenaline) A catecholamine secreted by the adrenal gland and by fibers of the sympathetic nervous system. It is responsible for many of the physical manifestations of fear and anxiety.

Ethics The discipline concerned with standards of values, behaviors, or beliefs adhered to by individuals or groups.

Eustress A positive emotion that demonstrates a person's confidence in the ability to master given demands or tasks with success.

Euthymia A normal mood state.

Extrapyramidal side effects A variety of signs and symptoms that are often side effects of the use of certain psychotropic drugs, particularly the phenothiazines. Three reversible side effects include acute dystonia, akathisia, and pseudoparkinsonism. A fourth, tardive dyskinesia, is most serious and is not reversible.

Family system Those individuals who make up the family unit and contribute to the functional state of the family as a unit.

Family therapy A treatment modality that focuses on the relationships within the family system.

Family triangle A dysfunctional phenomenon in which a third person in brought into a family system to help relieve anxiety or stress between two family members. Triangles are dysfunctional because the lowering of anxiety comes from *diversion* from the conflict rather than from *resolution* of the conflict between the two members.

Fantasy A retreat from reality and an attempt to solve problems in a private world. The difference between a healthy person and a schizophrenic, for example, is that a schizophrenic may not know where fantasy leaves off and reality begins.

Fear A reaction to a specific danger.

Feedback Communication of one person's impressions of and reactions to another person's actions or verbalizations.

Fellatio Oral sexual contact with the penis.

Fetish An object or part of the body to which sexual significance or meaning is attached.

Fight-or-flight response (sympathetic response) The body's physiological response to fear or rage that triggers the sympathetic branch of the autonomic nervous system as well as the endocrine system. This response is useful in emergencies; however, a sustained response can result in pathophysiological changes such as high blood pressure, ulcers, and cardiac problems.

Flight of ideas A continuous flow of speech in which the person jumps rapidly from one topic to another. Sometimes the listener can keep up with the changes; at other times, it is necessary to listen for themes in the incessant talking. Themes often include grandiose and fantasied estimation of personal sexual prowess, business ability, artistic talents, and so on.

Formication Tactile hallucination or illusion involving insects crawling on the body or under the skin.

Frustration Curtailment of personal goals, satisfaction, or security by conditions of external reality or by internal controls.

Fugue An altered state of consciousness involving both memory loss (as does psychogenic amnesia) and traveling away from home or from one's usual work locale. Therefore, fugue involves flight as well as forgetfulness (psychogenic fugue).

General adaptation syndrome (GAS) The body's organized response to stress, as demonstrated by Hans Selye. It progresses through three stages: (1) the stage of alarm, (2) the stage of resistance, and (3) the stage of exhaustion.

Genogram A systematic diagram of the three-generational relationships within a family system.

Grandiosity Exaggerated belief in or claims about one's importance or identity.

Grief The subjective feelings and affect that are precipitated by a loss.

Group Two or more individuals who have a relationship with one another, are interdependent, and may share some norms.

Group dynamics The interactions and interrelations among members of a therapy group and between members and the therapist. The effective use of group dynamics is essential in group treatment.

Group process Interaction continually taking place among members of a group.

Group therapy Psychotherapy based on the examination of group interaction with a view toward understanding and eventually changing the ways in which clients interact with others.

Hallucination A sense perception (seeing, hearing, tasting, smelling, or touching) for which no external stimulus exists (e.g., hearing voices when none are present).

Health Maintenance Organization (HMO) An organization that contracts with a group or individuals to offer designated health care services to plan members for a fixed, prepaid premium (an example of a managed care program).

Hippocrates (460–377 BC) Known as the Father of Medicine, he devised a code of ethical behavior that continues to guide physicians. He advocated the belief that mental illness was the result of natural causes rather than supernatural causes.

Histrionics A dramatic presentation of oneself with pervasive and excessive emotionality in order to seek attention, love, and admiration.

Homelessness—chronic The final stage in a lifelong series of crises and missed opportunities. It is the culmination of a gradual disengagement from supportive relationships and institutions.

Homosexual panic An acute and severe attack of anxiety based on unconscious conflicts involving gender identity.

Homosexuality Sexual attraction to or preference for persons of the same sex.

Hopelessness The belief by a person that no one can help him or her; extreme pessimism about the future.

Hospice philosophy A philosophy characterized by the acceptance of death as a natural conclusion to life, with clients rather than health care providers making the decisions how they want to live and die.

Hostility Anger that is destructive in nature and purpose.

Hotline A telephone crisis counseling service often used in crisis intervention centers to provide immediate contact between a person in crisis and a counselor.

Hypermetamorphosis The need to touch everything in sight.

Hyperorality The need to taste everything, chew everything, and put everything in one's mouth.

Hypersomnia Increased time spent in sleep, possibly to escape from painful feelings; however, the increased sleep is not experienced as restful or refreshing.

Hypochondriasis Excessive preoccupation with one's physical health, without the presence of any organic pathology.

Hypomania An elevated mood with symptoms less severe than those of mania. A person in hypomania does not experience impairment in reality testing, nor do the symptoms markedly impair the person's social, occupational, or interpersonal functioning.

Hysterical personality disorder A disorder characterized by dramatic, emotionally intense, unstable behavior.

Id One of three psychological processes that make up the Freudian system of personality (id, ego, and superego). The id is the source of all primitive drives and instincts and is thought of as the reservoir of all psychic energy.

Ideas of reference False impressions that outside events have special meaning for oneself.

Identification Unconsciously taking on the thoughts, mannerisms, or behaviors of a person or group, in order to decrease anxiety.

Identity The sense of one's self based on experience, memories, perceptions, and emotions.

Illusion An error in the perception of a sensory stimulus. For example, a person may mistake polka dots on a pillow for hairy spiders.

Impotence The inability to achieve or maintain a penile erection of sufficient quality to engage in successful sexual intercourse.

Impulsiveness An action that is abrupt, unplanned, and directed toward immediate gratification.

Incest A sexual relationship between persons related biologically.

Insight Understanding and awareness of the reasons for and meanings behind one's motives and behavior.

Insomnia Inability to fall asleep or to stay asleep, early morning awakening, or both.

Intellectualization The use of thinking and talking to avoid emotions and closeness.

Intimacy Emotional closeness.

Intoxication Excessive use of a drug or alcohol that leads to maladaptive behavior.

Intrapsychic Within the self.

Introjection Process by which a person incorporates or takes into his or her own personality qualities or values of another person or group with whom or with which intense emotional ties exist.

Intuition Emotional knowing without thinking or talking.

Isolation Separation of thoughts, ideas, or actions from their emotional aspects.

Johann Weyer (1515–1588) Known as the Father of Modern Psychiatry, Weyer made the greatest contributions to psychiatry during the Renaissance. He is identified with the humane treatment of the mentally ill.

Judgment The ability to make logical, rational decisions.

La belle indifference The affect or attitude of unconcern about a symptom that is used when the symptom is unconsciously used to lower anxiety. The lack of concern is thought to be a sign that the primary gain has been achieved.

Labile Having rapidly shifting emotions; unstable.

Lesbian A female homosexual.

Libido Sexual drive.

Limbic system The part of the brain that is related to emotions and referred to by some as the "emotional brain." It is associated with fear and anxiety; anger and aggression; love, joy, and hope; and sexuality and social behavior.

Limit setting The reasonable and rational setting of parameters for client behavior that provide control and safety.

Lithium carbonate This agent is known as an antimanic drug because it can stabilize the manic phase of a bipolar disorder. When effective, it can modify future manic episodes and protect against future depressive episodes.

Living will An expression by a person, while competent, that states the individual's preference that life-sustaining treatment be withheld or withdrawn if he or she becomes terminally ill and no longer able to make health care decisions.

Looseness of association A state in which thinking is haphazard, illogical, and confused, and connections in thought are interrupted; it is seen mostly in schizophrenic disorders.

Magical thinking The belief that thinking something can make it happen; it is seen in children and psychotic clients.

Malingering A conscious effort to deceive others, often for financial gain, by pretending physical symptoms.

Managed care A term that refers to an organized system that integrates the issues of cost management and health care. Health maintenance organizations (HMOs), preferred provider organizations (PPOs), and managed care options from government and private indemnity health insurance plans are the basic types of managed care organizations.

Mania An unstable elevated mood in which delusions, poor judgment, and other signs of impaired reality testing are evident. During a manic episode, clients have marked impairment in their social, occupational, and interpersonal functioning.

Manipulation Purposeful behavior directed at getting needs met. According to Chitty and Maynard (1986), manipulation is maladaptive when (1) it is the primary method used for getting needs met, (2) the needs, goals, and feelings of others are disregarded, and (3) others are treated as objects in order to fulfill the needs of the manipulator.

Masochism Unconscious or conscious gratification obtained when a person experiences mental or physical pain; often used to refer to deviant sexual behaviors.

Maturational crisis Normal state in growth and development in which specific maturational tasks must be learned while old coping mechanisms are no longer acceptable.

Mental status exam A formal assessment of cognitive functions such as intelligence, thought processes, and capacity for insight.

Milieu The physical and social environment in which an individual lives.

Milieu therapy Therapy focused on positive environmental manipulation (both physical and social) in order to effect positive change.

Mnemonic disturbance Loss of memory.

Modeling A technique in which desired behaviors are demonstrated. The client learns to imitate these behaviors in appropriate situations.

Mood A "pervasive and sustained emotion that, in the extreme, markedly colors the person's perception of the world" (APA 1987).

Mood syndrome An alteration in mood along with associated symptoms that occur for a minimal period.

Mourning The processes (grief work) by which grief is resolved.

Multiple personality disorder A severe dissociative disorder in which one or more distinct subpersonalities exist within an individual, each of which may be dominant at different times. Each subpersonality is a complex unit with its own memories, behavioral patterns, and social relationships, which may be very different from those of the primary personality.

Narcissism (narcism) Self-involvement with lack of empathy for others; the narcissistic person is very self-centered and self-important; it is normal in children but pathological when experienced in adults to the same degree.

Narcissistic personality disorder A disorder characterized by a pervasive pattern of grandiosity, need for admiration, and lack of empathy for others.

Negativism Opposition or resistance, either covert or overt, to outside suggestions or advice.

Negligence The act, or failure to act, that breaches the duty of due care and results in or is responsible for a person's injuries.

Neologisms Words a person makes up that have meaning only for that person; often part of a delusional system.

Neuroleptic malignant syndrome A rare and sometimes fatal reaction to high-potency neuroleptic drugs. Symptoms include muscle rigidity, fever, and elevated white blood cell count. It is thought to result from dopamine blockage on the basal ganglia and hypothalamus.

Neurons Specialized cells in the central nervous system. Each neuron has a cell body, an axon, and a dendrite.

Neurotransmitter A chemical substance that functions as a neural messenger. Neurotransmitters are released from the axon terminal of the presynaptic neuron when stimulated by an electrical impulse.

Nihilism A delusion that the self or part of the self does not exist.

No-suicide contract A contract made between a nurse or counselor and client, outlined in clear and simple language, in which the client states that he or she will *not* attempt self-harm and in which specific alternatives are given for the person instead.

Nonverbal communication Communication without words, such as body language, facial expressions, or gestures.

Nursing The diagnosis and treatment of human responses to actual or potential health problems.

Nursing informatics The study of information science applied to nursing and health care. The formation of nursing informatics has "building blocks" of knowledge that include basic computer literacy and the ability to access information-management systems such as the Internet and Medline.

Obesity A weight gain of at least 20% over the acceptable standard or ideal weight.

Obsession An idea, impulse, or emotion that a person cannot put out of his or her consciousness; it can be mild or severe.

Organic mental disorders Specific brain syndromes in which an etiology is known; for example, alcohol withdrawal delirium and Alzheimer's disease (APA 1987).

Orientation The ability to relate the self correctly to time, place, and person.

Overt anxiety Anxiety in which the attendant physical, physiological, and cognitive symptoms are evident and may be assessed.

Panic Sudden, overwhelming anxiety of such intensity that it produces disorganization of the personality, loss of rational thought, and inability to communicate, along with specific physiological changes.

Paranoia Any intense and strongly defended irrational suspicion. These ideas cannot be corrected by experiences and cannot be modified by facts or reality.

Passive-aggressive behavior Indirect expression of anger. Behavior may seem passive but is motivated by unconscious anger, often triggering anger and frustration in others. Examples of passive-aggressive behavior include lateness, forgetting, "mistakes," and obtuseness.

Peer review Review of clinical practice with peers, supervisors, or consultants.

Perception Mental processes by which intellectual, sensory, and emotional data are organized logically or meaningfully.

Perseveration The involuntary repetition of the same thought, phrase, or motor response (e.g., brushing teeth, walking); it is associated with brain damage.

Personality Deeply ingrained personal patterns of behavior, traits, and thoughts that evolve, both consciously and unconsciously, as a person's style and way of adapting to the environment.

Philippe Pinel (1745–1826) A reformer and humanitarian who introduced psychotherapeutic methods in the treatment of the mentally ill.

Phobia An intense irrational fear of an object, situation, or place. The fear persists even though the object of the fear is harmless and the person is aware of the irrationality.

Physical restraints Any manual method or mechanical device, material, or equipment that inhibits free movement.

Pierre Janet (1859–1947) Janet advanced the knowledge of the functioning of the mind. By the use of hypnosis, he was the first to demonstrate that many symptoms of "neurosis" lie in the unconscious mind.

Play therapy An intervention that allows a child to symbolically express feelings such as aggression, self-doubt, anxiety, and sadness through the medium of play.

Pleasure principle A tendency to seek immediate gratification of impulses and tension reduction; the id operates according to the pleasure principle.

Polydrug abuse The pathologic use of more than one drug.

Polypharmacy The taking of more than one drug at any given time.

Postvention Therapeutic interventions with the significant others of an individual who has committed suicide.

Poverty of speech Speech that is brief and uncommunicative.

Pressure of speech Forceful energy heard in a manic individual's frantic, jumbled speech as he or she struggles to keep pace with racing thoughts.

Primary anxiety Anxiety that is due to intrapersonal or intrapsychic causes, such as a phobia.

Primary depression A depressive mood episode that *is not* due to a known organic factor and *is not* part of another psychotic disorder, such as schizophrenia (APA 1987).

Primary gain The anxiety relief resulting from the use of defense mechanisms or symptom formation, such as somatizing (e.g., getting a headache instead of feeling angry).

Primary process A primitive and unconscious psychological activity in which the id attempts to reduce tension through formation of an image or by hallucinating the object that would satisfy its need.

Projection The unconscious attributing of one's own intolerable wishes, emotional feelings, or motivation to another person.

Projective identification A primitive form of projection used to externalize aggressive feelings. Once projection has occurred, fear of the person who is the object of the projection is coupled with a desire to control the person.

Prolonged grief A dysfunctional reaction to grief in which the bereaved remains intensely preoccupied with the memories of the deceased many years after the person has died.

Psychiatric liaison nurse A master's prepared nurse with a background in psychiatric and medical-surgical nursing. The liaison nurse functions as a nursing consultant in the management of psychosocial concerns and as a clinician in helping the client deal more effectively with physical and emotional problems.

Psychiatry The science of treating disorders of the psyche. It is the medical specialty that is derived from the study, diagnosis, treatment, and prevention of mental disorders.

Psychoeducational therapy A strategy of teaching clients and their families about disorders, treatments, coping techniques, and resources. It helps empower clients and families by having them become more involved and prepares them to participate in their own care once they have the knowledge.

Psychogenic Physical conditions affected by psychological factors.

Psychogenic amnesia The loss of memory for an event or period of time that contains overwhelming anxiety and pain. The loss of memory is related to psychological stress.

Psychomotor agitation The constant involvement in some tension-relieving activity, such as constantly pacing, biting one's nails, smoking, or tapping one's fingers on a tabletop.

Psychomotor retardation Extremely slow and difficult movements that in the extreme can entail complete inactivity and incontinence.

Psychophysiological A term that refers to all physical symptoms in which psychic elements play a significant role in initiating or maintaining chemical, physiological, or structural alterations responsible for the client's complaint. Referred to in DSM-II.

Psychosexual development Emotional and sexual growth from birth to adulthood.

Psychosis An extreme response to psychological or physical stressors that affects a person's affective, psychomotor, and physical behavior. Evidence of impairment in reality testing is evident by hallucinations or delusions.

Psychosocial rehabilitation The development of the skills necessary for people with chronic mental illness to live independently.

Psychosomatic An older term describing the interaction of the mind (psyche) and the body (soma). The term was used in reference to certain diseases thought to be caused by psychological factors. Referred to in DSM-I.

Psychotherapy A treatment modality based on the development of a trusting relationship between client and therapist for the purpose of exploring and modifying the client's behavior in a satisfying direction.

Psychotropic Affecting the mind.

Psychotropic drugs Drugs that have an effect on psychic function, behavior, or experience.

Racism A belief that inherent differences between races determine one's achievement and that one's own race is superior.

Rape See *Sexual assault/rape.*

Rape-trauma syndrome This syndrome comprises the acute phase and the long-term reorganization process that occurs after an actual or attempted sexual assault. Each phase has separate symptoms.

Rational emotive behavioral therapy (REBT) The first cognitive therapy model, developed by Albert Ellis in the 1950s; it combines aspects of cognitive as well as behavioral techniques to help people change self-defeating thoughts and behaviors and decrease painful feelings such as depression and anxiety. It is based on risk-taking and the assumption of responsibility for one's behavior.

Rationalization Justifying illogical or unreasonable ideas, actions, or feelings by developing acceptable explanations that satisfy the teller as well as the listener.

Reaction-formation (overcompensation) The process of keeping unacceptable feelings or behaviors out of awareness by developing the opposite emotion or behavior.

Reality principle The gradual development of the ability to delay immediate gratification and modify desires in accordance with the demands of society and external reality.

Receptors Protein molecules located in the cell membrane of neurons, muscles, and blood vessels. Receptors receive chemical stimulation that causes a chemical reaction resulting in either stimulation or inhibition of activity of the neuron, muscle, or blood cell.

Reframing A technique of changing the viewpoint of a situation and replacing it with another viewpoint that fits the facts equally well but changes the entire meaning.

Regression In the face of overwhelming anxiety, the ego returns to an earlier, more comforting (although less mature) way of behaving.

Relapse The process of becoming dysfunctional in sobriety that ends in a return to chemical use.

Relaxation response The opposite of the fight-or-flight response. This response is synonymous with the functioning of the parasympathetic branch of the nervous system. The relaxation response has a stabilizing effect on the nervous system.

Repression The exclusion of unpleasant or unwanted experiences, emotions, or ideas from conscious awareness; thought of as the first line of psychological defense.

Respite care Temporary supervision and care of a client who lives with his or her family. The purpose of respite care is to provide the family with some relief from the demands of the client's needs for continuous care.

Restraints See *Physical restraints* and *Chemical restraints.*

Reticular activating system (RAS) Nerve pathways of the reticular formation of the medulla oblongata. These cells control the overall degree of central nervous system activity such as wakefulness, attentiveness, and sleep.

Reuptake The process of neurotransmitters' returning to the presynaptic cell after communication with receptor cells.

Rigid or disengaged boundaries Those boundaries in which the "rules and roles" are adhered to no matter what the situation. Rigid boundaries prevent family members from trying out new roles or taking on more mature functions.

Rituals Repetitive actions that a person must do over and over until he or she is exhausted or anxiety is decreased; they are often done to lessen the anxiety triggered by an obsession.

Role playing A technique used in individual, group, or family therapy in which the therapist or a group member acts out the behavior of another member in order to increase the other person's ability to see a situation from another point of view. It is also a useful tool that therapists, teachers, and others use to help people practice skills in a safe environment before they try them in real-life situations, such as practicing asking for a raise, discussing a crucial topic with a person in authority, or saying no to someone without getting defensive or angry.

Sadism Sexual pleasure and erotic gratification obtained by inflicting pain, abuse, or humiliation on another.

Scapegoat A member of a group or family who becomes the target of aggression from others but who may not be the actual cause of hostility or frustration in them.

Schizoaffective disorder A disorder that includes a mixture of schizophrenic and affective symptoms (i.e., alterations in mood as well as disturbances in thought); it is thought by some to be a severe form of bipolar disorder.

Schizoid personality disorder A personality disorder in which there is a serious defect in interpersonal relationships. Other characteristics include lack of warmth, aloofness, and indifference to the feelings of others.

Schizophrenia A severe disturbance of thought or association, characterized by impaired reality testing, hallucinations, delusions, and limited socialization.

Seasonal affective disorder (SAD) A recently studied syndrome that appears to affect mostly women. It is characterized by hypersomnia, fatigue, weight gain, irritability, and interpersonal difficulties during the winter months. It has been successfully managed with daily treatments of 2 to 3 hours of bright light.

Seclusion The last step in a process to maximize safety to a client and others whereby a client is placed alone in a specially designed room for protection and close observation.

Secondary anxiety Anxiety that is due to physiological abnormalities such as certain medical disorders (e.g., neurological, endocrine, or circulatory) or is secondary to a pervasive psychiatric disorder such as depression.

Secondary dementia A result of some other pathological process, such as a metabolic, nutritional, or neurological process. AIDS-related dementia is an example.

Secondary depression A depressive mood syndrome that is caused by a physical illness or another psychiatric disorder or is part of an organic mental disorder; essentially, it is depression secondary to other causes.

Secondary gain Those advantages a person realizes from whatever symptoms or relief behaviors he or she employs. These advantages include increased attention from others, getting out of expected responsibilities, financial gain, and the ability to manipulate others in the environment.

Secondary process A process consistent with the reality principle: that is, realistic thinking.

Selective inattention Characterized by not noticing an almost infinite series of more-or-less meaningful details of one's own living that might cause anxiety. A concept articulated by H. S. Sullivan.

Selective serotonin reuptake inhibitors (SSRIs) First-line antidepressants that block the reuptake of serotonin, permitting serotonin to act for an extended period at the synaptic binding sites in the brain.

Self-concept A person's image of the self.

Self-esteem Feelings individuals have about their own worth and value.

Self-help group An organization of people who share similar problems who meet to receive peer support and encouragement and work together using their strengths to gain control over their lives.

Self-mutilation The act of self-induced pain or injury without the intent to kill oneself.

Sexual assault/rape Forced and violent vaginal or anal penetration against the victim's will and without the victim's consent. Legal definitions vary from state to state.

Situational crises Crises arising from external sources, as opposed to internal sources; most people have them to some extent during the course of their lives (e.g., with the death of a loved one, marriage, divorce, or a change in health status).

Social phobias These include phobias of an interpersonal nature, such as fear of public speaking, fear of eating in front of others, or fear of writing or performing in public.

Social skills training Training that utilizes the principles of guidance, demonstration, practice, and feedback to enhance a client's skills in community living. Training focuses on skills such as introducing oneself, starting and ending a conversation, asking for assistance, and other simple yet essential social interactions; it is often helpful in combating the negative symptoms of schizophrenia.

Somatic therapy Treatment that involves manipulations of the body, such as the use of medications or electroconvulsive therapy.

Somatization The expression of psychological stress through physical symptoms.

Somatizing Experiencing an emotional conflict as a physical symptom.

Specific phobias These are very common in the general population; essentially, a specific phobia is fear and avoidance of a single object, situation, or activity.

Spirituality The devotion or receptiveness to religious/moral values.

Splitting A primitive defense in which persons see themselves or others as all good or all bad, failing to integrate the positive and negative qualities of the self and others into a cohesive whole.

Spouse abuse The intentional act or perceived intention of physically injuring one's spouse. It is an act of mental cruelty.

Stereotype The assumption that all people in a similar cultural, racial, or ethnic group think and act alike.

Stereotyped behaviors Motor patterns that originally had meaning to the person (e.g., sweeping the floor or washing windows) but have become mechanical and lack purpose.

Stress The body's arousal response to any demand, change, or perceived threat.

Stupor A state in which a person is dazed and awareness of reality in his or her environment appears deadened. For example, a person may sit motionless for long periods of time and in extreme cases may appear to be in a coma.

Subconscious Often called the preconscious; includes experiences, thoughts, feelings, and desires that might not be in immediate awareness but can be recalled to consciousness. The subconscious mind helps repress unpleasant thoughts or feelings.

Subintentioned suicide Term used by Schneidman to describe self-destructive behaviors people employ that could hasten their own death, such as compulsive use of drugs, hyperobesity, and medical noncompliance (Schneidman 1963).

Sublimation The unconscious process of substituting constructive and socially acceptable activities for strong impulses that are not acceptable in their original form, such as strong aggressive or sexual drives.

Suicidal ideation Thoughts a person has regarding killing him- or herself.

Suicide The ultimate act of self-destruction in which a person purposefully ends his or her own life.

Suicide attempt Any willful, self-inflicted, life-threatening attempt that has not led to death.

Suicide gesture A suicide attempt that is planned to be discovered and is made for the purpose of influencing or manipulating others.

Sundown syndrome Increasing destabilization of cognitive abilities (e.g. confusion, lability of mood) during the late afternoon, early evening, or night. Seen in people with cognitive disorders.

Superego One of three psychological processes that make up the Freudian system of personality (id, ego, and superego). The superego is the internal representative of the values, ideals, and moral standards of society. The superego is said to be the moral arm of the personality.

Support groups Groups that help people during stressful periods using a variety of modalities in order to overcome overwhelming situations or unwanted behaviors.

Suppression The conscious putting off of awareness of disturbing situations or feelings; the only defense mechanism that operates on a conscious level.

Symbolization The process by which one object or idea comes to represent another. For example, the nurse's keys on a locked unit may represent power and autonomy, or a fancy house may represent prestige and power.

Synapse The gap between the membrane of one neuron and the membrane of another neuron. The synapse is the point at which the transmission of nerve impulses occurs.

Synesthesia A phenomenon experienced by people on hallucinogenic drugs; described as hearing colors or seeing sounds.

Tangentiality An association disturbance in which the speaker goes off the topic. When it happens frequently and the speaker does not return to the topic, interpersonal communication is destroyed.

***Tarasoff* decision** A California court decision that imposes a duty on the therapist to warn the appropriate person or persons when the therapist becomes aware that a client may present a risk of harm to a specific person or persons.

Tardive dyskinesia A serious and irreversible result of the use of phenothiazine-like drugs. It consists of involuntary tonic muscular spasms typically involving the tongue, fingers, toes, neck, trunk, or pelvis.

Therapeutic encounter A brief, informal meeting between nurse and client in which the relationship is useful and important for the client.

Therapeutic index The ratio of the lethal dose to the effective dose of a drug. It represents the safety of a drug. For example, a low therapeutic index means that the blood level of a drug that can cause death is not far removed from the blood level required for the drug to be effective. The higher the therapeutic index, the safer the drug.

Therapeutic nurse-client relationship A therapeutic relationship requiring that the nurse maximize his or her communication skills, understanding of human behaviors, and personal strengths in order to enhance personal growth in the client. This relationship applies to *all* clinical settings, not just those on a psychiatric unit.

Time out Removing or disengaging a child from a situation so that the child might regain self-control.

Token economy A behavioral approach to eliciting desired behaviors involving the application of the principles and procedures of operant conditioning; it is usually used in the management of a social setting such as a ward, classroom, or halfway house. Targeted behaviors are awarded "tokens" that can be exchanged for desired goods or privileges.

Tolerance A need for higher and higher doses of a drug in order to achieve intoxication or the desired effect.

Torts Civil wrongs for which money damages are collected by the injured party (plaintiff) from the wrongdoer (defendant).

Transference The experiencing of thoughts and feelings toward a person (often the therapist) that belong to a significant person in one's past. Transference is a valuable tool used by therapists in psychoanalytical psychotherapy.

Transsexuals People who have an early and persistent feeling that they are trapped in a body with the wrong genitals. They believe they are, and were always meant to be, of the opposite sex.

Triangle See *Family triangle.*

Type A personality Personality characteristics such as excessive competitiveness, strong sense of time urgency, irritability, authoritarianism, and distrust of others' motives. Type A people were once thought to be at high risk for coronary artery disease. However, a type A personality alone is no longer thought to be a risk factor. The trait thought to have a high correlation to coronary artery disease, however, is hostility.

Unconscious Repressed memories, feelings, thoughts, or wishes that are not available to the conscious mind. Usually, these unconscious memories, feelings, thoughts, or wishes harbor intense anxiety and can greatly affect an individual's behavior.

Undoing An act or behavior unconsciously motivated to make up for or negate a previous act or behavior (e.g., bringing the boss a present after talking about him or her unfavorably to co-workers).

Validate See *Consensual validation.*

Values clarification A process of self-discovery whereby a person can explore and determine his or her personal values and identify what priority these values hold in personal decision making. The result of this process can increase awareness about why the person behaves in certain ways.

Vegetative signs of depression During a depressive episode, these represent a significant change from normal functioning of those activities necessary to support physical life and growth, such as eating, sleeping, elimination, and sex.

Waxy flexibility Having one's arms or legs placed in a certain position and holding that same position for hours.

Withdrawal symptoms The negative physiological and psychological reactions that occur when a drug taken for a long period of time is reduced or no longer taken.

Word salad A mixture of phrases meaningless to the listener and to the speaker as well.

APPENDIX H

Answers to Self-Study Questions

Chapter 1

1. B (as of 1998)
2. D
3. Matching
   A. C/CS
   B. CS
   C. C/CS
   D. C/CS
   E. CS
   F. C/CS
   G. C/CS
   H. CS
   I. C
   J. C
4. Matching
   A. L
   B. O
   C. O
   D. L
   E. O
   F. L
   G. L
   H. O
   I. O
   J. L
5. True or False
   A. True
   B. True
   C. True
   D. True
   E. True
   F. False (Critical/clinical pathways include the entire health care team, identifying the tasks and expected outcomes of each service, e.g., nurse, activities/occupational therapists, psychologists, physicians, and case manager, and their responsibilities.)
   G. True
6. Refer to page 16.
7. On page 12.
8. Review page 18.
9. Refer to pages 18–20.

10,11,12. These are exercises. Use your instructor as a reference for computer instruction if you don't already have access to the Internet.

Chapter 2

True or False

1. True
2. True
3. True
4. True
5. False (All health care professionals constantly need to monitor their own cultural filters and seek to understand the client's experience from his or her cultural perspective. Refer to Chapter 5.)

Matching

6. C
7. E
8. G
9. H
10. B
11. F
12. A
13. D

Completion

14. Behavioral
15. Classical Psychoanalysis
16. Psychoanalytic Psychotherapy
17. Short-Term Dynamic Psychotherapy

Multiple Choice

18. D
19. A
20. C
21. C
22. D
23. A
24. C
25. D
26. A
27. C
28. B
29. D

Critical Thinking

30. Use Table 2–1 on page 32 as a guide.
31. Refer to pages 32–33.
32. Refer to Table 2–2 on page 35.

33,34. Process with a classmate/colleague.

Chapter 3

Multiple Choice

1. A
2. B
3. A
4. A
5. C
6. C
7. D
8. B
9. D
10. C

Short Answer

11. Refer to Box 3–1, page 66.
12. Refer to Table 3–1, page 70
13. Review Box 3–3, page 79.
14. Study Figure 3–3, page 72, and Box 3–2, page 71.
15. See page 69.
16. Page 80.
17. Page 83 and Table 3–3.

Critical Thinking

18. Refer to pages 68–69.
19. Page 78 and Box 3–3.
20. Page 80.

Chapter 4

Matching

1. D
2. C
3. A
4. E
5. F

True or False

6. True
7. True

For Discussion

8. See page 98.
9. See page 104.
10. See page 108.
11. See pages 112–114.

Critical Thinking

12. • Legally practice? The nurse's license allows her to practice in an ICU, *but* it is unreasonable to expect a psychiatric nurse to understand all of the equipment. It would probably be found to be negligent to place a psychiatric nurse in an ICU.
    - Yes
    - Yes, as far as medical-surgical expectations. If unfamiliar with current practice, the RN should seek continuing education prior to working with patients in a specialty area. To avoid insubordination charges, the nurse must clarify the expectations and areas of care to which he or she will be assigned when hired.
    - Harm to patient, negligence, liability if patient injured, misrepresentation.
    - Insubordination; charges of abandonment.
    - Clarify expectations with employer when being hired (in writing).
    - Request the assistance of another professional (nurse, supervisor, doctor) during nurse B's absence.
    - Both the hospital and nurse A will likely be named as defendants. The hospital breached its duty to provide competent care providers, especially if they knew of nurse A's limited scope of practice abilities.
13. • Yes, but the nasal packs in this case call for a higher standard of care, e.g., more frequent checks. The question will revolve around what behavior was/is reasonable and prudent to protect the client (Negligence Standard).
    - No. Nasal packing increases the need to check more often.
    - No. The doctor does not avoid any responsibility, but nurses are licensed professionals and as such are expected to exercise their own sound judgment when a client's safety is jeopardized.
    - No, the order for the restraint was inappropriate.
    - (a) The client is in a private room (isolated, where there is less opportunity for observation), and (b) this client could go into delirium tremens, which is a contraindication for restraints. The client could have had seizures with nasal packs in place.
    - No. Closer observation was warranted. The statute identified a standard found acceptable by the state, but more frequent checks (every 15 to 30 minutes) are generally recommended. Federal regulations would overrule less restrictive state regulations.
    - No restraints. Check the client more frequently. Don't place the client in an isolated private room. Question the doctor on the order to restrain and refuse to place the client in an unsafe position. (Don't confront the doctor, but rather share your concerns in a professional manner.)
14. Consult the supervisor first. A protected incident report might be filed until the allegations can be investigated.
    - Follow agency protocols for incident reporting. The nurse along with the supervisor would inform the admitting physician.
    - Yes!
    - With the supervisor, if the agency policies suggest this chain of communication. The client's rights must also be considered.
    - Follow agency policy for channels of communications.
    - Again, follow agency policy for channels of communications.
    - If the allegations have foundation, the agency should report the incident, especially if the State Medical Practice Act directs reporting.
    - The nurse should allow the agency administrators to follow necessary procedures for reporting.
15. • Yes, even if Beth denies taking the medications, Joe should discuss the problem with the supervisor.
    - The supervisor and agency will report after investigating.
    - If Beth has admitted it, Joe should identify Beth.
    - Yes, most state boards do mandate reporting, although often the agency will accept this responsibility (not suspicions, but admitted facts).
    - No. This is a legal duty to intervene.
16. • Not keeping a safe environment (e.g., introducing the bed frame, locking the room with the knowledge that the client is hearing command hallucinations to harm herself and therefore is at high risk for hurting herself).
    - Remove the bed frame from the room, frequently check on the client, notify the doctor of the client's statements, provide nursing interventions and support by staying with the client.
    - NEVER FALSIFY RECORDS. Fraudulent change to records could result in criminal as well as civil charges. The act is both unethical and illegal.
17. • No, the nurse has a legal duty to notify the boy's therapist, who, in turn, should warn the boy's mother.
    - Ethical principles cannot be valued over a human life that is threatened. The client will be in greater trouble if the nurse does not intervene and allows the boy to harm his mother. Preventing this legal and human dilemma is more ethical toward the client than maintaining confidentiality. Preventing a crime is in the client's best interest (beneficence); justice could not allow harm to an innocent victim; our society cannot allow total autonomy or we'd have no law and order.
    - The "special relationship" is recognized by the law as with the therapist, whom the nurse must notify, who in turn should warn the mother.
    - Would need to warn in either case.
    - No difference when discussing legal duty to warn and ethics.
    - Talk to the supervisor to have discharge reconsidered and to decide who should warn the mother.
18. • Statutes require child abuse to be reported. However, to avoid violating federal confidentiality laws, do not share the information that the abuser is in an alcoholic treatment program. It was not the client who shared the information, but nevertheless the nurse must avoid disclosing that the abuser is in treatment.

Chapter 5

1. B
2. B
3. *Explanatory models* is a term used by Kleinman (1980) to describe the cultural explanations about the causes and cures of illness. It affects how nurses and clients diagnose and treat health problems, and how they promote health.
4. Acceptance of, and adherence to, role expectations is a cooperative effort among both men and women within any culture. Arabic women can be virtuous, modest, and proper while also being proud, strong, and courageous.
5. African Americans can display intense affect in social situations. Indeed, to hide or deny feelings in a trusting relationship is considered inappropriate and dishonest. This is in sharp contrast to the European American ideals of emotional self-control.
6. The self is a central organizing feature in one's psychological life. The self is hypothesized to form in the context of cultural beliefs and values. Therefore, one's "self" is the way that one sees oneself in relationship to others. This will vary depending on the expectations and values of a culture. Some cultures expect this "self" to focus on individual goals, whereas others expect the larger group to be that focus.
7. There are essential conflicts between the individualistic, materialistic, and future-orientated values of the European American and the value orientations of the Native American. This, along with cultural extermination efforts, poverty, and alcoholism, has created alientation from both native and mainstream societies for many Native American peoples that for some have ended in attempted and completed suicides. Claiming native ways allows the Native American person to feel belonging and reduces some of this stress.

Critical Thinking

8. The Chinese tend to view the world in a holistic manner, seeing the mind, body, spirit, and environment as interrelated. Therefore, social sources of stress may become "somatized." The client and his or her family expect the person to perform in socially prescribed roles and interpret "individualistic" behaviors such as speaking one's mind as "outside of role expectations." Therefore, the family might expect this woman to pursue self-fulfillment outside the context of the family setting, instead of using assertion within the family for such self-expression. Assisting the client to determine all of her needs, which probably include role performance, would be useful. The nurse and client can work together to determine how she can meet her needs for self-expression and fulfillment.

Chapter 6

S (social), I (intimate), T (therapeutic)

1. S
2. I
3. I
4. T
5. S
6. T
7. I
8. I

True or False

9. True
10. True

O (orientation), W (working), T (termination)

11. T
12. O
13. W
14. T

Multiple Choice

15. A/C
16. B
17. C

18. How would you alter your answers after reading Chapter 7?
19. How would you alter your answers after reading Chapter 7?

Chapter 7

True or False

1. False; refer to Figure 7–1.
2. True
3. True
4. False; they all play a part.
5. True
6. True

V (verbal) or N (nonverbal)

7. N
8. V
9. N
10. N

11 through 17. Answer questions 11 through 17 by referring to Tables 7–2 and 7–3 (pages 188–190 and 191–193). This exercise can help you review more thoughtfully why techniques are either helpful or not helpful in a therapeutic setting.

Multiple Choice

18. C
19. D
20. C
21. B
22. D
23. D
24. D
25. Table 7–6 will give you some guidelines.
26. Table 7–6 will give you some guidelines.

Chapter 8

Multiple Choice

1. C
2. A
3. B
4. A
5. B
6. D

Chapter 9

Matching

1. A
2. B
3. C
4. F
5. D
6. E

Multiple Choice

7. C
8. A
9. A
10. C

11. Use the chapter as your guide.
12. Use the knowledge from all chapters to this point to give an informed and thoughtful reply.
13. Refer to Box 9–1.
14. Refer to Box 9–4.
15. Use what you have learned from Chapter 8 as well as from this chapter to answer this question.
16. F
17. Refer to Box 9–2. What other attributes can you think of?

True or False

18. True
19. False
20. False
21. False
22. False
23. True
24. False
25. Refer to pages 225–227.

Chapter 10

Matching

1. H
2. F
3. E
4. D
5. A
6. B
7. C
8. G
9. E
10. D
11. C
12. A
13. B
14. F

True or False

15. True
16. True
17. False
18. False; always take seriously and let the client know you need to share this information with all other staff members.
19. True
20. True

Multiple Choice

21. D
22. B
23. D
24. D

Chapter 11

1. Refer to Table 11–2.

Chapter 12

Short Answers

1. Predictability addresses patients' concerns about being neglected or having needs go unmet. Predictable contacts can act to reassure patients and decrease their anxiety. Regularly scheduled contacts also provide patients with nursing attention that is not contingent on the patients' behaviors; thus the contacts do not reinforce maladaptive coping behaviors such as yelling, demanding, and intimidating. Predictability in the inpatient psychiatric milieu provides stability. A clinical example might include regular contacts with patients and family members waiting in the emergency department; regular prescheduled contacts with patients who have been admitted to a medical or surgical unit, who are using ineffective ways of coping, and who have a pattern of maladaptive coping behaviors; predictable structure on inpatient psychiatric units.
2. Positive reinforcement—even social reinforcement—of more appropriate behaviors when they are present.
3. Sensory stimulation should be increased when patients have been hospitalized on a medical or surgical unit for a period of time such that they have experienced significant decreases in stimulus heterogeneity, social isolation, and diminished kinesthetic input. Sensory stimulation should be decreased for patients who are actively psychotic, patients on psychiatric or medical-surgical units, and patients suffering from cognitive deficits.
4. A. The patient presents a clear and present danger to self.
   B. The patient presents a clear and present danger to others.
   C. The patient has been legally detained for involuntary treatment and is thought to be an escape risk.
   D. The patient requests to be secluded or restrained.

5. A. Patients are doing the best they can.
   B. Patients want to improve.
   C. Patients' behaviors make sense within their world view.
6. A. Behavioral theory: anger and aggression are, in part, learned responses to environmental stimuli. These stimuli include observed responses in others and reinforcement of responses in the individual.
   B. Cognitive theory: anger is a function of an individual's cognitive appraisal of an event as threatening.
   C. Biological theory: anger and aggression are complex and not completely understood biological phenomena involving neurotransmitters (particularly serotonin), specific brain sites (such as the limbic system and the temporal lobe), and genetics.
7. A. Emotional lability.
   B. Inability to accurately receive verbal and written information.
   C. Inability to accurately perceive the extent of the illness or injury.

True or False

8. False
   False
   True
   False
9. False; expressing can escalate anger.
   True/False
   True
   False
   False
   True

Multiple Choice

10. C/D
11. A/B/C

Long Answers

12. Greet the patient by name, establish eye contact, acknowledge her distress, remind her of where she is.

    Offer to take the patient to the bathroom, offer a cup of tea, offer to walk with or sit with the patient, ask the patient to talk about herself.

    Assessment of possible worsening physiological status, assessment of the antecedents to the patient's distress.

    Ideally, no medications. Sedating medications could both worsen the patient's pulmonary status and increase her confusion by clouding her sensorium further.
13. Gathering additional information about the circumstances of the patient's previous assaults—using this if possible to decrease similar events on the unit; low stimulation protocol; structuring the patient's day for maximum predictability; use of prn medication for signs of increasing distress or irritability; collaborating with the patient to determine if he is aware of his warning signs when beginning to feel out of control; providing the patient with options when he is feeling worse (e.g., asking for medication, self-seclusion, asking for seclusion); teaching the patient management techniques for auditory hallucinations; assessing the patient's level of control with each contact: seclusion and restraint as necessary for staff and patient safety.
14. Allowing the nurse to stop caring for that patient; teaching the nurse the normal signs of post-trauma response (PTR), including nightmares and intrusive images; assessing for other signs of PTR; teaching the normal time lines for PTR; providing for discussion and debriefing of what has occurred; offering similar debriefing to the remainder of the staff; providing ongoing emotional support for the nurse for the duration of these signs.

Chapter 13

True or False

1. True
2. False; it is from biological theory.
3. False; it is part of learning theory.
4. F
5. H
6. C
7. G
8. D

9. Severe
10. Moderate
11. Panic
12. Mild
13. Moderate level; refer to Table 13–7 for interventions.
14. Severe level; refer to Table 13–8 for interventions.

Chapter 14

Matching

1. B
2. C
3. A
4. B
5. C
6. A
7. A
8. C
9. B
10. A

True or False

11. False; it takes 4–6 weeks, and then resolution of same, lower, or higher level is made. That is why early intervention is essential.
12. False; same level.
13. True
14. False; anyone can face a crisis situation.
15. True
16. False; the sooner the better the chances of a positive outcome.
17. True
18. False; however, the nurse counselor will be active in planning with the client.

Completion

19. Refer to pages 372–374.
20. Refer to pages 372–374.
21. Refer to Table 14–1.
22. Refer to page 375.
23. Use the text, plus think of types of situations you will encounter on a surgical unit, on a maternity unit, in the emergency department, on a pediatric unit, and on a psychiatric unit.
24. Refer to pages 370–371.

Chapter 15

Completion

1. Competent nursing extends into people's homes (e.g., home health nursing). Assessment of family needs and safety issues is part of our responsibility.
2. 1. Always consider family violence a possibility.
   2. Learn clues; conduct interview in private, asking questions in a direct, honest manner using language the client will understand.
   3. Assess safety. Does the client believe it is safe at home? Is reporting indicated?
3. 1. Acknowledge their response and ask for more information.
   2. Assess for safety.
   3. Offer resources and referrals.
   4. If appropriate, report to the appropriate agency.

Multiple Choice

4. E
5. F

Matching

6. G
7. A
8. F
9. C
10. E
11. B
12. D
13. E

Multiple Choice

14. A
15. A/B/C
16. A

17. Refer to pages 400-401.
18. 1. "Blame the victim."
    2. Discouragement.
    3. Anger.
19. 1. Is the violence acknowledged?
    2. Is there willingness to accept intervention?
    3. Is safety ensured (e.g., is the victim removed from the situation)?

Chapter 16

1. A. Verbatim statements by the survivor.
   B. Detailed observations of emotional status.
   C. Detailed observations of physical status and injuries (draw a body map).
   D. Any ordered lab tests and results.
2. A. Provide psychological and emotional support.

B. History taking, especially gynecological history.
C. Facilitate privacy to minimize the trauma of the examination.
D. Explain each step of the examination and provide reassurance.

Multiple Choice

3. D
4. B
5. D
6. D
7. D
8. D

Chapter 17

Multiple Choice

1. C
2. A
3. A
4. D
5. D
6. B

7. N
8. Y
9. Y
10. Y
11. Y
12. N
13. N

Matching

14. B
15. A
16. C

17. N
18. N
19. Y
20. Y
21. N
22. Y
23. N
24. Y
25. N

Critical Thinking

26. Application of hand cream after washing episode. Application of white cotton gloves over cream.
27. See Interventions 1a-1l listed in Nursing Care Plan 17–1.

    Relate appointment to preventing/treating the symptoms he experienced during his three recent attacks.

    Possible outcome: Client will use effective coping methods to deal with anxiety.

    Interventions: Teach cognitive-behavioral techniques to relieve anxiety: relaxation techniques; visualizing a pleasant scene; regular exercise; abdominal breathing; meditation; caffeine reduction; positive self-talk.
28. Explain to Mr. Zeamans that some authorities believe it is unwise for a recovering substance abuser to take a cross-addicting drug. Explain that there are other highly effective techniques for reducing anxiety. With Mr. Zeamans' input, develop a plan to teach selected anxiety control techniques.
29. Culturally determined symptoms of anxiety.

    Stoicism as a culturally determined response.

    Cultural preference for physical solutions to emotional problems.

    Traditional relationships of male to female and physician to client.

Chapter 18

Multiple Choice

1. C
2. A
3. C
4. C
5. C

6. Y
7. Y
8. Y
9. Y
10. Y
11. Y
12. A. Y
    B. Y
    C. Y
    D. Y
    E. Y
13. A. N
    B. N
    C. H
    D. N
14. A. N
    B. H
    C. H
    D. H

Critical Thinking

15. Plan should consider:
    Restriction to unit
    Removal of harmful objects
    Constant observation
    Establishing a relationship
16. Avoidance is based on frustration experienced by the staff.

Interventions:	*Rationales:*
Determine how all staff are to respond to requests associated with somatic complaints, and be consistent.	Consistency reduces anxiety.
Schedule frequent visits with client at times when she is not offering somatic complaints.	Shows positive regard for the client as a person. Avoids reinforcing symptoms.

17. Plan should contain interventions such as:

    No naps during day

    Keep as active as possible

    Provide an environment conducive to sleep

    Teach relaxation methods to employ at h.s.

    Drink warm milk at h.s.
18. Help client reevaluate the accuracy of ideas such as:

    Others being offended by her nose

    Negative effects of appearance on her employment

    Negative effects of appearance on her social life.

    Ask for actual instances and examples. If none can be given, point out that the idea has no basis in fact. If an example is given, help client see that the size of her nose is not the only possible explanation for the occurrence. Explore if others with large noses have been able to be successful, looking at the importance of other attributes.

Chapter 19

Multiple Choice

1. D
2. C

True or False

3. True
4. False; often need long-term treatment in community setting.
5. True
6. True
7. True
8. False

Multiple Choice

9. C
10. A/B/D
11. B
12. D
13. A
14. C
15. A
16. B
17. A
18. A
19. D
20. D

Chapter 20

1. Develops awareness.
2. Restitution.
3. Shock.

True or False

4. False; takes 1–2 years or longer.
5. True
6. False; nurses, like all humans, are profoundly affected by multiple losses. That is why inservice, conferences and staff meetings, and support are vital to help staff grieve when faced with losing client(s) staff were close to.

Matching

7. D
8. C
9. A
10. E
11. B
12. F

13. U
14. S
15. U
16. S

Multiple Choice

17. C
18. C
19. Refer to pages 550–551.
20. Refer to pages 550–551.
21. Refer to pages 550–551.
22. MD
23. D
24. MD
25. D
26. B
27. C
28. P
29. L
30. See page 558.
31. See page 558.
32. See page 558.
33. See page 559.
34. See page 559.
35. See page 559.
36. Refer to pages 559–561.
37. Refer to pages 559–561.
38. Refer to pages 559–561.
39. NP
40. P
41. P
42. NH; minimizes person's feelings.
43. NH; discourages person from evaluating his situation and finding alternative ways to deal with feelings and issues.
44. NH; value judgment.
45. H
46. NH; can increase feelings of alienation.
47. NH; help look at feelings and find ways to deal with them.
48. Refer to Table 20–6.
49. Refer to Table 20–6.
50. Refer to Table 20–6.
51. Refer to Table 20–6.

Multiple Choice

52. C
53. A
54. C
55. D
56. C
57. B

Chapter 21

Multiple Choice

1. D
2. C

Completion

3. Refer to page 603.
4. Refer to page 603.
5. Refer to page 603.
6. Refer to pages 603–604.
7. Refer to pages 603–604.
8. Refer to pages 603–604.
9. Refer to Table 21–4 for suggestions.
10. Refer to Table 21–4 for suggestions.
11. Refer to Table 21–4 for suggestions.
12. Refer to Table 21–4 for suggestions.
13. Use Box 21–1 as a guide.
14. Use Box 21–1 as a guide.
15. Use Box 21–1 as a guide.
16. Refer to page 611.
17. Refer to page 611.
18. Refer to page 611.
19. H
20. H
21. NH; can escalate excitement.
22. NH; loosening limits can increase the client's manipulation and anxiety.
23. NH; value judgments and belittling comments can lower self-esteem and escalate the client's out-of-control behaviors.
24. H

Chapter 22

1. Review pages 632 and 634.
2. Loss of ego boundaries.
3. A. See page 634.
   B. See page 634.
   C. See page 634.
4. A. See page 638.
   B. See page 638.

True or False

5. False
6. True
7. False; all relationships have some ambivalence.
8. True

Multiple Choice

9. A/B/D
10. A/B/C/D/E
11. A/B/C—the atypical antipsychotics. D/E—particularly the atypical antipsychotics.

12. D
13. H
14. D
15. D
16. H
17. H/D
18. D
19. D

True or False

20. False; tardive dyskinesia is not reversible.
21. True
22. False
23. True
24. True
25. False
26. True
27. True and False; true for standard, the atypical antipsychotics target the negative symptoms as well.
28. True
29. True
30. True
31. True
32. True
33. False

Multiple Choice

34. C
35. C
36. C
37. C
38. D
39. B

Chapter 23

Matching

1. DEL
2. DEM
3. DEM
4. DEL
5. DEM
6. DEL
7. DEM
8. DEL
9. G
10. F
11. D
12. C
13. B

Short Answer

14. Refer to pages 687–688 for guidance in answering this question.
15. A review of pages 696–698 will prepare you to identify the stages of Alzheimer's.

Chapter 24

True or False

1. True
2. False
3. False
4. False
5. False
6. True
7. True

Multiple Choice

8. C
9. D
10. D
11. C
12. C

Completion

13. T
14. S
15. S
16. T
17. P
18. S
19. Please refer to page 732.
20. Please refer to page 733.

Chapter 25

True or False

1. True
2. True

Short Answer

3. A. Sobriety.
   B. Alternatives to drug use.
   C. Nurture relationships with family and friends.
   D. Obtain a job.
4. A. Communicate observations openly and honestly.
   B. Focus on work-related behavior, not analysis of causation.
   C. Maintain a neutral demeanor.
   D. Expect the same work performance from chemically dependent person as from other workers.
   E. Focus on tangible results, not promises to do better.
   F. Face the problem head on.
5. Refer to pages 669–671 for guidance.
6. Refer to pages 669–671 for guidance.

Short Answer

7. A. Expect abstinence/sobriety.
   B. Individualize goals and interventions.
   C. Support and redirect defenses rather than remove them.
   D. Set limits on behavior.
   E. Recognize that the process of recovery is carried out in stages.
   F. Look for therapeutic leverage.
8. A. Any personal family history or other personal experiences with various substances.
   B. The fact that a substance abuser's behavior can be challenging and frustrating.
9. A. Individual.
   B. Group.
   C. Family.
   D. Marital.
   E. Relapse prevention.
10. A. Sobriety.
    B. Improved self-esteem.
    C. Enhanced coping abilities.
    D. Improved relationships with others.

Matching

11. I
12. W
13. O
14. I
15. B
16. C
17. C
18. B
19. B
20. G
21. F
22. E
23. C
24. B

Multiple Choice

25. D
26. D
27. B
28. D
29. D

Short Answer

30. C
31. C Cut down
    A Annoyed
    G Guilty
    E Eye-opener
32. A. Frame lapses and relapses into the program of treatment.
    B. Assist the client to learn from lapse so that a full-blown relapse can be avoided.
33. A. Offer support and kindness.
    B. Maintain consistency.
34. A. Point out relationship between drug use and consequences.
    B. Make appropriate referrals.
35. A. Person requires increased amounts to receive the desired effect.
    B. Withdrawal symptoms are experienced when the drug is stopped.
36. A. Ask the client what drugs he or she has recently taken and match with your knowledge of the drug's effect.
    B. Determine when the last dose was taken and the amount of the dose.

Chapter 26

Multiple Choice

1. D
2. C
3. B
4. C
5. D
6. D

Chapter 27

Multiple Choice

1. D
2. E
3. C
4. C
5. D
6. A

Chapter 28

Multiple Choice

1. What do your answers say about your spiritual self?
2. B
3. C
4. B
5. A
6. C

Chapter 29

1. A. Trusts others; sees world as safe and supportive (see Box 29–3).
   B. Can test reality.
   C. Masters developmental tasks.
   D. Expresses self in spontaneous, creative ways.
2.

Genetic	Parents with bipolar disorder or schizophrenia.
Prenatal	Exposure to drugs, alcohol, other toxins.
Psychosocial development	Failure to attach, failure to complete the separation/induration process.
Social/ environmental	Child abuse and neglect.
Cultural	Culture shock and cultural conflicts.

3. A. A temperament that can adapt to change. Ability to distance self from chaos in parent or family.
   B. Ability to form nurturing relationships.
4. A. History of present illness.
   B. Developmental history.
   C. Developmental assessment.
   D. Medical history.
   E. Family history.
   F. Mental status assessment/neurological assessment (see Box 29–4).
5. 4-year-old
   M
   E
   M
   E
   M
   E

   12-year-old
   E (see Table 29–1).
   M
   M
   E
   E
   M
6. F
   E
   C
   B
   D
   A
7. Mood/Affect Changes:
   A. Irritability.
   B. Sadness/crying.
   C. Apathy.
   D. Anhedonia; decreased self-esteem.

Physical Changes:

A. Physical complaints.
B. Insomnia/hypersomnia (see Box 29–7).
C. Loss of energy.
D. Appetite changes; weight gain/loss.

Cognitive Changes:

A. Boredom.
B. Decreased concentration.
C. Decreased school performance.
D. Preoccupation with illness/death; suicidal ideation.

Social/Behavior Changes:

A. Self-imposed isolation or rejection by peers.
B. Loss of boy friend/girl friend.
C. Drug/alcohol use.
D. Running away, truancy; interest in morbid music or literature.

8. All ages.
   All ages.
   Preschool, school-age.
   School-age, preadolescent.
   Preschool, school-age.
   School-age, preadolescent.
   All ages.
   All ages.
   Preschool, school-age, preadolescent.

9. A. Antipsychotic (risperidone, haloperidol).
   B. Tricyclic antidepressants (TCAs) and selective serotonin reuptake inhibitors (SSRIs).
   C. Psychostimulants (could be called "central nervous system stimulants"), TCAs, mood stabilizers.
   D. TCA (clomipramine), haloperidol.
   E. Antihistamines, anxiolytics, and antidepressants.
   F. Antipsychotic (risperidone), mood stabilizers (carbamazepine, valproic acid), antihypertensive (propranolol).
10. A. Assist the youth with new learning about self and the world.
    B. Assist the youth and family with relearning roles, relationships, and expectations.
    C. Assist in restoring those aspects of living that show deprivation.

Chapter 30

Multiple Choice

1. C
2. B
3. E
4. B
5. D
6. D

Matching

7. A
8. J
9. F
10. B
11. I
12. D

Chapter 31

True or False

1. True
2. False
3. True
4. False

Matching

5. REM
6. R
7. P

True or False

8. False
9. True
10. True
11. True
12. False
13. False
14. True
15. True
16. True
17. True
18. False
19. True

20. B
21. C
22. A
23. D

INDEX

Note: Page numbers in *italics* refer to illustrations; page numbers followed by b refer to boxed material, and those followed by t refer to tables.

NURSING DIAGNOSTIC CATEGORIES

Boldface type indicates diagnoses currently accepted by the North American Nursing Diagnosis Association (NANDA). Others are either diagnoses received by NANDA for development or not accepted by NANDA, but are found useful in clinical practice.

HEALTH PERCEPTION–HEALTH MANAGEMENT

Health-Seeking Behaviors (Specify)
Altered Health Maintenance (Specify)
Ineffective Management of Therapeutic Regimen (Specify Area)
Risk for Ineffective Management of Therapeutic Regimen (Specify Area)
Effective Management of Therapeutic Regimen
Ineffective Family Management of Therapeutic Regimen
Ineffective Community Management of Therapeutic Regimen
Health-Management Deficit (Specify Area)
Risk for Health-Management Deficit (Specify Area)
Noncompliance (Specify Area)
Risk for Noncompliance (Specify Area)
Risk for Infection (Specify Type/Area)
Risk for Injury (Trauma)
Risk for Perioperative Positioning Injury
Risk for Poisoning
Risk for Suffocation
Altered Protection (Specify)
Energy Field Disturbance

NUTRITIONAL METABOLIC PATTERN

Altered Nutrition: More Than Body Requirements or Exogenous Obesity
Altered Nutrition: More Than Body Requirements or Risk for Obesity
Altered Nutrition: Less Than Body Requirements or Nutritional Deficit (Specify Type)
Ineffective Breastfeeding
Interrupted Breastfeeding
Effective Breastfeeding
Ineffective Infant Feeding Program
Impaired Swallowing (Uncompensated)
Risk for Aspiration
Altered Oral Mucous Membrane (Specify Alteration)
Fluid Volume Deficit
Risk for Fluid Volume Deficit
Fluid Volume Excess
Risk for Impaired Skin Integrity or Risk for Skin Breakdown
Impaired Skin Integrity
Pressure Ulcer (Specify Stage)
Impaired Tissue Integrity (Specify Type)
Risk for Altered Body Temperature
Ineffective Thermoregulation
Hyperthermia
Hypothermia

ELIMINATION PATTERN

Colonic Constipation
Perceived Constipation
Intermittent Constipation Pattern
Diarrhea
Bowel Incontinence
Altered Urinary Elimination Pattern
Functional Incontinence
Reflex Incontinence
Stress Incontinence
Urge Incontinence
Total Incontinence
Urinary Retention

ACTIVITY EXERCISE PATTERN

Activity Intolerance (Specify Level)
Risk for Activity Intolerance
Fatigue
Impaired Physical Mobility (Specify Level)
Impaired Bed Mobility
Transfer Deficit
Impaired Locomotion
Impaired Ambulation
Risk for Disuse Syndrome
Risk for Joint Contractures
Total Self-Care Deficit (Specify Level)
Self-Bathing–Hygiene Deficit (Specify Level)
Self-Dressing–Grooming Deficit (Specify Level)
Self-Toileting Deficit (Specify Level)
Altered Growth and Development: Self-Care Skills (Specify Level)
Diversional Activity Deficit
Impaired Home Maintenance Management (Mild, Moderate, Severe, Potential, Chronic)
Dysfunctional Ventilatory Weaning Response (DVWR)
Inability to Sustain Spontaneous Ventilation
Ineffective Airway Clearance
Ineffective Breathing Pattern
Impaired Gas Exchange
Decreased Cardiac Output
Altered Tissue Perfusion (Specify)
Dysreflexia
Disorganized Infant Behavior
Risk for Disorganized Infant Behavior
Potential for Enhanced Organized Infant Behavior
Risk for Peripheral Neurovascular Dysfunction
Altered Growth and Development

Continued